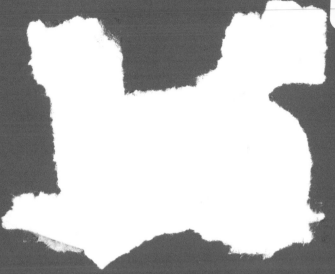

CLINICAL PRACTICE IN

Sexually Transmissible Infections

Commissioning Editors: Deborah Russell, Quincy McDonald
Project Development Manager: Sheila Black
Project Managers: Hilary Hewitt, Lewis Derrick
Design Manager: Jayne Jones
Designer: Keith Kale
Illustrator: Jenni Miller
Indexer: Hilary Tarrant

CLINICAL PRACTICE IN

Sexually Transmissible Infections

Commissioning Editors: Deborah Russell, Quincy McDonald
Project Development Manager: Sheila Black
Project Managers: Hilary Hewitt, Lewis Derrick
Design Manager: Jayne Jones
Designer: Keith Kale
Illustrator: Jenni Miller
Indexer: Hilary Tarrant

CLINICAL PRACTICE IN
Sexually Transmissible Infections

Alexander McMillan MD, FRCP, FRCP (Ed)
Consultant Physician, Department of Genito-Urinary Medicine,
The Royal Infirmary of Edinburgh, UK

Hugh Young BSc, PhD, DSc, FRCPath
Senior Lecturer, Medical Microbiology, The University of Edinburgh
Medical School; Director, Scottish *Neisseria gonorrhoeae*
Reference Laboratory, The Lothian University Hospitals NHS Trust,
Edinburgh, UK

Marie M Ogilvie MD, FRCPath
Senior Lecturer, Medical School, The University of Edinburgh, UK

Gordon R Scott MB, ChB, FRCP (Ed)
Consultant Physician, Department of Genito-Urinary Medicine,
The Royal Infirmary of Edinburgh, UK

SAUNDERS

SAUNDERS
An imprint of Elsevier Science Limited

First published 2002

ISBN 0 7020 2538 0

British Library Cataloguing in Publication Data
A catalogue record for this book is available from the British Library

Library of Congress Cataloging in Publication Data
A catalog record for this book is available from the Library of Congress

Drug Nomenclature

Directive 92/27/EEC requires use of the Recommended International Non-proprietary Name (rINN) for medicinal substances. In most cases the British Approved Name (BAN) and rINN are identical but where they differ the rINN has been used with the old BAN in parentheses.

There are two important exceptions: adrenaline and noradrenaline, where the BAN is used first followed by the new rINNS (epinephrine and norepinephrine) in parentheses.

Drug dosages

Medical knowledge is constantly changing. As new information becomes available, changes in treatment, procedures, equipment and the use of drugs become necessary. The editors and the publishers have taken care to ensure that the information given in this text is accurate and up to date. However, readers are strongly advised to confirm that the information, especially with regard to drug usage, complies with the latest legislation and standards of practice.

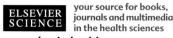

your source for books,
journals and multimedia
in the health sciences
www.elsevierhealth.com

The
publisher's
policy is to use
**paper manufactured
from sustainable forests**

Printed in China by RDC Group Ltd

Contents

List of Contributors

Professor Ron C Ballard MD PhD
Division of AIDS, STDs and TB, Centers for Disease Control and Prevention, Atlanta, Georgia, USA

Alexander McMillan MD, FRCP, FRCP (Ed)
Consultant Physician, Department of Genito-Urinary Medicine, The Royal Infirmary of Edinburgh, UK

Marie M Ogilvie MD, FRCPath
Senior Lecturer, Medical School, The University of Edinburgh, UK

Cornelis A Rietmeijer MD, MSPH
Director, HIV/AIDS Prevention, Denver Public Health Department, Colorado, USA

Gordon R Scott MB, ChB, FRCP (Ed)
Consultant Physician, Department of Genito-Urinary Medicine,
The Royal Infirmary of Edinburgh, UK

Hugh Young BSc, PhD, DSc, FRCPath
Senior Lecturer, Medical Microbiology, The University of Edinburgh Medical School;
Director, Scottish *Neisseria gonorrhoeae* Reference Laboratory, The Lothian University Hospitals NHS Trust, Edinburgh, UK

Preface

This book has been written primarily for doctors in training in genitourinary medicine, although we hope that more senior physicians in the speciality will also find some sections useful. We have attempted to bring together information that is widely scattered in the literature and to present an appreciation of clinical and laboratory aspects of the various subjects in a way that we believe will be useful to our colleagues. It is our hope that the book will be of value as a reference in teaching and also to the wider range of clinicians, for instance gynecologists and family planning specialists, who participate as we do in the practice of sexual and reproductive medicine and will therefore often require to consider the full range of sexually transmitted infections. General practitioners and other clinicians will find some answers to their questions, and physicians who may not ordinarily look after adolescents and young adults, may find the inclusion of sexually transmissible infections in their differential diagnosis a rewarding exercise.

Although this book is primarily for medical readers it is hoped that those involved in nursing or counseling patients, tracing contacts, or in health education will be able to obtain some of the factual information which they require. Barriers between disciplines are tending to become inappropriate and those who share objectives in patient care will need to pool their knowledge to obtain the best results possible.

In the past decade there have been considerable advances in molecular methods for the diagnosis of many of the sexually transmissible infections, particularly *Chlamydia trachomatis*, and we have attempted to incorporate discussion of these methods in the various relevant chapters. As the human immunodeficiency virus is a sexually transmissible organism, a chapter on this important infection has been included, although in a book of this size it is impossible to give an entirely comprehensive account, and the number of references has been limited.

Sound knowledge of the sexually transmissible infections and firm application of principles developed in this subject remain the indispensable essentials of medical practice.

Edinburgh 2002

A McMillan
H Young
M M Ogilvie
G R Scott

Acknowledgments

We wish to acknowledge the advice, help and discussion given by many friends and colleagues in the Royal Infirmary of Edinburgh and University of Edinburgh. We are particularly grateful to our colleagues in the Department of Genitourinary Medicine at the Royal Infirmary, Drs Carolyn Thompson, Dan Clutterbuck and Jaqueline Paterson, and to our Australian colleague Dr Robin Tideman, who read several chapters and offered excellent advice. Dr David Robertson, former Consultant Physician, Department of Genitourinary Medicine, very kindly agreed to the reproduction of material from the first and second edition of *Clinical Practice in Sexually Transmitted Diseases*. Dr Franklyn Judson, University of Colorado, Denver, offered helpful advice during the early period of the preparation of the volume, Dr Les Milne, Consultant Mycologist, Western General Hospital, Edinburgh, very kindly offered invaluable assistance in the preparation of the section on candidiasis, Chapter 17, and Dr P Allan, Consultant Radiologist, gave helpful service on scrotal ultrasonography (Chapter 13). We wish to give our appreciation and thanks also to: the Editor, *International Journal of Sexually Transmitted Diseases and AIDS* for permission to reproduce Boxes 4.2 and 4.3; Leeds University Press for permission to reproduce Figure 5.2; the Editor, *Sexually Transmitted Infections* for permission to publish Figure 5.25; Dr A Williams, Consultant Pathologist, University of Edinburgh for providing Figure 6.6, the Editor, *New England Journal of Medicine* for permission to reproduce Figure 6.18 and Table 15.11; Dr J Soul-Lawton and the American Society for Microbiology, and Dr RB van Dyke and the Editor, *American Journal of Medicine* for permission to reproduce Figure 6.19; Dr DA Collie, Consultant Neuroradiologist, Western General Hospital, Edinburgh for providing Figure 6.22; the British HIV Association for permission to reproduce the guidelines on recommendations for management of symptomless HIV-infected individuals, and for treatment regimens (Tables 7.8 and 7.9); Professor D Wray, Dental School, University of Glasgow for permission to reproduce Figures 7.19 and 7.20; Dr J Bell, Consultant Neuropathologist, Western General Hospital, Edinburgh for providing Figure 7.29; Dr B Dhillon, Consultant Ophthalmologist, Edinburgh Royal Infirmary for providing Figures 7.31 and 7.32; the Editor, *Science* for permission to reproduce Figure 7.33; Professor C Ludlam, Department of Haematology, Western General Hospital, Edinburgh for providing Figure 9.12; the Editor, *Journal of Urology* for permission to reproduce Table 13.1; the World Health Organization for their kindness in permitting the reproduction of the algorithms for the syndromic management of sexually transmitted infections (Chapter 2), and of Figure 15.35; Dr O Arya, former Consultant Physician, Department of Genitourinary Medicine, Liverpool, for providing Figures 15.36, 15.37 and 15.38; the American College of Physicians and the American Society of Internal Medicine for permission to reproduce Appendices 15.1 and 15.2; Prof VN Sehgal for providing Figures 16.3, 16.4 and 16.5; the Editor, *Journal of Parasitology* for permission to reproduce Figure 17.1; Dr T White and the American Society for Microbiology for permission to reproduce Figure 17.10; Dr RP Nugent and the American Society for Microbiology to reproduce Table 17.4; Professor J Ackers, London School of Hygiene and Tropical Medicine for providing Figure 18.3; the Editor *British Medical Journal* for permission to reproduce Figure 20.4; Professor J Hunter, former Professor of Dermatology, University of Edinburgh for providing Figures 20.3, 20.17 and 20.19.

The authors are also indebted to the staff of Elsevier Science, our publishers, for their encouragement and patience.

Section 1
Introduction

Human sexuality: the background to infection
C A Rietmeijer, A McMillan

The main reason that sexually transmitted infections (STIs) are grouped together is that they are linked to the most intimate behavior of humans. A discussion of sexual behavior and its social and societal contexts is therefore appropriate in a text on STIs, particularly where it helps us to understand the epidemiology of STIs and, more importantly, where it identifies ways in which these infections can be prevented.

Traditionally, disease surveillance has helped public health workers to target prevention interventions, for example by tracing contacts. Whilst not diminishing its worth, disease surveillance occurs after an infectious event has occurred which may have been years before the case is detected and reported, for example cases of human immunodeficiency virus (HIV) and AIDS, thus reducing the effectiveness of contact investigation. Furthermore, for the index (first reported) case, disease-based interventions may come too late because of the incurable nature of the infection, as in the case of HIV infection, or because complications may have already occurred, as in the case of pelvic inflammatory disease complicating untreated gonococcal or chlamydial infections. What is needed, therefore, are interventions that occur 'up stream' from the infectious event, that is, interventions altering the behavioral risk for infection. As a result, the collection of (sexual) behavioral data is currently seen as critical information for the development of effective 'upstream' behavioral interventions (see Chapter 2).

Analogous to disease surveillance, the term behavioral surveillance has been defined as the ongoing, systematic collection, analysis, and interpretation of behavioral data, closely integrated with the timely dissemination of these data to those responsible for preventing and controlling disease or injury[1]. In contrast to traditional disease surveillance, data sources for behavioral surveillance are not limited to surveillance systems, but may also include (periodic) surveys and results from research studies. Behavioral surveillance occurs at three levels

- general populations
- high-risk populations
- infected populations.

Surveillance of sexual behaviors among the general population yields temporal trends as well as identifying certain characteristics and sizes of high-risk populations (as defined by high-risk sexual behaviors). The availability of non-invasive STI screening methods (for example, urine-based screening for gonorrhea and chlamydial infections, and saliva-based screening for HIV) allows direct linkage of STI prevalence to behavioral indicators for use in general population surveys[2].

The weakness of general population surveys for STI prevention is that they yield limited information on populations at highest risk of STIs. These groups are often undersampled and the depth of STI-related information is limited, especially in surveys where sexual behavior is not the main focus. For example, from general population sex surveys, it appears that homosexual behavior is rather uncommon and that among homosexual men anal sex may not be the predominant type of sexual behavior. None the less, from a morbidity and mortality perspective, HIV infection transmitted sexually by men who have sex with men is the single most important STI in Europe and North America. Survey information relevant to the prevention of HIV must therefore come from these populations, often using convenience or purposive samples. Because the epidemiology of the different STIs varies, behavioral patterns underlying these infections among specific risk groups are also likely to be different. Studies specific to the sexual behavior of each risk group are therefore best suited for use in public health practice.

Sexual behavior and ecology

Disease has played an important part in the evolution of behavior. It is Freeland's hypothesis[3] that numerous behavior patterns in primates help individuals avoid new diseases and these behavior patterns play a part in controlling diseases the animals may harbor. Among other mechanisms, sexual fidelity by individuals to other members of their social group is the result of selection for the avoidance of new diseases. The maintenance of a home range or territory is also an effective disease-avoidance mechanism. Individuals mating within their own group have a higher probability of mating with animals carrying the same pathogens as themselves and a lower probability of acquiring new pathogens. Individuals having promiscuous sexual contact with animals outside the social group lower both the probability of surviving and of leaving offspring. In nature friendly or inter-group interactions are rare, although they do occur in particular situations. Although the admission of 'new blood' is occasionally favored to avoid excessive in-breeding, the introduction of an outsider to an established group is generally gradual allowing time for both the group and the new member to become immune to lethal or pathogenic doses of foreign disease-producing organisms. Therefore, changes in sexual behavior at the individual, group, or societal levels occurring over relatively short time periods may create an ecological 'niche' and an epidemiological starting point for old and new STIs. In his controversial book *Sexual Ecology*, Rotello makes a convincing case that sexual behavior changes occurring as part of the 'gay liberation' in the 1960s and 1970s effectively paved the way for the HIV epidemic among homosexual men[4]. Similarly, the sexual revolution in the western world also led to an increase in the incidence of 'old' STIs, including gonorrhea, syphilis, and chlamydia among both homosexuals and heterosexuals. More recently, broad societal changes in the former Soviet Union have led to significant changes in sexual morals in a previously restricted society, leading to a dramatic increase in the incidence of gonorrhea, syphilis[5], and HIV[6]; the extent of protective sexual behavior, however, is small[7]. The important lesson from considering STIs from an evolutionary or ecological perspective is that our current focus on treatment and vaccine-based prevention may be inadequate. Widespread antibiotic and antiviral use has already led to the selection of resistant strains of certain STIs, including gonorrhea and HIV. On the other hand, while effective vaccines have been developed for hepatitis A and B virus infections, and may be developed for HIV and other STIs, other pathogens may take advantage of the ecological niches created or sustained by certain sexual practices. The hope and expectations among many that safe sexual behaviors can be relaxed as soon as effective vaccines or treatments become available are unlikely to be fulfilled.

Sexual behavior and its relationship to sexually transmissible infections

A useful concept to frame the discussion on sexual behavior is the 'reproductive rate', or the number of new infections originating from one person infected with a given STI. Prevalence for this STI will increase if this rate exceeds 1, will hold steady if the rate equals 1, and will decrease if the rate falls below 1. The reproductive rate may be defined as the product of the average transmission efficiency of the pathogen (β), the rate of exposure of susceptible individuals to infectious sex partners (c), and the average duration of infectiousness (D)[8]. While the duration of infectiousness is largely defined by the type of pathogen and the availability and administration of treatment (influenced by health-seeking behavior), sexual behaviors are related to both transmission efficiency and rate of exposure. Clearly, this concept has major implications for STI prevention and will therefore again be considered in the discussion of primary and secondary STI prevention in Chapter 2.

Sexual behavior related to exposure to sexually transmissible infections

Exposure risks are defined by the time of sexual activity and the number of sexual partners during this interval. Thus the increasing rates of STIs starting in the late 1960s and 1970s were successfully linked to two factors
- earlier age of sexual debut
- increasing numbers of partners.

In the BBC Reith lectures for 1962 entitled 'This Island Now,' Professor Carstairs, Professor of Psychological Medicine of the University of Edinburgh, outlined many of the points of change which were occurring at that time in the UK[9]. He touched on the changing role of women and the abandonment of chastity as a supreme moral value.

He recognized that sexual experience before marriage with precautions against pregnancy would become a recognized preliminary to marriage. Changes in attitudes to sex have been profound and it is now commonplace to discuss openly subjects that were once taboo outside limited circles. In the UK, homosexual men have been freed from prosecution for sexual acts in private between adults; abortion has been legalized; contraceptives have been made very readily available and divorce is easier to obtain. The distinguished judge, Sir Leslie Scarman, pointed out[10] that with concepts derived from the human rights movement, men and women now expect to have opportunities of achieving personal happiness, unfettered by the views of others.

This 'sexual revolution' has been studied in many countries, particularly in the USA, although it is a difficult and costly subject to study, and the non-random nature and small sizes of the population samples studied[11] often make it uncertain to what extent the changes reported applied to society in general. Many of these reports, however, showed trends that were similar despite having geographical variation according to the predominant mores.

A number of reports on students supported the conclusion that, during the decade 1958 to 1968, there was a significantly greater change in the sexual experience of females than in that of males. Sexual intercourse was increasingly common during a 'going steady' relationship and the commitment of 'engagement' had become less important as a preliminary. Feelings of guilt connected with intercourse lessened. In a study of three different cultures; a highly restrictive Mormon culture in the inter-mountain region of the western USA, a moderately restrictive mid-western culture in central USA, and a highly permissive Danish Scandinavian culture; Christensen and Gregg[12] identified often marked changes in the attitudes of students over this decade, particularly in the female. Values for three items, selected to show trends in liberal attitudes, are given in Table 1.1. It was found that there was also a relationship between attitudes and behavior and, in particular, approval of coitus was a better

Table 1.1 Trends in three liberal attitudes found in three groups of students of various origins (adapted from Christensen and Gregg 1970 [12])

Attitudes	Year	Highly restrictive culture (USA)		Moderately restrictive culture (USA)		Very liberal culture (Denmark)	
		Males %	Females %	Males %	Females %	Males %	Females %
Opposition to censorship of pornography	1958	42	54	47	51	77	81
	1968	61	58	71	59	99	97
Acceptance of non-virginity in marital partner	1958	5	11	18	23	61	74
	1968	20	26	25	44	92	92
Approval of premarital coitus	1958	23	3	47	17	94	81
	1968	38	24	55	38	100	100
Total numbers in sample	**1958**	**94**	**74**	**213**	**142**	**149**	**86**
	1968	**115**	**105**	**245**	**238**	**134**	**61**

predictor of coital behavior for both males and females at the end of the decade than at the beginning. Attitudes towards sex had become more liberal and sexual intercourse was justified when there was commitment or affection between partners, this is a traditional Scandinavian pattern. There was also a suggestion in the Scandinavian sample that there was a trend for sexual intercourse not to be confined to one partner. Two negative accompaniments of premarital coitus were identified; the first was the feeling of yielding to force or to pressures other than personal desire, and the second was coitus followed by guilt or remorse. Both of these negative feelings were higher in restrictive than in permissive cultures, higher in females than in males, and higher in 1985 than in 1968[12].

The effects of the sexual revolution are reflected in a number of recent general population surveys from different countries. In the UK, for example, Johnson and colleagues, in a survey conducted in 1990 to 1991 among 18 876 individuals aged 16 to 59 years, found that age at first heterosexual intercourse decreased with the current age of the respondent. Among women aged between 55 and 59 years at the time of interview (born between 1931 and 1935), the median age at first sexual intercourse was 21 years. The median age at first sexual intercourse of the youngest women in the sample, aged 16 to 19 years,

however, was 17 years, 4 years earlier than for those born four decades previously. Likewise, compared with women aged 55 to 59 years, a substantial proportion of women aged 16 to 19 years had become sexually active when they were less than 16 years old (18.7% compared to 1%). Among men a similar pattern emerged: the median age at first heterosexual intercourse was 3 years earlier amongst men aged 16 to 19 years (17 years) than for those aged 55 to 59 years (20 years). Amongst the youngest men studied, 27.6% had had sexual intercourse before the age of 16 years, compared with only 18% of the oldest men[13]. Data from the USA yield similar, yet somewhat less profound, results. The National Health and Social Life Survey (NHSLS) was conducted in 1992 among a random sample of 3432 respondents. In this survey, age at first intercourse declined from 19 years among white women born between 1933 and 1944, to about 17.5 years among white women born between 1953 and 1962. Among white men these ages were 18 years and 17 years respectively. For black women and men there were no differences but black men had a lower mean age for all birth cohorts (15.5 years for those born between 1953 and 1962)[14]. In the UK, younger ages at first intercourse were also found among men and women of Afro-Caribbean descent compared to Caucasians or Asians[13]. Johnson *et al.*[13] also found an

association between age at first sexual intercourse and social class, the median age at first coitus for men in social class 1 (upper and middle-class background) was 19 years, compared with 16 years for those in social class 5 (working-class background). Similarly, the median age at first intercourse was significantly higher amongst women in social class 1 than in social class 5 (20 years versus 18 years)[13].

Another measure of changing sexual behavior is the number of reported lifetime partners. In the NHSLS, 41% of persons aged 55 to 59 years during the year of study (1999) reported no partner or one partner, this steadily decreased to 21% for ages 35 to 39 years, and then increased to 24% for ages 30 to 34 years, 27% for ages 25 to 29 years, and 40% for ages 18 to 24 years[14]. Clearly persons in the USA who became sexually active during the 1960s and 1970s were more likely to have greater numbers of sexual partners. The leveling off and increasing proportion of persons with no or one partner among younger cohorts may be the result of more conservative sexual morals (perhaps as a result of the HIV epidemic), but it may also be that younger individuals may not have had the time to accumulate larger numbers of partners.

As discussed at the beginning of this chapter, the number of sexual partners is an important parameter in the reproductive rate of STIs. Survey data indicate that the number of recent partners is largely a function of age and to a lesser extent of gender, race/ethnicity and social class. In the UK, Johnson et al.[13] found that men and women aged between 16 and 24 years reported having the greatest numbers of partners within the preceding 5 years, 11.2% of men and 2.5% of women had had at least 10 partners. Men of all ages reported higher numbers of sexual partners than women. Likewise, in the USA, 8.1% of respondents aged 18 to 24 years reported five or more sexual partners in the preceding 12 months; men were more likely to report five or more sexual partners than women (4.1% versus 1.6%), and blacks (5.5%) had more partners than whites (2.5%) or Hispanics (2.5%)[14]. While these proportions appear relatively low the absolute number of people in the USA who have five or more sexual partners is daunting at over 4 million people.

Marriage is the single most important factor related to having a single partner. In the UK, married men and women were less likely than single individuals to have had more than one heterosexual partner within the preceding year, only 1.2% and 0.2% of married men and women respectively had more than two partners, compared with 28.1% and 17.5% of single men and women respectively[13]. Individuals who were cohabiting occupied an intermediate position compared with the single and married individuals, a finding that may reflect the less committed nature of cohabiting relationships. Those consistently showing the highest prevalence of multiple partnerships were separated, divorced and widowed people, their levels of sexual activity exceeding those of single individuals; this was particularly marked in those aged 25 to 44 years[13]. The data presented suggested that the influence of a stable relationship is strong, regardless of the individual's age. In the USA the proportion of first partnerships that were marriages decreased from 93.8% and 84.5% among women and men born between 1933 and 1942, to 35.3% and 33.9% among women and men born between 1963 and 1974. However, once married, over 95% reported that they had had only one sexual partner in the previous 12 months, very similar to the UK data described above. In addition,

80% of women and 65% to 85% of men reported having only one partner for the duration of their marriage[14].

In summary, these data are consistent with the changing sexual norms during the 'sexual revolution'. The temporal changes in sexual behavior may, at least in part, be responsible for the increase in STIs during the time frames referred to. However, STIs are not equally distributed in the population and even among those with similar numbers of lifetime partners, certain populations appear to be disproportionately affected. For example, after controlling for the number of lifetime partners and other factors among participants of the NHSLS survey, African-Americans were five times more likely to report bacterial STIs compared to whites or Hispanics. These findings suggest that additional factors play a role in the unequal distribution of STIs[15].

Sexual networks and core groups

Recent research strongly suggests that the number of sexual partners a person has during a given time period may not be so closely associated with STI transmission as

- the way these partners are selected
- whether partnerships are sequential or concurrent
- how these sexual partners relate to one another.

This has led to the concept of *sexual networks*, and the sociological study of the dynamics of these networks has yielded important insights into STI epidemiology. Based on sexual activity, Laumann and Youm[15] distinguish three types of sexual network members

1. 'core group' members who have had at least four sexual partners in the previous 12 months and who are considered to be primarily responsible for the existence of STIs in the population over time

2. 'adjacents' who have had two or three sexual partners in the preceding 12 months

3. 'peripherals' who have had only one sexual partner in the 12-month period.

From an epidemiological point of view, persons in or close to the core group are the most important in fuelling the epidemic, while persons at the periphery seem to form an epidemiological 'dead-end'. The latter individuals may acquire the infection from a partner who is a member of the core group or adjacent to it, but they are less likely to continue transmission. In a further exploration of the NHSLS data, Laumann and Youm[15] provided empirical evidence for these hypothetical considerations by demonstrating that the disproportionate concentration of STIs among African-Americans was related to much greater sexual mixing patterns between 'core group' members and 'adjacents' and 'peripherals', compared to mixing patterns among whites and Hispanics. Persons who form the connection between the core and the periphery are referred to by some as 'bridging' populations. For example, Gorbach et al.[16] reported a study conducted in Cambodia, that showed that considerable proportions (15%–20%) of highly mobile groups, including the military, police, and motorcycle taxi-drivers were 'active bridgers', that is, they had sex with both high-risk and low-risk partners. Because the prevalence of STIs, including HIV, amongst high-risk groups in Cambodia is high, these groups may play a critical role in disseminating these infections into the general population.

Another form of bridging is found when STIs are transmitted between distinct geographical areas as a result of increased travel between these locations. The most dramatic example of this type of bridging is the probable role of truckers in disseminating HIV throughout central Africa. Before effective transportation between countries in this region STI epidemics may have gone unnoticed as they were limited to a few networks in a small geographic area. However, the construction of highways within and between these countries allowed for intensive traffic between these areas, often by male truckers who, during long absences from home, would engage in sexual relationships with prostitutes at truck stops, effectively setting up STI transmission chains 'along the way'[17].

In his discussion of the HIV epidemic among gay men, Rotello argues that the rapid rise in HIV infections in this group during the 1970s was the result of a number of network events. First, the existence of a highly sexually active 'core group' of men who have sex with men with a high rate of HIV infection. Second, a large number of less sexually active gay men adjacent to the core or at the periphery, who occasionally interacted with the core group in environments conducive to sexual behavior (for example, bath houses). As the prevalence of HIV infection among core group members was high, these men were at high risk of becoming infected themselves. Third, the extensive mixing and bridging across gay networks favored by anonymous sex, travel, etc.[4].

CONCURRENCY AND THE 'GAP'

Within sexual networks an additional behavioral feature deserves separate attention as it favors efficient STI transmission. Persons within networks who have similar numbers of partners in a given time period may differ in the timing of these partnerships. One person may have sequential monogamous relationships, while another person may have multiple partnerships concurrently. Let us assume that two men have four partners during a year. One has four sequential partnerships, each lasting 2 months with an interval between partnerships of 1 month. The other man also has four partners, but concurrently during the year. Let us assume further that both men become infected with an STI with a very high transmission efficiency (that is, one exposure will result in infection) in the middle of the year, and that the duration of infectiousness for this STI is 3 months. It follows that for the person with concurrent relationships, all four partners will become infected because he has sex with all of them during the time he is infectious. The man with sequential relationships, however, will only infect one other person, because

- he discontinued having sex with the first two partners before he became infected, and

- his infectiousness had ceased by the time he was engaged with the fourth partner, therefore only exposing the third partner.

There are a number of studies supporting the importance of concurrent partnerships. For example, Potterat et al.[18] analyzed chlamydia-contact tracing data collected in 1996 and 1997 in Colorado Springs, and found that concurrency was the most powerful predictor of transmission. Similarly, concurrency was associated with a high prevalence and incidence of HIV in a social network study by Rothenberg et al. in Atlanta[19]. Using stochastic simulation models, Morris and Kretschmar[20] concluded that concurrent partnerships may be as important as multiple partnerships or cofactor infection in amplifying the spread of HIV. Finally, Ferguson and Garnett[21], also using simulation models, demonstrated that even modest amounts of concurrency have an enormous impact on disease prevalence and persistence. They argue that an important reason for this finding is that in the absence of concurrency, the infectious period of any STI must be longer than the time between dissolution of one partnership and the formation of another. This leads us into the discussion of yet another phenomenon. While sequential partnerships are less efficient than concurrent partnerships in promulgating STIs, the timing between partnerships also influences epidemiological dynamics. The person with sequential partnerships in our example above had intervals of 2 months between partnerships, if the interval between the third and fourth partner for this person had been shorter, say 2 weeks, then the fourth partner would have also been infected. Therefore, the intervals between partnerships, referred to by some researchers as the 'gap', will also play an important role in transmission dynamics[22]. An 'unsafe gap' for a specific STI would exist if the interval between sequential partnerships was shorter than the duration of infectiousness. When evaluating the relative importance of concurrency and unsafe gaps in the epidemiology of specific STIs, it can be argued that concurrency is more important for STIs with a relatively short duration of infectiousness

(for example gonorrhea and chlamydia), while unsafe gaps will be more important for STIs of longer duration (for example genital herpes).

In summary, the dynamics within and between sexual networks play a very important role in STI epidemiology. Further network studies will undoubtedly yield even more insight into the roles and behavior of individuals within networks. Clearly, this information cannot be obtained from surveys of general populations but instead must target populations with, or at risk for, STIs. Furthermore, because the epidemiology for distinct STIs is different, it follows that network dynamics for each of these STIs may also be different and that such studies must be specific to the STI they are targeting. Ultimately, this information should prove essential for the development of prevention strategies. Clearly, from a prevention perspective, especially when only limited resources are available, it would be desirable to target efforts to those network links that are epidemiologically the most important. The problem, however, is that network investigations, for example through contact tracing, are costly and therefore limited, and that information may be collected for only a small number of network members. Furthermore, information may be collected by a number of different investigators who may not be able to share information in a timely fashion, or may lack the analytic tools to identify the most important leads from ongoing investigations. As a result, 'core transmitters' may only be identified long after exposure at a time when this information is no longer relevant. This process may be greatly aided by recent innovations in information technology. For example, contact investigators may conduct field investigations using hand-held computer devices that are directly linked to a central computer, while specialized software may be developed to conduct 'real-time' network analyses integrating all currently available data. These developments could prove to be of important use in the timely identification, evaluation, and treatment of core transmitters, and thus sever transmission pathways in an efficient manner. The availability of non-invasive, urine-based, screening technology will further assist in this process.

Sexual behavior related to transmission efficiency

Certain STIs such as gonorrhea and syphilis are more readily transmitted than others such as HIV, but sexual practices play an important role in enhancing or reducing the chance that exposure will result in infection or whether infection will result in complications. For example, receptive anal intercourse is a much more efficient route of HIV acquisition than insertive anal or vaginal intercourse and receptive vaginal intercourse is less likely to result in HIV infection than receptive anal intercourse. Changes in sexual practices among gay men in the latter half of the last century, favoring anal intercourse over oral sex and mutual masturbation, has likely played an important role in setting the stage for HIV infection[4].

Preventive behavior, particularly the correct and consistent use of condoms, has been shown to be very effective against the transmission or acquisition of bacterial and viral STIs, including HIV infection (Chapter 2). This message has been at the core of 'safe sex' messages since the beginning of the HIV epidemic and as a result condom use has steadily increased over time. Data from the USA National Survey of Family Growth have shown that amongst women, aged 15 to 19 years, the proportion who used a condom on the first occasion of vaginal intercourse increased from 28% during 1980 to 1982, to 55% during 1988 to 1990[23]. Similarly, amongst the high-school youth in the USA, condom use at the last time of intercourse increased from 46.2% to 56.8% between 1991 and 1997. Other encouraging trends in other sexual behaviors during that period included older age of sexual debut and fewer sexual partners[24]. While virtually non-existent before the HIV epidemic, condom use among gay men has also increased particularly for anal intercourse. For example, in a large cohort study of homosexually active men in England and Wales in 1987–1988, Hunt et al.[25] found that 38.9% of respondents used condoms consistently for insertive anal sex, and 42.5% used condoms consis-

tently for receptive anal sex. As in other studies, these authors also found that condom use was more prevalent with casual than with regular sexual partners. About the same time, similar findings were reported from San Francisco[26]. However, there are real problems in relying on condom use alone to reduce the spread of STIs. First, despite impressive preventive efforts, condom use is still far from universal. Second, incorrect use as well as condom breakage and slippage results in a 10% failure rate of condoms, an unacceptable risk when it relates to the potential transmission of a lethal virus such as HIV. Third, protection against the transmission of pathogens other than HIV is less certain (Chapter 2), particularly as condoms are used predominantly for penile–anal and penile–vaginal intercourse, but less often for penile–oral sex. Oral–anal and oral–vaginal sex typically occurs without barrier protection, allowing for exposure to a number of pathogens that are transmitted via the oral–anal route, such as *Giardia duodenalis*.

Despite the publication of a large body of literature, the influence of the intake of alcohol and other recreational drugs on sexual behavior remains controversial. Studies using the critical-incident technique have failed to support a link between alcohol intake at the time of sex and that sex being unsafe[27, 28]. However, others have suggested that an association does exist but it depends upon the situation and partner type[29].

Frequent use of marijuana and its use prior to sex have been associated with a risk of acquiring sexually transmitted infections in heterosexual populations[30, 31]. Amongst men who have sex with men, the use of marijuana and nitrites ('poppers') has been shown to have independent and similar effects on the likelihood of the occurrence and maintenance of unsafe sexual behavior[32, 33].

Conclusions

Although we are considered to live in the 'safe sex' era, 12 million cases of STIs still occur annually in the USA alone, including

20 000 new HIV infections (an additional 20 000 HIV infections occur as a result of needle-related practices)[34]. While most people would agree that safe sex practices, including condom use, have reduced the number of STIs, there is considerable debate as to whether these practices go far enough. Moreover, the focus on the 'Condom Code' has led many to dissociate STIs from their ecological context[4]. Rather, the use of condoms and other safer sex measures have been considered as a temporary inconvenience that could be lifted as soon as effective treatment and/or vaccines become available. In this regard, it is sobering to see that the perception that HIV may now be a treatable condition has led many to abandon safe sex behavior. In a survey among high-risk groups in the USA, for example, 31% of respondents stated that they were less concerned about HIV, and 17% stated that they were less concerned because of the availability of new treatments. Amongst gay men who were less concerned, the practice of unprotected anal sex was significantly higher[35]. As a result of relaxing safe sex behaviors, the prevalence of gonorrhea and syphilis amongst gay men has increased in many USA cities[36, 37], and the incidence of HIV infection has increased recently in San Francisco[38].

While these rates are still much lower than they were in the early part of the 1980s, these trends are troublesome. Clearly, a more sustained behavioral response will be necessary to control HIV and other STIs with their associated morbidity and mortality. Rotello[4] argues that such a response should transcend the technical 'fixes' such as condom use, but should instead be based on a comprehensive ecological and epidemiological understanding of STIs.

Referring to what has been discussed in this chapter, the following 'hierarchy of safety' may be proposed.

1. Nothing will be as safe as sexual abstinence and, whenever feasible, this behavior should be promoted. Unfortunately, abstinence is often offered as a single option because it is felt that the discussion of other options will undermine the abstinence message. However, there is no proof of

this, while at the same time the prevention message for those individuals who, for a variety of reasons, choose not to be abstinent will be lost.

2. Short of abstinence, the focus should be on the avoidance of concurrency, ideally by only engaging in mutually monogamous relationships. Within these relationships, both partners should be aware of each other's previous risk of exposure to STIs, and whether or not screening for these infections has been undertaken since the last risk activity. Young couples who want to be 'checked' out are often encountered in sexual health clinics, as they want to start a relationship and/or want to stop using condoms. While this will not always be easy, such behavior does show mutual care and respect and should therefore be encouraged. Detection of curable STIs allows for treatment before transmission occurs, while disclosure of infection status of incurable STIs such as HIV, herpes simplex virus (HSV), or human papillomavirus (HPV) allows partners to make informed decisions about engaging in sex or using condoms.

3. For those who choose to have concurrent partners, the focus should be on reducing the number of concurrent partners, to substitute less risky (for example, mutual masturbation or oral sex) for riskier (anal or vaginal) sex, and to use condoms consistently when engaging in anal or vaginal sex. Interventions that may help encourage these behaviors will be discussed in Chapter 2.

References

1 Rietmeijer C, Lansky A, Anderson J, Fichtner R. Developing standards in behavioral surveillance for HIV/STD prevention. *AIDS Educ Prev* 2001; In Press.

2 Mertz KJ, McQuillan GM, Levine WC, *et al.* A pilot study of the prevalence of chlamydial infection in a national household survey. *Sex Transm Dis* 1998; **25**: 225–228.

3 Freeland W. Pathogens and the evolution of primate sociality. *Biotropica* 1976; **8**: 12–24.

4 Rotello G. *Sexual Ecology.* New York, NY; Penguin Group: 1997.

5 Borisenko K, Tikhonova L, Renton A. Syphilis and other sexually transmitted infections in the Russian Federation. *Int J STD AIDS* 1999; **10**: 665–668.

6 UNAIDS. *AIDS epidemic update: December 1999.* Geneva: UNAIDS/WHO Joint United National Programme on HIV/AIDS: 1999.

7 Amirkhanian Y, Kelly J, Issayev D. AIDS knowledge, attitudes, and behaviour in Russia: results of a population-based, random-digit telephone survey in St Petersburg. *Int J STD AIDS* 2001; **12**: 50–57.

8 May RM, Anderson RM. Transmission dynamics of HIV infection. *Nature* 1987; **326**: 137–142.

9 Carstairs G. *This Island Now.* The BBC Reith Lectures, 1962. London; The Hogarth Press: 1963.

10 Scarman SL. English law – the new dimension. London; Stevens and Son: 1974.

11 Farkas G, Sine L, Evans I. Personality, sexuality and demographic differences between volunteers and non-volunteers for a laboratory study of male sexual behavior. *Arch Sex Behavior* 1978; **7**: 283–289.

12 Christensen H, Gregg C. Changing norms in America and Scandinavia. *J Marriage Family* 1970; **32**: 616–627.

13 Johnson A, Wadsworth J, Wellings K, Field J. *Sexual Attitudes and Lifestyles.* London; Blackwell Scientific Publications: 1994.

14 Michael R, Gagnon J, Laumann E, Kolata G. *Sex in America.* Boston; Little, Brown and Co.: 1994.

15 Laumann E, Youm Y. Racial/ethnic group differences in the prevalence of sexually transmitted diseases in the United States: a network explanation. *Sex Transm Dis* 1999; **26**: 250–261.

16 Gorbach P, Sopheab H, Phalla I, *et al.* Sexual bridging by Cambodian men. Potential importance for general population spread of STD and HIV epidemics. *Sex Transm Dis* 2000; **27**: 320–326.

17 Piot P, Gowman J, Laga M. The epidemiology of HIV and AIDS in Africa. In: Essex M, Mboup S, Kanki P, Kalengayi M (eds) *AIDS in Africa.* New York, NY; Raven Press: 1994, pp. 157–172.

18 Potterat J, Zimmerman-Rogers H, Muth S, *et al.* Chlamydia transmission: concurrency, reproduction number and the epidemic trajectory. *Am J Epidemiol* 1999; **150**: 1–10.

19 Rothenberg R, Long D, Sterk C, *et al.* The Atlanta Urban Networks Study: a blueprint for endemic transmission. *AIDS* 2000; **14**: 2191–2200.

20 Morris M, Kretschmar M. Concurrent partnerships and the spread of HIV. *AIDS* 1997; **11**: 641–648.

21 Ferguson N, Garnett G. More realistic models of sexually transmitted disease dynamics. Sexual partnership networks, pair models, and moment closure. *Sex Transm Dis* 2000; **27**: 600–609.

22 Aral S, Adimora A, Manhart L, Gorbach P, Koumans E, Kraut J. *Temporal ordering of sex partnerships: concurrence and the 'GAP' as factors fueling or limiting the spread of STIs.* Paper presented at the 2000 National STD Prevention Conference, 2000; Milwaukee, WI.

23 Peterson L. *Contraceptive use in the United States: 1982–90. Advance data, No. 260,* pp 1–15. Hyattsville, MD: National Center for Health Statistics, February 14, 1995.

24 Centers for Disease Control and Prevention. Trends in sexual risk behaviors among high school students – United States, 1991–1997. *MMWR* 1998; **47**: 1–5.

25 Hunt A, Weatherburn P, Hickson F, Davies P, McManus T, Coxon A. Changes in condom use by gay men. *AIDS Care* 1993; **5**: 439–448.

26 Catania J, Coates T, Stall R, *et al.* Changes in condom use among homosexual men in San Francisco. *Health Psychol* 1991; **10**: 190–199.

27 Weatherburn P, Davies PM, Hickson FCI, *et al.* No connection between alcohol use and unsafe sex among gay and bisexual men. *AIDS* 1993; **7**: 115–119.

28 Perry MJ, Solomon LJ, Winett RA, *et al.* High risk sexual behaviour and alcohol consumption among bar-going gay men. *AIDS* 1994; **8**: 1321–1324.

29 Seage GR, Mayer KH, Wold C, *et al.* The social context of drinking, drug use and unsafe sex in the Boston young men study. *J Acquir Immune Defic Syndr Hum Retrovirol* 1998; **17**: 368–375.

30 Simeon DT, Bain BC, Wyatt GE, *et al.* Characteristics of Jamaicans who smoke marijuana before sex and their risk status for sexually transmitted diseases. *West Ind Med J* 1996; **45**: 9–13.

31 Boyer CB, Shafer M, Teitle E, *et al.* Sexually transmitted diseases in a health maintenance organization teen clinic. *Arch Pediatr Adolesc Med* 1999; **153**: 838–844.

32 McCusker J, Westenhouse J, Stoddard AM, *et al.* Use of drugs and alcohol by homosexually active men in relation to sexual practices. *J Acquir Immune Defic Syndr* 1990; **3**: 729–736.

33 Calzavara LM, Coates RA, Raboud JM, *et al.* Ongoing high-risk sexual behaviors in relation to recreational drug use in sexual encounters: analysis of 5 years of data from the Toronto Sexual Contact Study. *Ann Epidemiol* 1993; **3**: 272–280.

34 Cates W. Panel at ASHA. Estimates of the incidence and prevalence of sexually transmitted diseases in the United States.

Sex Transm Dis 1999; **26** (Suppl.): S1–S7.

35 Lehman J, Hecht F, Wortley P, Lansky A, Stevens M, Fleming P. *Are at-risk populations less concerned about HIV infection in the HAART era.* Paper presented at the 7th Conference on Retroviruses and Opportunistic Infections; San Francisco: 2000.

36 Centers for Disease Control and Prevention. Increases in unsafe sex and rectal gonorrhea among men who have sex with men – San Francisco, CA, 1994–1997. *MMWR* 1999; **48**: 45–48.

37 Centers for Disease Control and Prevention. Resurgent bacterial sexually transmitted diseases among men who have sex with men – King County Washington, 1997–1999. *MMWR* 1999; **48**: 773–779.

38 McFarland W, Schwarcz S, Kellogg T, Hsu L, Kim A, Katz M. *Implications of highly active antiretroviral treatment for HIV prevention: the case of men who have sex with men in San Francisco.* Paper presented at the XIII International Conference on AIDS; Durban, South Africa: 2000.

Chapter 2

Some aspects of the prevention of sexually transmissible infections
C A Rietmeijer, A McMillan

The control of sexually transmissible infections (STIs), including HIV, is dependent on the identification and treatment of infected individuals, on a change in sexual behavior, on the use of barrier or chemical methods to prevent transmission of pathogens, and, for a small number of STIs, on vaccination. Developments in primary and secondary prevention are discussed here, together with the syndromic approach to the management of STIs. The use of condoms and microbicides is also discussed here. Methods of reducing the parenteral spread of blood-borne viral infections are discussed in Chapter 8 in relation to viral hepatitis. The reader is referred to individual chapters for a discussion on vaccines that are available for the prevention of spread of some STIs.

Developments in primary and secondary prevention

INTRODUCTION

The goal of prevention of STIs is to reduce the incidence of these infections such that their respective epidemics are brought into decline, leading either to the elimination of the infection from the population or to a phase in which the infection persists at low endemic levels. In technical terms this implies that the reproductive rate of the infection (that is, the average number of new infections originating from one infected individual) falls below one[1]. The reproductive rate (R_0) in a susceptible population is defined as the product of the average transmission efficiency of the pathogen (β), the rate of exposure of susceptible individuals to infectious sex partners (c), and the average duration of infectiousness (D)[2]. Potentially therefore, STI prevention programs have three distinct targets to break the chain of infection of STIs.

1. First, they may aim to reduce 'c' by delaying sexual exposure or by reducing the number of partners.
2. Second, they can attempt to reduce (β), for example, by promoting the use of condoms, with the understanding that certain STIs (for example HIV, chlamydia, and gonorrhea), because of their anatomical location, may be better prevented this way than others (for example HPV or HSV).
3. Third, prevention efforts can be targeted at early case recognition and treatment, thereby reducing the duration of potential infectiousness (D).

Traditionally, STI prevention programs have been largely limited to the last approach, that is, they have focused on testing and treating symptomatic individuals, often in a specialized clinical environment (for example in STI or genitourinary medicine (GUM) departments, or in adolescent health and family planning clinics). While this approach is still valuable, and continues to play a major role in STI prevention, there are a number of drawbacks if prevention efforts are restricted to this type of intervention. For example, case recognition and treatment is of limited use for STIs that have no curative treatment, for example HIV, HSV, and HPV. While treatment theoretically could reduce the amount of infectious organisms and hence infectivity of these infections, the effectiveness of such an approach for transmission prevention remains to be established. Furthermore, many people with STIs are asymptomatic and will therefore not access specialized clinical services. Even people with symptoms of an STI may avoid specialized clinics and rather seek the services of their primary care provider. In a recent survey in the USA, 49% of respondents who had ever had an STI had gone to a private practice for treatment. In comparison only 5% of respondents had sought treatment at an STI clinic[3]. However, private practices may not be comfortable in managing these patients and many do not pro-actively offer STI prevention services to people who are at risk of STIs but who access these providers for other reasons[4].

The recent development of nucleic acid amplification tests (NAAT), which allow non-invasive, urine-based testing for chlamydia and gonorrhea, may help lower the threshold at which the primary care provider will screen for these pathogens among high-risk, asymptomatic populations. These tests also allow the combination of 'traditional' case finding with primary prevention programs (for example in schools or combined with street outreach) as well as providing such services in clinical settings where the primary focus may not be on STIs (for example in youth detention centers). Since many of the persons screened in such settings are asymptomatic, these approaches, if acceptable and targeted to populations with the highest prevalence, may have a profound impact on chlamydia and gonorrhea epidemiology.

Historically, behavioral interventions to reduce transmission efficacy (β) and exposure to infected partners (c) have been limited to targeted poster campaigns (for example the syphilis and gonorrhea prevention campaigns during World War II) and counseling in the context of STI-specific clinical encounters. Until the early 1980s there had been little research to evaluate the efficacy of these efforts at prevention, or to develop new science-based prevention interventions. Because of the incurable nature of HIV, the HIV epidemic caused a shift of interest to primary prevention. During the mid- to late 1980s substantial funding was allocated to research on the prevention of HIV resulting in a number of well-evaluated interventions. These developments have expanded the range of primary prevention interventions to 'STI prevention program[s] beyond the traditional biomedical alternatives of antimicrobials and vaccines to include behavioral "virtual vaccines" to increase condom use and promote other healthy sexual behaviors'.[1]

ENHANCING SCREENING FOR SEXUALLY TRANSMISSIBLE INFECTIONS

In health-care settings outside clinical environments where screening for STIs among asymptomatic persons has been the norm for many years (for example in STI and GUM departments, family planning clinics, and adolescent health clinics), testing for STIs has historically been limited to individuals presenting with STI-related symptoms or to those who presented as contacts to infected persons. Barriers to expanded screening in these settings included

- discomfort in performing a sexual risk assessment
- perceived objections by patients to invasive examinations (including pelvic examination and urethral swabbing)

- the lack of STI-specific diagnostic capability.

The latter two barriers have now largely been overcome by the availability of urine-based NAAT, including polymerase chain reaction (PCR) and ligase chain reaction (LCR) assays. The sensitivity of these tests is superior to culture assays. For instance, it has been estimated that NAAT may be detecting 20% more chlamydial infections compared to older technology[5]. In fact, as the proportion of persons asymptomatically infected with *Chlamydia trachomatis* and *Neisseria gonorrhoeae* may be larger than previously suspected, the importance of screening high-risk, asymptomatic populations is emphasized. However, while these tests have specificities of 95% and above, their predictive value may fall below 50% in low-prevalence communities. This should be considered when counseling people who test positive on these tests, when confirmatory (culture or other) tests are not available, such as in street outreach settings.

A number of studies have investigated the feasibility and cost-effectiveness of urine-based chlamydia screening in primary care settings. For example in a study from The Netherlands opportunistic urine screening was offered to 3689 asymptomatic heterosexual individuals aged between 15 and 40 years who visited a general practice in Amsterdam for reasons unrelated to STIs. Of these people only 215 (5.8%) refused testing for STIs, and among the remainder a chlamydia prevalence of 4.9% was found[6]. In a subsequent analysis of these data, this approach was found to be cost effective provided that there is a prescreening prevalence of at least 1.8% of STIs and the program lasts for 10 years[7]. In another study, also from The Netherlands, a letter was sent out to 11 005 patients registered at 15 general practices, inviting them to mail a urine specimen for chlamydia testing. The overall response was 41% and the chlamydia prevalence was 2.6%[8, 9]. These and other studies demonstrate the acceptability of screening for STIs among providers and clients in primary care settings, and can serve as models that may be further tailored to individual practice settings.

SCREENING IN NON-TRADITIONAL SETTINGS

In public health, a distinction is usually made between primary prevention (i.e. preventing disease from occurring) and secondary prevention (i.e. preventing complications from disease after it has occurred). In STI prevention this distinction is blurred; treating a person for gonorrhea or chlamydia may be considered as secondary prevention for the patient (i.e. to prevent pelvic inflammatory disease), but as primary prevention of ongoing transmission to future uninfected partners. The availability of non-invasive screening methods for the detection of chlamydial infection and gonorrhea has further reduced the differences between primary and secondary prevention. Where prevention programs among at-risk populations were traditionally limited to education and other behavioral interventions (see pp. 13–16), these programs can now easily be supplemented with screening. The feasibility of such approaches has been demonstrated in a number of settings where high-risk populations congregate but where STI services have not traditionally been offered. These approaches have included screening in school-based settings[10], juvenile detention centers[11], drug treatment programs[12], community clinics[13], and street outreach in high-risk communities[14, 15]. Most of these studies have demonstrated high prevalence of chlamydia and, to a lesser extent, gonorrhea in these populations. Since most chlamydial infections and many gonococcal infections (particularly among women) are asymptomatic and are thus unlikely to come to the attention of clinical care providers, these types of screening programs appear to be very promising in the prevention and ultimate control of these STIs. However, while these studies serve as a 'proof of concept', the performance of these types of screening programs in 'real world' settings as well as their cost effectiveness remains to be established. In this context it will be important to select high-prevalence populations as well as to integrate screening with existing services, such as intake into drug treatment or juvenile detention, or as part of a street outreach program.

THE ROLE OF THE PRIMARY CARE PROVIDER IN THE PREVENTION OF SEXUALLY TRANSMISSIBLE INFECTIONS

Over the past decade the role of the health-care provider has shifted from being primarily reactive to the needs and complaints of patients, to being increasingly proactive in offering preventive services based on scientific evidence and promulgated through advocacy groups and professional organizations. These services are based on the concept that many diseases are characterized by initial asymptomatic stages of different durations, and that diagnosing diseases in these stages through screening may lead to interventions that could improve health outcomes. In addition, there is an increased focus on the evaluation of behaviors that are linked to negative health outcomes, including smoking, alcohol consumption, diet, use of seat belts, and high-risk sexual behavior. Based on these considerations, strong arguments can be made for a more proactive approach for prevention of STIs in the primary care setting. Indeed, many organizations include recommendations for prevention of STIs. For example the United States Preventive Services Task Force recommends that persons aged 13 to 64 years should be evaluated for sexual development and behavior. Depending on the assessment they should then be screened for HIV, chlamydial infection, gonorrhea, and syphilis, and be counseled regarding STIs, partner selection, use of condoms, unintended pregnancies, and contraceptive options[16].

BEHAVIORAL INTERVENTIONS: THE CASE FOR CLIENT-CENTERED COUNSELING

Behavioral counseling for STI and HIV risk reduction has traditionally been recommended as an integral part of STI and HIV prevention activities. The United States Preventive Services Task Force is but one of many authoritative sources in recent years to stress the importance of risk assessment and counseling for STI and HIV prevention among the sexually active population. However, until recently, no controlled studies had been conducted to demonstrate the efficacy of behavioral counseling in reducing the incidence of STIs. This absence of scientific data has led to a lack of clear counseling protocols and has often left counseling up to the inclination of the clinician or counselor. Where, over the years, clinical guidelines for the treatment of STIs have become widely accepted[17], substantial variation exists in the quality and quantity of counseling available. However, recent research has started to address these issues, and one study, Project Respect, is particularly promising. In this multi-center, randomized, controlled trial, a total of 5758 heterosexual patients were recruited in five STI clinics in the USA and were randomized to one of the following face-to-face interventions. These interventions included

- enhanced counseling – four interactive theory-based interventions, a total of 4 hours and 20 minutes in duration
- brief counseling – two 20-minute interactive counseling sessions based on the Center for Disease Control's recommended HIV counseling for patients attending public clinics and HIV test sites
- two short 5-minute didactic messages – this approximates to the current intervention in most STI clinics.

All interventions were structured around pre- and post-test HIV counseling and testing sessions. Study subjects were actively followed up after enrollment with questionnaires and STI tests for 12 months. Self-reported use of condoms and new diagnoses of STIs (gonorrhea, chlamydia, syphilis, and HIV) were the main outcome measures. Compared to participants receiving didactic messages, participants in the enhanced and the brief counseling groups reported higher use of condoms at 3 and 6 months, and had a 20% reduction in new STIs at 12 months. Reductions were similar across study sites, and were greater for adolescents and for persons diagnosed with a STI at enrollment[18]. The fact that the brief counseling sessions achieved similar risk reductions as the enhanced intervention, was encouraging from a practical perspective as, obviously, two 20-minute counseling sessions will be easier to implement than four sessions each averaging more than an hour.

Nevertheless, even the shorter intervention may be difficult to implement in the schedule of a busy clinic, especially if the numbers of staff are limited and there is no reimbursement for counseling. Furthermore, many patients will not return to the clinic after the initial visit, potentially limiting the effectiveness of a two-session intervention. Besides confirming the efficacy of counseling, future studies should therefore also investigate whether one-session counseling interventions can also be effective, and how best to implement counseling in the context of clinic logistics.

CLIENT-CENTERED COUNSELING AND OTHER THEORETICAL CONSIDERATIONS IN BEHAVIORAL INTERVENTIONS

The 'brief counseling' sessions shown to be effective in the Project Respect intervention trial were based on what is known as 'client-centered counseling'. Client-centered counseling is comprised of the following steps[18–20].

- to assess actual and self-perceived HIV or STI risk
- to help the participant recognize barriers to risk reduction
- to negotiate an acceptable and achievable risk-reduction plan
- to support patient-initiated behavior change.

The basic premise of client-centered counseling is that it is the responsibility of the client to develop his or her own prevention plan, based on a thorough appreciation of their STI or HIV risk and taking into account the reality of what is achievable given their own set of circumstances. The task of the counselor is to give information and to assist the client in formulating the plan. One of the challenges for the counselor in this intervention is to be satisfied with a plan that may be perceived (by the counselor) as inadequate. However, the goal is to have the client achieve small prevention measures, which may lead to larger ones in the future, rather than be frustrated in the defeat of an overly ambitious plan.

Although the client-centered intervention is not itself based on formal behavior change theory, certain concepts of behavioral theory are very useful in helping counselors to master the skills required for this intervention. The Transtheoretical

Model as formulated by Prochaska and DiClemente[21], for example, posits that behavior change occurs along a fluid continuum of five different stages

- pre-contemplation – no intention to change
- contemplation – long-term intention to change
- ready-for-action or preparation – short-term intention to change
- action – short-term change
- maintenance – long-term change.

The theory posits that different psychological processes are invoked in the transfer from one stage to the next. It has been further suggested that 'influencing factors' as identified in a number of other behavioral theories may similarly have differential effects in the stage-of-change continuum. These factors include

1. the person's perceptions that he or she is personally susceptible to acquiring a given disease or illness (from the Health Belief Model[22])
2. the person's attitude toward performing the behavior, based upon beliefs about the positive and negative consequences of performing that behavior (from the Theory of Reasoned Action[23])
3. perceived norms, which include the perception that others in the community are also changing, and that those with whom the person interacts most closely support the person's attempt to change (from the Theory of Reasoned Action[23])
4. self-efficacy, which involves the person's perception that he or she can perform the behavior under a variety of circumstances (from the Social Cognitive Theory[24, 25]).

Interventions focusing on cognitive and emotional factors (for example risk education) may be more effective in the early stages, while action-oriented approaches (including skills building and other interventions enhancing self-efficacy) will be more effective in later stages[21]. However, while these factors focus on psychological processes that ultimately form intentions and actions, we need to be aware that behaviors take place in a social environment and that community norms and values, peer role models (both positive and negative), and community empowerment also play a role in shaping individual behaviors. In this context, client-centered counseling as well as other behavioral interventions can be viewed as pragmatic models that incorporate theoretical concepts into a combination that appears to be most effective for certain behaviors in certain populations.

GROUP-LEVEL INTERVENTIONS

Prompted by the need to develop effective behavioral interventions for HIV prevention, a number of studies have been conducted during the past decade, most of which have focused on small group interventions. Many of these interventions are based on concepts from behavioral science theory. For example Main et al.[26] developed a group-level intervention primarily based on Social Cognitive Theory and the Theory of Reasoned Action[23]. It comprised a 15-session skills-based curriculum in high schools in six Colorado school districts. Compared to other schools, students who participated in the intervention reported fewer sex partners and used condoms more often[26]. Similarly, St Lawrence et al. developed an eight-session group intervention based on Social Cognitive Theory with attention to informational needs, motivational influences, and behavior from the information, motivation, and behavioral skills risk-reduction model. The 'Becoming A Responsible Teen (BART)' curriculum included eight 90 to 120-minute group sessions which focused on giving information, making sexual decisions, and developing technical, social, and cognitive competency skills, as well as social support and empowerment, for African-American youths attending a public health clinic in Jackson, Mississippi. Youths who participated in the intervention reported significantly greater use of condoms and lower frequency of unprotected intercourse compared to youths in a comparison group who received only the first of the eight sessions[27].

While these and other group-level behavioral interventions demonstrated positive effects on sexual behavior, it might be argued that self-reported behaviors may not necessarily be predictive of reducing STIs and HIV. However, similar studies did evaluate the subsequent incidence of STIs. For example, in a study in a Los Angeles STI clinic, Cohen et al.[28] evaluated a single 30-minute condom-skills education session, including an introduction on effective condom use, a group discussion on how condoms should be used, and a demonstration on how to put on a condom. Persons who participated in the intervention were significantly less likely to return to the STI clinic within the next 12 months with a new STI than those in the comparison group[28]. Finally, a randomized controlled trial conducted by Shain et al.[29] among African American and Hispanic women with non-viral STIs is perhaps the most conclusive group-level intervention study to date showing a significant reduction in STIs among African-American and Hispanic women with non-viral STIs who participated in a multi-component small group intervention. This multi-component, small-group intervention was comprised of three 3 to 4-hour sessions actively involving participants in open discussion, games, watching videotapes, behavior modeling, and role play. Based on the AIDS Risk Reduction Model[30], the group sessions were designed to help women recognize personal susceptibility, commit to changing their behavior, and acquire the necessary skills. The control group received standard counseling. Compared to the control group, the intervention group had significantly lower rates of re-infection with chlamydia or gonorrhea[29].

In summary, these and other studies suggest that group interventions focusing on building skills, self-efficacy, and social support may be effective in reducing the incidence of STIs including HIV. From a practical perspective, this type of intervention may be most easily implemented in clinics or other facilities where persons at high risk for STIs are concentrated, such as schools, juvenile detention centers, or community-based organizations. It may be argued, however, that many individuals who avail themselves of group interventions are already susceptible to behavior change and are therefore self-selected or, borrowing from the Transtheoretical Model, they may already be in the 'preparation stage' and beyond the 'contemplative' or 'pre-contemplative' stages of behavior change. Hence, group-level interventions may be less effective in reaching people in the earlier stages of change.

COMMUNITY-LEVEL INTERVENTIONS

The basic concept in community-level interventions is that at-risk individuals are exposed to behavioral interventions through formal and less formal communication channels within the community, regardless of their 'readiness' to change. An added benefit of this type of intervention is that whole communities can be targeted with the intervention and in this way changes may be made in community norms and other social factors influencing individual behavior. Finally, even though the intensity of these interventions at the individual level is limited, the overall coverage of the intervention may result in considerable benefits at the community level. In addition to the above-mentioned psychological behavior change models, many community-level interventions are based on concepts from the Diffusion of Innovations theory as formulated by Rogers[31]. This theory posits that people are most likely to adopt new behaviors when favorable evaluations of the behavior are conveyed to them by peers whom they respect. Thus, in this model a major role is played by community leaders and other 'change agents'. Community-level interventions have been designed for a number of health problems and have had different levels of success in preventing cardio-vascular disease[32, 33], in helping smokers to stop[34, 35], and most recently in preventing alcohol-related injuries[36]. In the area of promoting safer sex practices for HIV prevention, Kelly et al.[37], using cadres of popular opinion leaders, pioneered this approach in developing interventions amongst men who have sex with men and who attend gay bars. In a two-part intervention, persons who were popular with others were nominated by bartenders at gay clubs and were enrolled in four 90-minute group sessions covering HIV education and communication strategies. Next, each opinion leader agreed to have at least fourteen conversations with peers in bars about AIDS risk reduction. The intervention was conducted in gay bars in one city, while gay bars in two other cities were assigned control status. Compared to men in the control cities, homosexual men in the intervention city had a significantly greater reduction in unprotected anal intercourse.

In a similar approach, Kegeles et al.[38] described an intervention developed by a core group of young gay men with input from a community advisory group. The intervention included two formal outreach components, one directed at venues where young gay men congregated and one comprising safe-sex promotional events at the center from which the intervention was conducted. In addition, informal outreach included peer-initiated communications, initiated by 3-hour small group sessions addressing safer sex and skills. Finally, a small publicity campaign was developed to reinforce safer sex norms and disseminate awareness of the project. The intervention was conducted in Eugene, OR, while a similar community in Santa Barbara, CA served as the comparison community. Men in the intervention community were significantly more likely to reduce their frequency of unprotected intercourse than men in the comparison community.

The largest community-level HIV-prevention study was conducted by the AIDS Community Demonstration Projects between 1991 and 1994 in five USA cities. These sites developed a common protocol based on the Transtheoretical Model and using concepts from a number of other behavior change theories, including the Theory of Reasoned Action, the Health Belief Model, and the Social Cognitive Theory. The intervention was aimed at increasing condom use for anal and vaginal sex among a variety of target populations, including non-gay-identifying men who had sex with men, injection-drug users, sex-industry workers, high-risk youths, and other high-risk populations; enhancing the use of bleach was an added goal among injection-drug users. The target populations varied by site but intervention and evaluation protocols were the same. Intervention messages comprised printed role model stories developed from real-life experiences of local community members. Stories were behavior specific, for example the use of condoms for anal sex among non-gay-identifying men who had sex with men. Ongoing surveys in the community identified the stage of change for this behavior of the majority of the community (for example the 'Action Stage'). Scenarios for the role model stories then focused on the next stage (in this example

'maintenance') and factors influencing the transition between these stages were highlighted. Role model stories were packaged into appealing 'intervention kits' that also included condoms, lubricant, and bleach (for injection-drug users only) and which were distributed by peer volunteers recruited from the target community. Peer volunteers were trained in small group sessions and encouraged to discuss the contents of the kits with their peers as well as model behavior changes they had already made. The main outcome of the project was a significantly increased and consistent use of condoms with non-regular partners among members of all target groups in all intervention sites compared to individuals in the matched comparison sites[39]. A significant increase in the use of bleach was also found in one of the intervention sites targeting injection drug users[40].

STRUCTURAL AND ENVIRONMENTAL FACTORS

Improving sexual health has been designated as one of the premier strategies to reach the long-term goal of sustained prevention of STIs. The underlying rationale for this is that many individuals cannot make healthy sexual decisions because of a number of factors, including lack of objective information, mixed messages in the media, and confusing social norms[41]. Interventions as described above may assist in improving sexual health, but will fall short if they are embedded in a social, cultural, and political environment that is at odds with the messages distributed through prevention programs. In this context, it is important to focus on the role of schools and school-based sexual education. Next to parental guidance, such curricula are widely recommended as being a key component in shaping children and young adults into individuals in whom sexuality has become integrated as a balanced component in optimal physical, psychological, and social functioning[41]. Obviously, the content of such curricula is not free of prevailing community norms and moral values. For example there still remains a rift between whether it is best to teach abstinence only or encourage condom use. However, a synthesis between these two apparently opposing approaches may be possible. For example, an 'abstinence plus' curriculum may be envisioned teaching abstinence as the preferred way to avoid negative psychological and physical health consequences from sexual intercourse, but also discussing the role of condom use as a means of reducing risks for those who choose to engage in sexual intercourse. However, confusion may arise if the curriculum content is in conflict with other environmental factors, for example when condom use is included in the curriculum as a means to prevent STIs, but the school authorities prohibit the distribution of condoms.

PREVENTION OF SEXUALLY TRANSMISSIBLE VIRAL INFECTIONS

The above discussion has largely involved treatable bacterial STIs and HIV. The prevention aspects of viral STIs, particularly genital herpes and HPV infections are currently receiving more attention, but the prevention messages are as yet unclear and more research in this area is necessary. For example, while testing and treating high-risk asymptomatic individuals for chlamydial infection, gonorrhea, and syphilis is widely recommended, such recommendations do not yet exist for screening for herpes simplex type 2 virus (HSV-2) and HPV infections. There remain a number of unresolved questions before such recommendations are likely to be made, including to what extent HSV-2 seropositive individuals will transmit the virus to uninfected partners and thus what the overall benefit will be of widespread screening on HSV-2 prevention. Similar questions also surround screening for genital HPV infections with the added caveat that different genital HPV types cause different diseases and complications and that HPV screening must be type-specific to yield optimal preventive outcomes (Chapter 5). In the absence of curative treatment for these conditions, the potential benefits of screening for HSV and HPV should also be weighed against the negative psychological impact and potential stigma that persons who test positive for these pathogens may experience.

SUMMARY, CONCLUSIONS, AND FUTURE DEVELOPMENTS

In public health a distinction is usually made between primary prevention (preventing disease from occurring) and secondary prevention (preventing complications from existing disease). In STI and HIV prevention this distinction has long had a corollary in the environment in which these different types of prevention activities took place, that is, diagnosis and treatment of STIs (secondary prevention) in clinical settings and education and other behavioral interventions (primary prevention) in non-clinical sites. However, in STI prevention the distinction between primary and secondary prevention has not been so clear since secondary prevention at the individual level (for example treating gonorrhea to prevent pelvic inflammatory disease), is also primary prevention of transmission to future, uninfected partners. Recent developments in behavioral interventions as well as technical advances in testing and treatment are further blurring the difference. We now know that counseling in clinic settings, when conducted properly, can reduce the incidence of STIs, while screening for STI pathogens using non-invasive methods is now feasible in conditions that only 5 years ago would be viewed as the typical domain of behavioral interventions. Further feasibility and cost-effectiveness studies will determine the future extent of the 'cross-over' of primary and secondary prevention activities. There are a number of anticipated developments that will serve to further enhance their integration. First, advances in testing techniques are continuing. As discussed earlier (see pp. 11–12) urine-based NAAT for chlamydial and gonococcal infections has already made such testing available in a wide variety of non-clinical setting. Still, the currently approved tests require laboratory processing and results are generally not known until 24 hours or longer after the specimen has been collected. Particularly in outreach settings this may be a costly delay if the person cannot be contacted and treated after the result is known. Tests that can be administered as well as processed quickly in the field would constitute an enormous advantage as persons testing positive can

be treated in the field immediately. In this respect, a number of promising tests are currently being developed for gonorrhea and chlamydia urine testing, while rapid saliva and blood tests for syphilis and HIV are also anticipated. Secondly, advances in drug treatment also help to make community-based secondary prevention more feasible. For example, with the availability of azithromycin for the treatment of chlamydial infection (Chapter 10), we are now able to provide directly observed treatment in the field. More effective treatments for HIV also have a profound effect on HIV prevention. As viral loads decrease due to highly active antiretroviral therapy (HAART), HIV-infected patients may become less infectious and thus, again, treatment may provide both secondary as well as primary prevention benefits. However, these positive effects may be offset by increased sexual risk taking as sexual activity increases with improvements in physical well being. Also, decreased adherence to safe sexual practices may be accompanied by decreased adherence to HAART regimens and associated higher viral loads. Thus, the potential arises for increased HIV transmission in this group of patients. Because of the potential emergence of drug-resistant viruses among these less-adherent individuals, the spread of resistant HIV strains is likely. Therefore, increasingly, HIV treatment should go hand-in-hand with prevention of ongoing transmission and HIV care providers must be involved in this process. Conversely, HIV prevention case management must also involve treatment and adherence issues.

The integration of primary and secondary prevention may have a number of potential disadvantages. The implementation of screening and treatment of STIs outside clinical settings involves personnel, including outreach staff, who are not traditionally trained in performing these tasks. This may jeopardize the quality of the services delivered and therefore, before starting such programs, assurance must be given that participating staff will have received appropriate training. Partnerships with health departments and associated training centers will be needed in this process.

Persons receiving limited, urine-based, screening may also misinterpret these tests as a comprehensive evaluation for any STI. They should be informed about the limitations of these tests and should be referred to a clinic where comprehensive STI evaluations are available should they have symptoms or should they request a full evaluation. It might be argued that offering field-based testing, in fact could serve as a disincentive to obtain clinic-based evaluations. However, even though clinical services may be easily available, many at-risk individuals, particularly adolescents, will not access these services even while acknowledging their risks and for these persons field-based testing may be all that is acceptable[4].

In conclusion, developments in behavioral interventions as well as technical advances in STI testing have had and will continue to have a profound impact on the continuum of STI and HIV prevention both inside and outside the clinical environment. While the individual provider of STI services will continue to play a major role in STI prevention, this role can no longer be seen separately from other primary and secondary prevention efforts. Together, these efforts may ultimately lead to a comprehensive STI and HIV prevention system.

Syndromic management of sexually transmissible infections

The control of sexually transmitted infections relies on the prompt recognition and effective treatment of these infections, thereby reducing the risks of complications in an individual, and limiting the transmission of the infection in the community[42]. Traditionally, the management of sexually transmitted infections has relied on the laboratory diagnosis of the causative organism, and an appropriate treatment for the organism. Although this is still the preferred option in industrialized countries, this approach is costly, and, as there may be delays in treating infected individuals, it does not lend itself easily to the management of STIs in the developing world. The

World Health Organization has developed and promoted a syndrome management approach in many developing countries[43, 44]. Syndromic management is based on the identification of groups of symptoms and easily recognized signs (syndromes), and the provision of treatment to cover the pathogens likely to cause the syndrome in that geographical area. Flow charts or algorithms for the management of urethral discharge, genital ulceration, inguinal bubo, scrotal swelling, vaginal discharge, lower abdominal pain, and neonatal conjunctivitis have been devised to guide health workers in the implementation of syndromic management[45] (see Figures 2.1–2.10). In the algorithms for vaginal discharge, socio-demographic and behavioral factors are included*, and where possible,

---

* Risk assessment factors (point value) include: having a symptomatic partner (2), age less than 21 years (1), unmarried (1), more than one sexual partner (1), and having a new partner in the preceding 3 months (1). A score of 2 is high risk.

simple laboratory tests (Gram-smear and saline-mount microscopy).

STUDIES TO EVALUATE THE PERFORMANCE OF THE ALGORITHMS

Several studies have compared the outcomes of syndromic management with the more traditional laboratory-based approach to prevention of STIs. The syndromic management of men with *urethritis* has high sensitivity and positive predictive value. For example, in a study of 105 men who attended a primary health-care facility in Benin, Africa, the sensitivity, specificity and positive predictive value for the simple algorithm for the detection of gonococcal and chlamydial infection were 91.5%, 60.3%, and 65.2% respectively[46]. It was also noted that when Gram-smear microscopy was undertaken as an additional procedure in men with urethral discharge, the specificity and positive predictive value increased only modestly to 82.8% and 79.6% res-

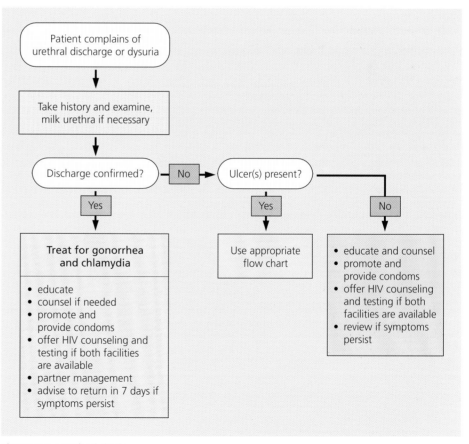

Figure 2.1 Urethral discharge

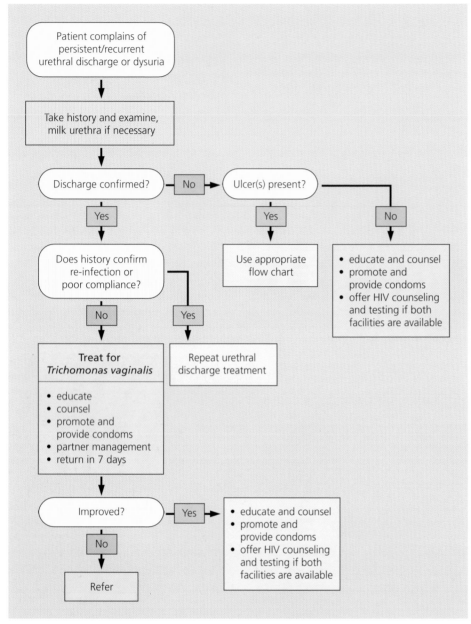

Figure 2.2 Persistent/recurrent urethral discharge in men. This flowchart assumes effective therapy for gonorrhoea and chlamydia to have been received and taken by the patient prior to this consultation.

pectively, but sensitivity fell to 83.0%[46]. Although sensitivity, specificity, and predictive values are poor when a disease-specific protocol is used, syndromic management of *genital ulcer disease* provides adequate treatment for more than 90% of patients[47]. Recent studies have called into question the validity of the WHO algorithms for the management of *vaginal discharge* for the detection of cervical infection with *Neisseria gonorrhoeae* and *Chlamydia*

trachomatis because specificity and positive predictive values are low[42]. For example, Daly *et al.*[48] found that for an algorithm for the diagnosis and treatment of cervical gonococcal and chlamydial infections that considered historical variables only, the sensitivity, specificity and positive predictive value were 43.0%, 73.4% and 28.1% respectively. Such findings are not surprising as the majority of women with uncomplicated chlamydial or gonococcal

infections are asymptomatic (Chapters 10 and 11). Ryan *et al.*[49] found that the symptom of lower abdominal pain also had a low positive predictive value (8.7%) in the detection of cervical infection. However, the combination of a positive risk assessment plus signs of cervicitis or pelvic inflammatory disease increase the positive predictive value, albeit at the cost of sensitivity[42]. The algorithms are more sensitive and specific for vaginal infections than for cervical infections. Ryan *et al.*[50], using an algorithm based on risk assessment and symptoms alone, found that the sensitivity, specificity and positive predictive value for the diagnosis of trichomoniasis or bacterial vaginosis were 67.8%, 49.6%, and 49.6% respectively. When a speculum examination was included in the assessment of the patient, the specificity and positive predictive value increased to 94.9% and 58.9% respectively; the sensitivity, however, declined to 10.0%.

Sexually transmitted infections are important cofactors in the transmission of HIV (see Chapters 6, 10, 11, 15, 16, and 17). In the case of urethritis or cervicitis, an increased level of shedding of HIV in genital secretions may lead to increased infectiousness and a greater possibility of HIV-1 transmission. Treatment of such conditions, however, should reduce the infectiousness of the HIV-infected individual. Cohen *et al.*[51] showed that the median concentration of HIV-1 RNA in cell-free seminal plasma from men with urethritis was eight times higher than that in HIV-seropositive men without urethritis (12.4 versus 1.51×10^4 copies/mL), but that the concentration of HIV-1 RNA decreased significantly within 1 week of successful treatment. Similarly, treatment of women with cervicitis caused by *N. gonorrhoeae* or *C. trachomatis* has been shown to reduce the HIV-1 RNA concentration in cervical secretions, and to reduce the prevalence of HIV-1-infected cells in these secretions[52]. The impact of treatment of STIs in reducing the incidence of HIV-1 was shown clearly in the Mwanza, Tanzania study[53]. This was a randomized trial to evaluate the impact of improved sexually transmitted disease case management on the incidence of HIV-1. The incidence of this infection was compared in six intervention com-

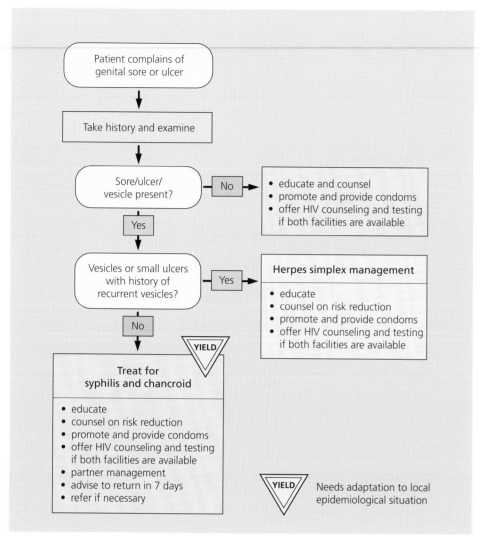

Figure 2.3 Genital ulcers.

for cervical infection where the prevalence exceeds 6%[45]. For the treatment of suspected pelvic inflammatory disease see Chapter 12. Infants with neonatal conjunctivitis should be treated for both gonococcal and chlamydial infection (Chapter 10). Criteria for the selection of drugs for the syndromic management of STIs are shown in Box 2.1[45]. In choosing drugs, consideration should be given to the capabilities and experience of the health worker.

The use of condoms in the prevention of sexually transmissible infections

A review of all aspects of condoms – their manufacture, quality control, efficacy as a contraceptive, and their role in the prevention of sexually transmissible infections – has recently been published[54], and the interested reader is referred to this excellent monograph.

MALE CONDOMS

The use of condoms, in the form of linen sheaths, for protection against sexually transmitted infections was first reported in the 16th century by the Italian anatomist, Fallopio. Most condoms are made of latex, but sheaths made from sheep intestine and, more recently, from polyurethane, are also marketed. In general there has been a

munities and six pair-matched comparison communities. The study focused on enhanced syndromic diagnosis of symptomatic sexually transmitted infection, based on the WHO algorithms. Of those individuals who were initially HIV-1 seronegative, 1.2% of 4149 in the intervention communities and 1.9% of the 4400 in the comparison communities seroconverted, a reduction of 40%.

TREATMENT OF SYNDROMES ASSOCIATED WITH SEXUALLY TRANSMISSIBLE INFECTIONS

In the management of a man with urethral discharge or a scrotal swelling, therapy should be for gonorrhea and chlamydial infection (see Chapters 10 and 11). Recommended syndromic management of genital ulceration includes therapy for syphilis, *plus* treatment for chancroid, *or* for donovanosis, *or* for lymphogranuloma venereum (LGV) where these infections are prevalent[45]. Inguinal and femoral buboes are most commonly associated with chancroid and LGV, and treatment for both infections is indicated (Chapter 16). Women presenting with vaginal discharge should be treated for trichomoniasis and for bacterial vaginosis (Chapter 17). The decision as to whether or not to treat a woman with vaginal discharge for gonorrhea and/or chlamydial infection depends on the prevalence of these infections in the community; it is said to be cost-effective to treat

Box 2.1 Criteria for the selection of drugs for the management of sexually transmissible infections

Drugs selected for treating STIs should meet the following criteria:

high efficacy, at least 95%
low cost
acceptable toxicity and tolerance
organism resistance unlikely to develop or likely to be delayed
single dose
oral administration
not contraindicated for pregnant or lactating women.

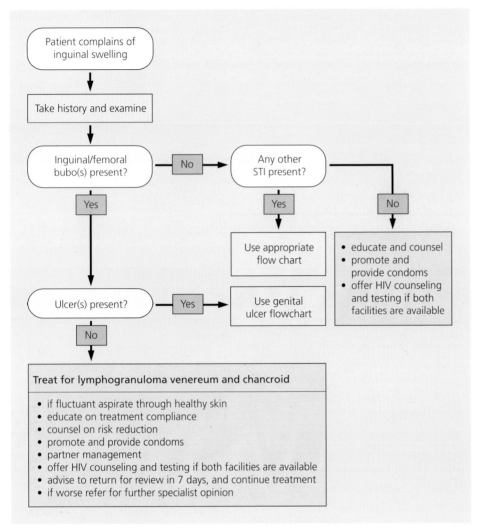

Figure 2.4 Inguinal bubo.

recent increase in the frequency of condom use at the time of first intercourse, but it is clear that individuals under the age of 16 years are less likely than older people to use condoms[55]. There is also some evidence that they are used more often than previously by men and women who have multiple partners. A recent study has shown that consistent condom use decreases in partnerships that change from new to regular[56].

Male latex condom

The latex condom is essentially a cylindrical tube with a hemispherical closed end that often has a protruding reservoir for ejaculated semen. These condoms, however, are marketed in a variety of sizes, shapes and colours, and some have surface protrusions. Although there is no clear evidence that they are more suitable for anal intercourse, thicker condoms are available. Condoms that are lubricated with spermicide such as nonoxynol-9 are also marketed.

In a series of ingenious experiments, it has been shown that latex condoms are impermeable to HIV, HSV, hepatitis B virus, and *Chlamydia trachomatis*[57, 58]. Although the pores in the natural condoms (for example those made of sheep intestine) are small enough to prevent passage of spermatozoa, they are sufficiently large to allow the passage of viruses. Their use in the prevention of sexually transmitted infections,

then, cannot be recommended[59]. Cross-sectional, case-control, and intervention studies have shown that consistent use of condoms reduces, but does not eliminate, the risk of transmission of many sexually transmitted infections. Condom breakage during intercourse is estimated to be less than 1%[60], and may result from perforation by fingernails, poor fitting because of the circumference of the penis, or the use of an oil-based lubricant. Although the use of stronger condoms has been promoted for anal intercourse between men, there is no significant difference in the failure rate between these and standard strength condoms[61].

Viral infections

Several studies have shown that consistent use of condoms for vaginal intercourse reduces the risk of acquisition of HIV infection. For example, Saracco et al.[62] prospectively studied 343 women who were HIV-seronegative at study entry and who were the monogamous partners of HIV-infected men. Nineteen seroconversions were noted in 529.6 person years of observation; the incidence of HIV infection was 7.2 per 100 person years in those women whose partners did not use condoms, compared with 1.1 amongst those who said that they always used condoms (relative risk was 6.6, 95% confidence interval 1.9–21.9). Similarly, de Vincenzi and colleagues[63] reported that there were no instances of seroconversion amongst 124 HIV-seronegative heterosexual individuals who consistently used condoms during vaginal or anal intercourse with an infected partner. In contrast, among the 121 couples who reported inconsistent condom use, the rate of seroconversion was 4.8 per 100 person-years (95% confidence interval 2.5–8.4). Using a mathematical model based on data included in a meta-analysis of studies in which condom use was stratified into consistent and inconsistent use, Pinkerton and Abramson[64] estimated that condom use reduced the per-contact probability of male to female HIV transmission by 95%. The use of condoms by men who have had anogenital sex with other men has also been shown to reduce the risk of HIV infection. Williams

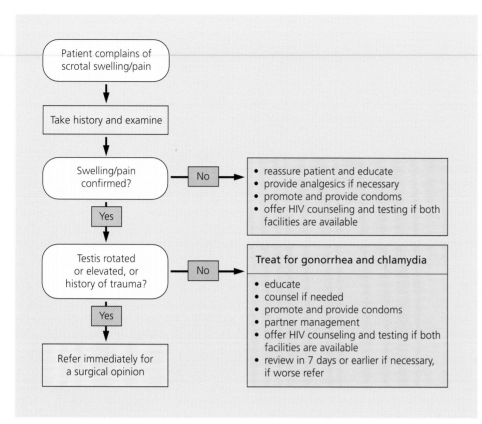

Figure 2.5 Scrotal swelling.

control study from Baltimore, condom use during the preceding month reduced the risk of gonococcal infection (odds ratio 0.4, 95% confidence interval 0.19–0.87). In Schwartz and colleagues' study, a history of condom use was also negatively associated with non-gonococcal urethritis (odds ratio 0.59, 95% confidence interval 0.43–0.79) and chlamydial infection (odds ratio 0.67, 95% confidence interval 0.44–1.03). Amongst women the use of a condom by a partner appears to protect against chlamydial infection. In a large, cross-sectional study[72] that identified *Chlamydia trachomatis* infection in 9.2% of 13 204 female military recruits, the adjusted odds ratio for having a partner who did not use condoms consistently was 1.4 (95% confidence interval 1.1–1.6). There have been relatively few studies on protection against *Treponema pallidum* infection. Indirect evidence comes from an intervention study that showed that the prevalence of syphilis amongst 824 female sex-industry workers in Fukuoka, Japan, fell from 7.5% to 0.5% in a 3-year period during which condom use by these women increased from 6.3% to 25.3%[73].

et al.[65] reported that the odds ratios for seroconversion for men who sometimes or never used condoms for anal intercourse were 7.9 (confidence interval 2.2–28.9) and 16.2 (confidence interval 3.0–86.0) respectively.

The public health impact of condom use has been clearly shown in studies from Thailand[66]. In 1991 the '100% Condom Program' was launched. In addition to a mass communication program to increase awareness of the need to reduce high-risk sexual behavior, condoms were supplied free of charge to commercial sex establishments and to female sex-industry workers. The incidence of HIV infection amongst young male conscripts in northern Thailand declined from a rate of 2.48 per 100 person years during 1991 to 1993, to 0.55 per 100 person years during 1993 to 1995. Together, these various studies show that it is reasonable to conclude that male condom use reduces the risk of HIV transmission. Condom use does not appear to protect against HSV infection[67] and the

evidence for protection against HPV is controversial[68]. Lack of protection against these viruses is not surprising as skin areas that are not covered may harbor infectious viruses. There are no published data on the protection afforded by condoms against hepatitis B, and only one study has shown lack of protection against hepatitis C[69]. Amongst female sex-industry workers in Lima, Peru, condom use for more than 50% of all sexual exposures reduced the risk of infection with human T cell lymphotropic virus type 1 (odds ratio 0.34; 95% confidence interval 0.13–0.89)[70].

Bacterial infections

Consistent use of condoms can protect against gonorrhea in both sexes. In the study reported by Schwartz *et al.*[71], consistent condom use was negatively associated with the acquisition of gonorrhea by men (odds ratio 0.31, 95% confidence interval 0.17–0.56). The use of the male condom can also protect women. In a case–

Trichomoniasis

A study amongst female prostitutes in Amsterdam showed that women whose partners did not always use condoms were at increased risk of trichomoniasis compared with women who reported consistent condom use (relative risk 1.7, 95% confidence interval 1.4–2.1)[74].

Male non-latex condoms

Three types of material are used in the production of non-latex condoms, polyester polyurethanes, polyether polyurethanes, and styrene-based elastomers[75]. They are said to be stronger than latex condoms, to give more sensation, to be odourless, to be more stable under adverse storage conditions, and to be less likely to provoke hypersensitivity reactions[75]. Data on the efficacy of these non-latex condoms in the protection against acquisition of sexually transmitted pathogens are currently lacking, but *in vitro* studies have shown that

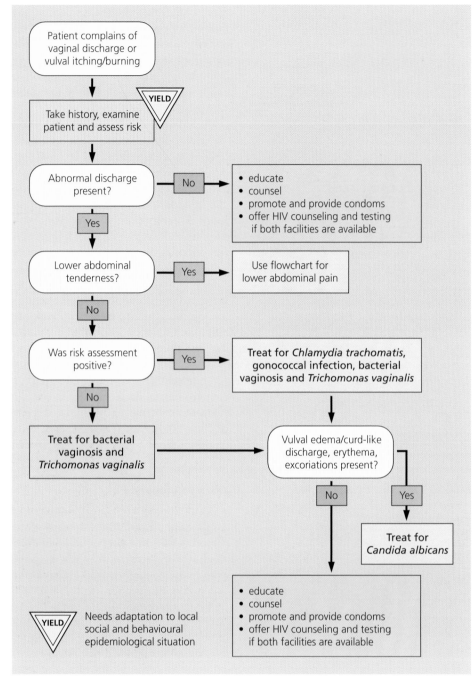

Figure 2.6 Vaginal discharge.

used it more often with regular partners than with new or casual partners[56]. It was also noted that women with multiple partners were more likely to use the female condom than those who had few different partners[56].

Microbicides in the prevention of sexually transmissible infections

There has been much interest in microbicides as a means of reducing the risk of transmission of HIV and other sexually transmitted infections. The global public health implications of an effective and cheap agent that would prevent transmission of HIV are self-evident. In addition, microbicides would provide women with a means of personal and covert protection, in areas where the use of condoms by men is deprecated.

Nonoxynol-9 was first proposed as a microbicide in 1976, and has been the most extensively evaluated agent. *In vitro* this agent inactivates *Neisseria gonorrhoeae*, *Chlamydia trachomatis*, *Haemophilus ducreyi*, *Trichomonas vaginalis* and HSV[78–80]. In addition, several workers have shown that nonoxynol-9 inactivates HIV-1 *in vitro*[81]. The intravaginal installation of the microbicide has been shown to protect macaque monkeys from infection with simian immunodeficiency virus[82]. Similarly, a single intravaginal dose of nonoxynol-9 protected four of six pig-tailed macaques from infection by *C. trachomatis*[83]. The use of nonoxynol-9 in women alters the vaginal microflora transiently[84]. After a single intravaginal application of the agent, lactobacilli concentrations decrease, but the proportion of hydrogen peroxide-producing organisms does not change. The proportion of women with *Gardnerella vaginalis*, and the concentration of *G. vaginalis* decrease transiently, and although the proportion of women with anaerobic Gram-negative bacilli increases, concentrations are decreased[84].

Efficacy trials on the use of nonoxynol-9 to reduce the risk of transmission of HIV have yielded mixed results. The microbicide has been used in different formulations,

polyurethane condoms allow some virus penetration that is somewhat higher than that for latex condoms[76].

FEMALE CONDOMS

The female condom is a soft, transparent, lubricated polyurethane sheath, 17 cm long and 7.8 cm at its widest diameter.

There is a flexible ring at either end. After insertion, the closed end of the condom covers the uterine cervix and is anchored behind the pubic bone. The larger, outer ring remains outside the vagina so that the sheath covers the labia. Acceptability of the female condom appears to vary from culture to culture[77]. In a study from Alabama, USA, it was found that women

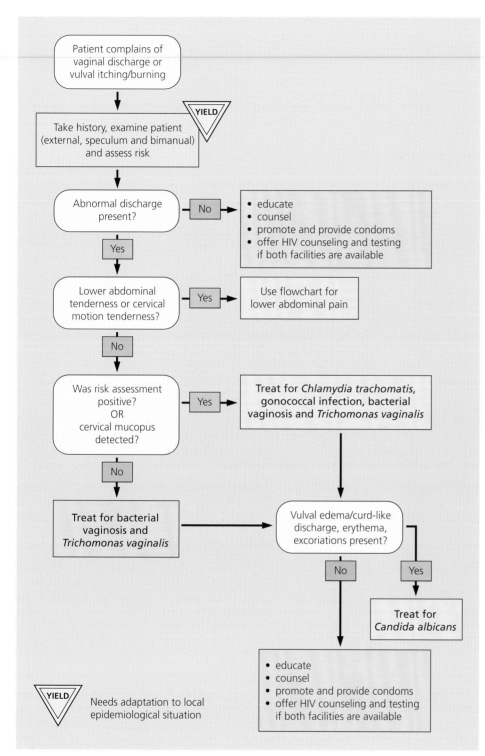

Figure 2.7 Vaginal discharge (speculum and bimanual).

however, found that the use of sponges containing nonoxynol-9 enhanced the risk of HIV acquisition. In contrast, Roddy and colleagues[87] failed to show a difference in HIV infection rates between women who used nonoxynol-9 films, each containing 70 mg of active agent, and those who used condoms only.

The use of nonoxynol-9 is not without adverse events. The repeated application of the agent to the macaque vagina results in cervical erythema and epithelial disruption, and there is histological evidence of acute inflammation with polymorphonuclear leukocyte infiltration and lymphoid follicle formation[88]. Similar adverse events have been reported in humans. For example Stafford et al.[89] noted erythema of the cervix in nine women who had received 100 mg nonoxynol-9 daily for 7 days, and in seven women there was focal infiltration of the lamina propria of the cervix with CD8+ lymphocytes and macrophages. The effect of nonoxynol-9 on the epithelium may be dose or vehicle related. For example, van Damme et al.[90] found that the incidence of genital lesions with or without epithelial disruption in women who used a vaginal gel containing 52.5 mg nonoxynol-9 several times per day was similar to that in women who received a placebo.

Unprotected receptive anal intercourse is a significant risk factor for acquisition of HIV, and it had been hoped that microbicides might offer some protection from infection. However, studies in mice have shown that installation of nonoxynol-9 into the rectum before exposure to HSV-2 increased the risk of infection and shortened the time until establishment of infection[91]. These workers also showed that this agent caused exfoliation of rectal epithelium, exposing the underlying connective tissue, and they concluded that the use of nonoxynol-5-containing products during anal intercourse might increase the risk of infection with sexually transmissible pathogens.

With the present formulations, nonoxynol-9 does not appear to be an ideal microbicide. Lower doses of this agent, however, may be more acceptable, and clinical trials of such preparations are in progress. Other agents are currently under evaluation as potential microbicides for the prevention of HIV infection. When select-

making it difficult to compare studies directly. As all the published studies to date have involved sex-industry workers, it is also uncertain how relevant the findings are to the general population. Amongst 273 female prostitutes in Cameroon, consistent use of a suppository containing 100 mg nonoxynol-9 resulted in a significantly lower rate of infection with HIV-1 than inconsistent use[85]. Kreiss et al.[86],

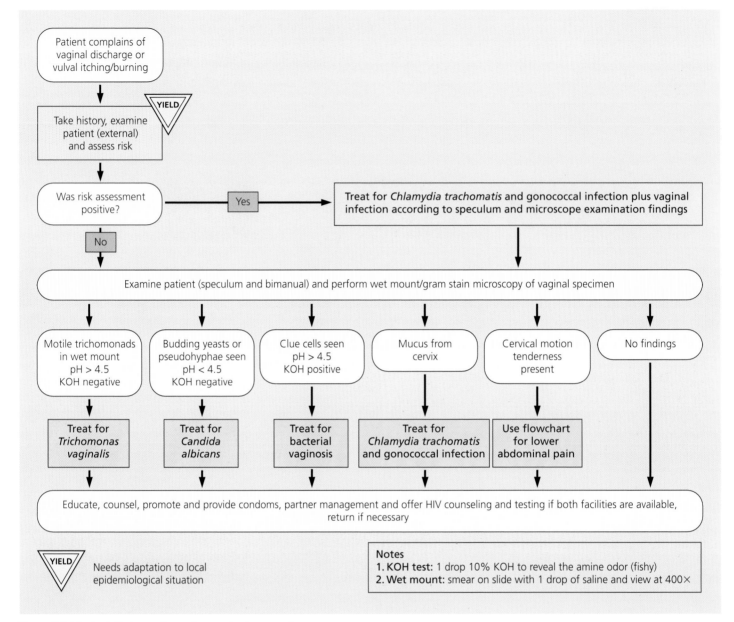

Figure 2.8 Vaginal discharge (speculum and microscope).

ing a candidate microbicide, certain criteria must be fulfilled. They should
1. kill HIV and, ideally, other sexually transmitted pathogens
2. be safe
3. be cheap
4. feel good.

However, they should not
1. kill lactobacilli
2. enhance growth of bacterial vaginosis-related bacteria (see Chapter 17 for association between bacterial vaginosis and HIV)

3. damage the epithelium
4. be obvious to the partner
5. cause symptoms to the woman or her partner.

Potential microbicides that are currently under evaluation include
- *cell surface disruptive agents* such as sodium dodecyl sulfate or benzalkonium chloride
- *acid-buffering agents* such as vaginal capsules containing hydrogen peroxide-producing lactobacilli and acid-buffering gels

- *attachment inhibitors* such as dextran sulfate that block attachment of pathogens to mucosal surfaces in a nonspecific manner
- *fusion inhibitors* such as cyanovirin that prevent essential interactions between the envelope glycoprotein and target cell receptors[92]
- *antiviral drugs* such as a combination of nevirapine with a nucleoside analogue reverse transcriptase inhibitor (Chapter 7).

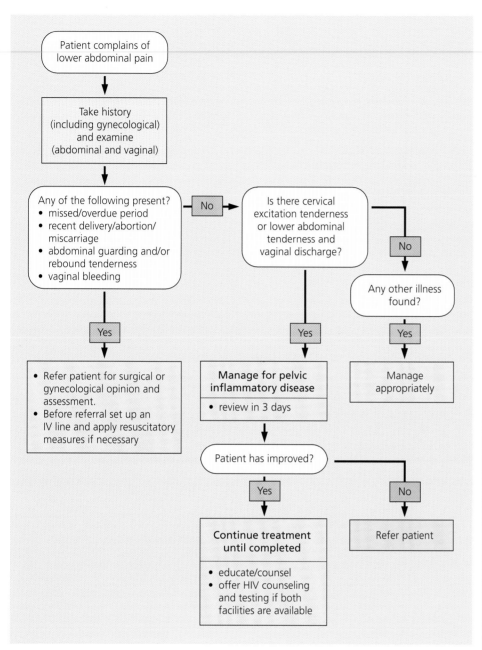

Figure 2.9 Lower abdominal pain.

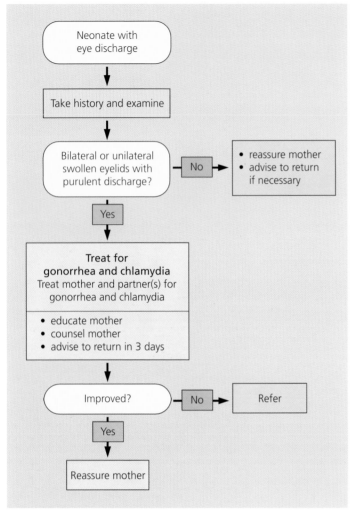

Figure 2.10 Neonatal conjunctivitis.

References

1 Wasserheit J, Valdiserri R, Wood R. Assessment of STD/HIV prevention programs in the United States: national, local, and community perspectives. In: Holmes KK, Mardh P-A, Sparling F, Lemon SM, Stamm W, Piot P, *et al.* (eds) *Sexually Transmitted Diseases*, 3rd edn. New York: McGraw-Hill: 1999.

2 May RM, Anderson RM. Transmission dynamics of HIV infection. *Nature* 1987; 326: 137–142

3 Brackbill RM, Sternberg MR, Fishbein M. Where do people go for treatment of sexually transmitted diseases? *Fam Plann Perspect* 1999; 31: 10–15.

4 Rietmeijer C, Bull S, Ortiz C, Leroux T, Douglas J. Patterns of general health care and STD services use among high-risk youth in Denver participating in community-based urine chlamydia screening. *Sex Transm Dis* 1998; 25: 457–463.

5 Schachter J. *Chlamydia trachomatis*: the more you look, the more you find – how much is there? *Sex Transm Dis* 1998; 25: 229–231.

6 Van den Hoek J, Mulder-Folkerts D, Coutinho R, Dukers N, Buimer M, van Doornum G. Opportunistic screening for genital infections with *Chlamydia trachomatis* among the sexually active population of Amsterdam. *Ned Tijdschr Geneeskd* 1999; 143: 668–672.

7 Welte R, Kretzschmar M, Leidl R, van den Hoek A, Jager JC, Postma MJ. Cost-effectiveness of screening programs for *Chlamydia trachomatis*: a population-based dynamic approach (in process citation). *Sex Transm Dis* 2000; 27: 518–529.

8 Van Valkengoed I, Boeke A, van den Brule A, *et al.* Systematic home screening for *Chlamydia trachomatis* infections of asymptomatic men and women in family

practice by means of mail-in urine samples. *Ned Tijdsch Geneeskd* 1999; 143: 672–676.

9 Morre SA, Van Valkengoed IG, Moes RM, Boeke AJ, Meijer CJ, Van den Brule AJ. Determination of *Chlamydia trachomatis* prevalence in an asymptomatic screening population: performances of the LCx and COBAS Amplicor tests with urine specimens. *J Clin Microbiol* 1999; 37: 3092–3096.

10 Cohen DA, Nsuami M, Etame RB, *et al.* A school-based Chlamydia control program using DNA amplification technology. *Pediatrics* 1998; 101: El.

11 Oh MK, Smith KR, O'Cain M, Kilmer D, Johnson J, Hook EW, 3rd. Urine-based screening of adolescents in detention to guide treatment for gonococcal and chlamydial infections. Translating research into intervention. *Arch Pediatr Adolesc Med* 1998; 152: 52–56.

12 Kelly PJ, Bair RM, Baillargeon J, German V. Risk behaviors and the prevalence of Chlamydia in a juvenile detention facility (in process citation). *Clin Pediatr* 2000; 39: 521–527.

13 Marrazzo JM, White CL, Krekeler B, *et al.* Community-based urine screening for *Chlamydia trachomatis* with a ligase chain reaction assay. *Ann Intern Med* 1997; 127: 796–803.

14 Rietmeijer CA, Yamaguchi KJ, Ortiz CG, *et al.* Feasibility and yield of screening urine for *Chlamydia trachomatis* by polymerase chain reaction among high-risk male youth in field-based and other non-clinic settings. A new strategy for sexually transmitted disease control. *Sex Transm Dis* 1997; 24: 429–435.

15 Gunn RA, Podschun GD, Fitzgerald S, *et al.* Screening high-risk adolescent males for *Chlamydia trachomatis* infection. Obtaining urine specimens in the field. *Sex Transm Dis* 1998; 25: 49–52.

16 US Preventive Services Task Force. *Guide to Clinical Preventive Services*, 2nd edn. Alexandria, VA: International Medical Publishing: 1996.

17 Centers for Disease Control and Prevention. 2002 Guidelines for treatment of sexually transmitted diseases. *MMWR* 2002; 51: RR-6.

18 Kamb ML, Fishbein M, Douglas JM, Jr. *et al.* Efficacy of risk-reduction counseling to prevent human immunodeficiency virus and sexually transmitted diseases: a randomized controlled trial. Project RESPECT Study Group. *JAMA* 1998; 280: 1161–1167.

19 Centers for Disease Control and Prevention. *HIV counseling, testing, and referral standards and guidelines.* Atlanta, GA: US Dept of Health and Human Services, Centers for Disease Control and Prevention: 1994.

20 Centers for Disease Control and Prevention. Technical guidance on HIV counseling. *MMWR* 1994; **42**: 11–17.

21 Prochaska JO, DiClemente CC (eds). *Toward a Comprehensive Model of Change*. New York, NY; Plenum Press: 1986.

22 Rosenstock IM. The health belief model and preventive health behavior. *Health Education Monographs* 1974; **2**: 354–385.

23 Fishbein M, Ajzen I. *Belief, Attitude, Intention and Behavior: an Introduction to Theory and Research*. Boston, MA; Addison-Wesley; 1975.

24 Bandura A. Exercise of personal agency through the self-efficacy mechanism. In: Schwartzer R, (ed.) *Self-efficacy: Thought Control of Action*. Washington, DC; Hemisphere: 1992.

25 Fishbein M, Guinan M. Behavioral science and public health: a necessary partnership for HIV prevention (editorial). *Public Health Rep* 1996; **111** (Suppl. 1): 5–10.

26 Main DS, Iverson DC, McGloin J, *et al.* Preventing HIV infection among adolescents: evaluation of a school-based education program. *Prev Med* 1994; **23**: 409–417.

27 St Lawrence J, Brasfield T, Jefferson K, Alleyne E, O'Bannon R, Shirley A. Cognitive-behavioral intervention to reduce African American adolescent's risk for HIV infection. *J Consult Clin Psychol* 1995; **63**: 221–237.

28 Cohen D, Dent C, MacKinnon D. Condom skills education and sexually transmitted disease reinfection. *J Sex Research* 1991; **28**: 139–144.

29 Shain RN, Piper JM, Newton ER, *et al.* A randomized, controlled trial of a behavioral intervention to prevent sexually transmitted disease among minority women. *N Engl J Med* 1999; **340**: 93–100.

30 Catania JA, Kegeles SM, Coates TJ. Towards an understanding of risk behavior: an AIDS risk reduction model (ARRM). *Health Educ Q* 1990; **17**: 53–72.

31 Rogers E. *Diffusion of Innovations*. New York and London: The Free Press: 1971.

32 Puska P, Nissines A, Tuomilehto J, *et al.* The community-based strategy to prevent coronary heart disease: conclusions from the ten years of the North Karelia Project. *Annual Review of Public Health* 1985; **6**: 147–193.

33 Farquhar JW, Fortmann SP, Flora JA, *et al.* Effects of community-wide education on cardiovascular disease risk factors: the Stanford Five-City Project. *JAMA* 1990; **264**: 359–365.

34 Community Intervention Trial for Smoking Cessation (COMMIT): II. Changes in adult cigarette smoking prevalence (see comments). *Am J Public Health* 1995; **85**: 193–200.

35 Community Intervention Trial for Smoking Cessation (COMMIT): I. Cohort results from a four-year community intervention (see comments). *Am J Public Health* 1995; **85**: 183–192.

36 Holder ID, Gruenewald PJ, Ponicki WR, *et al.* Effect of community-based interventions on high-risk drinking and alcohol-related injuries. *JAMA* 2000; **284**: 2341–2347.

37 Kelly JA, St. Lawrence JS, Stevenson LY, *et al.* Community AIDS/HIV risk reduction: the effects of endorsements by popular people in three cities. *Am J Public Health* 1992; **84**: 2027–2028.

38 Kegeles SM, Hays RB, Coates TJ. The Mpowerment project: a community-level HIV prevention intervention for young gay men. *Am J Public Health* 1996; **86**: 1129–1136.

39 The CDC AIDS Community Demonstration Projects Research Group. Community-level HIV intervention in five cities: final outcome data from the CDC AIDS Community Demonstration Projects. *Am J Public Health* 1999; **89**: 336–345.

40 Rietmeijer CA, Kane SM, Simons PZ, *et al.* Increasing the use of bleach and condoms among injecting drug users in Denver: outcomes of a targeted, community-level HIV prevention program. *AIDS* 1996; **10**: 291–298.

41 Institute of Medicine. *The Hidden Epidemic. Confronting Sexually Transmitted Diseases*. Washington, DC; National Academy Press: 1996.

42 Dallabetta GA, Gerbase AC, Holmes KK. Problems, solutions, and challenges in syndromic management of sexually transmitted diseases. *Sex Transm Infect* 1998; **74** (Suppl. 1): S1–S11.

43 World Health Organization. Management of patients with sexually transmitted diseases. WHO Technical Report Series 810. Geneva; WHO: 1991.

44 World Health Organization. Global programme on AIDS. *Management of Sexually Transmitted Diseases*. WHO/GPA/TEM/94.1. Geneva; WHO: 1994.

45 Uuskula A, Plank T, Lassus A, Bingham JS. Sexually transmitted infections in Estonia —syndromic management of urethritis in a European country? *Int J Std AIDS* 2001; **12**: 493–498.

46 Alary M, Baganizi E, Guedeme A, *et al.* Evaluation of clinical algorithms for the diagnosis of gonococcal and chlamydial infections among men with urethral discharge or dysuria and women with vaginal discharge in Benin. *Sex Transm Infect* 1998; **74** (Suppl. 1): S44–S49.

47 Htun Y, Morse SA, Dangor Y, *et al.* Comparison of clinically directed, disease specific, and syndromic protocols for the management of genital ulcer disease in Lesotho. *Sex Transm Infect* 1998; **74** (Suppl. 1): S23–S28.

48 Daly CC, Wangel A-M, Hoffman IF, *et al.* Validation of the WHO diagnostic algorithm and development of an alternative scoring system for the management of women presenting with vaginal discharge in Malawi. *Sex Transm Infect* 1998; **74** (Suppl. 1): S50–S58.

49 Ryan CA, Zidouh A, Manhart LE, *et al.* Reproductive tract infections in primary heath-care, family planning, and dermatovenereology clinics: evaluation of syndromic management in Morocco. *Sex Transm Infect* 1998; **74** (Suppl. 1): S95–S105.

50 Ryan CA, Courtois BN, Hawes SE, Stevens CE, Escenbach DA, Holmes KK. Risk assessment, symptoms, and signs as predictors of vulvovaginal and cervical infections in an urban US STD clinic: implications for use of STD algorithms. *Sex Transm Infect* 1998; **74** (Suppl. 1): S59–S76.

51 Cohen MS, Hoffman IF, Royce RA, *et al.* Reduction of concentration of HIV-1 in semen after treatment of urethritis: implications for prevention of sexual transmission of HIV-1. *Lancet* 1997; **349**: 1868–1873.

52 McClelland RS, Wang CC, Mandaliya K, *et al.* Treatment of cervicitis is associated with decreased cervical shedding of HIV-1. *AIDS* 2001; **15**: 105–110.

53 Grosskurth H, Mosha F, Todd J, *et al.* Impact of improved treatment of sexually transmitted diseases on HIV infection in rural Tanzania: randomised controlled trial. *Lancet* 1995; **346**: 530–536.

54 Mindel A (ed.). *Condoms*. London; British Medical Journal: 2000.

55 Grunseit AC, Johnson AM. Use of condoms: data from population surveys. In: *Condoms*, Mindel A (ed.) London; British Medical Journal: 2000.

56 Macaluso M, Demand MJ, Artz LM, Hook EW. Partner type and condom use. *AIDS* 2000; **14**: 537–546.

57 Minuyk GY, Bohme CE, Bowen TJ, *et al.* Efficacy of commercial condoms in the prevention of hepatitis B virus infection. *Gastroenterology* 1987; **93**: 710–714.

58 Judson FN, Ehret JM, Bodin GF, Levin MJ, Rietmeijer CAM. *In vitro* evaluations of condoms with and without nonoxynol 9 as physical and chemical barriers against *Chlamydia trachomatis*, herpes simplex virus type 2, and the human immunodeficiency virus. *Sex Transm Dis* 1989; **16**: 51–56.

59 Centers for Disease Control and Prevention. Update: barrier protection against HIV infection and other sexually transmitted diseases. *MMWR* 1993; **42**: 589–591.

60 Kestelman P. International quality standards: unfinished evolution. In: *Condoms*, Mindel A (ed.) London; British Medical Journal: 2000.

61 Golombok S, Harding R, Sheldon J. An evaluation of a thicker versus a standard condom with gay men. *AIDS* 2001; **15**: 245–250.

62 Saracco A, Musicco M, Nicolosi A, *et al.* Man-to-woman sexual transmission of HIV: longitudinal study of 343 steady partners of infected men. *J Acquir Immune Defic Syndr* 1993; **6**: 497–502.

63 De Vincenzi I, for the European Study Group on Heterosexual Transmission of HIV. A longitudinal study of human immunodeficiency virus transmission by heterosexual partners. *N Engl J Med* 1994; **331**: 341–346.

64 Pinkerton SD, Abramson PR. Effectiveness of condoms in preventing HIV transmission. *Soc Sci Med* 1997; **44**: 1303–1312.

65 Williams DI, Stephenson JM, Hart GJ, Copas A, Johnson AM, Williams IG. A case control study of HIV seroconversion in gay men, 1988–1993: what are the current risk factors? *Genitourin Med* 1996; **72**: 193–196.

66 Celentano DD, Nelson KE, Lyles CM, *et al.* Decreasing incidence of HIV and sexually transmitted diseases in young Thai men: evidence for success of the HIV/AIDS control and prevention program. *AIDS* 1998; **12**: F29–F36.

67 Olivarius F de F, Worm AM, Petersen CS, Kroon S, Lynge E. Sexual behaviour of women attending an inner city STD clinic before and after a general campaign for safer sex in Denmark. *Genitourin Med* 1992; **68**: 296–299.

68 Mindel A, Estcourt C. Condoms for the prevention of sexually transmitted infections. In: *Condoms*, Mindel A (ed.) London; British Medical Journal: 2000.

69 Osmond DH, Padian NS, Sheppard HW, Glass S, Shiboski SC, Reingold A. Risk factors for hepatitis C virus seropositivity in heterosexual couples. *JAMA* 1993; **269**: 361–365.

70 Gotuzzo E, Sanchez J, Escamilla J, *et al.* Human T cell lymphotropic virus type 1 infection among female sex workers in Peru. *J Infect Dis* 1994; **169**: 754–759.

71 Schwartz MA, Lafferty WE, Hughes JP, Handsfield HH. Risk factors for urethritis in heterosexual men. The role of fellatio and other sexual practices. *Sex Transm Dis* 1997; **24**: 449–455.

72 Gaydos CA, Howell MR, Pare B, *et al.* *Chlamydia trachomatis* infection in female military recruits. *N Engl J Med* 1998; **339**: 739–744.

73 Tanaka M, Nakayama H, Sakumoto M, Matsumoto T, Akazawa K, Kumazawa J. Trends in sexually transmitted diseases and condom use patterns among commercial sex workers in Fukuoka City, Japan 1990–93. *Genitourin Med* 1996; **72**: 358–361.

74 Fennema JSA, van Ameijden EJC, Coutinho RA, van den Hoek A. Clinical sexually transmitted diseases among human immunodeficiency virus-infected and noninfected drug-using prostitutes. *Sex Transm Dis* 1997; **24**: 363–371.

75 Farr G. Design and manufacture of male non-latex condoms for prevention of pregnancy and STIs. In: *Condoms*. Mindel A (ed). London. British Medical Journal. 2000.

76 Lytle CD, Routson LB, Seaborn GB, Dixon LG, Bushar HF, Cyr WH. An in vitro evaluation of condoms as barriers to a small virus. *Sex Transm Dis* 1997; **24**: 161–164.

77 Young AM. The female condom. In: *Condoms*. Mindel A (ed). London. British Medical Journal. 2000.

78 Bolch OH, Warren JC. In vitro effects of Emko on *Neisseria gonorrhoeae* and *Trichomonas vaginalis*. *Am J Obstet Gynecol* 1973; **115**: 1145–1148.

79 Benes S, McCormack WM. Inhibition of growth of *Chlamydia trachomatis* by nonoxynol-9 in vitro. *Antimicrob Agents Chemother* 1985; **27**: 724–726.

80 Jones BM, Geary I, Lee ME, Duerden BI. Susceptibility of *Haemophilus ducreyi* to spermicidal compounds, in vitro. *Genitourin Med* 1991; **67**: 268–269.

81 Hicks DR, Martin LS, Getchell JP, *et al.* Inactivation of HTLV-III/LAV-infected cultures of normal human lymphocytes by nonoxynol-9 in vitro. *Lancet* 1985; **ii**: 1422–1423.

82 Miller CJ, Alexander NJ, Gettie A, Hendrickx AG, Marx PA. The effect of contraceptives containing nonoxynol-9 on the genital transmission of simian immunodeficiency virus in rhesus macaques. *Fert Steril* 1992; **57**: 1126–1128.

83 Patton DL, Kidder GG, Sweeney YC, Rabe LK, Clark AM, Hillier SL. Effects of nonoxynol-9 on vaginal microflora and chlamydial infection in a monkey model. *Sex Transm Dis* 1996; **23**: 461–464.

84 Watts DH, Rabe L, Krohn MA, Aura J, Hillier SL. The effects of three nonoxynol-9 preparations on vaginal flora and epithelium. *J Infect Dis* 1999; **180**: 426–437.

85 Xekieng L, Feldblum PJ, Oliver RM, Kaptue L. Barrier contraceptive use and HIV infection among high-risk women in Cameroon. *AIDS* 1993; **7**: 725–731.

86 Kreiss J, Ngugi E, Holmes KK, *et al.* Efficacy of nonoxynol-9 contraceptive sponge use in preventing heterosexual acquisition of HIV in Nairobi prostitutes. *JAMA* 1992; **268**: 477–482.

87 Roddy RE, Zekeng L, Ryan KA, Tamoufe U, Weir SS, Wong EL. A controlled trial of nonoxynol 9 film to reduce male-to-female transmission of sexually transmitted diseases. *N Engl J Med* 1998; **339**: 504–510.

88 Patton DL, Kidder GG, Sweeney YC, Rabe LK, Hillier SL. Effects of multiple applications of benzalkonium chloride and nonoxynol-9 on the vaginal epithelium in the pigtailed macaque (*Macaca nemestrina*). *Am J Obstet Gynecol* 1999; **180**: 1080–1087.

89 Stafford MK, Ward H, Flanagan A, *et al.* Safety study of nonoxynol-9 as a vaginal microbicide: evidence of adverse effects. *J Acquir Immune Defic Syndromes* 1998; **17**: 327–331.

90 Van Damme L, Chandeying V, Ramjee G, *et al.* Safety of multiple daily applications of COL-1492, a nonoxynol-9 vaginal gel, among female sex workers. COL-1492 Phase II study group. *AIDS* 2000; **14**: 85–88.

91 Phillips DM, Zacharopoulos VR. Nonoxynol-9 enhances rectal infection by herpes simplex virus in mice. *Contraception* 1998; **57**: 341–348.

92 Esser MT, Mori T, Mondor I, *et al.* Cyanovirin-N binds to gp120 to interfere with CD4-dependent human immunodeficiency virus type 1 virion binding, fusion, and infectivity but does not affect the CD4 binding site on gp120 or soluble CD4-induced conformational changes in gp120. *J Virol* 1999; **73**: 4360–4371.

Chapter 3

Some social, ethical, and medico-legal aspects of sexually transmissible infections
A McMillan

A number of social, ethical and medico-legal aspects of sexually transmissible infections (STIs) are given consideration in the following ten sections in this chapter.

1. Confidentiality and STIs.
2. Medical advice and treatment in young persons.
3. Tracing of contacts and the case against compulsion, lessons from history.
4. Child abuse and STIs.
5. Testing for antibodies to human immunodeficiency viruses (HIV), its limitations, indications and restraints.
6. Homosexuality in males.
7. Prostitution in females.
8. Sexual assault.
9. Self-help groups.
10. Companionship, marriage and divorce.

1. Confidentiality and sexually transmissible infections

CONSENT AND CONFIDENTIALITY

In medical practice in the treatment of STIs there are two ethical principles, namely

1. voluntary consent to medical investigation and treatment, and
2. medical confidentiality

which deserve special attention. The argument against legal compulsion, if applied to investigation and treatment, is discussed in a historical context in Section 3 of this chapter and it again receives attention in relation to testing the blood of individuals against human immunodeficiency viruses (HIV) where explanation to the patient beforehand, and obtaining truly informed consent to the test, are regarded as essential preliminaries (Section 5). These ethical principles can only be maintained under circumstances where respect for the individual is given its due importance.

In both law and ethics medical confidences are regarded as sacred, with certain exceptions. It is a complicated subject with an extensive bibliography, including the following

- Lord Mansfield's ruling in The Duchess of Kingston Case of 1776 in Melville (1927)[1]
- *AB* v. *CD* (1851)[2]
- *Garner* v. *Garner* (1920)[3]
- Birkenhead (1922)[4]
- Riddell (1929)[5]
- *Henley* v. *Henley* (1955)[6]
- Bernfeld (1967; 1972)[7, 8]
- Mason and McCall Smith (1983)[9]

The questions are 'what the exceptions are?'[5] and 'when may the doctor tell, when should he tell and when must he tell?'. In the case of STIs, eminently treatable conditions, such as syphilis and gonorrhea, often present a dilemma to doctors. Although 'to tell' without the consent of a patient in this case may well secure virtually certain cure to a given partner, medical secrecy from the point of view of both the index patient and prospective patients, however, should not be broken without consent, and confidentiality should be secure. Otherwise doubt and fear of its breach might dissuade those needing medical attention from attending as patients in the first place. Mere statement of this viewpoint, however, and a negative attitude with lack of concern about the sexual partner of the index patient may lead to omission and development of preventive action by tracing of contacts. Such action should be based on persuasion and encouragement to patients. Legal coercion has no place as it leads to unwanted changes in attitudes to patients (see Section 3). Confidentiality, in England and Wales, is expressly demanded in two Ministerial Regulations (Notes 3.1 and 3.2). To encourage the tracing of contacts information may be passed in confidence to those responsible for the process.

In the case of infection with immunodeficiency viruses (HIV) continued unprotected sexual intercourse with a sexual partner as yet uninfected may bring to the latter catastrophic illness, even more

---

Note 3.1 National Health Service (VD) Regulations

(Applicable only to England and Wales.) 1968:

(1968 No. 1624) National Health Service (Venereal Diseases) Regulations 1968

(coming into operation December 1, 1968).

The Minister of Health, in exercise of his powers under Section 12 of the National Health Service Act 1946 and of all other powers enabling him in that behalf, hereby makes the following regulations:

3. Every Regional Hospital Board and every Board of Governors of a teaching hospital shall take all necessary steps to secure that any information obtained by officers of the Board with respect to persons examined or treated for venereal disease in a hospital for the administration of which the Board is responsible shall be treated as confidential except for the purpose of communicating to a medical practitioner, or to a person employed under the direction of a medical practitioner in connection with the treatment of persons suffering from such disease or the prevention of the spread thereof, and for the purpose of such treatment or prevention.

Note 3.2 National Health Service (VD) Regulations

1974: (1974, No. 29) National Health Service (Venereal Diseases) Regulations 1974 (coming into operation April 1, 1974).

Confidentiality of information

2. Every Regional Health Authority and every Area Health Authority shall take all necessary steps to secure that any information capable of identifying an individual obtained by officers of the Authority with respect to persons examined or treated for any sexually transmitted disease shall not be disclosed except:

a. for the purpose of communicating that information to a medical practitioner, or to a person employed under the direction of a medical practitioner in connection with the treatment of persons suffering from such a disease or the prevention of the spread thereof, and,

b. for the purpose of such treatment or prevention.

---

serious in pregnancy when there is also involvement of the fetus. The view that has gained acceptance is based on the value and effectiveness of persuasion tempered with respect for individual privacy. Failure to persuade should be a rare event that is not made rarer by the availability of a legal threat. The doctor cannot escape the nature of a moral dilemma. Professor Emmett[10] in her book *The Moral Prism*, clarifies the nature of the dilemma and in her opening chapter writes

> Ideally moral judgment might be a white light showing clearly what action would be best in any situation but just as light coming through a prism is refracted into a spectrum of different colors, so our moral thinking shows a range of different features, and attention can fasten now on one and now on another.

Morality is clearly a contestable concept. Respect for the patient, the value of persuasion and concern are likely to continue to yield more than the use of legal coercion which so profoundly alters the clinical atmosphere. Legal compulsion or threats, we maintain, should have no place in the tracing of contacts. These measures are discredited and were first rejected in England by the repeal of the Contagious Diseases Acts in 1886; later such measures in the UK were proved useless again by the failure more than 45 years ago of Regulation 33B (Defence Regulations 1939) described in Section 3 of this chapter.

Relaxation of the rule of medical secrecy is permissible with the patient's consent, but how much information and to which members of the clinical team it may be released is a complex question. Release of information may be permissible within a department but not to other hospital staff outside the department. To act on occasions in the patient's interests when consent to communicate information has not been specifically obtained may be justified. Consent from the patient certainly

should be sought whenever possible. If 'dysplasia' is reported in a cervical cytology smear and a patient fails to return, it is proper, if the patient cannot be found and asked for permission directly, to communicate the results to her general practitioner. The concept of informed consent, however, is a good one, and together with the giving of explanations is an ever increasing and necessary part of present-day medical practice.

Young people must be encouraged to attend if they have run risks of acquiring a STI. In those under the age of 16 years it is important to ask if they have told one or other parent and to suggest to them that they should do so. If they choose not to confide in their parents then confidences should be kept although the young person may agree to have a letter sent to their general practitioner. At no age should legal rules prevent the doctor from examining the patient, with his or her consent, in the manner indicated as necessary by the medical history, or from treating an infection provided the patient is capable of understanding the situation. If a girl is under 12 years of age the doctor has a responsibility to report what may have been a serious crime. In all cases the doctor's acts should be governed by what is considered to be best for the patient and medical attitudes should be protective in order to avoid damaging disclosures.

Disclosure of confidential medical information may be required by statute as in the requirements for reporting infectious diseases by the doctor. Again no immunity is granted to the doctor when a statutory duty is imposed on 'any person' to provide information in relation to the Prevention of Terrorism (Temporary Provisions) Act 1976, Section II and the doctor must provide on request any evidence which he has which may lead to the identification of a driver involved in an accident. Courts of law are empowered to order disclosure as they see fit either to the applicant, the applicant's legal advisers, or to his medical advisers. Medical confidences will always be broken in British courts of law in the interest of securing justice although in Belgium and France such confidences are absolute and are protected by their respective penal codes[9].

Confidences, however, are protected in a British court of law where they are part of a discourse between a person and his advocate or solicitor in connection with legal proceedings[4, 5]. Privilege is also given to those acting as conciliators in a matrimonial dispute (*Henley v. Henley* 1955)[6] on the basis that the State is more interested in reconciliation than divorce. The case of *Garner v. Garner* (1920)[3] is important with regard to 'venereal diseases'. In this case the petitioner was 'praying for the dissolution of her marriage' and relied on the fact that 'syphilis had been communicated to her by her husband'. The doctor, called to give evidence, claimed that his knowledge of the case had been obtained in the course of treatment of a venereal disease under the Public Health (Venereal Diseases) Regulations 1916 and was therefore confidential and not to be disclosed in a court of law. These Regulations expressly provided that 'all information obtained in regard to a person treated under the scheme approved by the Board in pursuance of the Regulations shall be regarded as confidential'. The doctor concerned was, however, being called as a witness by the woman upon whom he had attended; no question of 'privilege' therefore arose and Mr Justice McCardie decided that evidence must be given.

The provision of the Regulations of 1916 did not affect the question of medical privilege. Any attempt to treat and control venereal diseases, or using the term sexually transmitted infections to include infections caused by agents from viruses to eukaryotes, is often bedeviled by fear of disclosure of information on the part of those who might need such treatment. For this reason confidentiality has always been accorded great importance and at the present time when irrational fears of infection with the human immunodeficiency viruses (HIV) are prominent in the minds of the public, it is very important to maintain confidentiality. In British courts of law such confidentiality may be broken but, in contrast, in French law no witness is obliged in a civil case to give evidence against his will and by Article 378 of the Penal Code a doctor who does so in a case of any sort is guilty of an offense and is liable to punishment. What action would be best in many situations is contestable and the matter of medical confiden-

tiality is no exception. Professor Ian Kennedy, Director of the Centre for Medical Law and Ethics, King's College, London, it is reported (*The Independent*, 26th March, 1987), gave to members of the Social Services Select Committee as his belief that if doctors have an HIV-infected patient and fail to inform a wife or husband, then they may be open to challenge in the courts. Clearly the doctor must make every endeavor to persuade an HIV-infected patient to bring his or her sexual partner for treatment, but the need for special coercive legislation in this regard is questionable. There is a view, however, that the criminal law might play a small part in protecting those at risk from a carrier. In the case where an individual, fully aware of the danger and nature of his infection, willfully continues to put his sexual partner at risk then it is possible, in present English law, that a prosecution might be brought under the Offences Against the Persons Act 1861, if transmission of HIV-infection were covered by Section 23 'maliciously administering any poison or destruction or noxious thing'. If any such prosecution were to be brought and were to succeed the victim would then have the possible additional benefit of access to the Criminal Injuries Compensation Board[11].

2. Medical advice and treatment in young persons

At puberty, and particularly when sexual intercourse takes place at an early age, the questions of providing necessary advice on contraception and on STIs inevitably arise and bring with them problems such as the validity of consent to medical examination and treatment. In England and Wales for girls over the age of 16 no legal problem arises as the Family Reform Act 1969 provides by Section 8(1) that a person of 16 years can give his or her own consent to medical treatment. For those under 16 years it was considered that if the girl understood the nature of the treatment then she could validly consent to contraceptive advice. This view was specifically confirmed by a court of law for the first time[12] when Mr Justice Woolf decided the case of *Gillick* v. *West*

Norfolk and Wisbeck Area Health Authority 1983. Mrs Victoria Gillick had sought a declaration from the court that the advice, given by the Department of Health and Social Security to area health authorities, that contraceptive and abortion advice and treatment might exceptionally be provided for children under the age of 16 years, at a doctor's clinical discretion and without parental consent, was illegal. Mr Justice Woolf rejected her claim on the grounds that there was nothing in law to show that a person under the age of 16 years could not give personal consent to medical treatment and that the validity of such consent depended upon the person's intelligence and understanding of the proposed treatment. The Court of Appeal overruled the decision and granted Mrs Gillick the declaration asked for[13–16]. In October 1985, however, the decision of the Court of Appeal was reversed by the House of Lords. Lord Fraser considered

the only practical course was '... to entrust the doctor with a discretion to act in accordance with his view of what was in the best interests of the girl who was his patient.

He should, of course, always seek to persuade her to tell her parents that she was seeking contraceptive advice, and the nature of the advice that she received. At least he should seek to persuade her to agree to the doctor's informing the parents.

But there may well be cases where the girl refused either to tell the parents herself or to permit the doctor to do so and in such cases, the doctor would . . . be justified in proceeding without the parents' consent or even knowledge, provided he was satisfied that:

1. the girl would although under 16 years understand his advice;
2. he could not persuade her to inform her parents or to allow him to inform the parents that she was seeking contraceptive advice;
3. she was very likely to have sexual intercourse with or without contraceptive treatment;
4. unless she received contraceptive advice or treatment her physical or mental health or both were likely to suffer; and

5. her best interests required him to give her contraceptive advice, treatment or both without parental consent[17].

In Scottish law the concept of parental rights over children is fundamentally different and follows Roman law in distinguishing between the pupil child and the minor child. The pupil child is the girl below 12 years and the boy below 14 years, the minor child is the one above those ages and below 18 years. Although the parent of a pupil has power both over the person and property of the pupil the traditional long-accepted view in Scots law is to the effect that the parent of a minor has no power over the actual person of a minor and only certain powers of consent over the minor's dealing with his or her own property. Medical treatment concerns one's own body and the minor child, the girl over 12 years and the boy over 14 years, therefore needs no consent from her or his parent before accepting medical treatment, contraceptive or otherwise. A doctor must of course be very wary about treating a very young patient without parental consent, for he may only do so if convinced that the patient understands the nature of the treatment, otherwise the patient's own consent will not be valid. The determination of the girl's understanding is a matter for the doctor's judgment. It was the then Secretary of State for Scotland's opinion that the provision of contraceptive abortion advice and treatment to patients under the age of 16 years is a matter which 'rests with the doctor concerned, in light of the individual patient's needs and circumstances'[13, 14].

As the age of consent varies from country to country, and in the USA from state to state, the physician must be aware of the prevailing laws.

3. Tracing of contacts and the case against compulsion, lessons from history

Although males may have an asymptomatic gonococcal infection, the majority (85%–90%) tend to develop an obvious urethral discharge which makes them seek medical help. In contrast, in females the infection is frequently inapparent or asymptomatic (75%–85%) so it is essential to ensure that the female consort is investigated and treated. The process of securing the attendance of a sexual contact is known as contact tracing and to be successful depends upon the trust of the patient and contact(s) in the confidentiality of the process.

The necessary interviewing of the index patient is a matter of great delicacy, it is time-consuming and it must be carried out in privacy. It depends essentially upon the regard and respect of the interviewer for the patient. There is no place for hostility and everything must be done to encourage rapport. Gently, the patient must be persuaded that he or she is the only person who can ensure that the one or more consorts are treated. It is explained how effective treatment is and how helpful it would be for all concerned if the sexual partner could attend. Irrespective of the length of the list of recent consorts, irrespective of the varied character of those involved and irrespective of the form of sexual behavior, the patient must not be allowed to feel stigmatized or allowed to feel unworthy. If the patient's memory is faulty and the relationship has been casual, details are often hazy. At the best a note giving the index case number, date, diagnosis in code and clinic address, can be delivered by the patient to a consort to bring as an introduction to the clinic. If the patient fears to make the approach, the person responsible for contact tracing, say a health visitor, involved also in the clinic with counseling and all aspects of health education, will take the necessary steps. Sometimes, but not often, the description of a tattoo, a scar or a dress may help in the tracing. Information about haunts, about friends, or about work may also be of value. The patient must be assured of the tact and experience of the staff involved and of their skills in avoiding embarrassing situations. A good guide to the essentials of contact tracing containing useful reference material was published jointly by the Health Education Council and The Department of Health and Social Security[18]. Reference has been made in Section 1 of this chapter to the two Ministerial Regulations (Notes 3.1 and 3.2) which demand confidentiality in the contact-tracing process.

In Edinburgh it has been found generally that about half of the female contacts acknowledged by male patients with gonorrhea as possible sources of infection (source contacts), are unknown and therefore untraceable. The other half of source contacts are mostly traced and treated without great difficulty unless they belong to a floating population or change their address frequently. The secondary contacts with whom the index patient may have a long-term relationship and who may have been infected are traced and treated in nearly every case. In spite of the nature of the careful approach needed in contact tracing and the few, known insufficiently well to be described, who are missed, some still feel that legal compulsion is necessary. In the authors' opinion such compulsory measures are inappropriate and the power to use them inevitably changes attitudes of those working in clinics and discourages attendance in those whose need is greatest; persuasion and voluntary compliance are keywords to the procedures.

History is revealing. In the British army of the middle of the nineteenth century, more than 90% of the soldiers were unmarried as they were not permitted to marry until they had 7 years' service and had one good conduct badge. Many in the lower socioeconomic groups married early, but it was common for marriages to breakdown because of poverty. Women were particularly vulnerable as it was difficult for them to find employment and female servants were sacked without a 'character reference' if they became pregnant. In these circumstances prostitution was often the only alternative to destitution or the harsh environment of the workhouse. There were, too, more women than men because of the higher death rate of male children.

In 1860 about 25% of soldiers in London suffered from syphilis, and the Contagious Diseases Acts[19] were introduced with the object of checking the spread of venereal disease in the armed forces. These Acts applied to garrison towns and provided for the examination of prostitutes and their detention in hospital if diseased. The regulations were oppressive and extraordinarily bureaucratic in form. Every move in the appalling process required a certificate, duly listed in the Acts which were administered by officers drawn from the Metropolitan Police.

Josephine Butler opposed and vigorously campaigned against these Acts, forming a Ladies National Association for the repeal of the Contagious Diseases Acts. Her case was based on the fact that certain women, usually poor, were robbed of their civil rights and this violated the constitution. Among other objections she showed how these Acts were designed for the benefit of soldiers or sailors but applied only to civilian women who could be unjustifiably persecuted by officials administering the Acts. The opening shots in the campaign against the Contagious Diseases Acts include a protest in the *Daily News*, 31st December 1869, signed by Harriet Martineau, Florence Nightingale, Josephine Butler, and more than 100 other women. Although the statement provoked much abuse it effectively launched the vigorous debate which led, 17 years later, to the repeal of the Acts[20]. Although medical opinion of the day supported the legislation it provided no evidence that the diseases were checked in any way. The main attack was directed also against the double standard of morality in a male-dominated society which condoned the sexual activities of the male and persecuted the female, applied legislation against the prostitute but ignored her client. The evils of prostitution, including recruitment of girls to the trade, were under attack at a time when a virgin could be bought for a few shillings and the age of consent to sexual intercourse (until 1885) was only 12 years[21–23]. The Acts were finally repealed in 1886.

Further attempts to introduce coercive Acts have been made in the UK. In 1917 a Criminal Law Amendment Bill was introduced in the House of Commons by which it was proposed to make it penal for a person suffering from venereal disease in a communicable form to have sexual intercourse with any other person. The maximum penalty provided was 2 years imprisonment with hard labor. Power was to be given to the court to order a medical examination of the person charged. As the

existence of the infection could only be provable by medical evidence it was a matter of close concern to doctors. By November the opposition to the Bill in the House of Commons, which preferred a policy of persuasion to a policy of penalty, led to its being abandoned.

As the Criminal Law Amendment Bill failed to reach the statute book because of opposition inside and outside Parliament, and as there was a demand from Dominion Armed Forces' representatives, the Army Council in May 1918 passed Regulation 40D[24] imposing punishment for the offense of communicating venereal disease to soldiers, although the Regulation did not proceed as far as to make it compulsory for women arrested for this offense to subject themselves to a medical examination. The basis of the Regulation was similar to that of the Contagious Diseases Acts of 1864, 1866 and 1869, in that it was directed against civilian women with the intention of protecting soldiers[24].

The Regulation was not effective as a public health measure and women against whom no charge had been established were arrested, imprisoned and remanded for examination (201 prosecutions, 101 convictions). By the end of 1918, Regulation 40D was suspended as valueless and other more helpful measures were being suggested by the Royal Commission on Venereal Diseases, 1913–1916[25] at a time when an estimated 300 000 men, still infectious, of the navy and army were actually under treatment and might be due to return to their homes. As a result of these enlightened recommendations the Local Government Board developed an organization with clinics providing free diagnosis and treatment of persons suffering from venereal disease[26].

Compulsory powers were sought unsuccessfully by the Edinburgh Corporation Bill 1928[27]. The proposers believed that it was those who discontinued treatment while still infective who were the chief cause for the failure of medical control of these diseases.

Regulation 33B (Defence Regulations 1939) was brought in during the fourth year of World War II. It extended its compulsion, as a war-time measure only, to a group of persons, small in number, who

refused to attend voluntarily. In this Regulation specialists were required to pass on to the Medical Officer of Health the name of the contact thought by a patient to be responsible for passing on the venereal infection. The Medical Officer of Health would serve a notice on the contact if he received two or more notifications relating to him (or her) requiring him (or her) to attend a specialist and submit to an examination. If infected he (or she) would be required to have treatment.

Inevitably the Regulation restarted the controversy which raged at the time of the Contagious Diseases Acts and its inefficiency was shown by a reply given by the Minister of Health in Parliament (see Note 3.3)[28, 29].

In 1962 and again in 1967 attempts were made to restore the provisions of Regulation 33B in Bills introduced by Mr Richard Marsh and Sir Myer Galpern respectively.

Proposals of this kind are no doubt well meaning but legislation of this kind is an ineffective, discredited public health measure. It is the policy of persuasion backed up by a humane approach, careful techniques in clinics and good antibiotic and chemotherapy with contact tracing that is the mainstay of control. In the case of persistent virus infections, such as that of the human immunodeficiency viruses, when neither curative treatment nor vaccination are available, the problem of control is more complex. However, the present

---

Note 3.3 Results of Regulation 33B (1943)

In England and Wales 36 men and 475 women had been reported to a Medical Officer of Health as alleged sources of venereal infection of which 1 man and 27 women have been the subject of more than one report. Of these 28 persons two women have refused treatment, one expressly, and one by default, and have been prosecuted and imprisoned. No civilian voluntarily undergoing treatment for venereal disease is subject to compulsion to complete it.

authors believe that legal compulsion is not likely to be successful as a means of applying any control measures. In Japan AIDS has become a notifiable disease but it is claimed that the new law will protect the privacy of AIDS sufferers as long as they follow the doctor's advice[30].

In practice, a very small proportion of contacts, less than 1% of those who are found, refuse or fail to attend and about half of female contacts of men attending with gonorrhea cannot be traced because of a genuine lack of information. In the case of homosexually acquired infection, the proportion of contacts seen is often very low (about 14% in a recent study), probably because, in some individuals at least, the hostility of society makes the individual afraid to surface for help.

Although international action is envisaged by Resolution (74)5, adopted by the Committee of Ministers at Strasbourg in 1974, the greater the distance involved and the larger the number of administrative, political and geographical barriers, the less effective is contact tracing. The concept of international contact tracing would, to be effective, depend upon confidence that a humane system free from threats would be used to secure the necessary high standard of medical investigation and treatment. In the case of early syphilis and gonorrhea, efforts to achieve these aims on an international basis are laudable[31], but when a patient knows a contact sufficiently well to give an adequate description more can often be achieved at a personal level by letter.

4. Child abuse and sexually transmissible infections

In industrialized countries in the last two decades there has been a huge increase in the number of documented cases of child abuse, much of it occurring within the home, and an increasing proportion of this abuse is sexual. In developing countries too there are specific patterns of sexual abuse to children and worldwide there is much concern about the many facets of the

problem.[32]. Recognizing that boys are more likely to be physically injured or fail to thrive and that girls are more likely to be sexually abused[33, 34] it is necessary for doctors to take steps beyond those required for making a diagnosis of STI, administering specific antibiotic or chemotherapy and ensuring follow-up with tests of cure. Sexual abuse may include anal penetration with or without resultant injury[35] and in prepubertal girls *Neisseria gonorrhoeae*, for example, may be shown to be the cause of vulvovaginitis. When sexual abuse is considered to be possible the following approach, based on Clayden[36] is recommended.

1. A history should be obtained and if this includes that of emotional disturbance or if the child hints or states that sexual abuse has happened this should be regarded as a warning symptom.
2. The detection or exclusion of sexually transmissible infection is important. An organismal diagnosis must be substantiated in the laboratory (see Chapter 4). A recent study from the USA[37] found a high prevalence of unsuspected gonorrhea in prepubertal girls with vaginal discharge. In a group of 87 girls who were referred to a pediatric clinic on account of symptoms of vaginal discharge, burning, pain or itching, *N. gonorrhoeae* was isolated from 4 (9%) of the 43 girls with vaginal discharge. Before the diagnosis of gonococcal infection, sexual abuse had not been considered in any of these girls.
3. It is a warning sign if the child lies passively on the examining couch and does not resist anal inspection by tightening the levator ani or external sphincter muscles.
4. Signs of anal relaxation in the absence of abdominal distention are suspicious, especially if anal relaxation diminishes when a child is away from the abusing suspect.
5. Excoriation or bruising around the anus or inner aspects of the buttocks or thigh suggests assault.

The absence of anal signs cannot exclude sexual abuse[36] and gaping of the anal canal is seen in children with significant constipation. Referral of the child

for early expert pediatric assessment is mandatory in those where sexual abuse is either suspected or proved[38] and in response to the whole problem of non-accidental injury to children guidelines for action have been put together for use by practitioners in the disciplines concerned. These guidelines have been developed in various geographical localities in response to the problem and include a number of important points. In the case of hospitals, medical staff should take immediate action *to safeguard the child*. First the family doctor should be informed and the hospital social worker notified who will in turn, in the author's locality, inform the social work area officer. The latter will call a case conference when the circumstances indicate that this is necessary. Consideration should also be given to reporting the circumstances to the police who will report all cases of non-accidental injury (NAI) giving rise to concern to the Procurator Fiscal. When the clinical investigations are completed they should be signed by the examining doctor giving the date and time of examination and witnessed by a qualified nurse or doctor.

In the case of children who have been abused or are at risk of being abused 'NAI at risk' registers have been set up. These are maintained centrally by the social work departments and access for the purposes of consultation and registration is limited to those professions which require information as a necessary part of their responsibility to prevent or treat child abuse.

Allegations of sexual abuse in children are easy to make but difficult to prove. There is difficulty too in obtaining disclosure from a child who may have been long silenced by guilt or fear. The child abuse clinic at Great Ormond Street Hospital for Sick Children, led by the psychiatrist Bentovim, has pioneered an interview technique to overcome this problem using anatomically correct dolls to help to tease out details from a child who may lack the words to describe her experiences. The growing use of the technique, not just for treating victims but for diagnosing whether abuse has happened, has sparked off controversy. There is conflict, clearly, between the needs of clinical and therapeutic methods and the 'evidential' requirements of the courts in legal proceedings. The use of video recording and full transcripts in the case of the diagnostic interviews and expert evidence, together with limitation in the use of leading questions at the interviews, are modifications which are being added to what is seen as a constructive attempt to enable the courts to grapple with the problem of handling an allegation of sexual abuse[39, 40]. It has been considered, too, that protection of the child from further abuse and his or her future care are more in the interests of justice than the prosecution of the abuser.

In the case of children considered to be 'in need of compulsory measures of care' in Scotland there has been a break with the traditional law court setting since 1971 when a system based on 'Children's Hearings' was set up by the Social Work (Scotland) Act 1968. Under this Act the post of Reporter to the Children's Panel was established with the basic task of deciding whether or not cases notified should be brought before a Children's Hearing. If the reporter initiates proceedings he has to satisfy a lower standard of proof which is 'the balance of probabilities' rather than the high standard of proof, namely 'that of beyond reasonable doubt', required by the Procurator Fiscal when a person is accused in criminal proceedings. Child–adult sexual contact is a complex subject deserving attention. Additional informed and fully referenced discussion is available in the report of a working party of the Howard League for Penal Reform[41].

5. Testing for antibodies to human immunodeficiency viruses (HIV), its limitations, indications and restraints

A confirmed positive result in the HIV antibody test is a marker of infection with the retrovirus. The antibody response and seroconversion usually develops 2 to 3 months after exposure to the virus. The test does not measure infectiousness although the potential for this must be assumed. False negative and false positive results occur and

necessitate further tests for confirmation. HIV infection is discussed in detail in Chapter 7. The test should be carried out by a trained medical or nursing practitioner with sufficient knowledge and experience to give correct information and understand the implications of an HIV antibody test. The test can be undertaken in the following centers.

- Departments of Genitourinary Medicine or Sexual Health clinics, these departments offer testing within a confidential setting, patients can self-refer, and follow-up treatment for HIV-seropositive individuals is available.
- Special testing centers, these are sometimes attached to Infectious Diseases Units where treatment for HIV seropositive individuals is also available.
- General practitioners, although the service offered by GPs is confidential, insurance companies may require medical details from the GP with the patient's permission, for this reason some patients may prefer to have a test performed elsewhere.
- Other centers such as needle exchange sites and family planning clinics.
- In hospital while the patient is undergoing a diagnostic work-up. Support may be available from Departments of Genitourinary Medicine or Infectious Diseases units in the form of pre- and post-test counseling.

Counseling beforehand and informed consent are essential before testing. An outline of the issues discussed in the author's clinic is set out in Appendix 3.1. There are a number of contexts in which the use of the test is considered medically valuable[42, 43].

1. In the case of donations of tissue or body fluid, for the *benefit of the recipient* testing the donor's blood is important to ensure that HIV-negative materials are used, for example, in proposed donations of blood for transfusion or the manufacture of blood products such as Factor VIII; organs for transplant (kidneys, livers, hearts, lungs, cornea, bone marrow); semen[44]; milk; or postmenopausal urine for the manufacture of follicle stimulating hormone. In the case of Factor VIII concentrated heating inactivates HIV. Most blood transfusion centers operate a self-exclusion policy to

reduce the risk of a potentially infected individual donating blood. The message issued by the Scottish Blood Transfusion Service is shown in Note 3.4. Such policies significantly reduced the risk of transmission of HIV even before the virus was identified.

2. In the case of *patients* the result of the test has a *medical benefit* in determining treatment in specific instances such as in recipients of hemodialysis where the therapeutic use of immunosuppressive drugs may bring risk of clinical deterioration in HIV positive patients.

3. As there is now good evidence that the use of antiretroviral therapy during pregnancy and parturition significantly reduces the risk of maternofetal transmission of HIV (Chapter 7), there is a strong case for screening all pregnant women. As antibodies to HIV may not be detectable in the serum for months after exposure, repeat testing may be indicated in pregnant women who may be at continued risk

---

Note 3.4 Scottish National Blood Transfusion Service message

AIDS – PEOPLE WHO MUST NOT GIVE BLOOD:

1. Anyone who has AIDS or the AIDS antibody.

2. Any man who has had sex with another man since 1977.

3. Anyone who has EVER injected themselves with drugs.

4. Anyone who has lived in or visited Africa South of the Sahara at anytime since 1977 and has had sex with men *or women* living there.

5. Anyone who has had *regular* treatment with blood products since 1977.

6. Anyone who is, or has been, a prostitute.

7. Anyone who has ever had sex with a person in the above groups *even on a single occasion.*

of infection and in whom the initial antibody test is negative.

4. In the case of patients with, or suspected as having, AIDS the test is indicated. To confirm infection with HIV, or to reassure in connection with non-infection, the HIV antibody tests are available.

5. In the case of individuals at high risk some advocate the use of this test as a stimulus to changing sexual behavior. Advice about 'safe sex techniques' should, however, be given irrespective of whether individuals are seropositive or seronegative (Note 3.5). Considerable psychological and emotional morbidity may occur in a patient on learning that he or she is seropositive to HIV, particularly when the test has been conducted without consent or pre-counseling. Psychological shock, uncertainty over prognosis and the reaction of others may lead to severe anxiety, depression, obsessive disorder and sometimes suicidal acts. Broken relationships, unemployment and social dysfunction add to these burdens. Specific difficulties have been encountered – difficulties in obtaining dental or medical treatment, dismissal or premature retirement, financial and accommodation problems – in Saudi Arabia, for example, compulsory screening for immigration and employment has been introduced.

6. Anxious patients frequently refer to their wish for testing and counseling and a negative result may relieve the anxiety. Time must be allowed for a patient to make a decision whether or not to have a test.

7. With syphilis routine screening is justifiable as effective antibiotic remedy is to hand. In HIV infection no vaccine is available and positive results of the test have profound consequences on the individual in a situation where supporting services are limited and individual response to information of this kind may have serious consequences. Essentially counseling and education on 'safe sex' and positive behavioral change are necessary to limit spread of the retrovirus infection.

Note 3.5 The American Association of Physicians for Human Rights' specific suggestions to reduce the risk of acquiring HIV

1. Decrease the number of different partners with whom one has sex, and avoid men who have many different sex partners.

2. Do not inject *any* drugs not prescribed and avoid sexual contact with intravenous drug users.

3. Avoid one-time encounters with anonymous partners and/or group sex.

4. Avoid oral–anal contact ('rimming').

5. Avoid 'fisting' (both giving and receiving).

6. Avoid active or passive rectal intercourse (use of condoms may be helpful).

7. Avoid fecal contamination through scat.

8. An additional probable risk factor may be mucous membrane (mouth or rectum) contact with semen or urine.

9. Take care of your general health (get adequate rest, good food, physical exercise, reduce stress, and reduce toxic substances such as alcohol, cigarettes).

10. If you know or suspect that you may have any transmissible disease do not risk the health of others.

11. Sexually active homosexual men should *not* donate blood for blood transfusion.

12. If you need help attend or telephone a clinic.

---

6. Homosexuality in males

Homosexuality is often a 'stigma label'[45]. To be called homosexual is to be degraded, denounced, devalued or treated as different.

It may well mean shame, ostracism, discrimination, exclusion or physical attack. It is the knowledge of the cost of being publicly recognized as homosexual that leads many to conceal their sexual identity.

In western society, hostility towards the homosexual male by the heterosexual majority has ancient origins. In the first century AD the sin of Sodom (Genesis; XIX, 5) became closely identified with homosexual behavior[46]. Later, in the sixth century, Justinian admonished homosexuals and a thousand years later, in the England of Henry VIII, buggery was deemed a felony punishable by death. After repeals and re-enactments Queen Elizabeth I fixed death as the penalty which remained on the statute book until 1861, when it was replaced by a term of imprisonment of 7 years liable to be extended to penal servitude for life. Later in more modern times, the well-known Labouchere amendment (named after a Member of Parliament), to the Criminal Law Amendment Act 1885, brought homosexual acts in private expressly within the scope of the criminal law.

A less repressive approach developed with time and in 1944 in Sweden, for example, homosexual acts between consenting adults in private ceased to be criminal offenses. A reasoned view that this should be so also in England and Wales was set out in the Report of the Committee on Homosexual Offences and Prostitution, chaired by Sir John Wolfenden and known by his name[47]. An important issue in jurisprudence was raised in this Report, namely that 'unless society made a deliberate attempt to equate the sphere of crime with that of sin, there must remain a realm of private morality which is, in brief and crude terms, not the law's business'. In the high-level debate that followed, Lord Devlin[48], a Judge of the Queen's Bench, believed, on the one hand, that the law should indeed enforce morality, whereas Professor Hart[49] maintained that deviations from sexual morality such as homosexuality did not harm others and were therefore not a matter for the law. The liberal argument was based on the theme set out by John Stuart Mill in his famous essay 'On Liberty', published in 1859[50], in which he gave reasoned defense of individualism as an element of permanent importance to society and opposed coercion to enforce moral values. The Wolfenden Committee recommended 'that homosexual behavior between consenting adults in private be no longer a criminal offence'. Ten years later the Sexual Offences Act 1967 came into force and laid down that a homosexual act in private shall not be an offense 'provided that the parties consent thereto and have attained the age of twenty-one years'. A discriminatory clause, introduced by those who opposed the Bill, defined and restricted the meaning of the term 'in private' (see Note 3.6). This change had an unexpected effect. In 1946 the figure for convictions for homosexual acts in public in places such as lavatories was 561; it rose to a peak of 2322 in 1955 before falling in 1967 to 840 and for the

four years from 1973 to 1976 it averaged just under 1660. Although there may have been a real increase in this kind of behavior the increase may have been a result of the Sexual Offences Act 1967 which distinguished homosexual acts in private from those committed in public, the Act re-affirmed this aspect of the law. Variations in numbers in some areas may have been due to increased police surveillance and action[51, 52].

The phenomenon discussed is widespread. The majority of arrests in the USA related to homosexual behavior are made in public toilets or restrooms in city parks or, in the language of the homosexual subculture of the time, in 'tea rooms'[53]. Here are to be found the furtive, impersonal sexual encounters, where the participants may obtain sexual satisfaction anonymously without obligation or commitment, and where in silence and secrecy they may also, albeit with the risk of public exposure, protect their other identities, for example as a husband, a father, a respected member of the community (Note 3.7). Most sexual encounters in these circumstances are of an oral–genital nature and in only 1% is anal intercourse the objective. Conviction in open court for an offense of the kind already outlined[54–56] will bring publicity, stigmatization and can lead to dismissal from employment as a result (see Note 3.8).

Homosexual acts in private by consenting males have been legal in England and Wales since 1967. A similar result was achieved in Scotland by discretion not to prosecute until the Criminal Justice (Scotland) Act 1980 brought Scottish Law into line with Crown Office practice. In July 1978 the UK government published draft legislation to alter Northern Ireland law which, however, it dropped in view of the storm of protest in the Province. A complaint, however, was made by a homo-

---

Note 3.6 Definition of 'privacy' and other restrictions in the Sexual Offences Act 1967, applicable to England and Wales

An act which would otherwise be treated for the purposes of this Act as being done in private shall not be so treated if done:

a. when more than two persons take part or are present; or,

b. in a lavatory to which the public have or are permitted to have access, whether on payment or otherwise.

There are important exceptions to these provisions:

(i)   If one of the individuals is suffering from severe mental subnormality (Mental Health Act 1959) then his consent in law cannot be valid.

(ii) If one of the individuals is on the staff of the hospital having responsibility of the other then he would be excluded.

(iii) Members of the Armed Forces are excluded.

(iv) The homosexual acts among individuals on merchant ships are excluded also.

Note 3.7

54% of the males studied by Humphreys[53] were married and living with their families.

Note 3.8 Effect of conviction (Sexual Offences Act 1967)

a. *N County Council* v. *B* (1978) Industrial Relations Law Reports, 7, 252–255

A school teacher for almost 30 years was convicted after a plea of guilty of an offence of gross indecency with a man in a public lavatory and was as a result dismissed in accordance with the decision of a disciplinary committee. Although an Industrial Tribunal found in his favour that he had been unfairly dismissed, the local education authority appealed to the Employment Appeal Tribunal who set aside the decision of the Industrial Tribunal. The conviction provided evidence of homosexual inclinations which the teacher was not always able to resist or control and was the basis of the decision by the Disciplinary Sub-Committee. This body, acting on behalf of the Education Committee was entrusted with power of decision to dismiss or not to dismiss.

b. *B* v. *X Police Authority* (1978) Industrial Relations Law Reports, 7, 283–285

A chef in a canteen used by police and civilians admitting to being bi-sexual, was arrested and charged with two acts of gross indecency. Prosecution failed on technical grounds and he was acquitted. He had been arrested and charged in 1976 following police investigation into homosexual activities in the locality when a large number of people were interviewed and ultimately 15 or 16 of them faced prosecution at a Crown Court. Following discovery of his homosexual activities he was dismissed from his employment but he appealed to the Industrial Appeal Tribunal (*B* v. *X Police Authority* 1978), who decided that his dismissal was unfair on a number of counts including the tribunal's expressed surprise that it had been apparently accepted that 'seven police officers should all feel so strongly on the subject of homosexuality that they were not prepared to eat food cooked by a homosexual'.

sexual that the proscription of homosexual acts was an infringement of the respect for his private life guaranteed by Article 8 of the European Convention on Human Rights ('Everyone has the right to respect for his private and family life, his home and his correspondence'). The European Court of Human Rights agreed[57]. The direct result was the Homosexual Offences (Northern Ireland) Order of 1982, which brought the provinces into line with the rest of the UK[58]. Although Northern Irish opinion may regard homosexuality as immoral behavior, the Court considered it to be a matter of private behavior and only very serious reasons could justify State intervention involving criminal penalties. The Convention does not 'allow a majority an unqualified right to impose its standards of private morality on the whole of society'. Protection of the rights of others, however, justifies the prohibition of homosexual relations between an adult and a youth under 18 even though heterosexual relations with a young person of the same age are not punishable. Legislation is tending, however, to move in the direction of abolition of discrimination[59].

After some 60 hours of debate, at an estimated cost of more than $6 million and after having sparked off a petition of 835 000 signatures, the New Zealand Parliament passed their Homosexual Law Reform Bill where the consenting age was set at 16 years (*New Zealand News* UK 23/7/1986).

Although changes in laws that discriminate against homosexual males have been made in many countries, in modern times there is still a worldwide veto on homosexuality. Even when laws are changed the traditional moral viewpoint may not be as easily altered. Professor Hart[60] pointed out that moral rules are not immediately altered by a 'human fiat' and discriminatory pressures remain in the form of hostility, contempt or ostracism. Between 1983 and 1985 a change has been found in British attitudes to homosexual relationships[61]. The proportion saying that such relationships are always or mostly wrong has increased from 62% to 69% with a smaller decline in the proportion saying they are not wrong at all. Such a shift might be due to public concern about AIDS

and its association with the male homosexual community. No such parallel shift has occurred in the USA, where the proportion of the population considering homosexual relationships to be 'always' or 'mostly' wrong has been virtually stable for the past 3 years at around 75% and the proportion considering such relationships to be wrong 'only sometimes' or 'not at all' has remained at around 20%[62]. Moral rules are not immune from criticism, however, and in a democracy experimentation with alternatives can be tried and revised if need be[63].

Homosexuality, first labeled as sinful and criminal, came to be equated, at least in some quarters, with disease. This medical model was fostered, no doubt, by Freudian concepts of 'arrested development' or 'irrational phobias' and homosexuality was thought to be *ipso facto* pathological and chiefly the result of abnormal family circumstances. This stereotype was first seriously challenged by the work of Kinsey and his colleagues who pointed out the considerable incidence of such behavior and concluded that it was simply a natural variation of sexual expression[64].

That a homosexual – man or woman – is neither a sinner nor a sick person is the thesis of Bancroft's paper[65]. 'Homosexuality is not an illness but an alternative life style which may be and often is compatible with normal health and with those interpersonal and social values that we hold most high.' There is, as Bancroft writes, a duty for the right minded, and for the medical practitioner in particular, to encourage a climate of opinion, more positive and less repressive than that which has unjustly given rise to the social stigma associated with homosexuality, the repression that stems from it and the suffering that often results.

From the individual patient's point of view his sexual identity is crucially important to his adjustment and whether he sees himself as homosexual or heterosexual is more important than, say, his place in the Kinsey scale. Bancroft[64] goes on to identify three ways in which an individual with homosexual problems may need help from doctors

1. facilitating the individual's adaptation to a homosexual role

2. assisting those who have either a homosexual or uncertain sexual preferences to explore and establish heterosexual relationships
3. helping the individual to gain control over certain aspects of behavior which may bring him into conflict with the law.

Although the help given is not necessarily medical, the medical profession is one of the important sources of such help. To these undoubtedly important issues there is also added the important matter of prevention and treatment of STI.

Bell and Weinberg[62] admit that although they have taken a step forward in delineation of types of homosexuals their study failed to capture the full diversity that must be understood if society is ever fully to respect and appreciate the way in which individual homosexual men and women live their lives. In the lives of all, as in the most distinguished, there is much to reflect upon[65].

7. Prostitution

PROSTITUTION IN WOMEN

Sexually transmitted infection is an indisputable occupational hazard for prostitutes. Figures for infection rates have been collected of, for example, about 20% in Atlanta, GA[66] and 9% in Singapore[67] but clearly these will vary geographically according to prevailing circumstances. For example, gonococcal and chlamydial infections were diagnosed over a 2.5 year period in only 1 and 11 of 152 women respectively, screened at an outreach clinic in Edinburgh[68]. Infection rates in particular will tend to be greater in prostitutes in areas, particularly of the third world, where access to medical care and specific therapy is poor. The number with STI will be a function of the frequency with which they are tested, the sensitivity and specificity of the diagnostic tests used and the effectiveness of the therapy given, as well as the number of unprotected exposures they have, the prevalence of disease in their partners and the rates of transmission from hosts to susceptibles.

In many areas of Africa, HIV-1 infection is common in female sex-industry workers, and even where the prevalence of infection in the general population is high, that amongst prostitutes is even higher. For example, in Nairobi, 44% of 2162 prostitutes were seropositive for HIV, compared with 17.2% of 5033 pregnant women[69]. In Thailand in the late 1980s, high rates of infection had been recorded amongst female prostitutes, but there was considerable geographical variation within the country. The highest rates of infection were found in northern Thailand, with 37% of 238 women in Chiangmai being seropositive[70]. Clients of prostitutes in geographical areas where HIV is prevalent are at risk of infection. In northern Thailand in 1991, 12% of 2417 young male military recruits were identified as being infected with HIV. Just over 80% of the seropositive men had had sexual contact with a female prostitute, and there was a linear relationship between the prevalence of HIV infection and the number of visits to sex-industry workers[71]. Condom use by these men was inconsistent, only about one-quarter of men reporting the use of condoms[72]. Much lower prevalence rates of infection, however, have been reported in Europe. For example, only 2 of 228 sex-industry workers who were tested in London between 1989 and 1991 were HIV infected[73], and about the same period, in Glasgow, Scotland, 4 of 159 women, each an injecting drug user, were infected[74]. In general, the rate of condom use by female sex workers in Europe is high with 98% of 255 women in London reporting use of condoms for vaginal sex with their clients[73]. Data from the USA have shown similar levels of condom use[75]. In contrast to consistent use of condoms during sex with clients, relatively few women use such protection with their private partners – only 12% of the women studied by Ward et al[73].

Prostitution in women is defined most precisely by Paul Gebhard[76] who emphasizes its two essential elements

1. the exchange of money or valuable materials in return for sexual activity with physical contact
2. the relatively indiscriminate availability of such a transaction to individuals other than spouses or friends.

Sexual activity with strangers or with persons for whom there is no affectionate feeling does not itself constitute prostitution if the economic element is absent. The definition represents one end of a continuum ranging from the socially accepted arrangement of marriage, where one male is morally and legally entitled to sexual gratification in exchange for support, to the other extreme where the arrangement is of a very brief duration and involves numerous males.

The complexity of modern life, with accelerated cross-cultural diffusion made possible by rapid transportation, makes a brief description of prostitution in any given nation quite impossible. With reference to the nature of the sexual interaction itself, Gebhard[76] comments that in female prostitution the prostitute rarely or never reaches orgasm whereas the client almost invariably does. In contrast, in male homosexual prostitution the prostitute almost invariably reaches orgasm but the client frequently does not.

Cunnington[77] was able in 1979 to study in London the circumstances of thirty women convicted, at Bow Street Magistrates Court, of soliciting close to the West End and the street walkers' beats off Soho and Mayfair. In contrast to those in escort agencies and the like, street walkers could make contact with and choose clients quickly and, as accommodation was normally provided by the client, overheads were low. Half of the women had procurers, euphemistically called boyfriends, mostly from an ethnic sub-culture other than their own, who had a role partly personal and partly as business managers and who would generally 'manage' several women. For the prostitute, her work is described as hard, negotiating with a dozen or so men daily, getting them into a hotel room, avoiding sadists, having sex and avoiding the police. A secondary category of the women interviewed[77] did not think of themselves as prostitutes and had other jobs as barmaids, waitresses or shop assistants. This second category were part-time and included those who engaged in isolated acts of prostitution.

On conviction leading to imprisonment, the prostitute would often be abandoned by the procurer and precipitated into seeking female companionship with the more experienced and later into habitual prostitution. Cunnington's views were that penalties were ineffective, probation effective only when the order was in force and a prison sentence inappropriate, tending itself to produce serious effects on the family and an embittered victim.

Elsewhere in the series of reports, Trott[78] refers to the fact that prostitution is grossly under-researched. Studies involving the rich and transient population of large hotels, gaming clubs with satellite illegal or semi-legal entertainments bring risks also to a researcher. Reference is also made to the fact that the Street Offences Act 1959 (Note 3.9) clears prostitutes off the streets but drives prostitution underground into the clutches of criminal elements. In another context, the cohabitation ruling in the UK, denying state support in the case of a single woman, may drive her into prostitution[79]. Little is known of the lives of former prostitutes because those who have adequately coped with the transition back into society are anxious to conceal their past; one tends to see the failures rather than the successes[76].

There exists a socioeconomic demand for prostitution among travelers and military personnel, for example, who may have temporary difficulty in building relationships. There are those, too, who do not wish to become emotionally involved or who may wish to enjoy techniques that their customary partners refuse them, oral–genital contact being a prime example. It appears impossible to suppress prostitution in a complex society, particularly one in which sexual gratification is made difficult by mores and law. In large urban centers anonymity is easily achieved and many people are temporary visitors. In a small community, however, where secrecy

---

Note 3.9

Street Offences Act (applicable to England and Wales) (1959) S1(1) makes it an offence for a common prostitute to loiter or solicit in a street or public place for the purpose of prostitution.

is difficult and where life depends upon mutual cooperation, social sanctions, say in the form of ridicule and ostracism, are extremely effective in controlling prostitution[76].

Toleration with some degree of stigma is a common posture in many societies. In such, prostitution is often the resort of disadvantaged females for whom it may be a solution to the economic problem of survival without husbands.

In the context of modern times sex tourism has become targeted on a number of eastern countries such as Thailand, the Philippines and South Korea. In Bangkok, for example, some 100 000 individuals are engaged in prostitution, and STIs are a massive problem. Women arriving from impoverished rural areas are often forced into the prostitution business, and Japanese and European men appear to be among the large number of tourists who exploit the situation[80].

PROSTITUTION IN MEN

In contrast to female prostitution, much less has been written about male prostitution. Men who sell sex may work on the streets, work within agencies, meet clients in bars or through advertisements in papers, often masquerading as masseurs. Why a man becomes a prostitute is unclear, but Earls and David[81] found that influences related to financial gain, homosexual orientation and early sexual experiences were potential determinants for entry into prostitution. Most studies have reported that these men are young and are homosexual or bisexual in sexual orientation[82, 83]. The number of different partners varies widely, but amongst men working in brothels in Amsterdam Coutinho et al.[82] reported a mean annual number of partners of 147. In this series of fifty men, masturbation was the most common form of sexual activity with clients, anal intercourse occurred in only a minority of men. There appear, however, to be differences in sexual behavior between street workers and those working from home. In a study from The Netherlands of twenty-seven men[84], it was found that the former group of men were more likely than the latter to use hard drugs, to have a heterosexual preference,

and to have more clients but less regular ones. Although manual and oral contacts were the techniques practiced most commonly, insertive anal sex was also performed, and, particularly amongst men who identified themselves as homosexual, receptive anal sex occurred. These men were more likely to have anal intercourse with steady clients or with those they found sexually attractive. They were also more likely to have anal sex if there was an urgent need for drugs. Only a minority of men reported consistent condom use. Estcourt et al.[85], however, reported that 86% of forty-nine male sex workers used condoms consistently for anal sex with clients, but that they were less likely to have protected sex with non-paying male partners. Male workers who had non-paying female partners were significantly less likely to use condoms for vaginal or anal sex than men who had sex with men.

A high prevalence of sexually transmissible infections was found in male prostitutes in London in the early 1990s[83]: of the 57 men reported, 18% and 13% had urethral or rectal gonorrhea respectively, and 27% were seropositive for HIV. A high prevalence of HIV amongst male sex workers was also found by Elifson et al.[86] in Atlanta, GA, 29% of 235 actively working men were HIV seropositive. However, in Sydney, the prevalence of HIV infection in male sex workers (6.5% of 62) was found to be considerably less than that in non-working homosexual men (23.9% of 1885)[85].

There have been few studies on the clients of male prostitutes. One report of 15 clients of male sex workers in New Orleans showed that they were predominantly hetero- or bisexual, and that despite knowledge of HIV infection and its transmission, engaged in high-risk sexual behavior[87]. Elifson et al.[88], from Atlanta, GA, reported that 37% of 82 clients of male prostitutes were HIV-infected, a major risk factor for infection being receptive anal intercourse with a male sex worker.

Most reports on male prostitutes have concerned sex with other men, but Estcourt et al.[85] noted that 10% of 94 male sex workers had male and female clients. There is therefore a risk that male

sex workers may transmit infection to women either directly, or indirectly.

8. Sexual assault

SEXUAL ASSAULT OF WOMEN

Sexual assault is a crime which has multiple motivations, but in general has been shown to be more about the exertion of power and control and the expression of anger, than about sexual need[89]. Although the legal definition of sexual assault varies somewhat from country to country, most definitions include 'genital, anal, or oral penetration, by a part of the accused's body or by an object, using force or without the victim's consent.'[89]. In a charge of rape, penile penetration must be proved. Even partial penetration between the labia is sufficient to constitute penetration. Ejaculation of semen, however, is irrelevant. Non-consenting victims include minors, as well as victims who are intoxicated, drugged, asleep, have severe mental impairment, or who are otherwise impaired.

In the UK the age of consent for heterosexual intercourse is 16 years, and below the age of consent, sexual intercourse is always 'unlawful'. However, if a man is under the age of 24 years, and has not been charged previously with a similar offense, and the girl is younger than 16 years but older than 13 years and has such a physical appearance as to suggest that she may be older, the courts are likely to deal with him leniently. English law presumes that a boy under the age of 14 years is incapable of rape; this is not the case in Scotland. Although it was previously held that a man could not be charged with raping his wife, this is no longer the case in the UK.

As many cases – about 35% of women who attend STIs clinics[90] – are not reported to the police, the incidence of sexual assault in a community is difficult to determine. Although the incidence in the USA has been declining over the past 25 years (Figure 3.1), in Scotland and elsewhere, the number of cases of rape is increasing (Figure 3.2). This may reflect a true increase in incidence, a higher rate of

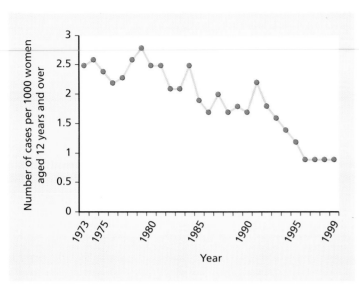

Figure 3.1 Rape rates in the USA 1973–1999 (National Crime Victimization Survey, Bureau of Justice Statistics 1999)

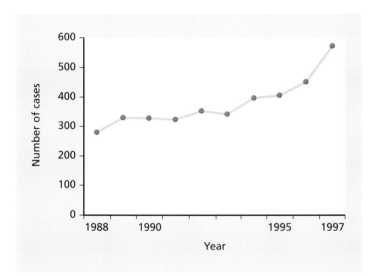

Figure 3.2 Number of cases of reported rape in Scotland 1988–1997 (The Scottish Office Statistical Bulletin 1997).

reporting to the police, or both. Many victims do not disclose the attack to anyone because of fear of being disbelieved, feelings of guilt and shame, uncertainty of the outcome of legal proceedings, and of concern about further violence by the assailant or his associates.

In up to 80% of women the assailant is an acquaintance of the victim[91]. 'Date rape' is a subset of acquaintance rape where non-consensual sex occurs between two people in a romantic relationship. In reported series, the lifetime prevalence of date or acquaintance rape amongst college-aged students ranges from 13% to 27%, and from 20% to 68% in adolescents[92]. Increased vulnerability to date rape includes

- younger age sexual debut
- earlier menarche
- early sexual activity
- being more accepting of violence towards women[92].

Individuals who have consumed alcohol before the assault appear to be at increased risk. Cues are misinterpreted as sexual invitations and the individual's coping responses and ability to defend herself are diminished. In a study from the USA, ethanol was found in as many as 38% of 1179 samples from victims of sexual assault[93]. The use of other drugs to facilitate sexual assault is also well recognized, and in the latter study cannabinoids (19%), benzodiazepines (8%), amphetamines (4%) and gamma-hydroxybutyrate (4%) were detected in the submitted samples. About 35% of samples contained multiple drugs.

In Riggs *et al.*'s large series of cases of sexual assault, vaginal penetration was the most common form of assault in women (83% of 1076 victims), with oral or anal penetration being reported by 25% and 17% of individuals respectively[94]. The sexual assault may involve more than one assailant (20% of cases in Rigg's series). During the assault threats are often made, and the victim fears for her/his life; in many cases, a weapon is present at the time of the assault.

The initial reactions that last for several hours or days after sexual assault are shock and disbelief. This phase is followed by one of denial and non-specific anxiety. During this period sleep disturbance, change in appetite and, in those who resume sexual relations, sexual dysfunction are common[95]. An adjustment phase follows in which depression and anger are features[89]. In some women there is spontaneous resolution of these reactions, but difficulties with social adjustment may persist indefinitely. Post-traumatic stress disorder* develops in a substantial proportion of victims; in the report by Petrak and Campbell[96], 17 of 19 women who were interviewed at a mean of 12 weeks from the assault had features of this disorder. The symptoms of post-traumatic stress disorder include intrusive recollections, distress occasioned by external and internal cues, exaggerated startle attack, isolation, hypervigilance, numbing, avoidance of anything related to the attack, isolation and depression[89]. There may also be somatic symptoms that include

---

* It should be noted that the DSMIV diagnosis of post-traumatic stress disorder requires that the stress has persisted for 6 months.

dysmenorrhea, menorrhagia, and sexual dysfunction. Golding et al.[97] found that in pre- and post-menopausal women, particularly those with more than one gynecological symptom, these features were associated with an increased likelihood of a history of assault. Other somatic symptoms include headaches and gastrointestinal symptoms. There is evidence that women who have been sexually assaulted or abused more than once are at particular risk of poorer social adjustment and of experiencing delayed reactions[98, 99]. A history of psychiatric illness is associated with the development of depression after the assault[100].

In addition to the psychological sequelae of sexual assault, the individual is at risk of pregnancy and of the acquisition of STIs. The prevalence of infection in victims has varied from series to series[101]. In some cases, acquisition of the infection had antedated the assault, but in others, the infection could be attributed to the incident. Jenny et al.[102] found that the risk of infection with *Neisseria gonorrhoeae* and *Chlamydia trachomatis* was 4.2% and 1.5% respectively. The risk of infection with *Trichomonas vaginalis* was higher (12.3%). These estimates were derived by determining the number of new infections present at follow-up among individuals who were not given prophylactic antimicrobial therapy and who were not found to be infected at the initial assessment. Where the prevalence of HIV infection is low, the risk of transmission of the virus at the time of sexual assault is also likely to be low. This may not, however, be the case where infection rates are high, and there have been case reports of the acquisition of HIV through sexual assault[103, 104].

SEXUAL ASSAULT OF MEN

Although it has long been known that male prisoners may be sexually assaulted, it has only recently become recognized that men outside prison may also be attacked. The number of recorded assaults in the UK is increasing, but many assaults are not reported and the true incidence is unknown. In a large cross-sectional survey of men attending general practices in England, seventy-one (2.89%, 95% confidence interval 2.21–3.56) of 2468 gave a

history of non-consensual sex as adults[105]. Forty of these men reported non-consensual sex with another male, thirty-two had had sex with a woman (one man had had non-consensual sex with a man and a woman). A woman cannot be charged with having forcible sex with a male, although she could be charged with indecent assault. Most studies on the effect of non-consensual sex on men have concerned assault by other men, and the following discussion concerns such individuals. Little is known about the psychological effects on men of forced sexual acts by women.

In the case of sexual assault by men, one or more males who may be homosexual or heterosexual carry out assaults, and the victim may be heterosexual or homosexual, though attacks against homosexual men are proportionately more common[106, 107]. Force or the threat of force or the transmission of a STI are often features of an assault. Alcohol or drugs are sometimes used to lower resistance.

Five major psychological components of the motivational intention of the assault have been documented[108]

1. conquest and control – the assault serves as an expression of power
2. revenge and retaliation – in some cases the offense is triggered by anger towards a victim
3. sadism and degradation – the act of aggression may become erotic
4. conflict and counteractions – the assailant attempts to punish the victim as a means of coping with his unresolved sexual interest
5. status and affiliation – some assailants feel pressurized to participate in 'gay rape' to maintain status amongst their peers.

The victim of the assault is often young and may be too embarrassed or ashamed to report the incident, even though he seeks treatment for non-genital injuries. The reporting of the sexual assault is difficult, probably because of society's mistaken belief that a man is capable of defending himself against such a attack or because the victim's sexuality may be questioned. Many men blame themselves.

The sexual acts that the victim is forced to endure[106] include receptive anal intercourse, with or without the performance of

fellatio, masturbating the assailant, or being masturbated, even to the point of ejaculation (the fact that the individual develops an erection during the attack often leads to feelings of embarrassment and guilt[108] and may contribute to non-reporting of the assault).

Major injury to the anal canal or rectum of the victim is uncommon, but STIs, including HIV, can be acquired at the time of the assault[109]. Of great concern, however, is the psychological effect. The rape itself is stressful, and, as in assault of women, the situation may often appear life-threatening to the victim.

Mood disturbance, especially fear, is common and depression, sometimes with a suicidal component, is well recognized Increased anger is common, and is sometimes expressed as generalized hostility towards homosexual men, with thoughts of revenge.

Somatic disturbances include sleep disorders and nightmares, reduced appetite and digestive difficulties. Sexual disturbances include decreased libido, retarded ejaculation, decreased interest in sex, and difficulty in relating to and having physical contact (for example hugging) with a partner. Interpersonal relationships may also suffer and there may be a feeling of unease and suspicion in all male company. Amnesia may also be a feature[110].

Many men sustain short-term or long-term damage to their sense of masculinity that is equated with loss of power, control, identity, confidence and independence. Problems with self-esteem and self-confidence are also common.

9. Self-help groups

Among the options in health care that are available, for example in Britain, to individuals Kelnan[111] identified three main sectors

- popular
- folk
- professional.

Choices are, however, restricted by law (Venereal Diseases Act 1917), in so far as the legally defined *venereal diseases* are concerned, to the professional sector. In the case of the wider range of diseases, covered by the term sexually transmissible infection, there may be no legal prohibitions but open discouragement against self-diagnosis and self-medication is one facet of health education generally agreed as correct. Among components of the popular sector is a wide range of self-help groups – 335 groups have been listed for the year 1982 – which can be classified on the basis of why people join them. The long list includes associations such as Alcoholics Anonymous, Lesbian Line, Gay Switchboard, National Council for the Single Woman and her Dependants, Women's Health Concern, Rape Crisis, Back Pain Association, Psoriasis Society, and Herpes Association. These self-help groups undertake a number of activities

1. information and referral
2. counseling and advice
3. public and professional activities
4. political and social activities
5. fund-raising for research or services
6. providing therapeutic services under professional guidance
7. mutual supportive activities.

Many groups are 'communities of suffering' where experience of a type of misfortune is a credential for membership. The reasons for the growth in the number of these groups include

- the perceived failure of existing medical and social services to meet people's needs
- the recognition by members of the value of mutual help
- the role of the media in publicizing the extent of specific difficulties.

These groups also have a role as a coping mechanism for individuals with conditions which carry a 'stigma' and provide a means of combating the latter difficulty[111].

The Terence Higgins Trust, another self-help group, was first formed and so named following the death of Terence Higgins from the Acquired Immune Deficiency Syndrome (AIDS). Saddened and alarmed at that time by the failure of official services and by the ignorance in the community of the threat of this disease, a group of his friends banded together to form this Trust. The activities of the Trust, now a registered charity, range from working with

people with HIV, through health education, to advising government, trade unions and professional groups. There are many people working as volunteers for the Trust as well as doctors, nurses and health advisers that are part of the medical group of the Trust. With the objectives to inform, advise and help on HIV the Trust prepared a number of booklets that addresses such issues as living with HIV when the partner is HIV seronegative, and HIV issues for African families. The address is The Terence Higgins Trust, 52–54 Grays Inn Road, London WC1X 8JU, telephone helpline 020 7242 1010 or view the website: http://www.tht.org.uk/.

10. Companionship, marriage, and divorce

It is clearly important for the doctor to avoid adding to a patient's difficulties by an approach which might upset the relationship between one partner and the other. The doctor must not divulge the confidences of one partner by giving information to the other, although there are clearly difficulties, not insurmountable, when he/she is responsible for the medical care of both. An attempt must be made to elicit what one partner has told the other and to determine the attitudes of the patient to his or her situation. An individual patient has a right to know the nature of any infection discovered and if asked directly the doctor should not prevaricate further but tell the truth, although he/she can do this in a reassuring and conciliatory way emphasizing the good parts of a relationship. Often a patient will convey without words an attitude to the situation and the doctor should try to interpret the patient's feelings and match his/her approach to them.

In divorce proceedings the acquisition of gonorrhea or syphilis has implications regarding adultery and as such the doctor should know something about the law of marriage and divorce and, as in both England and Scotland, its recent changes[112, 113]. In companionate relationships, as well as in marriage, STIs including gonorrhea and syphilis may contribute to a breakdown and the doctor should not feel

he is entitled to be more considerate to married partners and less so to those who are not.

Essentially marriage is maintained by the continued consent of each partner. The law itself does not necessarily help in maintaining such person-to-person relationships and in childless marriages the interest of the secular state is clearly more limited than in those with children. Tensions and difficulties are common, and counseling and family services are more important than legalities provided there is a willingness to use such services. In Scotland, at least, where safeguards to individual rights are necessary, in companionate childless relationships, so common among young people today, recognition might become possible by the Scottish method where 'by habit and repute' the legal validity of such marriages can be established[114].

The grounds for divorce in Scotland until 1st January 1977, were adultery, cruelty, desertion, incurable insanity, sodomy, and bestiality. In the case of the first four grounds the courts were, in effect, looking to see whether 'matrimonial offenses' had been 'committed'. In recent times attempts have been made to get away from ideas of fault and guilt, and the new Act allows divorce by consent after 2 years separation[113]. There is still a clear difference between Scotland and England at the present time in regard to divorce. In England and Wales (Divorce Reform Act 1969) 'irretrievable breakdown' of marriage is the only reason for dissolving it. Although such a description has a complex meaning the lawyer tends to look for evidence or a clear definition. For example, if the respondent has committed adultery and the petitioner finds life with the respondent intolerable as a result then this is a ground for divorce. A petitioner cannot now have an impulsive divorce on sole proof of adultery.

In the case of Scotland, Divorce (Scotland) Act 1976, although 'irretrievable breakdown' of marriage is the sole ground for divorce, proof of adultery establishes this 'irretrievable breakdown' and it is therefore still possible to have an 'impulsive divorce' in Scotland.

From the point of view of the events leading up to divorce proceedings solicitors may seek information from STI clinics to be used as evidence of adultery. Generally such an imputation from the legal point of view may be made only in the case of gonorrhea or syphilis, acquired after marriage. The doctor is required to give whatever information a solicitor may ask for on behalf of the client regarding the client's medical findings. He is not entitled to be given information about the client's partner without the consent of the party concerned unless the doctor receives an order by the Court, in Scotland that is the Court of Session at Edinburgh. It is important to maintain these safeguards and to avoid passing on information that the doctor is not entitled to give. Records on contact-tracing information are probably a separate issue to be excluded from case records.

Medical evidence in the UK is not privileged and the doctor must divulge his information if ordered to do so in court. Where litigation is imminent, however, between a husband and wife, as soon as a doctor or other counselor is asked by either the wife or husband to act as an intermediary between them with a view to reconciliation, any statement, either written or oral, made by either party is privileged. The law favors reconciliation and a person acting as a conciliator will not be compelled to give evidence as to what was said in the course of negotiation[6].

References

1 Melville L (ed.). *Trial of the Duchess of Kingston*. Hodge; Edinburgh: 1927, p. 243.

2 *AB v. CD* 1851 Cases decided in the Court of Session. Scotland 177–180.

3 *Garner v. Garner*. Medico-legal, medical professional privilege. *Br Med J* 1920; **i**: 135–136.

4 Birkenhead Viscount, Lord Chancellor of England. *Should a doctor tell?* London; Hodder and Stoughton: 1922, pp. 33–76.

5 Riddell Lord. The law and ethics of medical confidences. In: *Medico-legal problems*. London; H K Lewis: 1929, pp. 45–69.

6 *Henley v. Henley* 1955 Law reports, Probate Division 202–204.

7 Bernfeld WK. Medical professional secrecy with special reference to venereal diseases. *Br J Venereal Dis* 1967; **43**: 53–59

8 Bernfeld WK. Medical secrecy. *Cambrian Law Rev* 1972; **3**:11–26.

9 Mason JK, McCall Smith RA. Medical confidentiality. In: *Law and Medical Ethics*, London; Butterworth: 1983, p. 95–110.

10 Emmet D. *The Moral Prism*. London; MacMillan Press: 1979.

11 Forlin G, Wauchope P. AIDS and the criminal law. *Law Soc Gaz* 1987; 25/3/87, pp. 884–885.

12 Norrie KMcK. Contraceptives, consent and the child. *Scots Law Times* 1983, 16/12/1983, pp. 285–288.

13 Norrie KMcK. A comment on the Gillick case. *Br J Fam Plann* 1985 **11**: 1–4.

14 Norrie KMcK. The Gillick crusade ill-conceived under Scots law. *Scotsman*, 1985, 23/3/1985, p. 7.

15 Norrie KMcK. The Gillick case and parental rights in Scots Law. *Scots Law Times* 1985, pp. 157–162.

16 Brahams D. Parental consent – does doctor know best after all? The Gillick case. *New Law J* 1985; **135**: 8–10.

17 Times Law Report, House of Lords 1985 DHSS contraceptive guidance to doctors is lawful. *Times* 1985, 18/10/85.

18 Hunter I, Jacobs J, Kinnell H, Satin A. *Handbook on Contact Tracing in Sexually Transmitted Diseases*. London; Health Education Council: 1980.

19 Contagious Diseases Acts (1864, 1866, and 1869) respectively: 27 & 28 Victoriae, Cap 85. An Act for the Prevention of Contagious Diseases at certain Naval and Military Stations (1864) 29 Victoriae, Cap 35. An Act for the better Prevention of Contagious Diseases at certain Naval and Military Stations (1866) 32 & 33 Victoriae, Cap 80. An Act to amend the Contagious Diseases Act (1866, 1869).

20 Blom-Cooper L, Drewry G (eds). Law and morality. In: *Human Sexuality* 4.7, 4.8, 4.9. London; Duckworth: 1976, pp 114–121.

21 Bell E . *Josephine Butler, Flame of Fire.* London; Constable: 1962.

22 Rover C. *Love, Morals and the Feminists.* London; Routledge and Kegan Paul: 1967.

23 Petrie G. *A Singular Iniquity: the Campaigns of Josephine Butler.* London; Macmillan: 1971.

24 Venereal Disease and the Defence of the Realm Act. *Lancet* 1917; **ii**: 23.

25 Cd 8189 & 8190. *Final Report and Appendix to Final Report of the Commissioners.* Royal Commission on Venereal Diseases, London; HMSO: 1916.

26 Leading Article. The control of venereal disease. *Lancet* 1917; **i**: 309.

27 Statement for the Corporation 1928 Edinburgh Corporation Bill 1928 (Venereal Diseases). City and Royal Burgh of Edinburgh.

28 Results of Regulation 33B. *Br J Vener Dis* 1943; **19**: 92.

29 Shannon N P. The compulsory treatment of venereal diseases under Regulation 33B. *Br J Vener Dis* 1943; **19**: 22–23.

30 Swinbanks D. AIDS becomes a notifiable disease in Japan despite protests. *Nature* 1987; **326**: 232.

31 Willcox RR. International contact tracing in venereal disease. *WHO Chronicle* 1973; **27**: 418.

32 Leading Article. Ill-treatment of children. *Lancet* 1987; **i**: 367–368.

33 Notes and News. Increase of abuse in children. *Lancet* 1986; **ii**: 1473.

34 Creighton S. Child abuse in 1985 – initial findings from NSPCC register research. *Fam Law* 1987; **17**: 117–118.

35 Hobbs CJ, Wynne JM. Buggery in childhood – a common syndrome of child abuse. *Lancet* 1986; **ii**: 792–796.

36 Clayden G. Anal appearances and child sex abuse. *Lancet* 1987; **i**: 620–621.

37 Shapiro RA, Schubert CJ, Siegel RM. *Neisseria gonorrhoeae* infections in girls younger than 12 years of age evaluated for vaginitis. *Pediatrics* 1999; **104**: 72.

38 Hey F, Buchan PC, Littlewood J M, Hall R. Differential diagnosis in child sexual abuse. *Lancet* 1987; **i**: 283.

39 Douglas G, Willmore C. Diagnostic interviews as evidence in cases of child sexual abuse. *Fam Law* 1987; **17**: 151–154.

40 Dyer C. The dolls of Great Ormond Street. *Law Mag* 1987 1/5/1987, pp. 22–24.

41 Howard League for Penal Reform. *Unlawful Sex*. The Report of a Howard League Working Party; Waterlow Legal and Social Policy Library: 1985.

42 Miller D, Green J. Psychological support and counselling for patients with acquired immune deficiency syndrome (AIDS). *Genitourin Med* 1985; **61**: 273–278.

43 Miller D, Weber J, Green J (ed.). *The Management of AIDS Patients*. Basingstoke; Macmillan Press: 1986, pp. 131–173.

44 Stewart GJ, Tyler JPP, Cunningham AL, *et al.* Transmission of human T-cell lymphotropic virus type III (HTLV-III) by artificial insemination by donor. *Lancet* 1985; **ii**: 581–584.

45 Plummer K. *Sexual Stigma: an Interactionist Account*. London; Routledge and Keegan Paul: 1975.

46 Bailley DS. *Homosexuality and the Western Christian Tradition*. London; Longmans: 1955.

47 Wolfenden Report. *The Report of the Committee on Homosexual Offences and*

Prostitution, Cmnd. 247. London; Her Majesty's Stationery Office: 1957, pp. 131–137.

48 Devlin P. *The enforcement of morals*. London; Oxford University Press: 1959, cli. 1, pp. 1–25.

49 Hart HLA. *Law, Liberty and Morality*. London; Oxford University Press: 1963.

50 Mill JS. On liberty. In: *On Liberty, Representative Government and the Subjection of Women*, 1912 edition. The World's Classics; Oxford University Press: 1859, p. 15.

51 Walmsley R. Indecency between males and the Sexual Offences Act 1967. *Criminal Law Rev* (July): 1978, pp. 385–452.

52 Walmsley R, White K. *Sexual Offences, Consent and Sentencing*. Home Office Research Study No. 54. London; Her Majesty's Stationery Office: 1979. pp. 38–46.

53 Humphreys RA Laud. *Tearoom Trade (Impersonal Sex in Public Places)*. Chicago; Aldine: 1975.

54 Honoré T. *Sex Law*. London; Duckworth: 1978, pp. 84–110.

55 Crane P. *Gays and the Law*. London; Pluto Press: 1983, pp. 8–39.

56 Galloway B. The police and the courts. In: Galloway B (ed.) *Prejudice and Pride*. London; Routledge and Kegan Paul: 1983, pp. 102–106.

57 *D v. UK* Judgement of 22/10/81. European Court of Human Rights (ECHR).

58 Finnie W. *Domestic Effects of the European Convention on Human Rights*. Background paper. Information conference; Edinburgh University: 1983.

59 Jacque Jean-Paul. Forum. Council of Europe: 1983, 2/83, pp. VII–IX.

60 Hart HLA. *The Concept of Law*. London; Oxford University Press: 1961, pp. 168–176.

61 Jowell R, Witherspoon S, Brook L. *British Social Attitudes, the 1986 Report*. Vermont; Gower: 1986, pp. 151–156.

62 Bell AP, Weinberg MS. Homosexualities. *A Study of Diversity among Men and Women*. London; Mitchell Beazley: 1978, pp. 229–231.

63 Bancroft J. Homosexuality and the medical profession: a behaviourist's view. *J Med Ethics* 1975; **1**: 176–180.

64 Bancroft J. *Human Sexuality and its Problems*. Edinburgh; Churchill Livingstone: 1981, Ch 6, pp. 165, 171.

65 Hodges A. *Alan Turing: the Enigma*. London; Burnett Books: 1983.

66 Conrad GL, Kleris GS, Rush B, Darrow W. Sexually transmitted diseases among prostitutes and other sexual offenders. *Sex Transm Dis* 1981; **8**: 241–244.

67 Khoo R, Sng EH, Goh AJ. A study of sexually transmitted diseases in 200 prostitutes in Singapore. *Asian J Infect Dis* 1977; **1**: 77–79.

68 Scott GR, Peacock W, Cameron S. Outreach STD clinics for prostitutes in Edinburgh. *Int J STD AIDS* 1995; **6**: 197–200.

69 Kitabu M, Maitha G, Mungai J, *et al. Trends and Seroprevalence of HIV among Four Population Groups in Nairobi in the Period 1989–1991*. Eighth International Conference on AIDS/Third STD Congress. Amsterdam, July 1992. Abstract POC 4018.

70 Siraprapasiri T, Thanprasertsuk S, Rodklay A, *et al.* Risk factors for HIV among prostitutes in Chiangmai, Thailand. *AIDS* 1991; **5**: 579–582.

71 Celentano DD, Nelson KE, Suprasert S, *et al.* Behavioral and sociodemographic risks for frequent visits to commercial sex workers among northern Thai men. *AIDS* 1993; **12**: 81–102.

72 Nelson K, Celentano D, Suprasert S, *et al.* Risk factors for HIV infection among young men in northern Thailand. *JAMA* 1993; **270**: 955–960.

73 Ward H, Day S, Mezzone J, *et al.* Prostitution and risk of HIV: female prostitutes in London. *Br Med J* 1993; **307**: 356–358.

74 McKeganey N, Barnard M, Leyland A, Coote I, Follett E. Female street-working prostitution and HIV infection in Glasgow. *Br Med J* 1992; **305**: 801–804.

75 McKeganey NP. Prostitution and HIV: what do we know and where might research be directed in the future? *AIDS* 1994; **8**: 1215–1226.

76 Gebhard P. Human sexuality. *Encyclopaedia Britannica* 15th edn. Chicago; Encyclopaedia Britannica: 1982, pp. 75–81.

77 Cunnington S. Some aspects of prostitution in the West End of London in 1979. In: West DJ (ed.) *Sex Offenders in the Criminal Justice System*. Cropwood Conference Series No. 12. Cambridge: Institute of Criminology: 1980, pp. 121–130.

78 Trott L. On understanding prostitution and its problematic sources of information, with particular reference to Mayfair, London. In: West DJ (ed.) *Sex Offenders in the Criminal Justice System*. Cropwood Conference Series No. 12. Cambridge; Institute of Criminology: 1980.

79 Vickers J. Prostitution in the context of the Street Offences Act. In: West DJ (ed.) *Sex Offenders in the Criminal Justice System*. Cropwood Conference Series No. 12. Cambridge. Institute of Criminology; 1980: pp. 114–120.

80 Change International Reports Providence and Prostitution. *Image and Reality for Women in Buddhist Thailand*. London; Women and Society: 1980.

81 Earls CM, David H. A psychosocial study of male prostitution. *Arch Sex Behav* 1989; **18**: 401–419.

82 Couthino RA, van Andel RL, Rijsdijk TJ. Role of male prostitutes in the spread of sexually transmitted diseases and human immunodeficiency virus. *Genitourin Med* 1988; **64**: 207–208.

83 Tomlinson DR, Hillman RJ, Harris JR, Taylor-Robinson D. Screening for sexually transmitted disease in London-based male prostitutes. *Genitourin Med* 1991; **67**: 103–106.

84 De Graff R, Vanwesenbeeck I, van Zessen G, Starver CJ, Visser JH. Male prostitutes and safe sex: different settings, different risks. *AIDS Care* 1994; **6**: 267–268.

85 Estcourt CS, Marks C, Rohrsheim R, Johnson AM, Donovan B, Mindel A. HIV, sexually transmitted infections, and risk behaviours in male commercial sex workers in Sydney. *Sex Transm Infect* 2000; **76**: 294–298.

86 Elifson KW, Boles J, Sweat M. Risk factors associated with HIV infection among male prostitutes. *Am J Public Health* 1993; **83**: 79–83.

87 Morse EV, Simon PM, Balson PM, Osofsky HJ. Sexual behavior patterns of customers of male street prostitutes. *Arch Sex Behav* 1992; **21**: 347–357.

88 Elifson KW, Boles J, Darrow WW, Sterk CE. HIV seroprevalence and risk factors among clients of female and male prostitutes. *J Acquir Immune Defic Syndr* 1999; **20**: 195–200.

89 DeLahunta EA, Baram DA. Sexual assault. *Clin Obstet Gynecol* 1997; **40**: 648–660.

90 Ross JDC, Scott GR, Busuttil A. Rape, sexually transmitted diseases: pattern of referral and incidence in a department of genitourinary medicine. *J R Soc Med* 1991; **84**: 657–659.

91 Warshaw R. *I Never Call it Rape: the MS. Report on recognizing, fighting and surviving date and acquaintance rape*. New York; Harper and Row: 1988.

92 Rickert VI, Wiemann CM. Date rape among adolescents and young adults. *J Pediatr Adolesc Gynecol* 1998; **11**: 167–175.

93 El Sohly MA, Salamone SJ. Prevalence of drugs used in cases of alleged sexual assault. *J Anal Toxicol* 1999; **23**: 141–146.

94 Riggs N, Houry D, Long G, Markovchick V, Feldhaus KM. Analysis of 1.076 cases of sexual assault. *Ann Emerg Med* 2000; **35**: 358–362.

95 Holmes MM, Resnick HS, Frampton D. Follow-up of sexual assault victims. *Am J Obstet Gynecol* 1998; **179**: 336–342.

96 Petrak JA, Campbell EA. Post-traumatic stress disorder in female survivors of rape attending a genitourinary medicine clinic: a pilot study. *Int J STD AIDS* 1999; **10**: 531–535.

97 Golding JM, Wilsnack SC, Learman LA. Prevalence of sexual assault history among women with common gynecologic

symptoms. *Am J Obstet Gynecol* 1998; **179**: 1013–1019.

98 Frank E, Anderson BP. Psychiatric disorders in rape victims: past history and current symptomatology. *Compr Psychiatry* 1989; **28**: 77–85.

99 Ruch LO, Leon JJ. Sexual assault trauma and trauma change. *Women Health* 1983; **8**: 5–21.

100 Resick PA. The psychological impact of rape. *J Interpersonal Violence* 1993; **8**: 223–255.

101 Beck-Sague CM, Solomon F. Sexually transmitted diseases in abused children and adolescent and adult victims of rape: review of selected literature. *Clin Infect Dis* 1999; **28** (Suppl. 1): S74–S83.

102 Jenny C, Hooton TM, Bowers A, *et al.* Sexually transmitted diseases in victims of rape. *N Engl J Med* 1990; **322**: 713–716.

103 Murphy S, Kitchen V, Harris JRW, *et al.* Rape and subsequent seroconversion to HIV. *Br Med J* 1989; **299**: 718.

104 Gutman LT, St Claire KK, Weedy C, *et al.* Human immunodeficiency virus transmission by child sexual abuse. *Am J Dis Child* 1991; **145**: 137–141.

105 Coxell A, King M, Mezey G, Gordon D. Lifetime prevalence, characteristics, and associated problems of non-consensual sex in men: cross-sectional study. *Br Med J* 1999; **318**: 846–850.

106 Hillman RJ, O'Mara N, Taylor-Robinson D, Harris JRW. Medical and social aspects of sexual assault of males: a survey of 100 victims. *Br J Gen Pract* 1990; **40**: 502–504.

107 Hickson F, Davies P, Hunt A, Weatherburn P, McManus TJ, Coxon APM. Gay men as victims of non-consensual sex. *Arch Sex Behav* 1994; **23**: 281–294.

108 Groth AN, Burgess AW. Male rape: offenders and victims. *Am J Psychiatry* 1980; **137**: 806–810.

109 Hillman RJ, Tomlinson D, McMillan A, French PD, Harris JRW. Sexual assault of men: a series. *Genitourin Med* 1990; **66**: 247–250.

110 Kaszniak AW, Nussbaum PD, Berren MR, Santiago J. Amnesia as a consequence of male rape: a case report. *J Abnormal Psychol* 1988; **97**: 100–104.

111 Kelnan C. *Culture, Health and Illness.* Bristol; Wright PSG: 1984, pp. 54–57.

112 Grant B, Levin J. *Family Law.* London; Sweet and Maxwell: 1973.

113 Keith RM, Clark GV. *The Layman's Guide to Scots Law, vol. 2, Divorce.* Edinburgh; Gordon Bennett: 1977.

114 Willock ID. A new approach to divorce; irreconcilable break-up. *J Law Soc Scotland* 1974: 223–225.

APPENDIX

APPENDIX 3.1: HIV antibody testing

HIV antibody testing should always be undertaken with the informed consent of the patient, involving pre- and post-test counseling.

PRE-TEST COUNSELING

The principal issues to cover are as follows.

Confidentiality

This should be assured in all clinical settings. Increased anonymity is possible at Departments of Genitourinary Medicine and some specialist centers where names and addresses may be withheld.

An assessment of the risk

Levels of risk will vary depending on the prevalence of HIV in a given population.

1. Very high risk activities
   - unprotected vaginal and/or anal sex with a known HIV seropositive partner
   - sharing injecting equipment with a known HIV seropositive person.

2. High risk activities
   - unprotected anal sex between men
   - sharing injecting equipment
   - unprotected vaginal and/or anal sex with an injecting drug-using partner
   - unprotected vaginal and/or anal sex with a resident of a country where the E serogroup of HIV is prevalent (such as Thailand).

3. Moderate risk activities
   - protected anal sex between men
   - unprotected anal sex between a man and a woman in a western country
   - unprotected vaginal and/or anal sex between men and women in areas where there is a high prevalence of HIV.

4. Low risk activities
   - non-penetrative sexual contact between men
   - oral sex
   - unprotected vaginal sex in western countries
   - needle-stick injuries.

A discussion of the test itself to ensure that the patient is aware of the following points

1. The test detects antibodies to HIV, and it does not tell whether an individual has AIDS.

2. A period of 3 months after exposure is required before the test result can be considered accurate.

Implications of the test

1. Ascertain why the patient wants to know his/her status.

2. Use the opportunity to provide health education about on-going risks for HIV and other STIs.

3. Who to tell, discuss the impact the result may have on partners and family members.

4. Coping with a positive result, consider personal circumstances.

Advantages and disadvantages of having a test

The advantages are

1. Eligibility for medical monitoring and treatment, this is often offered to asymptomatic individuals.
2. The patient can make choices about his/her future.
3. The patient can take steps to avoid transmission of the virus to others.

The disadvantages are

1. Stress associated with experiencing an HIV-positive diagnosis.
2. The results may affect the patient's perception of the future, and their relationships and work.

Other points to consider

1. After the patient has consented to the test it is important to give clear information about when the result will be available.
2. Offer post-test counseling.

3. If the test is negative
   - reinforce risk-reduction strategies
   - if necessary, refer to appropriate agencies to assist with this
   - offer further tests if necessary
   - correct misconceptions, for example in an on-going relationship, if the patient is HIV antibody negative, this is not an indication of his/her partner's status.
4. If the test is positive
   - provide emotional support while the patient reacts to the information
   - give basic information about HIV
   - discuss whom to tell – the patient may need help to consider this issue carefully and to resist the temptation to tell people whom he/she may subsequently regret having told
   - discuss the patient's immediate plans for the period after he/she has left the unit – focus on support available such as the National AIDS Helpline
   - give an early follow-up appointment.
5. At follow-up
   - refer, with the patient's permission, to a center where medical monitoring and support for HIV infection can be provided, for example a Department of Genitourinary Medicine or an Infectious Diseases unit
   - if necessary refer for counseling and support
   - reinforce safer sex and risk reduction with written information if possible
   - discuss contraception
   - if appropriate give information about welfare rights
   - give written information about local services and agencies for HIV-positive individuals.

Chapter 4

Clinical investigation of the patient
A McMillan

Under the circumstances of rising demand for clinical, laboratory and other services, coupled with restrictions on the availability of these resources, clear objectives have to be defined for medical services, in particular out-patient departments. To secure minimum standards appropriate to the economies of the society being served and to avoid the omission of important steps, it is necessary to develop a structured approach to history taking and clinical examination. Although inappropriate for some patients this will involve focus of attention on those anatomical sites where implantation of the infecting organism or agent is likely to occur, namely the lower urogenital tract, the oropharynx and anorectum. Extension of the normal history taking and physical examination may be necessary for those with more serious disease, and underlying psychosexual difficulties should not be ignored.

It has been clear for a very long time that the straightforward, immensely successful idiom in medicine, and particularly in genitourinary medicine, namely 'identify the cause and remove it', is no longer adequate[1]. Although its extension to involve tracing and treatment of contacts is successful in immediately curable diseases such as gonorrhea it is clear that progress in genitourinary medicine is slowed and made more complex by a number of interacting factors. First and foremost is the increasing incidence of persistent viral infection due, for example, to papillomavirus, herpes simplex virus (HSV) and human immunodeficiency viruses (HIV). In all of these diseases medical intervention is not curative and there is likely to be a long-term, often lifetime, follow-up requirement. The first step outlined in this chapter will be effective when it is possible to identify the cause, remove it, and trace and, if necessary, treat contacts. In dealing with the persistent infections, however, all cannot be offered within the context of a single specialty and indeed the problems can surface in almost any medical setting. Thus it will not be enough to focus solely on the patient's immediate problem but in many cases it will be necessary to plan for follow-up and care in the long term. The potential need for help is staggering in its size but realizable goals can be defined and will always need resources outside the confines of the clinic.

In designing the approach the clinical and laboratory investigations undertaken must be in proportion to

1. the degree of risk in the individual patient

2. the likelihood of investigations bringing benefit.

In relation to the first the assessment will depend to a great extent on the sexual behavior of the individual, namely sexual

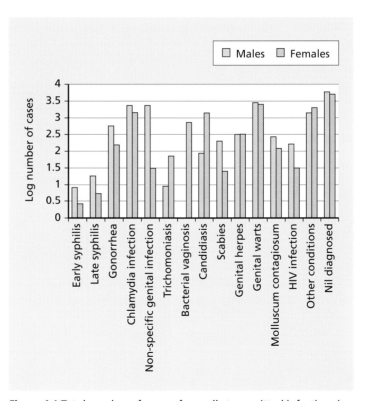

Figure 4.1 Total number of cases of sexually transmitted infections in males and females for the Department of Genitourinary Medicine, Edinburgh Royal Infirmary, 1995–1999. The totals are shown on a logarithmic scale.

orientation, sexual practices and degree of sexual mixing (promiscuity). 'At-risk' grouping of patients will take into account also the geographical location of the sexual encounter(s) and the practice or otherwise of drug abuse whether intravenous or not. In relation to the second it is clear that the detection or exclusion of hepatitis B surface antigen (HBsAg), for example, will enable decisions to be made on vaccination whereas the detection or exclusion of antibody to HIV in the serum will not. Specific diseases will vary geographically and in any given locality data keeping is necessary for the design of services (Figure 4.1).

Reception

The quality of reception is important and peremptoriness is to be deplored at all stages. Privacy is highly desirable for patients when personal details are being recorded for registration, reassurance about the confidentiality of the consultation may be given at the same time. Reception of patients is always important but particularly so in departments of genitourinary medicine specializing in sexually transmissible infections. Those responsible for design of out-patient departments have often failed to give these matters sufficient consideration.

Objectives of the clinical investigation

In any clinic four main objectives should form the framework for investigation of the patient.

1. First, it is important to make a clinical and microbial diagnosis of the wide variety of specific sexually transmissible infections, based on the identification of the organism or agent that is considered to be the cause. Limitations in resources may set limits to these investigations and some selection in the use of tests may often have to be imposed. In clinics in industrialized countries, laboratory tests for the detection of the causative organism should be available for the following sexually transmissible infections (STIs)

   - *Chlamydia trachomatis*
   - *Neisseria gonorrhoeae*
   - *Treponema pallidum*
   - *Trichomonas vaginalis*
   - *Candida albicans* and other yeasts
   - Human immunodeficiency viruses types 1 and 2 (HIV-1, HIV-2)
   - Hepatitis B virus (HBV)
   - Hepatitis C virus (HCV)
   - Herpes simplex virus (HSV)
   - *Giardia duodenalis*.

   Contact-tracing will be important in some infections, for example *Chlamydia trachomatis*, but much less so in others, for example bacterial vaginosis.

2. The second objective covers the detection of other medical problems and their resolution when possible. Some of the main aims may be summarized as follows

   - the encouragement in the use of contraception in those at risk of unwanted pregnancy
   - the detection of pregnancy
   - arrangement for antenatal care when necessary
   - assistance for those seeking help or advice in connection with continuation or termination of a pregnancy
   - detection of any psychosexual dysfunction
   - other medical issues which can conveniently be described as falling within the primary medical care of adolescents and young adults.

3. The third objective involves the clinic in medico-social work such as the detection and search for relief of homelessness, marital stress, and poverty. Those with problems and difficulties in establishing and maintaining relationships are of special concern to the clinician. Offering to put individual patients in touch with self-help groups may be appropriate. The doctor–patient relationship is an important one. Patients may fear that the stigma of a venereal disease will lower them in the opinion of their fellows. Doctors particularly must look at persons from the point of view of their whole personality. They must not allow deviance, deformity or difference to overshadow the fact that patients are human beings with qualities and faults similar to those in whom no stigma is recognized. It is in hospitals, and in clinics in particular, that doctors are privy to the sexual behavior of the individual. Doctors are, or should be, 'wise persons – before whom the individual with a fault need feel no shame nor exert self control, knowing that in spite of his failing he will be seen as an ordinary other'[2].

4. A fourth objective has to be introduced now and relates to infection or risk of infection by human immunodeficiency viruses (HIV). Although this is discussed more fully in Chapter 7, it will be necessary in localities of low incidence of infection, both in at-risk groups and in individuals anxious about their own situation, to begin the process of giving explanations and counseling before raising the question of testing for antibody to HIV. Appendix 4.1 summarizes some of the issues that should be discussed with the patient.

Taking the patient's history

History taking is an extension of the clinical skills required in any branch of medicine. A patient attending a clinic on his own account, on advice from a sexual contact, or after an explanation and referral by his general practitioner, will generally expect a series of questions relating to his or her recent sexual contacts. In some cases, however, the doctor might ask first about the patient's main complaints and their duration or, in the case of females, begin to consider and record the menstrual history and contraceptive practice of the patient.

Data about sexual intercourse are best obtained after the doctor has obtained rapport with the patient. For convenience, and to ensure that the main medical objectives are secured in every case, a pro forma is used in busy clinics, this provides a framework for the history taking and examination. Main details, therefore, will be rapidly apparent in the follow-up of the case by the doctor, who may not be the same one on every occasion.

SEXUAL HISTORY TAKING FROM A HETEROSEXUAL MAN

The following symptoms that may be volunteered by the patient or be elicited through specific enquiry, may indicate the presence of an STI.

Urethral discharge and dysuria

The symptoms of urethritis are variable in severity from person to person and do not reliably differentiate gonococcal from nongonococcal urethritis.

Genital ulceration

Genital herpes causes painful and tender genital ulceration. In the UK, the painful, tender genital ulceration and lymphadenitis of chancroid or lymphogranuloma venereum is found almost exclusively in individuals who have returned from geographical areas where these infections are common. Primary syphilis must always be considered in the individual who has a painless genital ulcer. Other causes of anogenital ulceration are shown in Table 4.1.

Sore throat or mouth

Pharyngeal gonorrhea is usually asymptomatic but sometimes produces a sore throat. Herpes simplex virus can cause painful oral ulceration.

Skin rash

Scabies is associated with an itchy skin rash occurring about 5 to 6 weeks after contact with an infected person or earlier if there has been previous exposure to the mite. Primary HIV, Epstein–Barr virus, and cytomegalovirus infections, and acute hepatitis A and B may all be associated with a transient and usually non-pruritic, generalized skin rash, the rash of secondary syphilis is usually more persistent. Persistent, itchy skin lesions may also be a feature of HIV infection.

Lymphadenopathy

Localized or generalized lymph node enlargement may be noticed by the patient infected with conditions such as those shown in Table 4.2.

The date of last coitus and the number of sexual partners of either sex in the last month and in the last year are noted. Notes should be made of whether or not the patient has a regular sexual partner and when he last had sex with her. In addition it is important to ask about other sexual partners within the preceding 3 to 6 months, and, if relevant, when sex with these partners occurred. He should be asked specifically if a sexual partner has told him that she has an infection. The use of barrier methods of contraception with any partner should be asked about. Information on antibiotic or chemotherapy received during the last month or longer will be relevant, particularly as it may obscure diagnosis or, at least, diminish the effectiveness of methods for the isolation of specific organisms. The doctor should ask specifically about known hypersensitivity to antimicrobial agents.

In connection with the past history, information should be obtained about previous sexually infectious diseases as well as previous illness of a medical or surgical nature. A history of hepatitis should be noted, and a record should be made of previous vaccination against hepatitis A and B viruses. Overseas visits, whether recent or remote, are relevant and enquiry should be made about sexual contact there, and, if relevant, the country of residence of the contact(s). The patient should be asked about past or present drug abuse and whether or not these drugs have been taken intravenously. In those with a history of injecting drug use, specific enquiry should be made about the sharing of injection equipment. When a blood-borne virus infection is suspected, inquiry should be made about tattooing, body-piercing, and medical procedures such as acupuncture.

Family history is often restricted in the male to those questions of sexual relationships, unless more detail on social

Table 4.1 Conditions that may be associated with anogenital ulceration or apparent ulceration

Infections	Dermatological conditions	Systemic diseases
Herpes simplex virus	Trauma	Erythema multiforme
Treponema pallidum	Chemical burns	Pyoderma gangrenosum
Chlamydia trachomatis	Lichen sclerosis et atrophicus	Behçet's syndrome
Lymphogranuloma venereum serovars	Balanitis xerotica obliterans	Reiter's disease (sexually acquired reactive arthritis)
Haemophilus ducreyi	Lichen simplex with excoriation	Crohn's disease
Klebsiella granulomatis	Lichen planus	
Pyogenic ulceration	Fixed drug eruption	
Mycobacterium tuberculosis	Other drug reactions (e.g.	
Trichomonas vaginalis	to foscarnet)	
Entamoeba histolytica	Erythroplasia of Queyrat	
Candida spp.	Vulval intraepithelial neoplasia	
Sarcoptes scabiei	Squamous cell carcinoma	

Table 4.2 Some causes of inguinal or femoral lymph node enlargement (greater than 1 cm in diameter)

Generalized lymphadenopathy	Localized lymphadenopathy

Systemic infection
For example STIs
    Epstein–Barr virus infection
    HIV infection
    Cytomegalovirus
    Hepatitis A virus infection
    Hepatitis B virus infection
    Primary herpes simplex virus infection
    Secondary syphilis
	Local infection
	Primary syphilis
	Primary and, less frequently,
	recurrent herpes simplex infection
	Chancroid
	Lymphogranuloma venereum
	Suppurative lesions of the
	anogenital region or lower limb

Immunologically based Collagen diseases Rheumatoid arthritis Drugs	*Neoplasm* Spread from, e.g. a squamous cell carcinoma of the penis
Neoplasm Primary Lymphomas Leukemias Secondary Carcinomatosis Melanoma	
Other Sarcoidosis	

background is required. Narrowing of the scope of the investigation is often a result of limited time and a patient's apparent wish to be cured quickly with the least possible intrusion into their personal affairs. In the case of patients with symptoms but no objective signs the possibility of psychosexual difficulties should be remembered and questions asked in explicit terms about matters such as premature ejaculation.

SEXUAL HISTORY TAKING FROM MEN WHO HAVE HAD SEX WITH MEN

The principles of history taking are as described for the heterosexual man, but, as certain infections are more prevalent amongst men who have had homosexual contact, a few additional points are worth considering.

1. A history of a sore throat developing within a few days of receptive orogenital contact is common and is often not associated with detectable infection.

2. There may be symptoms of viral hepatitis (Chapter 8).

3. Constipation, a mucopurulent anal discharge, anal bleeding, perianal discomfort or pruritus ani, and, in severe cases, pain and tenesmus are symptoms of proctitis caused, for example, by *Neisseria gonorrhoeae*. Many men with proctocolitis, such as results from campylobacter infection, have similar symptoms but in some, diarrhea with abdominal cramping, bloating, and fever are the principal features.

4. Diarrhea, epigastric fullness, abdominal cramps, increased flatulence, and nausea may be features of enteritis caused by *Giardia duodenalis*.

5. Perianal pain may be a feature of proctitis but is also a symptom of localized disease such as traumatic anal fissure and perianal hematoma.

6. A common cause of pruritus ani is threadworm infestation.

7. As syphilis was previously common in homosexual men and some tests, for example the *Treponema pallidum* hem-

agglutination assay, often remain positive for years after successful treatment, the proper interpretation of serological tests requires that specific inquiry is made about previous infections.

8. As a significant number of homosexual men have psychological problems, careful enquiry should be made into, for example, problems with sexual identity.

SEXUAL HISTORY TAKING FROM A HETEROSEXUAL WOMAN

The details in taking the sexual history of a heterosexual woman do not differ significantly from those described above for the heterosexual man. Note should be made, however, of her last menstrual period and of her menstrual cycle. The method of contraception used should be noted, and the number of pregnancies, whether full-term or aborted, should be recorded. Children's needs may make her attendance difficult. Judicious questions will often elicit symptoms of family stress.

Clinical examination: special features

Initial examination of both males and females can conveniently include inspection of the skin surface above the waist. This can be carried out having due regard to the patient's sense of privacy and feelings. Examine the cervical, axillary and epitrochlear and inguinal lymph nodes. The axillary region and scalp should be inspected. Careful examination of the wrist creases, the webs between the fingers, and the back of the elbow is necessary for the detection of scabies. The presence of old self-inflicted scars, marks of intravenous injections, tattoo marks and signs of uncleanliness should be noted.

In the inspection of the skin surface below the waist and of the anogenital region in particular, attention should be paid to the abdomen, inguinal lymph nodes, liver and spleen. Examination of the anogenital region with gloved hands is the correct procedure and is mandatory where moist, infective or potentially infective lesions are present. Disposable latex examination gloves are satisfactory.

The question of the presence of a chaperone during a genital examination has recently been addressed[3]. It is imperative that a chaperone is present when a male physician undertakes a genital examination of a woman, and a working party of the Royal College of Obstetricians and Gynaecologists[4] concluded that a chaperone should be offered to all women having an intimate examination in gynecology and obstetrics, irrespective of the sex of the gynecologist. A female nurse is the preferred choice as a chaperone; not only can she safeguard against abuse, but also she can assist in the examination and provide support for the anxious patient. If the patient declines a chaperone, this fact should be recorded in the patient's notes. Unlike women, men seldom express a need for the support of a chaperone, and indeed the presence of a female nurse may cause embarrassment to young men. Nevertheless, a chaperone of the sex preferred by the patient should be offered. Young people may prefer a relative to be present at the examination and this should be encouraged.

EXAMINATION OF THE HETEROSEXUAL MALE

The following is a method for the investigation of the heterosexual man who is at risk of an STI.

1. In contacts of gonorrhea or in those with anogenital gonorrhea, a cotton-wool swab should be passed over the pharynx and both tonsils or tonsillar beds and plated directly on medium selective for the gonococcus. The microscopic examination of smears from the pharynx for the gonococcus is not useful as a diagnostic procedure.
2. The pubic area should be inspected, for example, for *Phthirus pubis* or molluscum contagiosum.
3. The genitocrural folds should be inspected for lesions such as warts or tinea cruris.
4. Inguinal or femoral lymph node enlargement, with or without tenderness, should be sought. Lymph-adenopathy (individual nodes larger than 1 cm in diameter) may be found in conditions such as those shown in Table 4.2.
5. The scrotum and its contents should be examined next. The testes, epididymies, and spermatic cords and coverings are palpated. Epididymitis, for example, may complicate untreated gonococcal or chlamydial infections.
6. The shaft of the penis is inspected for lesions such as herpes and scabetic papules.
7. The prepuce, if present, is retracted, and the glans penis, frenum, coronal sulcus, prepuce, shaft and median raphe are examined.
8. The urethral meatus is examined carefully for urethral discharge, and the lips of the meatus should always be everted to identify warts. An attempt should be made to milk any discharge from the penile urethra. If a discharge is present, the urethral meatus should be cleansed with a saline-soaked gauze swab and the discharge obtained by means of a disposable plastic inoculating loop. The 10 μL loop, blue in color (Nunc products, Kamstrup, DK–Roskilde, Denmark), is inserted past the everted lips of the meatus and gently passed for 2 to 3 cm within the urethra. Where even minor urethral symptoms are present in the male a scraping should be taken, smeared on a microscope slide for Gram-staining, and then plated directly on to a selective medium for the gonococcus even if there is no visible discharge. If direct plating is impossible transport medium should be used (Chapter 11). It is a useful procedure in such cases to ask patients to return the following morning after retaining urine overnight. The patient should empty his bladder late at night before retiring and come to the clinic in the early morning. Such early morning urethral smears, examined by microscopy and culture, are useful in the detection of minimal degrees of urethritis, whether non-gonococcal or gonococcal. To avoid missing asymptomatic cases, there is a strong case for the routine culture of urethral scrapings in all cases where there has been a risk of acquiring gonorrhea. Facilities may, however, be restricted, in which case contacts should be examined to exclude the presence of the gonococcus.
9. Where facilities exist for the detection of chlamydial DNA by amplified molecular methods, a first-voided 20 mL specimen of urine is obtained in a sterile universal container. Alternatively, urethral material can be collected for the detection of chlamydial nucleic acids by passing an endo-urethral swab into the anterior urethra for 5 cm, withdrawing it and placing it in the buffer solution provided by the manufacturer of the test kit, before transporting it to the laboratory. Many clinics still rely on antigen-detection methods, and some clinicians use culture methods for the diagnosis of chlamydial genital tract infection. In the enzyme immunoassay systems, for which collection kits are available, urethral material is obtained as for PCR or LCR methods, and the swab is sent in the transport fluid provided. Alternatively, and when patient numbers are small, direct immunofluorescence for the detection of antigen is sometimes used (for example, the 'Microtrak' *Chlamydia trachomatis* direct specimen test, Syva, California, USA). In this test a urethral swab is rolled on to a slide and fixed in acetone. Urethral material for culture is obtained as above, and the endo-urethral swab is cut off into 2SP transport medium*.
10. In the case of men who are named contacts of women with trichomoniasis, it is helpful to examine a urethral scraping taken as above and suspended in isotonic saline.

---

* Transport medium for *Chlamydia*. '2SP' is a sucrose-phosphate solution, i.e. 0.2 M sucrose in 0.02 M phosphate buffer pH 7.2 with 50 μg/mL of streptomycin, 100 μg vancomycin, and, except for 2SP to be used for conjunctive specimens, 25 units/mL of nystatin. Specimens may be stored at −70°C before culture.

11. The perineum, perianal region and anus are examined, for example, for warts or anal fissure.

12. Direct visual examination of the urine is necessary as the urine will contain exudate from the urethra in the case of urethritis. In anterior urethritis, the initial 20 mL of urine passed will contain many pus cells, causing a turbidity that is not cleared by the addition of 10% acetic acid, it will be less in the second portion of urine passed. This crude test has value in detecting obvious urethritis. In subacute or chronic urethritis, casts consisting of mucopus from urethra and urethral glands, may sink as threads and deposits in the specimen. In anterior urethritis exudate will tend to be passed mainly in the first urine voided, in posterior urethritis or prostatitis the first and second specimens may contain such deposit. The clinical value of this so-called 'two-glass test', however, is extremely limited as treatment decisions are seldom made on these findings.

13. Examination of urine for protein, sugar, and blood is essential. The most widely used tests for these are the dipstick tests.
    - *Glucose* A qualitative test based on glucose oxidase that is practically specific for glucose.
    - *Protein* A semi-quantitative test, most sensitive for detection of albumin (Appendix 4.1). This test is very insensitive for Bence-Jones protein.
    - *Blood* This is a semi-quantitative test for heme derivatives. The test does not differentiate between hematuria, hemoglobinuria and myoglobinuria. A false-positive result can be seen when the urine is contaminated (1/1000) with povidone-iodine (Betadine®). For the investigation of microscopic hematuria see Appendix 4.2.

14. A specimen of venous blood is taken in every case for serological tests for syphilis and, when appropriate, for HSV and hepatitis B virus infections. Serological tests for hepatitis B (Hepatitis B surface antigen, HBsAg, and core antibody against the virus, anti-

HBc,) should be carried out in cases of intravenous drug misuse, in those with tattoos, and in those who have had sexual contact with individuals from geographical areas where hepatitis B virus is endemic. After counseling, serological screening for hepatitis C virus infection (anti-HCV) may be considered in those who have injected drugs intravenously, or whose sexual partners have hepatitis C virus infection. The question of testing for HIV infection should be raised and, if, after counseling (Appendix 3.1), the patient wishes to be tested, a blood sample should be obtained for this purpose.

EXAMINATION OF THE MAN WHO HAD SEX WITH MEN (MSM)

The clinical examination of the anogenital region of men who have had sex with other men is as described for the heterosexual man, but additional investigations are usually necessary.

Gonorrhea in MSM

As the urethra may be involved in 60%, the anorectum in 40% and the pharynx in about 7% of cases of gonorrhea amongst MSM, sampling from *all* these sites should be a routine in every case. In gonococcal urethritis there are generally, but not always, symptoms. In anorectal gonorrhea symptoms may be present only in one-third of cases and in the pharynx the infections tend to be asymptomatic. It is recommended that samples for *Neisseria gonorrhoeae* be taken from these sites as follows.

1. Urethral smear and culture.
2. Anorectal cultures. Because the lubricants used contain antibacterial agents, proctoscopy should be postponed until after the anorectal culture has been taken by passing a swab, moistened if necessary with sterile saline, through the anal canal towards the rectum. On proctoscopy, when there is evidence of inflammation with erythema, mucosal edema, mucopus and blood, it may be possible to obtain a sample of pus in which the gonococcus can be seen on microscopy although diagnosis will require confirmation by culture.
3. Pharyngeal cultures. A swab is passed over the tonsillar area and the back of the pharynx and plated directly on to medium selective for the gonococcus.

Two sets of samples from anorectal and pharyngeal sites at consecutive follow-up attendances are required before a gonococcal infection is discounted.

Chlamydial infection in men who have had sex with men

1. For the detection of urethral infection, obtain specimens as detailed above.
2. Rectal chlamydial infection is often symptomless, and material for the detection of chlamydiae by amplified molecular methods should be taken routinely by inserting the swab provided with the collection kit about 2.5 cm into the anal canal, rotating, and, after withdrawal, placing in the transport medium. Alternatively, specimens, obtained in the manner may be sent for culture. Direct immunofluorescence testing can be undertaken on rectal material, obtained as before and smeared on a specilly-prepared microscope slide, before fixing in acetone. EIA are unsuitable for the detection of chlamydial infection at this anatomical site.
3. Although chlamydial infection of the pharynx is apparently uncommon, specimens for the detection of infection by amplified molecular methods or by culture may be obtained by passing a swab over the tonsillar area and the back of the pharynx and placing in the appropriate transport medium.

Proctoscopy

Proctoscopy should always be undertaken at the initial clinic attendance of a man who has been the recipient partner during anal intercourse. Asymptomatic lesions of the anal canal such as warts will be readily identified and the appearance of the distal 5 cm of the rectum should be recorded. As the number of polymorphonuclear leukocytes in a Gram-stained smear of rectal material is highly variable, the authors do not recommend enumeration of these cells in the diagnosis of proctitis. Inflammatory changes associated with gonococcal, chlamydial and herpetic infections are generally limited to the distal 10 cm of the rectum, whereas those caused by *Shigella* spp., *Campylobacter* spp. and *Salmonella* spp. at sigmoidoscopy are seen to extend more proximally. As a routine diagnostic procedure, the authors do not advocate sigmoidoscopy unless there has been either unexplained rectal bleeding or an organismal cause has not been found for altered bowel habit, anorectal discharge, a sensation of incomplete defecation or pain. With the exception of infection with *Chlamydia trachomatis* lymphogranuloma venereum immunovars, the histology of the proctitis associated with the sexually transmissible enteric pathogens is non-specific, and rectal biopsy is unlikely to be helpful in diagnosis. This procedure, which is only rarely complicated by hemorrhage or perforation, may be indicated if the patient's symptoms do not resolve after successful antimicrobial therapy.

Proctitis

In the investigation of patients with symptoms of proctitis, in addition to obtaining material for culture for *N. gonorrhoeae*, and for the detection of *C. trachomatis* (see above). Rectal specimens taken with a cotton wool-tipped applicator stick that is broken off into a tube of viral transport medium (for example Hank's medium) should be cultured for HSV or tested for HSV DNA by PCR.

Diarrhea

A stool sample should be examined for bacterial pathogens and protozoa (Chapter 18). Infection with *Giardia duodenalis* is usually asymptomatic but can produce diarrhea without evidence of proctitis. In the case of patients with symptoms suggestive of protozoal infection, at least three stool samples should be examined before the diagnosis is excluded. It should be remembered that the use of antimicrobial agents, kaolin and other antidiarrheal preparations may suppress the excretion of cysts.

Serological tests

In addition to undertaking serological tests for syphilis, serum should be examined for hepatitis B surface antigen (HBsAg) and antibody against HBV core antigen (anti-

HBc), and if serological markers are absent the man should be offered immunization. In many clinics, screening for immunity to hepatitis A virus (anti-HAV IgG) is also undertaken and non-immune individuals are offered vaccination (see Chapter 8 for discussion on the need to pre-test individuals before offering vaccination).

EXAMINATION OF THE FEMALE

The physical examination of the anogenital region should be performed with the woman in the semi-lithotomy position on a couch in a warm and well-lit room.

1. If the woman has been at risk of pharyngeal gonorrhea, material from the tonsils or tonsillar fossae is taken for culture for the gonococcus.
2. The abdomen is inspected and palpated for tenderness, guarding, and masses.
3. The pubic area is inspected for *Phthirus pubis*, warts and molluscum contagiosum.
4. The inguinal and femoral lymph nodes are palpated, and note made of enlargement with or without tenderness (Table 4.2).
5. The labia majora are inspected, for example for warts.
6. The labia minora are gently separated and, after gently wiping with a cotton wool ball, the introitus is inspected, looking particularly for warts and the lesions of genital herpes.
7. A finger should be inserted into the vaginal orifice and the contents of the urethra and its para-urethral glands massaged towards the orifice. Smears for Gram-staining and microscopy, and cultures for *Neisseria gonorrhoeae* are taken from this site in all cases using a 10 μL plastic inoculating loop. Orifices of the distal pair of paraurethral glands open on either side of the urethral meatus (Skene's glands). Smears and cultures can be taken from this site specifically or added to the urethral swab when pus is seen at the duct orifice.
8. The greater vestibular glands (Bartholin's glands) lie in the posterior half of the labia majora and the orifices of the ducts open external to the hymen on

the inner side of the labia minora. The gland (1 to 1.5 cm in diameter) may be examined by passing a finger into the vagina and hooking it behind a point in the substance of the labium majus at the junction of the anterior two-thirds and posterior one-third. It cannot be palpated unless enlarged or fibrotic. By gently massaging the gland and expressing the mucous secretion towards the duct orifice, material may be collected in a loop or cotton-wool applicator for the immediate preparation of a smear and culture. Bartholinitis may complicate gonococcal and chlamydial infections.

9. A speculum is then passed, the character of any vaginal discharge fluid is noted, and the appearance of the walls of the vagina is recorded. (It is not usually necessary to lubricate a speculum, but if this is required, isotonic saline should be used in preference to lubricating gels that may contain substances that inhibit growth of gonococci). Vaginitis, for example, may be a feature of candidiasis when a curdy, white discharge adhering to the mucosa may also be found. In bacterial vaginosis, however, a homogeneous white discharge is seen, but the vaginal walls appear normal or mildly edematous.
10. Using narrow-range pH paper held in a pair of forceps, it may be useful to measure the pH of the secretions in the posterior vaginal fornix (avoid the alkaline cervical secretions). In bacterial vaginosis, for example, the pH is ≥ 5.0.
11. Vaginal material obtained from the posterior fornix with a cotton wool-tipped applicator stick is suspended in a drop of isotonic saline (0.154 M NaCl) on a microscope slide, and covered with a cover-slip. The slide is examined microscopically (magnification × 400) for *Trichomonas vaginalis*, fungal hyphae, and the 'clue cells' of bacterial vaginosis (Chapter 17). Sometimes the flagellated bacteria, *Mobiluncus* spp. may be recognized by their rapid forward motion.
12. A Gram-stained smear of material similarly obtained from the posterior fornix is prepared and examined at a

magnification of × 1000 for 'clue cells' and for spores and hyphae of *Candida* spp.

13. The appearance of the ectocervix and the character of any discharge from the endocervical canal is noted: in chlamydial and gonococcal infections, for example, there *may* be a muco-purulent discharge.

14. If the woman, aged 21 years or over, has not had a cervical smear taken within the preceding 3 years, this should be undertaken using an Ayles-bury or similar spatula *before* taking the endocervical specimens detailed below. Using Ayre's method, the spatula is used to scrape the superficial cells from the external os and lower end of cervix. The scrapings from the squamocolumnar junction are taken throughout an arc of 360° and a slide prepared and fixed immediately in 95% v/v ethanol.

15. For the detection of infection with *Chlamydia trachomatis*, specimens from the endocervical canal are obtained using one of the following methods.

    ● *Methods based on the detection of chlamydial nucleic acids*. A cotton wool-tipped wire swab is inserted about 1 cm into the endocervical canal, rotated several times, and, after withdrawal, is cut off into a tube of the buffer fluid provided by the kit manufacturer.

    ● *Culture methods*. A cotton wool-tipped applicator stick is used as above, but after withdrawal, it is agitated in the 2SP transport medium in which the specimen is transported to the laboratory.

    ● *Antigen detection methods*. For the detection of chlamydial antigens by enzyme immunoassay, endo-cervical material is obtained as before with a swab similar to that used for the detection of nucleic acids. The swab is cut off into a tube of buffer provided by the manufacturer of the test kit. Endocervical specimens can also be examined by direct immuno-fluorescence, the material being rolled on a slide and fixed in acetone before transport to the laboratory.

● NB Although the examination of urine or of tampon or vaginal flush specimens by PCR or LCR for chlamydial DNA may be used for chlamydial detection (Chapter 10), in the setting of a sexually transmitted infections clinic, the authors consider it better to obtain cervical specimens directly. In other settings, such as community clinics, self-obtained specimens may be examined for chlamydial DNA (Chapter 10).

16. Material from the endocervical canal is obtained using a cotton wool-tipped applicator stick, for Gram-smear micro-scopy and culture for *N. gonorrhoeae*.

17. The perineum, perianal region and anus are examined for lesions such as warts or anal fissures.

18. Anorectal specimens for culture for *N. gonorrhoeae* are obtained by passing a cotton wool-tipped applicator stick about 3 cm into the anal canal, with-drawing it and either plating it directly on to culture medium or inserting it into a tube of transport medium (see above). If skin tags or hemorrhoids make this process difficult a child's proctoscope may be slightly lubricated with saline and passed into the rec-tum. The swab may now be passed beyond the tip of the proctoscope that is then itself withdrawn first and the swab withdrawn gently afterwards. If there are anorectal symptoms, a proc-toscope should be passed and the anal canal and distal rectum examined, for example for warts or a distal proc-titis. In the latter case, the patient should be investigated as described on page 55 for the homosexual man.

19. In women with pelvic symptoms, a bimanual vaginal examination should be carried out gently. The lubricated (K-Y water-soluble lubricating jelly) index and second finger of the right hand are used to separate the labia and are then passed into the vagina. Gently pressing backwards the fingers are gradually passed towards the ante-rior fornix when the uterus can be pal-pated by the fingers of the left hand placed well above the symphysis pubis. The fundus of the retroverted uterus can be felt through the posterior

fornix. The uterine appendages may be examined through the lateral fornix and a swelling outlined between the fingers of the two hands. Tender-ness in the fornices, with or without swelling of the Fallopian tubes or on movement of the cervix, are signs elicited in inflammatory disease such as gonococcal infection of the upper genital tract. Inflammatory swellings may also be felt in the rectovaginal pouch (pouch of Douglas).

20. A sample of urine for analysis for protein, blood, and glucose should be obtained (see 'Examination of the heterosexual man', pp. 53–54). Pronounced dysuria or frequency tends to be associated more often with a urinary tract infection caused by coliform organisms, than by the gono-coccus.

21. If there is a risk of pregnancy perform a urine pregnancy test (Appendix 4.3).

22. Serological tests for syphilis (see pp. 407–414) should be taken in every case, and if the woman is at risk of hepatitis B or C virus infections, sero-logical screening should be offered (see pp. 221–222 and 237–239). If there is a risk of continuing exposure to hepatitis B virus, for example if she is a sex-industry worker, vaccination should be considered if she lacks immunity. The issue of HIV should be discussed and, if requested after coun-seling, blood is obtained for HIV anti-body testing (Appendix 3.1).

EXAMINATION OF ULCERS (see Chapter 20)

Table 4.1 shows some causes of anogenital ulceration.

Syphilis

Syphilis must be excluded as a cause of any sore in the anal or genital region. Although it is likely that the detection of specific DNA sequences by PCR will replace the earlier laboratory methods for the diagnosis of primary syphilis, the methods are not yet generally available and many clinics rely on dark-ground microscopy. This procedure is therefore considered in detail. After cleans-ing the surface with a swab soaked in sterile saline, serum is squeezed by gentle pressure from the depth of the lesion. This serum may be collected directly on a cover-slip or, if this is difficult, in a capillary tube. If collected in a glass capillary, one end of the capillary can be sealed in a gas microburner. The column of air beyond the seal is then heated to expel fluid neatly on to the center of a cover-slip which is then positioned on a slide. After firmly pressing the glass cover-slip and slide between pieces of filter paper, the preparation can be examined by dark-ground illumination. It is useful in a clinic to have the microscope arranged with an automatic focusing device so the chances of damaging the oil-immersion lens may be minimized and rapid examination made easy.

Dark-ground examination of serum from all ulcers on genital mucosa or at mucocutaneous junctions is a policy that should be adopted routinely so that a diagnosis of early syphilis may not be missed. Three sets of tests should be taken if syphilis is suspected. Lymph node puncture may occasionally yield *Treponema pallidum*. Monoclonal antibodies directed against a specific surface exposed antigen of *T. pallidum* should facilitate the development of diagnostic tests that may supplement or, in the interests of laboratory safety, replace dark-ground examination (see Chapter 15).

In homosexual men, typical anal chancres are uncommon, although dark-ground examination of radial linear anal fissures, seen in early syphilis in such cases, will sometimes reveal *T. pallidum*.

Herpes simplex virus infection

Direct diagnosis of HSV infection by a rapid antigen detection test (immuno-fluorescence or enzyme-immunoassay) should be requested when there is any doubt as to the clinical diagnosis, or where rapid confirmation is required to support the choice of therapy or other management. It is also more likely to give an answer than virus culture when the lesion is crusting. Electron microscopy of scrapings from lesions can also be used to detect HSV, but is largely superseded by immuno-fluorescence. Nucleic acid amplification by PCR is not routine for most samples for HSV, but is widely available in specialist

centers for CSF particularly. It can also be usefully applied to samples from atypical lesions. Virus isolation for confirmation and typing is suitable for most common herpes infections, especially if treatment has been started on clinical grounds. In all cases swabs from lesions should be submitted in a virus transport medium to preserve infectivity, maintain cells and inhibit microbial growth. Isolation of HSV is only available usually from virus laboratories with cell culture facilities, although the commercially produced Enzyme-Linked Virus Inducible System (ELVIS®, BioWhittaker) could be used in any microbiology laboratory to process substantial numbers of samples for HSV detection. This ingenious system has an HSV promoter gene in cells in prepared culture vials, any HSV infection induces the promoter and consequently expression of a linked enzyme that is detected by a blue stain. The newest version incorporates fluorescent staining method to type the virus (Chapter 6). Herpes simplex virus cytopathic effects in standard human fibroblast cell cultures appear from 1 to 7 days after inoculation, depending on the starting virus titer.

Culture of fluid from ulcers may yield HSV although such a finding does not exclude the possibility of coexisting syphilis.

Chancroid

Chancroid is an uncommon condition in industrialized countries, most cases having been acquired in parts of the world where infection is prevalent. Even where infection with *Haemophilus ducreyii*, the causative organism, is common the diagnosis of chancroid by clinical appearance is unreliable, the sensitivity being, at best, between 75 and 80% (Chapter 16). Microscopy of Gram-stained smears from the base of the ulcer or from material aspirated from a bubo fails to identify the organism in at least 50% of cases, and, as the organism is difficult to culture, up to 50% of infections are not identified by this method. Although not yet available widely, tests based on the detection of specific nucleic acids appear to be useful and will probably become the diagnostic methods of choice where resources permit. In the attempted laboratory diagnosis of chancroid, material

should be taken from the base of the ulcer or aspirated from a bubo.

Lymphogranuloma venereum

Giemsa-stained smears of scrapings from a suspected primary lesion and pus aspirated from a lymph node may be examined by microscopy for inclusions. Attempts should also be made to isolate the organism in tissue culture. *Chlamydia* spp., however, are only isolated in about 30% of cases. The lymphogranuloma venereum complement fixation test can be useful in diagnosis. The test generally becomes positive during the initial 4 weeks of infection and the titer rises during this period in the untreated patient. Titers of $\geq$ 1:64 are considered positive.

Donovanosis

This infection is also rarely seen in industrialized countries, but it is common in developing nations. A diagnosis of donovanosis is based on the microscopic demonstration of the causative organism – *Klebsiella* (*Calymmatobacterium*) *granulomatis* – in tissue smears taken from the lesions. A specimen of granulation tissue is obtained from the edge of the lesion using a curette or scalpel. The tissue is spread between two microscope slides and the resultant smear is stained with Giemsa's stain. Repeat examinations are often necessary. Histological examination of a wedge-shaped excision biopsy of the margin of the ulcer can be helpful.

Tracing contacts

It is essential that personnel involved in tracing contacts are adequately trained for their task. It is the authors' view that this aspect of the clinical task should fall on those who have had training in the care of patients as well as in community health. When interviewing patients a deep appreciation of the medical and social consequences of the various sexually transmissible infections is essential. An ability to give reasoned explanations about health matters which the patient may have been unable to comprehend when seen by the doctor, is one of the essential educational priorities of this type of work. An open mind, knowledge of sexually transmitted infections and an awareness of the varied nature of human sexuality are essential. Experience in the local community and in the homes of patients are the leavening of experience which will help to prevent or mitigate the sometimes serious social catastrophes. Where appropriate, conciliation should be possible in difficult situations that arise between partners, whether married or not. The diagnosis of gonorrhea and syphilis, and by implication the diagnosis of other STIs may be regarded as defamatory, so there are legal and social obligations requiring the exercise of care and consideration. It is the patient's cooperation which must be sought, and everything should be done to mitigate not only the medical but the social consequences arising from the diagnosis.

In the tracing of contacts, as in the UK, it is useful to have some procedures common to all clinics in the country, although methods of approach acceptable in one city may not be appropriate in another. At its simplest, a patient may be asked to give his or her consort a personal note, usually called a contact slip, to bring to the clinic. This note may be headed with the name of the clinic and contain a record of the patient's case number, his or her diagnosis in the code used in the locality or that to be found in the International Classification of Diseases, and the date of the diagnosis. Such a personal note can be readily interpreted in any clinic using the code, and the patient's anonymity is secure in the event of its loss.

If a contact is to be looked for in another part of the UK then a special contact tracing form (e.g. Special Clinic Contact Report; Department of Health and Social Security) may be sent to the physician in charge of the clinic serving the area concerned. When the name and address of the contact is known, limited additional details of description are needed. If only a forename is known and descriptions are inadequate, successful contact tracing is rare. Recognizing that these forms, together with the necessary searching, may be regarded as defamatory, personnel responsible for the process, including the medical staff, must exercise care and judgment in every case. In the process of tracing contacts the patient may be persuaded to help but it is not permissible to use any form of trick or coercion to obtain information. It is essential to

Table 4.3 Some priorities in tracing contacts

Diagnosis	Degree of danger to a sexual partner (+ to +++)	Degree of priority for rapid contact tracing (+ to +++)	Comment on priority
Acquired early-stage syphilis	+++	+++	Essential
Acquired late-stage syphilis	0	0	Except in a long-term partner
Gonorrhea	+++	+++	Essential
Non-gonococcal urethritis in the male. Chlamydial infection in male/female	++	++	Highly desirable
Lymphogranuloma venereum	++	++	Highly desirable
Trichomoniasis	+	+	Desirable in regular partner
Candidosis	+	+	Desirable in regular partner if patient has recurrent infection
Scabies	+	+	Treatment of household or family mostly advisable
Phthirus pubis	+	+	Desirable in partner(s)
Herpes genitalis	Uncertain	Varies	
Cytomegalovirus infection	+	+	Primary infection in pregnancy may be a danger to the fetus
Genital warts	+		Highly desirable
Hepatitis B virus infection	+++	+++	Tracing of contacts justified, particularly in pregnancy. Vaccination available Counseling in carrier and others
Molluscum contagiosum	+	+	Desirable in regular partner
Marburg disease, Lassa and Ebola fever	+++	+++	Essential to prevent spread of these rare epidemic diseases with a high mortality. Sexual intercourse is not the main method of spread
HIV infection	+++	a	Counseling essential to prevent spread of this dangerous infection.

a See text, Chapter 7 especially

treat individuals with respect and make sure that confidential information is not communicated to others. Threats are never justified. The exercise demands persuasion by explanation, kindness and tact. Initial failures may be rewarded by patience, and delays are preferable to the harmful effects of threats.

In the context of this chapter an attempt has been made to put together a working guide as an indicator of priorities in the tracing of contacts (Table 4.3).

Social aspects

Those involved in helping patients to resolve their social and personal problems, a regular feature of STI clinical work, whether clinician or health visitor, should be alert to possible needs of the patient, particularly financial or interpersonal, which may fall within the ambit of medical social work. Specific matters are given fuller consideration in Chapter 3 but, in particular, all patients of 16 years of age or less require special attention in every case and an endeavor should be made to allow young patients to reconsider their lifestyle in relation to the risks that are taken. This gives an opportunity for individuals to express their anxieties and problems as well as a chance for the medical staff to offer advice.

Management of the survivor of sexual assault

The role of the health care professional is
1. to assess and manage the survivor's physical and psychological well being
2. to provide treatment for and prevention of STIs and pregnancy as desired or requested
3. to collect necessary evidence and document pertinent data for criminal investigation and legal proceedings[5].

The collection of evidence of sexual assault is generally outwith the remit of the specialist in sexually transmitted infections, and should only be undertaken by physicians trained in forensic medicine; details are provided in standard texts. An inte-

grated clinical service for victims of sexual assault, however, is highly desirable. In such a setting, forensic specimens can be obtained, the individual can be screened for infection and offered antimicrobial prophylaxis, emergency contraception can be provided if appropriate, and psychological support offered promptly[6].

WOMEN

When an individual attends a STI clinic and indicates that she wants to report the assault to the police – and she should be specifically asked if she wants to do so – it is important to postpone the examination

for STIs until the necessary forensic examination has been completed[7].

Taking a sexual history from a survivor of a sexual assault is similar to that described on page 52. There is a particular need, however, for privacy and a gentle, supportive and non-judgmental approach; the patient should be offered the choice of a male or female physician or nurse. The history should include details of the assault, and the sexual history before and after the incident. The physical examination is as described on pp. 53–54, but it is important to make accurate notes in which details of injuries are recorded. It may be some time later that the individual reports

Table 4.4 Microbiological tests in female survivors of sexual assault

Specimen	Microbiological test
Pharyngeal	Culture for *Neisseria gonorrhoeae*[a]
Urethral	Gram-stained smear microscopy and culture for *N. gonorrhoeae*[a]
Endocervical	Culture for *Chlamydia trachomatis*, or PCR or LCR for chlamydial DNA[b] Gram-stained smear microscopy and culture for *N. gonorrhoeae*[a]
Vaginal	Saline mount preparation for *Trichomonas vaginalis*[a] Gram-stained smear microscopy for *Candida* spp. and 'clue cells'[a]
Anorectal	Gram-stained smear microscopy and culture for *N. gonorrhoeae* Culture for *C. trachomatis*, or PCR or LCR for chlamydial DNA
Blood	1. Serological test for syphilis at first attendance and repeated 4 and 12 weeks after the assault. 2. Serological tests for hepatitis B virus (HBsAg, anti-HBc, and anti-HBs) and for hepatitis C virus (anti-HCV) infections at first attendance and repeated at 12 and 24 weeks after the assault. 3. Serological tests for HIV infection at initial visit, 12 and 24 weeks after the incident[c]

[a] Repeat test if the assault had occurred within 2 weeks of clinic attendance, and if woman was not given antimicrobial prophylaxis.
[b] Diagnosis by culture is the only currently recognized evidence of chlamydial infection in UK courts. In the USA, if chlamydial culture is unavailable, FDA-approved nucleic acid amplification methods are acceptable if confirmation is available. A positive test in the latter should be verified by a second test based on a different diagnostic principle (Centers for Disease Control and Prevention 2002[11]).
[c] Only after appropriate counseling. If blood is not tested the serum should be stored for future testing if required.
PCR: polymerase chain reaction. LCR: ligase chain reaction. HBsAg: hepatitis B surface antigen. Anti-HBc: antibody against hepatitis B core antigen. Anti-HBs: antibody against hepatitis B surface antigen.

the assault to the police by which time there may be little evidence of injury and the examining physician's records then become extremely important.

Table 4.4 outlines the microbiological tests that should be undertaken in the survivor of sexual assault. It should be noted that in the UK, **isolation** of *Chlamydia trachomatis* **in culture** is the only evidence of chlamydial infection that is accepted by the courts. At the initial clinic attendance, serological testing for HIV and hepatitis B and C viruses should be discussed with the patient and undertaken if requested. In any case it is useful to obtain a serum sample for storage for future testing for these viruses should a subsequent test yield positive results. The transmission of STIs through sexual assault influences the sentencing of the assailant, and can result in substantial compensation for the survivor. It is, however, sometimes difficult to prove that an individual has acquired an STI through sexual assault, and the presence of an infection may not always be considered evidence of such assault. In some cases, however, the isolation of a pathogen from both assailant and survivor, and its subsequent molecular characterization may link both parties and be of forensic value.

Postcoital contraception should be discussed with the woman and prescribed if desired[8].

Hepatitis B vaccination should be offered at the individual's initial attendance, and the authors favor an accelerated schedule (Chapter 8). There is evidence that vaccination is protective at least up to 3 weeks after exposure to the virus[9].

The offer of post-exposure prophylaxis against the bacterial sexually transmitted infections and *Trichomonas vaginalis* is controversial. Many individuals present within a few days of the sexual attack before there are sufficient numbers of organisms to detect by culture. A substantial number of people fail to re-attend for follow-up – only 53% of women in one series[10] – and, if infected and untreated they may be at risk of complications. It is for this reason that post-exposure prophylaxis should be considered in individuals who attend within 2 weeks of the assault. This is particularly so in the case of individuals who de-cline further physical examination. When the insertion of an intra-uterine contraceptive device is required for emergency contraception, prophylaxis should also be given. Box 4.1 indicates the recommended regimen[11].

The question as to whether or not to offer post-exposure prophylaxis against HIV infection has not been fully answered. Although the *overall* probability of HIV transmission from a single episode of sexual assault is probably low, the risk of infection will depend on

1. the prevalence of HIV infection in the population of which the assailant is a part
2. the type of assault – vaginal, oral or anal – and whether this was associated with trauma, including bleeding
3. the presence of another STI in the assailant or survivor[11].

Although post-exposure prophylaxis with zidovudine has been shown to be effective in reducing the risk of HIV infection amongst health-care workers who have sustained a needle-stick injury from an HIV-infected patient (Chapter 7), the efficacy of prophylaxis following sexual exposure remains unknown. However, if there is a clear history of exposure to an assailant known to be HIV infected or at

---

Box 4.1 Post-exposure prophylaxis against gonococcal, chlamydial, and trichomonal infection in victims of sexual assault (Centers for Disease Control and Prevention 2002[11])

Ceftriaxone 125 mg as a single intramuscular injection

plus

Azithromycin 1 g as a single oral dose, or, doxycycline 100 mg every 12 hours by mouth for 7 days

plus

Metronidazole 2 g as a single oral dose

Table 4.5 Treatment regimens for post-exposure prophylaxis after sexual assault of adults (adapted from Centers for Disease Control and Prevention 2002[11])

Drug	Dosage (all drugs given orally)
Zidovudine	300 mg every 12 hours, or 200 mg every 8 hours for 28 days
and	
Lamuvudine	150 mg every 12 hours for 28 days
or	
Didanosine	400 mg once daily for 28 days
and	
Stavudine	40 mg every 12 hours for 28 days
If the assailant is known to be infected with HIV resistant to non-nucleoside reverse transcriptase inhibitors, consider adding	
Nelfinavir	1250 mg every 12 hours for 28 days
or	
Indinavir	800 mg every 8 hours for 28 days

NB Non-nucleoside reverse transcriptase inhibitors may have a role in post-exposure prophylaxis. Nevirapine, however, has been associated with severe hepatitis, and its routine use in post-exposure prophylaxis cannot be recommended.

Box 4.2 Impact scale. Each item on the impact score is rated from 'not at all' (0 points), to 'rarely' (1 point), 'sometimes' (3 points) and 'often' (5 points). The intrusion and avoidance items are treated separately and scores of around 17/35 (intrusions) and 20/40 (avoidance) indicate referral to a clinical psychologist.

Date: Clinic no:

Please indicate how often these comments are true for you:
e.g. not at all/rarely/sometimes/often

(1) I think about it when I don't mean to
(2) I avoid letting myself get upset when I think about it or am reminded of it
(3) I try to remove it from memory
(4) I have trouble falling asleep or staying asleep because of pictures or thoughts about it that come into my mind
(5) I have waves of strong feelings about it
(6) I have dreams about it
(7) I stay away from reminders of it
(8) I feel as if it hadn't happened or it wasn't real
(9) I try not to talk about it
(10) Pictures about it pop into my mind
(11) Other things keep making me think about it
(12) I am aware that I still have a lot of feelings about it, but don't deal with them
(13) I try not to think about it
(14) Any reminder brings back feelings about it
(15) My feelings about it are kind of numb

Intrusion subset = 1, 4, 5, 6, 10, 11, 14; avoidance subset = 2, 3, 7, 8, 9, 12, 13, 15

high risk of being infected, antiretroviral therapy should be offered. Treatment should be initiated as soon as possible, and not later than 72 hours, after the assault[12]. The survivor should be counseled about the uncertainties regarding efficacy of post-exposure prophylaxis and the toxicities of the drugs used. In the management of women who opt for prophylaxis (see Table 4.5 for currently recommended regimens), it is important to emphasize the importance of adhering to the therapy, and that close follow-up with anti-HIV testing at 6 weeks, 12 weeks and 6 months after the assault, is necessary.

Psychological support is necessary and health advisers within the clinic usually undertake this. More expert help, however, may be required and Harrison and Murphy[13] have developed a protocol for the identification of individuals in need of referral to a clinical psychologist (see Boxes 4.2 and 4.3).

MEN

The principles of management are similar to those for female victims of assault.

Management of sexual assault or abuse of children

Genitourinary physicians may be called upon to investigate a child for the presence of an STI. A purpose of the examination is to obtain evidence of an infection that is likely to have been sexually transmitted[11]. In the post-neonatal period, the presence of certain STIs such as gonorrhea, *Chlamydia trachomatis* infection and trichomoniasis are considered to be evidence of probable sexual abuse. Infection of children with individual agents, and their likelihood of acquisition as a result of sexual abuse, is considered in the relevant chapters of this textbook.

The child may have symptoms or signs suggestive of an STI, or he/she may be referred for diagnosis or exclusion of an STI following actual or suspected sexual abuse. Investigation of the latter cases is particularly important when the assailant has, or is suspected of having, an STI, or when the prevalence of infection in the community is high. Occasionally, a child may be brought for investigation after the discovery of an infection in a sibling.

Unless the physician is trained in the interpretation of signs of child sexual abuse, an experienced pediatrician or police surgeon should manage this aspect of the evaluation of a child. As it is important to avoid subjecting the child to undue psychological and physical trauma, it is preferable to hold a single medical consultation in which a genitourinary physician, police surgeon, and a pediatrician participate. If the abuse has occurred over a prolonged period, a single examination is usually sufficient. If the abuse is more recent, however, a further examination for STIs should be undertaken about 14 days after the most recent sexual exposure. This allows the organism to develop to a sufficient concentration to give positive test results[11].

The following sections outline the investigations for STIs that have been used successfully by the authors in most cases of suspected child sexual abuse.

IN BOTH SEXES

Inspect the mouth and pharynx for ulceration or condylomatous lesions. A cotton wool-tipped applicator stick should then be passed over the pharynx and both tonsils or tonsillar beds, and plated directly on medium selective for the gonococcus (attempted isolation of *C. trachomatis* from the pharynx is *not* recommended because

- the isolation rate is low
- the organism can be acquired perinatally and persist for an undefined period (Chapter 10)
- some laboratories may lack the facilities to differentiate *C. trachomatis* from *C. pneumoniae* isolates[11]).

IN GIRLS

1. In girls inspect the labia and introitus for erythema, ulceration, and condylomata, and note any vaginal discharge. Examine the perineum and perianal area for similar signs.
2. An endourethral swab is gently passed into the vagina, withdrawn, and a smear is prepared on a microscope slide

Box 4.3

All women take time to deal with an assault. I would like to take some time to talk about how you are at the moment, because it is important to recognize what the main issues are for you. Then if necessary we can offer you further help. Of course people react very differently, but there are some experiences that many women share after an assault. Perhaps we could start with talking about how you are with other people.

(1 **Behavior**
Extent of acknowledgment, support available?

Have you been able to tell anyone?
Yes/No comments:

(2) **Feelings**

Changes in intimacy, feelings of isolation?

Do you feel any closer or less close to family or friends?
Is there anyone you anticipate will be or has been unsupportive?
Yes/No comments:

(3) **Behavior**

Restriction because of fear, depression, lack of trust?

Has there been any change in your work or social life? (Have there been any other changes in your work/social life?)
Yes/No comments:

(4) **Behavior**

Social withdrawal, unable to trust self/others, low self-esteem?

Has there been any change in the way you get to know new people? e.g. 'Are you any more trusting or less trusting than before?'
Yes/No comments:

(5) **Behavior**

Any unreasonable avoidance?

If any difficulty is expressed, elicit the context, e.g. 'Are you able to go out alone at night?'
Yes/No comments:

(6) **Feelings**
Lack of trust, reduced sense of safety or control?

Do you think your feelings about men in general have changed?
Yes/No comments:

(7) **Behavior**

Behavioral example of above

When was the last time you felt comfortable with a man socially? or at work?
Comments:

(8) **Behavior**

Loss of desire, lack of enjoyment?

Has there been any change for the better or worse in your sexual relationships?
Yes/No comments:

(9) **Feelings**
Dislike of body, feelings of looking like a 'target'?

Has there been any change in how you feel about your appearance?
Yes/No comments:

(10) **Feelings**

Low self-esteem, avoidance of interaction?

Do you ever feel like you don't want to be noticed or wish you could disappear?
Yes/No comments:

(11) **Other**
Note degree of insight, avoidance.

Is there anything else that has changed for you since it happened?
Yes/No comments:

If the score is 4 or more, suggest referral for ways of coping with these.

---

for subsequent Gram-staining. The swab is then used to inoculate selective medium for culture of *Neisseria gonorrhoeae*. It is imperative that any presumptive isolate of *N. gonorrhoeae* is identified correctly (Chapter 11). Molecular characterization of the isolate may be helpful in suggesting or eliminating a possible source of infection (Chapter 11). The Gram-stained smear and the isolate should be preserved.

3. Another endourethral swab is passed, withdrawn, and used to inoculate transport medium for subsequent culture of *C. trachomatis* (Chapter 10). The isolate should be confirmed by the microscopic identification of the inclusions by direct immunofluorescence, using a monoclonal antibody specific for *C. trachomatis*. Isolates should be preserved. Currently in the UK and in many other countries, only the isolation of *C. trachomatis* is accepted as legal proof of infection. However, it is likely that nucleic acid amplification tests with confirmation using a second test based on a different diagnostic principle[11] will supersede these methods.

4. Another swab is used to make a saline mount preparation for microscopical examination for *Trichomonas vaginalis* and 'clue cells' suggesting a diagnosis of bacterial vaginosis. A Gram-stained smear should also be prepared and examined for clue cells (Chapter 17). When facilities are available, culture for trichomonads should also be attempted (Chapter 17).

5. Material for culture for *N. gonorrhoeae* should also be taken from the anal canal. A cotton wool-tipped applicator stick is gently inserted into the anal

canal to a distance of about 2.5 cm, withdrawn, and used to inoculate culture or transport medium. Another swab is used to inoculate transport medium for the attempted culture for *C. trachomatis*.

IN BOYS

1. Inspect the shaft of the penis, prepuce if present, urethral meatus and scrotum.

2. When there is a urethral discharge, a sample is taken from the urethral meatus using a disposable plastic inoculating loop. This specimen is said to be an adequate substitute for an endourethral swab[11]. When there is a urethral discharge, an endourethral specimen, obtained with an endourethral swab should be taken for culture for *C. trachomatis*. As limited data suggest that the prevalence of asymptomatic infection with *C. trachomatis* in prepubertal boys is low, testing by culture of asymptomatic boys is not justifiable[11].

3. Examine the perineum and perianal area for lesions such as condylomata, and obtain anorectal specimens for culture for *N. gonorrhoeae* and for *C. trachomatis*, as described above.

SEROLOGICAL TESTING

Serological tests for syphilis (Chapter 15) and hepatitis B (Chapter 8) should be undertaken on a blood sample collected at the time of presentation, and about 12 weeks after the most recent sexual exposure. Serological testing for HIV infection should be *considered* in all sexually abused children, but a final decision on whether to undertake the test should be made on the likelihood of infection in the assailant(s). In all cases, a sample of serum should be reserved in case further tests are needed. When the clinical investigations are completed they should be signed by the examining doctor giving the date and time of examination and witnessed by a qualified nurse or doctor.

PROPHYLAXIS AGAINST STIs

Because of the low risk of complications of gonococcal and chlamydial infection in prepubertal children, presumptive treatment before the results of laboratory tests are available is generally not indicated. The concerns of parents or guardians may influence the decision on whether or not to give such treatment. There may be pressure on the physician to give prophylactic treatment for bacterial and trichomonal infec-

tion if the prevalence of that infection in the community is high, and this should only be prescribed after the collection of the appropriate specimens for microbiological examination.

In all cases of child sexual abuse, psychological support is necessary, and the child should be referred to a health care professional skilled in this field.

Post-exposure prophylaxis against HIV infection in the child who has been sexually abused should be considered if the assailant(s) is (are) at high risk of HIV infection. Data on efficacy of such prophylaxis are lacking, but when the child presents within 48 to 72 hours of exposure to an individual whose behavior is believed to have placed him at increased risk of HIV infection, prophylaxis is probably justified. The toxicity of antiretroviral drugs in children seems to be low. Zidovudine, given in an oral dose of 160 mg/m^2 every 4 hours, with lamivudine, given orally in a dose of 4 mg/kg every 12 hours, both drugs being administered for 28 days, has been recommended by the Centers for Disease Control and Prevention[11]. If an assailant is known to be infected with HIV strains resistant to the nucleoside reverse transcriptase inhibitors, nelfinavir should be added to this regimen.

References

1 De Bono E. *Conflicts, a Better Way to Resolve Them*. London; Harrap: 1985, pp. 39–41 and throughout book.

2 Goffman E. *Stigma: Notes on the management of spoiled identity*. Prentice-Hall, New Jersey, and Penguin Books, Harmondsworth: 1963, pp. 28, 160, 175, 189, 193.

3 Bignell CJ. Chaperones for genital examination. *Br Med J* 1999; **319**: 137–138.

4 Royal College of Obstetricians and Gynaecologists. *Intimate Examinations: Report of a Working Party*. London; RCOG: 1997.

5 DeLahunta EA, Baram DA. Sexual assault. *Clin Obstet Gynecol* 1997; **40**: 648–660.

6 Bottomley CPEH, Sadler T, Welch J. Integrated clinical service for sexual

assault victims in a genitourinary setting. *Sex Transm Infect* 1999; **75**: 116–119.

7 Clinical Effectiveness Group (Association of Genitourinary Medicine and the Medical Society for the Study of Venereal Diseases). National guideline for the management of adult victims of sexual assault. *Sex Transm Infect* 1999; **75** (Suppl. 1): S82–S84.

8 Galsier A, Gebbie A (eds) *Handbook of Family Planning and Reproductive Heathcare* 4th edition. Edinburgh; Churchill Livingstone: 2000.

9 Crowe G, Forster GE, Dinsmore WW, Maw RO. A case of acute hepatitis B occurring four months after multiple rape. *Int J STD AIDS* 1996; **7**: 133–134.

10 Jenny C, Hooton TM, Bowers A, *et al.* Sexually transmitted diseases in victims of rape. *N Engl J Med* 1990; **322**: 713–716.

11 Centers for Disease Control and Prevention. 2002 Guidelines for treatment of sexually transmitted diseases. *MMWR* 2002; **51**: RR-6.

12 Bamberger JD, Waldo CR, Gerberding JL, Katz MH. Postexposure prophylaxis for human immunodeficiency virus (HIV) infection following sexual assault. *Am J Med* 1999; **106**: 323–326.

13 Harrison JM, Murphy SM. A care package for managing female sexual assault in genitourinary medicine. *Int J STD AIDS* 1999; **10**: 283–289.

14 National Clinical Guideline for investigation of aymptomatic proteinuria in adults. Scottish Intercollegiate Guidelines Network 1997.

15 Blacklock NJ. Bladder trauma in the long-distance runner: '10,000 metres haematuria'. *Br J Urol* 1977; **49**: 129–132.

16 Fairley KF, Birch DF. Haematuria – a simple method for identifying glomerular bleeding. *Kidney Int* 1982; **21**: 105–108.

17 Iseghem Ph Van, Hauglustaine D, Bollens W, Michielsen P. Urinary erythrocyte morphology in acute glomerulonephritis. *Br Med J* 1983; **287**: 1183.

18 Shichiri M, Oowada A, Nishio Y, Tomita K, Shiigai T. Use of autoanalyser to examine urinary-red-cell morphology in the diagnosis of glomerular haematuria. *Lancet* 1986; **ii**: 781–782.

19 Leading Article. Removing the guesswork from diagnosis in ectopic pregnancy. *Lancet* 1980; **i**: 188.

APPENDIX 4.1: *Proteinuria*

The urine 'stick' test (e.g. the multiple reagent strips, Multistix, Ames, Stoke Poges, UK) is good for screening for proteinuria. The strip is impregnated with tetra-bromphenol blue and buffered at pH 3.5. Based on the 'protein error of indicators' principle, the presence of protein results in the development of a green color. The test yields negative results with normal urine, so any positive result greater than 'trace' indicates significant proteinuria. Clinical judgment is necessary in the interpretation of trace results which may occur in urines of high specific gravity with non-significant proteinuria. The 'trace' result corresponds to 0.05 to 0.2 g/L albumin, but the test is less sensitive to globulin, Bence-Jones protein and microproteins, so that a negative result does not rule out the presence of these proteins. False positive results may occur with alkaline, highly buffered urine, or in the presence of contaminating quaternary ammonium compounds. Contamination of the urine sample with chlorhexidine antiseptic will give a false positive reading for protein (manufacturer's data).

Although the rate of protein excretion rather than the urinary concentration is more relevant in determining pathological states, and the sensitivity of the stick test depends upon the rate of urinary flow, the discovery of a positive result greater than trace necessitates referral for fuller renal investigation. A National Clinical Guideline for the investigation of asymptomatic proteinuria in adults has been produced by the Scottish Intercollegiate Guidelines Network[14], and the following recommendations are based on this report. When proteinuria (+) is found on dipstick testing, the test should be repeated on two morning urine samples, taken a week apart. Orthostatic proteinuria should be excluded by testing the first sample of urine passed after an overnight rest: this sample will yield negative results despite positive tests during the day. Functional proteinuria may occur in, for example, febrile states, and will remit with the resolution of the underlying disorder. Persistent proteinuria needs confirmation, for example, by estimation of the protein in a 24-hour collection. Referral to a nephrologist is necessary if

- the protein concentration is greater than 500 mg/L or the protein:creatinine ratio is greater than 30 mg/mmol, or
- the protein concentration is greater than 250 mg/L or the protein:creatinine ratio is greater than 20 mg/mmol with co-existent raised serum creatinine or hypertension.

Referral is also necessary if there is co-existent hematuria. Before referral, however, urinary tract infection should be excluded.

APPENDIX 4.2: *Asymptomatic microscopic hematuria*

Urine 'stick' tests (e.g. the multiple reagent strips, Multistix, Ames, Stoke Poges, UK) for detecting the presence of blood in the urine are very sensitive, they detect 150–620 μg/L free hemoglobin (or 5–20 $\times$ 10^6 intact red blood cells per liter) in urines with a specific gravity of 1005 and ascorbic acid concentrations of less than 0.28 mmol/L. They are less sensitive in urines with higher specific gravity or greater ascorbic acid content. The test is slightly more sensitive to free hemoglobin and myoglobin than to intact red cells. The appearance of green spots on the reacted reagent used indicates the presence of intact red cells in the urine. Certain oxidizing contaminants, such as betadine lotion, hypochlorite, and microbial peroxidase associated with urinary tract infection, may cause false positive results. Blood is often, but not always, found in the urine of menstruating females.

The test is based on the peroxidase-like activity of hemoglobin which catalyzes the reaction of cumene hydroperoxide and 3, 3', 5, 5'-tetramethylbenzidine. The resulting color ranges from orange through green to dark blue. When using the stick test, all reagent areas on plastic strips should be immersed in a freshly voided, well-mixed, uncentrifuged urine specimen collected in a clean container. If testing is not possible within 1 hour after voiding, the urine should be refrigerated and returned to room temperature before testing. After immersion the edge of the strip should be tapped against the side of the container to remove excess urine and afterwards the strip should be held horizontally to prevent possible mixing of chemicals from adjacent reagent areas and soiling of the hands. The test areas should then be compared with corresponding color charts on the bottle label at the reading times specified for each area. The strip should be held close to the color blocks and the colors matched carefully. *Accurate timing is essential for reliable quantitative results.* All reagent areas may be read between 1 and 2 minutes for qualitative results. The reagent strips should be stored at temperatures under 30°C only in the original bottles containing the desiccant which should not be removed (manufacturer's data, Ames Division, Miles Laboratories Ltd, Stoke Poges, Slough, SL2 4LY, England).

Microscopy of centrifuged urine sediment will reveal some red cells in all specimens of urine and this reflects the small but continuous loss of blood from the urinary tract (namely less than 0.5×10^6 red blood cells per liter). In many laboratories it is usual to express hematuria as the number of cells seen per high power field (HPF) but the HPF covers a variable volume of urine and this method fails to reveal half of the cases of microscopic hematuria in patients with known renal disease. To obtain accurate results the urine should be centrifuged in tubes with pointed bottoms, the sediment re-suspended in a known volume of fluid and the cells counted in a counting chamber.

With respect to the stick test, any positive result is indicative of microscopic hematuria well above the suggested normal count. Occasionally the blood will be a contaminant from the vagina, hyperplastic intrameatal warts, or in some cases in urethritis. Although in patients under the age of 40 years only 2% of those with asymptomatic microscopic hematuria will have a lesion that is life threatening or requires major surgery, full investigation is essential.

Preliminaries will have included examination of the urethral meatus and of any urethral discharge. Tests will have been taken to exclude *Neisseria gonorrhoeae* and *Chlamydia trachomatis*. Inspection of the urine microscopically for white cells and culture of a clean-catch specimen of urine are necessary at this stage. Proteinuria, red cell casts and renal impairment indicate renal disease and a referral to a nephrologist for further investigation should be made. In other cases, a full clinical examination should follow and include taking the blood pressure. For the patient under the age of 40 years the following conditions will be considered.

Bacteriuria

Bacteriuria in a young man is an indication for referral to a urologist for a full investigation including radiological imaging of the urinary tract and cystoscopy. In a young woman with hematuria, signs and symptoms of cystitis, and a positive urine culture, treatment should be given for the cystitis and, if on follow-up urinalysis is normal, no further investigation is needed. Evaluation will be needed should the hematuria persist after antibiotic or chemotherapy.

Exercise-related hematuria

A specific syndrome known as '10 000 meter hematuria' has been described by Blacklock[15] in the long-distance runner who runs over distances of 10^5 meters or longer. It occurs at the first voiding of urine after completion of the run and is typically profuse, sometimes with the passage of clots. Usually painless, there is sometimes suprapubic discomfort with some reference of pain to the tip of the penis. Cystoscopy within 48 hours reveals localized contusions with loss of epithelium and fibrinous exudate on the interureteric bar with extension laterally overlying the intramural ureter on each side. The posterior rim of the internal meatus has shown similar changes. The 'mirror image' lesions seen suggest that repetitive impact, minor in itself, produces the injury during a long run and it has been postulated that if there is sufficient urine within the bladder its cushioning effect prevents the apposition of the posterior bladder wall and the trigone. The lesion is superficial and theoretically could be preventable by the intake of fluid before running or the omission of bladder emptying before each run commences. Neither recommendation is easily acceptable by the dedicated athlete for fear of interfering with running performance[15].

In sports, including those involving minimal trauma (e.g. swimming, lacrosse, track-running, football, and rowing) hematuria is directly related to the duration of exercise and the energy consumed. During exercise blood is shunted from the splanchnic area and other organs including the kidneys, and reduction in blood flow in these areas may lead to hypoxia. This exercise-related hematuria appears to be

a frequent (9 of 50 marathon runners tested), self-limiting and benign condition and patients should be spared invasive testing unless its occurrence persists beyond 48 to 72 hours. Hemoglobinuria occurs with prolonged trauma to the feet or hands in susceptible individuals. There is a raised serum hemoglobin, lowered serum haptoglobin and methemalbuminemia. If the hemolysis is sufficient to exceed the hemoglobin-binding capacity of the haptoglobins hemoglobinuria results. This 'march' hemoglobinuria may be prevented by wearing thick-soled shoes.

Schistosomiasis

Hematuria, often at the end of micturition, is a characteristic early feature of infection with *Schistosoma haematobium*. The principal means of diagnosing all human schistosome infections remains the detection of ova in urine and feces. In *Schistosoma mansoni* infection diagnosis is reached by demonstrating the ova in the stool, but intestinal biopsy through a proctoscope or sigmoidoscope is also an effective means of finding eggs; such biopsy may also be positive in *S. haemotobium* or *S. japonicum* infections. In *S. japonicum* infection eggs are more commonly deposited in ectopic sites than those of other schistosome species.

Immunological methods are available and the circumoval precipitation technique (COPT) remains popular. Competitive micro-enzyme linked immunosorbent assay (micro-ELISA) and radioimmunoassay (RIA) are additional techniques available.

Hemoglobinopathies

Unexplained hematuria in West Africans may be associated with hemoglobin SC disease, detected readily in the laboratory by starch gel electrophoresis of hemoglobin.

MORPHOLOGY OF ERYTHROCYTES IN HEMATURIA
Glomerulonephritis

Although patients with proteinuria and accompanying hematuria – discovered by the stick test – are likely to be investigated for glomerular disease, those with hematuria and normal urinary protein may be subjected to extensive urological investigations when a more appropriate line of investigation would be renal function testing and renal biopsy.

The morphology of red cells found in the hematuria due to glomerular injury differs from that of non-glomerular bleeding. Damage to the erythrocytes in glomerular disease may be caused by a distortion during passage through the glomerular basement membrane or, more likely, by osmotic changes in the distal nephron. Red cells in urine in non-glomerular diseases (NG) have normal erythrocyte morphology, whereas those in glomerular disease (G) are markedly dysmorphic. The dysmorphism ranges widely

- red cells may show extruded phase-dense blobs of cytoplasm
- there may be granular deposits of phase-dense material around the inner aspect of the cell membrane, or
- red cells may have the appearance of 'doughnut cells' with cytoplasm extrusions[16].

Morphological changes can be seen by phase-contrast microscopy, but staining techniques have been advised as useful simpler routine procedures.

The site of urinary bleeding has been predicted in 85% of patients for whom a definite diagnosis was possible, in 11% hematuria was mixed, and an incorrect assessment of the site of bleeding was made in only 4%. The assessment of urinary red-cell morphology by means of phase-contrast microscopy can add importantly to clinical information and, together with the presence of red-cell casts and protein in the urine, can help the clinician decide on initial investigations in patients with hematuria. In patients presenting with gross hematuria, changes in red-cell morphology may not be clear cut and repeated examination of the urinary sediment may be necessary to avoid unnecessary urological investigations[17]. Examination of urinary casts for immunoglobulins, complement, and fibrin provides a further non-invasive method for distinguishing patients with active glomerular disease[16].

The phase-contrast microscopy required for determining red-cell morphology in urine requires individual skill and experience, and as a result is not easy to set up as a service. It has been shown that a urinary-cell-size distribution curve can be obtained with speed and clarity with the use of an autoanalyzer. In this procedure about 10 mL of urine (from a midstream urine sample) is centrifuged at 600 g for 5 minutes. The supernatant is removed and the re-suspended deposit analyzed by means of the autoanalyzer with the X–Y recorder attachment. Large differences in size distribution are seen in glomerular and non-glomerular cells. Patients with glomerular-cell-size distribution can be spared needless urological examinations and can be directly referred to a renal physician for consultation about renal biopsy. Those with a non-glomerular distribution can be referred for the essential urological investigations[18].

Calculi, congenital anomalies, tumor, damage to renal papillae

In patients with hematuria apart from

- individuals with proven glomerulonephritis
- females with proven cystitis
- young patients with hematuria that is clearly exercise-related

radiological imaging of the urinary tract is mandatory. The finding of a congenital anomaly or stone necessitates referral since surgical judgment is required regarding further investigation and management. Retrograde ureteropyelogram will enable delineation of a filling defect in the renal pelvis or ureter, whether due to tumor, blood clot, sloughed renal papilla, or non-opaque stone, and a cystoscopy will enable a coexistent bladder lesion to be excluded. Ultrasound, arteriograms and computed axial tomography (CAT) scanning are other techniques available to the urological surgeon.

APPENDIX 4.3: Pregnancy tests

Pregnancy tests are sometimes required to confirm immediately whether or not an individual is pregnant, this is done by measuring chorionic gonadotropin. Early diagnosis makes it easier to secure the social and medical support required in antenatal care. If the test is positive the pregnancy may be terminated for social or therapeutic reasons, and the earlier in the pregnancy this is done the less danger there is to the woman. Urine tests, normally an immunological test, are used.

Immunological tests for pregnancy react positively when chorionic gonadotropin (hCG) is present in the urine. A positive result indicates the secretory activity of trophoblastic tissue usually associated with the presence of a viable fetus. There is a close parallel between trophoblastic mass and hCG levels in the maternal serum which double every 36 to 48 hours during early pregnancy. Chorionic gonadotropin is produced before the missed but expected menstrual period in increasing amounts until a peak is reached about 8 weeks after conception. There is a dramatic fall after this peak but the hormone is excreted throughout normal pregnancy and into the post-partum period. Most immunological tests on urine do not distinguish between pituitary luteinizing hormone (LH) and hCG, but results of these tests are correctly positive in the absence of a fetus when a hydatidiform mole, chorioadenoma or choriocarcinoma is present. Similarly, urine from men with testicular tumors containing trophoblastic tissue will evoke a positive reaction. To exclude pregnancy as a cause of secondary amenorrhea, particularly in women approaching the menopause, quantitative determination of whole hCG and free beta-subunit in serum should be used, since such women may excrete enough LH to produce a false positive result with the latex agglutination test whereas such cross reaction does not occur with the former test. In a disturbed or ectopic pregnancy the results of the tests may either be positive or negative, indicating the secretory activity of the trophoblast and not necessarily the viability of the fetus.

Whereas a latex agglutination test in urine gives a positive result in only 50% of ectopic pregnancies, the hCG beta-subunit radioimmune assay is positive in 95% of such patients[19]. Although referral to a gynecologist is indicated when ectopic pregnancy is being considered as a possibility, the hCG measurement is a useful initial step to rule out the non-pregnant patient namely when hCG levels are lower than 6000 mIU/mL.

Many clinics use an immunoassay for hCG that yields results within 3 minutes (QuickVue, hCG urine test, QUIDEL Corporation, 10165 McKellar Court, San Diego, CA, USA). Urine specimens containing hCG concentrations as low as 25 mIU/mL will yield positive results. Often, a hCG level of 25 mIU/mL can be detected as early as 2 to 3 days before the expected menses. By the first day of the missed menses, concentrations often exceed 100 mIU/mL (manufacturer's data).

Section 2
Viral infections

Chapter 5

Human papillomavirus infection
A McMillan, M M Ogilvie

Not only are genital warts caused by human papillomavirus (HPV) unsightly, but their persistence and inconstant response to treatment cause anxiety and introspection in the patient, and give the patient the burden of multiple clinic attendances. Their high prevalence, high infectivity, long pre-patent period (average 3 months, range 2 weeks to many months), and often poor response to treatment all make effective control by therapy and contact tracing possible only to a limited extent. Until relatively recently genital warts had been regarded virtually as wholly benign growths that regress spontaneously. However, human papillomaviruses are not solely causes of benign tumors of skin and mucosa, in the longer term, and possibly in association with factors such as cigarette smoking, some types of HPV are recognized as the causative agents in the development of cancer, particularly of the cervix uteri.

Virology

Human papillomavirus (HPV) or, in colloquial terms, the wart virus, is one genus of a group of double-stranded DNA viruses now designated as an independent family, Papillomaviruses. Previously classified as two subfamilies of Papova viruses (pa = papilloma; po = polyoma; va = vacuolating agent), Papillomaviruses are separated from Polyomaviruses on the basis of size of their icosahedral capsid (45 nm average for polyomavirus, 55 nm on average for papillomavirus), genome length, gene organisation and other features. Examination of genital warts (condylomata acuminata) and common skin warts (verrucae vulgares) showed that both types of lesions contain morphologically identical virus particles (although much reduced in genital lesions) but with the methods using immune electron microscopy it was clear that the viruses were antigenically distinct.

Since papillomaviruses cannot be easily propagated *in vitro*, progress in research has, until recent years, been difficult and unrewarding. The quantities of virus in the lesions were so low that their characterization directly from such material was not possible. The extraction of virus DNA from warts and its molecular cloning has now enabled the preparation of quantities sufficient to develop methods for the classification of the papillomaviruses from a variety of lesions in a variety of anatomical sites. Papillomavirus DNA is a double-stranded circular molecule which can now be identified in minute traces, as little as one copy per cell, in human tissues. Not only can it be detected but the DNA can be ascribed to a specific type or subtype even when the presence of virus is undetectable by electron microscopy or existing immunoassays.

Classification of HPV into separate types was initially based on nucleic acid hybridization studies: a virus was considered to be a separate HPV type if such DNA studies revealed less than 50% homology with known virus types. Subtypes were those that showed more than 50% cross hybridization but differed in their restriction endonuclease cleavage patterns. This definition of a papillomavirus type, however, was changed in 1991: for an isolate to be recognized as a new type the entire genome had to be cloned and the nucleotide sequences of its major capsid protein gene (L1) open reading frame had to share less than 90% identity with the homologous sequences of other papillomaviruses[1].

On the basis of these nucleic acid studies, more than 100 types of HPV have been reported. Table 5.1 indicates the associations of some of these types with human lesions, however it is not intended to be an exhaustive list of associations. Four of the most common HPV types that infect the genital tract are HPV-6, HPV-11, HPV-16, and HPV-18. The first two types are found in the exophytic lesions of the external genitalia, vagina, uterine cervix, and anus, and, as they are not associated with cervical cancer, are designated 'low-risk' types. HPV types 42, 43, and 44 that are also found occasionally in the genital tract are also considered 'low-risk' types. Types 16 and 18, however, are frequently detected in anogenital cancers, and are classified as 'high-risk' types. Other, less common, HPV types, 31, 33, 35, 39, 45, 55, 56, 58, 59, 66, and 68, are also considered 'high-risk' types[2].

Although propagation of HPV in cultures of cell lines is impossible at present, the organotypic or raft culture system has been used to study viral replication and HPV-cell interactions[3]. In this system the *in vivo* physiology of the epidermis is mimicked by raising cells to a liquid–air interface. The dermal equivalent of the skin is provided by a collagen matrix with fibroblasts (plug). After seeding epidermal cells on top of this lattice to form a monolayer, the plug is placed on a metal grid supported over liquid medium so that only the bottom of the grid comes in contact with

Table 5.1 Human papillomavirus types in some human lesions

Lesion	Associated HPV types	
	Common	Less common
Skin warts		
Common or mosaic warts	2, 27	1, 4, 7, 26, 28, 29, 57, 60, 65
Plantar warts	1	2, 4, 63
Flat warts	3, 10	2, 26, 27, 28, 29, 41, 49
Anogenital lesions		
Condylomata acuminata	6, 11	16, 30, 40, 41, 42–44, 54, 55
Squamous intraepithelial lesions of cervix, vagina, vulva, penis, anus	6, 11, 16, 18, 31	30, 33, 34, 35, 56–59, 61, 62, 64, 67–70
Carcinomas	16, 18, 31, 45	33, 35, 39, 51, 52, 54, 56, 66, 68
Head and neck lesions		
Oral papillomata	2, 6, 11, 16	
Focal epithelial hyperplasia	13, 32	
Laryngeal papillomata	6, 11	30
Carcinomas		6, 11, 16, 18, 33, 57

the medium. Over the following 2 to 3 weeks, the epidermal cells stratify and differentiate. Human foreskin keratinocytes transfected with HPV have been extensively studied in this system.

The nude mouse xenograft system has also given invaluable information on the patterns of viral transcription and replication[4]. In this system, developed by Kreider and colleagues[5], fragments of human neonatal foreskin were incubated with an extract from a condyloma containing HPV-11, and then grafted under the renal capsule of nude mice. Condylomatous cysts developed, from which virions could be extracted and used to initiate new cycles of cyst formation. It has not been possible, however, to make a tissue extract containing a high-risk HPV type that could initiate infection in this model, nor to achieve virus production in nude mice using keratinocytes into which HPV DNA sequences have been introduced[6]. The system is therefore restricted to a single isolate of HPV-11.

The use of virus-like particles (VLPs) has given much valuable information on early events in HPV infection. In the absence of other viral proteins, the major capsid protein of papillomaviruses assembles into VLPs that are indistinguishable from virions. L1 alone from all papillomavirus types assembles into capsid-like structures when expressed at sufficiently high levels in eukaryotic cells[7]. Unlike virions, however, VLPs can easily be generated in a variety of eukaryotic expression systems, and they have been used to examine the humoral immune response to HPV infection. For this purpose capsids purified from lysed cells are used mainly in enzyme immunoassays.

The papillomavirus virion (Figure 5.1) is 55 nm in diameter and the capsid, which has an icosahedral symmetry, is made up of 72 individual capsomeres, composed principally of L1 protein. The genome is double-stranded, supercoiled, circular DNA of 7.2 kilobases (kb)[8], and the organization of the genomes is well conserved between types. The genomic map of HPV-18 is shown in linear form in Figure 5.2. The open reading frames (ORFs) E6, E7, E1, E2, E4, and E5 are designated as early, and L1 and L2 as late. Between L1 and E6 is a segment (non-coding region (NCR) or long control region (LCR)) that does not contain ORFs but, nevertheless, possesses sequences required for viral replication and regulation of transcription.

VIRAL LIFE CYCLE

HPV can adhere to and enter several cell types, and it is possible that α6 integrin may act as the cell receptor[9]. The mechanisms of virus entry into the cell and its translocation to the nucleus are unknown.

Viral DNA replication and transcription of the capsid genes is closely related to the differentiated state of the cell. Although the

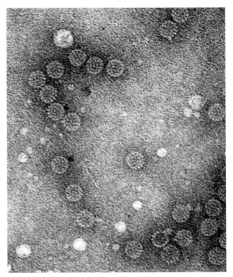

Figure 5.1 Virions of human papillomavirus (tungstophosphoric acid stain, × 100 000) (reproduced from Greenwood *et al.* 2000[223])

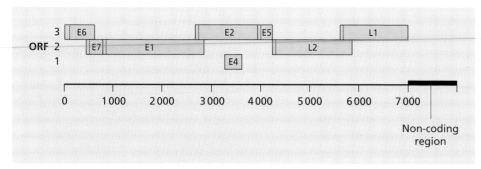

Figure 5.2 Genetic map of HPV-18 (adapted from Thierry 1996[14])

virus does not replicate in the basal cells of the epithelium, expression of E1 and E2 occurs here to maintain the viral genome as an episome. In the parabasal cells, there is transcription of E6 and E7 to permit subsequent HPV DNA replication. In HPV-infected cells, the major viral transcript encoding the first few codons of E1 fused to the E4 ORF appear to be the major transcript, encoding the viral protein, E1^E4. The E1^E4 promoter is used for the transcription of the late gene products, L1 and L2. E1^E4 and the capsid proteins are only expressed in the most differentiated layers of the epithelium.

Productive replication to generate virus progeny takes place in the more differentiated epithelial cells. The origin of replication is found in the NCR in a region to which E1 binds, and an adjacent E2-binding sequence[10, 11]. E1 interacts with the cellular polymerase–primase complex[12]. After the origin-dependent initiation of replication, the cell encodes all other factors for viral replication. Release of viral particles results from desquamating cells.

HPV and carcinogenesis

Certain HPV types have been implicated in the causation of cervical and other anogenital carcinomas (see pp. 79–80). *In vitro*, transforming and immortalizing activities are displayed only by the high risk viral types such as HPV-16 and HPV-18. This activity has been localized to two early proteins, E6 and E7, that interact with host proteins whose normal role is to regulate cell proliferation[13]. Such interactions are

weaker with the low-risk HPV types such as HPV-6. Expression of E6 and E7 is necessary for keratinocyte immortalization and for the maintenance of the cancer phenotype. Cancer may be a consequence of inactivation of tumor suppressor genes, as evidenced by the association of certain malignancies with mutations in the RB and p53 genes. Inactivation of the protein products of these genes probably plays an important role in HPV-induced carcinogenesis. Before considering some possible mechanisms of this, it is necessary to have some knowledge of the role of tumor suppressor genes in the control of the normal cell cycle.

The RB gene, located on chromosome 13, encodes a nuclear protein, pRB, that interacts with the cellular transcription factor E2F in the G1 phase of the cell cycle[*], thereby inhibiting E2F-induced transcription of genes involved in proliferation and DNA replication such as cyclin A, cyclin D, *c-myc*, thymidine kinase, and DNA polymerase α. Before entry into the S phase, pRB is phosphorylated by cyclin-dependent kinases, leading to disruption of the E2F/RB complex, and to E2F-activated cell cycle progression. The p53 gene, located on chromosome 17, activates genes that maintain genomic stability. When cellular DNA is damaged, p53 gene expression is enhanced, resulting in expression of the

cellular genes: p21, GADD45 (growth arrest on DNA damage) and bax. The gene products from p21 inhibit the cyclin-dependent kinases that are needed for cell cycle progression, and also interact with proliferating cell nuclear antigen, as do the products of GADD45. These interactions with an essential cofactor for DNA replication block DNA synthesis. There is therefore arrest of the G1 phase until damaged DNA is repaired and the cell cycle can progress. Bax expression is believed to induce apoptosis.

In cervical cancers, the HPV genome is integrated into the cellular genome at random positions. Integration often leads to disruption of the genome, including E1 and E2 ORFs, but the integrated part contains conserved sub-regions of the genome, including invariably the E6 and E7 genes. The subjects of HPV transcription and HPV oncoprotein function have been reviewed by Thierry[14] and by Crook and Vousden[13].

Transcription of the viral mRNAs coding for the two transforming proteins, E6 and E7, initiates at single promoters contained in the integrated HPV-16 or HPV-18 regulatory regions: P_{97} and P_{105} respectively; these promoters can be activated by an array of cellular factors. *In vitro*, the co-expression of E6 and E7 proteins has been shown to be sufficient to immortalize human keratinocytes.

The E6 proteins complex the p53 protein, resulting in ubiquitin-dependent proteolysis of p53[†]. Although the interaction between the E6 and p53 proteins interferes with some p53 functions such as DNA binding, abrogation of p53-induced G1 arrest requires the degradation of that protein. Oligomeric p53 is important for some of the transcriptional and growth inhibitory functions of p53, but monomeric p53 retains the ability to induce apoptosis. E6 targets both oligomeric and monomeric p53, enabling E6 to inhibit apoptosis by both forms of p53. E6 protein from low-risk HPV types binds weakly to p53, and does not lead to degradation of the protein.

---

* The cell cycle is divided into four main stages: (1) the *M phase*, consisting of mitosis and cytoplasmic division, (2) the *G_1 phase* in which there is a considerable degree of biosynthesis and growth, (3) the *S phase* in which there is doubling of the cellular DNA and replication of the chromosomes, and (4) the *G_2 phase* that precedes cell division.

† Ubiquitin is a cellular basic protein that marks other proteins for degradation by binding to lysine side chains or to terminal amino groups.

Phenotypic studies have shown that the expression of high-risk E6 in normal diploid fibroblasts results in genomic instability, probably by interfering with p53 function. Low-risk E6 does not induce such changes. It has been postulated that the accumulation of genetic changes contributes to malignant progression. There is some experimental evidence that the level of E6 expression may be a critical determinant of the activity in HPV-infected cells, and, although interference with p53 function may occur in the initial stages of oncogenesis, fully malignant cells may not show this phenotype[13]. Additional functions of E6, unrelated to its interaction with p53, may contribute to carcinogenesis. The expression of E6 protein from HPV-16 has recently been shown to activate telomerase, a ribonucleoprotein complex that synthesizes telomere repeat sequences, and is linked to cell immortalization[15]. Although keratinocytes that express HPV-16 E6 have an extended life span, they are not immortal, indicating that neither telomerase activation or degradation of p53 are sufficient for their immortalization.

High-risk E7 proteins bind to pRB, and the expression of E7 proteins interferes with pRB/E2F complexes, resulting in increased levels of free, transcriptionally active E2F. E7 proteins encoded by low-risk HPV types show a much lower affinity for binding to pRB. Binding of phosphorylated E7 protein of high-risk HPV types to pRB/E2F complexes results in release of E2F which then activates the E2F-dependent genes necessary for DNA synthesis. Binding to pRB may not be the only mechanism by which high-risk E7 contributes to deregulation of the cell cycle. E7 can bind to cyclins and to cyclin-dependent kinases, thereby disturbing normal cell growth.

The E2 gene of the genital HPV types encodes a transcriptional transactivator that inhibits transcription from the E6/E7 genes. The full length E2 protein binds to E2 binding sites close to the TATA box of the promoters P_{97} (HPV-16) and P_{105} (HPV-18), possibly resulting in steric hindrance at the site of formation of the transcriptional initiation complex. Disruption or deletion of the E2 ORF may therefore result in derepression of P_{97} or P_{105} transcription and over-expression of the oncoproteins E6 and E7.

It is therefore clear that deregulation of proliferation is facilitated in cervical carcinogenesis by the interaction between E6 and E7 and the cellular proteins that regulate the cell cycle. However, immortalized human epithelial cells are not tumorigenic, but oncogenesis can be induced by carcinogens, or may develop with long-term passage in culture[16, 17]. Further progression to malignancy is the diploid to aneuploid switch, signaling the acquisition of genetic instability and increased probability of other genetic mutations that ultimately lead to malignancy[18].

Pathology

CONDYLOMATA ACUMINATA

The basal cells of all warts are intact and the stratum spinosum is hyperplastic (acanthosis) (Figure 5.3). The stratum granulosum may be many cells thick and the stratum corneum hyperkeratotic or parakeratotic. Dermal papillae are elongated but the underlying dermis may be normal. In some cases, however, marked fibrosis of the dermis is a feature (Figure 5.4)[19]. In the stratum granulosum and adjacent prickle cells, large vacuolated cells are seen, known as koilocytes, in which the nuclei are surrounded by an apparently structureless halo; the nuclei are deeply basophilic and are the site of formation of mature virus. Hyperkeratosis is not a feature of condyloma acuminatum of the genital area where the stratum corneum consists as a rule of only one or two layers of parakeratotic cells. In these warts, acanthosis combined with extensive papillomatosis

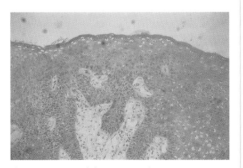

Figure 5.3 Condyloma acuminatum (hematoxylin and eosin × 60)

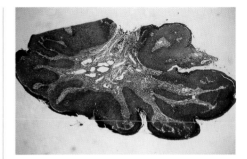

Figure 5.4 Condyloma acuminatum showing marked fibrosis of the stroma (Masson's trichrome stain × 60)

results in layers of the wart that consist entirely of sheets of hyperplastic prickle cells showing multiple mitotic figures. As the condylomata age, hyperkeratosis may develop. As a feature hyperkeratosis is more characteristic of plantar or palmar warts than plane warts. In genital condylomata acuminata wart virus particles are scanty.

SQUAMOUS INTRAEPITHELIAL LESIONS

With the advent of cervical cytology screening in the 1950s, it became clear that there was a group of cervical lesions that had some of the cytological and histological features of carcinoma-in-situ (CIS) but to a lesser degree. The term dysplasia was introduced to refer to these lesions[20]. As laboratory studies showed that all grades of dysplasia and CIS had an abnormal nuclear DNA content[21], and prospective clinical studies suggested that dysplasia and CIS constituted a histological continuum, Richart[22] introduced the term cervical intraepithelial neoplasia (CIN) to refer to this continuum. CIN I corresponded to mild dysplasia, CIN II to moderate dysplasia, and CIN III to severe dysplasia and CIS. With the recognition of the central role of HPV in the pathogenesis of cervical carcinoma, it is now evident that the CIN continuum concept of cervical cancer precursors is incorrect. The spectrum of histological changes represents two distinct entities

1. a productive HPV infection, and
2. a cancer precursor[21].

To reflect better the biological processes that underlie the histological appearances, the Bethesda System terminology[23] for cytological diagnosis uses the terms

1. low-grade squamous intraepithelial lesion (L-SIL), and
2. high-grade squamous intraepithelial lesion (H-SIL).

Many pathologists now use this system in reporting biopsy material.

Low-grade SILs previously classified as mild dysplasia, CIN I, flat condyloma, or koilocytosis, denote productive HPV infection that can be associated with a variety of different HPV types. The cell nuclei are enlarged, often angulated and hyperchromatic, and multinucleated cells may be seen. The cytoplasm is often vacuolated (these cells are termed koilocytes from the Greek word koilos, meaning empty), the koilocytes being found in the most superficial layers of the cervical epithelium. The cells comprising L-SILs have a diploid* or polyploid DNA content.

High-grade SILs are composed of proliferating, basal-type cells that have a high nuclear to cytoplasm ratio. In H-SILs the cytopathic effects associated with productive HPV infection are absent or less pronounced than in L-SIL. The lesions are usually aneuploid. H-SILs were previously referred to as moderate dysplasia, severe dysplasia, CIN II, CIN III, and CIS.

Immunology of HPV infection

CELLULAR IMMUNITY: REGRESSION OF CONDYLOMATA ACUMINATA

In the majority of immunocompetent individuals with anogenital warts, spontaneous regression eventually occurs. Biopsies of condylomata that are undergoing sponta-

---

* Haploid describes a nucleus with a single set of unpaired chromosomes (n). Diploid describes a nucleus with twice the haploid number of chromosomes (2n). A nucleus that has more than twice the number of haploid chromosomes is described as polyploid (for example 5n). An aneuploid nucleus, however, is one in which chromosomes have been added or deleted from the complete set, the total number of chromosomes not being an exact multiple of the haploid number (for example 2n–1).

---

neous regression show stromal edema and a dense sub-epithelial and epithelial infiltrate of T lymphocytes in which CD4+ cells outnumber CD8+ cells (Figures 5.5–5.9)[24, 25]. Macrophages are prominent in the stroma of regressing lesions, comprising up to 20% of the mononuclear cell population[25]. Infiltrating cells have increased expression of CD25 (the α chain of the interleukin-2 receptor) and HLA-DR. The majority of the T cells express the CD45RO isoform (memory cells), but 10–15% express the CD45RA isoform, indicating that naïve T cells are being recruited into regressing lesions. Keratinocytes in regressing warts show expression of HLA-DR and ICAM1, probably as a result of the production of cytokines such as interferon-γ (IFN-γ) and tumor necrosis factor-α (TNF-α) by infiltrating and activated CD4+ cells and macrophages. The endothelial cells in the blood vessels of the stroma show up-regulation of ICAM1, E-selectin and VCAM1, adhesion molecules that are important in lymphocyte homing to sites of inflammation. These immunohistochemical studies suggest that spontaneous regression of condylomata acuminata results from a T_{H1}-type response[‡].

---

‡ There are two types of adaptive immune responses, types 1 and 2. Type 1 responses involve the production of T_{H1}-type lymphocytes that are MHC class II restricted, CD4+ cells that secrete IFN-γ. The effector cells in this response are activated macrophages, MHC class 1 restricted CD8+ T cells, natural killer (NK) cells, and cytotoxic antibodies. Type 2 responses involve T_{H2}-type MHC class II restricted CD4+ T cells that secrete interleukin 4 (IL-4) and induce humoral immunity by helping antigen-primed B cells to differentiate and secrete non-cytotoxic antibodies[26]. Activation of tissue macrophages results in the secretion of IL-12 and TNF-α, the IL-12 inducing differentiation of naïve T cells to the T_{H1} pathway by maximizing IFN-γ production. Antigen-activated T cells express the CD40 ligand and binding of this to CD40 on the macrophage stimulates secretion of IL-12 and TNF-α. There is synergy between these cytokines and IL-2 and IL-15 secreted by T cells and macrophages respectively to induce further IFN-γ from NK cells and T cells which in turn enhances IL-12 from macrophages. There is thus macrophage activation, T cell differentiation, and amplification of NK cell activity.

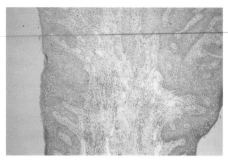

Figure 5.5 Spontaneously regressing condyloma acuminatum, showing dermal edema and mononuclear cell infiltrate of the stroma and epithelium (hematoxylin and eosin × 60)

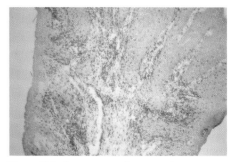

Figure 5.6 Spontaneously regressing condyloma acuminatum, showing dermal and stromal infiltration with CD3+ T lymphocytes (immunoperoxidase stain, × 60), compare with Figure 5.7

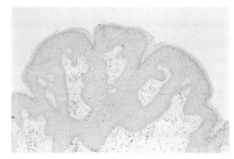

Figure 5.7 Condyloma that is not undergoing spontaneous regression, showing sparse infiltrate of stroma with CD3+ T lymphocytes (immunoperoxidase stain, × 60)

HUMORAL IMMUNITY

Animal model studies have shown that antibodies against HPV can neutralize infectious virus. In the nude mouse xenograft system, it has been shown that virus-specific neutralization of infectivity can be achieved with HPV-specific polyclonal antibody[27]. Using the same model system,

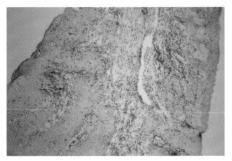

Figure 5.8 Spontaneously regressing condyloma acuminatum, showing dermal and stromal infiltration with CD4+ T lymphocytes (immunoperoxidase stain, × 60)

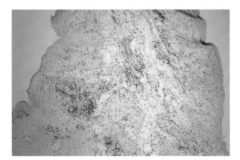

Figure 5.9 Spontaneously regressing condyloma acuminatum, showing dermal and stromal infiltration with CD8+ T lymphocytes (immunoperoxidase stain, × 60)

Christensen et al.[28] showed further that the majority of human sera, reactive against disrupted HPV-11 antigens in an enzyme immunoassay, neutralized HPV-11 infectivity. Monoclonal antibodies that neutralize infectivity have also been identified[29]. It has been shown further that these sera recognize a conformational epitope on the L1 protein[30], and that a neutralizing monoclonal antibody can prevent HPV-11 infection as late as 8 hours after addition of the virus[31]. As women with persistent infection with HPV-16 harbor the same variant over time but can become co-infected with additional variants, it is postulated that protection by neutralizing antibodies is type-specific.

In a cohort study of men and women who attended a STIs clinic in Amsterdam, The Netherlands, serum antibodies against several antigens became detectable at the time of a new HPV infection[32]. In contrast to men, in whom the antibody responses were mostly transient and disappeared during follow-up, women infected with HPV-16 tended to have a more sustained

antibody response. Although most cross-sectional studies have shown that the prevalence of type-specific serum antibodies is higher in women than in men[30, 33], the reasons are uncertain, but may reflect differences in the number of sexual partners between the sexes. Serological studies have shown that in men IgG antibodies to capsids of HPV-6 develop late during the course of condylomatous disease[34]. Amongst a cohort of 588 college women Carter et al.[35], however, noted that of the 69% of those with incident HPV-6 infection who seroconverted, antibodies became detectable at the time of detection of HPV DNA in genital specimens. Transient HPV infection was associated with a failure to seroconvert. They, and others, also noted that seroconversion for HPV-16 occurred most frequently between 6 and 12 months after infection and that serum IgG against HPV-16 was more likely to persist than reactivity with other types[35, 36].

Specific IgA against HPV types 6, 11, 16, and 18 is frequently detected in the serum of women who become infected with the corresponding HPV types[37], but in those with transient infection it does not persist for long. There is only a weak correlation between IgA and IgG seropositivity: Wang et al.[38] found that 46% of IgG positive women had detectable IgA, and that 55% of IgA seropositive individuals were IgG positive. As the detection of type-specific IgA is associated with the number of recent sexual partners[38], it is likely that its presence indicates recent or ongoing infection. Shortly after infection with HPV-6, type-specific IgM antibody responses are also induced transiently, sometimes simultaneously with IgG and IgA, but occasionally preceding the detection of these antibodies[39].

A local immune response to HPV has also been shown. Wang et al.[40] detected IgA reactive with capsids of HPV-16, HPV-18, and HPV-33 in cervical mucus from women infected with the corresponding type of HPV. This antibody response is independent of that in the serum. Antibodies of the IgG and secretory IgA classes reactive with capsids of HPV-16 are found in cervical secretions, and as with serum antibodies, they are found several months after HPV infection[41].

Epidemiology

The true prevalence of HPV anogenital infection in the community is unknown because

1. many individuals do not seek medical help
2. symptomless and subclinical infection is common
3. in most STI clinics, from which accurate data are generally available, the diagnosis is only made when condylomata are seen
4. many individuals with genital warts consult general practitioners, who are not obliged to notify this infection to public health authorities.

PREVALENCE

Based on condylomata acuminata

Anogenital warts are common amongst men and women who attend STI clinics, and in many countries, including the UK, the number of affected patients is increasing (Figure 5.10). Not surprisingly, lower prevalence rates have been reported in

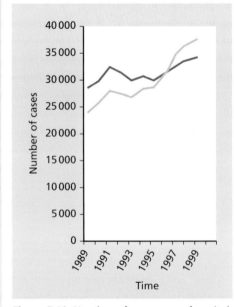

Figure 5.10 Number of new cases of genital warts diagnosed in genitourinary medicine clinics in the UK 1990–1999, the top line is male cases, the lower line is female cases (data from PHLS, DHSS&PS and the Scottish ISD(D)5 Collaborative Group 2000[221])

surveys of women attending other health care facilities, for example in women undergoing routine medical examination in Washington State, USA, only 0.8% of women aged 21 to 29 years of age, and 0.6% of women aged 30–39 years had genital warts[42].

Based on cytological evidence of human papillomavirus

Cytological changes associated with HPV infection in a cervical (Pap) smear, including koilocytosis and changes indicative of L-SIL, are often found in the absence of macroscopic HPV lesions. The results of cervical cytology screening can therefore provide additional information on the prevalence of HPV in a community. It must be noted, however, that there is considerable inter-observer variation in the interpretation of the smears[43]. In a large Finnish study, undertaken between 1985 and 1986, the crude annual incidence of cervical HPV infection was 7% amongst over 1000 women aged 22 years who participated in a mass cervical cytology screening program[44]. A very similar estimate for the rate of infection (8%) was found amongst college women in the USA[45]. As is the case with other sexually transmitted infections, for example, HSV-2, cytological evidence of HPV infection is detected more frequently in young women from the inner cities of the USA[46]. More limited data are available on the prevalence of HPV in men as detected by cytological methods. Using brushings from the urethral meatus and external genitalia, Hippelainen et al.[47], found that 6.5% of 201 specimens from Finnish conscripts, mean age 19.8 years, had evidence of HPV infection (koilocytosis). Direct examination of the skin and mucous membranes with an operating microscope or colposcope, before and after the application of acetic acid, appears to be more sensitive than cytological methods for the detection of HPV infection. Because of inter-observer variation in the interpretation of the findings, and because it does not lend itself to mass screening for infection, however, this method is unsuitable for epidemiological studies.

Based on detection of human papillomavirus nucleic acid

Human papillomavirus DNA can now be reliably detected by PCR, and this can be used to identify different HPV types in clinical specimens, including exfoliated cells. Several studies have shown the superiority of PCR over other methods for the detection of infection, and a few prevalence studies have been reported using this approach. For example, Bauer et al.[48] found that 33% of 467 women who attended a university health service in the USA for routine gynecological examination were infected with at least one known type of HPV. In The Netherlands, HPV DNA of any type was detected in cervical smears from about 14% of 156 women aged between 15 and 34 years, who attended their general practitioner for routine examination and who had normal cytology; a similar prevalence (13.9% of 2320 women) was found in individuals who attended a gynecology out-patient department. DNA of HPV types 16 and 18 were detected in 3.8% and 3.3% of the women who attended their general practitioner or the gynecology clinic respectively[49]. The prevalence of genital HPV in men appears to be similar to that of women. Using consensus primers in the PCR, Hippelainen et al.[47] detected HPV in exfoliated cells from the distal urethra or skin of the penis in 16.5% of 285 Finnish conscripts. Two years earlier, Kataoka et al.[50] reported the detection by PCR of HPV DNA in 44% of aceto-white lesions found on the external genitalia of 39 of 108 healthy Swedish men, aged 18 to 23 years, and in urethral brushings from 12% of the men who did not have apparent HPV-related lesions on the penis. HPV infection of the anal region is common amongst men who have sex with men. In a recent study, HPV DNA was detected by PCR in anal material collected from 93% of 346 HIV-seropositive men, and 61% of 262 HIV-non-infected men[51]. HPV-16 was the most common type detected in both groups, but multiple types were found more frequently in HIV-infected men (73% versus 23%).

Influence of age on detection of human papillomavirus genital tract infection

Women with genital warts who present to STI clinics for the first time tend to be younger than men: the peak age group at

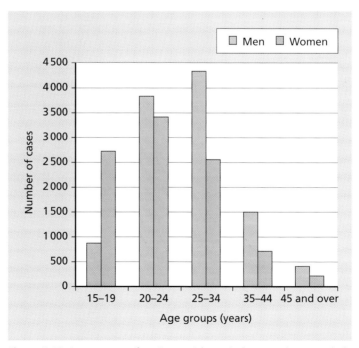

Figure 5.11 Age groups of patients with genital warts who attended genitourinary medicine clinics in Scotland 1996–1999 (data from Information and Statistics Division Scotland)

which the diagnosis was made in women and men who attended clinics in Scotland was 20 to 24 years and 25 to 34 years respectively (Figure 5.11). This observation in women is consistent with reports that the highest rates of HPV infection, as judged by the presence of koilocytes and/or changes suggestive of intraepithelial neoplasia in cervical cytology (Pap) smears, is found in sexually active women under 30 years of age[52]. The age-dependent prevalence of HPV was shown clearly in the Dutch studies reported by Melkert et al.[49]

- the rate of detection of HPV DNA was significantly lower amongst women aged between 35 and 55 years, than in younger women
- HPV DNA of any type was found in 13.9% of 2320 women aged 15 to 34 years
- HPV DNA of any type was found in only 6.6% of 1826 older women
- this age-dependent relationship was maximum in women aged 20 to 24 years.

These findings suggest that many HPV infections acquired by young women are transient, possibly being limited by acquisition of immunity or hormonal changes as the woman becomes older. Such a conclusion is supported by short-term cohort studies that show a decrease in prevalence of HPV over time. Evander et al.[53], for example, found that in a cohort of 276 young women the total prevalence of HPV infection decreased from 21% to 8.3% during a mean interval of 2 years. In a small proportion of women, however, there is persistent infection, and in Evander and colleagues' study[53], the same type of HPV persisted in only two women. The transient nature of most HPV infections as shown in studies of prevalent infection was shown further for incident infection by Ho et al.[54]. In a cohort study of 608 college women, followed at 6-monthly intervals, they showed that the median duration of incident infections was 8 months (95% confidence interval 7–10 months). Persistence of infection for more than 6 months correlated with older age, infection with multiple types of HPV, and infection with high-risk HPV types (relative risk 37.2; 95% confidence interval 14.6–94.8).

SEXUAL TRANSMISSION OF HUMAN PAPILLOMAVIRUS INFECTION

Oriel[55] found that 22 (71%) of 31 men and 31 (54%) of 57 women who had been sexual contacts of individuals with genital warts developed condylomata acuminata after a pre-patent period that varied from 3 weeks to 8 months (average 2.8 months).

The sexual transmission of genital HPV infection is supported by several epidemiological studies. Amongst women who had not had vaginal intercourse, Fairley et al.[56] did not detect HPV DNA in any of 23 individuals, and Rylander et al.[57] found HPV DNA type 6 in only 2 of 130 preparations of vaginal epithelial cells. There is a good correlation between the number of lifetime sexual partners and the detection of HPV DNA. For example, amongst women aged 16 to 29 years who had normal cervical cytology and who attended gynecology clinics in Portland, OR, HPV DNA was detected by PCR in 3.8% of 107 women who had only one lifetime sexual partner, but in 26.0% in those who had between six and nine partners[58]. HPV DNA is found in exfoliated skin cells from men who are the sexual partners of women with HPV infection of the cervix. Using filter *in situ* hybridization, a method that is less sensitive than PCR, viral DNA was found in 39% of 61 male contacts[59]. The relationship between the number of sexual partners and the prevalence of HPV infection in women is also true for men. Hippelainen et al.[47] did not detect viral DNA in any of 38 Finnish conscripts who had never had sexual contact, but, amongst those who were sexually active, they noted that the prevalence of HPV was related to the number of lifetime partners. In addition, they showed a clear relationship between HPV infection and failure to use a condom consistently.

Serological studies provide further supportive evidence of sexual transmission of the genital types of HPV. There is a correlation between the presence of type-specific IgG and IgG1 and the number of sexual partners. In Wang's study[38], 9% of 75 monogamous women but 36% of 191 women with more than five lifetime partners were seropositive for IgG against HPV-16 (odds ratio 5.3; 95% confidence interval 2.3–12.3).

Studies show that concordance between the infecting types in sexual partners is better than could have occurred by chance[60]. Schneider and colleagues[59] found that amongst the sexual partners of 156 women with HPV infection, the infecting viral type was identical in 87% of cases. This is not always the case, however, and Ho et al.[61] noted that only 4 of 8 couples who had HPV-16 shared the same HPV subtypes.

Whether or not infection with one type of HPV confers immunity against either infection with other types, or re-infection with the same type, is uncertain. Co-infection with different types, however, is common. Xi et al.[62] found that in women with persistent HPV-16 infection, one major variant predominated over time, and that minor variants of the virus appeared transiently.

Smoking tobacco may also be a risk factor for the development of genital warts. In a prospective study of 576 women living in an inner city and followed for an average of 14 months, Feldman et al.[63] found that current smokers were 5.2 times more likely to develop warts than non-smokers (95% confidence interval 1.02–26.0). The reasons for the association of cigarette smoking with increased risk of infection are uncertain.

NON-SEXUAL TRANSMISSION OF HUMAN PAPILLOMAVIRUS INFECTION

Although the majority of genital HPV infections in adults are acquired through sexual intercourse, the recent finding of HPV DNA in brushings from the fingers of patients with genital warts, has rekindled the argument that infection can be acquired through digital–genital contact. Sonnex and colleagues[64] detected HPV DNA on the fingers of 12 of 22 patients with genital warts, the skin and genital DNA types being identical (types 6 and 11) in six cases. This finding, however, does not necessarily indicate that infection can be transmitted from contaminated fingers to genitals[65]. Sometimes anogenital warts are caused by HPV types 1, 2 or 4, the types associated with common skin warts[66], and have most likely been acquired through auto-inoculation.

HUMAN PAPILLOMAVIRUS LESIONS OF THE ORAL CAVITY

Squamous cell papillomata are found at all ages, and HPV types 6 and 11 are found in about two-thirds of such lesions[67]. These types and HPV-16 have been found in about 4% and 2% of samples respectively from individuals with clinically normal oral mucosa[68]. Although concurrent infection of the oral cavity and genital tract, sometimes with discordant types, has been found in some women[69], the prevalence of upper respiratory tract papillomatosis amongst individuals with anogenital warts is low. In a study of 53 adults with genital warts who attended a STI clinic in the UK, Clarke et al.[70] found only two patients with HPV-related lesions of the oropharynx or larynx; 70% of the 53 patients had had orogenital contact.

ASSOCIATION OF HUMAN PAPILLOMAVIRUS INFECTION WITH SQUAMOUS INTRAEPITHELIAL LESIONS AND CARCINOMAS OF THE ANOGENITAL REGION AND OF THE HEAD AND NECK

In their large study of more than 1000 invasive cancer specimens from twenty-two countries, Bosch and colleagues[2] detected HPV DNA in about 93% of cervical carcinomas. Worldwide, with the exception of Indonesia where HPV-18 was more common, HPV-16 was the predominant type being found in about 50% of lesions[2]. HPV-18 was detected in 12%, HPV-45 in 8%, and HPV-31 in 5% of specimens. There was clustering of HPV-45 in western Africa, and HPV-39 and HPV-59 were almost exclusively found in specimens from Central and South America. Squamous cell carcinoma of the uterine cervix is thought to arise from SILs. The presence of HPV precedes and predicts the development of SIL, and HPV-16 is the most predictive type for SIL, including low-grade SILs. This was shown clearly in the nested case-control study reported by Liaw et al.[71]. They found

that, compared with initially HPV-negative women, individuals who were positive for HPV DNA at entry into the study, were 3.8 times (95% confidence interval 2.6–5.5) more likely to develop low-grade SILs subsequently and 12.7 times (95% confidence interval, 6.2–25.9) more likely to develop high-grade SILs. Fewer than 1% of women infected with the high-risk HPV types, however, develop cervical cancer[2, 72], and cofactors are probably important. The amount of HPV might also be an important factor in determining the outcome of infection. Josefsson et al.[73] estimated the amount of HPV 16 DNA extracted from archived cervical cytology preparations (3835 samples) from 478 Swedish women with cervical cancer, and from 608 individually matched control subjects. They found that the risk of H-SIL increased with the amount of HPV DNA detected. In a parallel report from the same group, it was noted that 25% of women with a high viral load before the age of 25 years developed H-SIL within 15 years[74]. The early cervical smears were often normal despite a high HPV viral load. These workers also showed that women with a persistently high viral load, and who develop H-SIL, have significant increases in the amount of HPV DNA over time.

Serological studies also support an association between SILs, cervical carcinoma and HPV-16 infection. In a prospective study from Sweden of over 15 000 women who were followed for a mean of 34.9 months, those who had antibodies against HPV-16 capsids had a threefold increased risk of developing SILs[75]. Similarly, Lehtinen et al.[76] who undertook a nested case-control study (27 women with invasive carcinoma, 45 women with SILs, and 143 matched controls) found a significant relationship between HPV-16 seropositivity and cervical cancer (odds ratio 12.5, 95% confidence interval 2.7–57).

Earlier studies that did not control for number of sexual partners or for HPV infection suggested that current cigarette smoking was a significant risk factor for cervical cancer. More recent cross-sectional studies, however, have not confirmed this risk[77]. These observations should lead the physician to question the epidemiological data. It is known, however, that current

smokers have a reduced population of Langerhans cells in the cervix[78], and it might be speculated that local immuno-deficiency may result in the persistence of HPV infection. When tested by the Ames-Salmonella microsomal test, cervical mucus from smokers is much more likely to be mutagenic than that from non-smokers[79]. Recently infection with Chlamydia trachomatis has been proposed as a possible co-factor in the pathogenesis of cervical cancer (Chapter 10).

Some, but by no means all, cases of vulval carcinoma are associated with HPV infection. An increased prevalence of HPV DNA has been found in basaloid carcinoma and warty carcinoma compared with the conventional type of keratinizing squamous cell carcinoma. Basaloid carcinomas are characterized by a uniform population of small, ovoid cells with a high nuclear: cytoplasm ratio. Warty carcinoma is similar to typical squamous cell carcinoma but contains many squamous cells that show marked nuclear pleomorphism, enlargement, atypia, and multinucleation in association with cytoplasmic cavitation resembling koilocytosis[80]. In Kurman and colleagues' study the majority of women with basaloid and warty carcinomas were under 60 years of age. Women with keratinizing squamous cell carcinoma, and the proportion of women of Afro-Caribbean origin was higher compared with women with keratinizing squamous cell carcinoma. In just over 75% of 35 cases of basaloid and warty carcinomas, tissue adjacent to the tumor showed SILs, suggesting that these were precursors. Further evidence for an association between HPV and vulval carcinogenesis comes from the detection by PCR of HPV types 16, 18, or 33 in 61% of vulval squamous cell carcinomas with adjacent H-SILs, but in only 13% of tumors without adjacent H-SILs, and in none of 101 normal vulval tissue specimens[81]. An additional observation in that study was the association of HPV with multicentric anogenital neoplasia.

HPV DNA has been found in 75% of men with L-SIL of the penis, and in all patients with H-SIL[82]. However, variable proportions of invasive penile cancers have been reported as being associated with HPV DNA. Most penile cancers are squamous cell carcinomas but there are subtypes that are morphologically different. It is now evident that penile squamous cell carcinomas exhibiting basaloid changes (nests of small basophilic cells with numerous mitoses) are more likely to be associated with HPV 16 than the typical carcinoma of the penis. Gregoire and colleagues[83] showed that 9 of 12 specimens showing basaloid features were positive for HPV-16. In contrast, HPV DNA was found in only 5 of 45 cases of typical squamous cell carcinoma of the penis.

Epidemiological data have shown that in men, receptive anal intercourse may be a risk factor for squamous and transitional-cell carcinomas of the anal canal. Parallels have been drawn between the etiology of anal cancer in men and cervical cancer in women. HPV types associated with the former cancer, particularly HPV-16, have been detected in anal squamous-cell carcinomas[84]. Recent epidemiological data have also provided evidence that anal cancer in women is associated with an STI. An increased risk of anal cancer was found in women who had had receptive anal intercourse, particularly before the age of 30 years, multiple sexual partners, and a history of a variety of STIs in themselves and their male partners[85].

Anal SILs (or, as it was originally designated, anal intraepithelial neoplasia (AIN)) were first described in 1986 and are most commonly found at the transitional zone of the anal canal, that is, at the junction of the squamous epithelium of the anal canal and the columnar epithelium of the rectum. Low-grade SILs tend to be associated with HPV types 6 and 11 and H-SILs with HPV types 16 and 18[86]. The association of anogenital SILs, HPV, and HIV infection is discussed on page 81.

HPV has also been implicated in the etiology of cancers of the head and neck. Overall, Gillison et al.[87] identified HPV DNA in 62 (25%) of 253 cases. Interestingly, HPV was detected in 57% of 60 oropharyngeal or tonsillar tumors. In about 90% of these HPV-positive cancers, high-risk HPV types were identified. Southern blot hybridization studies suggested that viral DNA had become integrated into the host cell genome. Compared with HPV-negative tumors, these tumors were less

likely to have p53 mutations, and affected patients had a better prognosis.

HUMAN PAPILLOMAVIRUS INFECTION IN THE IMMUNOCOMPROMISED PATIENT

Persistent HPV infection is common in patients with immunodeficiency states associated with depressed cell-mediated immunity such as lymphoma and leukemia. The prevalence of HPV infection in organ transplant recipients is high. Rudlinger et al.[88], for example, found warts in 48% of 120 renal allograft recipients. The longer the period of immunosuppression after transplantation, the greater the risk of developing viral warts. Barr et al.[89] noted that 20% of 133 patients who had had a graft within the preceding 5 years had warts, compared with 77% of 69 individuals whose graft survival time was over 5 years. Organ transplant recipients are at increased risk of skin cancer, particularly squamous cell carcinoma, and again the risk is directly proportional to the graft survival time[89]. Viral warts often show dysplastic changes in immunocompromised individuals, and the clinical and histological overlap between viral warts and squamous cell carcinoma suggests a possible link between the two conditions[89]. A variety of different types of HPV have been identified in skin squamous cell carcinomas with no real pattern of involvement. High exposure to ultraviolet radiation predisposes to the development of viral warts in transplant recipients. It has been suggested that many HPVs may act as promoters of carcinogenesis, by stimulating squamous cell proliferation in a variety of lesions, allowing mutations induced by ultraviolet radiation to become fixed by forced cell replication, thereby driving tumor progression[90].

Anogenital warts are also common in renal allograft recipients. The prevalence of cervical and anal SILs is significantly higher in women who have had renal allografts than in non-immunocompromised patients. For example, SILs were found by colposcopy in 24 (49%) of 49 transplant recipients, compared with 7 (10%) of 69 non-immunocompromised subjects[91]. In several studies HPV-16 and HPV-18 DNA

was found more often in immuno-suppressed women than in the control population[91, 92].

The prevalence of HPV infection in HIV-seropositive women is increased compared with HIV-non-infected women. For example, in a study of 220 HIV-infected and 231 HIV-non-infected women reported by Sun et al.[93], after four examinations the cumulative prevalence of HPV, as detected by PCR on cervicovaginal washings was 83% in the seropositive patients, and 62% in the HIV-seronegative group, a significant difference. The prevalence of infection was higher in HIV-infected women whose CD4+ cell count in the peripheral blood was less than 500 per mm^3. These authors also found that the prevalence of the high-risk HPV-16-associated types (16, 31, 33, 35, and 38), the high-risk HPV-18-associated types (18 and 45), and the intermediate risk types (51 and 53) was significantly higher amongst HIV-seropositive women than amongst HIV-seronegative individuals. In addition, the same group of workers had shown previously in a cross-sectional study that infection with multiple types of HPV is more frequent in HIV-infected women than in uninfected women[94]. Twenty per cent of the HIV-infected women who were studied prospectively by Sun et al.[93] had persistent infection with the high-risk HPV types, compared with only 3% of HIV-non-infected subjects; persistence was found particularly in those women whose CD4+ cell counts were less than 200 per mm^3.

In cross-sectional studies, it has been found that women with HIV infection and a peripheral blood CD4+ cell count of less than 500 per mm^3 are some four to five times more likely to have cervical low or high-grade intraepithelial lesions than HIV-seronegative women. Amongst these women there is a significant association between SIL and persistent infection with HPV, including high-risk types of HPV[95]. During a 1-year follow-up of 278 HIV-infected women, the cumulative incidence of SILs was 21%[95]. The incidence of SILs in this French study was somewhat higher than in the study reported from New York in which the incidence was 8.3 and 1.8 cases per 100 person-years of follow-up in HIV-infected and uninfected women respectively[96]. Progression from low-grade to

high-grade SIL seems to occur more commonly in HIV-infected women with a CD4+ cell count of less than 500 per mm^3 than in HIV-non-infected women, or in HIV-seropositive women with a CD4+ cell count of more than 500 per mm^3[95]. Cervical cancer, however, had not developed in any of the women studied by either Six et al. [95] or Ellerbrock et al.[96]. In Ellerbrock's study[96], only 6 (9%) of the incident SILs, however, were high grade. Risk factors for incident SILs identified in the latter study were

- HIV infection
- transient HPV DNA detection
- persistent HPV infection.

The association between HIV infection and SILs, however, is complex and not fully understood. For example, Ellerbrock et al.[96] found a higher incidence of SILs in women even after controlling for the presence or persistence of HPV[96]. Although the incidence of SILs in Ellerbrock's study appeared to be unaffected by antiretroviral therapy, most women had only received dual combination treatment and it is premature to draw conclusions regarding the influence of highly active antiretroviral treatment on the development of SILs.

In the USA it has been shown convincingly that the numbers of HPV-associated cancers amongst patients with symptomatic HIV infection occur in excess of those expected. For invasive cancers in women, the overall risks are significantly increased for cervical (relative risk 5.4, 95% confidence interval 3.9–7.2), vulvar/vaginal (relative risk 5.8, 95% confidence interval 3.0–10.2), and anal (relative risk 6.8, 95% confidence interval 2.7–14.0) cancers. In men the risks are increased for anal (relative risk 37.9, 95% confidence interval 33.0–43.4), penile (relative risk 3.7, 95% confidence interval 2.0–6.2), tonsillar (relative risk 2.6, 95% confidence interval 1.8–3.8) and conjunctival (relative risk, 14.6 95% confidence interval 5.8–30.0) cancers[97].

In the USA, the prevalence of invasive cervical cancer has been shown to be higher in young (20–34 years old) HIV-infected black (relative risk 3.8, 95% confidence interval 1.7–8.5) and Hispanic women (relative risk 7.3, confidence interval 1.4–37.1) than in non-infected individuals[98].

High-grade SILs of the vulva have also been described in immunocompromised patients[99].

The development of anal squamous-cell carcinomas in HIV-infected individuals is now well recognized[100]. In women, anal cytological abnormalities are common. In one study, 26% of 102 HIV-seropositive women, but only 7% of 96 HIV-seronegative women, had abnormal anal smears[101]. Squamous intraepithelial lesions of the anal canal are also common in HIV-infected homosexual men. Palefsky et al.[51] identified such lesions in 36% of 346 HIV-seropositive men and in only 7% of 262 non-infected homosexual men. H-SIL was found in 5% of the latter and in 1% of the former group. The most important risk factors for high-grade SILs have been shown to be

- low CD4+ cell count
- persistent HPV infection
- infection with multiple types of HPV
- high-level HPV infection with the more oncogenic types of HPV[102].

The pathogenesis of anal SIL in HIV-infected patients is complex and not properly understood[103]. As the prevalence of HPV is inversely related to the number of CD4+ cells in the peripheral blood, it has been postulated that the immune deficiency associated with HIV infection permits reactivation of latent HPV resulting in epithelial abnormalities. The situation may be analogous to the development of cancers at other sites in iatrogenically immuno-suppressed patients. Certainly, positive T cell proliferative responses to HPV-16 E6 or E7 peptides appear to be less common in HIV-seropositive homosexual men with low CD4+ cell counts compared with infected men with higher CD4+ cell counts or HIV-non-infected men[103]. In addition, a higher proportion of men with low-grade anal SILs have positive cytotoxic T cell responses to HPV E6 (but not to E7) than men with high-grade lesions[103]. Another mechanism of HIV–HPV interaction may be the effect of secreted HIV-1 proteins on HPV-infected keratinocytes. The tat protein may potentiate expression of E6 and E7 that may eventually result in chromosome changes that are responsible for malignant transformation[103].

Patients with HIV infection commonly develop papilliferous lesions of the oral cavity. HPV is often found in these lesions. Volter et al.[104] detected HPV DNA in 67% of 67 samples. HPV types 7 and 32 predominated (19% and 28% respectively), but other types, including HPV 2a, 6b, 13, 16, 18, 55, 59, 69, 72, and 73, were also found.

HUMAN PAPILLOMAVIRUS INFECTION IN PREGNANCY

Although an increased prevalence of HPV infection in pregnant women has been reported[105], more recent data have failed to confirm this finding[106, 107]. Anogenital warts may appear for the first time during pregnancy either as a result of recent infection or, in many cases, re-activation of latent HPV infection.

Clinical features and diagnosis of human papillomavirus infections

GENITAL WARTS

Various clinical types of wart can be distinguished. In men the fleshy hyperplastic warts (condylomata acuminata), either one or many, occur most often on the glans penis and on the inner lining of the prepuce. The appearance depends on the location, although moisture and accompanying inflammation may enhance the size and tendency to coalesce. Warts in the terminal urethra in particular have a bright red color. Hyperplastic warts also occur in women. Genital warts may occur at several sites in the same patient, the distribution as recorded by Oriel[55] was as follows.

In men

- frenum, corona, and glans, 52% (Figure 5.12)
- prepuce, 33%
- urethral meatus, 23% (Figure 5.13)
- shaft of penis, 18%
- scrotum, 2%
- perianal region, 8% (Figure 5.14).

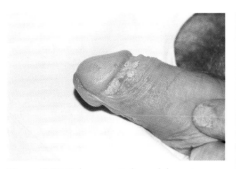

Figure 5.12 Sub-preputial condylomata acuminata

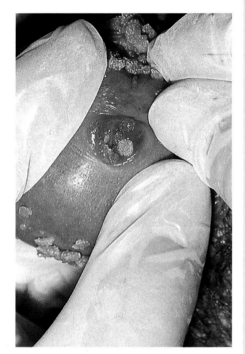

Figure 5.13 Intra-urethral condyloma (reproduced from McMillan and Scott 2000[224])

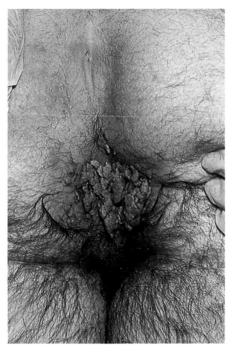

Figure 5.14 Perianal condylomata acuminata (reproduced from McMillan and Scott 2000[224])

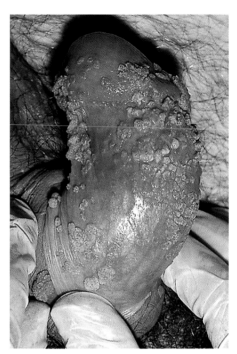

Figure 5.15 Extensive sub-preputial condylomata in an uncircumcised male (reproduced from McMillan and Scott 2000[224])

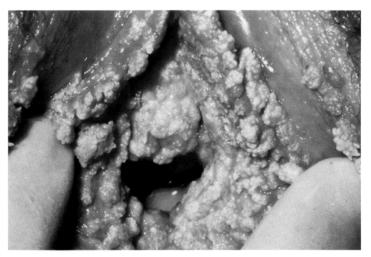

Figure 5.16 Condylomata acuminata at the vaginal introitus (reproduced from Rein 1996[225])

Genital warts are sometimes very extensive in the uncircumcised male (Figure 5.15).

In women

- posterior part of the introitus, 73% (Figure 5.16)
- labia minora and clitoris, 32%
- labia majora, 31%
- urethra, 8%
- vagina, 15% (Figure 5.17)
- cervix, 6% (Figure 5.18)
- perineum, 23%
- perianal region, 18%.

Most often warts first appeared at or near the posterior part of the vaginal introitus and on the adjacent labia majora and minora. They tend to cluster at the orifices of the greater vestibular glands (Figure 5.19).

In both sexes, condylomata acuminata may be found in the anal canal (Figure 5.20) and can cause bleeding during defecation. Occasionally this may be the only site of HPV condylomatous lesions.

In pregnant women, condylomata may become large and extensive (Figure 5.21), but rarely cause difficulty in delivery.

Other sites include the urethra, and bladder. Urethral condylomata can spread proximally from the common sites of predilection, namely the fossa navicularis and perimeatal portions of the urethra, to involve any part of the urethra and, rarely,

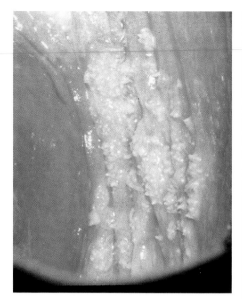

Figure 5.17 Condylomata of the vaginal mucosa (reproduced from Rein 1996[225])

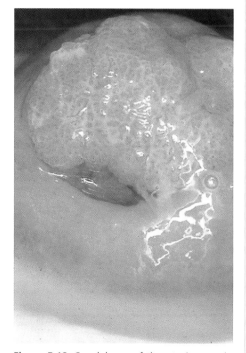

Figure 5.18 Condyloma of the uterine cervix (reproduced from McMillan and Scott 2000[224])

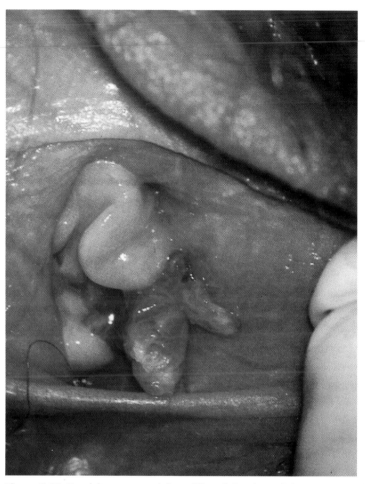

Figure 5.19 Condyloma around the orifice of the duct of the greater vestibular gland (reproduced from Rein 1996[225])

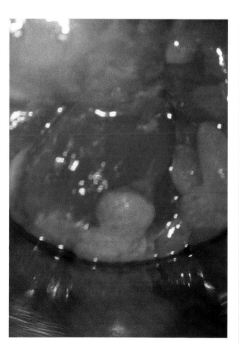

Figure 5.20 Condylomata acuminata of the anal canal (reproduced from McMillan and Scott 2000[224])

the bladder. These condylomata have been recognized by a voiding cystourethrography[108] following intravenously administered contrast. Although excretory voiding cystourethrography will avoid the need for urethral instrumentation, which itself may contribute to the retrograde spread of condylomata, it carries a recog-

nized risk (a mortality rate of 1/20 000) and therefore is not indicated in the vast majority of cases of urethral meatus warts. The place of ultrasonography in the diagnosis of urethral condylomata remains to be established.

Sessile warts, resembling plane warts on the non-genital skin, tend to be seen on the shaft of the penis (Figure 5.22), and although often multiple they do not coalesce. Sessile warts do not seem to occur on the vulva. Clear differentiation from the common wart is not always possible. Multiple common skin warts (verrucae vulgares) present as raised lesions; they occur only on the shaft of the penis and occasionally on the vulva and perianal skin.

The differential diagnosis of condylomata acuminata includes penile papillae (page 556), vestibular papillae, pilosebaceous and Tyson's glands, molluscum contagiosum, skin tags, and condylomata lata (page 420).

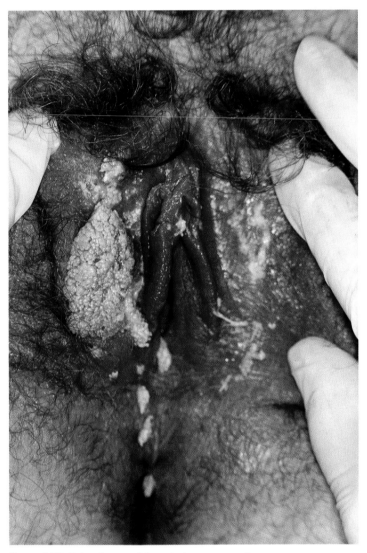

Figure 5.21 Extensive condylomata in a pregnant woman

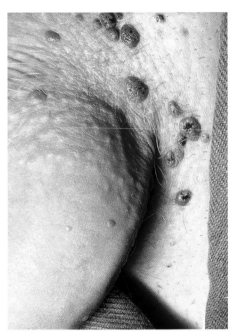

Figure 5.22 Sessile warts in the pubic area

SQUAMOUS INTRAEPITHELIAL LESIONS

Of the uterine cervix

Non-condylomatous HPV lesions of the cervix are common, and most HPV-associated cervical intraepithelial lesions appear during the metaplastic process within the transformation zone. Screening for these lesions is by cytology, with colposcopy as required. The appearance of these lesions is variable, and a detailed description lies outwith the scope of this textbook. The interested reader is referred to one of the standard texts on colposcopy.

Of the vagina

Metaplasia extending from the cervix into the vagina may become atypical. Squamous intraepithelial lesions may arise within this area, usually in association with cervical SILs. Isolated SILs may also present particularly in the upper third of the vagina. Punctation and mosaicism may be seen, and the surface is usually granular.

Of the vulva

Women with SILs of the vulva usually complain of pruritus vulvae with soreness,

but others have noticed an abnormal swelling[109]. The most common finding is a slightly elevated irregular white lesion sharply demarcated from the surrounding tissues and measuring on average 2.5 cm[110]. In patients under the age of 40 years the lesions are usually multiple, sometimes coalescing into plaques, whereas in older women single lesions are more common. Less frequently, the lesions are red or brown and sometimes eroded.

Although most vulval SILs are detectable on close naked-eye examination, the use of the colposcope is sometimes useful in defining the extent of an individual lesion. In some cases only areas of hyperkeratosis with normal surrounding tissues are visible with the colposcope, but in others there are sharply defined punctate or mosaic changes.

The differential diagnosis includes melanocytic nevi, pigmented warts, and rarely, seborrheic warts and malignant melanoma. Red lesions need to be differentiated from candidiasis, eczema, psoriasis, and lichen planus.

Although cytological examination is useful in the detection of cervical SILs, its value in vulval SILs is more limited as the exfoliation of underlying cells may be prevented by an area of hyperkeratosis. In areas of the skin in which punctation or mosaicism can be detected with the colposcope, cytological examination may be helpful. Histological examination of biopsy specimens, however, is essential for diagnosis.

Of the penis

Subclinical HPV lesions of the penis can be identified with the aid of a colposcope or hand lens, before and after the application of acetic acid to the skin*. The most common lesions are sharply demarcated, elevated, aceto-white areas[111]; the normal branching vascular network is not seen within the lesion because the epithelium is thicker than normal, but capillary loops are prominent. Lesions vary in size from less than 0.1 to 10 mm in diameter. Papular lesions (well-circumscribed, elevated lesions with a smooth surface and clearly distinct form condyloma acuminatum) are also common. Multiple sites are often affected but lesions are most frequently found on the prepuce, frenum, and shaft of the penis[111]. Diffuse aceto-white areas are common in balanoposthitis, but the vascular pattern of HPV-associated lesions is usually absent. Penoscopic appearances, however, cannot predict the presence of SIL with certainty, and histological examination is essential for diagnosis[47]†. For example, plasma cell balanitis of Zoon, a condition of unknown etiology, that presents as large red areas on the mucous membranes, needs to be differentiated from SILs by biopsy.

Of the anal canal

Squamous intraepithelial lesions of the anal canal are most commonly found at the transitional zone, that is, at the junc-

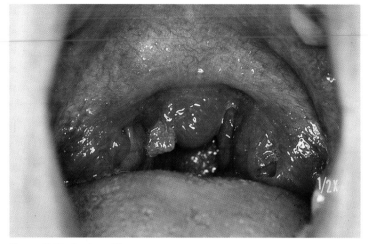

Figure 5.23 Oral papilloma

tion of the squamous epithelium of the anal canal and the columnar epithelium of the rectum. With the operating microscope, after the application of acetic acid, H-SILs appear as irregular white areas with cobblestoning and mosaicism, and corkscrew vessels[86].

ORAL WARTS

Squamous cell papillomas are benign tumors that usually affect the soft palate (Figure 5.23), but are sometimes found on the lateral border, frenulum or dorsum of the tongue. The lesion is usually solitary and presents as a white or pink, broadbased or pedunculated swelling. The surface often appears verrucous.

Screening for cervical squamous intraepithelial lesions and HPV infection

Squamous intraepithelial lesions in the epithelium of the uterine cervix can be detected by examining microscopically cells obtained by scraping the squamocolumnar junction with a wooden spatula, the Ayre spatula is the best known and others such as the Aylesbury and Lerner, and when the junction is within the endocervical canal, the cytobrush. In the interpretation of cervical smears, the Bethesda System ter-

minology for cytological diagnosis is being increasingly adopted[23]. In the UK, initiation of screening for SILs is recommended after a woman's 20th birthday and before her 25th birthday[112]. The interval between cytological screening of women who have had normal smears varies between 3 and 5 years. Referral for colposcopy should be made[112]

- after one smear showing H-SLI or glandular abnormality
- after two smears showing L-SLI
- after three smears described as inadequate or showing borderline nuclear change unless the cytopathologist specifies difficulty in distinguishing the borderline changes from H-SLI, in which case colposcopy may be indicated earlier
- when cervical cancer is suspected but is not clinically overt.

Colposcopy should be considered the first time a woman has a smear that is consistent with L-SIL if that smear follows treatment for SIL or if it is anticipated that the woman will not comply with smear follow-up. Colposcopy in addition to cytology is recommended at the first follow-up visit if excision has been used to eradicate SIL and the margins are doubtful, or if H-SIL has been treated by excision of the transformation zone.

As noted previously, the presence of HPV precedes and predicts the development of SIL and, although HPV-16 appears to be the most predictive type for SIL of any grade, less than 1% of women develop

---

* This is conveniently undertaken by soaking a surgical swab in acetic acid, 5% v/v, followed by wrapping the entire penis with the prepuce retracted, if applicable, and leaving for 5 minutes; additional application of acetic acid may be necessary during the procedure.
† Lignocaine, 1% w/v is used to infiltrate the sub-epithelial tissues. The lesion is then biopsied using a scalpel or 4 mm punch. A small absorbable suture may be necessary to close the defect in the epithelium.

cervical cancer. Screening to detect high-risk HPV types has been proposed, but there are many uncertainties about such a screening program[113]

- there seems to be a relationship between the amount of HPV-16 DNA and the subsequent development of cervical cancer, but the viral load that defines high risk has not yet been determined
- the management of the woman with high levels of HPV-16 DNA but without SIL is uncertain
- the population at which such screening should be targeted is not clear
- whether or not accessibility to HPV typing leads to substantial improvement over standard cervical cytology screening is unknown.

Although it is our routine clinical practice to offer colposcopic screening for cervical SILs at annual intervals to *immunocompromised women*, including those infected with HIV, a mathematical model has shown that amongst HIV-infected women, annual cervical cytology after two negative smears obtained 6 months apart resulted in a gain in quality adjusted life expectancy, but that colposcopy provided no additional benefit[114].

Screening for anal squamous intraepithelial lesions and anal cancer

There is good evidence for an increased risk of anal cancer amongst immunocompromised individuals (see pp. 80–81), and the authors' current practice is to undertake cytological examination at annual intervals. This is done by inserting a Cytobrush® (Medscand, Sweden) into the anal canal to a distance of about 2.5 cm, rotating 360° several times within the canal, and, immediately after withdrawal, preparing a smear by rotating the brush over almost the entire length of a clean microscope slide. The smear should be immediately placed in fixative to reduce the risk of producing drying artefacts. Anal cytology is a sensitive but non-specific method for identifying patients with SILs. When compared with anoscopy and histology, the sensitivity in one series was 87.5%,

but the specificity was only 16.3%[115]. In the authors' clinical practice, patients with an abnormal smear are offered anoscopic examination, using a colposcope before and after the application of acetic acid to the anal canal. Aceto-white areas are biopsied using punch biopsy forceps (for example, modified Young's forceps).

In a mathematical model, screening for SIL in HIV-seropositive homosexual men has been shown to lead to an increased quality adjusted life expectancy by about 3 months at all stages of HIV disease[116]. The question of whether or not to undertake regular screening for SILs and anal cancer in men who have had receptive anal intercourse has recently been addressed by Goldie et al.[117]. In their mathematical model, cytological screening at 2 to 3 year intervals increased the discounted quality adjusted life expectancy by 1.8 months. They showed further that life-expectancy benefits were comparable with other preventive health measures. Whilst such screening may be a laudable goal, lack of resources in many countries preclude this undertaking.

Treatment of anogenital warts

GENERAL CONSIDERATIONS

Although most anogenital warts in immunocompetent patients eventually undergo spontaneous regression, treatment is offered to the majority of affected individuals with moist hyperplastic condylomata acuminata to reduce the risk of secondary infection and to alleviate anxiety. It is the latter consideration that is most important in deciding on treatment of dry, keratinized warts that can prove refractory to treatment. Soon after diagnosis of anogenital warts, all patients should be counseled carefully about the infection; some of the issues that should be addressed are discussed below.

The exclusion, detection and, if required, treatment of other STIs in the affected individual and the sexual contact(s) are essential first steps. Before initiation of wart therapy, it is important to attend to any other local infection whether sexually transmitted or not. In the case of men a balanoposthitis should be treated as described on pp. 552–

553, and in women any cause of vaginitis or discharge must be discovered and eradicated, particularly candidiasis or trichomoniasis. Sometimes warts regress after local inflammation has been controlled.

In the absence of curative antiviral therapy the management of anogenital warts is often difficult because of recurrences so commonly observed following all forms of therapy. Human papillomavirus is frequently present in clinically and histologically normal skin adjacent to the condylomata acuminata. In a study, 9 of 20 biopsies of clinically normal skin obtained from within 10 mm of the margin of laser-treated lesions showed evidence of HPV DNA sequences. Although recurrence did not occur in all cases these studies[118] suggest that the latent HPV may be responsible for recurrences. The choice of the initial wart treatment depends on several factors, including patient choice, the duration, physical characteristics, and anatomical sites of the warts, and the personal experience of the physician. The efficacy of the various treatments available for use in the treatment of external anogenital warts has recently been reviewed by Beutner and Wiley[119] who have produced a very detailed literature summary that can be downloaded from the *Papillomavirus Report* World Wide Web page (http://www.leeds.ac.uk/lmi/pvr/pvrmain.html).

PODOPHYLLIN AND PODOPHYLLOTOXIN

Podophyllin

Podophyllin deserves full consideration because of its widespread clinical use and its often spectacular initial effects, particularly when applied to hyperplastic condylomata acuminata of the genital skin. The authors, however, consider it outdated and prefer to use podophyllotoxin.

Preparation and contents

Podophyllin is an ethanol extract prepared from the dried rhizome and roots of the plant *Podophyllum* spp. (Greek *podos* – a foot, *phyllon* – a leaf), so named as the leaf has a fancied resemblance to a webbed foot (Figure 5.24). The American species, *Podophyllum peltatum* (Botanical Magazine, 1816, vol. 43,

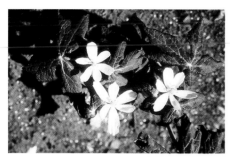

Figure 5.24 *Podophyllum peltatum*

1819) grows in moist shady places from New England to Carolina; a second species of therapeutic interest, *P. emodi*, occurs in the Himalayan mountains and Kashmir. In its preparation the syrupy ethanol extract is poured into cold water then acidified with hydrochloric acid to form a precipitate which is dried and powdered. Light brown to greenish yellow in color, it darkens on exposure to light and heat. This extract contains, among other compounds, colorless lignans, insoluble in water, which vary quantitatively between the species and from batch to batch. In a study by von Grogh[120] in the case of *P. peltatum* the lignan content of samples was found to consist of podophyllotoxin 10%, and alpha- and beta-peltatin 13%; in extracts from *P. emodi*, podophyllotoxin 40% and 4'-demethyl-podophyllotoxin 2% were found.

Mode of action

In rabbit and mouse model systems, podophyllotoxin has been shown to be the most active lignan contained in podophyllin resin[121, 122] and has a destructive effect on keratinocytes and dermal cells. At low concentrations (1 mmol) podophyllotoxin acts in a similar manner to colchicine and binds specifically at the same (or greatly-overlapping) site to tubulin, a component protein of the microtubules* but, in contrast to colchicine, this binding is reversible[123].

---

* Microtubules form the principal fibrous protein of the mitotic spindle and are an essential component of the biological machinery that moves chromosomes and other cytoplasmic constituents. They act by providing directionality to intracellular movement but not the compelling force. The disorder of microtubular function produced by substances which bind to tubulin affects cells generally and is seen, for example, where bidirectional fast axon transport is blocked by agents that bind to tubulin.

Cell division is arrested at the metaphase stage. At higher concentrations (10–100 mmol) podophyllotoxin inhibits nucleoside transport and leads to cell destruction[124].

Clinical effects

For many years the topical application of podophyllin has been used in the treatment of anogenital warts with various formulations being used in clinical practice[125]. Intervals between treatment have been variously studied and it is generally recommended that a week should elapse between applications of podophyllin.

About 4 to 6 hours following the application of podophyllin (20% w/v in 95% ethanol), treated condylomata show blanching and later a drying effect is seen when the pink or red moist warts appear white, gray, and dry; sometimes there is dark brown discoloration. In 4 to 24 hours the condylomata decrease in size, and in 48 hours there is complete involution[126]. The authors of the study just described also noted failures in the treatment of chronic perianal condylomata where penetration of podophyllin was prevented by the dry keratinized surface.

Sullivan and King[126] recorded also the histological changes and observed the disintegration of the chromatin content and aborted mitoses produced by podophyllin and colchicine. They contrasted these effects with those of salicylic acid (30% in liquid paraffin) in which the superficial skin retained its normal nuclear structure and the subtle cytolytic action of podophyllin was not seen.

Unwanted effects

Unwanted local effects of podophyllin, even with the washing off of the preparation after an interval, vary from local itching, burning, tenderness, and erythema to pain, swelling, and ulceration. Balanoposthitis may be severe – associated with phimosis that can, if neglected, lead to a necrotizing balanitis. The skin of the scrotum and vulva may show erythema and scaling.

When podophyllin has been used aggressively and in quantities beyond that now recommended, systemic ill effects have been recorded including dizziness, lethargy, pre-coma, nausea, vomiting, abdominal

pain, respiratory distress, and cold clamminess of the skin. Reversible bone marrow suppression with thrombocytopenia and leukopenia have been recognized[127] and irreversible peripheral neuropathy may be followed by systemic toxicity[128].

In *pregnancy* podophyllin should not be used as it has an antimitotic effect which, although mainly local, is better to avoid. In one case reported in the literature, where a very large amount of podophyllin in tincture of benzoin compound was applied to florid vulval warts, the patient developed a severe peripheral neuropathy and intrauterine death of the fetus (32 weeks) occurred[128].

Recommendations for the use of podophyllin

If the use of podophyllin is necessary, say for reasons of cost, the authors recommend dispensing about 0.5 mL quantities to be used for once-only applications given by trained personnel within the clinic; the use of single containers for repeated applications in the clinics is condemned as it may bring risks of cross-infection. Ordinarily, a few warts should be treated at a time, the adjacent skin being protected by yellow or white soft paraffin (BNF), powder or both. It is good practice to treat, with due regard to any local reaction produced, at frequent intervals (every 3 to 7 days) with small amounts of 25% podophyllin in liquid paraffin or methylated spirit (not more than 0.3 mL at a time). In the case of the preparation in spirit, time should be given to allow drying. The patient should be advised to wash off the podophyllin after an interval of about 6 hours.

The application of podophyllin to large condylomata (≥ 10 cm^2 in area) often results in extensive tissue necrosis with pain and swelling, and caution should be exercised in using podophyllin in the treatment of such lesions. Although some physicians use these agents in the treatment of cervical, vaginal, and intra-anal warts, podophyllin and podophyllotoxin are probably best avoided in these situations. Sustained disappearance of warts with podophyllin treatment is not certain, and even 3 months after initiation of therapy, many patients have recurrent or persistent lesions. As, probably, there is continued viral activity in the area, recurrence at the initial site or in adjacent skin or mucosa is not unexpected. Despite treatment, persistence is particularly noted with warts that have been present for more than 3 months and that have a dry keratinized surface. Such warts are better treated initially by ablative methods.

Efficacy

At least 3 months after cessation of therapy, the reported clearance rate of anogenital warts has varied between 22% and 73%[119], reflecting the differences between studies in trial design, the formulation of the agent, and the duration and anatomical site of the lesions. Three months after clearance of warts with podophyllin, the recurrence rate has ranged from 23% to 55%[119].

Podophyllotoxin

Preparations

Podophyllotoxin is available as an acidic solution in ethanol (0.5% w/v, Warticon®, Perstorp Pharma Limited; Condyline®, Ardern; Podofilox®) and as a cream or gel (0.15% w/w, Warticon®; Podofilox®).

Mode of action

See page 87.

Clinical effects

The effect on condylomata acuminata is similar to podophyllin (see page 87).

Unwanted effects

Mild tenderness, burning, and pain are common, being described by about 60% of patients, and erythema, edema, and minor erosions are also frequently seen[119]. The highest incidence of these effects is seen during the first week of treatment[129]. The safety of podophyllotoxin in pregnancy remains to be established and it is probably best avoided.

Recommendations for the use of podophyllotoxin

Using the plastic applicators provided by the manufacturers, the solution is applied twice daily for 3 consecutive days. The cream or gel is also applied twice daily with a finger. The volume of solution applied should not exceed 0.5 mL or 50 single applications per session, and the area treated per session with solution, cream, or gel should not exceed 10 cm^2. It is recommended that the physician or nurse should apply the first treatment to demonstrate the method of proper application and to identify which warts should be treated[130]. It is also recommended that the health care professional should treat warts that exceed 4 cm^2 in area. If the warts persist, treatment should be repeated at weekly intervals for a total of four treatment cycles.

Efficacy

From the results of placebo-controlled trials, there is no doubt that podophyllotoxin is superior to placebo in producing remission of external genital warts[131, 132]. Compared with podophyllin, podophyllotoxin is more effective in producing complete clearance of warts after 6 weeks of treatment. For example, Edwards *et al.*[133] reported that 28 (88%) of 32 men treated with podophyllotoxin solution were wart-free at assessment compared with 12 (63%) of 19 men who had been given podophyllin (20%). Good results have also been recorded in the treatment of external warts in women. Hellberg and colleagues[134] found that 23 (82%) of 28 patients treated with podophyllotoxin cream but only 16 (59%) of 27 given podophyllin (20%) had complete clearance of warts within 6 weeks of initiation of therapy.

5-FLUOROURACIL

5-fluorouracil (5-FU) is a pyrimidine analog that is incorporated into RNA in preference to the natural substrate uracil. It inhibits thymidylate synthetase thereby impairing RNA and DNA synthesis. It becomes effective in the S phase of the cell cycle (page 73) and causes disturbance of cell growth and division. The drug is available as a 5% w/w cream that is applied topically. In animal studies, less than 10% of the agent is absorbed systemically, and what is absorbed is apparently metabolized by routes similar to those for endogenous uracil[135]. The cream is applied once or twice per day to the warts until they regress or until pain or ulceration necessitates cessation of treatment. Reasonably good results in the treatment of extensive vulval lesions have been reported by Krebs[136] who observed a complete response in 41% of 49 women. It was also noted that the application of 5-FU on two consecutive nights per week for 10 weeks was as effective as continuous therapy, but there were fewer side effects. The daily installation of 5-FU cream into the vagina has been used for many years in the management of vaginal condylomata. Using a plastic applicator, 5-FU cream is inserted into the vagina before retiring to bed, twice weekly for 3 to 10 weeks. A tampon is inserted after the cream has been applied, and the introitus is protected by the application of yellow soft paraffin. The cream is washed off in the morning. Nine months after a single course of treatment, Ferenczy[137] noted that 10% of women had persistence of warts. Condylomata at the urethral meatus can be difficult to treat, but von Krogh[138] reported clearance of warts from this site in 13 of 14 men within an average of 3 weeks from initiation of treatment with 5-FU cream applied twice daily.

After application of 5-FU cream, there is transient erythema of the surrounding skin, but ulceration may be a troublesome complication. Amongst a group of 220 women who had been treated for HPV-related lesions of the vagina, Krebs and Helmkamp[136] found that about 8% had chronic ulceration of the vaginal fornices or ectocervix 6 months after completion of therapy.

A gel, containing a combination of 5-FU and adrenaline (epinephrine), in a formulation for intralesional injection had been developed for the treatment of genital warts. By providing sustained drug release, the gel increased the exposure of diseased tissue to high drug concentrations for extended periods. The drug combination was injected into the lesion once weekly for up to 6 weeks. Preliminary results in a phase III placebo-controlled trial were good, with a complete response rate at the end of treatment of 77% of the 801 condylomata treated, compared with only 12% of 241 warts treated with placebo; 50% of lesions recurred, however, within 3 months[139]. Almost every patient had transient burning, stinging, or pain at the injection site, and ulceration was noted in 48% of individuals treated with the agent. This preparation is no longer available in the UK.

CRYOTHERAPY

Principles of treatment

Cryotherapy destroys warts by cytolysis, directly as the result of the formation of intracellular ice crystals and their later thawing, and from injury to the micro-circulation. As a result of vasoconstriction and damage to the endothelium, thrombosis develops in the arterioles and venules of the tissue. Scoular[140] has reviewed the mechanism of action and the choice of equipment for this procedure. The optimum temperature required to induce cell death is unknown, but it is likely to be −50°C or lower. Not surprisingly, there is a marked subdermal temperature gradient below a cryotherapy probe, with the temperature ranging from −120°C at the skin surface to −26°C a few millimeters deeper. According to Scoular[140], the main criterion used to assess effectiveness of cryotherapy is formation of an ice ball 1 to 2 mm beyond the periphery of the lesion. Freezing should continue for an adequate time, depending on the size of the wart. For example, Zacarian[141] recorded temperatures 5 mm below a 16 mm cryoprobe of 0°C after 30 seconds, −8°C after 60 seconds and −23°C after 120 seconds freezing.

Within 30 seconds of freezing, cells begin to show pyknotic nuclei, edema and other cytoplasmic changes. At the edge of the frozen area cells have eosinophilic cytoplasm and basophilic nuclei. Later changes are those seen in any acutely ischemic area. The cellular infiltrate is mainly of polymorphonuclear leukocytes with some lymphocytes and plasma cells most obvious at the edge of the frozen area. Destruction of epidermal cells is associated with vesiculation followed by sloughing. Resolution begins within 3 days and healing usually occurs without scarring[142].

Cryotherapy methods

1. The application of liquid nitrogen (boiling point −195.8°C) to discrete warts is often used. The aim should be to freeze the wart until a halo of frozen skin is just visible at the base. A cotton wool-tipped applicator can be immersed in a vacuum flask of liquid nitrogen and then applied to the wart, exposed and immobilized by stretching the skin between the fingers.

2. A hand-held insulated and pressurized flask filled with liquid nitrogen and with a control valve to which a range of sprays of different diameter may be fitted is satisfactory for the treatment of most external genital warts. Very effective freezing can be achieved with such equipment, and the risks of cross-infection are minimal. As the flasks are somewhat bulky, however, accuracy in freezing small lesions or urethral warts may be suboptimal. Another disadvantage of the cryospray is the need to refill the container at frequent intervals*, thereby adding to the costs of the procedure.

3. Closed cryotherapy systems operate by providing a continuous supply of liquid nitrous oxide or carbon dioxide from a cylinder to a 'gun' that controls the flow of liquid gas to a removable probe. A range of probes is available facilitating accurate freezing of warts of different sizes. To prevent cross-infection, probes must be autoclaved before use on different patients.

Unwanted effects

About 20% of patients have mild pain during and for a few hours after the procedure; more severe pain and ulceration at the treated site has been reported as occurring in up to a further 20% of patients[143]. Treatment of perianal warts is more painful and when cryotherapy for large condylomata is required, consideration should be given to the topical application of Emla cream for 15 minutes followed by infiltration of lidocaine (lignocaine) solution[144]. The treatment of perianal

---

* The refilling of flasks should be undertaken with great care. Thermal gloves and a protective perspex face shield should be worn, and, as the gas is an asphyxiant, refilling from a main container must be undertaken in a well-ventilated room.

warts by cryotherapy is more likely to be associated with ulceration and secondary infection than that of genital warts[145].

Efficacy

Three or more months after initiation of cryotherapy, 63% to 92% of patients have clearance of external genital warts[119]. Perianal warts do not respond as well as genital warts to freezing[146].

ELECTROCAUTERY

Thermal damage to wart tissue results from the application of a resistance wire heated with an electric current. It is an effective treatment in the case of genital warts that are discrete, and especially if they are also pedunculated. A 1% solution of lidocaine (lignocaine) is used as a local anesthetic and the wart removed with the cautery. The aim should be to coagulate the wart down to the basement membrane and cause minimal damage to the surrounding skin. When there are multiple warts, it may be necessary to undertake electrocautery on several occasions before total clearance is achieved. In the case of intrameatal warts, lidocaine (lignocaine) gel (20 mg/mL) may be instilled into the terminal urethra and the wart cauterized after 5 to 10 minutes. In the case of treated small warts, postoperative pain is minimal and the ulceration that inevitably follows electrocautery usually heals within 7 to 10 days with little scarring. When larger areas have been treated, analgesia may be required for several days after the procedure, and some scarring may result.

Efficacy

There have been few studies on treatment efficacy with electrocautery, but Simmons et al.[147] reported good results in a small series: 10 of 11 men had complete clearance of warts 3 months after treatment.

ELECTROSURGICAL METHODS

In these methods, reviewed by Scoular[140], heat is produced in tissue at the point of entry of high-frequency currents. Several methods may be useful in the treatment of genital warts:

1. *Electrofulguration.* High voltage, low amperage current sparks across an air gap between the electrode and the wart without touching it. There is little dermal damage and healing is rapid.

2. *Electrodessication.* This method is similar to electrofulguration, except that the electrode is in direct contact with the tissue.

3. *Cutting.* In addition to the cutting modality, a coagulating current is usually blended in. Electrosurgical cutting occurs under conditions of very high current density when the temperature rises rapidly and sufficiently to damage tissue[148]. Arcs form when the electric field between two electrodes becomes strong enough to ionize the particles in the space between the electrodes. Cutting diathermy is generally used in the treatment of large condylomata, and its use may require general anesthesia. Large loop excision of the T zone of the uterine cervix is used extensively in the management of suspected SILs and sometimes in the treatment of cervical condylomata. Local anesthesia for the procedure is necessary, and prilocaine hydrochloride 30 mg/mL with felypressin 0.03 unit/mL (Citanest® with Octapressin injection 3%) injected into the cervix with a dental syringe and needle is most satisfactory for this purpose.

Unwanted effects

Intensive coagulation can result in slow wound healing, secondary hemorrhage 10 to 14 days later, infection and scarring[140]. Bleeding during and after loop diathermy complicates up to 7% of women, and secondary hemorrhage occasionally occurs. Minor infection after the latter procedure is also common, but, although preterm birth and low birth weight in subsequent pregnancies were thought to be important complications, more recent data do not support this assumption. As burns, electrocution, fire, and interference with cardiac pacemakers are potential hazards of electro-

surgery, all precautions should be taken to prevent these[140].

Efficacy

Stone and colleagues[149] found that 94% of 88 patients had complete clearance of external genital warts within 6 weeks of initiation of weekly treatment by electrofulguration, and that 3 months later, 78% of 46 patients followed for that period were wart free. Few other studies on the efficacy of electrosurgery have been reported.

SCISSOR EXCISION

In the original descriptions of the method of scissor excision of perianal and intra-anal warts under general anesthesia, the wart-bearing area is infiltrated with saline adrenaline (epinephrine) solution (1/300 000); quantities of about 20 to 150 mL are required. The warts that have separated and become discrete are then removed with fine-pointed curved scissors by cutting at the base of the wart from back to front so that exudate and blood do not obscure progress[150, 151]. The method can be modified as an out-patient procedure for smaller warts in the perianal region, on the vulva and on the penis, only a local anesthesia being required[152]. The use of adrenaline (epinephrine) on the penis, however, is contraindicated. Postoperative pain is common but usually of mild-to-moderate severity and only requiring simple analgesia. Bleeding is minimal and healing is usually complete within 10 to 14 days, with little scarring.

Efficacy

Scissor excision is highly effective in removing external genital warts. In Jensen's study[153] of 30 patients with perianal warts, there were only two treatment failures when the individuals were assessed 1 week after the procedure, and the recurrence rate 12 months post-treatment was 29%, compared with 65% of 30 subjects whose warts had been treated with podophyllin. Khawaja[154] also noted a low recurrence rate of 19% of 16 patients at 42 weeks after scissor excision.

TRICHLOROETHANOIC ACID AND BICHLOROETHANOIC ACID

In the treatment of external genital warts, some physicians use trichloroethanoic acid (TCA) or bichloroethanoic acid (BCA) alone or in combination with podophyllin. The acid acts by coagulating the tissue proteins, with resultant necrosis. The acid in an 80% to 90% w/v solution in water is applied once weekly to the warts, using a wooden applicator stick or a plastic probe. Care should be taken to avoid contact with surrounding normal skin, and the solution should be allowed to dry before the patient sits or stands[130]. If pain is intense, the acid can be neutralized by dusting with sodium bicarbonate. There have been few studies on the efficacy of these acids, but Abdullah *et al.*[155] compared the results of weekly application of TCA solution (95% w/v) for up to 6 weeks with cryotherapy for the same time period. They noted that 21 (70%) of 30 patients whose warts had been treated with TCA and 37 (86%) of 43 individuals who had had cryotherapy had complete resolution of the warts 3 months after completion of treatment. Although they concluded that cryotherapy was more effective than TCA, the difference in resolution rates between the two regimens was not statistically significant. However, local ulceration was noted only in patients who had been treated with TCA.

Gabriel and Thin[156] found that patients who were treated with a combination of TCA and podophyllin (dispensed as a mixture of TCA 50% w/v and podophyllin resin 25% w/v) required fewer treatments (mean number of treatments was 2.9 (SD 1.1)) than those given podophyllin alone (mean number of treatments was 4.0 (SD 1.6)). They noted, however, more unwanted effects in the former group. It is stated that TCA is of limited value in the treatment of dry warts.

LASER THERAPY

The carbon dioxide laser is the most widely used for the treatment of anogenital warts. Infrared radiation produced by the laser is focused by a series of mirrors and lenses, all types of tissue absorb this energy. Different power densities produce different biological effects. A beam of about 0.1 mm in diameter is suitable for incising tissue, whereas a defocused beam of about 2 mm spot size can be used to vaporize tissue. Around the zone of vaporization, there is a margin of coagulation[148]. As thermal necrosis of healthy tissue is limited to about 50 μm beneath the zone of vaporization, areas treated with the carbon dioxide laser heal well. Laser treatment is performed with a hand piece or a micromanipulator, and the use of a smoke evacuator is necessary during vaporization.

Bar-Am and colleagues[157] found that 82% of 119 men treated for genital warts had complete clearance after one session of laser therapy; after three treatment sessions the condylomata of all patients had been removed. Fourteen weeks following the procedure, however, recurrence was noted in 9% of the men. Healing time ranged from 3 to 6 weeks, the longer healing time being observed in men who had diffuse lesions. Of 20 women with extensive vulval condylomata treated by laser ablation, Reid et al.[158] reported that 60% had had recurrence within 18 months of the procedure.

Laser therapy is seldom used as a first-line treatment of anogenital warts. As there is perfect control of tissue destruction and a reduced risk of hemorrhage, this form of treatment may be preferable to diathermy, electrocautery, or scissor excision in the management of extensive lesions that are considered only suitable for surgical removal. Improper power settings may damage normal tissues, and the authors consider that only physicians who are skilled in the use of lasers should undertake this procedure. As general anesthesia is often required when the condylomata are extensive, laser therapy has a limited role in the outpatient management of anogenital warts.

INTERFERONS

Because of their direct and indirect activity against viruses, interferons (INFs) have been assessed as treatments for HPV-related conditions of the anogenital region. Interferons, produced in response to viruses or double-stranded RNAs, fall into three groups

1. IFN-α, of which there are at least 20 variants, made by leukocytes,
2. IFN-β, a single protein produced by fibroblasts
3. IFN-γ made by activated T cells and natural killer cells.

The α- and β-interferons have antiviral and anti-proliferative activity and, although the antiviral activity of IFN-γ is less than that of the other two interferons, IFN-γ is a potent inducer of macrophage activation and of the expression of class II molecules on tissue cells, thereby allowing them to act as antigen-presenting cells.

Mode of action

Interferons act against viral infections in two ways.

1. *A direct antiviral effect.* Interferons activate two genes that code for proteins that have antiviral activity
   - a 67 kDa protein kinase that inhibits phosphorylation of e 1F-2 and blocks translation of proteins
   - 2'5' oligoadenylate synthetase that activates a latent endonuclease involved in degrading viral RNA. IFN-β, but not IFN-α or IFN-γ, has a marked and specific cytopathic effect on the HPV-infected human diploid keratinocyte cell line HPK-1A.
2. *Immune modulation.* In order that HPV-infected cells can be identified and an immune response elicited, viral epitopes must be presented to T cells in the context of expression of MHC class I and MHC class II molecules on the cell surface. The effects of systemic IFN-α and IFN-γ on the levels of mRNA of the genes of cytokines, accessory molecules, and infiltrating cells of the immune system has been investigated by Arany and colleagues[159, 160]. Interferons induce activation of MHC class II (HLA-DR) genes whose product presents antigen to CD4$^+$ T cells. In individuals who respond to interferon therapy, HLA-DR levels in condylomata are greatly up regulated[159], and the predominantly CD4$^+$ T cell infiltrate in regressing warts probably reflects this up regulation. As IL-1α (a stimulator of T$_{H1}$ cell

proliferation), IL-2, and IFN-γ (both cytokines are released from T$_{H1}$ cells) are up regulated in condylomata removed from patients responding to therapy, interferons appear to induce a T$_{H1}$ response. T$_{H1}$ cells activate macrophages as is seen in Type 1 responses, and clearance of virus results. The immune response in condylomata undergoing spontaneous regression in which CD4$^+$ T cells and macrophages predominate (see page 75) is consistent with that of delayed-type hypersensitivity. The up regulation of HLA-DR is not found in patients whose warts fail to respond, and as a result, the ability of keratinocytes (non-professional antigen-presenting cells) to function as antigen-presenting cells is impaired[160].

Class I MHC molecules and β_2-microglobulin form a complex on the surface of keratinocytes, and viral epitopes, processed by the infected keratinocyte, are presented to CD8$^+$ (cytotoxic) T cells in association with these molecules. Interferons activate the expression of MHC class I and β_2-microglobulin genes that ultimately results in the CD8$^+$ T cell infiltrate seen in warts that are regressing[159]. There are deficits in MHC class I expression in condylomata that fail to respond to treatment.

Up regulation of IL-1β and GM-CSF is found both in condylomata that respond to interferon therapy and those that do not, probably explaining the CD16 (natural killer cell/macrophage) infiltrate seen in both responders and non-responders[159].

The epithelium of condylomata is depleted of Langerhans cells, and this is particularly noted in those lesions that fail to respond to interferons. These cells are the professional antigen-presenting cells in the skin and their depletion may result in inappropriate antigen processing and immune response.

Different responses to interferon treatment may result from differential expression of different HPV genes. There is an inverse relationship between the inducibility of HLA-DR and the expression of E7 genes: condylomata that fail to respond to treatment have higher expression of E7 genes[160]. Higher capsid protein levels (L1 expression) may be associated with a better response to interferon[161].

Clinical efficacy

All three classes of interferons, used as single agents or as adjuvant therapy, and administered by either the systemic route, intralesional injection, or topically, have been studied in the treatment of anogenital warts. It should be noted that because criteria for patient selection, the duration of warts, and the extent of previous therapy have varied considerably, it is difficult to compare the results of different trials.

Interferon-α

Systemic interferon-α

As single agent therapy

The Condylomata International Collaborative Study Group reported in 1991[162] that in the treatment of warts of less than 6 months duration, IFN-α given subcutaneously in a dose of 1.5 MIU three times per week for 4 weeks was not as effective as podophyllin in producing clearance of the lesions. Only 15 (23%) of 64 patients treated with interferon had complete resolution of their warts 3 months after completion of therapy, compared with 31 (45%) of 69 individuals who had used podophyllin.

The Condylomata International Collaborative Study Group[163] reported the results of a double-blind placebo-controlled trial of IFN-α given by subcutaneous injection of 1.5 MIU three times per week for 4 weeks to patients whose anogenital warts had failed to respond to standard therapy. Three months after completion of treatment there was no significant difference in the complete or partial response rate between the interferon and placebo groups.

As adjuvant to other treatments

Conflicting results from different studies on the use of systemic IFN-α as adjuvant therapy have been published. Reid et al.[158] reported favorable results of interferon treatment following surgery. After laser removal of extensive anogenital warts, recombinant IFN-α was given by subcutaneous injection in a dose of 1 MIU three times per week for 10 weeks. Eighteen months after surgery, 21 (82%) of 27 women who had been treated in this way had complete resolution of warts, compared with only 17 (45%) of 38 patients treated by laser alone or by laser and the topical application of 5-fluorouracil cream. Less satisfactory results were reported by Armstrong et al.[164] who undertook a similar study. They found that IFN-α as adjuvant to surgery was no better than placebo in achieving complete regression of warts. Sixty-five (50%) of 131 patients treated by ablative therapy and IFN-α, and 29 (43%) of 67 treated by ablation only had complete response 38 weeks after initiation of treatment. Systemic IFN-α has also been used in cycles[165]. Three cycles, consisting of a subcutaneous injection of 1 MIU daily for 5 days, with a 4-week interval between each cycle, has been shown to be superior to continuous therapy in achieving resolution of anogenital warts.

The efficacy of combination treatment with systemic IFN-α given three times per week for 6 weeks and podophyllin applied twice weekly has been compared with podophyllin alone[166]. Complete disappearance of warts (that had been present for less than 6 months) by week 10 was found in 36% of 42 patients treated with interferon, and 26% of the 43 treated with podophyllin alone, a difference that was not significant. In addition, it was shown that there was no significant difference in the recurrence rate between the two treatment groups.

Eron et al.[167] studied the effect of subcutaneously administered IFN-α given three times per week for 8 weeks, on the recurrence of warts after clearance by cryotherapy. Over 60% of these patients had been treated previously for condylomata. At 6 months follow-up, 69% of the 36 patients who had received interferon, and 73% of the 37 who had been given placebo, had had recurrence, a difference that is not significant. A year earlier Handley et al.[168] had reported similar findings.

Intralesional interferon-α

As single agent therapy

The first large double-blind, placebo-controlled trial of intralesional IFN-α in the treatment of anogenital warts was published by Eron et al.[169]. Interferon-α, in a dosage of 1 MIU, was injected directly into one to three warts three times per week for 3 weeks.

Thirteen weeks after completion of treatment 36% of the interferon-treated warts, and 17% of the placebo-treated warts had cleared, a significant difference. The maximal clinical response was noted 1 week after completion of therapy, when 69% of the 124 interferon-treated individuals, and 15% of the 128 placebo-treated patients, had had at least a 50% reduction in wart area. Thereafter, the mean wart area in the interferon-treated group increased at a rate that was lower than that of the placebo group. Of 24 interferon-treated patients who had cleared their warts and who were followed-up, 5 (21%) had recurrence after more than 9 months. The rates of clearing of untreated warts in the interferon group and the placebo group were identical to the rate of clearing of placebo-treated warts. These authors also noted that the response to interferon therapy of both treated and untreated lesions was inversely related to wart age. A difference in regression rate was also noted in the placebo recipients, and older warts (more than 3 months duration) were more likely to persist. The response to interferon was also found to be inversely related to the pre-treatment size of the warts. Treatment response, however, was independent of previous treatment.

Compared with placebo, Friedman-Kien[170] found a significant difference in the response rate of patients treated with IFN-αn3 injected into the condylomata in a mean dose of 0.92 MU per treatment for up to 8 weeks. Twelve weeks after completion of therapy, 59% of 81 interferon-treated patients had complete resolution of warts, compared with 20% of 75 patients given placebo. Ten months later, however, recurrence was found in 10 of 41 interferon-treated patients and in 3 of 14 placebo recipients.

The response to IFN-α is reduced in HIV-infected individuals[171].

As adjuvant therapy

Douglas et al.[172] described the results of treatment of warts (three in each patient) with intralesional IFN-α as an adjuvant to podophyllin and with podophyllin alone. Sixty-seven percent of the 49 patients who received combination therapy had complete clearance of the three treated warts compared with 42% of the 48 who had been treated with podophyllin alone, a difference that was considered significant. Most (86%) of the study group of patients had been treated previously for warts. The duration of warts was associated with outcome; subjects that had had warts for less than 12 months responded better than those whose warts had been present longer. Unfortunately, recurrence at the test site was found in about 65% of patients who had had either treatment schedule.

Topical interferon-α

Good results were observed in the treatment of genital warts in men with human leukocyte IFN-α, 2 MIU/g cream, applied topically three times per day on 3 days per week for 4 weeks[173]. It was found that there was complete clearance of lesions in 18 of 20 men treated with interferon cream, but in only 12 of 20 men given podophyllotoxin cream, and 4 of 20 men who received placebo cream. Little detail on recurrence, however, was given, and an insufficient number of patients was studied to allow conclusions to be drawn on the efficacy of this treatment modality.

Interferon-β

Systemic interferon-β

Interferon-β has been evaluated as a potential treatment for anogenital warts and encouraging results were reported by Olmos et al.[174]. An intramuscular injection of 2 MIU of natural IFN-β or placebo was given daily for 10 days to 53 and 47 patients respectively. Eight weeks after completion of the injections, 51% of the evaluable subjects who had received interferon had had a complete response, compared with 29% of 45 placebo recipients, a difference that was statistically significant. The median time to disappearance of lesions was 1.56 months. The use of systemic IFN-β as adjuvant therapy has not been adequately investigated.

Intralesional interferon-β

Dinsmore and others[175] reported the results of a multicenter, placebo-controlled trial of recombinant human IFN-β1a, injected directly into the condyloma in a dosage of 1 MIU per lesion. Up to six warts in each patient were treated three times per

week for 3 weeks; the majority of these patients had been treated previously without success. Three weeks after the completion of therapy, treatment was significantly more successful, as defined by the complete disappearance of the treated warts or at least a 50% reduction in their area, in those patients who received interferon; this effect was particularly noticeable in women. A similar study was undertaken by Bornstein et al.[176] who noted complete clearance at 3-month follow-up in 12 of 30 patients treated with interferon, compared with 8 of 30 individuals given placebo. They also showed that the reduction in area of treated warts was significantly greater in those who had had an incomplete response to interferon than in those who had been given placebo (73% versus 33%).

Interferon-β gel

As an adjuvant to ablative therapy, Gross and colleagues[177] studied the effect of topical IFN-β gel, applied to the ablated area and adjacent skin or mucosa, five times per day for 4 weeks. After 24 weeks of follow-up, there was a significant difference in relapse rate between patients treated with interferon gel at a concentration of 0.15 MIU/g and those patients given placebo: 46% of 35 patients treated with interferon gel had had no relapse, compared with only 25% of 36 placebo recipients. For reasons that are incompletely understood, the response rate was lower in patients who had been treated with gel containing a higher concentration of interferon. Currently, IFN-β is not generally available in the UK or in the USA.

Interferon-γ

There have been comparatively few studies on the use of IFN-γ. Kirby and colleagues[178] reported on an open-labeled, dose-response trial in patients with refractory anogenital warts that had been present for a mean of 11.8 months (range 2 to 36 months), and who had had a mean of 2.1 prior treatment types (range 1 to 3 types). Overall, with one treatment course, complete remission was achieved in only 2 of 28 patients and partial remission in 46% of these individuals assessed 8 weeks post-treatment. Zouboulis[179]

showed no significant difference in the cure rates of warts in patients who had been given IFN-γ by subcutaneous injection for 7 days as adjuvant therapy to electrocautery or laser. These results suggest that, at present, there is no place for IFN-γ in the treatment of recalcitrant warts.

Adverse effects of interferons

The severity of side effects in patients treated with systemic or intralesional interferons is dose dependent. Most patients develop influenza-like symptoms, including fever, chills, headache, malaise, myalgia, and arthralgia within a few hours of parenteral injection, and nausea, vomiting, and diarrhea may all complicate treatment. These symptoms usually diminish with continued therapy after the first 2 to 3 days, although weakness, lethargy and fatigue may persist for the duration of therapy. Dizziness, vertigo, insomnia, depression, drowsiness, and confusion are uncommon side effects. Transient episodes of hypertonia or severe muscle weakness have been reported during the first few days of initiation of systemic IFN-β therapy (Biogen Europe Data Sheet 2000). Pain at the injection site is common, particularly when the intralesional route is used, but systemic side effects are fewer with this form of therapy. Transient leukopenia and, less often, thrombocytopenia, may occur, particularly in individuals who receive more than 3 MIU IFN-α per day. Plasma enzyme tests of liver function may rise transiently and, rarely, decreased renal function has been described (Roche Products Limited Data Sheet 2000). Although neutralizing antibodies are detected in about 20% of patients treated with IFN-α, especially recombinant IFN-α2a and in some treated with IFN-β[180], their significance is uncertain. The development of autoantibodies during treatment with interferons has been observed, and autoimmune disease has occurred in those with a predisposition to such disorders.

Interferon therapy is contraindicated in individuals with
- known hypersensitivity
- cardiac disease
- severe renal, hepatic, or myeloid dysfunction

- severe depression
- poorly controlled epilepsy.

The safety of interferons in pregnancy has not been established. Spontaneous abortion has been reported in pregnant rhesus monkeys that had been given very high doses of IFN-α and IFN-β during the early to mid-fetal period. The authors recommend that the interferons be avoided during pregnancy and lactation.

Conclusions on interferon therapy

The various studies on the efficacy of the interferons in the treatment of anogenital warts have yielded divergent results, probably because of the different inclusion criteria, formulation of the drug, mode of application, dose, treatment regimen, and follow-up period. Overall, however, there has been a failure to show a clear advantage of interferon treatments over conventional therapy with respect to efficacy. Although the local and systemic adverse events are usually mild to moderate in severity, the high frequency of these events, and the need for care in administration of the drug, particularly when intralesional injections are made, do not commend interferons for routine use in the management of anogenital warts.

IMIQUIMOD

Imiquimod is an immune-response modifier that has potent anti-tumor and antiviral activity. As it modulates innate immunity by activating macrophages and thereby inducing the Type 1 response considered responsible for wart regression, the drug has been evaluated for the treatment of condylomata.

Mechanism of action

Stanley[26] has recently reviewed imiquimod's mode of action. When given by mouth to primates or rodents, imiquimod induces high serum levels of IFN-α, tumor necrosis factor-α (TNF-α) and interleukin-6 (IL-6), and the topical application of imiquimod to the skin of hairless mice induces IFN-α and TNF-α. When human peripheral blood mononuclear cells are incubated in the presence of imiquimod a range of cytokines are produced: IFN-α, TNF-α, IL-1α, IL-1β, IL-6, IL-8, IL-10, IL-12, GM-CSF, G-CSF, MIP-1α and the IL-1 receptor antagonist. The efficiency of interferon production is dose-related. The principal source of IFN-α induced by imiquimod is a member of the macrophage/monocyte lineage, and it has been shown that the induction of several IFN A genes as well as IFN B, TNF-α, IL-6 and IL-8 genes occurs only in monocytes/macrophages[181]. IFN-γ is also produced when human peripheral blood mononuclear cells are incubated with imiquimod, and this can be inhibited by antibody against IL-12. Imiquimod treatment induces cytokine expression in keratinocytes: the expression of mRNAs for IFN-α, IL-6, and IL-8 is up regulated in neonatal foreskin cells cultured in the presence of imiquimod.

Spontaneous regression of anogenital warts is associated with a T_{H1}-type response (see page 75) and, as imiquimod activates macrophages and induces T_{H1}-type cytokines, it is the drug's ability to generate and maintain effective cell mediated immunity that probably explains its efficacy in clinical practice. This hypothesis is supported by the study reported by Tyring et al.[182]. Imiquimod or vehicle was applied to condylomata three times per week for up to 16 weeks. Biopsies of a treated wart or from skin from which a lesion had been cleared, were taken before treatment, 6 weeks later and at 16 weeks or the end of treatment. Tissue was analyzed for mRNA for several cytokines and for HPV DNA. Messenger RNAs for IFN-α, IFN-β, IFN-γ, TNF-α and IL-2 were increased in regressing lesions compared to non-regressing warts. It is likely that Langerhans cells or infiltrating monocytes are the source of this INF-α and TNF-α; imiquimod can certainly stimulate cytokine secretion from monocyte-derived dendritic cells and Langerhans cells[183]. There were significant decreases in HPV DNA that correlated with decreases in mRNA levels for L1 and E7. In turn, the reduction in levels of these viral proteins correlated with increases in IL-12, IFN-γ and TNF-α. A further property of some of these cytokines that may be important in producing wart regression is their effect on Langerhans cells. It is known that TNF-α and INF-γ activate these cells and induce migration. In regressing warts, the ratio of CD1a positive cells in the epidermis (Langerhans cells) to that in the stroma is lower than that seen in persisting warts and it has been suggested that this change results from activation of cells in the epidermis followed by their migration to the draining lymph nodes where antigen presentation to naïve T cells can occur[26].

Pharmacokinetic properties

Less than 0.9% of topically applied imiquimod cream is absorbed from the skin. The small quantity that is absorbed into the systemic circulation is rapidly excreted by both urinary and fecal routes (3M Health Care Data Sheet 2000).

Recommendations for use of imiquimod

Imiquimod, available as a cream (5% w/w) in single-use sachets, is currently licensed for use only on external genital or perianal warts. A thin layer of cream is applied to the wart area and allowed to remain on the skin for between 6 and 10 hours (preferably overnight) before washing with soap and water. The cream is applied three times per week, say on Monday, Wednesday, and Friday of each week, until the warts have regressed completely, or, as drug safety beyond this period has not been established, for a maximum of 16 weeks (3M Health Care Data Sheet 1999). If the patient develops marked pain or discomfort, it may be necessary to discontinue therapy. When symptoms have resolved, however, the drug can be re-introduced, although it may be helpful to reduce the frequency of applications, for example, by instructing the individual to apply the cream once in the first week, twice in the second, and three times per week thereafter. The use of imiquimod in the treatment of internal warts has not been evaluated and currently its application to urethral, cervical, intravaginal, and anal warts is not recommended. Inflammatory skin conditions may be aggravated by imiquimod, and its use should be avoided in patients with such genital conditions. As the cream may weaken condoms and diaphragms, alternative means of contraception should be considered until treatment has been completed (3M Health Care Data Sheet 1999).

Efficacy

In a recent double-blind, placebo-controlled trial of 5% imiquimod cream, applied three times per week for 8 weeks, Beutner and others[184] found complete resolution of warts in 37% of 51 imiquimod-treated patients and 0% of the 57 placebo recipients (by intent-to-treat analysis). The median time to complete clearance was 7 weeks. Thirty-four (76%) of the 45 imiquimod and 4 (8%) of the 50 placebo recipients experienced a 50% or more reduction in wart area by the end of the treatment period (by on-treatment analysis). Three of 16 patients who had complete resolution of warts developed recurrence during a 10-week follow-up.

In a further multicenter study with imiquimod being used daily for a maximum of 16 weeks, Beutner et al.[185] reported similar results with respect to complete wart clearance (Table 5.1). The clearance rate for female patients was significantly higher than that for males, and the median time to clearance was shorter for women (8 weeks) than for men (10 weeks). They also noted that 93% of 69 patients in the imiquimod group but only 23% of 75 placebo-treated patients had at least a 50% reduction in wart area. Of the 48 patients who had complete wart clearance and who were followed-up for 12 weeks after completion of therapy, 19% had recurrence.

Edwards et al.[186] reported on the use of 5% imiquimod cream applied three times per week for up to 16 weeks. In an intent-to-treat analysis, 54 (50%) of 109 patients had complete wart clearance compared with 11 (11%) of the 100 individuals given vehicle alone. Of those who had cleared the warts, 13% had recurrence.

Adverse events

Erythema develops in the majority of individuals treated with imiquimod, but excoriation and erosion are found in just under 50% of patients. Induration, vesiculation, scabbing, and ulceration occur less commonly.

Although teratogenic or embryo-toxic effects have not been observed in animal studies, the safety of imiquimod in the treatment of genital warts in pregnancy has not been established, and it is recommended that the drug should only be used in pregnant or lactating women if the benefits of treatment are likely to outweigh any risk (3M Health Care Data Sheet 1999).

Conclusions on use of imiquimod

Compared with other wart treatments imiquimod is expensive, and although its use may be cost-effective, its place as first-line management of condylomata is not yet established. From a consideration of its mode of action, however, it is not suitable for the treatment of long-standing, fibrotic warts.

OTHER IMMUNOMODULATORY AGENTS

Inosine pranobex

Inosine pranobex is an immunomodulatory agent that has been evaluated in the treatment of anogenital warts[187, 188], but, as efficacy has not been shown convincingly, it has no place in routine treatment.

An approach to treating anogenital warts in the immunocompetent patient

Patients with anogenital warts present the health care professional with two major problems: *recurrence* and *persistence*. These problems occur because of persistence of HPV in keratinocytes, defective immune responses in individuals with persistence and recurrence of warts, and the lack of specific antiviral therapy.

A scheme of management that has been found helpful is shown in Figure 5.25.

The hyperplastic condylomata acuminata that have been present for less than 3 months, often clear quickly after treatment with podophyllotoxin, imiquimod, podophyllin, or cryotherapy. Podophyllo-

toxin appears to be more effective than podophyllin in clearing warts and it has the added advantage that the patient can apply it. Recurrence, either at the site of the initial lesions or on adjacent skin or mucosa, is common, and probably indicates active viral activity in that area. Therefore, repeated cycles of treatment are often necessary before there is complete eradication. As surrounding tissue necrosis may occur, podophyllin or podophyllotoxin should not be used for the treatment of warts in the vagina, anal canal, or on the uterine cervix. Spontaneous regression of condylomata at these sites often occurs, and unless there are associated symptoms such as anorectal bleeding or troublesome vaginal discharge, they may be left untreated. If considered necessary, intravaginal warts can be treated by laser or by the installation of 5-fluorouracil cream. Loop diathermy for ectocervical warts has the advantage that histological examination for SIL is possible, and is the treatment of choice for cervical warts. Intra-anal warts are conveniently treated by scissor excision under local or general anesthesia.

Treatment with podophyllin or podophyllotoxin is less successful for sessile warts or lesions on dry skin surfaces, such as the shaft of the penis, and these are best treated by ablative methods. Extensive hyperplastic anogenital warts are often refractory to podophyllin, podophyllotoxin, and cryotherapy, and are best managed surgically or by the topical application of 5-fluorouracil cream.

Persistence at the same site for at least 6 months despite regular conventional treatment is common and, in only very few cases, is a feature of immunodeficiency. A special case, however, is that of pregnancy (see below).

In deciding on the treatment of persistent lesions it is worth considering the following.

1. *The size and number of the lesions.* Many individuals have few warts that are less than a millimetre in diameter and reassurance that spontaneous regression will eventually occur, together with counseling (see below), may be all that is necessary. In addition to the psychological morbidity, larger and more numerous warts, however, can

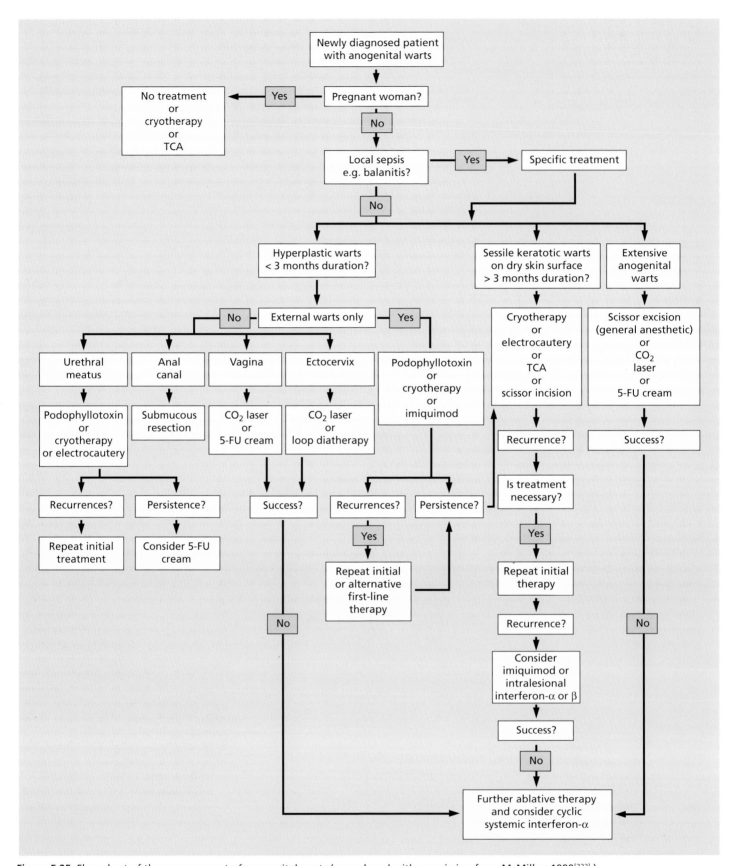

Figure 5.25 Flow chart of the management of anogenital warts (reproduced with permission from McMillan 1999[222])

cause discomfort, and, particularly at the urethral meatus and in the perianal region, they may bleed and become secondarily infected.

2. *How the patient perceives his or her infection.* Many patients seek some form of treatment because the presence of even the smallest wart causes considerable anxiety. In one study, about one-third of women with anogenital warts continued to worry about ever being cured[189], and many men also voice concern about the uncertainty of cure and lack of infectivity to partners[190].

In counseling the patient, it is helpful to discuss the following

- the benign nature of the lesions
- feelings of guilt about having acquired a STI
- the long pre-patent period, thus not necessarily indicating infidelity on the part of a partner in a monogamous relationship, it is sometimes helpful to discuss this issue with both partners.
- the natural history of HPV infection
- treatment that is not curative
- the possible adverse effects of treatment of small lesions; there may be damage to surrounding, latent virus-containing tissue with the subsequent growth of warts at that site (Koebner phenomenon)
- methods for reducing the risk of transmission of HPV to a sexual partner (see Prevention of transmission of human papillomavirus infection, p. 100). Whether or not infection with one type of HPV confers immunity against infection with other types or reinfection with the same type is uncertain. However, the use of condoms has been shown to improve the clearance rate in males with genital warts[191], and, although there is no clear evidence that their use reduces the risk of re-infection from a sexual partner, it is best perhaps to advocate the use of condoms until the lesions have been cleared for, say, 3 months.

Sometimes such reassurance is all that is required, but some patients are not satisfied with this approach and demand treatment.

Cryotherapy can be very successful in clearing warts that have failed to respond to podophyllin: perianal warts, however, do not respond very well. However, scissor excision, either under local or general anesthetic, is particularly helpful in the management of perianal warts and for sessile lesions of the labia majora and shaft of the penis. The results are generally good with little scarring at the excision site. Circumcision may be necessary in diabetic men with preputial warts and phimosis. Electrocautery and, where available, diathermy and laser therapy are alternative treatment methods, but, if the lesions are extensive, there may be considerable pain at the operation site and the wounds may heal more slowly than after scissor excision.

The topical application of tri- or bichloroethanoic acid may be successful in the treatment of small persistent lesions, but painful ulceration may result.

Some physicians use two or more treatment modalities on a single wart, for example, cryotherapy followed by the topical application of podophyllin or podophyllotoxin. Other than the combination of podophyllin and trichloroethanoic acid (see page 90), however, there is little evidence that these regimens are more effective than single agent therapy, and, in the authors' experience, there is an increased frequency of discomfort and pain.

The topical application of 5-fluorouracil (5%) cream may be useful in the treatment of refractory condylomata of the urethral meatus and of the perianal area. Local adverse effects, particularly ulceration, are common and the patient should be warned about these.

Even with ablative methods, recurrence is not uncommon and, if further ablative treatment fails, immunomodulatory therapy may be tried to reduce the risk of further recurrence.

Treatment of warts in pregnancy

In pregnant women, spontaneous regression of condylomata acuminata warts often occurs during the first few weeks after delivery, but sometimes they do not disappear completely[192]. During the pregnancy, when the lesions are small and symptomless, the authors favor a non-intervention approach. The woman should be reassured that spontaneous regression within several weeks of delivery is the usual outcome, and that any persistent warts can be treated as described earlier. There is no evidence that eradication of warts during pregnancy reduces the risk of perinatal transmission which, in any case, is low (see page 99). When treatment is indicated, for example, because of discomfort or patient choice, options are somewhat limited. The use of podophyllin, podophyllotoxin, and 5-fluorouracil cream should be avoided, and the safety of imiquimod in pregnancy has not been established. Scissor excision of extensive lesions may result in severe hemorrhage, and diathermy may cause considerable postoperative pain. Cryotherapy, electrocautery, or the cautious application of trichloroethanoic acid can be used to treat small condylomata but recurrence or persistence is common during the pregnancy. Good results have been reported in the treatment of condylomata by laser vaporization, with no recurrences being observed in a group of 16 women treated at gestational ages between 13 and 35 weeks[193]. When warts are extensive, however, this method will necessitate general anesthesia.

As the risks of cesarean section are likely to outweigh the possible benefits of reducing the risk of perinatal transmission of HPV to the neonate, this method of delivery is not indicated in the management of women with condylomata acuminata unless there are other obstetric indications. Cesarean section, however, may be indicated in the rare instances when the condylomata are so large that they obstruct labor or are thought likely to cause significant hemorrhage during vaginal delivery.

Treatment of warts in the immunocompromised patient

The response to treatment with the modalities described above is often unsatisfactory. Repeated treatments are almost always required. In the management of anogenital warts in HIV-infected patients, imiquimod has been useful. Gilson et al.[194] conducted a prospective, randomized, double-blind, vehicle-controlled trial in 100 HIV-infected patients, 65 given imiquimod and 35 treated with vehicle alone. They found that, although there was no significant difference between vehicle and drug with respect to complete clearance of warts, a reduction more than 50% in the area of the warts was noted in significantly more imiquimod recipients (38% versus 14%).

Treatment of squamous intraepithelial lesions

CERVIX

It is generally agreed that all patients with H-SIL should be treated once diagnosed, while patients with L-SIL may be treated or followed up carefully[112]. Squamous intraepithelial lesions of the uterine cervix are now most commonly treated by loop electrosurgical excision procedure. Laser conization or vaporization are alternative treatment methods. For detailed descriptions on treatment, the interested reader is referred to one of the excellent text books on colposcopy. Following treatment, the first smear should be taken at 6 months and if normal repeated at 12 months[112].

VAGINA

The relationship between vaginal SILs and invasive disease is not well defined. In a study of 23 women with such lesions, vaginal carcinoma developed in two cases, lesions persisted in three women, and spontaneous regression occurred in 18 cases[195]. Vaginal SILs can be treated by excisional biopsy or laser vaporization.

VULVA

The risk of progression of vulval SILs to carcinoma in young women (under the age of 30 years) is very low, but about 30% of older women have progression of the disease. In younger women, however, progression may occur in those who are immunocompromised. Spontaneous regression of the lesions in untreated women has been described[109] but the mechanisms are

uncertain. For small localized lesions, simple excision, laser vaporization, or electrosurgery are the treatments of choice. Recurrence after local excision is common (about 30% of cases) and most likely to occur if the edges of the excised tissue show, histologically, SIL[110]. As about 30% of patients with vulval SIL have concomitant cervical SILs or lower genital tract malignancy, in each patient a thorough gynecological examination is essential.

PENIS

The risk of progression of penile SILs to malignancy is low in young men, but over the age of 50 years the risk increases. Spontaneous regression of the lesions has occasionally been described[196], but cryotherapy, laser vaporization, and local excision have been used successfully in the treatment of this condition.

ANUS

It is common experience that L-SIL of the anal canal in immunocompetent individuals often regresses spontaneously. High-grade lesions should, however, be excised[197]. *NB In the absence of coexisting SILs, screening for and treatment of subclinical HPV infection is not recommended*[198].

Human papillomavirus infection in children

JUVENILE-ONSET LARYNGEAL PAPILLOMATOSIS (RECURRENT RESPIRATORY PAPILLOMATOSIS, RRP)

The incidence and prevalence of juvenile-onset laryngeal papillomatosis are essentially unknown. Kashima *et al.*[199] estimated that the proportion of infants who subsequently develop the condition varies between 1 in 80 and 1 in 1500 live births, with children born to mothers with condylomata being at greatest risk (1 in 400). Despite the increase in the incidence of HPV infection, there has not been a parallel

rise in that of juvenile-onset laryngeal papillomatosis.

Juvenile-onset laryngeal papillomatosis is almost always associated with infection with HPV types 6 and 11[200], rarely type 16 has been identified in lesions[201]. Studies suggest that there is maternal transmission of HPV to the child

- up to 60% of mothers whose children are affected have a history of genital warts[202]
- Kashima *et al.*[203] noted that cases were more likely to be first-born, to have been delivered vaginally and to have been born to young mothers than a control group of children.

As affected children have been born to mothers delivered by cesarean section, it is probable that some infants become infected through ascending infection[201].

Juvenile-onset disease presents before the age of 16 years, with the majority (75% to 83%) presenting between 3 to 4 months and 5 years of birth[204]. Hoarseness is the first symptom in 90% of cases. The sites of predilection are the ciliated and squamous epithelial junctions, namely the laryngeal surface of the epiglottis, the upper and lower margins of the ventricles, the under surface of the vocal cords, and the carina[205]. Between 2% to 17% of cases of juvenile-onset laryngeal papillomatosis involve the distal trachea and bronchi. Untreated, there is progressive respiratory obstruction with stridor, and possibly death. Malignant transformation may develop, either in association with smoking and irradiation, or spontaneously with an incidence of 2% to 3%[204]. Although spontaneous regression of juvenile-onset laryngeal papillomatosis has been noted at puberty, this is certainly not always the case, and recurrences have been observed in about 50% of individuals 6 to 12 years after puberty[206].

Treatment is aimed at ensuring a safe airway, and this necessitates the removal of the papillomata using a carbon dioxide laser. Although systemic, topical, and intralesional chemotherapy has been studied, the general conclusion is that these treatments are unsatisfactory[204]. The same conclusion has been reached with respect to interferons as adjuvant therapy.

ANOGENITAL WARTS

As in the case of juvenile-onset laryngeal papillomatosis, the incidence and prevalence of anogenital warts in children is unknown. Serological studies, however, suggest that HPV infection with the anogenital types is uncommon. For example, af Geijerstam *et al.*[207] detected antibody against capsids of HPV 16, 18, and 33 in the sera of only 3.0%, 0.6%, and 2.7% respectively from 1031 Swedish children aged 0 to 13 years.

Although HPV-associated lesions in prepubertal children cannot be regarded as a definite indication of sexual abuse, it is a possibility that requires to be taken into account by the clinician. In just over three-quarters of children, these warts are caused by the same HPV types, 6 and 11, that cause condylomata acuminata in adults, but the source of infection is often in doubt.

Perinatal transmission is, of course, a possibility. The transmission of HPV, including types 16 and 18, from mother to child has been described. An important factor in transmission is the viral load in cervical/vaginal cells; women with a high viral load as determined by laser densitometry of PCR products, are more likely to transmit infection to their infants than those with a low viral load[208]. Confirmation of the maternal origin of infant infection comes from the work of Kaye and colleagues[209] who showed that concordant HPV-16 variants or prototypic sequences were detected in 9 of 13 mother/infant samples. The rare reports of condylomata acuminata in the neonate[210], and the development of lesions in infants born by cesarean section[211], suggest that intra-uterine infection is also possible. Support for this hypothesis comes from the detection of viral DNA in the amniotic fluid of 24 of 37 pregnant women with cervical HPV infection[212], and transplacental transmission of HPV is suggested by the finding of HPV DNA in the cord blood of infants born to mothers with known HPV infection[213]. A child can therefore become infected *in utero* or during parturition. The risk of neonatal infection, however, appears to be low. Watts and colleagues[214] identified 112 women who had historical, clinical, or DNA evidence of HPV infection, and assessed infants at regular intervals for 36 months after birth. Using a

PCR with HPV L1 consensus primers, they detected viral DNA in only 5 (1.5%) of 335 genital specimens from the infants, 4 (1.2%) of the 324 anal specimens, and none of the 372 oro-pharyngeal specimens; none of the children developed anogenital warts. The pre-patent period for anogenital warts acquired through vertical transmission is difficult to assess, but some clinicians consider an upper limit of 2 to 3 years from birth[215].

Transmission of HPV through sexual abuse most certainly occurs, but the proportion of cases of anogenital warts that result from abuse is uncertain. Robinson[216] reviewed all the reported studies since 1976 and concluded that about 50% of cases are related to sexual abuse. The detection of child sexual abuse is often difficult, but other clinical and social findings may indicate the possibility (see Chapter 3).

Inoculation of the anogenital skin of young children (aged 18 months to 5 years) with HPV (types 2a/27/57) from the hand warts of a mother is well documented, and in older children, auto-inoculation from the child's own hands is described[215].

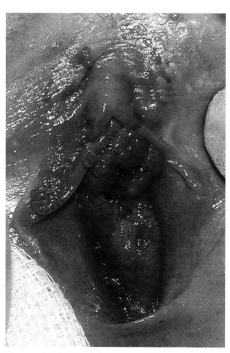

Figure 5.26 Condylomata at the vaginal introitus of an 18-month old girl (reproduced from McMillan and Scott 2000[224])

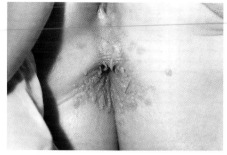

Figure 5.27 Condylomata acuminata of the perianal region in a 2-year-old girl

Condylomata acuminata in children resemble those of the adult, and are found

- *in girls* at the vaginal introitus (Figure 5.26), and in the urethral, perineal and perianal areas (Figure 5.27), in the perianal region, warts are often confluent, forming a mat around the anus
- *in boys* in the perianal and perigenital areas, penile condylomata are uncommon[192].

Sessile (papular) warts are found on the fully keratinized epithelium of the anogenital region. They are usually multiple, raised papules with a smooth surface (Figure 5.28).

In the management of the child over the age of 1 year with anogenital warts, it is important to consider the possibility of sexual abuse and to exclude other STIs in

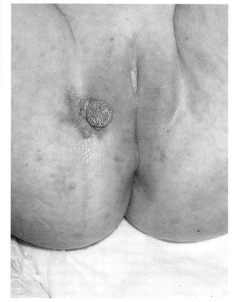

Figure 5.28 Sessile warts in a 13-month-old girl

such children. It has been suggested that the screening should include an HIV antibody test, particularly when a concurrent STI has been diagnosed[217]. A more detailed discussion on the investigation of the sexually abused child is found in Chapter 4.

TREATMENT

As spontaneous regression occurs within 1 year of their appearance in over 75% of cases[218], it has been suggested that symptomless anogenital warts in children should be left untreated for at least 1 year. The treatments recommended for adults can be used but imiquimod and podophyllotoxin are not recommended for use in children. Podophyllin may be used to treat small, soft condylomata, but it should be applied cautiously as a 10% w/v suspension, because of possible damage to surrounding skin. As systemic absorption may occur when this agent is applied to large condylomata, podophyllin is best avoided in these circumstances[192]. Ablative methods under general anesthesia may be necessary for refractory warts or for keratinized lesions.

Prevention of transmission of human papillomavirus infection

Prevention of HPV infection is difficult. Genital warts are contagious, and, although lesions can be eradicated by treatment, there is no certainty that the patient is no longer infectious to others. HPV is transmitted by direct skin-to-skin or mucosa contact, and it is unlikely that even consistent use of condoms will eliminate the risk of infection. There is now good evidence, however, that the risk can be reduced by condom use. In a case-control study, Syrjanen *et al.*[219] found that women whose partners did not use condoms were at increased risk of cervical HPV infection: partners of 16% of 146 women with cervical HPV compared with 12% of 146 women with no clinical evidence of infection. A more recent case-control study from Sydney, Australia[220] showed that men who used condoms consistently were much less likely to have genital warts than those who did not (odds ratio 0.7, 95% confidence interval 0.3–0.9). Women whose partners always used condoms were also less likely to have genital warts (odds ratio 0.7, 95% confidence interval 0.4–1.0).

References

1 Van Ranst M, Tachezy R, Burk RD. Human papillomaviruses: a never-ending story? In: Lacey C (ed.) *Papillomavirus Reviews: Current Research on Papillomaviruses.* Leeds; Leeds University Press: 1996.

2 Bosch FX, Manos MM, Munoz N, *et al.* Prevalence of human papillomavirus in cervical cancer: a worldwide perspective. *J Natl Cancer Inst* 1995; **87**: 796–802.

3 Meyers C, Laimins LA. *In vitro* model systems for the study of HPV induced neoplasias. In: Lacey C (ed.) *Papillomavirus Reviews: Current Research on Papillomaviruses.* Leeds; Leeds University Press: 1996.

4 Stoler MH, Whitbeck A, Wolinsky SM, *et al.* Infectious cycle of human papillomvirus type 11 in human foreskin xenograffts in nude mice. *J Virol* 1990; **64**: 3310–3318.

5 Kreider JW, Howett MK, Leure-Dupree AE, Zaing RJ, Weber JA. Laboratory production *in vivo* of human papillomavirus type 11. *J Virol* 1987; **61**: 590–593.

6 Hagensee ME, Galloway DA. Growing human papillomaviruses and virus-like particles in the laboratory. In: Lacey C (ed.) *Papillomavirus Reviews: Current Research on Papillomaviruses.* Leeds; Leeds University Press: 1996.

7 Schiller JT, Roden RBS. Papillomavirus-like particles: basic and applied studies. In: Lacey C (ed.) *Papillomavirus Reviews: Current Research on Papillomaviruses.* Leeds; Leeds University Press: 1996.

8 Howley PM. Papillomavirinae: the viruses and their replication. In: Fields BN, Knipe DM, Howley PM (eds) *Fields Virology* 3rd edition. Philadelphia; Lippincott-Raven: 1996.

9 Evander M, Frazer IH, Payne E, Qi YM, Hengst K, McMillan NA. Identification of the alpha6 integrin as a candidate receptor for papillomaviruses. *J Virol* 1997; **71**: 2449–2456.

10 Chiang CM, Ustar M, Stenlund A, Ho TF, Broker TR, Chow LT . Viral E1 and E2 proteins support replication of homologous and heterologous papillomavirus origins. *Proc Natl Acad Sci USA* 1992; **89**: 5799–5803.

11 Del Vecchio AM, Romanczuk H, Howley PM, Baker CC. Transient replication of human papillomavirus DNAs. *J Virol* 1992; **66**: 5949–5958.

12 Yang L, Mohr I, Fouts E, Lim DA, Nohaile M, Botchan M. The E1 protein of bovine papillomavirus 1 is an ATP-dependent DNA helicase. *Proc Natl Acad Sci USA* 1993; **90**: 5086–5090.

13 Crook T, Vousden KH. HPV oncogene function. In: Lacey C (ed.) *Papillomavirus Reviews: Current Research on Papillomaviruses.* Leeds; Leeds University Press: 1996.

14 Thierry F. HPV proteins in the control of HPV transcription. In: Lacey C (ed.) *Papillomavirus Reviews: Current Research on Papillomaviruses.* Leeds; Leeds University Press: 1996.

15 Klingelhutz AJ, Foster SA, McDougall JK. Telomerase activation by the E6 gene product of human papillomvirus type 16. *Nature* 1996; **380**: 79–82.

16 Hurlin PJ, Kaur P, Smith PP, Perz-Reyes N, Blanton RA, McDougall JK. Progression of human papillomavirus type-18 immortalised cells to a malignant phenotype. *Proc Natl Acad Sci USA* 1991; **88**: 570–574.

17 Garrett LR, Perz-Reyes N, Smith PP, McDougall JK. Interaction of HPV-18 and nitrosomethylurea in the induction of squamous cell carcinoma. *Carcinogenesis* 1993; **14**: 329–332.

18 Stanley M, Sarkar S. Genetic changes in cervical carcinoma. In: Lacey C (ed.) *Papillomavirus Reviews: Current Research on Papillomaviruses.* Leeds; Leeds University Press: 1996.

19 McMillan A, Bishop PE, Fletcher S. An immunohistological study of condylomata acuminata. *Histopathology* 1990; **17**: 45–52.

20 Reagan JW, Seidemann IL, Saracusa Y. Cellular morphology of carcinoma in situ and dysplasia or atypical hyperplasia of uterine cervix. *Cancer* 1953; **6**: 224–225.

21 Wright TC, Kurman RJ. A critical review of the morphologic classification systems of preinvasive lesions of the cervix: the scientific basis for shifting the paradigm. *Papillomavirus Rep* 1994; **5**: 175–182.

22 Richart RM. Natural history of cervical intraepithelial neoplasia. *Clin Obstet Gynecol* 1968; **10**: 748–784.

23 National Cancer Institute Workshop: the 1988 Bethesda System for reporting cervical/vaginal cytologic diagnoses. *JAMA* 1989; **262**: 931–934.

24 Bishop PE, McMillan A, Fletcher S. An immunohistological study of spontaneous regression of condylomata acuminata. *Genitourin Med* 1990; **66**: 79–81.

25 Coleman N, Birley HDL, Renton AM, *et al.* Immunological events in regressing genital warts. *Am J Clin Pathol* 1994; **102**: 768–774.

26 Stanley MA. Mechanism of action of imiquimod. *Papillomavirus Rep* 1999; **10**: 23–29.

27 Christensen ND, Kreider JW. Antibody-mediated neutralization in vivo of infectious papillomaviruses. *J Virol* 1990; **64**: 3151–3156.

28 Christensen ND, Kreider JW, Shah KV, Rando RF. Detection of human serum antibodies that neutralize infectious human papillomavirus type 11 virions. *J Gen Virol* 1992; **73**: 1261–1267.

29 Christensen ND, Kreider JW, Cladel NM, Patrick SD, Welsh PA. Monoclonal antibody-mediated neutralization of infectious human papillomavirus type 11. *J Virol* 1990; **64**: 5678–5681.

30 Carter JJ, Wipf GC, Hagensee ME, *et al.* Use of human papillomavirus type 6 capsids to detect antibodies in people with genital warts. *J Infect Dis* 1995; **172**: 11–18.

31 Christensen ND, Cladel NM, Reed CA. Postattachment neutralization of papillomaviruses by monoclonal and polyclonal antibodies. *Virology* 1995; **207**: 136–142.

32 Wikstrom A, van Doornum GJ, Quint WG, Schiller JT, Dillner J. Identification of human papillomavirus seroconversions. *J Gen Virol* 1995; **76**: 529–539.

33 Greer CE, Wheeler CM, Ladner MB, *et al.* Human papillomavirus (HPV) type distribution and serological response to HPV type 6 virus-like particles in patients with genital warts. *J Clin Microbiol* 1995; **33**: 2058–2063.

34 Wikstrom A, Eklund C, von Krogh G, Lidbrink P, Dillner J. Antibodies against human papillomavirus type 6 capsids are elevated in men with previous condylomas. *Acta Pathol Microbiol Scand* 1997; **105**: 884–888.

35 Carter JJ, Koutsky LA, Hughes JP, *et al.*. Comparison of human papillomavirus types 16, 18, and 6 capsid antibody responses following incident infection. *J Infect Dis* 2000; **181**: 1911–1919.

36 af Geijersstam V, Kibur M, Wang Z, *et al.* Stability over time of serum antibody levels to human papillomavirus type 16. *J Infect Dis* 1998; **177**: 1710–1714.

37 Van Doornum G, Prins M, Andersson-Ellstrom A, Dillner J. Immunoglobulin A, G, and M responses to L1 and L2 caspids of human papillomavirus types 6, 11, 18 and 33 L1 after newly acquired infection. *Sex Transm Infect* 1998; **74**: 354–360.

38 Wang ZH, Kjellberg L, Abdalla H, *et al.* Type specificity and significance of different isotypes of serum antibodies to human papillomavirus capsids. *J Infect Dis* 2000; **181**: 456–462.

39 Wikstrom A, van Doornum GJ, Kirnbauer R, Quint WG, Dillner J. Prospective study on the development of antibodies against human papillomavirus type 6 among patients with condyloma acuminata or new asymptomatic infection. *J Med Virol* 1995; **46**: 368–374.

40 Wang Z, Hansson BG, Forslund O, *et al.* Cervical mucus antibodies against human papillomavirus type 16, 18 and 33 capsids in relation to presence of viral DNA. *J Clin Microbiol* 1996; **34**: 3056–3062.

41 Hagensee ME, Koutsky LA, Lee SK, *et al.* Detection of cervical antibodies to human papillomavirus type 16 (HPV-16) capsid antigens in relation to detection of HPV-16 DNA and cervical lesions. *J Infect Dis* 2000; **181**: 1234–1239.

42 Koutsky LA, Galloway DA, Holmes KK. Epidemiology of genital human papillomavirus infection. *Epidemiol Rev* 1988; **10**: 122–163.

43 Ismail SM, Colclough AB, Dinnen JS, *et al.* Observer variation in histopathological diagnosis and grading of cervical intraepithelial neoplasia. *Br Med J* 1989; **298**: 707–710.

44 Syrjanen K, Syrjanen S. Epidemiology of human papillomavirus infections and genital neoplasia. *Scand J Infect Dis* 1990; **69** (Suppl.): 7–17.

45 Kiviat NB, Koutsky LA, Paavonen JA, *et al.* Prevalence of genital papillomavirus infection among women attending a college student health clinic or a sexually transmitted disease clinic. *J Infect Dis* 1989; **159**: 293–302.

46 Martinez J, Smith R, Farmer M, *et al.* High prevalence of genital tract papillomavirus infection in female adolescents. *Pediatrics* 1988; **82**: 604–608.

47 Hippelainen M, Syrjanen S, Hippelainen M, *et al.* Prevalence and risk factors of genital human papillomavirus (HPV) infections in healthy males: a study of Finnish conscripts. *Sex Transm Dis* 1993; **20**: 321–328.

48 Bauer HM, Ting Y, Greer CE, *et al.* Genital human papillomavirus infection in female university students as determined by a PCR-based method. *JAMA* 1991; **265**: 472–477.

49 Melkert PW, Hopman E, van den Brule AJ, *et al.* Prevalence of HPV in cytomorphologicaly normal cervical smears, as determined by the polymerase chain reaction, is age-dependent. *Int J Cancer* 1993; **53**: 919–923.

50 Kataoka A, Claesson U, Hansson BG, Eriksson M, Lindh E. Human papillomavirus infection of the male diagnosed by southern-blot hybridization and polymerase reaction: comparison between urethra samples and penile biopsy samples. *J Med Virol* 1991; **33**: 159–164.

51 Palefsky JM, Holly EA, Ralston ML, Jay N. Prevalence and risk factors for human papillomavirus infection of the anal canal in human immunodeficiency virus (HIV)-positive and HIV-negative homosexual men. *J Infect Dis* 1998; **177**: 361–367.

52 Meisels A. Cytologic diagnosis of human papillomavirus. Influence of age and pregnancy stage. *Acta Cytol* 1992; **36**: 480–482.

53 Evander M, Edlund K, Gustaffson A, *et al.* Human papillomavirus infection is transient in young women: a population-based cohort. *J Infect Dis* 1995; **171**: 1026–1030.

54 Ho GYF, Bierman R, Beardsley L, Chang CJ, Burk RD. Natural history of cervicovaginal papillomavirus infection in young women. *N Engl J Med* 1998; **338**: 423–428.

55 Oriel JD. Natural history of genital warts. *Br J Vener Dis* 1971; **47**: 1–13.

56 Fairley CK, Chen S, Tabrizi SN, Leeton K, Quinn MA, Garland SM. The absence of genital human papillomavirus DNA in virginal women. *Int J STD AIDS* 1992; **3**: 414–417.

57 Rylander E, Ruusuvaara L, Almstromer MW, Evander M, Wadell G. The absence of vaginal human papillomavirus 16 DNA in women who have not experienced sexual intercourse. *Obstet Gynecol* 1994; **83**: 735–737.

58 Bauer HM, Hildesheim A, Schiffman MH, *et al.* Determinants of genital human papillomavirus infection in low-risk women in Portland, Oregon. *Sex Transm Dis* 1993; **20**: 274–278.

59 Schneider A, Kirchmayr R, De Villiers EM, Gissman L. Subclinical human papillomavirus infections in male sexual partners of female carriers. *J Urol* 1988; **140**: 1431–1434.

60 Baken LA, Kooutsky LA, Kuypers J, *et al.* Genital human papillomavirus infection among male and female sex partners: prevalence and type specific concordance. *J Infect Dis* 1995; **171**: 429–432.

61 Ho L, Tay S-K, Chan S-Y, Bernard HU. Sequence variants of human papillomavirus type 16 from couples suggest sexual transmission with low infectivity and polyclonality in genital neoplasia. *J Infect Dis* 1993; **168**: 803–809.

62 Xi LF, Demers GW, Koutsky LA, *et al.* Analysis of human papillomavirus type 16 variants indicated establishment of persistent infection. *J Infect Dis* 1995; **172**: 747–755.

63 Feldman JG, Chirgwin K, Lehovitz JA, Minkoff H. The association of smoking and risk of condyloma acuminatum in women. *Obstet Gynecol* 1997; **80**: 346–350.

64 Sonnex C, Strauss S, Gray JJ. Detection of human papillomavirus DNA on the fingers of patients with genital warts. *Sex Transm Infect* 1999; **75**: 317–319.

65 Mindel A, Tideman R. HPV transmission – still feeling the way. *Br Med J* 1999; **354**: 2097–2098.

66 Krzyzek RA, Watts SL, Anderson DL, Faras AJ, Pass F. Anogenital warts contain several distinct species of human papillomavirus. *J Virol* 1980; **36**: 236–244.

67 Gonzalez-Moles MA, Ruiz-Avila I, Gonzalez-Moles S, Martinez I, Ceballos A, Nogales F. Detection of HPV DNA by in situ hybridization in benign, premalignant and malignant lesions of the oral mucosa. *Bull Groupment Int Rech Scient Stomatol Odontol* 1994; **37**: 79–85.

68 Lambropoulos AF, Dimitrakopoulos J, Frangoulides E, Katopodi R, Kotsis A, Karakasis D. Incidence of human papillomavirus 6, 11, 16, 18 and 33 in normal oral mucosa of a Greek population. *Eur J Oral Sci* 1997; **105**: 294–297.

69 Badaracco G, Venuti A, DiLonardo A, *et al.* Concurrent HPV infection in oral and genital mucosa. *J Oral Pathol Med* 1998; **27**: 130–134.

70 Clarke J, Terry RM, Lacey CJN. A study to estimate the prevalence of upper respiratory tract papillomatosis in patients with genital warts. *Int J STD AIDS* 1991; **2**: 114–115.

71 Liaw KL, Glass AG, Manos MM, *et al.* Detection of human papillomavirus DNA in cytologically normal women and subsequent cervical squamous epithelial lesions. *J Natl Cancer Inst* 1999; **91**: 954–960.

72 Parkin DM, Pisani P, Ferlay J. Estimates of the worldwide incidence of eighteen major cancers in 1985. *Int J Cancer* 1993; **54**: 594–606.

73 Josefsson AM, Magnusson PKE, Ylitalo N, *et al.* Viral load of human papilloma virus 16 as a determinant of cervical carcinoma in situ: a nested case-control study. *Lancet* 2000; **355**: 2189–2193.

74 Ylitalo N, Sorensen P, Josefsson AM, *et al.* Consistent high viral load of human papillomavirus 16 and risk of cervical carcinoma in situ: a nested case-control study. *Lancet* 2000; **355**: 2194–2198.

75 Chau KL, Wiklund F, Lenner P, *et al.* A prospective study on the risk of cervical intra-epithelial neoplasia among healthy subjects with serum antibodies to HPV compared with HPV DNA in cervical smears. *Int J Cancer* 1996; **68**: 54–59.

76 Lehtinen M, Dillner J, Knekt P, *et al.* Serological diagnosed infection with human papillomavirus type 16 and risk for subsequent development of cervical carcinoma: nested case-control study. *Br Med J* 1996; **312**: 537–539.

77 Nischan P, Ebeling K, Schindler C. Smoking and invasive cervical cancer risk. Results from a case-control study. *Am J Epidemiol* 1988; **128**: 74–77.

78 Barton SE, Maddox PH, Jenkins D, Edwards R, Cuzick J, Singer A. Effect of cigarette smoking on cervical epithelial immunity: a mechanism for neoplastic change? *Lancet* 1988; **ii**: 652–654.

79 Holly EA, Petrakis NL, Friend NF, Sarles DL, Lee RE, Flander LB. Mutagenic mucus in the cervix of smokers. *J Natl Cancer Inst* 1986; **76**: 983–986.

80 Kurman RJ, Toki T, Schiffman MH. Basaloid and warty carcinomas of the vulva. Distinctive types of squamous cell carcinoma frequently associated with human papillomaviruses. *Am J Surg Pathol* 1993; **17**: 133–145.

81 Hording U, Kringsholm B, Andreasson B, Visfeldt J, Daugaard S, Bock JE. Human papillomavirus in vulvar squamous-cell carcinoma and in normal vulvar tissue: a search for a possible impact of HPV on vulvar cancer prognosis. *Int J Cancer* 1993; **55**: 394–396.

82 Aynaud O, Ionesco M, Barrasso R. Penile intraepithelial neoplasia. Specific clinical features correlate with histologic and virologic findings. *Cancer* 1994; **74**: 1762–1767.

83 Gregoire L, Cubilla AL, Reuter VE, Haas GP, Lancaster WD. Preferential association of human papillomavirus with high-grade histologic variants of penile-invasive squamous cell carcinoma. *J Natl Cancer Inst* 1995; **87**: 1705–1709.

84 Zaki SR, Judd R, Coffield LM, Greer P, Rolston F, Evatt BL. Human papillomavirus infection and anal carcinoma. Retrospective analysis by in situ hybridization and the polymerase chain reaction. *Am J Pathol* 1992; **140**: 1345–1355.

85 Frisch M, Glimelius B, van der Brule, *et al.* Sexually transmitted infection as a cause of anal cancer. *N Engl J Med* 1997; **337**: 1350–1358.

86 Scholefield JH, Sonnex C, Talbot IC, *et al.* Anal and cervical intraepithelial neoplasia: possible parallel. *Lancet* 1989; **ii**: 765–768.

87 Gillison ML, Koch WM, Capone RB, *et al.* Evidence for a causal association between papillomavirus and a subset of head and neck cancers. *J Natl Cancer Inst* 2000; **92**: 709–720.

88 Rudlinger R, Smith IW, Bunney MH, Hunter JAA. Human papillomavirus infections in a group of renal transplant patients. *Br J Dermatol* 1986; **115**: 681–692.

89 Barr BBB, Benton EC, McLaren K, *et al.* Human papillomavirus infection and skin cancer in renal allograft recipients. *Lancet* 1989; **i**: 124–129.

90 Benton EC, Arends MJ. Human papillomavirus in the immunosuppressed. In: Lacey C (ed.) *Papillomavirus Reviews: Current Research on Papillomaviruses.* Leeds; Leeds University Press: 1996.

91 Alloub MI, Barr BBB, McLaren KM, Smith IW, Bunney MH, Smart GE. Human papillomavirus infection and cervical intraepithelial neoplasia in women with renal allografts. *Br Med J* 1989; **298**: 153–156.

92 Ogunbiyi OA, Scholefield JH, Raftery AT, *et al.* Prevalence of anal human papillomavirus infection and intraepithelial neoplasia in renal allograft recipients. *Br J Surg* 1994; **81**: 365–367.

93 Sun XW, Kuhn L, Ellerbrock TV, Chiasson MA, Bush TJ, Wright TC. Human papillomavirus infection in women infected with the human immunodeficiency virus. *N Engl J Med* 1997; **337**: 1343–1349.

94 Sun XW, Ellerbrock TV, Lungu O, Chiasson MA, Bush TJ, Wright TC. Human papillomavirus infection in human immunodeficiency virus-seropositive women. *Obstet Gynecol* 1995; **85**: 680–686.

95 Six C, Heard I, Bergeron C, *et al.* Comparative prevalence, incidence and short-term prognosis of cervical squamous intraepithelial lesions amongst HIV-positive and HIV-negative women. *AIDS* 1998; **12**: 1047–1056.

96 Ellerbrock TV, Chiasson MA, Bush TJ, *et al.* Incidence of cervical squamous intraepithelial lesions in HIV-infected women. *JAMA* 2000; **283**: 1031–1037.

97 Frisch M, Biggar RJ, Goedert JJ. For the AIDS-Cancer Match Registry Study Group. Human papillomavirus-associated cancers in patients with human immunodeficiency virus infection and acquired immunodeficiency syndrome. *J Natl Cancer Inst* 2000; **92**: 1500–1510.

98 Chin KM, Sidhu JS, Janssen RS, Weber JT. Invasive cervical cancer in human immunodeficiency virus-infected and hospital patients. *Obstet Gynecol* 1998; **92**: 83–87.

99 Chiasson MA, Ellerbrock TV, Bush TJ, Sun XW, Wright TC. Increased prevalence of vulvovaginal condyloma and vulvar intraepithelial neoplasia in women infected with the human immunodeficiency virus. *Obstet Gynecol* 1997; **89**: 690–694.

100 Melbye M, Cote TR, Kessler L, Gall M, Biggar RJ, and the AIDS/Cancer Working Group. *Lancet* 1994; **343**: 636–639.

101 Hillemanns P, Ellerbrock TV, McPhillips S, *et al.* Prevalence of anal human papillomavirus infection and anal cytologic abnormalities in HIV-seropositive women. *AIDS* 1996; **10**: 1641–1647.

102 Palefsky JM, Holly EA, Ralston ML, Jay N, Berry JM, Darragh TM. High incidence of anal high-grade squamous intra-epithelial lesions among HIV-positive and HIV-negative homosexual and bisexual men. *AIDS* 1998; **12**: 495–503.

103 Palefsky JM. Anal squamous intraepithelial lesions: relation to HIV and human papillomavirus infection. *J Acqu Immun Def Syndromes* 1999; **21** (Suppl. 1): S42–S48.

104 Volter C, He Y, Delius H, *et al.* Novel HPV types in oral papillomatous lesions from patients with HIV infection. *Int J Cancer* 1996; **66**: 453–456.

105 Schneider A, Hotz M, Gissman L. Increased prevalence of human papillomaviruses in the lower genital tract of pregnant women. *Int J Cancer* 1987; **40**: 198–201.

106 Kemp EA, Kakenewerth AM, Laurent SL, Gravitt PE, Stroeker J. Human papillomavirus prevalence in pregnancy. *Obstet Gynecol* 1992; **79**: 649–656.

107 DeRoda Husman AM, Walboomers JM, Hopman E, *et al.* HPV prevalence in cytomorphologically normal cervical scrapes of pregnant women as determined by PCR: the age-related pattern. *J Med Virol* 1995; **46**: 97–102.

108 Pollack HM, de Benedictis JJ, Marmar JL, Praiss DE. Urethrographic manifestations of venereal warts (condylomata acuminata). *Radiology* 1978; **126**: 643–646.

109 Bernstein SG, Kovacs BR, Townsend DE, Morrow P. Vulvar carcinoma in situ. *Obstet Gynecol* 1983; **61**: 304–307.

110 Andreasson B, Bock JE. Intraepithelial neoplasia in the vulvar region. *Gynecol Oncol* 1985; **21**: 300–305.

111 Hippelainen M, Yliskoski M, Saarikoski S, Syrjanen S, Syrjanen K. Genital human papillomavirus lesions of the male sexual partners: the diagnostic accuracy of penoscopy. *Genitourin Med* 1991; **67**: 291–296.

112 Duncan ID (ed.). *Guidelines for Clinical Practice and Programme Management*, 2nd edition. London; NHSCSP Publication No. 8: 1997.

113 Johnston C. Quantitative tests for human papillomavirus (editorial). *Lancet* 2000; **355**: 2179–2180.

114 Goldie SJ, Weinstein MC, Kuntz KM, Freedberg KA. The costs, clinical benefits, and cost-effectiveness of screening for cervical cancer in HIV-infected women. *Ann Int Med* 1999; **130**: 97–107.

115 De Ruiter A, Carter P, Katz DR, *et al.* A comparison between cytology and histology to detect anal intraepithelial neoplasia. *Genitourin Med* 1994; **70**: 22–25.

116 Goldie SJ, Kuntz KM, Weinstein MC, Freedberg KA, Welton ML, Palefsky JM. The clinical effectiveness and cost-effectiveness of screening for anal squamous intraepithelial lesions in homosexual and bisexual HIV-positive men. *JAMA* 1999; **281**: 1822–1829.

117 Goldie SJ, Kuntz KM, Weinstein MC, Freedberg KA, Palefsy JM. Cost-effectiveness of screening for anal squamous intraepithelial lesions and anal cancer in human immunodeficiency virus-negative homosexual and bisexual men. *Am J Med* 2000; **108**: 634–641.

118 Ferenczy A, Mitao M, Nagai N, Silverstein SJ, Crum CP. Latent papillomavirus and recurring genital warts. *N Engl J Med* 1985; **313**: 784–788.

119 Beutner KR, Wiley DJ. Recurrent external genital warts: a literature review. *Papillomavirus Rep* 1997; **8**: 69–74.

120 von Krogh G. Topical treatment of penile condylomata acuminata with podophyllin, podophyllotoxin and colchicine. A comparative study. *Acta Dermatovenereologica* 1978; **58**: 163–168.

121 von Krogh G, Maibach HI. Cutaneous cytodestructive potency of lignans. I. A comparative evaluation of influence on epidermal and dermal DNA synthesis and on dermal microcirculation in the hairless mouse. *Arch Dermatol Res* 1982; **274**: 9–20.

122 von Krogh G, Maibach HI. Cutaneous cytodestructive potency of lignans. II. A comparative evaluation of macroscopic toxic influence on rabbit skin subsequent to repeated 10-day applications. *Dermatologica* 1983; **167**: 70–77.

123 Wilson L, Bamburg JR, Mizel SB, Grisham LM, Creswell KM. Interaction of drugs with microtubule proteins. *Fed Proc* 1974; **33**: 158–166.

124 Mizel SB, Wilson L. Nucleoside transport in mammalian cells: inhibition by colchicine. *Biochemistry* 1972; **11**: 2573–2578.

125 Von Krogh G. Podophyllotoxin for condylomata acuminata eradication. Clinical and experimental comparative studies on *Podophyllum* lignans, colchicine and 5-fluorouracil. *Acta Dermatovenereologica* 1981; **98** (Suppl.).

126 Sullivan M, King L. Effects of resin of podophyllum on normal skin, condylomata acuminata and verrucae vulgaris. *Archives of Dermatology and Syphilology* 1947; **56**: 30–47.

127 Stoehr GP, Peterson AL, Taylor WJ. Systemic complications of local podophyllin therapy. *Ann Int Med* 1978; **89**: 362–363.

128 Chamberlain MJ, Reynolds AL, Yeoman WB. Toxic effect of podophyllum application in pregnancy. *Br Med J* 1972; **ii**: 391–392.

129 Kinghorn GR, McMillan A, Mulcahy F, Drake S, Lacey C, Bingham JS. An open, comparative study of the efficacy of 0.5% podophyllotoxin lotion and 25% podophyllotoxin solution in the treatment of condylomata acuminata in males and females. *Int J STD AIDS* 1993; **4**: 194–199.

130 Centers for Disease Control and Prevention. 2002 Guidelines for treatment of sexually transmitted diseases. *MMWR* 2002; **51**: RR-6.

131 Beutner KR, Conant MA, Friedman-Kien AE, *et al.* Patient-applied podofilox for treatment of genital warts. *Lancet* 1989; **I**: 831–834.

132 von Krogh G, Szpak E, Andersson M, Bergelin I. Self-treatment using 0.25%–0.50% podophyllotoxin-ethanol solutions against penile condylomata acuminata: a placebo-controlled comparative study. *Genitourin Med* 1994; **70**: 105–109.

133 Edwards A, Atma-Ram A, Thin RN. Podophyllotoxin 0.5% v. podophyllin 20% to treat penile warts. *Genitourin Med* 1988; **64**: 263–265.

134 Hellberg D, Svarrer T, Nilsson S, Valentin J. Self-treatment of female external genital warts with 0.5% podophyllotoxin cream (Condyline®) vs weekly applications of 20% podophyllin solution. *Int J STD AIDS* 1995; **6**: 257–261.

135 Miller E. The metabolism and pharmacology of 5-fluorouracil. *J Surg Oncol* 1971; **3**: 309–315.

136 Krebs HB, Helmkamp BF. Chronic ulcerations following topical therapy with 5-fluorouracil for vaginal human papillomavirus-associated lesions. *Obstet Gynecol* 1991; **78**: 205–208.

137 Ferenczy A. Comparison of 5-fluorouracil and CO_2 laser for treatment of vaginal condylomata. *Obstet Gynecol* 1984; **64**: 773–778.

138 von Krogh G. 5-fluoro-uracil cream in the successful treatment of therapeutically refractory condylomata acuminata of the urinary meatus. *Acta Dermatovenereol* 1976; **56**: 297–301.

139 Swinehart JM, Sperling M, Phillips S, *et al.*. Intralesional fluorouracil/epinephrine injectable gel for treatment of condylomata acuminata. A phase 3 clinical study. *Arch Dermatol* 1997; **133**: 67–73.

140 Scoular A. Choosing equipment for treating genital warts in genitourinary medicine clinics. *Genitourin Med* 1991; **67**: 413–419.

141 Zacarian SA. Is lateral spread of freeze a valid guide of depth of freeze? *J Dermatol Surg Onc* 1978; **4**: 561–563.

142 Dawber RPR, Wilkinson JD. Physical and surgical procedures. In: Rook A, Wilkinson DS, Ebling FJG, Champion RH, Burton JL

(eds) *Textbook of Dermatology* 4th edition. Oxford; Blackwell Scientific Publications: 1986.

143 Godley MJ, Bradbeer CS, Gellan M, Thin RNT. Cryotherapy compared with trichloroacetic acid in treating genital warts. *Genitourin Med* 1987; 63: 390–392.

144 Menter A, Black-Noller G, Riendeau LA, Monti KL. The use of EMLA cream and 1% lidocaine infiltration in men for relief of pain associated with the removal of genital warts by cryotherapy. *J Am Acad Dermatol* 1997; 37: 96–100.

145 Ghosh AK. Cryosurgery of genital warts in cases in which podophyllin treatment failed or was contraindicated. *Br J Vener Dis* 1977; 53: 49–53.

146 Balsdon MJ. Cryosurgery of genital warts. *Br J Vener Dis* 1978; 54: 352–353.

147 Simmons PD, Langlet F, Thin RNT. Cryotherapy versus electrocautery in the treatment of genital warts. *Br J Vener Dis* 1981; 57: 273–274.

148 Gross GE, Barrasso R. General principles of treatment. In: Gross GE, Barrasso R (eds) *Human Papillomavirus Infection. A Colour Atlas.* Berlin; Ullstein Mosby: 1997.

149 Stone KM, Becker TM, Hadgu A, Kraus SJ. Treatment of external genital warts: a randomised clinical trial comparing podophyllin, cryotherapy, and electrodesiccation. *Genitourin Med* 1990; 66: 16–19.

150 Thomson JPJ, Grace RH. The treatment of perianal and anal condylomata acuminata. *J R Soc Med* 1978; 71: 180–185.

151 Gollock JM, Slatford K, Hunter JM. Scissor excision of anogenital warts. *Br J Vener Dis* 1982; 58: 400–401.

152 McMillan A, Scott GR. Outpatient treatment of perianal warts by scissor excision. *Genitourin Med* 1987; 63: 114–115.

153 Jensen S. Comparison of podophyllin application with simple surgical excision in clearance and recurence of perianal condylomata acuminata. *Lancet* 1985; ii: 1146–1148.

154 Khawaja H. Podophyllin versus scissors excision in the treatment of perianal condylomata acuminata: a prospective study. *Br J Surg* 1989; 76: 1067–1068.

155 Abdullah AN, Walzman M, Wade A. Treatment of external genital warts comparing cryotherapy (liquid nitrogen) and trichloroacetic acid. *Sex Transm Dis* 1993; 20: 344–345.

156 Gabriel G, Thin RNT. Treatment of anogenital warts. Comparison of trichloracetic acid and podophyllin versus podophyllin alone. *Br J Vener Dis* 1983; 59: 124–126

157 Bar-Am A, Shilon M, Peyser MR, Ophir J, Brenner S. Treatment of male genital condylomatous lesions by carbon dioxide laser after failure of previous non-laser

methods. *J Am Acad Dermatol* 1991; 24: 87–89.

158 Reid R, Greenberg MD, Pizzuti DJ, Omoto KH, Rutledge LH, Soo W. Superficial laser vulvectomy. V. Surgical debulking is enhanced by adjuvant systemic interferon. *Am J Obstet Gynecol* 1992; 166: 815–820.

159 Arany I, Tyring SK. Activation of local cell-mediated immunity in interferon-responsive patients with human papillomavirus-associated lesions. *J Interferon Cytokine Res* 1996; 16: 453–460.

160 Arany I, Tyring SK. Status of local cellular immunity in interferon-responsive and nonresponsive human papillomavirus-associated lesions. *Sex Transm Dis* 1996; 23: 475–480.

161 Steinberg BM, Gallacher T, Stoler MH, Abramson AL. Relationship between human papillomavirus types in laryngeal papillomatosis and response to interferon-alpha. *Cancer Cells* 1987; 5: 403–409.

162 Condylomata International Collaborative Study Group. A comparison of interferon alfa-2a and podophyllin in the treatment of primary condylomata acuminata. *Genitourin Med* 1991; 67: 394–399.

163 Condylomata International Collaborative Study Group. Recurrent condylomata acuminata treated with recombinant interferon alpha-2a. *Acta Derm Venereol (Stockh)* 1993; 73: 223–226.

164 Armstrong DKB, Maw RD, Dinsmore WW, *et al.* Combined therapy trial with interferon alpha-2a and ablative therapy in the treatment of anogenital warts. *Genitourin Med* 1996; 72: 103–107.

165 Gross GR, Roussaki A, Baur S, *et al.* Systemically administered interferon alfa-2a prevents recurrence of condylomata acuminata following CO_2 laser ablation. The influence of the cyclic low-dose therapy regimen. Results of a multicentre double-blind placebo-controlled clinical trial. *Genitourin Med* 1996; 72: 71.

166 Armstrong DK, Maw RD, Dinsmore WW, *et al.* A randomised, double-blind, parallel group study to compare subcutaneous interferon alpha-2a plus podophyllin with placebo plus podophyllin in the treatment of primary condylomata acuminata. *Genitourin Med* 1994; 70: 389–393.

167 Eron LJ, Adler MB, O'Rourke JM, Rittweger K, DePamphilis J, Pizzuti DJ. Recurrence of condylomata acuminata following cryotherapy is not prevented by systemically administered interferon. *Genitourin Med* 1993; 69: 91–93.

168 Handley JM, Horner T, Maw RD, Lawther H, Dinsmore WW. Subcutaneous interferon alpha 2a combined with cryotherapy vs cryotherapy alone in the treatment of primary anogenital warts: a randomised

observer blind placebo controlled study. *Genitourin Med* 1991; 67: 297–302.

169 Eron LJ, Judson F, Tucker S et al. Interferon therapy for condylomata acuminata. *N Engl J Med* 1986; 315: 1059–1064.

170 Friedman-Kien A. Management of condylomata acuminata with Alferon N injection, interferon alfa-n3 (human leukocyte derived). *Am J Obstet Gynecol* 1995; 172: 1359–1368.

171 Douglas JM, Rogers M, Judson FN. The effect of asymptomatic infection with HTLV-III on the response of anogenital warts to intralesional treatment with recombinant alpha$_2$ interferon. *J Infect Dis* 1986; 154: 331–334.

172 Douglas JM, Eron LJ, Judson FN, *et al.* A randomized trial of combination therapy with intralesional interferon 2β and podophyllin versus podophyllin alone for the therapy of anogenital warts. *J Infect Dis* 1990; 162: 52–59.

173 Syed TA, Khayyami M, Kriz D, *et al.* Management of genital warts in women with human leukocyte interferon alpha vs podophyllotoxin in cream: a placebo-controlled, double-blind, comparative study. *J Mol Med* 1995; 73: 255–258.

174 Olmos L, Vilata J, Pichardo AR, Lloret A, Ojeda A, Calderon MD. Double-blind, randomised clinical trial on the effect of interferon-beta in the treatment of condylomata acuminata. *Int J STD AIDS* 1995; 5: 182–185.

175 Dinsmore W, Jordan J, O'Mahony C et al. Recombinant human interferon-β in the treatment of condylomata acuminata. *Int J STD AIDS* 1997; 8: 622–628.

176 Bornstein J, Pascal B, Zarfati D, Goldshmid N, Abramovici H. Recombinant human interferon-β for condylomata acuminata: a randomized, double-blind placebo-controlled study of intralesional therapy. *Int J STD AIDS* 1997; 8: 622–628.

177 Gross G, Rogozinski T, Schofer H, *et al.* Recombinant interferon beta gel as an adjuvant in the treatment of recurrent genital warts: results of a placebo-controlled double-blind study in 120 patients. *Dermatology* 1998; 196: 330–334.

178 Kirby PK, Kiviat N, Beckman A, Wells D, Sherwin S, Corey L. Tolerance and efficacy of recombinant human interferon gamma in the treatment of refractory genital warts. *Am J Med* 1988; 85: 183–188.

179 Zouboulis CC, Buttner P, Orfanos CE. Systemic interferon gamma as adjuvant therapy for refractory anogenital warts: a randomized clinical trial and meta-analysis of the available data. *Arch Dermatol* 1992; 128: 1413–1414.

180 Rockley PF, Tyring SK. Interferons alpha, beta and gamma therapy of anogenital

human papillomavirus infections. *Pharmacol Ther* 1995; **65**: 265–287.

181 Megyeri K, Au WC, Rosztoczy I, *et al.* Stimulation of interferon and cytokine gene expression by imiquimod and stimulation by Sendai virus utilize similar signalling transduction pathways. *Mol Cell Biol* 1995; **15**: 2207–2218.

182 Tyring SK, Arany I, Stanley MA, *et al.* A randomized, controlled, molecular study of condylomata acuminata clearance during treatment with imiquimod. *J Infect Dis* 1998; **178**: 551–555.

183 Wagner TL, Ahonen CL, Couture AM, *et al.* Modulation of Th1 and Th2 cytokine production with the immune response modifiers, R848 and imiquimod. *Cell Immunol* 1999; **191**: 10–19.

184 Beutner KR, Spruance SL, Hougham AJ, Fox TL, Owens M, Douglas JM. Treatment of genital warts with an immune-response modifier (imiquimod). *J Am Acad Dermatol* 1998; **38**: 230–239.

185 Beutner KR, Tyring SK, Trofatter KF, *et al.* Imiquimod, a patient-applied immune-response modifier for treatment of external genital warts. *Antimicrob Agents Chemother* 1998; **42**: 789–794.

186 Edwards L, Ferenczy A, Eron L, *et al.* Self-administered topical 5% imiquimod cream for external anogenital warts. *Arch Dermatol* 1998; **134**: 25–30.

187 Mohanty KC, Scott CS. Immunotherapy of genital warts with inosine pranobex (immunovir): preliminary study. *Genitourin Med* 1986; **62**: 352–355.

188 Davidson-Parker J, Dinsmore W, Khan MH, Hicks DA, Moris CA, Morris DF. Immunotherapy of genital warts with inosine pranobex and conventional treatment: double blind placebo controlled study. *Genitourin Med* 1988; **64**: 383–386.

189 Persson G, Dahlof LG, Krantz I. Physical and psychological effects of anogenital warts on female patients. *Sex Transm Dis* 1993; **20**: 10–13.

190 Voog E, Lowhagen G-B. Follow-up of men with genital papilloma virus infection. *Acta Derm Venereol* 1992; **72**: 185–186.

191 Hippelainen MI, Hippelaain M, Saarikoski S, Syrjanen K. Clinical course and prognostic factors in human papilloma-virus infections on men. *Sex Transm Dis* 1994; **21**: 272–279.

192 Oriel JD. Sexually transmitted diseases in children: human papillomavirus infection. *Genitourin Med* 1992; **68**: 80–83.

193 Adelson MD, Semo R, Baggish MS, Osborne NG. Laser vaporization of genital condylomata in pregnancy. *J Gynecol Surg* 1990; **6**: 257–262.

194 Gilson RJC, Shupack JL, Friedman-Kien AE, *et al.* A randomized, controlled, safety study using imiquimod for the topical treatment of anogenital warts in HIV-infected patients. *AIDS* 1999; **13**: 2397–2404.

195 Aho M, Vesterinen E, Meyer B, Purola E, Paavonen J. Natural history of vaginal intraepithelial neoplasia. *Cancer* 1991; **68**: 195–197.

196 Berger BW, Hori Y. Multicentric Bowen's disease of the genitalia. Spontaneous regression of lesion. *Arch Dermatol* 1978; **114**: 1698–1699.

197 Scholefield JH, Ogunbiyi OA, Smith JHF, Rogers K, Sharp F. Treatment of anal intraepithelial neoplasia. *Br J Surg* 1994; **81**: 1238–1240.

198 Centers for Disease Control and Prevention. 2002 Guidelines for treatment of sexually transmitted diseases. *MMWR* 2002; **51**: RR-6.

199 Kashima HK, Shah K, Goodstein M. Recurrent respiratory papillomatosis. In: Holmes KK, Mardh P-A, Sparling F, Weisner P (ed.) *Sexually Transmitted Diseases.* New York; McGraw-Hill Book Co: 1990.

200 Mounts P, Kashima H. Association of human papillomavirus subtype and clinical course in respiratory papillomatosis. *Laryngoscope* 1984; **94**: 28–32.

201 Bauman N, Smith R. Recurrent respiratory papillomatosis. *Pediatr Otol* 1996; **43**: 1385–1401.

202 Becker TM. Laryngeal papillomatosis. In: Hitchcock PJ, MacKay HT, Wasserheit JN (eds) *Sexually Transmitted Diseases and Adverse Outcomes of Pregnancy.* Washington DC; American Society for Microbiology: 1999.

203 Kashima H, Shah K, Lyles R, *et al.* A comparison of risk factors in juvenile onset and adult onset recurrent respiratory papillomatosis. *Laryngoscope* 1992; **102**: 9–13.

204 Clark IJ, MacKenzie K. Recurrent respiratory papillomatosis – current knowledge and treatment. *Papillomavirus Rep* 1996; **7**: 113–118.

205 Kashima H, Mounts P, Leventhal B, Hruban RH. Sites of predilection in recurrent respiratory papillomatosis. *Ann Otol Rhino Laryngol* 1993; **102**: 580–583.

206 Bomholt A. Laryngeal papillomas with adult onset. An epidemiological study from the Copenhagen region. *Acta Oto-laryngol* 1988; **106**: 140–144.

207 af Geijersstam V, Eklund C, Wang Z, *et al.* A survey of seroprevalence of human papillomavirus types 16, 18 and 33 among children. *Int J Cancer* 1999; **80**: 489–493.

208 Kaye JN, Cason J, Pakarian FB, *et al.* Viral load as a determinant for transmission of human papillomavirus type 16 from mother to child. *J Med Virol* 1994; **44**: 415–421.

209 Kaye JN, Starkey WG, Kell B, *et al.* Human papillomavirus type 16 in infants: use of DNA sequence analyses to determine the source of infection. *J Gen Virol* 1996; **77**: 1139–1143.

210 Tang C-K, Shermeta DW, Wood C. Congenital condylomata acuminata. *Am J Obstet Gynecol* 1978; **131**: 912–913.

211 Cohen BA, Honig P, Androphy E. Anogenital warts in children. Clinical and virologic evaluation for sexual abuse. *Arch Dermatol* 1990; **126**: 1575–1580.

212 Armbruster-Moraes E, Ioshimoto LM, Leao E, Zugaib M. Presence of human papillomavirus DNA in amniotic fluids of pregnant women with cervical lesions. *Gynecol Oncol* 1994; **54**: 152–158.

213 Tseng C-J, Lin CY, Wang R-L, *et al.* Possible transplacental transmission of human papillomaviruses. *Am J Obstet Gynecol* 1992; **166**: 35–40.

214 Watts DH, Koutsky LA, Holmes KK, *et al.* Low risk of perinatal transmission of human papillomavirus: results from a prospective cohort study. *Am J Obstet Gynecol* 1998; **178**: 365–373.

215 Lacey CJN. Genital warts in children. In: Lacey C (ed.) *Papillomavirus Reviews: Current Research on Papillomaviruses.* Leeds; Leeds University Press: 1996.

216 Robinson AJ. Sexually transmitted organisms in children and child sexual abuse. *Int J STD AIDS* 1998; **9**: 501–510.

217 Gutman LT, St Claire KK, Weedy C, *et al.* Human immunodeficiency virus transmission by child sexual abuse. *Am J Dis Child* 1991; **145**: 137–141.

218 Allen AL, Siegfried EC. The natural history of condyloma in children. *J Am Acad Dermatol* 1998; **39**: 951–955.

219 Syrjanen K, Vayrynen M, Castren O, *et al.* Sexual behaviour of women with human papillomavirus (HPV) lesions of the uterine cervix. *Br J Vener Dis* 1984; **60**: 243–248.

220 Wen LM, Estcourt CS, Simpson JM, Mindel A. Risk factors for the acquisition of genital warts: are condoms protective? *Sex Transm Infect* 1999; **75**: 312–316.

221 PHLS, DHSS&PS and the Scottish ISD(D)5 Collaborative Group. *Trends in Sexually Transmitted Infections in the United Kingdom, 1990–1999.* London; Public Health Laboratory Service: 2000.

222 McMillan A. The management of difficult anogenital warts. *Sex Transm Infect* 1999; **75**: 192–194.

223 Greenwood D, Slack R, Peutherer J (eds) *Medical Microbiology.* Churchill Livingstone; Edinburgh: 2000.

224 McMillan A, Scott GR. *Sexually Transmitted Infections, Colour Guide.* Churchill Livingstone; Edinburgh: 2000.

225 Rein MF (ed.). *Atlas of Infectious Diseases, Volume V. Sexually Transmitted Diseases.* Churchill Livingstone; Philadelphia: 1996.

Chapter 6

Herpes simplex virus infection

A McMillan, M M Ogilvie

Herpes simplex is an acute infectious disease, characterized by a vesicular eruption that sometimes recurs, occurring anywhere on the skin or mucosal surfaces, but most often on or near the lips or the genitals. Sometimes the infection involves the eye to cause a conjunctivitis with or without corneal involvement. The causative virus, herpes simplex virus (HSV) is divided into two distinct, but related, types. Modern HSV typing is based on detection of type-specific antigens or gene sequences. Herpes simplex virus type 1 (HSV-1) is commonly isolated from lesions around the mouth or eye and is transmitted by direct contact, for example kissing, by droplets from acute cases, or from the saliva of asymptomatic virus excretors. Herpes simplex virus type 1 is now an important cause of genital herpes and is most frequently transmitted sexually by direct orogenital sexual contact. Herpes simplex virus type 2 (HSV-2) is responsible for more than 50% of cases of genital tract herpes infections and is spread by direct contact during sexual intercourse. The high incidence of inapparent infections, whether of HSV-1 or HSV-2, is becoming better appreciated.

Biology of herpes simplex virus

(synonyms: α_1-*herpesvirus; human herpesvirus 1* and *human herpesvirus 2*)

The herpes virus particle (virion) has a characteristic appearance when viewed by electron microscopy. Heavy metal negative staining outlines an icosahedral capsid (diameter 100 nm), assembled from repeated protein units (capsomeres), surrounding the electron-dense core of viral DNA. The tegument, an amorphous layer around the capsid, in mature infectious virions is surrounded by a lipid envelope derived from host cell membranes. The enveloped herpes particles measure approximately 200 nm, and many short spikes of viral glycoproteins are seen projecting from the envelope[1] (Figure 6.1). This lipid envelope renders the herpesviruses relatively thermolabile and readily inactivated by lipid solvents such as alcohols and detergents.

Herpes simplex virus is in the genus *Simplexvirus*, a genus in the family Herpesviridae, in the subfamily Alphaherpesvirinae comprised of neurotropic

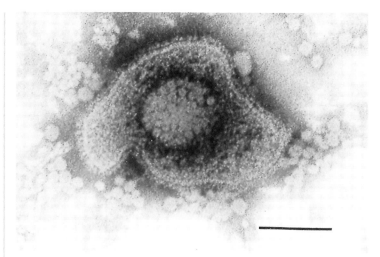

Figure 6.1 Herpes simplex virus virion. Scale, 100 nm

herpesviruses that grow quite quickly in epithelial or fibroblast cell cultures, and which include human herpesvirus 3, the varicella-zoster virus (VZV). The linear double-stranded herpesvirus DNA genome contains around 100 genes, coding, for example, for viral glycoproteins, capsid proteins, enzymes involved in DNA replication, and transcripts associated with latency[1]. Digestion of viral DNA by restriction endonucleases permits analysis of the resulting fragments of DNA, separated by electrophoresis, for epidemiological comparison of strains within herpes species – a technique sometimes referred to as 'fingerprinting'. Thus it has been possible to establish whether HSV isolates of one type from two patients are related or not[2]. The various envelope glycoproteins (termed gB, gD_1, gG_2, etc. with the source HSV type indicated) have been shown to have significant roles in attachment to cell receptors (gC, gD), and entry of virus into cells by membrane fusion (gB, gD, gH, gL), in addition to other activities[1].

Herpes simplex virus type-common and type-specific antigens are found on various HSV proteins, but the type-specific antibody tests that now provide important epidemiological information are based predominantly, but not exclusively, on detection of antibody to the HSV glycoprotein gG[3, 4]. Glycoprotein gG$_1$ and gG$_2$ have some homology, but gG$_2$ has a large extra sequence of amino acids making it nearly three times as long as the HSV-1 counterpart.

LIFE CYCLE OF HERPES SIMPLEX VIRUS

The life cycle of HSV is depicted in Figure 6.2. After attachment through surface glycoproteins (gC and gD) to receptors on epithelial cells, now more clearly identified[5, 6], the envelope of HSV fuses with the cell membrane. The viral capsid (nucleocapsid) with some tegument is transported across the cytoplasm to a pore in the nuclear membrane, where viral DNA and tegument proteins enter the nucleus. Replication of herpesviral DNA takes place within the nucleus, following an orderly cascade of events beginning with immediate early regulatory functions, then new viral DNA genomes are produced

about 6 hours after infection. The structural proteins of the capsid, and glycoproteins are made in the cytoplasm, but after nucleocapsid assembly in the nucleus, the viral envelope is acquired from stretches of nuclear membrane containing viral glycoproteins. Viruses then pass by membranous vesicles to the cell surface, are released after another fusion event, and can then infect neighboring cells or be shed in fluid from 12 to 18 hours after infection. Glycoproteins gB, gD, gK, and gL are all essential for replication, and so is gH which is necessary for release of infectious particles. Infected cells producing new HSV generally do not survive, becoming enlarged, sometimes fusing with neighbors to give characteristic multinucleated giant cells, and finally dying as a consequence of inhibition of cell metabolism[1].

Natural history of herpes simplex virus infection

In a discussion of the natural history of HSV infection it is necessary to define and name the various events that occur in the course of the infection.

The definitions given below are based on those of Wildy and his Cambridge colleagues[7] but are modified to take into account suggestions made by Rawls[8]; clinical and virological features in herpes genitalis at various stages in its natural history are represented diagrammatically in Figure 6.3. Figure 6.4 shows these features in a recurrent episode of orolabial herpes[9].

1. *Primary infection.* This is an infection that may be asymptomatic, remain localized, or become generalized in an individual who has not been previously infected with either type of HSV as shown by a lack of antibodies to any HSV type.

2. *Initial infection.* This denotes the first infection by one HSV type. It may be either a *primary infection* in individuals *without* serological evidence of a previous herpetic infection (seronegative by a sensitive assay) or a *non-primary infection* in those *with* evidence of previous infection (seropositive). Clinically primary and non-primary initial infections may be indistinguishable on physical examination.

3. *Latency.* There is apparent recovery but some virus remains dormant in nervous tissue, particularly in certain sensory ganglion cells; this is latency (latent means hidden).

4. *Reactivation.* Virus may be reawakened either spontaneously or as a result of external stimuli, so that infectious virus may once again be found.

5. *Recurrence.* The reactivated virus may on occasion initiate a peripheral lesion in the dermatome relating to the sensory ganglion. The lesion is referred to as a *recurrent lesion* and the phenomenon is *recurrence*. Wildy et al.[7] used the term 'recrudescence' to describe this phenomenon but since the term 'recurrence' is deeply embedded in the literature it is used here instead[8].

6. *Axonal transport.* The whole phenomenon requires translation of the virus from the periphery to the sensory ganglion and back again by way of, it is believed, the cytoplasm within the axon. The rate of translocation from the skin to the

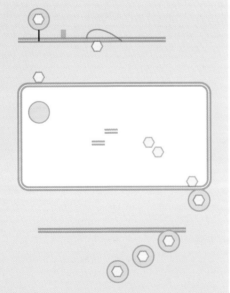

1. HSV attachment to cell receptor and entry mediated by co-receptors and viral fusion protein

2. Nucleocapsid (with some tegument proteins) moves to nuclear pore

3. Viral DNA circularizes in nucleus and early transcripts are formed

4. Viral DNA is replicated

5. Viral capsid proteins self-assemble to produce capsids in nucleus

6. ds viral DNA incorporated and nucleocapsis becomes enveloped at patch of nuclear membrane containing viral glycoproteins

7. HSV virions move to plasma membrane in vesicles and are released from cell

Figure 6.2 Life cycle of herpes simplex virus. ds, double stranded

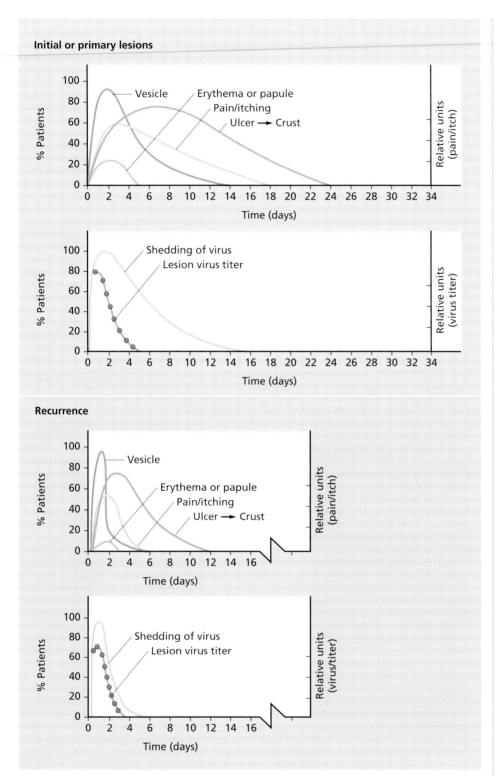

Figure 6.3 Diagrammatic representation of surface clinical and virological features in herpes genitalis at various stages in its natural history. The patterns evolve during the approximate times shown (based on Wildy *et al.* 1982[7], Spruance *et al.* 1977[26], Rawls 1985[8], and other sources, see text) (reproduced with permission from Robertson *et al.* 1989[204])

ganglion lies within the range of 2 to 10 mm/h.

7. *Asymptomatic virus shedding.* Sometimes the virus evidently reactivates and passes to a peripheral site but fails to cause a noticeable lesion, although it probably multiplies and can be isolated.

Box 6.1 summarizes the salient points in the natural history of genital HSV infection.

GENITAL HERPES

Initial infection

Notwithstanding the wide variation in the severity of clinical disease in *primary infection* the majority of cases appear to be asymptomatic. Less than 10% of individuals with HSV-2-specific serum antibody give a history consistent with genital herpes[10, 11], and recently it has been shown that nearly 60% of newly acquired HSV-2 infections and just over 35% of HSV-1 infections are symptomless[12]. Nevertheless, about 50% of women who have acquired HSV-2 subclinically subsequently develop symptomatic genital herpes[13].

In the majority of cases of clinically apparent disease the lesions are localized to the site of inoculation, the sensory neurons innervating that site, and the lymphatics draining it. Spread to contiguous areas or transfer to more distant sites by autoinoculation can also occur (see page 111). *Non-primary initial infections* with a heterologous type are less severe than *primary initial infections*[7, 14].

Clinical recurrence

After the primary or initial infection with HSV-1 and HSV-2, whether obvious or inapparent, there may be no further clinical manifestations throughout life. In the year following symptomatic primary genital herpes associated with *HSV-2*, however, recurrence is common. It has been shown that up to 89% of individuals have recurrences, with a median recurrence rate of 0.34 episodes per month or 4 to 5 episodes per year[15, 16]. Significantly fewer recurrences are found in those who have had symptomatic primary *HSV-1* genital infection: a median recurrence rate

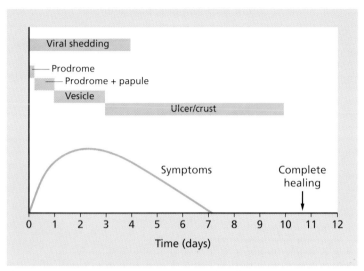

Figure 6.4 Diagrammatic representation of surface clinical and virological features of recurrent herpes labialis (after Fiddian *et al.* 1983[9])

of 0.08 episodes per month or one episode per year has been reported[15]. In people who have had a prolonged initial illness (lasting more than 35 days), the interval between primary infection and recurrence tends to be shorter and the recurrence rate to be twice as frequent as those with a less prolonged episode[15]. Significantly, from the public health aspect, men tend to have more recurrences than women. In the year following symptomatic primary infection, 74% of women and 92% of men have recurrences and the median recurrence rates amongst women and men are, respectively, 0.33 and 0.43 episodes per month[15]. In those patients who have had primary HSV-1 or HSV-2 infections, the recurrence rates in the second year after the initial infection are significantly less than during the first year[16]. There is, however, much variation in recurrence rates between individuals: one-third of individuals have at least two fewer recurrences in the second year than in the first year after primary infection, and one-third have more recurrences in the second year than in the first. Prior infection with HSV-1 does not appear to influence the recurrence rate in those who subsequently acquire HSV-2 infection[16]. In many patients there is a reduction in recurrence rate in subsequent years, suggesting that the pool of reactivatable virus in the ganglia dimin-

ishes with time; the rate of decrease in recurrences, however, tends to become smaller with the passage of time. For example, in Benedetti's study[16], a decrease of 0.2 recurrences per year was found in patients followed up for more than 8 years, compared with a decrease of 0.8 recurrences per year in patients followed for 4 years or less. Nevertheless, most patients seem to have a decrease of more than one recurrence per year between years 1 and 5 after initial HSV-2 infection. It should be noted, however, that about 25% of individuals have at least one more recurrence in year 5 than in year 1.

Subclinical recurrence in the anogenital region

Much of the available data on asymptomatic excretion of HSV originates from the elegant studies of Corey's group in Seattle. Women have been studied more intensively than men, and conclusions based on these data need not necessarily reflect the situation in men. Likewise, most studies have been performed on individuals who have had symptomatic genital herpes, and there are fewer data on asymptomatic shedding amongst asymptomatic patients. The rate of asymptomatic shedding of HSV after recovery from an initial episode of genital herpes depends on the type of HSV

and whether that episode was primary or non-primary infection. For example, Koelle and others[17] found that 10% of women who had had primary HSV-1 infection, 18% who had had primary HSV-2 infection, and 23% who had had non-primary HSV-2 infection had asymptomatic excretion of virus at some time during the first year after the initial episode of genital herpes. In women who had had primary or non-primary HSV-2 infection, the rate of shedding of virus from the cervix was higher than in those who had had HSV-1

Box 6.1 Natural history of genital herpes

- Majority of primary infections symptomless.
- About 90% of individuals with initial infection with HSV-2 have clinical recurrence in first year after episode.
- Fewer clinical recurrences if HSV-1 associated with initial infection.
- Clinical recurrence rate higher in those who had severe initial episode.
- Symptomatic recurrences more likely in men than in women.
- Tendency to fewer clinical recurrences after first year from infection.
- Symptomless recurrence more likely in women who have had HSV-2 initial infection than those who have had HSV-1 infection.
- Rate of symptomless shedding of HSV in women higher in first 3 months after initial episode than subsequently.
- Symptomless excretion of virus generally short-lived (< 2 days in 90% of women).
- 30% of women with subclinical recurrence shed virus within 7 days of, and 20% in 7 days after resolution of clinical recurrence.
- Rate of symptomless excretion higher in women who have frequent clinical recurrences.

Increased rate of subclinical virus shedding in HIV-infected men and women.

infection (3.1% and 2.6% versus 0.6% respectively). Virus was more commonly excreted during the first 3 months after the initial episode than during subsequent months. In a study in which women with a history of genital herpes obtained daily samples for at least 60 days from the genital tract and rectum for viral culture, subclinical shedding of HSV occurred in 55% of 65 women with HSV-2 infection, and 29% of 14 women with HSV-1 infection[18]. Many episodes of subclinical virus excretion involved more than one anatomical site. Irrespective of virus type, subclinical shedding of HSV lasted 1 day in 75% of women, 2 days in 14% of women, 3 days in 6% of women, and at least 4 days in 11% of women. Thirty per cent of episodes of asymptomatic virus shedding occurred in the 7 days preceding a symptomatic recurrence and 20% in the 7 days after such a recurrence. As has been noted with symptomatic recurrence (see pp. 109–110), subclinical shedding of virus is more likely to occur within 12 months of the initial episode of genital herpes than in subsequent years. Women who have frequent symptomatic recurrences (more than 12 per year) are also more likely to have subclinical shedding of HSV[18].

Nevertheless, when patients are educated about the clinical features of genital herpes, many describe symptomatic recurrence of HSV-2 infection. For example, after educational counseling of their patients, Wald et al.[19] noted that 61% of HSV-2 seropositive women without a history of genital herpes subsequently reported a clinical history consistent with genital herpes. It is probable, then, that the majority of HSV-2-infected individuals have, in fact, symptomatic disease.

Asymptomatic shedding of HSV-1 and HSV-2 from the rectums of HIV-seronegative homosexual men who give a history of anogenital herpes, or who are seropositive for HSV, is common[20]. The frequency and site of shedding of HSV-2 in 30 homosexual men, of whom 19 had a history of symptomatic disease, was investigated in a manner similar to that described above for women, samples being collected daily for 100 days. Overall, HSV-2 was isolated on 3.1% of the days, and viral shedding was predominantly perianal (65 of 78 isolates). Subclinical shedding of HSV-2 from the genitalia or perianal region occurred on 2.1% of the 2335 days, and on most days when this occurred, the participants were truly symptomless. The rate of viral excretion, however, was higher amongst men who experienced prodromal symptoms (6.6% on the days that the men reported prodromal features). The mean duration of viral shedding from the anogenital region was shorter in men who had subclinical viral excretion than in those who were symptomatic (1.4 days versus 2.2 days). An interesting observation was that men who were seropositive for both HSV-1 and HSV-2 were more likely to shed HSV-2 than those who were only HSV-2 seropositive.

Men and women infected with HIV are more likely to shed HSV than HIV-seronegative individuals. For example, in one cross-sectional study HSV-2 shedding was found in 13% and 4% of 106 HIV-seropositive and 70 HIV-seronegative women, and 79% of the HIV-seropositive group had symptomless excretion of the virus[21]. Similar findings were reported in a group of homosexual men who were HIV-seropositive. Schacker et al.[22] studied a group of 68 HIV-infected and 13 HIV-non-infected homosexual men and obtained daily cultures for HSV from the mouth, genitalia, and rectum. These men were followed up for a median of 57 days. Amongst HIV-infected men, HSV-2 was detected on 405 (9.7%) of 4167 days, compared with 24 (3.1%) of 766 days amongst HIV-seronegative men. They found that most reactivations were in the perirectal area and were subclinical (46 of 68 HIV-infected men). Men with a low CD4+ cell count were more likely to shed HSV than those with a high count, and increased shedding was more likely amongst men who were seropositive for both HSV-2 and HSV-1 than those who were seropositive for only HSV-2.

Extragenital herpes simplex virus infection

Lesions caused by HSV-1 or HSV-2 can occur at anatomical sites other than the oropharynx and the genitalia; these sites include the buttocks, trunk, fingers, and eyes. It has been postulated that infection at these sites occurs through auto-inoculation (eyes, fingers), direct contact with infected lesions (upper thighs, trunk), shared nerve supply (sacral skin, buttocks), or, rarely, by viremia. Primary genital HSV-1 infection is more often associated with non-genital lesions than primary genital HSV-2 infection (25% versus 9%), and the lesions tend to be on the face or fingers; non-genital lesions in individuals with primary HSV-2 infection tend to be on the buttocks or legs[23].

Overall, up to 21% of patients with primary genital herpes will subsequently develop a non-genital recurrence. The recurrence rate of HSV of either type at non-genital sites, however, is less frequent than that of genital herpes, and the interval between the initial episode and recurrence at the extragenital site is significantly longer than that of genital infection. Although the buttock lesions of HSV-2 recur less frequently, they last longer than genital lesions. Recurrence of HSV infection at non-genital sites may also occur in patients whose primary infection affected the genitalia alone[23].

OROLABIAL HERPES

The severity of signs and symptoms in *primary* infection appears to be age related; usually asymptomatic infections occur in the 2- to 3-year age group and symptomatic infections in the adolescent or young adult. Virus shedding continues on average for 14 to 21 days after the appearance of the lesions.

The prevalence of serum antibodies against HSV-1 in young adults in developed countries appears to be declining, indicating that infections in childhood are less common. In this situation, primary infections in adolescence become more common and, as in ocular infections[24], more severe clinical forms of the disease in this age group will be seen more often.

Herpes simplex virus type 1 may occasionally be isolated from saliva, tears, and the genital tract between clinical recurrences, and regularly from recurrent lesions.

Oral shedding of HSV-1 has been reviewed recently[25]. During recurrent herpes labialis. HSV-1 can be cultured from 89% of oral lesions and 25% of saliva samples[26]. The virus isolation rate, however, depends on the clinical stage when sampling is undertaken, for example HSV-1 can be cultured almost twice as often from oral secretions from individuals with vesicular lesions as from those with ulceration[27]. The duration of virus shedding appears to vary depending on the trigger for reactivation. In one study[28] the mean duration of HSV-1 shedding was 1.2 days for otherwise well individuals, 3 days for immunocompromised patients, and 5.8 days for those who had had oral surgery.

As detected by virus culture asymptomatic shedding of HSV-1 from the oral cavity mucosa or lips is found in 2% to 9% of individuals[29]. Using amplification methods for the detection of viral DNA increases the proportion of symptomless excreters of the virus detected in a given population: in a recent Japanese study, 2.7% of patients attending an oral surgery clinic had HSV-1 isolated from the oral cavity but specific DNA was detected by polymerase chain reaction (PCR) in 4.7% of the 1000 subjects[30]. An increased incidence of symptomless virus shedding has been reported in HSV-1 seropositive individuals who have sustained orofacial trauma, for example Kameyama et al.[28] cultured HSV from saliva collected over a 1-month period from 31% of individuals with facial fractures.

The frequency of recurrence of orolabial herpes associated with HSV-2 is significantly lower than that of HSV-1. In a small study the mean monthly recurrence rate of orolabial herpes caused by HSV-1 was 0.12 per month and that caused by HSV-2 was 0.001 per month[31].

Pathogenesis and pathology

The hallmark of alphaherpesviruses is their ability to establish a latent state in primary sensory neurons from whence they may be reactivated by various stimuli leading to a recurrent productive infection at the local site innervated. Whilst replicating in epithe-

lium, HSV (and VZV) virus particles enter through sensory nerve endings and are transported up the axon to the neuronal nucleus in the sensory (dorsal root) ganglion (Figure 6.5). Some of the virus reaching the ganglion cells is able to establish a latent infection in which a proportion of the neurons maintain several copies of non-replicating HSV genome. Herpes simplex virus type 1 is usually latent in the trigeminal ganglion and HSV-2 in the sacral ganglia. Either HSV type may become latent in other ganglia[32], and latent virus may also be recoverable from autonomic ganglia. This is truly a latent phase during which virus cannot be recovered from skin or mucosal sites where herpes lesions have previously occurred. There is, however, the possibility of reactivation, the mechanism of which is not understood. During this process the HSV returns to the nerve ending where infection of surrounding epithelial cells may occur, but does not always produce a recognizable lesion. There may be asymptomatic shedding of virus only detectable by the most sensitive detection method. Recurrences are associated with increased levels of mediators such as prostaglandins, and with a decrease in cell-mediated immune function, especially delayed hypersensitivity. Thus, even if the mechanism of reactivation is not understood, HSV recurrences can be predicted in those known to harbor latent virus.

Reactivation may be induced by trauma to the affected sensory ganglion, trauma or exposure to ultraviolet light at the previously affected epithelial surface site, immunosuppression by drugs, or by bacterial infections such as pneumococcal or meningococcal septicemia.

The HSV-infected host responds to a whole range of viral antigens, producing cytotoxic T cells (CTL) (especially and unusually CD4+) within 4 to 6 days, and helper T lymphocytes (CD4+) which activate primed B cells to produce specific antibodies later, and which are also involved in the induction of delayed hypersensitivity[32]. Viral glycoproteins are important immunogens, probably all of them inducing neutralizing antibody. However, non-structural antigens are presented early on at the infected cell surface by major histocompatability complex (MHC) class I molecules, and the ability of CTL to recognize these antigens and destroy the cell before new virions are released is probably significant for limiting infection. Neurons harboring latent HSV contain no virus-coded proteins. They do, however, contain latency-associated RNA transcripts that may code antisense proteins, which seem to be associated with maintenance of latency[35]. Neurons do not express MHC class I or II antigens to present herpesvirus antigens, so are not recognized by the immune system[36]. Other

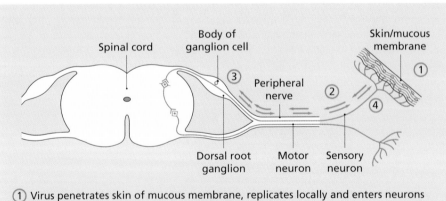

① Virus penetrates skin of mucous membrane, replicates locally and enters neurons
② Centripetal migration of nucleocapsid within axon
③ Synthesis of infectious virion in ganglion
④ Centrifugal migration of virions to skin or mucous membranes

Figure 6.5 Pathogenesis of herpes simplex virus infection

ways in which HSV evades immune recognition include binding to complement components, Fc receptors, and the peptide transporter TAP[37]. The particular MHC make up of individuals has been associated with their risk of HSV-2 infection, and with symptomatic infection[38]. Further understanding is needed of the factors operating at the cellular level, and particularly on mucosal surfaces, in order to elicit protective immune responses for control of genital HSV.

The nature of ganglionic latency is enigmatic and what controls that state is unknown.

The microscopical findings in primary and recurrent lesions of the skin and mucous membranes are identical, and resemble those of herpes zoster and varicella. The histopathology of genital herpes and orolabial herpes (the latter has been studied the most) is identical[33, 34]. During the evolution of the lesion the earliest changes, which are often focal but become more pronounced in later stages, are found in the keratinocytes, particularly in the basal-cell layer. Within the nuclei there is peripheral margination of the chromatin and homogeneous, basophilic material with a 'ground-glass' appearance distends the nucleus; this material contains viral DNA. Later this mass appears to retract from the nuclear margin. Ballooning of the nuclei with disappearance of the nucleoli is prominent in the crusted lesions and eosinophilic inclusions (Cowdry A inclusions), that contain little viral DNA and are probably artifacts, are sometimes seen at this late stage. Cytoplasmic changes lag behind those of the nuclei. The earliest change is vacuolization of the cytoplasm of the basal layer, followed by dyskeratosis and acantholysis. A serous exudate separates damaged keratinocytes and gradually a vesicle forms under the stratum corneum. The margins of the vesicles are usually clearly demarcated, showing an abrupt transformation from normal epithelium to balloon degeneration. Multinucleated giant cells are found in papules and vesicles, but are most commonly found in crusted lesions, particularly in the differentiating epidermal cell layers. In early lesions and in papules and vesicles, there is a minimal inflammatory response with infiltration with neutrophils and mononuclear cells. Neutrophils are the predominant cell type in the epidermis, dermis, and crust of the crusted lesion. Virus-induced changes are also found within sebaceous glands and hair follicles.

HERPETIC PROCTITIS

In herpetic proctitis, there may be focal ulceration of the epithelium with microabscess formation extending into the submucosa. Lymphocytic infiltration around the submucosal blood vessels may be seen, as may multinucleated cells and intranuclear inclusions[39].

HERPETIC ENCEPHALITIS

In encephalitis there is asymmetrical softening with numerous hemorrhages on the surface of affected areas. The inferior and medial parts of the temporal lobe, the insula and orbital part of the frontal lobe are involved. There is perivascular inflammation and hemorrhage, and the neurons, oligodendrocytes, and astrocytes show eosinophilic intranuclear inclusions. There is no demyelination.

CYTOLOGY OF HERPES SIMPLEX VIRUS INFECTION

In cytological preparations (Figure 6.6) from lesions[40], multinucleated giant cells are often seen together with nuclear changes: some nuclei contain small intra-

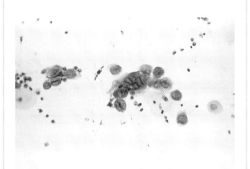

Figure 6.6 Cytological preparation from the cervix of a woman with genital herpes, showing multinucleated giant cells and eosinophilic inclusions (× 1000, Papanicolaou stain) (reproduced with permission from Dr A Williams, Department of Pathology, University of Edinburgh Medical School)

nuclear vacuoles with basophilic particles scattered within the nucleus, other nuclei have a homogeneous ground-glass appearance, and others have eosinophilic inclusion bodies surrounded by a clear 'halo'.

Immunology

Herpes simplex virus persists throughout the life of the infected individual and achieves this by mechanisms that enable it to avoid host responses, namely the ability of the virus to

- pass from cell to cell by a fusion process circumventing the need to emerge into the extracellular environment
- secure latent infection of a neuronal cell by a mechanism as yet not precisely known,
- evade natural defense systems of the host, i.e. macrophages, natural killer cells, and interferon.

Evidence about humoral immunity can be obtained from the study of infection in man but most data on other aspects of its natural history or cell-mediated immunity are obtained from animal studies, particularly in mice, where supplementary evidence indicates that the mouse is a useful model for studying the infection.

Following infection there are both humoral and cell-mediated immune responses lasting many years. Herpes simplex virus types 1 and 2 possess shared antigenic determinants so that infection with one results in the production of antibodies and lymphocytes which will react with the other.

Primary infection yields a rise in antibody titers reaching a peak in about 4 to 6 weeks and remaining stable afterwards. Virus-specific IgM antibodies are produced in the early stages and persist for 6 to 8 weeks.

In individuals with pre-existing antibodies recurrence is not associated with a marked change in antibody titer; similarly re-infection with the same or different type of the virus produces little change. In neither recurrence nor re-infection is there an IgM response unless the infection is extensive, when there may be an IgM and an IgG response.

In the newborn passively transferred maternal antibodies are often present but are gradually lost during the first 6 months of life. Herpes simplex virus type 1 antibodies appear in childhood more often in the lower socioeconomic groups than in the higher; in the latter group, therefore, HSV-1 and HSV-2 are more likely to produce a primary infection during adolescence and early adult life.

Interferon, macrophages, and natural killer (NK) cells are important in the immediate defense against HSV, and the neonate has a diminished capacity in this regard. Langerhans cells (dendritic antigen-presenting cells in the epithelium) are also important, and are known to be reduced by ultraviolet light exposure[41]. The cellular immune response to HSV infection is discussed above.

Epidemiology

The number of cases of genital herpes reported from STI clinics has been increasing over the past 20 years. Figure 6.7 shows the number of cases of first episode genital herpes reported from the clinics of the UK. As shown by the National Health and Nutrition Examination Surveys (NHANES II and III) undertaken between 1976 to 1980 and 1988 to 1994 respectively, the seroprevalence of HSV-2 infection in the USA has increased some 30% since the 1970s[42, 11]. The prevalence of antibodies against HSV-2 has been shown to vary between populations. In the USA, the seroprevalence of HSV-2 is higher amongst black people (45.9%) than amongst white people (17.8%), and this may reflect the poorer socioeconomic status of many blacks, and different sexual or health-related behavior. A striking increase in the prevalence of HSV-2 infection amongst whites was observed in the interval between the NHANES II and NHANES III studies. Amongst white teenagers, the prevalence of specific HSV-2 antibody increased fivefold and that amongst white men and women in their twenties doubled in that period. The change in seroprevalence of HSV amongst black people was less marked but this may reflect their already high seropositivity. On both sides of the Atlantic, specific antibody is found more frequently amongst women than heterosexual men: 12.4% and 3.2% of female and male blood donors respectively in London, UK[10], and 25.6% of women and 17.8% of men assessed in the NHANES III study[11]. This difference may reflect the higher efficiency of transmission of HSV-2 from a male to a female (see below). In the UK the seroprevalence of HSV-2 is higher amongst STI clinic attenders (24.5% of women and 17.3% of men in one London clinic[10]) than amongst blood donors. Men who have sex with men and who attend STI clinics have also been shown to have a higher prevalence of HSV-2 specific antibody than heterosexual men attending the same clinic (27.1% versus 17.3%[10]). The frequency of detection of specific antibody against HSV-2 increases with age up to about 40 years, and there is a strong correlation between its prevalence and both an increasing number of years of sexual activity, and an increasing number of sexual partners (particularly amongst whites in the USA)[10, 11]. Age at first sexual experience is not, however, associated with an increased seroprevalence of HSV-2[10, 11].

Over the past 15 years the proportion of individuals with initial genital herpes caused by HSV-1 has been increasing, and in some areas almost 50% of genital isolates are HSV-1 (Figure 6.8). It is presumed that the majority of these people have acquired the infection by orogenital contact.

Asymptomatic shedding of HSV-1 and HSV-2 from the genital tract is now well recognized but the prevalence of asymptomatic excreters varies depending on the setting of the study. For example, in a study from an STI clinic in the USA, 4% of 372 women with serological or virological evidence of genital herpes had asymptomatic shedding of virus at the time of sampling[43]. Shedding of HSV-2 was not found in any of 131 men and in only 2 of 401 women who attended clinics other than those for the management of STIs in Sweden[44]. Sometimes excretion of virus originates from lesions that are inaccessible, or, if on the uterine cervix, can only be seen by the use of a colposcope[45].

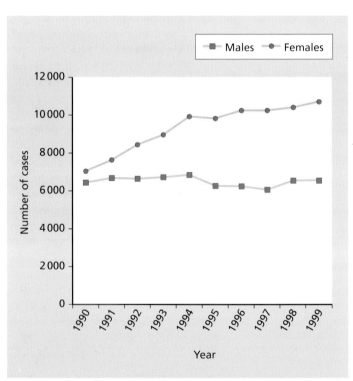

Figure 6.7 Number of cases of initial genital herpes reported from STI clinics in the UK 1990–1999 (from PHLS DHSS&PS and the Scottish ISD(D)5 Collaborative Group 2000[205])

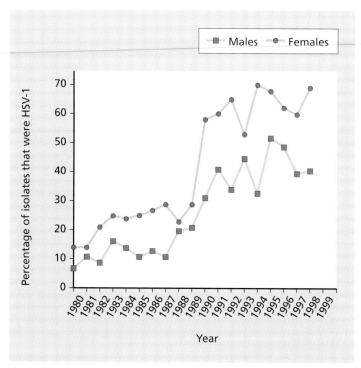

Figure 6.8 Proportion of individuals with initial genital herpes caused by HSV-1 who attended the Department of Genitourinary Medicine at Edinburgh Royal Infirmary 1989–1998

SEXUAL TRANSMISSION OF HERPES SIMPLEX VIRUS

Acquisition of HSV is through direct contact with infected tissue or secretions. As the virus is labile and readily inactivated at room temperature, the risk of transmission from fomites is very small. The virus can be transmitted from individuals who are symptomatic, although they may not recognize these symptoms as being those of HSV, or who are truly asymptomatic. The sexual transmission of HSV-2 from asymptomatic excreters of the virus has been recognized since the mid-1980s[46–48]. Mertz et al.[49] noted that 9 of 13 episodes of virus transmission related to sexual contact during asymptomatic viral shedding from a partner with known recurrent genital herpes; transmission to the other 4 individuals at risk occurred during the prodrome or just after lesions had been noted by the source partner. Although these authors reported that previous infection with HSV-1 appeared to reduce the risk for acquisition of HSV-2 among women, this has not been confirmed in recent studies[50, 51]. The overall risk of genital transmission of HSV between couples is low, about 10% per year, but the risk of acquisition of the virus appears to be higher in women than in men[49, 52]. In Mertz and colleagues' study[49], the risk of transmission from men to women was 17%, compared with 3% from women to men. This increased risk may reflect the larger surface area of the female genital mucosa, compared with the male, that may be exposed to infection, and the higher recurrence rate noted amongst men (see page 110). Another factor that may result in the observed increased transmission rate to women may be the lack of severity of the clinical features of recurrent disease in men. Symptoms of genital herpes in the male are often mild, and because they are not recognized as herpetic, sexual intercourse may occur when infectious lesions are present.

Herpes simplex virus appears to be transmitted relatively efficiently. In the study reported by Mertz et al.[46], the median interval between the first sexual exposure and the transmission of the infection to the index patient was 3 months (range 1 day to 14 years), and the median number of sexual exposures per couple prior to transmission was 24 (range 1 to 720).

ROLE OF HERPES SIMPLEX VIRUS IN THE TRANSMISSION OF HIV

In a prospective study of 62 men who developed HIV infection and 61 men who remained HIV-non-infected, Holmberg et al.[53] noted an increased prevalence of antibodies against HSV-2, but not against HSV-1, amongst men who seroconverted for HIV. They found that 68% of 47 HIV seroconverters had antibodies against HSV-2 compared with 46% of 57 men who remained HIV seronegative. Seroconversion to HSV-2 was found in 11 (42%) of 26 HIV seroconverters, compared to only 5 (14%) of 35 men who remained HIV seronegative. Similar findings were reported by Hook et al.[54] who undertook a case-control study amongst HIV-infected (179 individuals) and HIV-non-infected (367 individuals) heterosexual men and women. They noted that 62.7% of HIV-infected but only 46.7% of HIV-non-infected men were seropositive for HSV-2; the HSV-2 seroprevalence rates amongst HIV-infected and non-infected women were 78.7% and 57.7% respectively. The seroprevalence rate for HSV-1 was similar among both patient groups. These studies suggested that HSV-2 infection was a risk factor for subsequent or concurrent HIV infection.

Although previously considered to be an uncommon cause of genital ulceration in South Africa, HSV-2 has recently been shown to be the most frequent etiological agent in genital ulceration, having been detected in 36% of 538 affected men[55]. The frequent association of HSV-2 ulceration with HIV-1 infection is of great public health concern: HSV-2 was detected in 47.4% of ulcerated lesions in 215 HIV-1-infected men, compared with 28.2% of 323 HIV-1-non-infected men. Further evidence of an association between HSV-2 and HIV-1 comes from the cross-sectional study reported by Gwanzura et al.[56]: the seroprevalence of HSV-2 amongst 191 HIV-infected and 224 HIV-non-infected male factory workers in Zimbabwe was 82.7% and 35.7% respectively.

In an elegant study of 12 HIV-1 and HSV-2 seropositive homosexual men, Schacker *et al.*[22] examined HIV-1 viral shedding from anogenital ulcers caused by HSV-2. These 12 men were followed through 26 episodes of recurrence. Using PCR HIV-1 RNA was detected in lesions of 25 of the 26 episodes, sometimes at high titer and exceeding the patient's plasma RNA taken at the same time. The median percentage of days on which HIV was detected in the lesions sampled was 66.7%, but HIV-1 RNA became undetectable once the lesions had re-epithelialized. As the HIV-1 nucleic acid detected was virion associated, the infectious potential of such lesions is clear.

Clinical features of herpes simplex virus

The very common nature of inapparent infections whether by HSV-1 or HSV-2 is now well-recognized (see pp. 110–111). When apparent, the prepatent or incubation period lies between 3 and 9 days.

PRIMARY AND INITIAL INFECTIONS

Primary infections of the oral cavity and pharynx

Primary herpetic gingivostomatitis is the most common clinical manifestation of primary infection of HSV-1 in children between 1 and 5 years of age. The stomatitis begins with fever, malaise, restlessness, and excessive dribbling. Drinking and eating are very painful and the breath is foul. Vesicles containing high titers of virus appear as white plaques on the tongue, pharynx, palate, and buccal mucosa. The plaques are followed by ulcers with a yellowing pseudomembrane. Regional lymph nodes are enlarged and tender[57]. An identical clinical picture may be seen in young adults who escaped infection in childhood but acquired the infection by kissing someone with a primary infection or, most often, a reactivated lesion or 'cold sore'.

Herpes simplex virus infection of the pharynx is common in individuals with

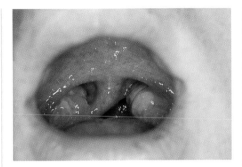

Figure 6.9 Primary HSV-2 infection of the tonsils

primary genital herpes. Corey *et al.*[58] isolated HSV-2 from the pharynges of 11% of individuals with primary HSV-2 genital herpes and HSV-1 from the pharynges of 20% of patients with HSV-1 genital infection. Primary herpetic pharyngitis causes a sore throat and is usually associated with fever, malaise, myalgia, headache, and tender anterior cervical lymphadenopathy; it may be difficult to distinguish from pharyngitis due to other causes. There may be mild erythema of the pharynx or diffuse ulceration, the ulcerated areas being covered with a white exudate (Figure 6.9).

Primary and initial genital herpes

The frequency of constitutional symptoms, the number of lesions, and the duration of symptoms are similar for HSV-1 and HSV-2 primary genital infections. In patients with non-primary first episode HSV-2 infections, the frequency of constitutional features, the severity of local pain, and the duration of lesions are less than in those who have primary infection[58]. Thus prior infection with HSV-1 appears to lessen the severity of first episode genital herpes.

Primary genital herpes in women

Symptoms and signs of primary genital herpes tend to be more severe in women than in men and are usually those of vulvovaginitis, often accompanied by systemic symptoms of fever and malaise, while local pain and dysuria can be severe. Systemic features appear early in the course of the illness and peak within 4 days of the onset of the lesions, thereafter receding during the remainder of the first week.

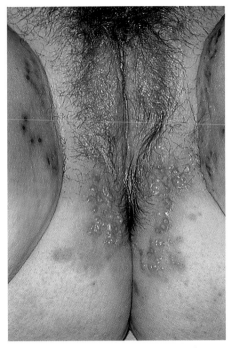

Figure 6.10 Primary HSV-2 infection of the vulva (reproduced from McMillan and Scott 2000[206])

Difficulty in starting micturition or retention of urine may be the presenting clinical feature and there may be increased vaginal discharge. White plaques are present on the red swollen mucosae of the vulva, cervix, and, occasionally the vagina (4%); scattered vesicles are seen on the labia and these may extend to involve the perianal skin and the skin of the thigh (Figure 6.10). During the second and third weeks of the illness, the regional lymph nodes become enlarged and tender, and are often slow to return to normal. Healing tends to take place over a period of 1 to 2 weeks, but new lesions sometimes continue to develop over a period of 6 weeks. Untreated, the mean time from the onset of the lesions to complete re-epithelialization has been reported as being 19.7 days[58]. Lesions on dry surfaces such as the mons pubis become crusted before re-epithelialization; mucosal lesions and those on moist skin re-epithelialize without crusting.

In primary cervicitis there may be only swelling and redness of the mucosa but sometimes there is a necrotic ulceration (Figure 6.11) and friability of the cervix which bleeds easily.

In view of the disparity between the frequency of HSV-2 antibody and that of

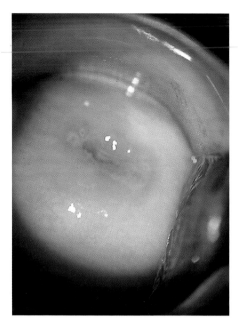

Figure 6.11 Primary HSV-2 infection of the uterine cervix (reproduced from McMillan and Scott 2000[206])

clinical features (see page 109), it is perhaps not surprising that primary or initial genital herpes is not always associated with the symptoms and signs just described. Koutsky et al.[43] reported that 4 (9%) of 44 women

with culture-proven initial symptomatic vulval herpes had an atypical presentation: vulval erythema, fissuring of the introitus, or an indurated lesion thought to be a furuncle. These workers also reported that HSV can be associated with cervical ulceration that may only be visible with the colposcope. It is our opinion that, as primary or initial genital herpes is under-diagnosed in many clinics, specimens for the detection of HSV should be taken from any vesicular or ulcerated lesion(s) of the genitalia.

Primary genital herpes in men

In primary genital herpes in men systemic features are less common than in women (39% versus 68%[58]). The lesions can involve the glans or coronal sulcus (Figure 6.12) and, if severe, there may be a phimosis with accumulation of secondarily infected exudate and occasionally a necrotizing balanitis (Figure 6.13). In rare instances, a necrotizing balanitis may develop without phimosis. In circumcised men, genital lesions are less common. Crops of vesicles may develop on the shaft of the penis, on the anterior aspect of the scrotum,

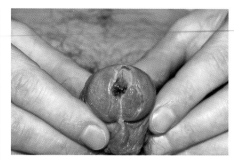

Figure 6.13 Necrotizing balanitis associated with HSV-2

and on the skin nearby. Crusting before re-epithelialization is seen on the shaft of the penis, the glans in the circumcised male, and the dry skin of the outer aspect of the prepuce; in the uncircumcised male, lesions of the glans and mucosal surface of the prepuce re-epithelialize without crusting. Untreated, the mean time from onset of the lesions to complete healing has been reported as 16.5 days[58].

Primary urethral herpes simplex virus infection in men and women

Although HSV can be isolated from the urethra of almost 30% of men and 80% of

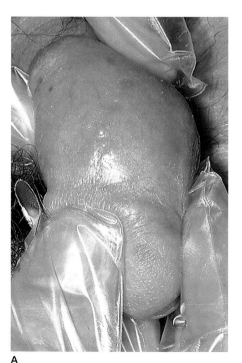

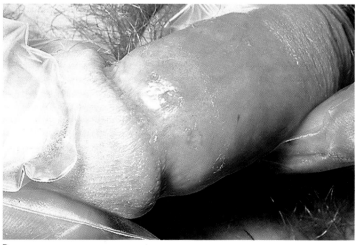

A   B

Figure 6.12 Primary HSV-2 infection of the coronal sulcus showing (A) vesicles, (B) 1 day later, ulceration (reproduced from McMillan and Scott 2000[206])

women with external lesions of primary genital herpes[58], the urethra in both sexes may, uncommonly, be affected in the absence of signs elsewhere. Dysuria is the most common symptom in men and can be severe. There may be a mucoid urethral discharge, and a Gram-stained smear of this shows significant numbers of polymorphonuclear leukocytes. Hematuria may be an additional feature. A clue to the diagnosis is the finding of tender inguinal lymph node enlargement and, sometimes, fever. Frequency, dysuria, and hematuria with fever and inguinal lymphadenitis are the most common features of urethral infection in women. When undertaken, urethroscopy has shown mucosal ulceration[59].

Primary anorectal herpes in men and women

Herpes simplex virus can also involve the anorectum. In men this may result from unprotected receptive anal intercourse, digitation with a contaminated finger, or receptive oral–anal contact. Women may be infected similarly, or at the time of vaginal intercourse. Anorectal pain, a mucoid or blood-stained discharge, constipation, tenesmus, anal pruritus, difficulty in starting micturition, paresthesiae in the

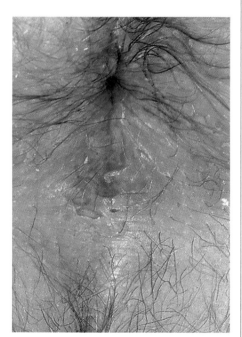

Figure 6.14 Primary perianal herpes in a young homosexual man (reproduced from McMillan and Scott 2000[206])

sacral area, pain in the back of the thigh, fever, and enlargement of the inguinal lymph nodes are more characteristic of proctitis due to HSV than that due to other causes[39]. Vesicles or shallow ulcers of the perianal or anal region (Figure 6.14) are seen in only 50% of cases. Through the proctoscope the rectal mucosa may be seen to be friable and petechiae may form on its surface when touched with a cotton wool swab. Occasionally there are vesicles and a diffuse ulceration of the distal 10 cm of the rectal mucosa, very seldom extending to the sigmoid colon[60].

Primary herpes simplex virus infection at other sites in men and women

Extragenital lesions may occur in areas near to the genitals, particularly in the buttocks, groin or thigh. Herpesvirus may be acquired at other sites by contact, as in herpetic whitlow (Figure 6.15) seen in patients and, in the past, in medical personnel, as 'scrumpox' in the case of rugby players, or even on the trunk among wrestlers. Other forms include keratoconjunctivitis and eczema herpeticum, where infection has become superimposed on eczematous skin (Kaposi's varicelliform eruption). These extragenital lesions result from autoinoculation rather than by viremia[58].

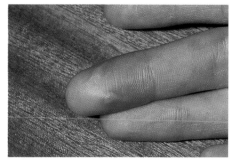

Figure 6.15 Herpetic whitlow

Complications of primary genital herpes in men and women (Table 6.1)

Secondary infection

Various species of pathogenic aerobic and anaerobic bacteria can be isolated from herpetic genital ulcers[67] but serious secondary infection is unusual. Although the time to healing is reported to be shorter in patients given cotrimoxazole in combination with aciclovir, than in those given the antiviral drug alone[68], there are insufficient data to support the routine use of antimicrobial therapy in patients with first episode herpes. Secondary infection with fungi, for example vulvovaginal candidiasis, has also been reported in 14% of women with primary genital herpes[58], with symptoms usually being experienced during the second week of the illness.

Table 6.1 Early complications of primary genital herpes

Early complications	Long term complications
Local complications: 　secondary bacterial infection 　phimosis/paraphimosis 　labial adhesions Extragenital complications: 　autoinoculation 　dissemination, especially in 　　pregnant women and the 　　immunocompromised 　neurological 　　meningitis 　　encephalitis 　　transverse myelitis 　　sacral autonomic neuropathy	recurrences psychosexual complications neonatal transmission

Genital adhesions

Fibrinous adhesions between ulcerated surfaces of the labia minora and under the clitoral hood are not uncommon[62], and unless the complication is recognized and treated early, fibrosis requiring surgery can develop. Rarely, preputial adhesions with phimosis complicate genital herpes in the male[63].

Upper genital tract infection

Lower abdominal pain and tenderness of the uterine adnexae accompany involvement of the urogenital tract, but, although herpetic endometritis has been described (rarely), it is uncertain whether this pelvic inflammation is caused by ascending HSV infection or to other sexually transmitted causes.

Aseptic meningitis

Fever, severe headache, malaise, photophobia, neck stiffness and the presence of Kernig's or Brudzinski's sign indicating meningeal involvement may occur within 6 to 12 days of onset in 36% of women and 13% of men with primary genital infection with HSV-2[58]. The cerebrospinal fluid (CSF) pressure is slightly increased and there is a lymphocytic pleocytosis (5 to 1000 per mm³) that diminishes spontaneously; the CSF glucose concentration may be normal, elevated in relation to the plasma level, or, less frequently, reduced. Symptoms usually recede within 72 hours of their onset. Herpes simplex virus meningitis is more commonly associated with genital herpes than with orolabial infection[61].

Sacral radiculomyelopathy

Sacral anesthesia, urinary retention requiring intermittent catheterization, and constipation may occur. The patient may complain of numbness and tingling in the buttocks or of perineal pain and there may be a decrease in perception of fine touch in these areas. Urinary retention and constipation may follow. In men impotence is associated with a decrease in the bulbocavernosus reflex. Uncommonly acute retention of urine may occur and persist for a week or more in association with an episode of anogenital herpes in women in particular and in homosexual men with

perianal herpes or herpetic proctitis[64, 65]. Although pain may be responsible, constipation, blunting of sensation over the sacral dermatomes and neuralgic pains in the same area, and sometimes absence of the bulbocavernosus reflex suggest involvement of the sacral nerve roots.

Other neurological complications

Rarely, transverse myelitis with rapidly progressive symmetrical paralysis of the lower limbs has been reported[66].

Disseminated infection

In immunocompetent individuals, dissemination of HSV is rare[69]. Visceral dissemination has been described mostly in pregnant women (see pp. 134–135), and vesicular or pustular cutaneous lesions (Figure 6.16).

Psychological complications

These are common and of great importance. After being diagnosed as having genital herpes, patients may go through several stages[70]

1. denial
2. belief that there is a cure
3. realization that they have HSV infection
4. loneliness
5. anger towards the individual from whom they suspect they have acquired the infection
6. fear of sexual deprivations
7. poor self-image.

RECURRENT HERPES SIMPLEX VIRUS INFECTION

Recurrent orolabial herpes

In the commonest form of herpes simplex of the face or lips, itching or burning precedes, by an hour or two, the development of erythematous macules, then papule formation and, within 1 day, vesicle formation. Ulcers or crusts form that persist for about 1 week (Figure 6.17) after which there is complete healing. Virus is detectable by culture for about 4 days after the onset of symptoms. Ordinarily healing is complete within 7 to 10 days. The shallow ulcers that develop may be very painful. Recurrent ulcers tend to be in the same region but not precisely in the same spot. Sometimes in otherwise healthy children and young adults, recrudescent herpes can resemble primary herpetic gingivostomatitis[71].

Recurrent genital herpes

In recurrent herpes simplex of the genitals, or indeed of any site, recurrences may be heralded by a prodromal sensation of tingling, occurring 30 minutes to 48 hours before the appearance of lesions. In some

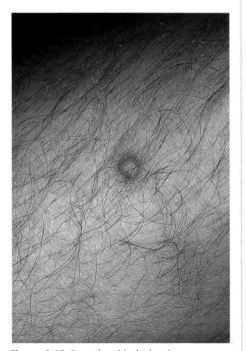

Figure 6.16 Pustular skin lesion in disseminated HSV-2 infection

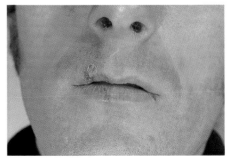

Figure 6.17 Recurrent, crusting lesion of orolabial herpes

patients, stabbing pains in the distribution of the sciatic nerve that last for several days may herald the recurrence (sometimes these prodromal features may develop without the subsequent appearance of lesions[72]). Several small vesicular lesions then appear and may coalesce. Lesions tend to increase in size over the first 3 days of the episode, remain static for about a week and resolve rapidly thereafter; the mean time from the appearance of vesicles to complete re-epithelialization has been reported as 10 days[58]. The symptoms are substantially milder than those of the initial episode and constitutional symptoms are infrequent. Symptoms, however, tend to be more severe in women than in men.

Complications of recurrent genital herpes

Physical complications and sequelae are uncommon. On the penis there may be some depigmentation and scarring of the affected site, particularly when there have been multiple recurrences over months or years. In the eye, repeated recurrences may result in corneal opacity. Psychological and psychosexual sequelae, however, are important complications. Patients with recurrent genital herpes may experience

- shame and guilt
- withdrawal from social interactions
- a shunning of intimate relationships because of fear of discovery of infection by a partner with disapproval and subsequent rejection
- depression
- fear of transmitting HSV to others.

As a result the individual can become increasingly isolated and withdrawn.

Rarely, recurrent erythema multiforme may complicate recurrent genital herpes[73], and recurrent aseptic meningitis (Mollaret's meningitis, presenting with features of acute meningitis, but resolving spontaneously within a few days) may be associated with HSV infection, particularly HSV-2 infection[74]. Evidence has been accruing that in at least some patients with peripheral 7th nerve palsy (Bell's palsy), HSV-1 may be causative, and that there is a rationale for antiviral treatment of affected individuals[75].

Diagnosis of herpes simplex virus infections

It is recommended that the clinician should investigate all cases where there is a possibility of genital herpes simplex infection, in order to confirm clinical diagnosis and to detect atypical infections. Inaccurate clinical histories are common: 11% of clinic attenders and 7% of blood donors thought incorrectly that they had had genital herpes[76]. Laboratories undertake both virus detection and serological studies for HSV, and each technique has a place in the diagnosis of HSV infection. Early in the treatment of any new patient with HSV infection, primary or recurrent, samples should be sent for virus detection, with an acute clotted-blood sample for storage or serology. Antibody responses will require time to develop, and a convalescent clotted blood sample 4 to 6 weeks after onset is best for detection of changes. Where type-specific serology is available, a baseline blood sample may be considered for screening in certain situations[77].

HERPES SIMPLEX VIRUS DETECTION

Material for the detection of HSV should be obtained from lesions by gently scraping with a cotton wool-tipped applicator stick. The specimen obtained is then agitated in a bijou bottle containing virus transport medium, for example, Hanks' balanced salt solution[78]. Direct diagnosis of HSV infection by a rapid antigen detection test (immunofluorescence or enzyme immuno-assay) may be useful when there is any doubt as to the clinical diagnosis, or where rapid confirmation is required to support the choice of therapy or other management. It is also more likely to give an answer than virus culture when the lesion is crusting (electron microscopy of scrapings from lesions can also be used to detect HSV, but is largely superseded by immunofluorescence). Nucleic acid amplification by PCR should be used routinely for most samples for HSV. It can also be usefully applied to samples from atypical lesions. Virus isolation for confirmation and

typing is suitable for most common HSV infections, especially if treatment has been started on clinical grounds. In all cases swabs from lesions should be submitted in a virus transport medium to preserve infectivity, maintain cells, and inhibit microbial growth.

Isolation of HSV is usually only available from virus laboratories with cell culture facilities, although the commercially-produced Enzyme-Linked Virus Inducible System (ELVIS™) could be used in any microbiology laboratory processing substantial numbers of samples for HSV detection. This ingenious system has an HSV promoter gene in cells in prepared culture vials; any HSV infection induces the promoter and consequently expression of a linked enzyme that is detected by a blue stain. The newest version incorporates a fluorescent-staining method to type the virus[79]. Herpes simplex virus cytopathic effects in standard human fibroblast cell cultures appear from 1 to 7 days after inoculation, depending on the starting virus titer. The virus may then be typed by staining the cells with fluorescent-labeled type-specific monoclonal antibodies[80]. Typing the virus is relevant to prognosis and epidemiology.

Detection of PCR amplified HSV DNA in CSF (or other samples) is proving a much more sensitive method of detection than virus isolation, the previous 'gold standard'[81]. The two HSV types can be differentiated either by using type-specific primers in the single or nested PCR, or using common primers followed by analysis with restriction enzymes or hybridization probes for each type. It is the greatly improved detection of HSV by PCR that has informed the re-assessment of CNS infections in particular[82].

SEROLOGY FOR HERPES SIMPLEX VIRUS

Complement fixation tests (CFT) for HSV antibody have little place now except in the diagnosis of primary infections when a significant change in antibody titer can be expected if paired serum samples taken at onset and 4 to 6 weeks later are examined in parallel. The CF titer of antibody measures total HSV antibody and does not differentiate either type-specific antibodies or IgM.

Enzyme immunoassays are much more sensitive than CFT. With HSV antigen from whole virus or infected cells, tests can reveal whether any HSV antibody is present, but do not give reliable type-specific data[83]. Western blotting has, for a long time, been the reference method used by few experts to establish the appearance of antibodies to different HSV antigens from both types. Recently validated type-specific antigen-based preparations have come on the market, allowing more widespread type-specific antibody detection[84]. These tests for type-specific HSV antibodies are being considered for screening in situations where a patient is at risk, as in pregnancy[77] (see also Prevention, pp. 132 and 137). Where seroconversion is looked for, it is important to remember that treatment often results in a delay in the appearance of these antibodies, and late convalescent samples, at 6 weeks, should

be included. A new point-of-care test (near-patient test) has been evaluated, with promising results for early detection of seroconversion to HSV-2 antibodies[85]. In a pre-market evaluation of this test, sera from 50 patients with culture-proven HSV-1 and from 253 patients with genital HSV-2 were tested. Compared with viral culture and Western blot analysis, the sensitivity and specificity of the test were 96% and 98% respectively[86]. An advantage of this test is that results are available in minutes.

Treatment

ANTIVIRAL DRUGS FOR HERPES SIMPLEX VIRUS INFECTION

Three antiviral agents – aciclovir, vala-ciclovir, and famciclovir – are generally

available for use in the treatment of HSV infection. In addition, penciclovir cream is used in the treatment of recurrent orolabial infections. Cidofovir and foscarnet are valuable in the therapy of infections caused by aciclovir-resistant HSV.

Aciclovir

Aciclovir (9-[2-hydroxyethoxymethyl]-guanine) is an analogue of 2'-deoxy-guanosine and is a potent inhibitor of HSV-1 (median 50% inhibitory concentration (IC_{50}) against HSV-1 = 0.1 μM), HSV-2 (median IC_{50} against HSV-2 = 0.4 μM), and VZV (median IC_{50} against VZV = 2.6 μM)[87, 88]. It was the first antiviral agent to show real benefit in the treatment of primary or initial herpes genitalis, and is still the most widely used agent. Unfortunately, aciclovir, like the other available antiviral agents, although giving some

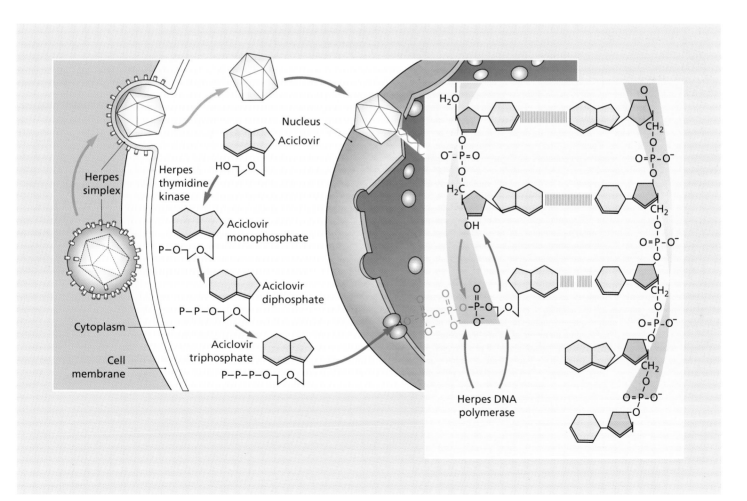

Figure 6.18 Mechanism of action of aciclovir in cells infected by herpes simplex virus (reproduced with permission from Balfour 1999[96])

temporary relief in recurrent herpes, does not affect ganglionic latency. In the treatment of primary or initial muco-cutaneous HSV infections, with or without dissemination or in recurrent herpes in the immunocompromised individual, aciclovir is highly effective and can be life saving.

Mode of action

In HSV-infected cells, aciclovir is phos-phorylated to its monophosphate by a viral-encoded TK (Figure 6.18). The mono-phosphate is then further phosphorylated by cellular enzymes to produce aciclovir triphosphate (ACV-TP), a more potent inhibitor of viral DNA polymerase than of cellular DNA polymerases, ACV-TP enters the nucleus of the cell and inhibits HSV DNA in a three-step mechanism[89]. In the first step ACV-TP binds to *pol*, the catalytic subunit of HSV DNA polymerase, where it can act as a competitive inhibitor of the natural substrate dGTP (2'-deoxyguanosine triphosphate). Aciclovir triphosphate then acts as a substrate when the pyrophosphate is cleaved from the ACV-TP; the resulting ACV monophosphate is incorporated into the chain and acts as a chain terminator. In the third step, the deoxynucleotide tri-phosphates complementary to the next template position acts as an inhibitor of the DNA polymerase binding it irrevers-ibly to the ACV-terminated primer/template complex.

Pharmacokinetics

Only some 10% to 20% of a 200 mg dose of aciclovir given by mouth is absorbed from the gastrointestinal tract[87]. In patients with genital HSV on an oral dose of 200 mg every 4 hours, five times per day (the standard oral treatment) peak levels are found 1.5 to 1.75 hours after the oral dose. Peak plasma aciclovir levels range from 1.4 to 4.0 μM with a mean of 2.5 μM (1 μM = 0.225 μg/mL)[90], greatly exceeding the IC_{50} for HSV-1 and HSV-2. The pharmacokinetics of aciclovir in late pregnancy are similar to those in the non-pregnant woman[91].

Aciclovir levels in saliva are well correlated with simultaneous plasma levels, saliva levels being approximately 13% of plasma levels. Simultaneous plasma and vaginal contents levels are poorly cor-related; peak levels in vaginal secretions range from 0.5 to 3.6 μM[92]. Aciclovir concentrations in the amniotic fluid of women given the drug during late pregnancy (mean concentration $\pm$ SD = 5.8 $\pm$ 2.7 μM) have been found to be higher than in the plasma (mean concen-tration $\pm$ SD = 0.9 $\pm$ 1.3 μM)[93] and aciclovir concentrations in breast milk are up to four times those of the plasma[94].

The peak aciclovir concentrations in plasma and vaginal fluid are in the range of the 50% inhibitory dose of 0.5 μM for HSV-1 and 1.62 μM for HSV-2 determined by Crumpacker *et al.*[95], with saliva levels at the lower end of this range.

With intravenous aciclovir (5.0 mg/kg) given every 8 hours, peak levels of 12.7 to 43.2 μM (mean 26.1 μM) have been found in 30 patients with genital herpes and the estimated half-life of aciclovir is said to be 3.3 hours[92]. These authors concluded that inhibitory levels of aciclovir could be achieved in plasma and body secretions with oral therapy without evidence of drug toxicity.

Excretion

Aciclovir appears to be excreted by glomerular filtration and renal tubular excretion. Clearance from plasma is relatively rapid and depends primarily on the efficiency of renal secretion. The clear-ance of aciclovir is substantially higher than the estimated creatinine clearance, indicating that not only glomerular filtration but also renal tubular excretion contributes to the elimination of the drug. If probenecid is given renal clearance falls but it remains twice the value of the estimated creatinine clearance[90].

Because of the route of elimination, the drug has the potential to crystallize out in the kidney tubules; this was noted in early days when the drug was given as a bolus injection intravenously and when the patient was not adequately hydrated. Patients should therefore be well hydrated and with slow intravenous infusion over approximately 1 hour this problem has not recurred (see below for details of intra-venous administration of aciclovir).

Metabolic elimination

Blum *et al.*[90] also found that 9-carboxy-methoxymethyl-guanine is the only signifi-cant metabolite of aciclovir, accounting for 8.5% to 14.1% of the dose. This metabolite has little anti-HSV activity. In those with moderately impaired renal function more drug is eliminated by metabolism as renal function decreases.

Plasma protein binding

At plasma concentrations of aciclovir of 1.8 to 22.2 μM only small amounts (15.4% $\pm$ 4.4%) of the drug are protein bound[90].

Aciclovir tolerance and unwanted effects

Among 350 patients with serious and potentially life-threatening HSV infections receiving rapid (bolus) intravenous injec-tions of aciclovir, raised plasma urea and/or creatinine levels were noted in 23 (6.5%); with local injection-site reactions in 6 (1.7%), these were the only adverse events considered to be caused by aciclovir. Overall, of 465 patients given intravenous aciclovir, only 9% showed renal side effects but these can be virtually eliminated when rapid intravenous injections are avoided, attention is paid to careful hydration of patients, and other renal damaging influences are controlled. Adverse side effects that have been reported are reversible neurological reactions such as confusion, hallucinations, and tremors, abnormalities of plasma enzyme tests of liver function, anemia, leukopenia, thrombocytopenia, rashes, and fevers. As these reactions have occurred in individuals with underlying medical conditions, however, it is unclear if the drug was causative.

Although gastrointestinal symptoms and headache have been recorded in patients given aciclovir, it is uncertain if the drug was responsible for these; a reduction in the dose of the drug, however, may be necessary. Skin rashes that have resolved after stopping the drug have been reported, and it is recommended that therapy should be discontinued in individ-uals with moderate to severe rashes[96].

Hypersensitivity reactions are rare, but aciclovir must not be given to an individual with such a history.

Aciclovir is not carcinogenic to either rats or mice. Results of tests in animals show no evidence of teratogenicity, nor is it carcinogenic, nor does it affect fertility[97]. Aciclovir does not appear to have immunosuppressive properties.

At therapeutic doses about 20% of aciclovir is absorbed from the gastrointestinal tract. Larger doses are absorbed less efficiently, and it is unlikely that serious toxic effects would occur if an entire treatment course of 25 tablets were taken at once.

Aciclovir resistance

In vitro studies have shown that serial passage of HSV in increasing concentrations of aciclovir can result in the development of resistance[98]. Resistance results from either deficiency in viral TK, from decreased TK activity, or, less commonly, from TK with altered substrate specificity[99]; resistance may also follow mutation in the genes encoding for viral DNA polymerase[100]. There has been much detailed work on the genetic mechanism of TK deficiency. Frameshift mutations are clustered within two long homopolymer nucleotide stretches with insertion or deletions of one or more nucleotides, especially within runs of guanosines and cytosines[101], and result in premature termination codons.

Aciclovir-resistant strains of HSV have only rarely been isolated from immunocompetent patients[102, 103], most affected individuals having some form of immunodeficiency, including HIV infection[104]. In a survey of HSV resistant to aciclovir in northwest England[105], 6% of isolates from 95 immunocompromised patients showed resistance (IC_{50} above 3 μM in a plaque-reduction assay), a finding that is in keeping with other published reports. Resistant isolates were found in 0.1% to 0.7% of immunocompetent individuals, with no apparent difference in prevalence between untreated patients and those treated previously with aciclovir.

Although TK-deficient isolates can establish and maintain latency, aciclovir-resistant strains reactivate less efficiently and show diminished neurovirulence in mice[106] (neurovirulence seems to be directly related to TK activity). In immunocompromised patients, however, aciclovir-resistant strains can cause disease, particularly mucocutaneous ulceration, encephalitis, and pneumonia. This discrepancy between impaired pathogenicity in the animal model and disease in the human is incompletely understood. One explanation may be that the strains isolated from clinical specimens might express low amounts of TK that are undetectable by current laboratory methods. An alternative explanation may be that TK function is supplied by a sub-population of TK-competent virus[107]. Clinical and virological clearing of mucocutaneous aciclovir-resistant viral shedding by foscarnet or alternative therapy, followed by no antiviral treatment may still lead to reactivation of aciclovir-resistant isolates in a subsequent episode. Complete withdrawal of aciclovir, however, may eventually lead to aciclovir-sensitive (wild type TK) reactivation[107]. This reversion of HSV over time to a sensitive population suggests that, at least in the short-term, aciclovir may become useful again.

Aciclovir-resistant strains of HSV remain sensitive to foscarnet, and this is the drug of choice in the treatment of infections caused by such strains.

Aciclovir formulations available

Aciclovir for intravenous infusion

Aciclovir by intravenous infusion is required for the treatment of infection in the immunocompromised, in pregnant women with disseminated infection, and in individuals with severe initial genital herpes. Details of the administration of this formulation are given in Appendix 6.1, and the dosage adjustment necessary in those with renal impairment in Appendix 6.2.

Aciclovir for oral use

Aciclovir by mouth is used in the treatment of initial episode and recurrent HSV infections, and to suppress recurrence in immunocompetent and immunocompromised individuals.

For oral use, aciclovir is available as 200 mg, 400 mg, and 800 mg tablets and as dispersible tablets. The dispersible tablets can be swallowed whole with a little water, or they may be dispersed in at least 50 mL of water. Aciclovir suspensions of 200 mg per 5 mL and 400 mg per 5 mL are also available, and may be preferred by individuals who have difficulty in swallowing tablets. In patients with HSV infection and with renal impairment, dosage adjustment is not usually required unless the creatinine clearance is less than 10 mg/min; in such individuals aciclovir may be given in a dosage of 200 mg twice daily at approximately 12 hour intervals.

Aciclovir for eye use

Aciclovir 3% w/v in a white soft paraffin base is available for ophthalmic use as Zovirax Eye Ointment, 4.5 g tubes (Glaxo Wellcome), and is used in the treatment of herpetic keratitis. The drug is absorbed from the ointment through the corneal epithelium and superficial ocular tissue, achieving antiviral levels in the aqueous humor. A 1 cm ribbon of ointment should be placed inside the lower conjunctival sac five times per day at approximately 4-hour intervals. Treatment should continue for at least 3 days after healing is complete. Local irritation and inflammation has been reported during use of the ophthalmic ointment, and superficial punctate keratopathy that has healed without scarring has occurred (Wellcome; ABPI Data Sheet Compendium 1999–2000).

Aciclovir for skin use

Aciclovir 5% w/w in a white aqueous cream base is available for use in recurrent oral and genital HSV infection. The cream is applied five times daily at approximately 4-hour intervals until the lesions have healed. Transient burning or stinging may occur following application. Erythema or mild drying and flaking of the skin has been reported in a small proportion of patients. Aciclovir cream is contraindicated in those with known hypersensitivity to aciclovir or to the excipient propylene glycol.

Valaciclovir

Valaciclovir is the 1-L-valyl ester of aciclovir.

Mode of action

As valaciclovir is almost entirely converted to aciclovir, the mode of action is that of aciclovir (see page 122).

Pharmacokinetics

When given by mouth the drug is well absorbed and 99% is rapidly converted to aciclovir from first-pass intestinal and hepatic metabolism by enzyme hydrolysis[108]. In volunteers given 1000 mg valaciclovir, the absolute bioavailability of aciclovir from the drug has been found to be 54.2% (range 42% to 73%), i.e. three to five times greater than that achieved following oral aciclovir, and similar to the exposure achieved with intravenous aciclovir[109]. After a single oral dose of 1000 mg valaciclovir, the mean peak concentration (± SD) of aciclovir was 29.53 (± 12.47) μM at a median time of 1.75 hours post-dosing, and the area under

the concentration-time curve was 89.37 (± 19.37) h/μM. The differences between the plasma concentrations of aciclovir between single oral doses of 1000 mg of valaciclovir and 200 mg of aciclovir are shown in Figure 6.19.

The pharmacokinetics of oral valaciclovir in late pregnancy have recently been studied[93] and compared with those of oral aciclovir. After a single oral dose of 500 mg of valaciclovir, the mean peak aciclovir concentrations (C_{max}) and the mean values for the daily area under the concentration–time curve (AUC) were significantly higher for valaciclovir recipients than for those given 400 mg aciclovir by mouth; there were similar findings at steady-state testing. Although there was no significant difference between the mean aciclovir concentration in amniotic fluid between those women given aciclovir and those given valaciclovir, the amniotic fluid concentrations were higher than in the plasma. After dosing with valaciclovir, aciclovir is found in human breast milk at a concentration 0.6 to 4.1 times that in plasma.

Excretion and metabolic elimination

Valaciclovir is eliminated as aciclovir and the principal aciclovir metabolite, 9-carboxymethoxy-methylguanine, in the urine.

Unwanted effects

These are mild and include nausea and headache. In clinical trials of valaciclovir in the treatment of herpes zoster, the frequency of side effects in patients given valaciclovir or placebo has been similar.

Valaciclovir for oral use

Valaciclovir, as hydrochloride, is available for oral use in the form of 500 mg tablets. In the treatment of primary or initial genital herpes the dose is 500 to 1000 mg twice daily for 5 to 10 days. In individuals with renal impairment, the dose of valaciclovir need only be adjusted to 1000 mg daily if the creatinine clearance is less than 15 mL/min. Valaciclovir has also proven useful in the treatment and suppression of frequently recurring genital herpes (see page 126).

Famciclovir

Famciclovir is the diacetyl-6-deoxy analog of penciclovir. Penciclovir, the active metabolite of famciclovir, is highly active against HSV-1 and HSV-2. Using a plaque reduction assay, Boyd et al.[110] showed that the IC_{50}s (± SD) of penciclovir against clinical isolates of HSV-1 and HSV-2 were 0.4 (± 0.1) and 1.5 (± 0.4) μg/mL respectively; these IC_{50}s were higher than those of aciclovir, 0.2 (± 0.2) and 0.6 (± 0.2) μg/mL respectively. These results appeared to indicate that penciclovir is less active than aciclovir and that it is less active against HSV-2 than against HSV-1. The same workers, however, found that in the virus yield reduction assay, penciclovir was more potent than aciclovir against HSV-1 and both drugs were equally active against HSV-2. In that assay, the IC_{99}s (i.e. the concentration of drug required to reduce the yield of infectious virus obtained 24 hours after infection by 99% relative to control cultures) of penciclovir for HSV-1 and HSV-2 were, respectively, 0.4

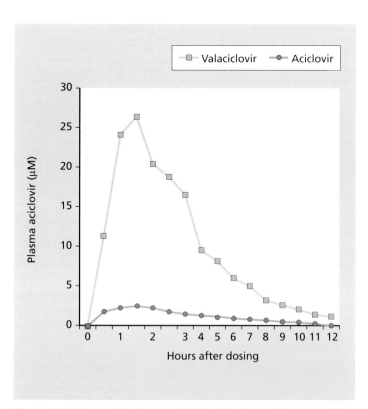

Figure 6.19 Mean aciclovir concentrations in plasma after an oral dose of 200 mg aciclovir or 1000 mg valaciclovir (reproduced with permission from van Dyke *et al.* 1982[92] and Soul-Lawton *et al.* 1995[109])

and 0.7 μg/mL, and of aciclovir 1.0 and 0.9 μg/mL respectively. In the treatment of primary or initial mucocutaneous HSV infections, famciclovir is highly effective. As shown in a mouse model system, there may be an effect on ganglionic latency[111, 112]. Animals were given a 5-day course of famciclovir or valaciclovir 1 to 5 days after oral infection with HSV-2. When animals were examined after cessation of treatment, infectious virus in the tissues was below the limits of detection. Rebound of virus replication in the ganglia and brain stems of mice that had been treated with valaciclovir but not with famciclovir, was found. When ganglia were explanted from survivors 6 weeks later, latent virus was reactivated in control animals, and in about two-thirds of mice treated with valaciclovir; no mice treated with famciclovir had evidence of latency by this test. If treatment with either compound was delayed for several months, however, neither drug affected latency. The authors concluded that the difference between these compounds reflected differences in the metabolism of penciclovir and aciclovir in infected neurons[112]. The clinical relevance of these findings is uncertain.

The place of famciclovir in the management of serious HSV infections remains to be established.

Mode of action

About 77% of an oral dose of famciclovir is absorbed and rapidly converted to penciclovir, the active drug. De-acetylation of famciclovir occurs in the duodenum, liver, and blood, and oxidation to penciclovir occurs in the liver[113].

Penciclovir is phosphorylated to the monophosphate by virus-induced TK and subsequently to the triphosphate by cellular enzymes. In HSV-1 and HSV-2-infected MRC-5 cells in tissue culture, penciclovir is phosphorylated more rapidly and to a greater extent than aciclovir[114, 115]. Very low concentrations of penciclovir are occasionally found in uninfected cells. Penciclovir is an inhibitor of viral DNA polymerase, competing with the natural substrate dGTP; it has very low levels of activity against cellular DNA polymerase[116]. Penciclovir is not, however, an obligate DNA chain terminator because of the availability of a hydroxyl group corresponding to the 3′ hydroxyl of the 2′ deoxyribose ring. The intracellular half-life of penciclovir triphosphate is long: 20 and 10 hours in HSV-2 and in HSV-1-infected MRC-5 cells respectively, compared with 0.7 hours in the case of aciclovir triphosphate[114, 115].

Pharmacokinetics

The mean peak plasma concentration of penciclovir following oral administration of 250 mg of famciclovir is 1.6 μg/mL and occurs at a median time of 45 minutes after the dose. Plasma concentration–time curves of penciclovir are similar following single and repeat dosing. The terminal plasma half-life of penciclovir after both single and repeat dosing with famciclovir is about 2 hours. In healthy young individuals, the plasma concentration–time curve (AUC) after oral administration of 250 mg of famciclovir is reported as 4.26 μg h mL^{-1}. Penciclovir is poorly bound to plasma proteins.

Excretion

Penciclovir is eliminated rapidly and almost unchanged by active renal tubular secretion and glomerular filtration. About 65% of the oral dose of famciclovir is excreted in urine as penciclovir and 5% as BRL 42359, its immediate precursor.

Unwanted effects

Famciclovir is well tolerated. In clinical trials, headache and nausea have been reported with equal frequency in those receiving famciclovir and those given placebo. Animal studies have not shown any embryotoxic or teratogenic effects with famciclovir or penciclovir. Famciclovir has no significant effects on spermatogenesis or sperm morphology and motility in man. At very high doses, impaired fertility has been observed in male rats but not in female rats (SmithKline Beecham Pharmaceuticals Data Sheet 1998). The development of mammary adenocarcinoma has been reported in female rats that received more than 50 times the therapeutic dose of famciclovir; male rats or mice of either sex did not develop this cancer (SmithKline Beecham Pharmaceuticals Data Sheet 1998). Penciclovir is excreted in the breast milk of lactating rats, but data in humans are unavailable.

Famciclovir for oral use

For oral use, famciclovir is available as 125 mg, 250 mg, and 500 mg tablets. In the treatment of primary or initial genital herpes, the usual dose is 250 mg three times per day, at approximately 8-hour intervals for 5 to 10 days. In the treatment of mucocutaneous HSV infection in the immunocompromised, the dose should be adjusted to 500 mg twice daily at approximately 12-hour intervals for 7 days. In individuals with impaired renal function, dosage modification is needed: when the creatinine clearance is 30 to 59 mL min^{-1} 1.73 m^{-2}, the dose of famciclovir should be 250 mg twice daily, and if there is more severe renal dysfunction, 250 mg should be given once daily. Famciclovir is also used in the treatment of recurrent HSV infection, and to suppress recurrence in immunocompetent and immunocompromised individuals.

Hypersensitivity reactions are rare, but famciclovir must not be given to a patient with such a history.

CLINICAL EXPERIENCE IN THE USE OF ANTIVIRAL DRUGS IN THE TREATMENT OF HERPES SIMPLEX VIRUS INFECTIONS IN IMMUNOCOMPETENT INDIVIDUALS

Primary or initial genital herpes

Aciclovir

In the early 1980s a randomized, double-blind, placebo-controlled trial showed the efficacy of aciclovir given by intravenous infusion in the treatment of individuals with primary or initial genital herpes[117]. The medians for healing time, duration of vesicles, new lesion formation, virus shedding, and all symptoms were significantly shorter than in controls. In half the patients treated with aciclovir all lesions had healed by the seventh day, compared with less than 10% in those who received placebo. No new lesions occurred 2 days after the initiation of aciclovir treatment. The most dramatic effect was the reduction in the duration of viral shedding, reported to have ceased by day 5 in all patients treated with aciclovir, whereas placebo-treated patients continued viral shedding for up to 20 days.

Intravenous administration of aciclovir, of course, is impractical for the treatment of the majority of immunocompetent patients with first episode genital herpes. Oral therapy, however, provides a similar level of effectiveness[118] without the disadvantage of admission to hospital and the administration of intravenous infusions. The duration of symptoms may be expected to be reduced by half or more providing treatment is started early enough. In Nilsen's cases all 17 aciclovir-treated patients were culture negative after 5 days of oral treatment, whereas over 75% of the 14 placebo patients were still shedding virus. Centers for Disease Control Guidelines[119] recommend a 7- to 10-day course of treatment. Occasionally, however, early recurrences occur. Unfortunately, the short 5-day course of aciclovir does not decrease the likelihood of subsequent recurrence[120]. There is no place for topical treatment in the management of primary genital herpes, and there is no benefit in prescribing topical agents in addition to oral treatment[121].

Valaciclovir

A major disadvantage of oral aciclovir therapy is its poor bioavailability and the need for frequent daily doses. Its pro-drug, valaciclovir, with a pharmacokinetic profile that allows less frequent dosing, has been evaluated in the treatment of primary and initial genital herpes[122]. This was a multicenter, randomized, double-blind trial that compared 10-day regimens of valaciclovir (1000 mg twice daily) and aciclovir (200 mg five times per day) in the treatment of 643 adults. There was no significant difference between the groups with respect to the duration of viral shedding, time to healing, duration of pain, and time to loss of all symptoms after initiation of therapy. The authors concluded that valaciclovir is a useful alternative to aciclovir with the advantage of more convenient dosing regimens and the potential for improved adherence. A decided disadvantage, however, is the increased cost

compared to aciclovir (the present cost of ten 500 mg tablets of valaciclovir is £23.50; whereas twenty-five 200 mg tablets of aciclovir cost £13.36).

Famciclovir

Although famciclovir in an oral dose of 250 mg three times per day at approximately 8-hour intervals for 7 to 10 days is indicated for the treatment of first episode genital herpes[119], adequate trial data on efficacy are lacking. Treatment of initial genital herpes with famciclovir is more expensive than with aciclovir (the current cost of fifteen 250 mg tablets is £84.35).

Recurrent genital herpes

Oral therapy

Episodic treatment

Aciclovir Although the formation of new lesions is usually inhibited when aciclovir is given by mouth to individuals with recurrent genital herpes, the effects on lesion progression are less pronounced than in initial disease. In a double-blind, randomized trial in which the results of treatment with aciclovir, given in a dosage of 200 mg five times per day for 5 days, were compared with those of placebo, significant differences were noted[118]. The healing time of lesions was significantly less in individuals given aciclovir (median 5 days, range 2 to 11 days) than in those treated with placebo (median 6 days, range 2 to 14 days). There was no difference, however, in the duration of all the symptoms of the recurrence. Viral shedding time was also significantly shorter in the aciclovir-treated group (median duration of shedding 1 day, range 1 to 4 days) than in the placebo group (median duration of shedding 2 days, range 1 to more than 7 days). In this study, lesions had been present for some time (mean 1.0 day) before initiation of therapy, and even better results have been reported in patients treated during the prodrome or within 24 hours of the onset of recurrence. Compared with delayed therapy, when aciclovir is given within 24 hours of the appearance of symptoms or signs, there is a shorter healing time, a reduction in the frequency of new lesion formation,

and an increased proportion of aborted episodes[123, 124]. Even when given early, unfortunately, aciclovir does not differ from placebo in its effect on the duration of itch and pain, and its use as an episodic treatment for recurrent genital herpes has been questioned[125].

Valaciclovir Because of its better pharmacokinetic profile, however, valaciclovir might be considered a better alternative in the acute management of a recurrent episode of genital herpes. In a large study, the development of vesicles or ulcers was prevented in 23% of men and 36% of women who were given valaciclovir (500 mg twice daily by mouth) within 24 hours of symptoms or signs of recurrence but in only 14% of men and 26% of women who received placebo[126]. The length of the episode was significantly shorter in the valaciclovir-treated group than in the placebo recipients (median 4.0 versus 5.9 days), as was the time to epithelialization of ulcers (median 4.1 versus 6.0 days). The median duration of virus shedding was also shorter in the valaciclovir recipients (2.0 days) than in those given placebo (4.0 days). The study also showed that there was no clear advantage in using a higher dose of valaciclovir. Aciclovir and valaciclovir have been shown to be comparable in terms of frequency of aborted recurrences, duration of symptoms, and healing time[127]. The principal advantage of valaciclovir over aciclovir treatment, however, is the twice-daily dosing regimen, the only disadvantage being its greater cost.

Famciclovir Famciclovir has also been evaluated in the treatment of recurrent genital herpes. In a double blind, placebo-controlled, dose-ranging study, famciclovir was given in oral doses of either 125 mg, 250 mg, or 500 mg twice daily for 5 days, treatment being initiated within 6 hours of the symptoms of recurrence appearing[128]. The time to complete healing of all lesions was significantly shorter amongst those who received famciclovir (median time at 250 mg regimen = 3.7 days) than amongst the placebo recipients (median time 4.8 days). The duration of all symptoms, including pain and itch, was also shorter in the famciclovir treatment group (median time = 3.1 days) than in those who were given placebo (median time = 3.7 days). The median time to cessation of virus shedding in patients given the 250 mg drug regimen was 1.5 days and 3.3 days in those given placebo, a difference that is highly significant. In addition, those individuals who initiated famciclovir therapy before virus shedding (as detected by culture) were less likely to shed virus during treatment than the placebo recipients. There was no significant difference between any treatment outcome and the dose of famciclovir.

For episodic treatment of recurrent genital herpes, the Centers for Disease Control and Prevention (2002) currently recommend aciclovir, given orally in doses of either 400 mg every 8 hours, or 200 mg five times per day, or 800 mg every 12 hours, treatment continuing for 5 days. Famciclovir, given by mouth in a dose of 125 mg every 12 hours for 5 days, is also recommended, as is valaciclovir in an oral dose of either 500 mg twice daily for 3 to 5 days, or 1.0 g once daily for 5 days.

Suppressive treatment

Aciclovir In individuals with very frequent recurrences of genital herpes, suppression with continuous oral medication is the most satisfactory approach to management. In a randomized, placebo-controlled trial, Mindel and colleagues[129] showed that, compared with placebo, aciclovir in a daily dosage of 200 mg four times per day for 12 weeks significantly reduced the frequency of recurrence: the mean recurrence rates per month were 1.4 and 0.05 in the placebo and aciclovir recipients respectively. In addition, the time to recurrence was significantly longer in the aciclovir-treated group (median 100 days) than in the placebo group (14 days). Similar results were reported simultaneously from workers in the USA[130, 131]. On cessation of therapy, however, all patients had recurrence with no reduction in the frequency of recurrences[131]. When suppressive therapy is extended to 1 year and longer, the efficacy of aciclovir is maintained[132–134]. In one study[134], when aciclovir was given in a dose of 400 mg twice daily by mouth to a group of individuals who had had frequent recurrences of genital herpes with a mean number of recurrences in the year

preceding enrolment of 12.8, the mean number of recurrences had fallen to 1.8 and 1.4 during the first and second years of suppressive treatment respectively. An interesting observation was made by Goldberg and colleagues[135] who noted that in individuals receiving suppressive treatment for 5 years, there was a gradual decrease in the number of recurrences per year for the first 3 years, after which there was no significant difference in the frequency of recurrences from year to year. They found that 46% of subjects had had no recurrences by the end of the first year, and that by years 3 to 5, 65% to 70% had had no recurrences. This and other studies showed that the drug was well tolerated without serious adverse effects and no evidence of cumulative toxicity. The optimum dose of aciclovir for suppressive treatment has been debated, but most consider a total daily dose of 800 mg to be superior to lower doses. Mindel et al.[136], however, found that about 20% of those receiving 800 mg as a single daily dose had recurrence within 30 days of initiation of therapy. They also noted that the time to first recurrence in patients who received 400 mg twice daily was significantly shorter than those on 200 mg four times per day. This difference, however, may be offset by better adherence to a twice daily than a four times per day regimen. An observation, that is difficult to interpret because there was no control group, was that, after cessation of treatment, the frequency of recurrences (0.71 per 28 days) was significantly less than in the pre-treatment period.

An important double-blind, placebo-controlled study on the effect of daily oral treatment with aciclovir (400 mg twice daily) on subclinical virus shedding was described by Wald and colleagues[137]. The study group consisted of 34 women who had become infected with HSV-2 within 2 years of initiation of the study. Material for culture for HSV was obtained daily from the vulva, cervix/vagina, and perianal areas of 17 women who received aciclovir and 17 women who were given placebo. There was a significant difference in the frequency of virus excretion between the two groups: 15 placebo recipients but only 3 aciclovir-treated women had at least 1 day of virus shedding. Subclinical

shedding occurred on 6 (0.37%) of 1611 days with aciclovir, compared with 83 (5.8%) of 1439 days with placebo. In all patients who received aciclovir, the frequency of subclinical shedding was reduced at all anatomical sites and in all patients.

Valaciclovir A clear disadvantage of suppressive therapy with aciclovir is the need for multiple daily dosing with attendant adherence difficulties. The pharmacokinetic profile of valaciclovir is such that once daily medication should be possible for the suppression of frequently recurring genital herpes. An international placebo-controlled trial[138] showed that once daily valaciclovir in an oral dose of 500 mg was highly effective: after 16 weeks therapy 69% of valaciclovir recipients were recurrence-free compared with 10% of those who had been given placebo. In a large, dose-ranging study, it was found that valaciclovir in doses of either 250 mg twice daily, 500 mg once daily, or 1 g once daily for 1 year were as effective in suppressing recurrent genital herpes as aciclovir given in a dose of 400 mg twice daily[139]. Suppressive valaciclovir treatment is well tolerated with few serious side effects. The most common unwanted effects were nausea and headache.

Famciclovir Famciclovir is also effective in suppression of recurrent genital herpes. In a double blind, placebo-controlled trial of famciclovir given as a daily oral dose of 125 mg or 250 mg three times per day or 250 mg twice daily to individuals with frequently recurring genital herpes, it was shown that the time to first recurrence was significantly longer in those who received the drug (median time to recurrence was 222 to 336 days) than in placebo recipients (median time to recurrence was 47 days). It was also reported that 79% to 86% of famciclovir recipients were recurrence-free at 6 months, compared with only 27% of placebo recipients[140]. This study confirmed the findings of a previous trial on the efficacy of famciclovir in the suppression of recurrences of genital herpes[141].

Topical therapy

Good results in the use of aciclovir cream were obtained by Kinghorn et al.[141a] who noted also the important point that aciclovir applied only to the external lesions was associated with a significant reduction of virus shedding and duration of lesions at all sites, including internal sites (31 of 36 women with HSV isolated from the cervix and 13 of 15 men who had positive urethral swabs for HSV, showed a significant reduction in virus shedding and duration of lesions after topical application of aciclovir cream to external lesions). In recurrent HSV infections early patient-initiated therapy with aciclovir cream appeared to be as effective as early oral therapy in recurrent genital herpes[141a].

Primary or initial orolabial herpes

There are few data on the treatment of primary or initial orolabial herpes. Amir et al.[142], however, reported the results of a double-blind placebo-controlled study on the use of aciclovir suspension in the treatment of herpetic gingivostomatitis in young children. The drug was given in an oral dose of 15 mg/kg five times per day for 7 days; 61 children with positive cultures for HSV completed the study. Compared with those receiving placebo there was a shorter duration of

- oral lesions (median 4 versus 10 days)
- fever (1 versus 3 days)
- eating difficulties (4 versus 7 days)
- viral shedding (1 versus 5 days).

The ideal dose and length of therapy, however, has yet to be determined.

Recurrent orolabial herpes

Twenty to forty per cent of the population of the UK at some stage has recurrent orolabial infection with HSV, although only 1% have severe recurrence that requires specific therapy[143]. Most recurrences can be managed by the topical application of an antiseptic cream to reduce the risk of secondary bacterial infection. Patients with more severe recurrences, however, may request specific therapy, and topical and oral antiviral drugs are available.

Topical therapy

The use of topical antiviral therapy remains controversial. Compared with placebo, topical treatment of recurrent orolabial HSV infection with *aciclovir ointment* (5% w/w in a polyethylene glycol base), applied five times per day for 5 days, reduces the time to complete healing (7 versus 8 days)[144], but this effect is of marginal benefit to most patients. There have been several trials of *aciclovir cream* (5% w/w in propylene glycol) which is said to penetrate the skin and mucosae better than ointment, but the results with respect to lesion healing have been inconsistent. Fiddian et al.[9] showed that the time to healing was reduced in those who received aciclovir compared to placebo recipients (4 versus 6 days). These results differ from those reported by Shaw et al.[145] who found that there was no significant difference between aciclovir and placebo-treated subjects (9 versus 10 days). Fiddian's group, however, showed that if treatment with aciclovir cream is initiated before the vesicular stage of the eruption, more than one-third of the lesions will be aborted. This finding has been confirmed in an elegant recent study that used electronic infrared thermography to recognize the prodromal phase of herpes labialis. It was found that the use of aciclovir cream within 12 hours of symptoms prevented the clinical development of herpetic lesions in 46% of 70 treated individuals with a history of recurrent disease[146]. In conclusion, topical aciclovir cream may have a role in the management of individuals with severe recurrent herpes labialis but treatment should be initiated before vesicles develop. There seems little advantage over placebo, however, in the treatment of individuals with more advanced lesions.

The use of *penciclovir cream* for the treatment of recurrent herpes labialis has been shown to be useful. When compared with placebo, penciclovir cream (1% w/w), applied every 2 hours during the day, decreases healing time (4.8 versus 5.5 days), and reduces the duration of pain and of viral shedding (median 3 days) in each arm of the study (but, using the Cox proportional hazard regression model, the hazard ratio was 1.35 with a 95% confidence interval of 1.10–1.64, $P < 0.003$)[147]. In contrast to aciclovir therapy, penciclovir seems to be effective even when initiated late in the course of the recurrence.

Oral therapy

Aciclovir given by mouth has been used for the treatment of recurrent orolabial herpes in the immunocompetent patient. As measured by the frequency of macular or papular (aborted) lesions, and the mean maximum lesion size, drug treatment does not appear to affect the development of lesions even when given within 1 hour of the symptoms of recurrence[148]. Compared with placebo-treated individuals, however, healing time is significantly shorter and the mean duration of pain is reduced. As these differences are marginal, oral aciclovir therapy probably has little place in the management of most immunocompetent individuals with recurrent orolabial HSV infection. There have been several studies on suppressive therapy of recurrent orolabial herpes[149]. Aciclovir given in a dose of 400 mg twice daily by mouth for 4 months has been reported to reduce the frequency of recurrence by 53% and to result in a 71% reduction in virus culture positive recurrences compared with placebo therapy[150]. Prophylaxis for recurrent herpes labialis with short-term oral treatment, however, seems less certain. Although an initial report of short-term prophylaxis in skiers indicated benefit in reducing recurrent lesions, a more recent study from Canada on the use of oral aciclovir (800 mg twice daily given 12 to 24 hours before outdoor activity) in a group of skiers showed that there was no significant difference between the drug and placebo in the prevention of recurrent orolabial HSV infection[151]. The benefit of suppressive therapy for herpes labialis is much less obvious than for genital herpes. In those with frequently recurring disease, or when the risk of transmission by oro–genital sex of HSV-1 to a sexual partner who is seronegative for HSV-1, should be minimized, such treatment may be warranted.

Herpetic conjunctivitis

Richards et al.[152] reviewed the trial data on the treatment of ocular herpes (herpetic keratitis) with aciclovir ophthalmic ointment (Zovirax Eye Ointment, Glaxo Wellcome) which has proved to be superior in comparison with other antiviral agents for the eye. Deeper infections are more difficult to treat than epithelial keratitis.

Suppressive therapy in the management of recurrent HSV eye disease was clearly shown in a placebo-controlled study of 703 immunocompetent patients[153]. The active drug was aciclovir, given in an oral dose of 400 mg every 12 hours for 12 months. Among the 337 patients with stromal keratitis, the most serious form of ocular HSV disease, the cumulative probability of recurrent stromal keratitis was significantly lower (14%) in those receivng aciclovir, than in the placebo group (28%).

An approach to the clinical management of genital herpes in immunocompetent individuals

THE PATIENT WITH PRIMARY OR INITIAL GENITAL HERPES

Counseling and support is essential in the management of the newly diagnosed individual with first episode genital herpes.

At the initial attendance, many individuals are anxious and may not fully comprehend all that is said by the health care worker, it is therefore helpful to give written information as well. A discussion of more emotive issues such as HSV infection in pregnancy is better postponed until resolution of the initial episode. Patients should be given the opportunity to return within a few days to discuss their anxieties and fears with the physician or health adviser and, when the individual is in a relationship, it is sometimes helpful to have a joint counseling session. Issues that should be discussed at the initial or subsequent consultation are shown in Box 6.2. Typing of the isolate can be of prognostic value, and the individual should be made aware of the infecting type, and the likelihood of recurrence (see pp. 109–110). Self-help groups can offer valuable support, and the individual should be given information on how to contact one of them (Appendix 6.3).

Consideration should be given to screening for other STIs that may have been acquired concurrently.

Antiviral therapy should be initiated as soon as possible after the development of symptoms, and certainly within 5 days if there is to be real benefit from treatment. Table 6.2 summarizes drug regimens[154, 155] that are useful in the treatment of primary or initial genital herpes. It should be noted that the drug regimens recommended in the US Guidelines for Treatment of Sexually Transmitted Diseases are slightly different from those recommended in the UK[154] in that treatment duration is longer (7 to 10 days); there are no data comparing the relative efficacy of the various recommended durations of treatment. The choice of agent should be one of personal preference and cost. There is no benefit in using topical therapy in addition to oral therapy.

In addition to specific antiviral treatment, mild analgesics should be prescribed for pain, and the individual should bathe the affected area frequently with physiological saline (9 g/L w/v). Fibrinous labial adhesions in women should be treated by gentle digital separation and paraffin gauze may be interposed between opposing surfaces. Acute retention of urine may be managed initially by the patient attempting micturition whilst in a warm bath in order to reduce the effect of external dysuria. If this procedure is unsuccessful, catheterization should be undertaken; in the case of women with introital herpes, a suprapubic catheter may be preferable to a urethral catheter to minimize discomfort.

Box 6.2 Issues to be discussed around the time of diagnosis of primary or initial genital herpes

- The nature of the infection and how the virus could have been acquired
- Virus latency and reactivation with or without clinical features even years after inapparent or apparent primary infection
- The possibility of recurrences
- The symptomless excretion of infectious virus and the possibility of onward transmission
- Risk reduction for transmission of the virus – condom use
- Risk of male transmitting infection to uninfected partner during pregnancy
- Risk of maternal transmission to the fetus, and need to inform obstetrician/midwife
- Autoinoculation e.g. to the cornea
- Antiviral therapy
- The possibility of partner notification

Table 6.2 Drugs regimens in the treatment of primary or initial genital herpes

Drug	Dosage (all drugs given orally)	Unwanted effects
Aciclovir	200 mg five times daily at approximately 4-hour intervals for 5 days *or* for 7–10 days[a] *or* 400 mg three times per day at 8-hour intervals for 7–10 days[a]	Gastrointestinal disturbances, headache, rarely rash.
Valaciclovir	500 mg two times per day at approximately 12-hour intervals for 5 days *or* 1 g twice daily at 12 hour intervals for 7–10 days[a]	As for aciclovir
Famciclovir	250 mg three times per day at approximately 8-hour intervals for 5 days *or* for 7–10 days[a]	Nausea, headache.

[a] These drug regimens are those recommended in the 2002 US Guidelines for Treatment of Sexually Transmitted Diseases (Centers for Disease Control 2002[155])

THE PATIENT WITH RECURRENT GENITAL HERPES

Between patients, there is much variation in the frequency and severity of recurrence and hence the need for specific antiviral therapy is not uniform. In some patients, the recurrent episode is short lived with few symptoms, and all that is required in management is careful attention to genital hygiene with saline bathing, the application of white soft paraffin BP, and, perhaps, the topical application of an antiseptic agent such as povidone iodine 10% in an alcoholic solution. Other patients, however, have frequently recurring lesions and/or severe, prolonged symptoms, and in many individuals recurrent genital herpes is associated with psychological disturbance.

An approach to the management of the immunocompetent patient with recurrent genital herpes who requires antiviral treatment is shown in Figure 6.20. The algorithm is only a guide and management must be tailored to the needs of the individual whose wishes must be taken into consideration. Although episodic treatment of patients with infrequent recurrences only confers marginal benefit, some clinicians find this approach helpful. If such therapy is used, treatment (Table 6.2) should be initiated during the prodrome (if there is one) or within 6 hours of the appearance of symptoms. Patients should therefore be given a supply of drug to have ready for immediate use. Sometimes patients with infrequent recurrences may require a short course of suppressive

therapy to prevent troublesome symptoms over a particular time, for example, students preparing for examinations.

In deciding on suppressive therapy, several factors should be considered (Box 6.3). First, it is essential that the diagnosis of genital herpes be confirmed. If a virological confirmation of genital herpes has not been made previously, and if lesions are absent at the time of first consultation for management of presumed recurrent herpes, it may be necessary to invite the patient to return to the clinic within 24 hours of the appearance of symptoms so that the appropriate investigations can be performed.

Although individuals who have six or more recurrences per year are likely to show the most benefit in terms of reduction in frequency of recurrences, other people with fewer but severe recurrences, including those with neuralgia or other prodromal symptoms but who fail to develop genital lesions, may also benefit from suppressive therapy. In addition to the physical effects of suppressive therapy, there is a significant reduction in anxiety about the illness[156]. After the initial episode of genital herpes, there is a variable period of up to 1 year when recurrences are more frequent than in later months or years. It is therefore better to postpone a decision about suppressive therapy until a pattern of recurrence can be established[157]. The choice of drug is one of personal preference but the most commonly used regimens[154, 155] are summarized in Table 6.3. Treatment should be initiated after a recurrence or when the

---

Box 6.3 Factors to be considered in deciding on need for suppressive therapy of recurrent genital herpes (Mindel 1993)

- Frequency of recurrences
- Severity of recurrences
- Duration of recurrences
- Prodromal symptoms
- Neuralgia
- Total duration of infection
- Psychological or psychosexual problems

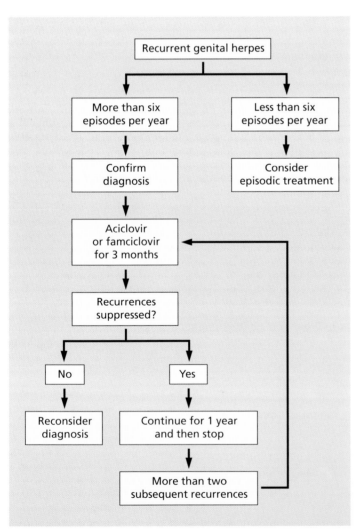

Figure 6.20 An approach to the immunocompetent patient with recurrent genital herpes

Table 6.3 Drug regimens for suppressive treatment of genital herpes

Drug	Dosage (all drugs given orally)
Aciclovir	200 mg four times per day at approximately 6-hour intervals[a] *or* 400 mg twice daily at 12-hour intervals for 1 year
Valaciclovir	250 mg twice daily at 12-hour intervals *or* 500 to 1000 mg once daily for 1 year
Famciclovir	250 mg twice daily at 12-hour intervals for 1 year

[a] Although this is the dose of aciclovir that has been shown to be most efficacious[136], the use of aciclovir (400 mg) twice daily may be more acceptable to the patient.

individual is symptomless[157]. Counseling of the individual who is about to initiate suppressive therapy is important, particularly with respect to adherence to the prescribed regimen, the possibility that recurrence is still possible, and the uncertainty about transmission of HSV to a sexual partner. Although patients who receive suppressive aciclovir have fewer days of subclinical HSV-2 shedding than placebo recipients[19], the effect on virus transmission is unknown. When the patient is taking suppressive therapy, it is helpful to review him/her at 3-monthly intervals to ensure efficacy of treatment, and, if suppression is inadequate, to consider possible reasons for treatment failure (Box 6.4). The daily drug dose or frequency of dosing may need to be changed to reduce further the frequency of recurrences. Malabsorption is less of a problem with valaciclovir and famciclovir than with aciclovir. In immunocompetent individuals, resistance, or reduced susceptibility to antiviral agents is rare (see page 123).

After 1 year of suppressive therapy the frequency of recurrences may be decreased compared with the pre-treatment period (see page 127). It is therefore useful to discontinue suppressive treatment after 1 year to assess the frequency of recurrences. If there is a return to frequent recurrences, suppressive treatment can be re-instituted, and, if need be, continued for several years. A decision on recommencing suppressive treatment, however, should not be made until the individual has had at least two recurrences[154]. The safety of long-term therapy with aciclovir seems to have been established, but there are insufficient data for valaciclovir and famciclovir. The development of mammary adenocarcinoma in female rats treated with very large doses of famciclovir, has led some physicians to caution against long-term use of this drug[96].

Herpes simplex virus infection in pregnancy

NEONATAL INFECTION

The incidence of neonatal herpes varies geographically. In the UK between 1986 and 1991, 76 infants with neonatal herpes were reported to the British Paediatric Association Surveillance Unit, the incidence of infection being 1.65 per 100 000 live births[158]. Twenty-five infants had HSV-1, 24 had HSV-2, and the infecting virus type in the other 27 cases was unknown. In the USA in 1984, the annual incidence of neonatal infection was estimated to be at least 4 per 100 000 live births[159]; HSV-2 was the infecting viral type in 71 (68%) of the 105 infants from whom HSV was cultured. Higher infection rates have been reported from Seattle, Washington State, USA, where the incidence is about 11 cases per 100 000 live births[160].

Herpes simplex virus can be transmitted to the neonate from a mother with primary or initial genital herpes at term. It has been estimated that the risk of neonatal herpes developing after vaginal delivery to a mother with primary or initial genital HSV infection is about 41%[50, 161–163]. The majority of women whose infants develop neonatal herpes have had symptomless seroconversion at or near term. In Brown's study[163], of the 94 women who seroconverted *by* the time of labor (60 and 34 women had subclinical and symptomatic infections respectively), there were no cases of neonatal herpes and no increased risk of complications of pregnancy such as intrauterine growth retardation or spontaneous abortion. Of the 9 mothers, however, who had acquired genital HSV *at or near to* time of delivery, 4 infants developed neonatal herpes.

Prematurity and intrauterine growth retardation have been described in infants of mothers who have acquired HSV-2 during the third trimester, and spontaneous abortion has followed seroconversion during the first trimester[50]. More recent studies, however, have shown that the frequency of complications of pregnancy amongst women who have seroconversion during gestation is low[163]. There is no evidence for a role for HSV in the development of complications of pregnancy in women with a history of recurrent genital herpes[164].

Not all infants exposed to HSV at birth become infected. It has been known for some time that neonates exposed to HSV during delivery to mothers with a history of recurrent genital herpes are at low risk for the development of neonatal herpes[165]. This was clearly shown in a study from

---

Box 6.4 Factors that should be considered in individuals who fail to respond to suppressive antiviral therapy

- Condition not herpes
- Inadequate dose
  - Frequency
  - Total daily dose
- Poor adherence to regimen
- Malabsorption
- Resistance

Seattle that examined the risks of neonatal transmission from mothers with initial genital herpes and those with a history of recurrent HSV infection who had subclinical shedding of HSV at term[166]. Eight of 20 infants born to women with initial genital herpes developed neonatal disease compared with only 1 of the 96 who had had recurrent infection. It would appear that babies whose sera contain type-specific antibodies against the homologous virus are at much less risk of acquisition of infection from mothers who are excreting the virus during delivery[163]. Neonatal infection, however, can be acquired from recurrent lesions at term, but the risk is estimated at being less than 8%[165].

The use of fetal scalp electrodes in mothers in labor, who have a history of recurrent genital herpes, may be a risk factor for neonatal herpes[166a] and the infant may also acquire the infection after delivery from maternal orolabial herpes or herpes infection in one of the medical or nursing attendants[167].

Women with HIV-1 infection are more likely to be seropositive for HSV-2, and it has been shown that, in pregnancy, the frequency of reactivation of HSV-2 is significantly higher in these women than in those who are not HIV-infected[168]. The significance of this finding is as yet unclear, but there is no evidence that the risk of HSV infection to the neonate is increased.

Clinical features of neonatal infection

Disseminated forms

The HSV infection usually affects the liver and adrenals, but other organs are commonly involved including the brain, trachea, lungs, esophagus, stomach, kidneys, spleen, pancreas, heart, and bone marrow. Low birth weight or prematurity are more common in this group than that expected in the population at large.

The illness may appear at birth or as long as 21 days after birth (average 6 days). There are a variety of clinical manifestations in disseminated infection including pyrexia or hypothermia, vomiting, loose stools, lethargy, convulsions, dyspnea, and jaundice. The illness is usually stormy, death occurring on average within 6 days of onset if untreated.

There are only a few cases linking HSV to the congenital defects of microcephaly, intracranial calcification, diffuse brain changes, chorioretinitis, retinal dysplasias, and microphthalmia associated with vesicular rash at birth.

Localized forms

Central nervous system Signs of meningoencephalitis indicate the need for lumbar puncture, which reveals a lymphocytic pleocytosis. In about half of untreated cases, death follows in 1 to 3 weeks and in the remainder there tend to be sequelae such as microcephaly, porencephaly, and varying degrees of psychomotor retardation. Eye effects are also seen.

Eye Conjunctivitis and keratitis develop early, and occasionally chorioretinitis develops slowly about a month after birth.

Skin Isolated vesicular lesions can occur as well as a more generalized rash. The vesicular lesions recur repeatedly up to 2 years after birth, becoming less extensive than the original eruption, but tending to be found at the same site. Although the skin lesions are sometimes benign, central nervous system and ocular sequelae may follow, so a prolonged follow-up is advised.

Oral cavity Vesicular lesions in the mouth are very rare and appear as a gingivostomatitis or involve the larynx. Diagnosis is dependent on recognition of the lesions and isolation of HSV.

MANAGEMENT OF HERPES SIMPLEX VIRUS IN PREGNANCY AND THE PREVENTION OF TRANSMISSION OF THE VIRUS TO THE FETUS AND THE NEWBORN

Guidelines for the prevention of acquisition of HSV in pregnancy have been published[154].

At the first antenatal clinic attendance, women should be asked if they or their partner has had genital herpes. As discussed above (page 131), neonatal herpes is most likely to be acquired from a mother who has recently become infected with HSV. Although not yet widely available, serological tests may be helpful in this regard. Type-specific testing of pregnant women presenting with first episode genital herpes may be useful in differentiating new infection from a recurrence. When there is a history of genital herpes in the male, it is therefore important that precautions be taken to reduce the risk of transmission of the virus to a woman lacking immunity to that HSV type. These issues should ideally be discussed with both partners before a planned pregnancy. When there is no history of orolabial or genital herpes in the woman, serological testing may be useful in identifying susceptibility to HSV. Unprotected intercourse should be avoided during recurrent genital herpes in the partner, even when the woman is seropositive for HSV: there is a small risk of superinfection. Although their use should be encouraged until after delivery, evidence to show that the consistent use of condoms during pregnancy reduces the risk of transmission of HSV is lacking. The risk of HSV-1 infection from oro–genital sex should also be discussed, and if a partner has a history of orolabial herpes, oral sex should be avoided, especially if oral lesions are present, or the use of barriers, such as dental dams, should be advised.

The vulva of all women, irrespective of a history of genital herpes should be examined at the onset of labor for signs of infection, and, if lesions are found, the patient should be managed as suggested below.

Medical and nursing staff, and friends and relatives with mucocutaneous herpetic lesions including herpetic whitlow, should take the appropriate precautions to avoid transmission of the virus while handling the child. In the case of orolabial or genital herpes, such precautions include careful hand washing before handling the child, and in cases of orolabial herpes, avoiding direct contact between the lesions and the baby. Personnel with herpetic whitlow should be excluded from the nursery until the lesion has healed.

Guidelines for the treatment of pregnant women with genital herpes have been developed and much of the following discussion is based on these[169].

There are no data to suggest the need for termination in women who acquire HSV during pregnancy[163]. Although aciclovir is not licensed for use in pregnancy, there has now been substantial use of the drug by pregnant women, and, in keeping with the results of tests on animals, there has been no evidence of teratogenicity. As aciclovir has not been shown to be teratogenic, termination of pregnancy is not indicated in women who have been treated inadvertently during early pregnancy. Women with primary or initial genital herpes often require specific treatment, but aciclovir should only be prescribed after careful discussion with the patient, and her partner, on the benefits and possible risks of the drug. The results of these discussions should be recorded in the patient's case notes. The drug may be given, in standard dosage, by mouth, or, if the episode is severe, by intravenous infusion. Unless labor ensues, the pregnancy should be managed as usual, with the probability that the baby will be delivered vaginally. Glaxo Wellcome ran a central registry of aciclovir use by pregnant women. This is now closed and the data are undergoing final analysis.

Women who have had primary genital herpes during pregnancy are more likely than those who have had non-primary infection to have symptomless viral shedding from the cervix or vulva in the remaining months of the pregnancy[50]. The rates of viral shedding of HSV-2 at weekly intervals were 5.6% in those who had primary infection and 2.1% in those with non-primary infection. Herpes simplex virus shedding is also more likely to occur at term in women who have had primary HSV infection during the last trimester[50]. There is then strong support for the recommendation that cesarean section should be the preferred method of delivery in women who have their first episode of genital herpes in the third trimester, particularly within 6 weeks of term[169]. These recommendations differ a little from

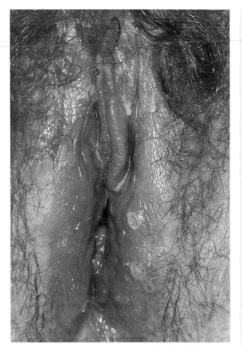

Figure 6.21 Primary HSV-2 infection in a woman at term

those recommended in the USA[155] where vaginal delivery is recommended unless the woman has symptoms or signs of genital herpes or its prodrome. Mothers with symptomatic primary or initial herpes at term (Figure 6.21) should be delivered by cesarean section before the membranes have ruptured or within 4 hours of their rupture. Performing a cesarean section beyond this time is not likely to protect the fetus. If vaginal delivery is performed, or if the membranes have been ruptured for more than 4 hours, the mother and infant should be treated with intravenous aciclovir. Vaginal procedures such as the application of scalp electrodes are best avoided to reduce the risk of damaging the baby's skin and allowing viral entry.

The management of women with recurrent genital herpes at the time of labor is controversial. Cesarean section has only been recommended for those with lesions at term[170], but this ignores the fact that infants born to mothers who have recurrent infection have neutralizing maternal antibodies in their sera that protect against infection with the homologous strain of HSV[163]. It has been estimated that if all women with recurrent herpes at term had delivery by cesarean section, 1583 opera-

tions would have to be performed to prevent one case of neonatal herpes[171]. The assumptions made in this cost–benefit analysis were based on small studies, and unless the issue is further clarified by randomized controlled studies, the decision on mode of delivery should be made by the mother with whom the risks and benefits of vaginal delivery and cesarean section have been discussed fully by her obstetrician.

The results of several small trials on the use of aciclovir in suppressing recurrence of genital herpes at term have been conflicting. Scott *et al.*[172] found that the incidence of both symptomatic recurrence and cesarean section were reduced. Brocklehurst and colleagues[173], in a placebo-controlled trial of aciclovir given orally in a dosage of 200 mg four times per day from 36 weeks of gestation, however, noted that, although the number of symptomatic recurrences was significantly reduced, the number of deliveries by cesarean section was not decreased. It was also shown that 2 of 31 women receiving aciclovir had asymptomatic excretion of virus from the cervix or vulva at the time of delivery. Until larger studies have been completed, it is impossible to give advice on the use of aciclovir to prevent transmission of HSV to infants of mothers with a history of recurrent genital herpes.

MANAGEMENT OF THE NEONATE

Guidelines on the management of babies born to mothers with primary or initial genital herpes have been published[169]. Box 6.5 shows the specimens for virus

---

Box 6.5 Specimens that should be obtained for virus culture from infants born to mothers with primary or initial genital herpes

- Urine
- Stool
- Oro-pharynx: secretions or swabs (in VTM*)
- Conjunctivae: swab
- Skin (if lesions present, swab in VTM)

*VTM = viral transport medium

culture that should be obtained from the infant. Intravenous aciclovir therapy should be initiated as soon as possible after delivery, but, if the child is well and virus has not been cultured from samples, the drug can be discontinued. When aciclovir is not given the child should be monitored closely for signs of infection (see page 132).

The place of virus culture of specimens from a baby born to a mother with recurrent genital herpes at term is uncertain, but it is recommended that one set of specimens should be obtained from the baby after delivery. When there are no lesions at the time of delivery of a mother with a history of genital herpes, culture of specimens from the baby is not necessary. In every case, however, parents should be advised on the signs of neonatal infection and, if found, medical advice should be sought as soon as possible.

Treatment of neonates with herpes simplex virus infection

Aciclovir is so well tolerated in infants that treatment of all neonates with HSV infection is recommended whether or not there is clinical evidence of systemic involvement. Lack of such evidence does not imply necessarily that the disease is limited to the skin or will remain so, and there are good grounds for believing that for benefit aciclovir should be given early[174]. Even with antiviral therapy, however, more than 40% of infants with encephalitis or disseminated infection still die or have sequelae[175].

The intravenous dose of 10 mg per kg body weight, given slowly, 8-hourly for 10 days is suggested for neonates. Since rises on days 2 and 3 may occur, it is wise to monitor plasma urea and creatinine. For children over 1 month of age a dose of 250 mg/mm^2 8-hourly is safe and effective. Solutions of up to 25 mg/mL of sodium salt in water have been given over a period of 1 hour by an infusion pump, although in older infants the drug reconstituted in this way has usually been further diluted with sodium chloride 0.18% w/v and dextrose 4% w/v intravenous infusion BP, to give a concentration of not more than 0.5%. When given in this way, rises in plasma urea and creatinine do not seem to occur.

DISSEMINATED HERPES SIMPLEX VIRUS INFECTION IN PREGNANCY

Although a rare complication in pregnant women, disseminated HSV infection can have devastating effects if untreated, with mortality among the mothers affected and their infants being 75% and 69% respectively. Fewer than 30 cases have been reported since the first description of the condition in 1969 and these have been reviewed recently[176]. Disseminated infection has been reported most commonly during the third trimester of pregnancy (70% of cases), and has been rarely described during the first trimester. About two-thirds of cases have been associated with HSV-2, and one-third with HSV-1. Unfortunately, in the majority of case reports it has been difficult to determine whether dissemination had occurred during primary or initial infection or during recurrence. It seems likely, however, that those with primary infection are at most risk because of the lack of antibody against either type of HSV. The probable

Table 6.4 Differential diagnosis of disseminated herpes simplex virus infection in a pregnant woman

Pre-eclampsia hepatic tenderness, nausea, vomiting, elevated plasma enzyme tests of liver function; later hypertension, proteinuria, cerebral disturbance	*Acute psychosis* *Cerebral neoplasm* *Delirium tremens* *Cerebral abscess* *Other causes of meningitis*
Acute fatty liver of pregnancy epigastric pain, jaundice, bleeding diathesis, proteinuria, hypertension, peripheral oedema; later hypoglycemia, coma, acute renal and liver failure, and bleeding diathesis	
HELLP syndrome microangiopathic hemolytic anemia, raised plasma enzyme tests of liver function, thrombocytopenia	
Cholestasis of pregnancy pruritus, jaundice, steatorrhea, elevated bilirubin and slightly elevated plasma enzyme tests of liver function	
Hepatitis A virus infection	
Hepatitis B virus infection	
Hepatitis C virus infection	
Hepatitis E virus infection	
Epstein–Barr virus infection	
Cytomegalovirus infection	
HIV infection	

sites from which dissemination has occurred have been the genitalia, the oropharynx, or both. In some pregnant women with encephalitis associated with oropharyngeal HSV-1, it is possible that the virus has reached the brain via the olfactory nerves, but in other cases, and in those following genital infection, visceral and skin lesions have resulted from blood-borne spread of the virus.

In the majority of patients fever, malaise, myalgia, and anorexia precede the development of the other features of dissemination by up to 1 week, and it should be noted that about 40% of patients do not have visible skin or mucosal lesions when the disease presents. Encephalitis is a common feature that may occur alone or, more commonly, be associated with hepatitis; the clinical features of encephalitis are described below. Acute hepatitis with extensive parenchymal necrosis, and coagulation defects (thrombocytopenia, prolonged prothrombin and partial thromboplastin times), sometimes with concurrent encephalitis, is more commonly associated with HSV-2 than with HSV-1 infection. In some cases vesicular lesions of the skin without visceral involvement have been the only signs of dissemination (HSV-2 in both reported cases). Rarely, a necrotizing bronchopneumonia has been reported.

The differential diagnosis is extensive (Table 6.4), and in the presence of coagulopathy, a definitive diagnosis by the detection of inclusion bodies in biopsy specimens may not be possible. As the use of intravenous aciclovir has been shown to be highly effective in treatment (see Treatment for details of administration, page 143), such therapy should not be withheld from a pregnant woman with features of possible disseminated disease and genital or oral lesions suggestive of HSV infection.

Herpes encephalitis

Although encephalitis may complicate primary HSV infection, most cases are thought to result from the reactivation of latent virus. Herpes simplex virus type 1 is the most common infecting type: HSV-2 was the cause in only 1 of 64 cases of herpes encephalitis in a series from Manchester, UK[177]. It is an uncommon disease with an estimated incidence in the USA of 1 in 400 000 persons per year. Any age group may be affected. The clinical features include

- disturbance of affect or consciousness
- loss of memory
- expressive aphasia
- behavior change
- olfactory or gustatory hallucinations
- temporal lobe seizures.

It should be noted that mucocutaneous lesions of HSV infection are not usually found.

Untreated, most patients become comatose by the end of the first week and death ensues within 2 weeks.

DIAGNOSIS

Imaging studies[178] Typically, CT and MRI studies show bilateral changes in the affected temporal lobes and adjacent posterior frontal region, usually with mass effect. In the very early stages of the disease, however, the changes may appear unilateral. On MRI examination (Figure 6.22), there is reduced density in the affected areas and there is contrast enhancement that may be patchy, peripheral, or gyral. It is important to note that there may be minimal changes in the first 2 to 3 days. Magnetic resonance imaging is more sensitive to white matter changes, the lesions appearing as high signals in T_2-weighted images and appear more extensive than by CT scanning; MRI therefore is more helpful in identifying disease in the early stages. Hemorrhage may cause an increased signal in T_1-weighted images and usually indicates extensive necrosis.

Neuroimaging, however, is neither sensitive nor specific, particularly in early disease, and other investigations are necessary to establish a diagnosis.

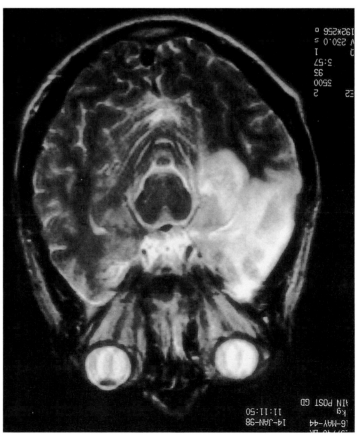

Figure 6.22 MRI scan of an individual with herpes encephalitis (reproduced with permission from Dr P Allen, Department of Medical Radiology, University of Edinburgh)

Biopsy Biopsy of the temporal lobe is both sensitive and specific, but the procedure may be associated with significant morbidity and is not the first investigation of choice.

Cerebrospinal fluid examination When there is no CT or MRI evidence of an intracranial mass, CSF examination can be helpful (Box 6.6). Many of the findings in the CSF are non-specific (Box 6.6) but the detection of HSV DNA by nested PCR amplification of HSV sequences offers a reliable method for diagnosis. In one study, the sensitivity and specificity of the test were 95% and 100% respectively, and the positive and negative predictive values were 100% and 97.8% respectively[81]. Herpes simplex virus DNA, however, may not be detectable more than 10 days after the onset of the illness, and in such cases immunological tests can be useful. Immunological diagnosis depends on the detection of intrathecal synthesis of antibody to HSV, using paired CSF and serum[179], and is particularly useful when neurological features have been present for at least 3 to 12 days.

TREATMENT

The treatment of herpetic encephalitis is with intravenous aciclovir.

Box 6.6 Cerebrospinal fluid findings in herpes simplex virus encephalitis

Pressure ↑

Xanthochromia

Cell count ↑ (initially polymorphonuclear leukocytes; later lymphocytes predominate; erythrocytes often present)

Total protein ↑

Glucose normal or ↑

Complement fixing antibody detectable[a]

HSV culture + in less than 5% of cases

HSV DNA +[b]

[a] Test may be negative in the first week of illness
[b] Test may be negative after 10 days of onset of illness
+ = positive
↑ = elevated

Herpes simplex virus infection in the immunocompromised host

Orolabial and genital herpes in HIV infection usually results from reactivation of latent infection. As the HIV infection progresses, recurrences become more frequent and, if untreated, last longer. Slowly progressive (sometimes over months), painful and tender, superficial ulceration of the perianal region (Figure 6.23), the genitalia, and the natal cleft is found in those individuals who are severely immunocompromised[180] and extensive facial ulceration with black eschar formation may also occur at this stage. Generalized papular eruptions and hyperkeratotic warty lesions, sometimes resembling condylomata acuminata, have also been noted in HIV-infected individuals[181, 182].

Chronic ulceration or verrucous (warty) lesions have also been described in individuals with other causes of immuno-deficiency, including immunosuppressive

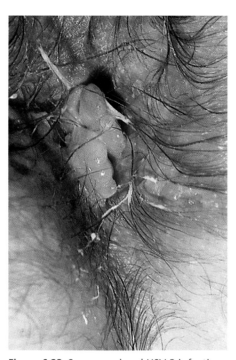

Figure 6.23 Severe perianal HSV-2 infection in a HIV-infected patient whose peripheral blood CD4 cell count was 1 cell/mm³ (reproduced from McMillan and Scott 2000[206])

therapy after solid organ transplantation, common variable immunodeficiency, and the Wiskott–Aldrich syndrome[183–185]. Therefore, HSV as a cause of vesicular, ulcerated, or verrucous lesions in an immunocompromised host should always be considered, and the appropriate laboratory tests undertaken. Disseminated disease has also been reported in the context of immunosuppression, and Seksik et al.[186] have recently reported a fatal case of HSV hepatitis in a young man that developed within 8 days of initiation of corticosteroid therapy for ulcerative colitis. The development of resistance to aciclovir in immunocompromised patients is well recognized and can cause difficulty in treatment (see page 123).

Oral HSV infection in immuno-compromised individuals, including those with HIV infection, affects the tongue (usually the lateral surface, although the dorsum may be involved with painful fissuring[187]), buccal mucosa, floor of the mouth, and the soft palate. The clinical features are variable but include diffuse erythema, crater-like ulceration, solitary ulceration resembling that caused by trauma, coalescing yellow papules, and exophytic nodules.

TREATMENT OF HERPES SIMPLEX VIRUS INFECTION IN IMMUNOCOMPROMISED INDIVIDUALS

Aciclovir, given by intravenous infusion in a dosage of 5 mg/kg every 8 hours is most commonly used in the treatment of severe HSV infections. A recent study, however, has shown that intravenous penciclovir in a dose of 5 mg/kg every 12 hours was as efficacious as aciclovir in healing lesions and stopping viral shedding[188] in immunosuppressed patients with muco-cutaneous herpes. Although penciclovir-resistant strains of HSV were not detected, data on the prevalence of aciclovir resistance in the study population were not given. Less severe mucocutaneous disease may respond to treatment with standard doses of oral aciclovir. In individuals treated for lesions associated with an aciclovir-resistant strain of HSV, recurrence at the same site may again be associated with resistant virus[189]. This, however, is not always so and, after obtaining material for culture and susceptibility testing, oral aciclovir should be given. Recurrent lesions at other locations in the same individual, however, are more likely to be sensitive to aciclovir. In individuals who have initially been treated with standard doses of aciclovir and who develop new lesions after more than 3 to 5 days of initiation of therapy, the dose of drug should be increased to 800 mg five times per day. Again, material from lesions that then fail to respond should be obtained for culture and susceptibility testing, and the treatment changed. Foscarnet (Appendix 6.4), given by intravenous infusion in a dosage of 60 mg/kg twice daily for either 10 days or until the lesions have healed[190], is the treatment of choice for most patients, but some with accessible lesions have been successfully treated with the topical application of either trifuridine ophthalmic solution every 8 hours[190] or cidofovir gel (0.1% or 0.3% w/v) daily. Lalezari and colleagues[191] found that almost 50% of patients treated with cidofovir gel had complete healing or a 50% reduction in area of the lesions within 5 days. Neither trifuridine nor cidofovir have been compared to foscarnet in clinical trials. There have been anec-dotal reports on the successful treatment with intravenous cidofovir of lesions caused by aciclovir and foscarnet-resistant HSV[192].

Aciclovir, valaciclovir, or famciclovir are useful in suppressive therapy of recurrent HSV infection, and should be given in the doses recommended for immunocompetent individuals (see page 131). For the episodic treatment of recurrent genital herpes, the Centers for Disease Control and Prevention[155] currently recommend aciclovir, given orally in doses of either 400 mg every 8 hours, or 200 mg five times per day, or 800 mg every 12 hours, treatment continuing for 5 days. Famciclovir, given by mouth in a dose of 125 mg every 12 hours for 5 days, is also recommended, as is valaciclovir in an oral dose of either 500 mg twice daily for 3 to 5 days, or 1.0 g once daily for 5 days[155]. Famciclovir has recently been shown to reduce the frequency of symptomatic recurrence and viral shedding in patients with HIV infection (median CD4 cell count of 384 cells/mm^3) and prior HSV-2 infections[193].

In this double-blind, placebo-controlled, crossover trial, HSV-2 was isolated on 122 (11%) of 1114 days when the patient was receiving placebo but on only 9 (1%) of 1071 days when taking famciclovir.

Prevention of genital herpes simplex virus infection

SEROLOGICAL TESTING AS PART OF A PREVENTATIVE STRATEGY

Although newer serological tests have increased sensitivity, specificity, and positive and negative predictive values compared with older tests (see pp. 120–121), their role in routine clinical practice is still not clearly defined. An advisory panel convened under the auspices of the Centers for Disease Control, USA, recommended the immediate implementation of several strategies to prevent the sexual transmission of HSV[194]. Included was a recommendation to offer serological screening, using type-specific tests, as part of the routine investigations to diagnose or exclude STIs. The rationale behind such a recommendation is that many individuals who acquire HSV-2 subclinically subsequently develop clinical recurrences[13], but are unaware that the symptoms are those of genital herpes. Patients who are identified as being seropositive for HSV-2 can be educated to recognize the clinical manifestations of the infection, to distinguish these features from those of other common conditions such as urinary tract infection and genital dermatoses, and to abstain from sexual contact during the recurrence. After educational counseling sessions with color illustrations of typical and atypical lesions, about two-thirds of patients have been able to identify recurrent disease[19]. Although this strategy will reduce the risk of transmission of HSV-2, it cannot eliminate it entirely, as a minority of individuals shed the virus even when they are symptomless (see pp. 110–111). A further use of serological testing is to identify sero-discordant couples, that is, one infected and one uninfected person. This may be particularly important in the pregnant female partner of infected men (see page 132).

Where the proportion of patients with HSV-1 genital herpes is high, however, serological screening is probably of less value in that a positive test neither confirms nor refutes a diagnosis of genital herpes.

The public health benefits of serological screening for HSV infection are unclear. In the absence of an effective prophylactic vaccine, reliable interventions to prevent the sexual transmission of HSV have not been established. Until such strategies have been formally evaluated, many experts believe that the widespread introduction of serological screening should be postponed[195].

CONDOMS AND SPERMICIDES

The use of condoms in preventing transmission of sexually transmissible pathogens is discussed in Chapter 2. With respect to HSV, it was shown several years ago that, in laboratory plunger tests, high concentrations of HSV-2 did not cross the latex condoms studied[196]. The degree of protection against transmission of the virus, however, is unclear. A cross-sectional study from Costa Rica showed that the seroprevalence of HSV-2 was significantly higher amongst women whose partners never used condoms than amongst those who had used condoms for at least 2 years before the study[197]. Data from other sources, however, have failed to show a significant protective effect of condoms in the transmission of HSV-2. Despite an increase in the proportion of women using condoms, the incidence of genital herpes amongst women who attended a STI clinic in Denmark remained unchanged over a 4-year period[198]. Similarly, in a study from Peru, there was no difference in the seroprevalence of HSV-2 between female sex industry workers who used condoms consistently and those who did not[199]. As condoms may not entirely cover the area of skin or mucosa from which HSV is being shed, and as the virus can be transmitted by close bodily contact, condom use may reduce but not eliminate the risk of viral transmission.

In vitro studies have shown that spermicides, including nonoxynol-9 decrease HSV-2 infectivity[200]. There is, however, no conclusive evidence that the use of such agents reduces the risk of HSV infection.

ANTIVIRAL DRUGS

Although suppressive treatment with antiviral drugs reduces the frequency of viral shedding (see page 127), it has not been shown conclusively that such therapy reduces viral transmission.

VACCINES FOR HERPES SIMPLEX VIRUS

Protection against HSV by active immunization is a major challenge in view of the lack of protection against naturally recurrent disease. There are concerns about using live herpesvirus or DNA, although that is the best method to achieve cellular immunity, on account of persistence and the potential for neurovirulence or oncogenicity[201]. There has been progress with experimental herpes simplex vaccines and one has recently been approved. This is a live but genetically disabled replication-incompetent virus, lacking gH, termed a DIsabled Single Cycle virus (DISC) vaccine[202]. Subunit vaccines based on the viral glycoproteins gD and gB induce high titers of neutralizing antibody, but one such vaccine used in large phase III trials gave very limited protection and failed to reduce acquisition of HSV-2 by seronegative sexual partners[51]. A recent double-blind, placebo-controlled study, using a recombinant glycoprotein D_2 (gD_2) and a novel adjuvant that has stimulated T_{H1} responses in volunteers, has shown more promise[203]. Amongst women who were seronegative for HSV-1 and HSV-2, but had sexual partners who had genital herpes, vaccination gave about 73% protection against infection. Protection was not found in male vaccinees, or in women who were seropositive for HSV-1 only.

References

1 Davison AJ and Clements JB. Herpesviruses: general properties. In: Mahy BWJ, Collier L, (eds) *Topley and Wilson's Microbiology and Microbial Infections, Virology* vol. 1, 9th edition. London; Arnold: 1998.

2 Umene K. Molecular epidemiology of herpes simplex virus type 1. *Rev Med Microbiol* 1998; **9**: 217–224.

3 Marsden HS, Stow ND, Preston VG, Timbury MC, Wilkie NM. Physical mapping of herpes simplex virus-induced polypeptides. *J Gen Virolgy* 1978; **28**: 624–642.

4 Grabowska A, Jameson C, Laing P, *et al.* Identification of type-specific domain within glycoprotein G of herpes simplex virus 2 (HSV-2) recognized by the majority of patients infected with HSV-2, but not by those infected with HSV-1. *J Gen Virol* 1999; **80**: 1789–1798.

5 WuDunn D, Spear PG. Initial interaction of herpes simplex virus with cells is binding to heparan sulphate. *J Virol* 1989; **63**: 52–58.

6 Cocchi F, Lopez M, Menotti L, *et al.* The V domain of herpesvirus Ig-like receptor (HIgR) contains a major functional region in herpes simplex virus –1 entry into cells and interacts physically with the viral glycoprotein D. *Proc Natl Acad Sci* 1998; **95**: 15700–15705.

7 Wildy P, Field HJ, Nash AA. Classical herpes latency revisited. In: Mahy BWJ, Minson AC, Darby GK (eds) *Virus Persistence.* Cambridge; Cambridge University Press: 1982.

8 Rawls WE. Herpes simplex virus. In: Fields BN (ed.) *Virology* 1st edition. New York; Raven Press: 1985.

9 Fiddian AP, Yeo JM, Stubbings R, Dean D. Successful treatment of herpes labialis with topical aciclovir. *Br Med J* 1983; **286**: 1699–1701.

10 Cowan FM, Johnson AM, Ashley R, Corey L, Mindel A. Antibody to herpes simplex virus type 2 as serological marker of sexual lifestyle in populations. *B Med J* 1994; **309**: 1325–1329.

11 Fleming DT, McQuillan GM, Johnson RE, *et al.* Herpes simplex virus type 2 in the United States, 1976 to 1994. *N Engl J Med* 1997; **337**: 1105–1111.

12 Langenberg AGM, Corey L, Ashley RL, Leong WP, Straus S. A prospective study of new infections with herpes simplex virus type 1 and type 2. *N Engl J Med* 1999; **341**: 1432–1438.

13 Langenberg A, Benedetti J, Jenkins J, Ashley R, Winter C, Corey L. Development of clinically recognizable genital lesions among women previously identified as having "asymptomatic" herpes simplex virus type 2 infection. *Ann Int Med* 1989; **110**: 882–887.

14 Klein RJ. The pathogenesis of acute, latent and recurrent herpes simplex virus infections: brief review. *Arch Virol* 1982; **72**: 143–168.

15 Benedetti J, Corey L, Ashley R. Recurrence rates in genital herpes after symptomatic first-episode infection. *Ann Int Med* 1994; **121**: 847–854.

16 Benedetti J, Zeh J, Corey L. Clinical reactivation of genital herpes simplex virus infection decreases in frequency over time. *Ann Int Med* 1999; **131**: 14–20.

17 Koelle DM, Benedetti J, Langenberg A, *et al.* Asymptomatic reactivation of herpes simplex virus in women after the first episode of genital herpes. *Ann Int Med* 1992; **116**: 433–437.

18 Wald A, Zeh J, Selke J, Ashley RL, Corey L. Virologic characteristics of subclinical and symptomatic genital herpes infections. *N Engl J Med* 1995; **333**: 770–775.

19 Wald A, Zeh J, Barnum G, Davis LG, Corey L. Suppression of subclinical shedding of herpes simplex virus type 2 with acyclovir. *Ann Int Med* 1996; **124**: 8–15.

20 Krone MR, Wald A, Tabet SR, Paradise M, Corey L, Celum CL. Herpes simplex virus shedding in human immunodeficiency virus-negative men who have sex with men: frequency, patterns, and risk factors. *Clin Infect Dis* 2000; **30**: 261–267.

21 Augenbraum M, Feldman J, Chirgwin K, *et al.* Increased genital shedding of herpes simplex virus type 2 in HIV-seropositive women. *Ann Int Med* 1995; **123**: 845–847.

22 Schacker T, Hu HL, Koelle DM, *et al.* Famciclovir for the suppression of symptomatic and asymptomatic herpes simplex virus reactivation in HIV-infected persons. A double-blind, placebo-controlled trial. *Ann Int Med* 1998; **128**: 21–28.

23 Benedetti J, Zeh J, Selke S, Corey L. Frequency and reactivation of non-genital lesions among patients with genital herpes simplex virus. *Am J Med* 1995; **98**: 237–242.

24 Darougar S, Wishart MS, Viswalingam ND. Epidemiologcial and clinical features of primary herpes simplex virus ocular infection. *Br J Ophthalmol* 1985; **69**: 2–6.

25 Scott DA, Coulter WA, Lamey P-J. Oral shedding of herpes simplex virus type 1: a review. *J Oral Pathol Med* 1997; **26**: 441–447.

26 Spruance SL, Overall JC, Kern ER, *et al.* The natural history of recurrent herpes simplex labialis: implications for antiviral therapy. *N Engl J Med* 1977; **297**: 69–75.

27 Spruance SL. Pathogenesis of herpes simplex labialis: excretion of virus in the oral cavity. *J Clin Microbiol* 1984; **19**: 675–679.

28 Kameyama T, Futami M, Nakayoshi N, Sujaku C, Yamamoto S. Shedding of herpes simplex virus type 1 into saliva in patients

with orofacial fracture. *J Med Virol* 1989; **28**: 78–80.

29 Wheeler CE. The herpes simplex problem. *J Am Acad Dermatol* 1988; **18**: 163–168.

30 Tateishi K, Toh Y, Minagawa H, Tashiro H. Detection of herpes simplex virus (HSV) in the saliva from 1,000 oral surgery outpatients by the polymerase chain reaction (PCR) and virus isolation. *J Oral Pathol Med* 1994; **23**: 80–84.

31 LaffertyWE, Coombs RW, Benedetti J, Critchlow C, Corey L. Recurrences after oral and genital herpes simplex virus infection. Influence of site and viral type. *N Engl J Med* 1987; **316**: 1444–1449.

32 Minson AC. Alphaherpesviruses: herpes simplex and varicella-zoster. In: Mahy BWJ, Collier L, (eds) *Topley and Wilson's Microbiology and Microbial Infections, Virology* vol. 1, 9th edition. London; Arnold: 1998.

33 Juel-Jensen, MacCallum FO. *Herpes Simplex Varicella and Zoster*. London; William Heinemann: 1972.

34 Huff JC, Krueger GG, Overall JC, Copeland J, Spruance SL. The histopathologic evolution of recurrent herpes simplex labialis. *J Am Acad Dermatol* 1981; **5**: 550–557.

35 Croen KD, Ostrove JM, Dragovic LJ, Smialek JE, Straus SE. Latent herpes simplex virus in human trigeminal ganglia. Detection of an immediate early gene "anti-sense" transcript by in situ hybridization. *N Engl J Med* 1987; **317**: 1427–1432.

36 Roizman B, Sears A. Herpes simplex viruses and their replication. In: Fields BN, Knipe DM, Howley P *et al*. (eds) *Field's Virology*. Philadelphia; Lippincott-Raven: 1996.

37 Hill A, Jugovic P, York I, *et al*. Herpes simplex virus turns off the TAP to evade host immunity. *Nature* (London) 1995; **375**: 411–415.

38 Lekstrom-Himes JA, Hohman P, Warren T, *et al*. Association of major histocompatibility complex determinants with the development of symptomatic and asymptomatic genital herpes simplex virus type 2 infections. *J Infect Dis* 1999; **179**: 1077–1085.

39 Goodell SE, Quinn TC, Mkrtichian E, Schuffler MD, Holmes KK, Corey L. Herpes simplex virus proctitis in homosexual men. *N Engl J Med* 1983; **308**: 868–871.

40 Ng ABP, Reagan JW, Lindner E. The cellular manifestations of primary and recurrent herpes genitalis. *Acta Cytol* 1970; **14**: 124–129.

41 Dittmar HC, Weiss JM, Termeer CC, *et al*. In vivo UVA-1 and UVB irradiation differentially perturbs the antigen-presenting function of human epidermal Langerhans cells. *J Invest Dermatol* 1999; **112**: 322–325.

42 Johnson RE, Nahmias AJ, Magder LS, Lee FK, Brooks CA, Snowden CB. A seroepidemiologic survey of the prevalence of herpes simplex virus type 2 infection in the United States. *N Engl J Med* 1989; **321**: 7–12.

43 Koutsky LA, Stevens CE, Holmes KK, *et al*. Underdiagnosis of genital herpes by current clinical and viral-isolation procedures. *N Engl J Med* 1992; **326**: 1533–1539.

44 Jeansson S, Molin L. On the occurrence of genital herpes simplex virus infection. clinical and virological findings and relation to gonorrhoea. *Acta Dermatovenereol* 1974; **54**: 479–485.

45 Barton S, Wright LK, Link CM, Munday PE. Screening to detect asymptomatic shedding of herpes simplex virus (HSV) in women with recurrent genital HSV infection. *Genitourin Med* 1986; **62**: 181–185.

46 Mertz GJ, Schmidt O, Jourden JL, *et al*. Frequency of acquisition of first-episode genital infection with herpes simplex virus from symptomatic and asymptomatic source contacts. *Sex Transm Dis* 1985; **12**: 33–39.

47 Rooney JF, Felser JM, Ostrove JM, Straus SE. Acquisition of genital herpes from an asymptomatic sexual partner. *N Engl J Med* 1986; **314**: 1561–1564.

48 Barton SE, Davis JM, Moss VW, Tyms AS, Munday PE. Asymptomatic shedding and subsequent transmission of genital herpes simplex virus. *Genitourin Med* 1987; **63**: 102–105.

49 Mertz GJ, Benedetti J, Ashley R, Selke SA, Corey L. Risk factors for the sexual transmission of genital herpes. *Ann Int Med* 1992; **116**: 197–202.

50 Brown ZA, Vontver LA, Benedetti J, *et al*. Effects on infants of a first episode of genital herpes during pregnancy. *N Engl J Med* 1987; **317**: 1246–1251.

51 Corey L, Langenberg ACM, Ashley R, *et al*. Recombinant glycoprotein vaccine for the prevention of genital HSV-2 infection: two randomized controlled trials. *JAMA* 1999; **282**: 331–340.

52 Bryson Y, Dillon M, Bernstein DI, Radolf J, Zakowski P, Garratty E. Risk of acquisition of genital herpes simplex virus type 2 in sex partners of persons with genital herpes: a prospective couple study. *J Infect Dis* 1993; **167**: 942–946.

53 Holmberg SD, Stewart JA, Gerber AR, *et al*. Prior herpes simplex virus type 2 infection as a risk factor for HIV infection. *JAMA* 1988; **259**: 1048–1050.

54 Hook EW, Cannon RO, Nahmias AJ, *et al*. Herpes simplex virus infection as a risk factor for human immunodeficiency virus infection in heterosexuals. *J Infect Dis* 1992; **165**: 251–255.

55 Chen CY, Ballard RC, Beck-Sague CM, *et al*. Human immunodeficiency virus infection and genital ulcer disease in South Africa: the herpetic connection. *Sex Transm Dis* 2000; **27**: 21–29.

56 Gwanzura L, McFarland W, Alexander D, Burke RL, Katzenstein D. Association between human immunodeficiency virus and herpes simplex virus type 2 among male factory workers in Zimbabwe. *J Infect Dis* 2998; **177**: 481–484.

57 Nagington J, Rook A, Highet AS. Herpes simplex. In: Rook A, Wilkinson DS, Ebling FJG, Champion RH, Burton JH, (eds) *Textbook of Dermatology* 4th edition. Oxford; Blackwell: 1986.

58 Corey L, Adams HG, Brown ZA, Holmes KK. Genital herpes simplex virus infections: clinical manifestations, course, and complications. *Ann Int Med* 1983; **98**: 958–972.

59 Person DA, Kaufman RH, Gardner HL, Rawls WE. Hepesvirus type 2 in genitourinary tract infection. *Am J Obstet Gynecol* 1973; **116**: 993–995.

60 Shah SJ, Scholz FJ. Anorectal herpes: radiographic findings. *Radiology* 1983; **147**: 81–82.

61 Craig C, Nahmias A. Different patterns of neurologic involvement with herpes simplex virus types 1 and 2: isolation of herpes simplex virus from the buffy coat of two adults with aseptic meningitis. *J Infect Dis* 1973; **127**: 365–372.

62 Walzman MW, Wade AAH. Labial adhesions after genital herpes infection. *Genitourin Med* 1989; **65**: 187–188.

63 White C, Sparks RA. Prepucial occlusion and circumcision after genital herpes infection. *Int J STD AIDS* 1991; **2**: 209–210.

64 Oates JK, Greenhouse PRDH. Retention of urine in anogenital herpetic infection. *Lancet* 1978; **I**: 691–692.

65 Samarasinghe PL, Oates JK, MacLennan IPB. Herpetic proctitis and sacral radiomyelopathy – a hazard for homosexual men. *Br Med J* 1979; **ii**: 365–366.

66 Klatensky J, Cappel R, Snoeck JM, Flament J, Thiry L. Ascending myelitis in association with herpes simplex virus. *N Engl J Med* 1972; **287**: 182–184.

67 Masfari AN, Ginghorn GR, Hafiz S, Barton IG, Duerden BI. Anaerobic bacteria and herpes simplex virus in genital ulceration. *Genitourin Med* 1985; **61**: 109–113.

68 Kinghorn GR, Abeywickreme I, Jeavons M, *et al*. Efficacy of oral treatment with acyclovir and co-trimoxazole in first episode genital herpes. *Genitourin Med* 1986; **62**: 33–37.

69 Safrin S. Acyclovir-resistant herpes simplex virus infection. *J Infect Dis* 1995; **172**: 603.

70 Luby ED, Gillespie O. Psychological responses to genital herpes. *Helper* 1981; **3**: 2–3.

71 Christie SN, McCaughey C, Marley JJ, Coyle PV, Scott DA, Lamey PJ. Recrudescent herpes simplex infection mimicking primary herpetic gingivostomatitis. *J Oral Pathol Med* 1998; **27**: 8–10.

72 Sacks SL. Frequency and duration of patient-observed recurrent genital HSV infections: characterization of the non-lesional prodrome. *J Infect Dis* 1984; **150**: 8873–8877.

73 Britz M, Sibulkin D. Recurrent erythema multiforme and herpes genitalis. *JAMA* 1975; **233**: 812–813.

74 Jensenius M, Myrvang B, Storvold G, Bucher A, Hellum KB, Bruu AL. Herpes simplex virus type 2 DNA detected in cerebrospinal fluid of 9 patients with Mollaret's meningitis. *Acta Neurol Scand* 1998; **98**: 209–212.

75 Steiner I, Mattan Y. Bell's palsy and herpes viruses: to (acyclo)vir or not to (acyclo)vir? *J Neurol Sciences* 1999; **170**: 19–23.

76 Cowan FM, Johnson AM, Ashley R, Corey L, Mindel A. Relationship between antibodies to herpes simplex virus (HSV) and symptoms of HSV infection. *J Infect Dis* 1996; **174**: 470–475.

77 Brugha R, Brown D, Meheus A, Renton A. Should we be screening for asymptomatic HSV infections? *Sex Transm Infect* 1999; **75**: 142–144.

78 Simmon A, Marmion BP. Rapid diagnosis of viral infections. In: Collee JG, Fraser AG, Marmion BP, Simmons A, (eds) *Practical Medical Microbiology* 14th edition. Edinburgh; Churchill Livingstone: 1996.

79 Turchek BM, Huang YT. Evaluation of ELVIS™ HSV/ID Typing System for the detection and typing of herpes simplex virus from clinical specimens. *J Clin Virol* 1999; **12**: 65–69.

80 Liljeqvist J-A, Svennerholm B, Bergstrom T. Typing of clinical herpes simplex virus type 1 and type 2 isolates with monoclonal antibodies. *J Clin Microbiol* 1999; **37**: 2717–2718.

81 Aurelius E, Johansson B, Skoldenberg B, Staland A, Forsgren M. Rapid diagnosis of herpes simplex encephalitis by nested primer polymerase chain reaction assay of cerebrospinal fluid. *Lancet* 1991; **337**: 189–192.

82 Tang YW, Mitchell PS, Espy MJ, Smith TF, Pershing DH. Molecular diagnosis of herpes simplex virus infections in the central nervous system. *J Clin Microbiol* 1999; **37**: 2127–2136.

83 Ashley RL, Wald A. Genital herpes: review of the epidemic and potential use of type-specific serology. *Clin Microbiol Rev* 1999; **12**: 1–8.

84 Eis-Hubinger AM, Daumer M, Matz B, *et al.* Evaluation of three glycoprotein G2-based enzyme immunoassays for detection of antibodies to herpes simplex virus type 2 in human sera. *J Clin Microbiol* 1999; **37**: 1242–1246.

85 Ashley RL, Eagleton M, Pfeiffer N. Ability of a rapid serology test to detect seroconversion to herpes simplex virus type 2 glycoprotein G soon after infection. *J Clin Microbiol* 1999; **37**:1632–1633.

86 Ashley RL, Wald A, Eagleton M. Premarket evaluation of the POCkit HSV-2 type-specific serologic test in culture-documented cases of genital herpes simplex virus type 2. *Sex Transm Dis* 2000; **27**: 266–269.

87 Balfour HH. Acyclovir. In: Peterson PK, Verhoef J (eds) *The Antimicrobial Agents Manual* vol. 3. New York; Elsevier Science: 1988, 345–360.

88 Cole NL, Balfour HH. Varicella-zoster virus does not become more resistant to acyclovir during therapy. *J Infect Dis* 1986; **153**: 605–608.

89 Reardon JE, Spector T. Herpes simplex virus type 1 DNA polymerase: mechanism of inhibition of acyclovir triphosphate. *J Biol Chem* 1989; **264**: 7405–7411.

90 Blum MR, Liao SHJ, De Miranda P. Overview of acyclovir pharmacokinetic disposition in adults and children. *Am J Med* 1982; **73**: 186–192.

91 Frenkel LM, Brown ZA, Bryson YJ, *et al.* Pharmacokinetics of acyclovir in the term human pregnancy and neonate. *Am J Obstet Gynecol* 1991; **164**: 569–576.

92 Van Dyke RB, Connor JD, Wyborny C, Hintz M, Keeney RE. Pharmacokinetics of orally administered acyclovir in patients with herpes progenitalis. *Am J Med* 1982; **73**: 172–175.

93 Kimberlin DF, Weller S, Whitley RJ, *et al.* Pharmacokinetics of oral valacyclovir and acyclovir in late pregnancy. *Am J Obstet Gynecol* 1998; **179**: 846–851.

94 Lau RJ, Emery MG, Galinsky RE. Unexpected accumulation of acyclovir in breast milk. *Obstet Gynecol* 1987; **69**: 468–471.

95 Crumpacker CS, Schnipper LE, Zaia JA, Levin MJ. Growth inhibition of herpesviruses isolated from human infections. *Antimicrob Agents Chemother* 1979; **15**: 642–645.

96 Balfour HH. Antiviral drugs. *N Engl J Med* 1999; **340**: 1255–1268.

97 Wellcome Medical Division. *Zovirax (acyclovir)*. Crewe, Cheshire; The Wellcome Foundation: 1984.

98 Larder BA, Darby G. Virus drug-resistance: mechanisms and consequences. *Antiviral Res* 1984; **4**: 1–42.

99 Gaudreau A, Hill E, Balafour HH, Erice A, Boivin G. Phenotypic and genotypic characterization of acyclovir-resistant herpes simplex viruses from immunocompromised patients. *J Infect Dis* 1998; **178**: 297–303.

100 Collins P, Larder BA, Oliver NM, Kemp S, Smith IW, Darby G. Characterization of a DNA polymerase mutant of herpes simplex virus from a severely immunocompromised

patient receiving acyclovir. *J Gen Virol* 1989; **70**: 375–382.

101 Sasadeusz JJ, Tufaro F, Safrin S, *et al.* Homopolymer mutational hot spots mediate herpes simplex virus resistance to acyclovir. *J Virol* 1997; **71**: 3872–3878.

102 Kost RG, Hill EL, Tigges M, Straus SE. Recurrent acyclovir-resistant genital herpes in an immunocompetent patient. *N Engl J Med* 1993; **329**: 1777–1782.

103 Swetter SM, Hill EL, Kern ER, *et al.* Chronic vulvar ulceration in an immunocompetent woman due to acyclovir-resistant, thymidine kinase-deficient herpes simplex virus. *J Infect Dis* 1998; **177**: 543–550.

104 Erlich KS, Mills J, Chatis P, *et al.* Acyclovir-resistant herpes simplex virus infections in patients with the acquired immunodeficiency syndrome. *N Engl J Med* 1989; **320**: 293–296.

105 Christophers J, Clayton J, Craske J, *et al.* Survey of resistance of herpes simplex virus to acyclovir in northwest England. *Antimicrob Agents Chemother* 1998; **42**: 868–872.

106 Coen DM, Kosz-Vnenchak M, Jacobson JG, *et al.* Thymidine kinase-negative herpes simplex virus mutants establish latency in mouse trigeminal ganglia but do not reactivate. *Proc Natl Acad Sci USA* 1989; **86**: 4736–4740.

107 Sasadeusz JJ, Sacks SL. Spontaneous reactivation of thymidine kinase-deficient, acyclovir-resistant type 2 herpes simplex virus: masked heterogeneity or reversion? *J Infect Dis* 1996; **174**: 476–482.

108 Weller S, Blum SR, Doucette M, *et al.* Pharmacokinetics of the acyclovir prodrug valaciclovir after single and multiple dose administration in normal volunteers. *Clin Pharmacol Exp Ther* 1993; **54**: 595–605.

109 Soul-Lawton S, Seaber E, On N, *et al.* Absolute bioavailability and metabolic disposition of valaciclovir, the L-valyl ester of acyclovir, following oral administration in humans. *Antimicrob Agents Chemother* 1995; **39**: 2759–2764.

110 Boyd MR, Bacon TH, Sutton D, Cole M. Antiherpesvirus activity of 9-(4-hydroxy-3-hydroxy-methylbut-1-yl)guanine (BRL 39123) in cell culture. *Antimicrob Agents Chemother* 1987; **31**: 1238–1242.

111 Thackray AM, Field HJ. Comparison of effects of famciclovir and valaciclovir on pathogenesis of herpes simplex virus type 2 in a murine infection model. *Antimicrob Agents Chemother* 1996; **40**: 846–851.

112 Thackray AM, Field HJ. Differential effects of famciclovir and valaciclovir on the pathogenesis of herpes simplex virus in a murine infection model including reactivation from latency. *J Infect Dis* 1996; **173**: 291–299.

113 Vere Hodge RA, Sutton D, Boyd MR, Harnden MR, Jarvest RL. Selection of an oral prodrug (BRL 42810; famciclovir) for the antiherpes-virus agent BRL 39123 [9-

(4-hydroxymethylbut-1-yl)guanine; penciclovir]. *Antimicrob Agents Chemother* 1989; **33**: 1765–1773.

114 Vere Hodge RA, Perkins RM. Mode of action of 9-(4-hydroxy-3-hydroxymethylbut-1-yl)guanine (BRL 39123) against herpes simplex virus in MRC-5 cells. *Antimicrob Agents Chemother* 1989; **33**: 223–229.

115 Earnshaw DL, Bacon TH, Darlison SJ, Edmonds K, Perkins RM, Vere Hodge RA. Mode of antiviral action of penciclovir in MRC-5 cells infected with herpes simplex virus type 1 (HSV-1), HSV-2, and varicella-zoster virus. *Antimicrob Agents Chemother* 1992; **36**: 2747–2757.

116 Vere Hodge RA, Cheng Y-C. The mode of action of penciclovir. *Antiviral Chem Chemother* 1993; **4**, Suppl. 1: 13–24.

117 Mindel A, Adler MW, Sutherland S, Fiddian AP. Intravenous acyclovir treatment for primary genital herpes. *Lancet* 1982; **I**: 697–700.

118 Nilsen AE, Aasen T, Halsos AM, *et al.* Efficacy of oral acyclovir in the treatment of initial and recurrent genital herpes. *Lancet* 1982; **ii** : 571–573.

119 Centers for Disease Control and Prevention. 2002 Guidelines for treatment of sexually transmitted diseases. *MMWR* 2002; **51**: RR-6.

120 Corey L, Holmes KK. Genital herpes simplex virus infections: current concepts in diagnosis, therapy and prevention. *Ann Int Med* 1983; **98**: 973–983.

121 Kinghorn GR, Abeywickreme I, Jeavons M, *et al.* Efficacy of combined treatment with oral and topical acyclovir in first episode genital herpes. *Genitourin Med* 1986; **62**: 186–188.

122 Fife KH, Barbarash RA, Rudolph T, *et al.* Valaciclovir versus acyclovir in the treatment of first-episode genital herpes infection. Results of an international, multicenter, double-blind, randomised clinical trial. The valaciclovir international herpes simplex virus study group. *Sex Transm Dis* 1997; **24**: 481–486.

123 Reichman RC, Badger GJ, Mertz GJ, *et al.* Treatment of recurrent genital herpes simplex infections with oral acyclovir. A controlled trial. *JAMA* 1984; **251**: 2103–2107.

124 Ruhnek-Forsbeck M, Sandstrom E, Andersson B, *et al.* Treatment of recurrent genital herpes simplex infections with oral acyclovir. *J Antimicrob Chemother* 1985; **16**: 621–628.

125 Whitley RJ, Gnann JW. Acyclovir: a decade later. *N Engl J Med* 1992; **327**: 782–789.

126 Spruance SL, Tyring SK, Degregorio B, Miller C, Beutner K. A large scale placebo-controlled trial of peroral valaciclovir for episodic treatment of recurrent herpes genitalis. *Arch Int Med* 1996; **156**: 1729–1735.

127 Bodsworth NJ, Crooks RJ, Borelli S, *et al.* Valaciclovir versus aciclovir in patient initiated treatment of recurrent genital herpes: a randomised, double-blind clinical trial. *Genitourin Med* 1997; **73**: 110–116.

128 Sacks SL, Aoki FY, Diaz-Mitoma F, Sellors J, *et al.* Patient-initiated, twice-daily oral famciclovir for early recurrent genital herpes. A randomized, double-blind multicenter trial. *JAMA* 1996; **276**: 44–49.

129 Mindel A, Weller IVD, Faherty A, *et al.* Prophylactic oral acyclovir in recurrent genital herpes. *Lancet* 1984; **ii**: 57–60.

130 Straus SE, Takiff HE, Seidlin M, *et al.* Suppression of frequently recurring genital herpes: a placebo-controlled double-blind trial of oral acyclovir. *N Engl J Med* 1984; **310**: 1545–1550.

131 Douglas JM, Critchlow C, Benedetti J, *et al.* A double-blind study of oral acyclovir for suppression of recurrences of genital herpes simplex virus. *N Engl J Med* 1984; **310**: 1551–1556.

132 Kinghorn GR. Long-term suppression with oral acyclovir of recurrent herpes simplex virus infections in otherwise healthy patients. *Am J Med* 1988; **85**, Suppl. 2A: 26–29.

133 Mertz GJ, Eron L, Kaufman R, *et al.* Prolonged continuous versus intermittent oral acyclovir treatment in normal adults with frequently recurring genital herpes simplex virus infection. *Am J Med* 1988; **85**, Suppl. 2A: 14–19.

134 Baker DA, Blythe JG, Kaufman R, Hlae R, Portnoy J. One-year suppression of frequent recurrences of genital herpes with oral acyclovir. *Obstet Gynecol* 1989; **73**: 84–87.

135 Goldberg LH, Kaufman RH, Kurtz TO, *et al.* Continuous five-year treatment of patients with frequently recurring genital herpes simplex virus infection with acyclovir. *J Med Virol* 1993; Suppl. 1: 45–50.

136 Mindel A, Faherty A, Carney O, Patou G, Freris M, Williams P. Dosage and long-term suppressive acyclovir therapy for recurrent genital herpes. *Lancet* 1988; **I**: 926–928.

137 Wald A, Kim M, Catlett L, Selke S, Ashley R, Corey L. Genital HSV-2 shedding in women with HSV-2 antibodies but without a history of genital herpes. *Thirty-sixth Interscience Conference on Antimicrobial Agents and Chemotherapy*; New Orleans, Washington DC: American Society for Microbiology: 1996, Abstract H80.

138 Patel R, Bodsworth NJ, Woolley P, *et al.* Valaciclovir for the suppression of recurrent genital HSV infection: a placebo controlled study of once daily therapy. *Genitourin Med* 1997; **73**: 105–109.

139 Reitano M, Tyring S, Lang W, *et al.* Valaciclovir for the suppression of recurrent genital herpes simplex virus infection: a large-scale dose range-finding study. *J Infect Dis* 1998; **178**: 603–610.

140 Diaz-Mitoma F, Sibbald RG, Shafran SD, Boon R, Saltzman RL. Oral famciclovir for the suppression of recurrent genital herpes: a randomized controlled trial. Collaborative Famciclovir genital herpes research group. *JAMA* 1998; **280**: 887–892.

141 Mertz GJ, Loveless MO, Levin MJ, *et al.* Oral famciclovir for suppression of recurrent genital herpes simplex virus infection in women. A multicenter, double-blind, placebo-controlled trial. *Arch Int Med* 1997; **157**: 343–349.

141a Kinghorn GR, Turner EB, Barton IG, Potter CCW, Burke CA, Fiddian AP. Efficacy of topical acyclovir cream in first and recurrent episodes of genital herpes. *Antiviral Res* 1983; **3**: 291–301.

142 Amir J, Harel L, Smetana Z, Varsano I. Treatment of herpes simplex gingivostomatitis with aciclovir in children: a randomised double blind placebo controlled study. *Br Med J* 1997; **314**: 1800–1803.

143 Higgins CR, Schofield JK, Tatnall FM, Leigh IM. Natural history, management and complications of herpes labialis. *J Med Virol* 1993; Suppl 1: 22–26.

144 Fiddian AP, Ivanyi L. Topical acyclovir in the management of recurrent herpes labialis. *Br J Dermatol* 1983; **109**: 321–326.

145 Shaw M, King M, Best JM. Failure of acyclovir cream in treatment of recurrent herpes labialis. *Br Med J* 1985; **291**: 7–9.

146 Biagoni PA, Lamey P-J. Acyclovir cream prevents clinical and thermographic progression of recrudescent herpes labialis beyond the prodromal stage. *Acta Dermatol Venereol (Stockh)*; **78**: 46–47.

147 Spruance SL, Rea TL, Thoming C, Tucker R, Saltzman R, Boon R. Penciclovir cream for the treatment of herpes simplex labialis. A randomized, multicenter, double-blind, placebo-controlled trial. Topical penciclovir collaborative study group. *JAMA* 1997; **277**: 1374–1379.

148 Spruance SL, Stewart JC, Rowe NH, McKeough MB, Wenerstrom G, Freeman DJ. Treatment of recurrent herpes simplex labialis with oral acyclovir. *J Infect Dis* 1990; **161**: 185–190.

149 Spruance SL. Prophylactic chemotherapy with acyclovir for recurrent herpes simplex labialis. *J Med Virol* 1993; Suppl. 1: 27–32.

150 Rooney JF, Straus SE, Mannix ML *et al.* Oral acyclovir to suppress frequently recurrent herpes labialis. *Ann Int Med* 1993; **118**: 268–272.

151 Raborn GW, Martel AY, Grace MG, McGaw WT. Oral acyclovir in prevention of herpes labialis. A randomised, double-blind, multicentered clinical trial. *Oral Surg Oral Med Oral Pathol Oral Radiol Endo* 1998; **85**: 55–59.

152 Richards DM, Carmine AA, Brogden RN, Heel RC, Speight TM, Avery GS. Acyclovir. A review of its pharmacodynamic properties and therapeutic efficacy. *Drugs* 1983; **26**: 378–438.

153 Herpetic Eye Disease Study Group. Acyclovir for the prevention of recurrent herpes simplex virus eye disease. *N Engl J Med* 1998; **339**: 300–306.

154 National guideline for the management of genital herpes. *Sex Transm Inf* 1999; **75**, Suppl. 1: S24–S28.

155 Centers for Disease Control and Prevention. 2002 Guidelines for treatment of sexually transmitted diseases. *MMWR* 2002; **51**: RR-6.

156 Carney O, Ross E, Ikkos G, Mindel A. The effect of suppressive oral acyclovir on the psychological morbidity associated with recurrent genital herpes. *Genitourin Med* 1993; **69**: 457–459.

157 Mindel A. Long-term clinical and psychological management of genital herpes. *J Med Virol* 1993; Suppl. 1: 39–44.

158 Tookey P, Peckham CS. Neonatal herpes simplex virus infection in the British Isles. *Paediatr Perinat Epidemiol* 1996; **10**: 432–442.

159 Stone KM, Brooks CA, Guinan ME, Alexander ER. National surveillance for neonatal herpes simplex virus infections. *Sex Transm Dis* 1989; **16**: 152–156.

160 Brown ZA. Genital herpes and pregnancy. In: Hitchcock PJ, MacKay HT, Wasserheit JN, (eds) *Sexually Transmitted Diseases and Adverse Outcomes of Pregnancy*. Washington DC: ASM Press: 1999.

161 Nahmias AJ, Josey WE, Naib ZM, Freeman MG, Fernandez RJ, Wheeler JH. Perinatal risk associated with genital herpes simplex virus infection. *Am J Obstet Gynecol* 1971; **110**: 825–836.

162 Arvin AM, Hensleigh PA, Prober CG, *et al*. Failure of antepartum maternal cultures to predict the infant's risk of exposure to herpes simplex virus at delivery. *N Engl J Med* 1986; **315**: 796–800.

163 Brown ZA, Selke S, Zeh J, *et al*. The acquisition of herpes simplex virus during pregnancy. *N Engl J Med* 1997; **337**: 509–515.

164 Vontver LA, Hickok DE, Brown Z, Reid L, Corey L. Recurrent genital herpes simplex virus infection in pregnancy: infant outcome and frequency of asymptomatic recurrences. *Am J Obstet Gynecol* 1982; **142**: 75.

165 Prober CG, Sullender WM, Yasukawa LL, *et al*. Low risk of herpes simplex virus infections in neonates exposed to the virus at the time of vaginal delivery to mothers with recurrent genital herpes simplex virus infections. *N Engl J Med* 1987; **316**: 240–244.

166 Brown Z, Hume S, Selke J, *et al*. Subclinical shedding of herpes simplex virus (HSV) at the time of labor. *Am J Obstet Gynecol* 1998; **178**: S3.

166a Brown ZA, Benedetti J, Ashley R, *et al*. Neonatal herpes simplex virus infection in relation to asymptomatic maternal infection at the time of labor. *N Engl J Med* 1991; **324**: 1247–1252.

167 Francis DP, Herrmann KL, McMahon JR, Chavigny KH, Sanderlin KC. Nosocomially and maternally acquired herpesvirus hominis infections. A report of four fatal cases in neonates. *Am J Dis Child* 1975; **129**: 889–893.

168 Hitti J, Watts DH, Burchett SK, *et al*. Herpes simplex virus seropositivity and reactivation at delivery among pregnant women infected with human immunodeficiency virus-1. *Am J Obstet Gynecol* 1997; **177**: 450–454.

169 Smith JR, Cowan FM, Munday P. The management of herpes simplex virus infection in pregnancy. *Br J Obstet Gynaecol* 1998; **105**: 255–260.

170 Lissauer T, Jeffries D. Preventing neonatal herpes infection. *Br Med J* 1989; **96**: 1015–1018.

171 Randolph AR, Washington E, Prober CG. Cesarean delivery for women presenting with genital herpes lesions: efficacy, risks and costs. *JAMA* 1993; **270**: 77–82.

172 Scott LL, Sanchez PJ, Jackson GL, Zeray F, Wendel G. Acyclovir suppression to prevent cesarean delivery after first-episode genital herpes. *Obstet Gynecol* 1996; **87**: 69–73.

173 Brocklehurst P, Kinghorn G, Carney O, *et al*. A randomised controlled trial of suppressive acyclovir in late pregnancy in women with recurrent genital herpes infection. *Br J Obstet Gynaecol* 1998; **105**: 275–280.

174 Gould JM, Chessells JM, Marshall WC, McKendrick GDW. Acyclovir in herpesvirus infections in children: experience in an open study with particular reference to safety. *J Infect* 1982; **5**: 283–289.

175 Whitley R, Arvin A, Prober C, *et al*. A controlled trial comparing vidarabine with acyclovir in neonatal herpes simplex virus infection. *N Engl J Med* 1991; **324**: 444–449.

176 Young EJ, Chafizadeh E, Oliveira VL, Genta RM. Disseminated herpes virus infection during pregnancy. *Clin Inf Dis* 1996; **22**: 51–58.

177 Dennett C, Cleator GM, Klapper PE. HSV-1 and HSV-2 in herpes simplex encephalitis: a study of sixty-four cases in the United Kingdom. *J Med Virol* 1997; **53**: 1–3.

178 Moseley I, Sutton D, Kendall BE, Stevens J. In: Sutton D, (ed.) *A Textbook of Radiology and Imaging* 5th edition. Edinburgh: Churchill Livingstone: 1993.

179 Levine DP, Laute CB, Lerner AM. Simultaneous serum and CSF antibodies in herpes simplex virus encephalitis. *JAMA* 1978; **240**: 356–360.

180 Siegal FP, Lopez C, Hammer GS, *et al*. Severe acquired immunodeficiency in male homosexuals, manifested by chronic perianal ulcerative herpes simplex lesions. *N Engl J Med* 1981; **305**: 1439–1444.

181 Langtry JAA, Ostlere LS, Hawkins D, *et al*. The difficulty in diagnosis of cutaneous herpes simplex virus infection in patients with AIDS. *Clin Exp Dermatol* 1994; **19**: 224–226.

182 Vogel P, Smith KJ, Skelton HG, *et al*. Verrucous lesions of herpes simplex in HIV-1+ patients. *Int J Dermatol* 1993; **32**: 680–682.

183 Burke EM, Karp DL, Wu TC, *et al*. Atypical oral presentation of herpes simplex virus infection in a patient after orthotopic liver transplantation. *Eur Arch Otorhinolaryngol* 1994; **251**: 301–303.

184 Beasley KL, Cooley GE, Kao GF, Lowitt MH, Burnett JW, Aurelian L. Herpes simplex vegetans: atypical genital herpes infection in a patient with common variable immunodeficiency. *J Am Acad Dermatol* 1997; **37**: 860–863.

185 Saijo M, Suzutani T, Murono K, Hirano Y, Itoh K. Recurrent aciclovir-resistant herpes simplex in a child with Wiskott-Aldrich syndrome. *Br J Dermatol* 1998; **139**: 311–314.

186 Seksik P, Gozlan J, Guitton C, Galaula G, Maury E, Offenstadt G. Fatal herpetic hepatitis in adult following short corticotherapy: a case report. *Intensive Care Med* 1999; **25**: 415–417.

187 Grossman ME, Stevens AW, Cohen PR. Herpetic geometric glossitis. *N Engl J Med* 1993; **329**: 1859–1860.

188 Lazarus HM, Belanger R, Candoni A, *et al*. Intravenous penciclovir for treatment of herpes simplex infections in immunocompromised patients: results of a multicenter, acyclovir-controlled trial. *Antimicrob Agents Chemother* 1999; **43**: 1192–1197.

189 Safrin S, Crumpacker C, Chatis P, *et al*. A controlled trial comparing foscarnet with viadarabine for acyclovir-resistant mucocutaneous herpes simplex in the acquired immunodeficiency syndrome. *N Engl J Med* 1991; **325**: 551–555.

190 Balfour HH, Benson C, Braun J, *et al*. Management of acyclovir-resistant herpes simplex and varicella-zoster virus infections. *J Acquir Immune Defic Syndr* 1994; **7**: 254–260.

191 Lalezari J, Schacker T, Feinberg J, *et al*. A randomised double blind controlled trial of cidofovir gel for the treatment of acyclovir-unresponsive mucocutaneous herpes simplex virus infection in patients with AIDS. *J Infect Dis* 1997; **176**: 892–898.

192 LoPresti AE, Levine JF, Munk GB, Tai CY, Mendel DB. Successful treatment of an

acyclovir- and foscarnet-resistant herpes simplex virus type 1 lesion with intravenous cidofovir. *Clin Infect Dis* 1998; **26**: 512–513.

193 Shacker T, Ryncarz AJ, Goddard J, Diem K, Shaughnessy M, Corey L. Frequent recovery of HIV-1 from genital herpes simplex virus lesions in HIV-1 infected men. *JAMA* 1998; **280**: 61–66.

194 Handsfield HH, Stone KM, Wasserheit JN. Prevention agenda for genital herpes. *Sex Transm Dis* 1999; **26**: 228–231.

195 Cowan F. Testing for type-specific antibody to herpes simplex virus – implications for clinical practice. *J Antimicrob Chemother* 2000; **45** Topic T3: 9–13.

196 Conant MA, Spicer DW, Smith CD. Herpes simplex virus transmission: condom studies. *Sex Transm Dis* 1984; **11**: 94–95.

197 Oberle MW, Rosero-Bixby L, Lee FK, Sanchez-Braverman M, Nahmias AJ, Guinan ME. Herpes simplex virus antibodies: high prevalence in monogamous women in Costa Rica. *Am J Trop Med Hyg* 1989; **41**: 224–229.

198 Olivarius F de F, Worm AM, Petersen CS, Kroon S, Lynge E. Sexual behaviour of women attending an inner-city STD clinic before and after a general campaign for safer sex in Denmark. *Genitourin Med* 1992; **68**: 296–299.

199 Sanchez J, Gotuzzo E, Escamilla J, *et al.* Gender differences in sexual practices and sexually transmitted infections among adults in Lima, Peru. *Am J Public Health* 1996; **86**: 1098–1107.

200 Singh B, Posti B, Cutler JC. Virucidal effect of certain chemical contraceptives on type 2 herpesvirus. *Am J Obstet Gynecol* 1976; **126**: 422–425.

201 Bernstein DI, Stanberry LR. Herpes simplex virus vaccines. *Vaccine* 1999; **17**: 1681–1689.

202 Roberts JFC, Uttridge JA, Hickling JK, *et al.* Safety, tolerability and viral containment of a disabled infectious single cycle HSV-2 vaccine evaluated in phase 1 clinical trials in HSV-2 seropositive and seronegative volunteers. *Abstracts of the 8th International Congress on Infectious Diseases*; Boston MA: May 1998, p. 89, Abstract 22 009.

203 Spruance SS. Herpes vaccine efficacy study group. Gender-specific efficacy of a prophylactic SBASA4-adjuvanted gD2 subunit vaccine against genital herpes disease (GHD): results of two efficacy trials. *Fortieth Interscience Conference on Antimicrobial Agents and Chemotherapy*; Toronto, Washington DC: 2000, Abstract L-4.

204 Robertson DHH, McMillan A, Young H. *Clinical Practice in Sexually Transmissible Diseases* 2nd edition. Edinburgh: Churchill Livingstone: 1989.

205 PHLS, DHSS&PS and the Scottish ISD(D)5 Collaborative Group. *Trends in Sexually Transmitted Infections in the United Kingdom, 1990–1999*. London: Public Health Laboratory Service: 2000.

206 McMillan A, Scott GR. *Sexually Transmitted Infections, Colour Guide*. Churchill Livingstone: Edinburgh: 2000.

APPENDICES

APPENDIX 6.1

ADMINISTRATION OF ACICLOVIR BY INTRAVENOUS INFUSION

Zovirax IV (Glaxo Wellcome), Aciclovir IV (Faulding DBL), and Aciclovir Sodium (Lennon) are available in the UK. The drug, as sodium salt, is dispensed in 250 mg or 500 mg vials. The following infusion fluids can be used: sodium chloride intravenous infusion 0.9% w/v, *or* sodium chloride and glucose intravenous infusion, *or* compound sodium lactate intravenous infusion (Hartmann's solution).

- After reconstitution in water for injection or sodium chloride 0.9% w/v to a concentration of 25 mg/mL (10 mL and 20 mL for the 250 mg and 500 mg vials respectively), Zovirax IV (Glaxo Wellcome) and Aciclovir Sodium (Lennon) are diluted further with infusion fluid to a final concentration not exceeding 5 mg/mL. The minimum volume must be greater than 50 mL and preferably 100 mL. Alternatively, these preparations can be given in a concentration of 25 mg/mL using a suitable controlled-rate infusion pump.
- For Aciclovir IV (Faulding DBL) the drug should be diluted to a concentration not more than 5 mg/mL with infusion fluid.

Rapid intravenous injection (bolus) of aciclovir (5 mg/kg) is associated with transient rises in plasma urea and creatinine levels, probably resulting from crystallization in the renal tubules, *the drug should be given by intravenous infusion over 1 hour*. It is also important that adequate hydration of the patient is maintained. In adults, intravenous aciclovir is given every 8 hours at a dose of 5 mg/kg usually for 5 days. In the case of herpes encephalitis, the dosage is 10 mg/kg, 8 hourly for 10 days. Caution should be exercised in giving aciclovir by the intravenous route to those with impaired renal function: Appendix 6.2, Table 6.5 gives a guide to dosage adjustment (Glaxo Wellcome).

APPENDIX 6.2

Table 6.5 Dosage of aciclovir to be given by intravenous infusion in patients with renal impairment (Glaxo Wellcome Data Sheet 1999)

Creatinine clearance	Dosage of aciclovir
25–50 mL/min	5 or 10 mg/kg body weight should be given every 12 hours.
10–25 mL/min	5 or 10 mg/kg body weight should be given every 24 hours.
Anuric to 10 mL/min	In patients on hemodialysis or receiving continuous ambulatory peritoneal dialysis 2.5 or 5 mg/kg weight should be given every 24 hours.

APPENDIX 6.3

SUPPORT ASSOCIATIONS

Support, advice, and information for patients with genital herpes are available from:
The Herpes Viruses Association, 41 North Road, London N7 9DP, UK.
Telephone number: 44 (0) 207 609 9061.
Website: www.herpes.org.uk

APPENDIX 6.4

Foscarnet (trisodum phosphonoformate) is a pyrophosphate analogue that attaches to the pyrophosphate binding sites of viral DNA and RNA polymerases. It is virustatic, and resistance to the drug can develop. In the treatment of aciclovir-resistant mucocutaneous lesions of HSV in those with normal renal function, it is administered as a slow (given over a period of one hour) intravenous infusion in a dosage of 40 mg/kg every 8 hours. The patient should be well-hydrated before the initiation of the infusion, a 0.5–1.0 L of normal saline should be given at each infusion (Astra Pharmaceuticals Ltd, Data Sheet, 2000). When renal function is impaired, dosage reduction is necessary: see Astra Pharmaceuticals Ltd, Data Sheet, 2000. Renal impairment is a comon adverse event, and it is recommended that serum creatinine should be monitored every second day, with adjustment of the dose of foscarnet as necessary. Electrolyte abnormalities also occur: hypocalcemia, hypo-magnesemia, hypokalemia, hypophosphatemia and hyperphosphatemia. Convulsions may also be an adverse event, and the hemoglobin concentration may fall. Genital ulceration reulting from the irritant effect of foscaret in the urine may occur. Foscarnet is contraindicated in pregnancy, and breast-feeding should be discontinued before initiation of therapy.

Chapter 7

Human immunodeficiency virus infection
G R Scott, A McMillan

Introduction

In 1981 cases of *Pneumocystis carinii* pneumonia were described in young gay men in the USA. The term 'acquired immunodeficiency syndrome' (AIDS) was coined and descriptions followed of other features of this syndrome such as Kaposi's sarcoma. A number of putative causes were proposed and rejected before the causative virus was identified in 1983. Montagnier's group in Paris named this virus lymphadenopathy associated virus (LAV)[1], whereas Gallo and his team identified a similar virus which they named human T-lymphotropic virus type 3 (HTLV-3)[2]. Levy's laboratory in San Francisco isolated retroviruses from AIDS patients and designated these as AIDS-associated retrovirus (ARV)[3]. In 1986, it was proposed that these variants should all be named human immunodeficiency virus (HIV)[4].

In the early stages of the epidemic, alterations in T-lymphocyte subsets, particularly depletion of CD4+ T cells, were recognized in association with the clinical features[5], and in 1984 the crucial role of the CD4 receptor in allowing viral entry was described[6, 7]. A test for antibodies to HIV became available in the UK in 1985. A related virus, HIV-2, was identified in 1985[8].

Zidovudine, also referred to as azido-thymidine, was the first antiretroviral drug to be introduced into clinical practice in 1987, and was followed by other reverse transcriptase inhibitors such as didanosine and zalcitabine. Prevention of opportunistic infections such as *P. carinii* also helped to reduce morbidity in HIV infection[9]. The failure of single agents (monotherapy) to confer lasting clinical benefit was demonstrated in a number of trials such as the Concorde study published in 1993[10]. Dual therapy showed more prolonged, but ultimately time-limited, benefit in trials such as Delta and ACTG 175[11, 12]. However it was not until Ho's seminal work on the dynamics of viral turnover in HIV infection, together with the availability of newer antiretroviral drugs in the form of protease inhibitors, that the optimal use of combination therapy became apparent[13, 14]. The availability of protease inhibitors allowed the use of triple antiretroviral therapy (ART). The possibility of achieving undetectable levels of proviral DNA (viral load) in the blood offered the chance of reversing the loss of immune function with the potential of long-term survival for patients with HIV/AIDS[15]. The recognition of significant morbidity from long-term use of ART[16], and the inability of current treatment modalities to eradicate HIV from the body[17] have tempered some of the optimism that followed these new developments. Studies involving therapies to boost immune control of HIV signaled a new phase in the battle for patients in the developed world.

After many years of uncertainty about the origins of HIV-1 and 2, 1999 saw clear evidence of crossover of these viruses from chimpanzees[18] and sooty mangabeys[19].

Politics have never been far removed from discussions involving HIV/AIDS and lack of access to ART, both for the treatment of infection and for reduction in materno–fetal transmission, became a crucial issue for the developing world.

In the year 2000, at least 30 million of the estimated 34 million HIV-infected people worldwide have no immediate prospect of access to ART[20].

HIV can infect children and cause disease. A consideration of pediatric issues, however, lies outwith the scope of this textbook and the interested reader is referred to one of several textbooks on this subject, such as Pizzo and Wilfert[21].

Biology of HIV

HIV belongs to the family of Retroviruses – so named because RNA is transcribed into DNA, using the enzyme reverse transcriptase, in contrast to the usual transfer of genetic information from DNA to RNA. The ability of retroviral DNA to integrate with the host cell DNA results in persisting infection. The oncogenic properties of retroviruses had been described as far back as 1911 by Rous, who demonstrated that a cell-free extract from chicken sarcoma could induce sarcoma in a recipient bird[22]. Further descriptions of animal retroviruses followed, before the first human retrovirus, human T-lymphotropic virus type 1 (HTLV-1), was isolated from a patient with lymphoma[23]. Many genera of human and animal retroviruses have now been described (www.ncbi.nlm.nih.gov/retroviruses).

HIV-1 and 2 belong to a subgroup of retroviruses called lentiviruses. These have also long been recognized in animals, and differ from other retroviruses in that chronic infection results in disease rather than malignancy. For example, visna maedi virus had been found to cause neurological and respiratory diseases in sheep in 1954[24]. A list of lentiviruses is shown in Box 7.1.

Crucially, lentiviruses can infect non-dividing cells in contrast to oncoretroviruses which can only integrate with cellular DNA as a result of mitosis.

Box 7.1 Lentiviruses

Bovine immunodeficiency virus

Jembrana disease virus

Feline immunodeficiency virus

Equine infectious anemia virus

Caprine arthritis-encephalitis virus

Ovine lentivirus

Visna maedi virus

Human immunodeficiency virus type 1

Human immunodeficiency virus type 2

Simian immunodeficiency virus

Lentiviruses can also infect cells of the macrophage/monocyte lineage, a crucial factor in evading immune destruction. All lentiviruses are neurotropic, probably as a result of trafficking of monocytes to the brain. The blood–brain barrier may offer additional sanctuary from the host immune response[25].

HIV-1

This virus was identified in several laboratories in 1983[1], and 1984[2, 3], and given a variety of names before universal adoption of the title 'human immunodeficiency virus' (HIV) in 1986[4].

With the exception of a few dissenters, it is accepted that this virus is the causative agent of AIDS. On the basis of genetic diversity three subgroups of HIV – M (main), O (outlier), and N (non-M non-O) – have been found to share common ancestry with strains of simian immunodeficiency virus (SIV) cpz that infect the chimpanzee *Pantroglodytes troglodytes* in Central and West Africa. It seems highly likely that HIV-1 crossed from chimpanzees to humans on at least three separate occasions in the 1920s or 1930s[18]. Group O strains are found in Cameroon and surrounding countries in West Central Africa, and group N was found initially in Cameroon. Group M has exploited the development of rapid international travel and is now found worldwide. Within group M there are further subdivisions into a number of subtypes (clades). Although eleven subtypes, (A–K) have been described, it is now recognized that many of these are in fact mosaics resulting from packaging of RNA from two or more co-infecting subtypes[26]. Such strains were named 'recombinants', although the term 'circulating recombinant forms (CRF)' is now favored[27]. Subtypes E and I have been reclassified as CRF.

Although subtype B is dominant in North and South America and Western Europe, subtype C is probably the most prevalent subtype worldwide.

There has been much debate as to whether or not subtypes differ in their properties, such as efficiency of transmission or replication kinetics[28–30]. Studies in Thailand suggest that CRF01_AE (previously referred to as subtype E) might be more easily transmitted heterosexually than subtype B[31]. Development work on assays for viral load estimation was initially carried out on HIV strains that were subtype B, and there has been concern that there may be poor quantitation of other subtypes[32, 33]. With respect to anti-retroviral therapy, there is evidence that Group O strains may be resistant to non-nucleoside reverse transcriptase inhibitors (NNRTI)[34].

Co-receptors for HIV entry

HIV usually gains entry to cells via the CD4 receptor. However, the presence on the cell membrane of one of a number of chemokine co-receptors is also required. Strains of HIV can be independently subdivided into distinct functional groups according to co-receptor affinity. Two main co-receptors for chemokines are recognized.

CXCR-4 (also sometimes referred to as *fusin*) is expressed by T lymphocytes and allows entry of syncitium-inducing strains[35]. CCR-5 is expressed by monocytes and is the receptor for chemokines such as Rantes, MIP-1α and MIP-1β. CCR-5 allows entry of non-syncitium inducing strains of HIV[36]. Additional chemokine receptors (CCR-2 and CCR-3) can also serve as co-receptors for HIV-1 under certain circumstances *in vitro*, but are not believed to function as co-receptors for primary isolates[37, 38].

Rantes, MIP-1α, and MIP-1β inhibit infection with monocytotropic strains. Ten per cent of caucasians carry an allele with a 32 base pair deletion in the CCR-5 gene; 1% of such a population will therefore be homozygous for the mutation (CCR-5Δ32) and, as a result, resistant to infection with monocytotropic strains. This may explain why some individuals remain HIV-negative despite repeated exposure to infection[39].

Individuals who are heterozygous for this deletion remain susceptible to HIV infection, but have a slower rate of progression[40, 41] and may have a better response to anti-retroviral therapy[42]. Other polymorphisms in CCR-5 are also associated with a reduced rate of progression[43]. Polymorphisms in stromal derived factor (SDF-1), the principal ligand for CXCR-4, may also influence disease progression in HIV-infected individuals[44].

Syncitium-inducing and non-syncitium-inducing phenotypes

During the course of HIV infection changes in the hypervariable V3 loop of the envelope glycoprotein gp120 result in a switch from virus that infects cells expressing CCR5 to infection of those expressing CXCR4, in particular T lymphocytes[45]. This viral phenotype is referred to as 'syncitium-inducing' (SI), and such viruses tend to grow more rapidly than non-syncitium inducing (NSI) viruses in tissue culture. Emergence of SI variants is associated with an accelerated decline in CD4+ T-cell count and more rapid progression of disease than for patients infected with NSI phenotypes[46, 47].

HIV-2

HIV-1 and HIV-2 are about 60% homologous within more conserved regions of the *gag* and *pol* genes, and only 30% to 40% within other viral genes including *env*[48]. Indeed, HIV-2 is more closely related to SIV than HIV-1. It seems highly likely that HIV-2 crossed from sooty mangabeys to humans living in West Africa, where this primate is found[19].

Six subtypes (A to F) of HIV-2 are described. Subtype A appears to be the most prevalent. It is uncertain if there are differences in pathogenicity or transmission dynamics between subtypes. As with HIV-1, HIV-2 strains can be divided into SI and NSI according to the preferred co-receptors CXCR-4 or CCR-5, although it appears that HIV-2 may also use other co-receptors[49].

STRUCTURE OF HIV-1 AND FUNCTION OF GENE PRODUCTS

Figures 7.1 and 7.2 are diagramatic representations of the viral genome, and the structure of a mature HIV virion for which the genome encodes. The viral genome contains three main open reading frames (ORFs) encoding for *gag*, *pol*, and *env* gene products.

Gag encodes the structural proteins, *pol* encodes for reverse transcriptase, as well as integrase, protease and RNase H, and *env* encodes the envelope proteins.

The gag precursor protein is cleaved by protease into CA, the capsid protein (p24), MA, the matrix protein (p17), NC, the nucleocapsid protein (p7), and protein p6 which has an attachment role for the accessory gene product vpr. The *env* gene product is a glycoprotein (gp160) that has two subunits, gp120 and gp41.

The viral genome of HIV-1 encodes for six supplementary genes – *vif, vpr, vpu, tat, rev*, and *nef. Tat* and *rev* gene products are regulatory proteins essential for viral replication. The remaining genes encode for proteins that appear to be less essential for viral expression and are therefore designated 'accessory' genes. None the less, the proteins encoded by these genes play important roles in viral pathogenesis[50, 51].

The vif protein (virion infectivity factor) enhances infectivity of virions released from non-permissive cells, possibly by regulating protease during virion assembly. As part of the pre-integration complex that enters the infected cell, vif protein is also likely to have an early role in the HIV life cycle, possibly related to nuclear import of viral DNA.[52]. Vpr protein facilitates nuclear import of the viral genome, and also inhibits cell proliferation by arresting the cell at the G2 phase of its cycle (see page 73), during which viral expression is maximal. In HIV-1, vpr plays an essential role in the infection of terminally differentiated macrophages[53]. Vpr requires p6 for incorporation into the virion. P6 also facilitates release of assembled particles from the cell surface.

Vpu and nef proteins downregulate surface expression of CD4. Vpu binds CD4 in endoplasmic reticulum, leading to proteolysis. Nef protein removes CD4 already on the cell surface. The reason for this may be to reduce the risk of env protein binding to CD4 following assembly/release of new virions. Vpu and nef proteins also reduce major histocompatibility complex class I (MHC-1) expression, thus helping to avoid cytotoxic T-lymphocyte (CTL) lysis of infected cells[54, 55]. Vpu may also increase viral release from infected cells[56].

Nef is unique to HIV and SIV. In addition to down regulating cell surface expression of CD4 and MHC-1, the nef protein also appears to increase T-cell activation, leading to an increase in Fas ligand (FasL) expression. The FasL expression by infected CD4+ T cells can trigger apoptosis of virus-specific CTL, which themselves express Fas. This situation thus mimics the expression of FasL at sites of immune privilege, or the up regulation of FasL by certain tumors. In this way the virus can evade the immune response by preventing the development of an effective CTL response. *Nef* also appears to have a role in increasing viral infectivity, although the mechanism is not clear. Many of its

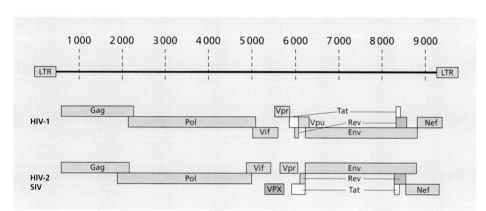

Figure 7.1 HIV-1 genome (reproduced from Mandell[428])

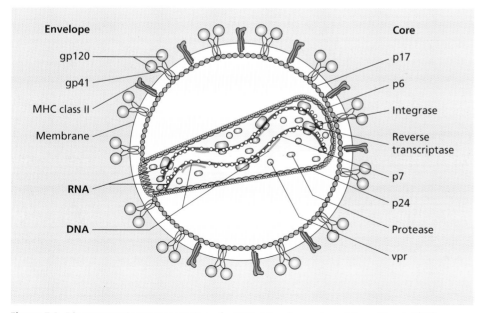

Figure 7.2 Diagrammatic representation of a HIV virion (reproduced from Mandell[428])

actions occur through interactions with proteins involved in cellular activation and signaling such as Src family tyrosine kinases[57]. Defects in the *nef* gene may be associated with long-term non-progression of HIV infection[58].

The tat protein is a potent activator of the viral long terminal repeat (LTR) promoter acting predominantly at the level of transcription elongation. The target sequence for tat is an RNA stemloop structure, termed TAR, located next to the LTR transcription start site. Tat acts in co-operation with a cellular kinase – human cyclin T1 (hCycT1) – a component of positive transcription elongation factor b (P-TEFb) that binds to TAR co-operatively with tat protein. Recruitment of hCycT1/P-TEFb to TAR enhances transcription elongation by allowing the CDK9 component of P-TEFb to phosphorylate the carboxyl-terminal domain (CTD) of initiated RNA polymerase II (Pol II) complexes, a modification required for efficient elongation by Pol II[59]. Other putative roles for tat are reviewed by Jeang *et al.*[60].

Rev facilitates export of retroviral RNA from the nucleus to the cytoplasm in conjunction with a cellular protein called exportin 1.

The core of a mature virion comprises two copies of viral genomic RNA and associated tRNA molecules, along with mature gag and pol protein products. The MA protein lies inside the lipid bilayer; the CA protein forms the structural core of the nucleoprotein complex; and the nucleocapsid NC protein binds viral genomic RNA. The mature pol proteins are the virus-associated enzymes protease, reverse transcriptase, and integrase. HIV-1 particles also contain the viral proteins Vpr (incorporated via its interaction with the p6 gag protein), nef and vif. The host cell protein cyclophilin A is also incorporated into HIV-1 particles by an interaction with the CA protein, and may play a role in attachment of HIV to the target cell[61]. The core is surrounded by a lipid envelope derived from the infected cell. Embedded in this lipid bilayer is the envelope glycoprotein (gp160) of HIV, which has two subunits: gp120 and gp41. Gp120 is on the exterior of the envelope and binds to the virion via the transmembrane subunit

gp41. In its native form, the envelope glycoprotein is a trimer of three gp120 subunits and three gp41 subunits.

STRUCTURE OF HIV-2 AND FUNCTION OF GENE PRODUCTS

In terms of viral structure there are two main differences between HIV-1 and HIV-2. The latter has no *vpu* gene, the lack of which may partially explain the reduced virulence of HIV-2. The vpr protein of HIV-2 is unable to fulfil all of the functions undertaken by HIV-1 vpr, and an alternative accessory protein, vpx, unique to the HIV-2/SIV lineage enables infection of macrophages[53].

Nef gene deletions seem to be more common in HIV-2 than in HIV-1, a factor that has been postulated to explain the reduced pathogenicity[62]. Differences in the LTR may reduce transcription in HIV-2[63].

VIRAL LIFE CYCLE

The viral life cycle is summarized in Figure 7.3. Gp120 binds to CD4 in conjunction with the CCR-5 co-receptor in monocytes, or the CXCR-4 co-receptor expressed by T lymphocytes. Structural

reconfiguration exposes the hydrophobic fusion domain on gp41, which inserts into the cell membrane and allows fusion of the lipid bilayers of both cell and viral membranes. A pre-integration complex consisting of reverse transcriptase (RT), integrase, nucleocapsid, matrix, vpr, tRNA(Lys) plus two copies of genomic viral RNA is then released into the cell. Reverse transcriptase synthesizes a complementary strand of DNA, the RNA template is then cleaved by RNase H, leaving a polypurine tract (PPT) that primes the synthesis of the second strand of DNA. The double-stranded DNA is imported into the cell nucleus where it integrates with cellular DNA. The matrix protein, vpr, and integrase participate in this process.

When the cell activates as part of its role in immune function, cellular proteins, nuclear factor kappa B (NF-KB) and nuclear factor of activated T cells (NFAT) enter the nucleus[64], but bind preferentially to the LTR of the integrated HIV DNA. HIV DNA is thus activated, and tat upregulates transcription to RNA via its interaction with a cellular kinase – human cyclin T1 (hCycT1) – a component of positive transcription elongation factor b (P-TEFb) that binds to TAR, an RNA stemloop structure

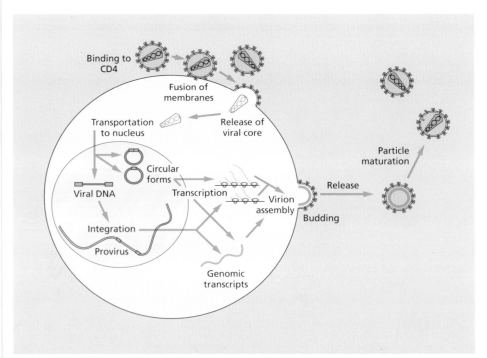

Figure 7.3 Diagrammatic representation of the life cycle of HIV (reproduced from Mandell[428])

located next to the LTR transcription start site.

Messenger RNA leaves the nucleus to begin the process of viral protein synthesis. Synthesized RNA may remain unspliced, or be spliced singly or multiply. Nuclear export of the larger unspliced or singly spliced RNA requires the rev protein, which binds to a region of the RNA called the Rev Response Element (RRE). Viral proteins are synthesized in the cytoplasm, apart from the env protein gp160 which is synthesized in the endoplasmic reticulum. The envelope lipid bilayer is derived from the infected cell. During viral assembly, the gag precursor protein is cleaved by protease, and the mature virion buds from the cell surface. Vif, nef, and vpu proteins contribute to the process of assembly and release.

PATHOGENESIS

Events during primary infection

Most sexually transmitted HIV strains are NSI, macrophage-tropic and use CCR5 chemokine co-receptor for cell entry. They are often referred to as R5 strains.

Mucosal surfaces such as the genital tract contain dendritic antigen-presenting cells (APC) – Langerhans cells. These cells express CCR-5. Also present on the cell surface is a type C lectin named DC-SIGN which binds HIV[65].

Following sexual exposure to HIV, mucosal Langerhans cells may either ingest virus, or bind to it via DC-SIGN[66]. Virus is then transported to regional lymphatic tissue where HIV antigens or the complete virion is presented to CD4+ T cells. These cells then activate to begin the generation of an immune response. However, activated CD4+ cells are more easily infected by HIV-1 because they express higher levels of the chemokine receptors that serve as co-receptors for the virus. High-level replication of virus thus ensues with infection of large numbers of CD4+ T cells. Although most of these cells die following productive HIV infection, some will become latently infected with HIV. This helps to protect the virus from the developing immune response, and also contributes to the long-liver reservoir of infection that militates against eradication of virus by highly active antiretroviral therapy (HAART). From the regional lymphoid tissue, infection spreads to the blood with high titers of viremia as a result. This is reflected in the high viral load that is usually seen in individuals identified during primary infection[67, 68].

Immune response to HIV infection

In any viral infection, cytotoxic T lymphocytes expressing CD8 on their surface (henceforth referred to as CD8+ CTL), recognize processed viral antigens (epitopes) when presented on the surface of the infected cell in conjunction with MHC-1 molecules. This recognition triggers the release of perforins and granzymes that mediate lysis of the infected cell. In chronic viral infections such as HIV, the role of immune-specific CD4+ T-helper (T$_h$) lymphocytes is crucial. Expression of endocytosed viral antigens on the surface of APCs in conjunction with class II MHC antigens stimulates CD4+ T$_h$ cells to release cytokines such as interleukin-2 (IL-2) that enhance the CD8+ CTL response. However, if these CD4+ cells are infected with HIV, the result of cellular activation will be to initiate new virion production rather than augmentation of the HIV-specific immune response. HIV-specific CD4+ T cells die, resulting in blunting of the CD8+ T-cell immune response during primary infection. This allows chronic productive infection to persist in the vast majority of cases. It was originally thought that all HIV-specific CD4+ T$_h$ cells were destroyed by HIV at this stage, but it is now recognized that some survive and maintain a degree of anti-HIV CTL activity[69]. The relative degree of preservation of this response determines the viral load 'set point', and the subsequent rate of loss of CD4+ T cells[69, 70].

In a few instances, strong HIV-specific CD4+ T$_h$ responses survive. Such individuals may be able to control HIV effectively during chronic infection allowing maintenance of a normal CD4+ T-lymphocyte count – a situation referred to as long-term non-progression[71]. Human leukocyte antigen (HLA) typing of HIV-infected individuals has shown an association between expression of the MHC class 1 allele HLA B*5701 and non-progression, indicating that genetic factors have a role in determining the outcome of the HIV–host interaction[72].

Chronic HIV infection

Initial thoughts that HIV infection was relatively quiescent in chronic infection, especially in asymptomatic patients, were dispelled by mathematical models devised in Ho's laboratory in the mid-1990s[14]. Calculations based on these models suggested a lifespan for productively infected cells of 2.2 days on average, and a lifespan for plasma virions estimated at a mean of 0.3 days. Approximately 10 billion (or 10^{10}) virions were predicted to be produced each day. A schematic summary of the dynamics of HIV infection was developed, and the role of long-lived, HIV-infected cell populations in preventing rapid elimination of infection by the use of HAART was acknowledged.

Newer methods have been introduced for measuring T-cell turnover such as determination of telomere lengths, Ki67 antigen expression, bromodeoxyuridine (BrdU) incorporation, and 2H-glucose labeling[73]. Studies using these methods suggest a lower rate of turnover of 7×10^7 cells/day.[74]

Theoretically, such high viral turnover would lead to the death of significant numbers of CD4+ T lymphocytes, and thus over time there would be a decline in the CD4+ T-lymphocyte count in the peripheral blood. There are a number of mechanisms by which this might be achieved

1. direct virus-induced cell lysis
2. induction of apoptosis (programed cell death) by virus following completion of replication
3. CTL-mediated immune killing of virally infected cells.

However, these theories are undermined by the observation that very few cells in the blood are infected with HIV[75]. The death of these HIV-infected cells alone would be insufficient to explain the decline in CD4+ T-cell count.

Many theories have been proposed to explain how HIV infection might lead to depletion of CD4+ T cells by killing un-infected cells. These include

1. membrane fusion between infected cells and uninfected 'bystander' cells – the 'kiss of death'
2. autoimmune killing of uninfected cells
3. HIV 'superantigen'-mediated deletion of certain T-cell sub-populations
4. induction of apoptosis in bystander cells by HIV proteins such as tat, or gp120 released from productively infected cells.

It appears that the critical events take place in lymphatic tissue rather than in blood. Only 2% of the total body pool of CD4+ T cells are in blood[76]. The number of CD4+ T cells in lymphoid tissues is not reduced; in fact it often increases in lymph nodes[77, 78]. In fact the increasing numbers of CD4+ T cells in lymph nodes in early disease might contribute to the common occurrence of lymphadenopathy in HIV-seropositive individuals. Only in late disease do CD4+ T cells disappear in lymph nodes. The inverted ratio of CD4+ T cells to CD8+ T cells seen in the blood in HIV infection does not occur in the lymph nodes until late in the disease.

Virus trapped in follicular dendritic cells acts as a persistent antigenic stimulus, driving activation, proliferation, and apoptosis of CD4+ T cells. These apoptotic cells have been shown to be bystander cells, not producing HIV RNA[79]. Thus, indirect killing of CD4+ T cells appears to be the major mechanism of CD4+ T-cell depletion. Initiation of HAART decreases HIV antigen expression by follicular dendritic cells, reducing the trapping and death of CD4+ lymphocytes, and resulting in redistribution of these cells into blood[74].

Progression to clinical disease

HIV-1

The rate of progression to overt immune deficiency reflects the interaction between the relative preservation of HIV-specific immune response, the genetically determined ease with which HIV infects target cells, the ability of the immune system to replenish CD4+ T-cell numbers, and the phenotype of virus (SI versus NSI). On average it takes 8 to 11 years from seroconversion to develop late-stage symptomatic disease, and a further 1 to 2 years to death in untreated individuals[80–83]. Increasing age is a major factor in a more

rapid progression to late-stage disease[84, 85]. Although there may be differences in plasma viral load between men and women, the rate of progression is similar[86].

HIV-2

HIV-2 is less virulent than HIV-1, with longer time to the development of late stage disease and a reduced mortality rate compared to HIV-1[87, 88]. As with HIV-1, plasma viral load of HIV-2 is predictive of CD4+ T-lymphocyte decline[89]. However, significant numbers of HIV-2-infected individuals have viral loads of less than 500 copies/mL, indicating a different equilibrium between the immune system and HIV-2 compared with HIV-1[90]. Strong CTL responses to HIV-2 give better immune control, and may contribute to slower progression to disease[48].

HIV-1–HIV-2 interactions

It has been postulated that prior infection with HIV-2 might protect against subsequent infection with HIV-1, in a fashion analogous to vaccination[91]. Although Travers et al.[92] found that HIV-2-infected Senegalese women appeared to be protected against HIV-1 infection, subsequent studies have not confirmed this finding[93–95]. Dual infection is well recognized, although diag-

nosis can be difficult to confirm because of cross-reacting antibodies[96, 97]. Infection with one type of HIV does not appear to increase the risk of disease progression by the other[98, 99].

Epidemiology

HIV-1

The reader is referred to the WHO/UNAIDS website which gives updated prevalence data by country (www.unaids.org). Figure 7.4 shows the global distribution of HIV infection at the end of the year 2000. The total number of people living with HIV is currently estimated to be 34.3 million, of whom 15.7 million are women and 1.3 million are children under 15 years of age. There have been approximately 19 million deaths since the beginning of the epidemic, 2.8 million of which occurred in 1999. Also during 1999, there were an estimated 5.4 million new infections, of which 2.3 million were in women and 620 000 were in children below the age of 15 years of age[20].

HIV-2

The highest prevalence of HIV-2 infection is found in Guinea Bissau, with lower rates

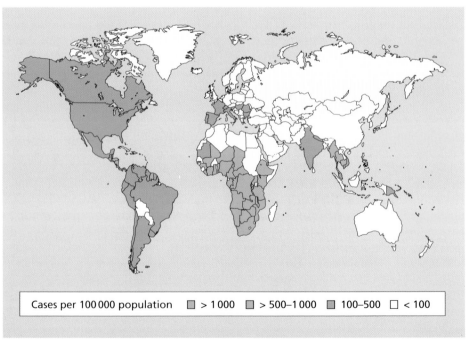

Figure 7.4 Estimated number of cases of HIV per 100 000 population (based on UNAIDS data 2001[429])

of infection in surrounding countries such as Senegal, Guinea, and the Gambia. The prevalence is stable or even declining in some countries, possibly as it is replaced by the more infectious HIV-1. In Europe, cases have been largely restricted to Portugal. Small numbers of cases have been reported in other European countries, as well as in North America and Asia.

PATTERNS OF TRANSMISSION OF HIV

In Africa, heterosexual and mother-to-child transmission of HIV infection has predominated. Many countries have experienced devastating epidemics, with 16 countries carrying a burden of infection of more than 10% of the entire adult population. Although some countries such as Uganda and Zambia have shown reductions in incidence, South Africa experienced an explosive rise in infection in the second half of the 1990s. In Asia, HIV is more sporadic, and only three countries have a prevalence among 15 to 49-year-olds of more than 1%. However, significant epidemics among intravenous drug users have occurred, and sex workers in parts of India and Thailand have high rates of infection.

In Central and South America, heterosexual sex is the main mode of transmission.

Many Caribbean islands have rates of infection which are only exceeded in Sub-Saharan Africa.

In most of North America and Europe, HIV infection has been largely concentrated among men who have sex with men, and intravenous drug users. In Southern European countries such as Italy, Spain, and Portugal, and in many countries of the former Soviet Union, HIV linked to injecting drug use has fuelled heterosexually transmitted infection. Given the high rates of STIs in many eastern European countries, further spread of HIV infection seems inevitable.

In the UK, men who have sex with men remain the largest risk group, both in terms of prevalence and new infections. Growing numbers of cases linked to Sub-Saharan Africa have been identified in the late 1990s. Prevention of mother-to-child transmission in this group has become a major challenge. Figure 7.5 shows the prevalence of infection in the UK. Current data are available from the PHLS website (www.phls.co.uk).

Individual risk groups and risks of specific practices for HIV-1

HIV-1 is not a highly infectious virus when compared to, for example, influenza viruses. Intact skin forms an effective barrier to infection, even if exposed to blood with high viral titers. Three main routes of transmission of HIV are recognized, these are sexual, blood-borne, and vertical (mother-to-child) transmission. Transmission can also occur by needle-stick injury.

Sexual transmission

The probability of transmission per act of sexual intercourse is low compared to other routes of exposure. This may reflect reduced infectivity of genital tract fluids, mucosal barriers to transmission, or reduced availability of the target cells for HIV infection[100]. Several factors influence transmission dynamics. These include genetic susceptibility to HIV infection, the viral load of the HIV-seropositive partner, local infection, cervical ectropion in women, circumcision status in men, the method of contraception used, and menstruation.

Genetic susceptibility

Ten per cent of Caucasians carry an allele with a 32 base pair deletion in the CCR-5 gene. About 1% of such a population will therefore be homozygous for the mutation (CCR-5Δ32) and, as a result, be resistant to infection with monocytotropic strains. This may explain why some individuals remain HIV-negative despite repeated exposure to infection[39].

Viral load and heterosexual transmission

Viral load appears to be the main determinant of heterosexual transmission of HIV[101]. In HIV-discordant couples in Uganda[102], a correlation was observed between the plasma HIV-1 RNA level and the probability of transmission. The probability of transmission per act from HIV-1-positive women to their HIV-1-negative male partners (0.0013) was similar to that of transmission per act from HIV-1-positive men to their HIV-1-negative female partners. With a viral load of less than 3500 copies/mL, the transmission probability was found to be 0.0001 (1 per 10 000 episodes of intercourse). When blood viral burden was greater than 50 000 copies/mL, the transmission probability was calculated to be 0.0051 (5.1 per 1000 episodes of intercourse). Earlier work from this group showed no transmissions

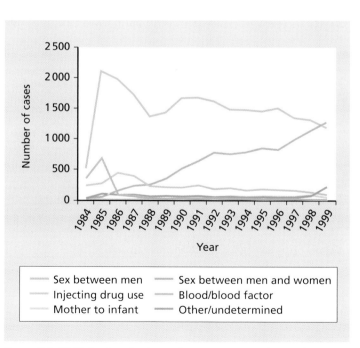

Figure 7.5 HIV infections in the UK between 1984 and 1999, by source of infection (data from PHLS, DHSS&PS and the Scottish ISD(D)5 Collaborative Group)

among fifty-one subjects with a serum viral load of less than 1500 copies/mL[103]. It is likely that the plasma viral load is a surrogate for HIV in genital tract fluids[104], although this is not an invariable finding[105]. Mathematical modeling suggests that when HIV RNA in semen is low (less than 5000 copies/mL) transmission is unlikely to occur, with a probability of 1 per 10 000 episodes of intercourse. Conversely, when the concentration of HIV in semen is high (more than 1 million copies/mL) the probability of transmission rises to 3 per 100 episodes of intercourse[106]. Such high concentrations of HIV RNA have been detected in semen specimens from HIV-positive men with a concomitant STI such as trichomoniasis or gonorrhea (see pp. 476 and 320–321). Late-stage infection and primary HIV infection[107] are both associated with an increased likelihood of HIV transmission. This is almost certainly a reflection of increased viral load at these times[104].

STIs and sexual transmission

Transmission dynamics can be altered dramatically by concomitant genital tract infection by other STIs. There are several potential mechanisms, for example increasing the concentration of HIV in genital secretions, increasing the number of cells receptive to HIV, or increasing the number of receptors per cell. The increased risk of transmission of HIV infection from individuals with gonorrhea, genital chlamydial infection, trichomoniasis, and genital ulcer disease such as HSV, chancroid, and syphilis is considered in Chapters 6, 10, 11, and 16. Intervention trials have also established the importance of STIs in HIV-1 transmission (Chapter 2).

Other factors

In women, other factors associated with increased HIV transmission through sexual contact include bacterial vaginosis (see Chapter 17)[108], cervical ectropion[109], anal sex[110], and sex during menstruation[111]. With regard to method of contraception used, there is evidence that use of depot medroxyprogesterone acetate or oral contraceptive pills increases the risk of both acquisition and transmission of HIV-1[112, 113].

In men, much debate has focused on the issue of circumcision. This issue is discussed in Chapter 20.

Sexual infectivity is not constant, and may vary considerably between and within couples[114]. Antiretroviral therapy is of benefit in reducing the risk of transmission[115], probably by reducing HIV in genital secretions[116]. Population modeling predicts significant reduction in HIV transmission through widespread access to ART[103]. The sexual transmission of HIV-1 with mutations associated with resistance to nucleoside reverse transcriptase inhibitors, to non-nucleoside reverse transcriptase inhibitors, to protease inhibitors, or to multiple antiretroviral drugs is now well recognized[117–119].

Male homosexual transmission

Some factors are clearly identical to those that apply to heterosexual transmission, for example seminal viral load and its relationship to concomitant STI, and ulcerative anogenital disease. Many cohort studies clearly identify receptive anal intercourse as the major risk factor for HIV seropositivity[120]. The risk of transmission from an HIV-positive man practising unprotected, insertive anal sex is estimated to be 0.8% to 3%[121]. The risk to an HIV-negative insertive man having anal sex with an HIV-positive partner is similar to that associated with heterosexual sex, although a study showing the presence of HIV DNA in the anorectal mucosa of men on combination therapy indicates that risk remains to the insertive partner[122]. Orogenital transmission was originally felt to carry a low risk of transmission, although anecdotal cases were occasionally reported[120]. A recent study, however, suggests that receptive oral sex can lead to HIV acquisition, the risk having been estimated at 0.0004 per contact[123].

Blood-borne transmission

Blood-blood transmission of HIV, either by needle-sharing intravenous drug use (IDU) or blood transfusion is much more efficient than sexual transmission. Explosive epidemics of HIV related to IDU have been observed in many parts of the world[124]. The importance of sexual acquisition of HIV-1 amongst injecting drug users, however, has been shown in a case-control study from San Francisco. Seroconversion amongst male IDUs was 8.8 times higher amongst men who had sex with men than amongst heterosexual men, and women who had engaged in prostitution within the preceding year were 5.1 times more likely as others to have seroconverted[125].

Mother-to-child transmission

HIV-1 infection acquired through mother-to-child transmission represents the second largest risk group worldwide. Transmission rates in untreated cases range from 15–45%. There are three components to mother-to-child transmission – intrauterine, intrapartum, and postpartum via breast-feeding. Intrauterine transmission is rare, and the relative contributions of intrapartum and postpartum transmission depend upon the frequency and duration of breast feeding[126, 127].

In populations where breast feeding is rare, the major determinant of mother-to-child transmission is maternal viral load at the time of delivery (Table 7.1). Transmission, however, has been observed across the entire range of HIV viral loads, and has

Table 7.1 Mother-to-child transmission of HIV-1: relationship between viral load at time of delivery and risk of neonatal infection (Blattner *et al.* 2000[426])

Plasma viral load at delivery (copies/mL)	Transmission rate
< 400	0.9%
400–2999	6.4%
3000–39 000	11.3%
40 000–100 000	21%
> 100 000	31.2%

been described rarely, even when there has been undetectable HIV RNA in the mother's plasma[128–130]. As there does not appear to be a threshold at which HIV transmission to a child does not occur, other uncertain factors also play a part in mother-to-child transmission[131].

There is also a correlation between the duration of rupture of membranes and the risk of transmission of HIV. Among mothers with membranes that had been ruptured for more than 4 hours before delivery, the rate of transmission to the neonate was 25%, compared with 14% amongst those women whose membranes had been ruptured for a shorter time[132]. It has been estimated that the risk of viral transmission increases by approximately 2% per additional hour of membrane rupture[133].

Several studies have shown that HIV can be transmitted to an infant through breast milk. For example, data from the European Collaborative Study[134] showed that the odds ratio of HIV transmission was 2.25 (95% confidence interval 0.97–5.23) in breast-fed infants compared with those who were not breast fed. This finding was substantiated by a systematic review of four studies in which mothers acquired HIV-1 postnatally, the estimated risk of transmission by breast feeding being 29%[135]. In a review of five studies in which the mother was infected prenatally, it was shown that breast feeding increased the risk of transmission to the child by 14%[135].

Although infants can be infected at any time during breast feeding, most breast-milk transmission occurs early[136]. There is a clear difference in the transmission rate between infants who are breast fed and those who receive formula food. In the series reported by Nduati et al.[136], the cumulative probability of HIV infection at 24 months of age was 36.7% (95% confidence interval 29.4–44.0%) in those infants who were breast fed, compared with 20.5% (95% confidence interval 14.0–27.0%) in those who were given formula food. The use of breast milk substitutes therefore prevented 44% of infant infections. Coutsoudis et al.[137] examined infant feeding practices in relation to infection during the first 3 months of life. Using Kaplan–Meier life tables, they estimated that the proportion of children who became infected from an HIV-infected mother was significantly lower amongst those who were exclusively breast fed (14.6%) than amongst those who received mixed feeds before 3 months (24.1%), or amongst those who were never breast fed (18.8%).

Infection can also occur in the late postnatal period. In a prospective cohort study from Rwanda[138], it was shown that HIV can be transmitted by breast feeding when mothers seroconvert at any time during lactation: at least 3 of 16 infants born to mothers who seroconverted after delivery became HIV-infected. The significance of breast feeding in late postnatal transmission of HIV was shown in an analysis by Leroy et al.[139]. They noted that none of 2807 children, born to HIV-infected mothers in industrialized countries, became infected; less than 5% of the children had been breast fed. In Africa, however, late postnatal transmission occurred in 5% of 902 children, almost all of whom had been breast fed.

HIV is present in breast milk, and the HIV RNA level does not appear to vary significantly during the postnatal period. The viral load in breast milk is directly related to the mother's plasma viral load, and it has been shown that the median HIV viral load in breast milk was significantly higher in women with mastitis than in those with normal breasts; an increased risk of HIV transmission is also associated with mastitis[140].

The rate of transmission may be reduced by a number of interventions including cesarean section, antiretroviral therapy, and avoidance of breast feeding. These are discussed on pp. 195–198.

Needle-stick injury

The risk to a health care worker (HCW) of acquiring HIV via a needle-stick injury or other percutaneous exposure is approximately 0.3%. This is much less than the risk of acquiring hepatitis B (approximately 30% from a HBeAg-positive source) or hepatitis C (approximately 3%)[141]. However this global figure conceals a wide spectrum of risk dependent upon a number of factors such as the viral load of the source, the nature of the penetrating object, for example hollow-bore or solid needle, depth of injury, and whether or not gloves were worn. Worldwide, re-use of injection equipment for medical procedures such as vaccination has also been associated with transmission of HIV[142].

HIV-2 transmission

The prevalence of HIV-2 infection is stable or may even be declining, implying lower transmissibility of HIV-2 compared to HIV-1. Modes of transmission are as for HIV-1, although the evidence is less conclusive. Shedding of HIV-2 in the genital tract appears to be less than in HIV-1-infected individuals[143].

Mother-to-child transmission occurs at a lower rate for HIV-2 (4% to 5%) than for HIV-1[144], almost certainly as a reflection of maternal viral load[145].

Clinical features of HIV-1 infection

CLINICAL FEATURES OF ACUTE SEROCONVERSION ILLNESS

(synonym: *primary HIV infection*)
Acute seroconversion illness was first described in 1985[146]. Although the proportion of patients who experience acute seroconversion illness (ASI) is uncertain, it is often stated that between 30% and 75% experience such an illness, reflecting the uncertainty. Undoubtedly, however, seroconversion can occur in the absence of symptoms. Minor symptoms compatible with a 'viral illness' are also possible.

The cardinal features of the complete seroconversion illness are sore throat, cervical lymphadenopathy, and maculopapular rash (Figure 7.6). Less frequently there may be arthralgia, myalgia, diarrhea, headache, nausea and vomiting, and aphthous ulceration. Acute neurological syndromes including encephalitis, meningitis, brachial neuritis, myelopathy, and Guillain–Barré syndrome have been described rarely[147]. Temporary immunosuppression may result in opportunistic

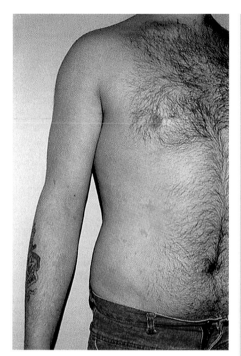

Figure 7.6 Maculopapular rash of primary HIV infection (reproduced from McMillan and Scott 2000[430])

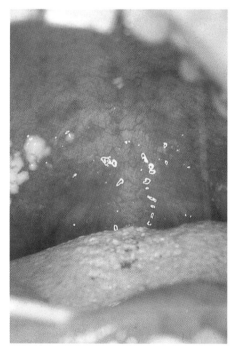

Figure 7.7 Pseudomembranous candidiasis of the mouth occurring in primary HIV infection (reproduced from McMillan and Scott 2000[430])

infections of which oral (Figure 7.7) or esophageal candidiasis is the most common described[148].

Laboratory features may show either lymphopenia, or lymphocytosis with atypical cells similar to infectious mononucleosis[149]. Thrombocytopenia is seen in up to 50% of patients with ASI. Elevation of hepatic enzymes occurs in 20% of cases[150].

Recognition of ASI is important, as current practice is to consider immediate ART with the hope that HIV-specific immune responses may be preserved. There is also evidence that patients with severe ASI have a more rapid progression to symptomatic disease[151, 152].

CLINICAL FEATURES OF CHRONIC HIV INFECTION AND AN OUTLINE OF THE MANAGEMENT OF OPPORTUNISTIC INFECTIONS

Following resolution of any seroconversion illness, patients enter a variable period of asymptomatic infection that can last between 1 and many years, but is on average between 5 and 8 years. The duration of this asymptomatic phase appears to be determined by the individual's immune response. With the passage of time, the CD4+ T-cell count in the peripheral blood declines at a rate that varies from individual to individual, but that is related to the plasma viral load. Patients with a high viral load tend to have CD4+ T-cell counts that decline more quickly than if the viral load is low. As the CD4+ T-cell count falls towards 200/mm³, there is an increasing risk of the development of minor symptoms relating to immunosuppression. These may be non-specific symptoms of a chronic viremic illness such as fatigue and fever or night sweats; or symptoms related to opportunistic viral or fungal infections. In addition there are a number of non-infectious manifestations of symptomatic HIV disease. In some cases referred to above as long-term non-progressors, individuals can remain asymptomatic for at least 20 years.

It is convenient to describe the more salient clinical features by system, although it is common, particularly in late-stage infection, for two or more systems to be affected.

Skin

Seborrheic dermatitis

Seborrheic dermatitis[153] is often the first dermatological manifestation of symptomatic HIV (Figure 7.8). It begins insidiously in the nasolabial folds and around the eyebrows. It usually responds well to topical imidazole-hydrocortisone creams. Later, the dermatitis and scaling may spread to the back, chest, and abdomen, and in such cases oral antifungals such as itraconazole and more potent topical corticosteroids may then be required.

Tinea pedis

This is caused by *Trichophyton rubrum* or *Epidermophyton floccosum*, with or without toe nail involvement, and can be severe (Figure 7.9). In extensive disease oral antifungal agents such as itraconazole are usually more effective than topical agents.

Extensive warts

Any individual may develop extensive warts, but facial warts should raise concerns about the possibility of HIV infection.

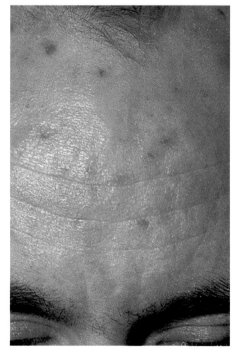

Figure 7.8 Seborrheic dermatitis of the forehead (reproduced from McMillan and Scott 2000[430])

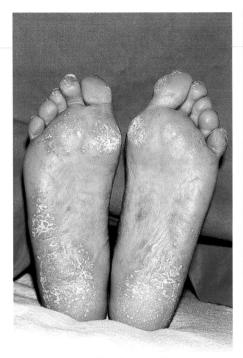

Figure 7.9 Extensive tinea pedis

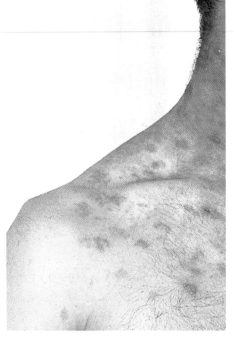

Figure 7.10 Herpes zoster (reproduced from McMillan and Scott 2000[430])

Molluscum contagiosum

These papular, umbilicated lesions may be found around the genital and lower abdominal regions in immunocompetent adults (Chapter 9). However the finding of lesions on the face or upper chest is very suggestive of immunosuppression. In late-stage HIV disease, giant forms may become extensive and secondary bacterial infection may supervene.

Frequently recurring genital herpes

This can be seen in any patient. However, the recurrence rate tends to decline over time in the immunocompetent patient. Increasing frequency, and especially episodes lasting for more than 1 month, should raise the possibility of HIV-related immunosuppression. Extensive orolabial and anogenital ulceration may occur, particularly in those who are severely immunocompromised (Chapter 6).

Herpes zoster

Herpes zoster, if multidermatomal, is again virtually pathognomonic of HIV infection. However, single dermatome disease is frequently seen (Figure 7.10) as part of the natural history of the developing immunodeficiency. Treatment with aciclovir or famciclovir for 10 days rather than the usual 5-day course is often required.

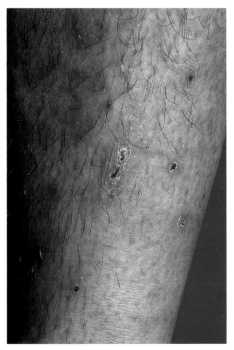

Figure 7.11 Eosinophilic folliculitis of the leg

Psoriasis

Although there is no specific association between HIV and psoriasis, the development of HIV-induced immune dysfunction may lead to the exacerbation of pre-existing psoriasis, or the unmasking of a hitherto unexpressed psoriatic predisposition. Lesions usually respond dramatically to the successful introduction of HAART and resultant suppression of viral load.

Eosinophilic folliculitis

Many patients have crops of intensely itchy, red papules, resembling insect bites, scattered over the body and face (Figure 7.11). Histology may reveal considerable numbers of eosinophils in an inflammatory infiltrate involving follicles, hence the name[154]. A number of treatments including antihistamines, antifungals, antibiotics, and topical corticosteroids can be tried, but often with disappointing results.

Xeroderma and telogen effluvium

Dry skin (xeroderma), and diffuse hair loss (telogen effluvium) have also been described in association with HIV infection.

Kaposi's sarcoma

Kaposi's sarcoma (KS) is caused by the human herpes virus type 8 (HHV-8) (see Chapter 9), and was first described as an indolent tumor amongst elderly Europeans by Kaposi in 1872. In the 1950s, a slightly more aggressive variant of the condition was recognized in African populations, and in the 1970s, KS was described in immunosuppressed patients, for example, following organ transplantation. The emergence of Kaposi's sarcoma as a feature of HIV infection in homosexual men was reported by Friedman-Kien and colleagues in 1981[155]. Four forms of KS are therefore recognized

1. classic 'Mediterranean'
2. endemic 'African'
3. immunosuppression-associated, or post-transplant
4. epidemic, or HIV-associated[156].

All are caused by HHV-8 and all share common histological features, although the clinical course is variable.

In HIV-associated KS, any anatomical site may be affected, but particularly the

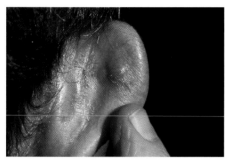

Figure 7.12 Kaposi's sarcoma of the ear

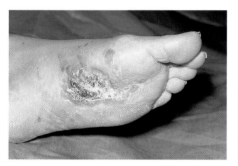

Figure 7.13 Kaposi's sarcoma of the sole of the foot

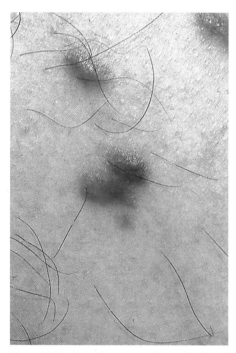

Figure 7.14 Kaposi's sarcoma (nodular form) (reproduced from McMillan and Scott 2000[430])

head and neck; the tumor, however, is rarely confined to one region. Common cutaneous sites that are affected include the tip of the nose, behind the ear (Figure 7.12), the soles of the feet

(Figure 7.13), and the penis. The nodular form of KS tends to predominate: the lesions vary in size from a few millimeters to several centimeters in diameter; they are brownish-red to blue in color (Figure 7.14), and, when palpated, they are firm. They are, however, usually painless and non-tender. Sometimes they are symmetrical and follow the cutaneous lymphatic drainage (Figure 7.15). Lymph node involvement is not uncommon. The diagnosis may be obvious, but in some cases, biopsy is required. In the dermis of early lesions ('patch lesions'), there are dilated and irregular vessels lined with abnormal endothelium. The later, plaque stage, is

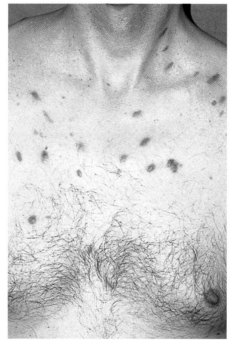

Figure 7.15 Kaposi's sarcoma of the chest wall (reproduced from McMillan and Scott 2000[430])

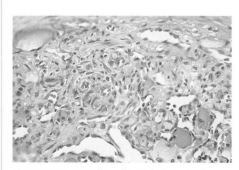

Figure 7.16 Spindle cells and abnormal endothelium in a section of a Kaposi's sarcoma nodule ($\times$ 25, hematoxylin and eosin)

associated with a proliferation of spindle cells together with abnormal endothelium (Figure 7.16)[157].

The management of Kaposi's sarcoma lies outwith the scope of this textbook but is reviewed by Antman and Chang[156].

Bacillary angiomatosis

Bacillary angiomatosis usually occurs in HIV-infected individuals who are severely immuncompromised. Many organs can be involved, including bone, skin, and brain. Cutaneous lesions develop over a short period of time as multiple, erythematous or purple, round papules, that become nodular, and sometimes pedunculated[158]. These nodules are often surrounded by a collarette of scales. Biopsies show a vascular tumor composed of cuboidal epitheloid cells with abundant, pale-staining cytoplasm[158], and after silver staining, bacilli are found in tissue sections. The condition is caused by either *Bartonella henselae* or *B. quintana*[159] that can be detected in biopsies by culture or by polymerase chain reaction (PCR). Treatment is with a prolonged course of erythromycin[160].

Oral cavity

Oral hairy leukoplakia

Oral hairy leukoplakia (Figure 7.17) is virtually pathognomonic of HIV infection, although it is occasionally seen in other settings of immunodeficiency, for example following bone marrow transplant. The lesion is caused by the Epstein–Barr virus (EBV), and reflects a loss of immune control of this virus as part of the developing immunodeficiency[161]. Oral hairy leukoplakia presents as a white patch, usually on the lateral border of the tongue, but sometimes on the buccal mucosa. It is usually symp-

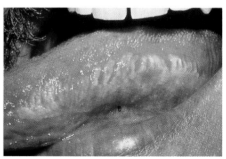

Figure 7.17 Oral hairy leukoplakia

tomless, unless there is candidal super-infection. A definitive diagnosis, which is seldom required in clinical practice, can be made by biopsy with the detection of EBV DNA by *in situ* hybridization.

Oral candidiasis

Oral candidiasis is the most common opportunistic infection seen in patients with HIV. Most cases are caused by *Candida albicans*, although other *Candida* species are implicated rarely. Four types of appearance are recognized

1. pseudomembranous, characterized by white plaques adherent to the oral mucosa (Figure 7.18)
2. angular cheilitis (Figure 7.19)
3. chronic hyperplastic candidosis, characterized by a red and white speckled appearance of the palate
4. erythematous, which often has super-imposed pseudomembranous plaques.

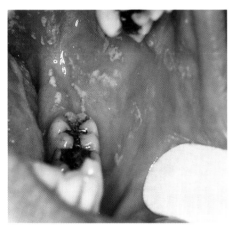

Figure 7.18 Pseudomembranous candidiasis of the buccal mucosa

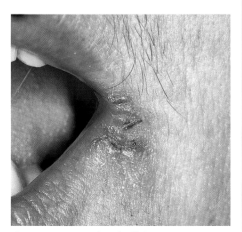

Figure 7.19 Angular cheilitis

Symptoms include pain, especially when consuming hot, spicy food or effervescent drinks, and altered taste. Laryngeal plaques may cause coughing and retching. Topical therapy with amphotericin, nystatin, or miconazole rarely gives symptomatic relief, but oral therapy such as flucaonazole or itraconazole is usually effective. In patients with CD4+ T-cell counts of less than 50/mm³ treatment should not be extended beyond this as resistance to oral antifungals can develop (Chapter 17).

Periodontal disease

Necrotizing ulcerative gingivitis, periodontitis with gingival recession (Figure 7.20), and stomatitis are all associated with HIV infection. Necrotizing ulcerative gingivitis is caused by infection with *Treponema vincentii*, *Fusobacterium nucleatum*, *Prevotella intermedia*, and sometimes *Candida* spp. Spread to the periodontal ligament and adjacent bone signals the deeper infection of periodontitis. Infection may then spread to soft tissue surrounding the gums (stomatitis). Specialist referral is required for debridement of diseased tissue and the use of metronidazole.

Aphthous ulceration of the oral cavity

Aphthous ulceration of the oral cavity or tonsils is not uncommon (Figure 7.21). These lesions tend to be painful. The use of thalidomide, given by mouth in a dosage of 200 mg once daily, has proved helpful in the management of persistent aphthous

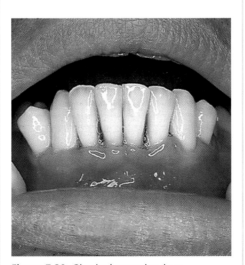

Figure 7.20 Gingival recession in a HIV-infected man (reproduced from McMillan and Scott 2000[430])

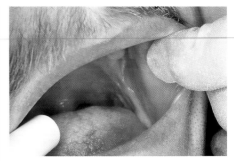

Figure 7.21 Aphthous ulceration of the pharynx

ulceration[162]. Herpes simplex virus infection should always be excluded as a cause of oral ulceration, and, as tonsillar lymphoma can occur, biopsy should be undertaken if lesions persist.

Kaposi's sarcoma

Oral Kaposi's sarcoma (Figure 7.22) has been found to be a poor prognostic indicator in the pre-HAART era, although it is not clear if the situation is still the same.

Salivary gland disease[161]

Diffuse enlargement, cysts, and lymphoid infiltration have all been described. Although the latter has similarities with Sjögren's syndrome, the infiltrating cells in HIV infection are CD8+ lymphocytes as opposed to the CD4+ cells seen in Sjögren's syndrome. Magnetic resonance imaging and biopsy may be required to exclude lymphoma.

Respiratory system

Recurrent upper respiratory tract infections

Recurrent upper respiratory tract infections, for example sinusitis or otitis, may

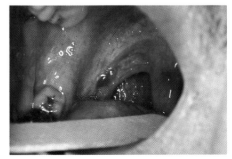

Figure 7.22 Kaposi's sarcoma of the buccal mucosa

sometimes be presenting features. CT scans of the head often show thickening of the mucosa lining the sinuses, with or without clinical disease. Nasal congestion and/or rhinorrhea may be troublesome, with limited response to topical steroid sprays such as fluticasone.

Pneumocystis carinii

Pneumocystis carinii is a ubiquitous organism that was originally thought to be a protozoan but is now regarded as more homologous with a fungal lineage. It is unclear whether latent infection reactivates as immune function deteriorates, or if there is exogenous infection from environmental exposure. The infection is rarely seen if the CD4+ T-cell count in the peripheral blood is greater than $200/mm^3$[163]. A high index of suspicion may be required in patients presenting with chest symptoms *de novo*. Pattern recognition is again important – minor opportunistic infections, such as one or probably more of the skin infections listed above, and mouth lesions such as oral hairy leukoplakia and/or oral candidiasis predate major opportunistic infection. Constitutional symptoms of HIV such as fever, night sweats, and weight loss will usually have been present for several weeks or months.

The characteristic symptoms of *P. carinii* pneumonia (PCP) are shortness of breath and a non-productive cough. As with many HIV-related syndromes the time-scale is gradual. Patients will often describe 4 to

6 weeks of shortness of breath, gradually increasing in severity, along with a dry non-productive cough. Examination of the chest may be unremarkable, or there may be bilateral crackles. In early cases, the chest radiograph may be normal, but later bilateral perihilar shadowing (Figure 7.23) may become more extensive. Nodules and cavitation may occur rarely. The diagnosis is made by finding *P. carinii* in broncho-alveolar lavage specimens, or in sputum induced by the inhalation of hypertonic saline. The organisms may also be detected in transbronchial lung biopsy samples (Figure 7.24), although this procedure is not the investigation of first choice.

The severity of PCP is determined by the Po_2. Mild PCP is defined as a Po_2 above 11 mmol/L, moderate PCP as a Po_2 of between 8 and 11 mmol/L, and severe PCP as a Po_2 of less than 8 mmol/L.

Patients with severe disease should be hospitalized; they usually require supplemental oxygen. High-dose cotrimoxazole is the drug of choice in the treatment of PCP. In those with mild to moderate disease it is given orally, but in severe cases it is best given by intravenous infusion, in each case for 14 to 21 days. The survival rate with

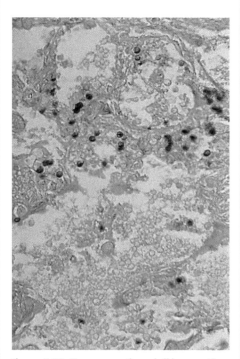

Figure 7.24 *Pneumocystis carinii* in a section of lung (× 60, silver methenamine stain) (reproduced from McMillan and Scott 2000[430])

such therapy is up to 90%. The development of a skin rash that may be severe, anaemia, leukopenia, or hepatitis may necessitate dose reduction or change of therapy. Pentamidine isetionate, given by the intravenous route is used in patients who cannot tolerate cotrimoxazole. It is also used in cases refractory to cotrimaxozole, but the survival rate is only in the order of 50%. Nephrotoxicity, hepatotoxicity and neutropenia are the most common adverse events with pentamidine, and hypoglycemia may develop. Although pentamidine isetionate when given by nebuliser has fewer side effects, the clinical response is slower, and it should only be used in mild cases. In the treatment of mild to moderate PCP, trimethorprim with dapsone, clindamycin with primaquine, and have all been used with similar success rates. Atovaquone given by mouth has also been shown to be effective in about 65% when used in patients with mild to moderate PCP. Trimetrexate is a potent inhibitor of the organism's dihydrofolate reductase, and has been used in the treatment of patients who have proved refractory to other drug regimens. In moderate and severe cases the patient should also be given corticosteroids, such as prednisolone by mouth or by intravenous infusion at the same time as initiation of specific therapy, as it has been shown that such adjunctive therapy reduces the risk of respiratory failure and of mortality. After successful treatment of PCP, prophylaxis with either cotrimoxazole, nebulised pentamidine isetionate, dapsone or atovaquone should be given until HAART has resulted in an increase in the CD4+ T-cell count in the peripheral blood to greater than 200 cells per mm^3 for at least three months. In the primary prevention of PCP, these drugs are given to individuals whose CD4+ count is < 200 per m^3. For details of the treatment of *P. carinii* pneumonia, the reader is referred to a textbook of HIV medicine/AIDS. Care should be taken to identify other infections, either secondary bacterial chest infections or other common opportunistic infections such as oral candida, with treatment prescribed as appropriate.

There is no consensus as to whether antiretroviral therapy should be instituted before or after the completion of PCP treatment. A natural desire to control HIV

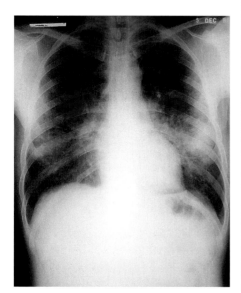

Figure 7.23 Perihilar shadowing in *Pneumocystis carinii* pneumonia

replication and thus bolster immune function is offset by concern about additive toxicity, especially dermatological and hematological.

Tuberculosis

Patients with HIV infection are at increased risk of tuberculosis, both primary and reactivation of pre-existing infection. One-third of the world's population was estimated to be infected with *Mycobacterium tuberculosis* in 1997. As there is considerable overlap in the geographical regions where HIV and tuberculosis are highly prevalent, interaction between the two infections is common. Most tuberculous infections are latent, and in the absence of HIV there would be a life-time risk of developing active disease of approximately 10%. However, studies in patients co-infected with HIV show a risk of re-activation of 5% to 10% per year of observation. The risk is related to the degree of immunosuppression. In a study from Italy, the annual incidence was 2.59 per 100 person years with a CD4+ T-cell count in the peripheral blood of more than 350/mm^3, 6.54 for CD4+ T-cell counts of 200–350/mm^3, and 13.3 if the CD4+ T-cell count was less than 200/mm$^{3[164]}$.

The clinical presentation of tuberculosis in HIV-infected patients depends upon the degree of immunosuppression[165]. If the peripheral blood CD4+ T-cell count is above 300/mm^3, the presentation is usually identical to that of an HIV-negative individual, with symptoms of productive cough, hemoptysis, fever, and weight loss. A chest X-ray shows infiltrates and cavities that tend to localize to the upper lobes. If the CD4+ T-cell count is less than 200/mm^3, there is a greater frequency of extrapulmonary involvement and diffuse pulmonary disease without cavitation. In late-stage HIV disease with a CD4+ T-cell count of less than 50/mm^3, there may be miliary disease and involvement of the lymphatic system, central nervous system (CNS) (parenchymal and meningeal), soft tissue, bone marrow, liver, and other viscera. Fever is common but cough may not be present. On the chest radiograph, any lobe of the lungs may be involved and the clinical presentation may be indistinguishable from community-acquired pneumonia. The diagnosis of

tuberculosis in patients with symptomatic HIV disease may be difficult. Only about 30% of these patients react to the tuberculin skin test[166]. Chest radiographs may not show classic upper-lobe infiltrates. Diffuse, interstitial, or lower-lobe infiltrates, often with prominent hilar and paratracheal enlargement, are common. In patients who are not severely immunocompromised, Ziehl-Neelsen-stained smears show acid-fast bacilli (AFB) in about 50% of cases, a similar proportion to that in HIV-non-infected patients with pulmonary disease. When there is more severe immuno-deficiency, fewer positive smear results are obtained[167]. At least 90% of cases of pulmonary tuberculosis will be identified by examination of three expectorated or induced sputum specimens obtained on separate days for smear microscopy and culture. The sensitivity of culture of specimens from other infected sites such as lymph nodes is between 80% and 90%. Nucleic acid amplification methods such as PCR and ligase chain reaction have high sensitivity (more than 75%), specificity (up to 100%), and positive predictive value (up to 100%) when applied to respiratory specimens; these parameters are lower in non-respiratory specimens[168].

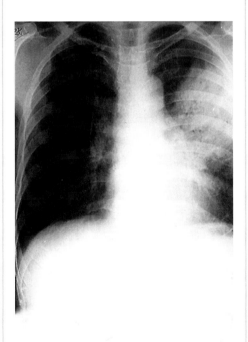

Figure 7.25 Pneumococcal pneumonia in a HIV-infected patient (reproduced from McMillan and Scott 2000[430])

The treatment of tuberculosis should only be undertaken in conjunction with advice from a respiratory physician experienced in the management of the condition. Multi-drug resistant (MDR) tuberculosis is common in many parts of the developing world. Any patient suspected of having MDR disease should be admitted immediately into a negative-pressure room without waiting for microbiological confirmation.

Because of interactions between anti-retroviral and anti-tuberculous drugs, specialist advice should be sought if both are to be prescribed together.

Bacterial pneumonia

Bacterial pneumonia (Figure 7.25) is common in HIV regardless of the CD4+ T-cell count in the peripheral blood. The risk, however, is highest in those with a CD4+ T-cell count of less than 200/mm$^{3[169]}$.

Pleural effusion

Causes of pleural effusion in the HIV-infected individual include bacterial infection, for example *Streptococcus pneumoniae*, tuberculosis, Kaposi's sarcoma, and lymphoma. Pleural aspiration should be undertaken. Bloody fluid may represent either malignancy or tuberculosis. Pleural biopsy should be performed.

Gastrointestinal tract

Esophageal disease

Esophageal candidiasis is the most common cause of upper gastrointestinal symptoms in HIV infection. Patients present with progressive dysphagia and/or retrosternal chest discomfort. Pseudomembranous candidiasis is often, but not invariably, found in the mouth of patients with esophageal candidiasis. The diagnosis may be suggested by the finding of filling defects in a barium swallow X-ray examination (Figure 7.26), but endoscopy is the definitive diagnostic investigation. Cytomegalovirus (CMV) infection can cause diffuse esophagitis or ulceration, the symptoms being similar to those of candidiasis. Biopsy is essential for diagnosis (Chapter 9). Kaposi's sarcoma can also affect the esophagus and cause dysphagia and chest discomfort; in many cases oral lesions are also noted.

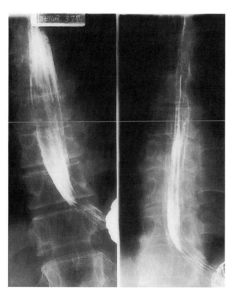

Figure 7.26 Barium swallow in a patient with esophageal candidiasis, showing filling defects in the lumen

Diarrhea

A wide range of organisms has been reported as causing diarrhea in HIV infection, including *Cryptosporidium parvum*, microsporidia, CMV, *Mycobacterium avium intracellulare*, *Giardia duodenalis*, *Entamoeba histolytica*, *Campylobacter* spp., *Salmonella* spp., *Shigella* spp., *Clostridium difficile*, *Enterocytozoon bieneusi*, *Isospora belli*, enteric viruses such as adenovirus, rotavirus, coronavirus, or small round structured viruses[170]. *Cryptosporidium* spp. and microsporidia are particularly common, causing illness in those with severe immunodeficiency. The side effects of drugs, especially protease inhibitors, and bacterial overgrowth in the small bowel, may also cause diarrhea. In up to 25% of patients with diarrhea, no pathogens can be identified despite intensive investigation, and the term 'HIV enteropathy' has been applied to this group of individuals. The pathogenesis of this condition is unknown, although lymphatic obstruction, villous atrophy with or without crypt hyperplasia, HIV infection of mononuclear cells in the lamina propria with the release of cytokines, and impaired epithelial barrier function may play a role[170, 171].

In the investigation of the HIV-infected patient with diarrhea, three to six consecutive stool samples should be examined by direct microscopy as a saline mount

preparation or after staining for protozoa; enzyme immunoassay may also be useful for the diagnosis of *G. duodenalis* (Chapter 18). A specimen should also be stained by the Ziehl-Neelsen method for *Mycobacterium* spp. Culture of the feces for bacterial pathogens should be undertaken routinely, and in the case of individuals whose CD4+ cell count is less than 100/mm³, blood and/or bone marrow should be cultured for *Mycobacterium* spp. If these tests yield negative results, flexible sigmoidoscopy with rectal biopsy should be performed. Microscopic examination of rectal specimens may reveal CMV disease, adenovirus, or *Cryptosporidium* spp. Upper gastrointestinal endoscopy with jejunal biopsy should follow if these investigations have failed to identify a pathogen. This procedure may assist in the diagnosis of previously unsuspected microsporidia, *G. duodenalis*, *M. avium intracellulare*, or *I. belli*.

Most individuals in whom no pathogens are found by these initial investigations have minor symptoms that usually resolve spontaneously. A few have continued large-volume diarrhea, and in some of these widespread Kaposi's sarcoma of the gut or lymphoma is subsequently diagnosed.

Wasting

Weight loss is common in late-stage HIV infection and is related to opportunistic infection[170], for example CMV and *M. avium intracellulare* infections increase resting energy expenditure and lead to loss of lean body mass.

Heart

Pericardial effusion

This is seen in approximately 20% of patients with late-stage disease, and is usually of no hemodynamic significance. Causes include infections such as tuberculosis, staphylococci, and pneumococci, and also malignancies including Kaposi's sarcoma and lymphoma[172].

Cardiomyopathy

Anderson and Virmani[173] found a lymphocytic myocarditis in 37 (52%) of 71 patients with AIDS who had died.

In a prospective study[174] of 952 initially asymptomatic HIV-infected patients, who were enrolled from 1992, 76 (8%) developed dilated cardiomyopathy during a mean follow-up period of 60 months, giving a mean annual incidence of 15.9 cases per 1000 patients. The incidence was higher in those with a CD4+ cell count less than 400/mm³. The same authors found myocarditis in myocardial biopsy specimens from 83% of patients, and detected HIV nucleic acids in a small number of monocytes, endothelial cell myocytes of 53 individuals[174]. The cause of HIV-related cardiac disease is probably multifactorial. It may be a direct action of HIV, but other potential pathogenic factors include nutritional deficiencies, opportunistic infections such as toxoplasma and CMV, and a cardiotoxic effect of antiretroviral drugs should be considered. Dilated cardiomyopathy in late-stage HIV infection has been seen less frequently since the advent of HAART.

Patients present with breathlessness and demonstrate typical clinical signs of heart failure. Chest radiographs may show a normal heart size, but echocardiography is usually diagnostic. Echocardiography may show dilatation of all four chambers, left ventricular hypokinesis, and decreased fractional shortening. The prognosis of HIV-related cardiomyopathy is poor, the median survival from diagnosis being 101 days[175]. It is unclear if the institution of HAART can lead to improvement of cardiac function with reduction in the mortality and morbidity rates.

Endocarditis

Acute or subacute infective endocarditis is classically associated with intravenous drug use, with *Staphylococcus aureus* and *Streptococcus viridans* the most common organisms cultured. Marantic (non-infectious endocarditis) has been described rarely, and systemic embolization is a recognized complication.

Pulmonary hypertension

This is more common in HIV infection than in the general population[176]. The pathogenesis is unclear and the main symptom is dyspnea. Right heart failure or respiratory failure may supervene.

Cancers

Disseminated Kaposi's sarcoma may involve the pericardium. This may be insignificant, although pericardial effusion with tamponade has been described. Cardiac involvement may be seen with disseminated lymphoma of any type. Patients present with cardiac failure, pericardial effusion, with or without tamponade, or with arrhythmia.

Drug-related toxicity

Drugs for treating malignancy such as doxorubicin have long been known to cause cardiomyopathy, and interferon and foscarnet have also been implicated.

Nucleoside reverse transcriptase inhibitors may cause mitochondrial dysfunction in muscle, and cases ascribed to zidovudine have been reported[177].

Coronary heart disease

This may become more common as a result of hyperlipidemia as a side-effect of HAART (see page 192).

Lymphatic system

Persistent generalized lymphadenopathy is defined as the presence of palpable lymph node enlargement (more than 1 cm in diameter) at one or more extra-inguinal sites for more than 3 months in the absence of another cause. Characteristically, the nodes are firm and non-tender. Common sites include the posterior and anterior cervical nodes, axillary, and inguinal nodes. Enlargement of nodes at one site, particularly if the onset is rapid and associated with pressure symptoms, should raise the possibility of lymphoma or Kaposi's sarcoma, and biopsy is recommended.

Blood and blood vessel disorders

Anemia

Anemia is the most common hematological abnormality found in HIV-infected patients, particularly in the later stages of the disease, when up to three-quarters of individuals are affected[178]. Amongst patients with late-stage HIV infection, non-specific abnormalities are found in the bone marrow, including dyserythropoiesis, erythroid hypoplasia and reticuloendothelial iron block[179]. The cause of anemia appears to be multifactorial, and includes a direct suppressive effect of HIV on erythropoiesis, and indirectly through an effect of the virus on the bone marrow stroma[180, 181]. Opportunistic infections, neoplasms, and antiretroviral drugs such as zidovudine and hydroxyurea, and other drugs may also play a role in the etiology of the anemia.

Neutropenia

Neutropenia occurs in about 10% of asymptomatic HIV-infected individuals, and in more than half of those with advanced disease[182]. In addition to the low numbers of cells, neutrophil function is also impaired, as evidenced by defective chemotaxis, leukocyte migration, granulation responses, bactericidal capacity, and superoxide generation[183]. The risk of bacterial infection more than doubles when the neutrophil count in the peripheral blood falls below 1000×10^9 cells/L[184]. Neutropenia may result from the direct effect of HIV on the bone marrow, or be secondary to opportunistic infection, neoplasms, particularly lymphoma, or drugs, including those used in antiretroviral therapy.

Thrombocytopenia

Thrombocytopenia is well described in patients with HIV infection[185], about 10% of infected individuals having a platelet count of less than 100×10^9 cells/L. The numbers of megakaryocytes in the bone marrow are normal or increased, and increased concentrations of platelet-associated IgG, IgM, C3, and immune complexes on autologous platelets have been found in patients with this condition[185, 186]. There is a moderate reduction in platelet survival, with depressed platelet production but no increased clearance of platelets by the liver or spleen, as is found in idiopathic thrombocytopenic purpura[187]. The pathogenesis of the thrombocytopenia is uncertain, but, as infection of the megakaryocyte occurs, it may be attributable to a direct effect of the virus. Treatment with zidovudine has been shown to increase the platelet count in HIV-infected patients[187]. Thrombocytopenia may also result from the effect of opportunistic infections or neoplasms on the bone marrow.

Coagulation abnormalities other than thrombocytopenia have been described, and include a prolonged activated thromboplastin time because of the presence of lupus anticoagulant, an increased prevalence of protein S and heparin cofactor II deficiency, and hypoalbuminemia-related fibrin polymerization defects[188]. In addition, a prethrombotic state may exist in patients with HIV infection: D-dimer levels have been found to be elevated in some individuals. This observation, and an association between HIV and endothelial dysfunction, may account for the occurrence of arterial and venous thrombosis, including acute brachial artery thrombosis, in these patients[189].

Joint and bone disorders

Reactive arthritis

Reactive arthritis may affect as many as 5% of HIV-infected patients at some time during their illness. Typically, large joints are affected. Occasionally, there is a classic trigger infection such as salmonella or campylobacter. The arthritis often improves following the introduction of ART. Patients with psoriasis may also develop an arthropathy.

Osteonecrosis or avascular necrosis

This has become increasingly recognized amongst HIV-infected individuals since the mid-1990s[190]. Prior use of corticosteroids, testosterone and anabolic steroids, hyperlipidemia, alcohol abuse, hemoglobinopathies, including sickle cell disease, and hypercoagulability have been associated with this condition. The head of the femur is the most commonly affected site. Although the condition may be asymptomatic, the patient often has pain that can be severe and disabling. The diagnosis is made by radiological examination or imaging by CT or MRI.

Liver and biliary tract

Pre-existing co-infection with hepatitis B virus or hepatitis C virus

As HIV and hepatitis B virus (HBV) have the same routes of transmission, co-infection is common. The influence of HIV on HBV infection is discussed in Chapter 9.

In a meta-analysis of the response to interferon therapy of HBV, it has been shown that HIV-infected patients, respond poorly to interferon[191]. This observation has been confirmed in a small controlled trial in which an 8% response was seen in HIV-positive subjects, compared with 39% in controls[192]. Newer antiviral drugs such as lamivudine, which directly inhibit HBV replication rather than modulating the immune response, may hold more promise for effective treatment of these patients in the future.

All HIV-positive patients should be screened for evidence of previous infection with hepatitis A virus (HAV) and current or past infection with HBV. Seronegative individuals should be given appropriate vaccination(s). Vaccination against HBV has been recommended for all patients infected with HIV. Unfortunately, HIV infection reduces the efficacy of vaccination in these patients. Several studies have demonstrated a sub-optimal response to plasma-derived vaccine in both magnitude and duration of the antibody response[193–195]. Lack of responsiveness does not clearly correlate with CD4+ T-cell count in the peripheral blood. Among those patients who do respond, loss of protective anti-HBs is seen in 43% at 4 years after vaccination, compared to 8% of immunocompetent controls.

Hepatitis C virus infection in HIV-infected individuals is discussed in Chapter 8.

Opportunistic infections of the liver

Opportunistic infections such as *M. avium intracellulare*, disseminated fungal infections, and disseminated *P. carinii* that cause liver dysfunction and raised alkaline phosphatase levels, tend to develop in the later stages of HIV infection[196, 197].

Peliosis hepatis, caused by the bacterium *Bartonella hensalae* may complicate cutaneous bacillary angiomatosis. In a case-control study, infection with *B. hensalae* was linked to exposure to cats[159]. Histologically, peliosis consists of blood-filled cystic spaces within the hepatic parenchyma. Serum transaminase levels are modestly elevated, with more prominent elevations of serum alkaline phosphatase. In addition to cutaneous lesions, patients may experience fevers, sweats, rigors, right upper quadrant pain, or pain from bony lytic lesions.

Neoplasms

Neoplasms may also affect the liver. Kaposi's sarcoma is found in the liver of about one-third of individuals with cutaneous disease at autopsy, and non-Hodgkin lymphoma may involve the liver[198].

Drug-induced liver disease

Drug-induced liver disease may be a complication of antiretroviral drugs (see pp. 181–182 and 191–192).

Splenomegaly

Splenomegaly in asymptomatic HIV infection is most commonly associated with liver disease. In a series of 70 consecutive, asymptomatic HIV-infected patients reported by Furrer[199], splenomegaly was found by physical examination in 23% of patients and by ultrasonography in 66%; patients with concurrent liver disease had a higher prevalence of splenomegaly.

In endemic areas, or in individuals returning from such areas, visceral leishmaniasis should be considered in the differential diagnosis of fever, splenomegaly, hepatomegaly, and pancytopenia[200].

Liver failure

In a study from Italy, 12% of 308 hospital deaths were associated with liver failure[201], this being the primary cause in just under half of these patients. There was an independent association between liver disease mortality, hepatitis B surface antigenemia, and heavy alcohol use.

Biliary tract disease

Acalculous cholecystitis is not common in patients with late-stage HIV infection, but it has been linked to infection with CMV or *Cryptosporidium* spp.[202, 203]. In contrast to immunocompetent patients with acalculous cholecystitis, these patients are young and ambulatory, and present with right upper quadrant pain and abnormal liver function tests. A history of prior infection with CMV or *C. parvum* is common, as is associated sclerosing cholangitis and/or papillary stenosis of the distal common bile duct. The diagnosis may be made by ultrasonography or technetium scintigraphy, and cholecystectomy is therapeutic.

As with other biliary manifestations, AIDS cholangiopathy presents as right upper pain and markedly elevated alkaline phosphatase levels. Serum bilirubin elevation is modest, however, and patients are rarely icteric. Sonography or CT reveal dilated intra- and/or extrahepatic bile ducts in 81% of patients[204]. On endoscopic retrograde cholangiopancreatography (ERCP), four patterns may be seen

1. papillary stenosis alone is seen in 28%
2. sclerosing cholangitis alone in 12%
3. papillary stenosis combined with sclerosing cholangitis in 49%
4. isolated long extrahepatic duct strictures in 10%.

Universal and sustained pain relief is achieved in patients with papillary stenosis who undergo sphincterotomy, regardless of whether sclerosing cholangitis is also present. Biochemical abnormalities are unaffected, however, as is overall survival[204]. The association of AIDS cholangiopathy with specific pathogens is less clear. Cryptosporidia and CMV have been described most frequently, with microsporidia and *M. avium intracellulare* also reported; however, no pathogens were isolated in more than 40% of reported cases[205–207].

Kidney

Acute tubular necrosis

This may be caused by a number of drugs used in HIV management, for example foscarnet and amphotericin. Interstitial nephritis may be caused by co-trimoxazole. Indinavir may crystallize in urine resulting in nephrolithiasis.

HIV-associated nephropathy (HIVAN)

This is probably the direct result of renal infection with HIV. The pathogenesis is, however, uncertain. HIV-related renal disease is more prevalent amongst African Americans, especially male injecting drug users, than white Americans or Hispanic people. It is characterized by proteinuria (more than 3.5 g of urinary protein per day), and focal and segmental glomerulosclerosis[208]. In the pre-HAART era, the syndrome was rapidly progressive with end-stage renal disease developing within a few weeks[208]. Although the use of corticosteroids was helpful in some cases, the response to such treatment was inconsistent. However, it appears that HIVAN can be reversed, and renal function improved following initiation of HAART[209].

Central nervous system

HIV encephalopathy and the AIDS-dementia complex

Evidence suggests that HIV infection of the CNS occurs early in the course of the infection[210], and the proviral load increases in both plasma and cerebrospinal fluid (CSF) as the disease progresses.

AIDS-dementia complex (ADC), or HIV-1-associated cognitive/motor complex, is common. Data from the MACS study in the USA have shown that the annual incidence is 7% with almost 20% of people with AIDS likely to develop dementia[211]. In about 6% dementia is the first AIDS-defining illness. Milder forms of cognitive impairment may affect up to 30% of symptomless HIV-infected individuals[212]. Although the incidence of dementia has decreased during the HAART era, dementia now accounts for a higher proportion of AIDS-defining illnesses, implying that the degree of protection may be less than for opportunistic infection.

AIDS-dementia complex is usually a late manifestation of HIV infection. The earliest symptoms of the condition, which resembles that of a subcortical dementia, are those of disturbances in concentration and memory[213]. Motor deficits include impaired fine motor movements, tremor, loss of balance, and, less frequently, leg weakness. Behavioral disturbances are common. More severe features include socially inappropriate behavior and acute mania. In the early stages there may be few abnormal neurological signs and the minimental examination is usually within normal limits. Untreated, there is rapid progression with global cognitive and motor impairment, often developing into a vegetative state, and accompanied by paraparesis or quadriparesis, myoclonus, and incontinence. Consciousness is rarely altered, unlike other causes of encephalopathy.

Neuropsychological testing is of particular value in the detection of early cognitive impairment. Defects are found in areas of sustained attention, mental flexibility, sequential problem solving and motor speed. These tests have proved useful in clinical trials on the effects of drug therapy on ADC.

The brain in HIV encephalitis shows a variety of histological changes[214]. The pathological process is multifocal and generally affects the subcortical white matter and deep gray matter. There may be diffuse areas of pallor, focal areas of rarefaction, and vacuolation (HIV leukoencephalopathy). The pallor does not result from demyelination, but from axonal and myelin damage, possibly related to disturbances in microcirculation and disruption of the blood–brain barrier. The inflammatory changes consist of foci of perivascular and parenchymal collections of lymphocytes and macrophages, often accompanied by reactive astrocytosis. Foamy macrophages and multinucleated cells are found in more severely affected individuals. Although it was thought initially that the cerebral cortex was unaffected, more recent studies have shown loss of large neurons in the frontal temporal and parietal lobes associated with gliosis. There is also loss of the complexity of the dendritic tree and a reduction in the number of presynaptic terminals.

HIV infection is limited to macrophages and microglia, capillary endothelium, and multinucleated giant cells, and it is probable that cerebral injury results from the secretion of neurotoxic and inflammatory factors by macrophages and microglia.

As neuropathological changes and the clinical features induced by HIV are not clearly overlapping, there is a clear need for specific markers of HIV-induced neuropathology. At present the diagnosis is a clinical one, aided by the use of tests to exclude other causes of observed neurological abnormalities and to strengthen the probability that these features are the direct result of HIV infection and not the result of an opportunistic infection or neoplasm.

Cerebral atrophy is the most common finding on CT scans; the predominant pattern of atrophy may be central (ventricular dilatation) or peripheral (sulcal dilatation) or a combination of both. Atrophy is found in most individuals with ADC and in a small proportion of individuals with an earlier stage of HIV infection. Serial studies have shown progressive atrophy in patients with ADC or encephalopathy. The finding of cerebral atrophy, of course, is not specific of ADC. The second most common abnormality on CT scanning in ADC patients is low-attenuation parenchymal lesions without mass effect; such lesions are found in up to one-third of cases. They are most obvious in late disease and are associated with marked cerebral atrophy and severe HIV encephalitis.

MRI shows atrophy and white matter lesions. The latter are usually diffuse and the MRI picture correlates with myelin pallor.

In general, the presence of central atrophy and symmetrical periventricular or diffuse white matter lesions in demented HIV-positive patients suggests the diagnosis of viral encephalitis, most probably HIV encephalitis. These changes, however, are not specific, and could equally well reflect CMV infection.

Positron emission tomography with fluorodeoxyglucose has shown relative hypermetabolism in the basal ganglia and thalamus in patients with early ADC and hypometabolism in cortical and subcortical areas of those with more severe dementia[213]. Positron emission tomography may be useful in the evaluation of the effect of treatment in the context of clinical trials.

Single photon emission tomography has shown focal areas of reduced cerebral perfusion in patients with ADC as well as in individuals with early HIV infection[215]. These decreases do not correlate with degree of immunosuppression or of cognitive function, and the underlying mechanism is uncertain. It is also clear that these changes are not specific for ADC, being found, for example, in individuals who abuse cocaine.

Magnetic resonance spectroscopy has been used to study brain metabolism in HIV-infected individuals[216]. There is a reduction in N-acetyl aspartate, a marker of mature neurons in patients with advanced dementia, and an increase in choline at all stages of infection, including people with no obvious neurological abnormalities. The changes in choline levels reflect gliosis even in early infection.

The CSF shows pleocytosis in about one-third of patients with ADC, mildly elevated protein in two-thirds, and oligoclonal bands in one-third. There are elevated levels of CSF β_2 microglobulin and neopterin, possibly reflecting microglial or macrophage activation. There is good correlation between the level of these substances and the severity of dementia[217]. HIV can be isolated from the CSF of people with HIV, who have neurological symptoms and signs[218]; the virus, however, can also be found in those with no such features. HIV-specific intrathecal IgG antibody is also found commonly in HIV-infected individuals, irrespective of clinical stage and neurological findings[219]. Proviral HIV DNA can be detected in the CSF of HIV-infected individuals[220]. The DNA viral load is significantly higher in the CSF than in the blood, is higher in individuals with AIDS than in asymptomatic persons, and loads tend to be higher in those with neurological disease. HIV RNA can also be detected in CSF; the viral load is less than that in the plasma, and there is no relationship between plasma and CSF concentrations. There is, however, a strong correlation between the CSF viral load and ADC[221], although its concentration can be elevated in other conditions such as cryptococcal meningitis. Cinque and colleagues from Italy[222] showed convincingly that quantitative PCR for HIV RNA in the CSF can be used as a specific marker for HIV encephalitis; a value above 4.5 log copies/mL was highly predictive of the condition.

Transverse vacuolar myelopathy

There is marked geographical variation in the prevalence of vacuolar myelopathy amongst HIV infected individuals, but in general it complicates about 1% to 2% of patients.

Histologically, the condition is indistinguishable from subacute degeneration of the cord[223]. The changes are most marked in the thoracic region. There is vacuolation throughout the white matter of the spinal cord, but is most extensive in the mid- and lower thoracic levels, and tends to be more numerous in the lateral than in the posterior columns. The vacuolation is not confined to anatomical tracts. The vacuoles develop within myelin and often contain lipid-laden macrophages many of which show activation markers; the axons are usually normal. The pathogenesis of vacuolar myelopathy is uncertain.

Vacuolar myelopathy is a late manifestation of HIV infection. It presents as a spastic paraplegia with sensory ataxia. There is often associated HIV dementia. Studies have shown that in up to 10% of HIV-infected individuals, there is evidence of subclinical myelopathy as suggested by the finding of abnormal evoked potentials.

Human T-lymphotropic virus type 1 infection is associated with a clinical syndrome that is similar to that caused by vacuolar myelopathy (Chapter 9). Recent studies have shown that amongst HIV-infected individuals with HTLV-1 co-infection, there is a higher frequency of myelopathy than in those who are not infected with HTLV-1. In Harrison's study of Brazilians, almost three-quarters of those with dual infection had myelopathy[224]. The reasons for this finding are uncertain. It may be that HIV increases the expression of HTLV-1-related conditions or accelerate the development of HTLV-1-associated myelopathy. HIV may increase the HTLV-1 viral load that has been shown to correlate with the expression of HTLV-1-related diseases. Conversely, HTLV-1 may increase the risk of development of vacuolar myelopathy.

Opportunistic infections

Protozoal infection

Toxoplasmosis Toxoplasmosis is the most common opportunistic infection to affect the CNS in patients with HIV infection and it accounts for up to 70% of cases of focal CNS disease. Most cases of cerebral toxoplasmosis result from reactivation of *T. gondii* infection acquired earlier in life. It has been estimated that about one-quarter of HIV-infected people who have a CD4+ T-cell count of less than 100/mm³, who are seropositive for *T. gondii* and who have not received prophylaxis will subsequently develop toxoplasma encephalitis[225]. The seroprevalence of toxoplasma infection amongst HIV-positive and negative individuals is high in some European countries such as France[226]. *Toxoplasma gondii* is a ubiquitous protozoan that may infect mammals, birds, and reptiles. It is an obligate intracellular parasite and may exist in three forms

1. trophozoite
2. cyst
3. oocyst.

Cysts may be found in meat for human consumption such as pork or lamb, and may not be killed if the meat is only partially cooked. Oocysts form only in the intestines of members of the cat family, and may be ingested via material contaminated by cat feces. Cysts or oocysts cross the gut wall with dissemination of infection throughout the body. In the immunocompetent individual infection is usually asymptomatic, although infection during pregnancy can result in significant fetal morbidity. Infection is lifelong, with cysts persisting in many tissues. As long as immune function remains, no adverse consequences result. However, in HIV-infected individuals whose peripheral blood CD4+ count falls to less than 200/mm³, there is an increasing risk of reactivation[227].

As the clinical features of cerebral toxoplasmosis are non-specific and include symptoms of CNS dysfunction and focal and non-focal signs, further investigations are required to confirm the diagnosis.

The typical findings on CT of the head are multiple, enhancing nodules or rings with a predilection for white matter, cortico-medullary junction and the basal ganglia (Figure 7.27)[227]. Areas of edema usually surround the lesions sometimes producing a mass effect and a shift of surrounding structures. Sometimes solitary and non-enhancing lesions may be found. For identification of lesions MRI is more sensitive than CT[227]; discrete areas of increased signal intensity are the characteristic findings. Positron emission tomography shows decreased glucose metabolism in toxoplasma abscesses, and this investigation may help to differentiate the infection from lymphoma[228], the second most common cause of a mass lesion in the brain of HIV-infected people. These imaging changes, however, are non-specific and additional diagnostic tests are necessary to make a definitive diagnosis.

In a patient with suggestive neuro-radiological signs, a negative serological test for serum IgG antibody against *T. gondii* does not preclude a diagnosis of cerebral toxoplasmosis, but a positive result is highly

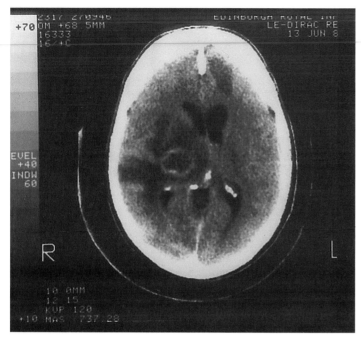

Figure 7.27 CT of the brain of a patient with toxoplasma encephalitis showing multiple, contrast-enhancing lesions

predictive of that diagnosis[229]. As blood culture lacks sensitivity and takes at least 4 days to yield results, it is not a helpful diagnostic test. Lumbar puncture is often contraindicated because of the mass effect. When it has been undertaken, the CSF pressure, white cell count, and glucose concentration are often normal, and the only, non-specific, abnormality is a slightly elevated total protein level. The protozoan can be cultured from the CSF in less than 40% of cases. Toxoplasma DNA can be detected by PCR in the CSF, the sensitivity of the test, however, being only 50% to 60%; the specificity of the test is high – between 96% and 100%, and the positive and negative predictive values have been reported as 100% and 87% to 92% respectively[230]. The sensitivity of the PCR on serum is low, varying between 13% and 50% in reported series, and is really only useful in disseminated infections.

Treatment of suspected cerebral toxoplasmosis is often initiated before a definitive diagnosis is made and, indeed, it is often the clinical and radiological response to therapy that confirms the diagnosis. Failure to respond to therapy should prompt further investigation including, possibly, stereotactic brain biopsy. The combination of sulfadiazine and pyrimethamine, given orally, is the usual treatment. Just over 70% of patients respond to treatment and, of these, more than 85% show a clinical response within 7 to 10 days, and in at least 90% of cases radiological improvement is seen within 14 days of initiation of therapy[227]. Side effects with this drug combination, however, are common and most are attributable to the sulfonamide component; in one series 70% of treated patients had adverse effects, particularly with skin rash and leukopenia. Such side effects may necessitate change of therapy to pyrimethamine and clindamycin. Alternative treatment regimens include the use of pyrimethamine (with folinic acid) and clarithromycin or azithromycin or atovaquone or dapsone, all given orally. In patients who respond to treatment, this should be continued for 6 weeks. As relapse may occur in up to 60% of patients after discontinuation of initial therapy, suppression with sulfadiazine and pyrimethamine (and folinic acid); or pyrimethamine (and folinic acid) and any one of azithromycin, clarithromycin, dapsone, or atovaquone is recommended thereafter. It is possible that this advice will change in individuals who are receiving highly active antiretroviral therapy and who show a sustained improvement in immune function.

Consideration should be given to the use of anti-toxoplasma primary prophylaxis in HIV-infected people with a low CD4+ T-cell count and specific serum antibody against the virus. There is clear evidence that the use of co-trimoxazole or dapsone with pyrimethamine significantly reduces the risk of development of cerebral toxoplasmosis[225].

Fungal infections

Cryptococcal infection Cryptococcus neoformans is an encapsulated yeast-like fungus of which there are two main variants, *C. neoformans neoformans* and *C. neoformans gatti*, that differ in their culture characteristics and geographical distribution[231]. The latter variety is more common in the tropics, but most isolates from HIV-infected individuals are *C. neoformans neoformans*. Before the widespread use of the azole antifungal agents, cryptococcosis was found in 5% to 10% of patients with an AIDS-defining illness. Inhalation is believed to be the usual mode of infection in humans.

Although disseminated disease may affect almost any organ meningoencephalitis or meningitis is the disease most frequently found. The clinical features of meningeal cryptococcosis include headache (73% of cases), malaise (76%), fever (65%), nausea and vomiting (42%), neck stiffness (22%), photophobia (18%), altered mentation (28%), focal deficits (6%), and seizures (4%)[232]. Most patients do not have the classic features of meningitis.

Up to 20% of individuals with cryptococcal meningitis have visual disturbances caused by increased intracranial pressure, infiltration of the optic nerves resulting in necrosis, or compression of the optic nerves with vascular compromise. Papilledema may be found in up to 12% of individuals, and visual field defects may also occur.

Cryptococcal meningitis may cause psychiatric symptoms that include behavioral disturbances and mania.

Not uncommonly, the diagnosis is made during routine investigation of an individual with unexplained fever.

Diagnosis can sometimes be difficult. As there is little inflammatory reaction in the meninges, CT and MRI usually fail to show meningeal enhancement. Cryptococcomas appear as solid, ring-enhancing lesions. It may be normal or there may be non-specific changes in the composition of the CSF[232]. The white cell count is raised in about one-fifth of patients and the total protein increased in about 50% of individuals; the glucose concentration may be reduced in 25% of cases. A positive India-ink test is found in only about 75% of patients, and the cryptococcal antigen test on the CSF is negative in up to 10% of cases. Tests for serum cryptococcal antigen are positive in over 95% of cases but, if the tests are negative and the clinician suspects the diagnosis, further investigations should be undertaken. For the diagnosis of cryptococcal meningitis it is the authors' routine practice to culture CSF in an appropriate medium, and to repeat lumbar puncture if necessary to obtain further specimens for culture if the first sample has yielded negative results.

Amphotericin B, either alone or in combination with flucytosine, is the treatment of choice. Fluconazole can be used in individuals who are intolerant of the latter agent. Initial treatment with any regimen should be continued for 2 to 3 weeks.

Mortality rates from cryptococcal meningitis have varied from series to series, but have ranged from 5% to about 15%, most deaths occurring in the first 2 weeks of therapy[233]. Later deaths have resulted from high intracranial pressures. Of the patients who respond to initial therapy, up to 50% have recurrence of cryptococcal infection unless they receive suppressive therapy. Recurrence is almost certainly because of persistence of the original infecting strain of the organism. Suppressive or consolidation treatment should be with fluconazole. Itraconazole, also given orally, can be used in those who cannot tolerate fluconazole or when there is treatment failure.

Despite suppressive treatment, 2% to 16% of patients relapse. In some cases this is because of poor compliance with therapy, but in others it may result from resistance to the antifungal agent. Certainly, resistance has been demonstrated to both fluconazole and amphotericin B. The authors have noted, however, that very high doses of fluconazole (800 mg/day) can be helpful even when there is drug resistance.

The role of primary prophylaxis against cryptococcal meningitis in individuals with a CD4+ T-cell count in the peripheral blood of less than 250/mm^3 is controversial[234].

Coccidiodomycosis, histoplasmosis, and blastomycosis These can all cause cerebral abscesses in AIDS patients, and need to be considered in the differential diagnosis of mass lesions in individuals from areas of the world where these infections are common[235].

Viral infections

JC virus infection Amongst people with AIDS there is about a 4% prevalence of progressive multifocal leukoencephalopathy (PML) caused by the ubiquitous DNA-containing polyomavirus, the JC virus, which has tropism for oligodendrocytes and astrocytes.

Although the cerebral hemispheres are most commonly affected, PML may develop anywhere in the white matter of the CNS[235]. As a result of lytic infection of the oligodendrocytes by the JC virus, there are multiple foci of loss of myelin and oligodendrocytes. At the margins of lesions, hyperchromatic, enlarged oligodendroglial nuclei with inclusion bodies are seen. There is reactive gliosis with multinucleated astrocytes. There is also infiltration with microglia.

Usually there is a subacute onset of unifocal or multifocal neurological abnormalities[235]. Multifocal involvement, however, always develops. The most common clinical features are hemiplegia, visual disturbances such as cortical blindness and homonymous hemianopia, altered mental state, personality change, memory dysfunction, and cognitive and speech disturbances. Cerebellar involvement can result in ataxia, dysarthria, and/or scanning speech.

The disease is progressive, and most patients die within 6 months of the onset. Remission, prolonged survival, and spontaneous recovery, however, have all been reported.

MRI is the imaging investigation of choice, although the features are non-specific[236]. There are areas of decreased T_1 and increased T_2 signal affecting white matter, usually asymmetrically, but with a predilection for the parietal and occipital lobes. There is no associated mass effect and usually no enhancement. On CT there are areas of decreased white matter density without mass effect or enhancement.

Although the routine examination of the CSF is generally unhelpful, the diagnosis of PML can be confirmed by the detection by PCR of JCV DNA in the fluid[230]. This test, although positive in only about 75% of autopsy or biopsy-proven PML, has proved helpful in confirming the radiological diagnosis; false positive results are rare. It is still uncertain if this test will eventually replace biopsy in the diagnosis of PML. In addition, measuring JC viral load in the CSF may be useful in the monitoring of the effect of antiviral therapy.

Stereotactic brain biopsy is the definitive diagnostic test, but there may be false negative results from inadequate sampling and it is not without its risks.

Until recently treatment of PML has been generally unsatisfactory. Although cytarabine has been used, a recent multi-center study showed that use of the drug, given either intravenously or intrathecally, does not improve prognosis. Cidofovir, a viral DNA polymerase inhibitor, has been used in the treatment of a small number of individuals with PML. In each case, there has been clinical and radiological improvement and loss of detection of JC DNA in the CSF. A randomized controlled trial is currently underway.

In vitro studies have shown that HIV-1 *tat* has the capacity to increase transcriptional activity of the JC viral genome in glial cells[237]. This would suggest that control of HIV infection by antiretroviral agents could have an effect on PML. This observation has been supported somewhat by recent reports on the effect on such individuals of highly active antiretroviral therapy[238, 239]. These have shown that, although complete remission may not be achieved, there may be an improvement in symptoms and a slower rate of progression. In addition, longer survival occurs in those patients who achieve an undetectable JCV DNA viral load in the CSF during treatment with HAART[239].

Cytomegalovirus Cytomegalovirus disease usually presents late in the course of HIV infection and produces encephalitis, myelitis, radiculitis, and multifocal neuropathy.

The most common pattern of encephalitis is of a subacute encephalopathy with confusion, delirium, impaired memory, inattention, ataxia, and weakness[235]. Focal encephalitis presents with fever, headache, and focal signs. Vasculitis resulting in cerebral infarction may be a complication of CMV infection. Ventriculitis with cranial neuropathies and nystagmus occurs in about 10% of patients with CMV encephalitis, and brain stem involvement with ophthalmoplegia and ataxia and quadriparesis has also been reported.

Imaging techniques have low sensitivity and specificity for the diagnosis of CMV encephalitis, although ependymal enhancement on MRI may raise suspicions; small focal lesions that may reflect parenchymal necrosis may be seen in some patients.

The CSF shows non-specific features with either a normal cell count or a mild lymphocytosis, a low glucose concentration, and a mildly elevated protein level. The most sensitive diagnostic test is the detection of CMV DNA in the CSF by PCR[230]. The sensitivity and specificity are high, in excess of 80%, and the positive and negative predictive values are between 86% and 92% and 95% and 98% respectively. The finding of CMV DNA is strongly suggestive of CMV lesions in the CNS but, as the test can be positive with minor lesions, quantitative testing may be helpful. Conversely, if CMV DNA is not detected in a patient with suggestive features, an alternative diagnosis such as HIV encephalopathy should be considered.

Herpes simplex virus This is an uncommon opportunistic infection amongst HIV-infected people. The clinical features and diagnosis are discussed in Chapter 6.

Varicella-zoster virus Although uncommon, varicella-zoster virus has been associated with multifocal leukoencephalitis and ventriculitis, with necrotizing vasculitis, and with vasculopathy and cerebral infarcts[235]. A necrotizing myelitis has also been described. Typical skin lesions often precede or appear at the same time as the onset of the neurological disease. The virus

has sometimes been cultured from the CSF of AIDS patients with neurological involvement, but no other reliable diagnostic test has been described. The value of PCR to detect viral DNA in the CSF of these individuals is uncertain.

Bacterial infections

Pyogenic abscesses are uncommon, but injecting drug users may be at risk from *Staph. aureus*. On CT scanning these abscesses have a smooth enhancing wall and a central area of necrosis may be found. *Nocardia* spp. infection can produce abscesses that are similar in appearance to those of pyogenic abscesses, but the detection of sub-ependymal nodules may suggest this diagnosis.

Tuberculosis The prevalence of tuberculous meningitis and cerebral abscess formation amongst HIV-infected individuals varies geographically.

The spectrum of CNS involvement includes abscesses, tuberculomas, and, most commonly, meningitis[240]. The onset of meningitis is subacute with headaches, altered mental state, and seizures. There may be meningismus and papilledema, but these are not constant features. Cranial nerve involvement is common, particularly of the 6th, 3rd, 7th, and 8th nerves. Basal meningitis may affect the circle of Willis with vasculitis and infarction resulting in ophthalmoplegias, hemiplegia, and movement disorders.

Intracranial tuberculomas and abscesses present with focal neurological abnormalities, headache, or obtundation resulting from increased intracranial pressure. Pulmonary findings may be absent.

Meningeal enhancement of contrast-enhanced CT scans or MRI is found in about 50% of cases of TB meningitis, often with communicating hydrocephalus[241]. Tuberculous abscesses and tuberculomas show as focal enhancing lesions that may resemble toxoplasmosis.

In tuberculous meningitis, the CSF pressure is usually, but not always, elevated. The total protein content of the CSF is often raised but, again, can be normal. There is usually an increased cell count, polymorphonuclear leukocytes initially predominating, then lymphocytes, however

there may be a normal cell count. The glucose concentration in the CSF tends to be low, as does the ratio of CSF to plasma glucose concentration. Direct microscopy for acid-fast bacilli is generally unhelpful, although the examination of multiple specimens from the same patient is likely to increase the diagnostic yield. Culture may be helpful, but results are not available for several weeks, and even this diagnostic test can yield negative results. The CSF is often normal in patients with tuberculomas or abscesses. The use of PCR-based methods for the diagnosis of tuberculous meningitis has proved useful, the sensitivity and specificity being over 90% and 97% respectively[230].

Treatment is with standard anti-tuberculous chemotherapy, although infection with multi-drug-resistant *M. tuberculosis* may pose particular problems.

Atypical mycobacteria Atypical mycobacteria infrequently cause CNS infection, but meningitis and cerebral abscess formation have been described.

Syphilis Although studies have yielded contradictory results, neurosyphilis, particularly meningitis, is more likely to develop more rapidly in immunocompromised individuals than in those who are not immune suppressed.

Cerebral gummas have been described in HIV-infected individuals, appearing as hypodense lesions that enhance with contrast.

Treatment of neurosyphilis in HIV-infected patients should be with intravenous benzylpenicillin, in the same dosage as in HIV-seronegative people (Chapter 15).

Neoplasms and the brain

B-cell lymphoma

Primary CNS lymphomas occur in between 2% and 13% of AIDS patients[242], and are usually found in late-stage infection with CD4+ counts of less than 100 cells/mm³. The majority are high-grade, diffuse, large cell, immunoblastic, B-cell lymphomas (Figure 7.28). They are monoclonal and invariably associated with Epstein–Barr virus[243]. Any area of the brain can be affected, but the periventricular areas are most commonly involved.

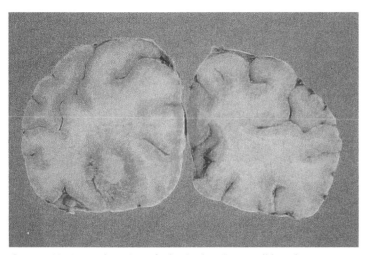

Figure 7.28 Coronal section of a brain showing B-cell lymphoma

The clinical picture is variable, depending on the area of brain affected, but may include focal neurological deficits, seizures, altered mental status, and signs of increased intracranial pressure.

Cerebral lymphoma is the second most common cause of a focal CNS mass lesion after toxoplasma encephalitis. CT scans may be normal or show multiple focal contrast-enhancing lesions with variable amounts of surrounding edema (Figure 7.29). The appearance on CT or MRI imaging, however, is non-specific, and is often indistinguishable from cerebral toxoplasmosis. Single lesions, or periventricular lesions, are more suggestive of lymphoma than toxoplasmosis, but such findings are only seen in a minority of patients. Single photon emission computerized tomography with quantification of thallium-201 uptake may aid differentiation of these conditions[228]. Lymphomas show active uptake; false negative results, however, may be obtained with small or necrotic lesions. These tumors that show increased glucose metabolism can also be differentiated from toxoplasma abscesses by positron emission tomography.

As malignant cells are only occasionally seen, cytological examination of the CSF is generally unhelpful, and lumbar puncture may indeed be contraindicated because of a mass effect or mid-line shift on CT or MRI. When it is possible to obtain CSF, the use of PCR for the detection of EBV DNA in the fluid, however, can be a valuable diagnostic tool. Studies have shown a sensitivity of 50% to 100%, a specificity of 94% to 100%, a positive predictive value of 90% to 100%, and a negative predictive value of 97% to 99%[230]. With the high negative predictive value, a negative result on CSF should prompt the clinician to consider alternative diagnoses, particularly toxoplasma encephalitis. It is also clear that the detection of EBV DNA can antedate the clinical and radiological appearance of lymphoma, making surveillance necessary in those individuals in whom it has been a coincidental finding.

The overall prognosis is poor with a median survival time of 2.5 to 4.8 months, despite treatment by whole-brain irradiation. Chemotherapy with low dose methotrexate, bleomycin, doxorubicin, cyclophosphamide, vincristine, and dexamethasone, or intravenous methotrexate as sole agent, may induce remission in up to 50% of patients. Anecdotal reports suggest that patients with cerebral lymphomas may benefit from a therapeutic regimen that includes highly active antiretroviral agents.

Cerebrovascular disease in HIV-infected individuals

Stroke in HIV-infected individuals may be embolic or thrombotic. Ischemic disease is more common than hemorrhagic. Cerebral embolism is usually from the heart[244], and non-bacterial thrombotic endocarditis and bacterial endocarditis, particularly in injecting drug users, have been well described. Cerebral vasculitis that may be associated

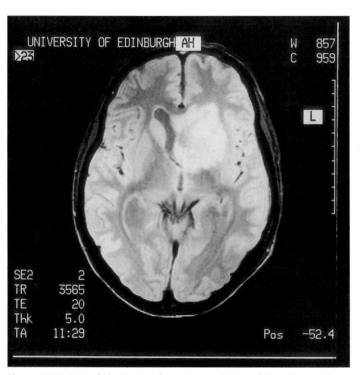

Figure 7.29 MRI of the brain of a patient with B-cell lymphoma (the same patient whose brain is shown in Figure 7.28)

with infection, including HIV itself, can result in stroke[244]. Hyperviscosity syndrome has been reported in AIDS patients and is another potential cause of ischemic cerebrovascular disease. Cerebral venous thrombosis as a result of cachexia and dehydration has also been described.

Intracranial hemorrhage can result from thrombocytopenia that may be autoimmune, drug induced, or secondary to disseminated intravascular coagulation. Hemorrhage may also be caused by vasculitis, mycotic aneurysm rupture, and intracranial malignancy.

Peripheral nervous system

Peripheral neuropathy in HIV infection

Distal sensory neuropathy

This is the most common form of peripheral neuropathy in infected individuals, and is diagnosed most frequently in late-stage infection. The onset is gradual, the feet being affected first with paresthesiae and, in about 10% of cases, pain. Ankle reflexes are absent and there is diminished sensation in the toes; vibration sense is the first to be lost. Spontaneous loss of the neuropathic pain may occur, but there continues to be loss of sensation in the feet.

Histologically, there is degeneration of the long axons in their distal regions, 'dying back', with loss of both large and small myelinated fibers, and of unmyelinated fibers[245]. There is sometimes infiltration of the epineurium with lymphocytes, but the predominant infiltration is with macrophages in relation to degenerating nerve fibers. The density of epidermal nerve fibers in the distal leg of individuals with AIDS-associated sensory neuropathy is reduced, and this decrease in density is greater distally than proximally. The pathogenesis is uncertain, but proposed mechanisms have included

- direct damage to nerves by HIV or its glycoprotein gp120
- the neurotoxic effects of cytokines such as tumor necrosis factor-alpha (TNF-α), IL-1, and IL-6
- malnutrition
- vitamin B12 deficiency
- other infections such as CMV.

Nucleoside analog reverse transcriptase inhibitors, particularly zalcitabine and didanosine may exacerbate the neuropathy, especially in late-stage disease. Other neurotoxic drugs include vincristine for the treatment of Kaposi's sarcoma and lymphomas, isoniazid for the treatment if tuberculosis, and thalidomide has been shown to cause or exacerbate distal sensory neuropathy.

Treatment is symptomatic and dependent on severity. In those with mild symptoms, a non-steroidal anti-inflammatory agent is often all that is necessary. Antidepressants may be useful in those with moderate symptoms and some functional impairment, and anticonvulsants such as carbamazepine and gabapentin may be useful. Opiates may be necessary in those with severe pain.

Chronic inflammatory demyelinating neuropathy

This form of peripheral neuropathy usually presents early in the course of HIV infection[245]. Moderate to severe weakness, both proximally and distally is the usual presenting feature. Sensory signs are mild – there is often some minor diminution of vibration sense – but there is widespread or global areflexia. Neuropathic pain is exceptional. Conduction velocities are reduced, there are prolonged F waves, and often prolonged distal latencies. If the CSF is examined, the total protein concentration is high and, in contrast to other chronic inflammatory demyelinating polyneuropathies, there is a lymphocytosis. Histologically, there is demyelination, remyelination, and axonal degeneration; there is often a mild lymphocytic infiltration.

Guillain–Barré syndrome Most reported cases have occurred at other times, but most commonly, early in the course of infection. The CSF changes are similar to those seen in HIV seronegative cases, but with the important exception, that there is lymphocytic pleocytosis[246].

Acute inflammatory demyelinating polyradiculopathy This is the most common form of Guillain–Barré syndrome to have been

described in HIV infected patients. There is early lymphocytic infiltration of the spinal roots and peripheral nerves and subsequent macrophage-mediated segmental stripping of the myelin; in many cases, but especially in those with severe disease, there is secondary disruption and loss of axons[246].

Acute motor-sensory axonal neuropathy This has also been described in association with HIV infection. There is severe axonal degeneration of motor and sensory nerve axons with minimal lymphocytic infiltration and little demyelination; neurons, however, are spared and are capable of regeneration. There are very reduced or absent evoked responses on distal supramaximal stimulation of motor and sensory nerves, progressing rapidly to total loss of electrical excitability.

The course and prognosis of the Guillain–Barré syndrome in HIV-infected individuals seems to be similar to or, possibly, milder than that in seronegative patients. Although there have been no formal studies, treatment with immunoglobulin or plasmapheresis is likely to be helpful.

Diffuse infiltrative lymphocytosis syndrome

This is an unusual complication of HIV infection that can be accompanied by a symmetrical or asymmetrical sensorimotor neuropathy[247]. The onset may be acute or subacute and can occur at any stage of infection. It is invariably accompanied by other features that include lymphadenopathy, salivary gland enlargement, and a sicca syndrome. There is a perivascular infiltration of CD8+ T cells in the epineurium and endoneurium. Antiretroviral therapy and steroids can ameliorate the features of this condition.

Vasculitic neuropathy

This is rare but may occur in early HIV infection and may be associated with renal or other organ involvement. The features are those of a multiple mononeuropathy[245]. Untreated the condition is progressive but it usually responds to immunosuppressive therapy.

Vitamin B12 and other vitamin deficiencies

These can result from malabsorption and anorexia and associated neuropathy may be seen in late HIV infection.

Mononeuropathies

Bell's palsy has been described in both early and late infection, and is possibly related to HSV-1 reactivation.

Herpes zoster, of course, is common, and results from varicella-zoster virus reactivation.

CMV polyradiculopathy

This is a late feature of HIV infection. There is sudden onset of pain in the lower back and legs, perineal paresthesiae, and a rapidly developing flaccid paraparesis associated with sphincter disturbances; if there is associated myelitis, there is a sensory level, and extensor plantar reflexes[245]. Histologically, there is a pronounced polymorphonuclear infiltration of the lumbosacral roots with necrosis. MRI shows thickened nerve roots that enhance with gadolinium. The CSF shows pleocytosis with polymorphs, the total protein concentration is raised, and the glucose concentration reduced.

CMV can also produce multiple mononeuropathy that evolves subacutely over a period of weeks or even months.

Treatment of both manifestations of CMV infection is with ganciclovir or foscarnet.

Tumor infiltration of nerves and nerve roots, for example with lymphoma, is rare.

Autonomic neuropathy

Histological abnormalities of the autonomic nervous system of the jejunum and rectum have been described in HIV-infected people and cardiovascular autonomic function, as tested by Ewing's method, has been shown to be abnormal in many patients, with the most severe abnormalities being found in those with late-stage infection. This may result in postural hypotension, vasovagal reactions, and may be associated with cardiorespiratory arrest following invasive procedures[248].

Myopathy

In HIV-infected patients myopathy may be primary, that is associated with HIV, or secondary to toxic, neoplastic, infectious, and metabolic processes.

HIV myopathy can occur at any time during the course of HIV infection and is not related to the degree of immunosuppression. It may be the presenting feature of the infection. There is slowly progressive weakness of proximal limb muscles, particularly the hip and neck flexors. There may also be fatigue, myalgia, and dysphagia[249]. Deep tendon reflexes are intact. Although it is not a specific marker of myopathy in HIV-infected individuals, the serum creatine kinase level is elevated in the majority of cases of HIV myopathy[250]. More than 90% of cases have electromyographic evidence of myopathy[250]. Histologically there may be myofiber necrosis and an interstitial and interfascicular infiltration of mononuclear cells (myositis), or there may be structural myofiber abnormalities with a less constant inflammatory cell infiltrate[249]. The pathogenesis of HIV myopathy is uncertain. The use of corticosteroids or non-steroidal anti-inflammatory drugs may be beneficial.

In the late 1980s an association between the use of zidovudine and a myopathy was noted[251], possibly as a result of inhibition of the mitochondrial enzyme DNA polymerase-γ. The myopathy may not be reversible on cessation of the drug, but high-dose steroid use may be helpful.

Toxoplasma gondii can cause acute painful myopathy, and rarely microsporidia may be causative. Other secondary myopathies include those associated with *Staph. aureus* infection (pyomyositis), and lymphomatous infiltration of the muscles (affecting about 9% of cases)[249].

Ocular disease

Anterior segment features

Keratoconjunctivitis sicca

This is common, particularly later in the course of immunodeficiency, and is associated with HIV-induced inflammation of the lacrimal glands.

Infectious keratitis

Herpes simplex and varicella-zoster viruses can cause keratitis. Bacterial and fungal infections are more prevalent amongst HIV-infected individuals than amongst non-infected persons, and microsporidia can cause a punctate keratitis[252].

Iridocyclitis

Iridocyclitis is most often associated with CMV or varicella-zoster virus infections, but other casues include *T. gondii*, syphilis, and drugs such as rifabutin.

Posterior segment features

HIV retinopathy

This condition is diagnosed in up to 70% of HIV-infected individuals, particularly as they become increasingly immunocompromised. Cotton-wool spots, intraretinal hemorrhages, and micro-aneurysms are the most common features[253] (Figure 7.30). The condition is usually asymptomatic, although a few patients may have visual field defects.

Cytomegalovirus infection

CMV retinitis, that had previously affected up to 40% of HIV-infected patients has become less common since the advent of HAART[254]. The disease typically occurs when the CD4+ cell count in the peripheral blood has fallen below 100 cells/mm³. The patient complains of blurred vision, 'floaters', or visual field loss. There is full-thickness retinal whitening with intraretinal hemorrhages (Figure 7.31). Ganciclovir and foscarnet, both given intravenously, are the mainstays of therapy, although cidofovir, also given by the intravenous route, is also a useful agent.

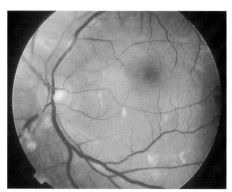

Figure 7.30 HIV retinopathy

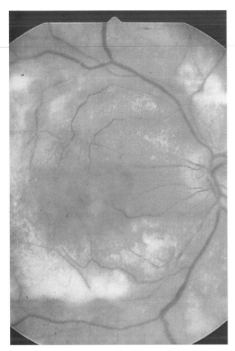

Figure 7.31 Cytomegalovirus retinitis (reproduced from McMillan and Scott 2000[430])

Treatment involves an induction period, followed by a maintenance regimen. Intravitreal injections or implants of ganciclovir have also been used successfully in therapy. There is now good evidence that amongst patients receiving HAART, if the CMV retinitis is stable and there is continued elevation of the CD4+ cell count in the peripheral blood, maintenance treatment with anti-CMV drugs is unnecessary[255]. If HAART is discontinued, however, and the CD4+ cell count falls below 50/mm³, prophylaxis should be re-introduced[256]. Transient intraocular inflammation may develop in patients with CMV retinitis who initiate HAART; this phenomenon is related to immune reconstitution[257].

Varicella-zoster virus infection

Retinal whitening with intraretinal hemorrhage is found in this condition[258]. The progress of the disease is more rapid than in the case of CMV infection, and the lesions are multifocal. There may be concurrent herpes zoster lesions on the skin.

Toxoplasma choroidoretinitis

Toxoplasma choroidoretinitis is characterized by moderate to severe inflammation of the anterior chamber and vitreous; there may be pigmented retinal scars but retinal hemorrhage is not a feature[258].

Syphilis

Syphilis may affect the eye in HIV-infected individuals, and may present as iridocyclitis or diffuse ocular inflammation.

Endocrine system

Hypogonatropic hypogonadism, the cause of which is unknown, is the most common abnormality amongst men who present with the clinical and biochemical features of hypogonadism, although complete anterior pituitary failure and primary hypogonadism have been reported[259].

Thyroid dysfunction amongst HIV-infected individuals is rare, and is usually caused by destruction of the thyroid gland by opportunistic infections or tumors[260]. The adrenal gland may be similarly affected[261].

Laboratory tests for HIV infection

ENZYME IMMUNOASSAY SCREENING TESTS

Screening for HIV infection is generally by tests for the detection of specific antibodies against the virus. Enzyme immunoassays (EIAs) are most commonly used, and those more recently developed have been designed to detect antibody against both HIV-1 and HIV-2. First and second generation assays employed whole virus lysate and recombinant proteins respectively. Third generation assays, the current recommendation, incorporate a mixture of recombinant antigens from the core (*gag*), *pol* (polymerase), and *env* products of HIV-1 and HIV-2, and synthetic peptides from immunodominant epitopes of *env*, adsorbed onto a solid phase (well or bead or microparticles). Many assays will include antigen from the outlier group (O) of HIV-1 with the M (major) group. Antibodies in the test serum bind to the antigens, and the reaction is then revealed by one of a variety of enzyme-linked detection stages[262]

1. indirect – the enzyme-labeled anti-human antibody binds to the bound patient serum
2. competitive – the patient serum competes with labeled antibody to bind to antigen
3. the antibody is sandwiched between the capture antigen and labeled antigen.

The tests that detect any class of antibody (IgM or IgA as well as IgG) may be positive slightly earlier during seroconversion than tests detecting IgG alone.

Sensitivity, specificity, and predictive value

The sensitivity of EIAs that incorporate at least one synthetic HIV antigen is high. In an assessment of twelve commonly used assays against a panel of 1902 anti-HIV positive sera, McAlpine *et al.*[263] found a sensitivity of greater than 99.9%. The third generation tests can detect low levels of antibody, including IgM and IgA, and hence yield positive results significantly earlier (on average about 5 days) than the second-generation tests[264, 265]. Most infected individuals will have seroconverted within 3 months when their blood is tested by these assays. The positive predictive value (over 80%) of these tests is dependent on the prevalence of HIV in the population screened, and all reactive results in the screening EIA should be confirmed by a second (different) EIA, and by supplemental testing.

In some centers, two EIAs are used for the serological diagnosis of HIV infection: one detects anti-HIV-1 and anti-HIV-2 and the other is a competitive EIA based on HIV-1 lysate[262]. This combination of tests can differentiate between HIV-1 subtype O and HIV-2, and can eliminate some false positive results. The use of recombinant or synthetic antigens also lead to a reduction in non-specific reactivity against cell-derived antigens.

Fourth generation screening tests for HIV have been developed that permit simultaneous detection of antigen and antibody. These assays incorporate HIV p24 antigen detection with that of anti-HIV-1, anti-HIV-2, and anti-HIV-1 group O, and detect infection, but not antibody, at an earlier stage than the third-generation tests described above. In one study[266] a total of 16 of 29 infections in seroconverting patients were detected an average of 8.5 days earlier with such an assay than with a third generation EIA. Similar findings were reported by van Binsbergen et al.[267].

Diagnosis based on detecting HIV antibodies is unlikely to be successful in the first few days of symptoms of a sero-conversion illness, and either a test for HIV-1 p24 antigen, viral RNA or HIV-1 proviral load should be performed[268]. Recognition of this condition is important as current practice is to consider immediate ART, with the hope that HIV-specific immune responses may be preserved.

There are rare instances of HIV-infected individuals with clinical features of late-stage HIV infection but with persistently negative serological tests for the virus[269]. Persistently negative serological tests are probably the result of immune dysfunction that may be caused by an imbalance in the T_{h1} and T_{h2} responses, selective loss of memory cells, a defect in the antigen-presenting cell, or induction of suppressor cells and factors[270]. When negative results are obtained in the EIA in a patient with symptoms or signs suggestive of HIV infection, testing for HIV p24 antigen, nucleic acid amplification, or co-culture for the virus should be undertaken to establish the diagnosis.

RAPID RESULTS FROM SEROLOGICAL TESTS

Rapid serological tests have been designed for use in the clinical setting. This is not synonymous with the 'same day' antibody testing that has proved a popular service within the authors' clinic, whereby results of serological testing by the standard assay of blood taken during a morning clinic are available that afternoon. Such a service is feasible in a large laboratory, particularly where an automated assay is in use, although there is pressure to complete the second test required for a reactive sample. The following rapid methods are used in practice in some instances.

Solid-surface dot-blot enzyme immunoassays

Synthetic or recombinant antigens are adsorbed on to a nitrocellulose membrane or on to microparticles. After incubation with the test serum, bound antibody is detected by anti-human antibody conjugated to an enzyme.

A widely used test has a sensitivity of 100%, and a specificity of 99.5% compared with EIA[271]. The positive predictive value when the test is used on STI clinic attenders is 88%, and 81% amongst individuals attending an HIV counseling and testing clinic[271].

Other assays that yield results in about 10 minutes have been shown to have high sensitivity (100%) and specificity (99.8%), and high positive (96.2%) and negative (100%) predictive values when used in routine screening in an accident and emergency department[272]. Some assays, however, yield negative results in early infection[273]. Positive tests must be confirmed by supplemental tests. False positive results may occur if the serum is kept at high temperature, or if there is inadequate separation of the serum.

Latex agglutination

Latex particles coated with recombinant or synthetic antigen are incubated with the patient's serum; a positive result is one in which there is agglutination of the particles as noted with the naked eye. Van Kerckhoven et al.[274] noted that the sensitivity and specificity of these tests varied from 71% to 99%, and 93% to 99% respectively.

DETECTION OF HIV-1 ANTIBODY IN SALIVA

HIV-1 antibodies can be detected in saliva, and EIAs modified to concentrate immunoglobulins by capturing IgG from whole saliva, performed on oral samples obtained with a collecting device, have been used for the diagnosis of HIV infection. The sensitivity, specificity, and positive and negative predictive values of these tests are high. For example, anti-HIV-1 was detected by EIA in the saliva of each of 195 HIV-1-infected individuals but in none of 198 non-infected military personnel, giving values for these parameters of 100%[275]. When a modified Western blot (see below) was used for confirmation of the results in the EIA, 190 saliva samples were positive, and 5 were indeterminate. Gallo et al.[276]

found that the sensitivity of the EIA used in their study of 3570 subjects who had been recruited from a variety of settings was 99.9% (672 of 673 HIV-1-infected patients). The Western blot was positive in 665 of these individuals and indeterminate in eight subjects. The EIA, followed by Western blot if positive results were obtained, was negative in 99.9% (2893 of 2897 subjects) and indeterminate in 4 individuals[276]. Studies in other settings have confirmed this high sensitivity and specificity[277].

SUPPLEMENTAL OR CONFIRMATORY TESTS

Immunoblot

The original HIV immunoblot, the Western blot, is derived from a lysate of HIV grown in cell culture. Electrophoresis of the lysate on polyacrylamide gel separates the proteins by molecular weight, and these are then transferred to nitrocellulose paper. Test sera are added, and any antibodies present will bind to the relevant proteins such as p17, p24, gp41, and gp120/160. The presence of bound antibody is detected with enzyme-labeled anti-human antibody and a chromogenic substrate. The presence of antibodies to at least two of p24, gp41, or gp120/160 is diagnostic of HIV-1 infection[278]. The positive predictive value of a positive EIA and Western blot is 99.99%[279]. When no bands are detected the result is negative. Indeterminate results are sometimes obtained in the immunoblot; in these cases there are one or two bands (most often p17, p24, and/or p55) but the diagnostic pattern is absent.

The second generation immunoblots are prepared from recombinant and synthetic antigens immobilized on nitro-cellulose strips, and may contain HIV-1 or HIV-2 specific antigens, or a mixture. There are less non-specific reactions as cellular proteins are not present. In the USA 0.3% of 48×10^6 blood donations gave positive results in the EIAs; 13.5% of these have an indeterminate immunoblot[280]. In some cases, seroconversion may be identified by the third generation EIAs, before a diagnostic pattern is seen in the immunoblot. Zaaijer et al.[264] noted that in 6 of 10 seroconversions, the EIA was positive before any band appeared in the Western blot. It should be noted that about 18% of individuals whose serum shows a p24 band in the immunoblot will seroconvert[281], and the use of detection methods for HIV RNA or for p24 antigen may be helpful in individuals who have a history of risk activity for HIV. In the absence of a history of exposure to risk of infection, most indeterminate immunoblots do not indicate HIV infection[280]. Indeterminate results in the Western blot have been associated with the presence of antinuclear antibodies and rheumatoid factor in the serum, and with recent immunization and sera from parous women[282].

As commercially available immunoblots are prepared with subtype B strains, some may fail to identify infection with subtype O strains[266].

Indirect immunofluorescence

The indirect immunofluorescence assay on HIV-producing cells permits the detection of antibodies to all HIV antigens, and was used as a confirmatory test for HIV-1 infection in the early years. Although results are concordant with Western blot[283], the test is subjective and labor intensive, and is seldom used now in practice.

Culture

Peripheral blood mononuclear cells are separated from heparinized or EDTA-treated blood by Ficoll-Hypaque gradient centrifugation, and co-cultured with phytohemagglutinin-activated cells from HIV-negative individuals in RPMI-1640 medium supplemented with fetal calf serum and IL-2[284]. Virus can be detected[285] by

1. the presence of p24 antigen in the supernate tested for by EIA
2. the presence of reverse transcriptase, detected by its activity or by EIA
3. indirect immunofluorescence for HIV antigens
4. Western blot
5. *in situ* hybridization
6. PCR for proviral DNA, a method that yields results within 48 hours[286].

This method for the detection of HIV infection, however, has largely been superseded by nucleic acid amplification methods. HIV culture requires containment level 3 facilities in specialist laboratories.

PLASMA HIV-1 RNA DETECTION AND QUANTIFICATION

Blood specimens for the detection of HIV RNA should be collected in EDTA-containing tubes and delivered very promptly to the laboratory so that plasma may be separated and stored within a few hours. Most assays use PCR amplification following conversion of HIV RNA into cDNA by reverse transcription (RT-PCR)[287]. The most widely used commercial PCR assay has a lower limit of detection of 400 copies of HIV-1 RNA/mL, but by introducing a high-speed centrifugation step, the test has an analytical sensitivity down to 50 copies/mL[288]. A branched DNA (bDNA) signal amplification assay is different in concept to the RT-PCR assay, with the reactions occurring at one temperature[289]. After hybridization of target HIV RNA to probes, it is adsorbed to a solid phase, then hybridized to a complex, multiply branched section of DNA bearing indicator compound, which in turn is labeled and detected by chemiluminescence. By controlling non-specific hybridization, a detection limit of about 50 copies/mL can be achieved[290]. A third assay, NASBA, is based on nucleic acid sequence-based amplification at one temperature using a mixture of enzymes and few manipulations. The limit of detection is higher than the other assays, being 80 copies/mL, however useful information regarding response to therapy and predicting progression can be obtained with this less-demanding assay. These 'viral load' assays are invaluable in the management of the patient who is being treated with antiretroviral drugs. As earlier assays used primers for HIV-1 subtype B, infection with other subtypes was sometimes not identified. Most commercial kits now incorporate primers that permit the amplification of all subtypes.

A patient presenting with a seroconversion illness may well have a negative antibody test. In these circumstances, a test for HIV RNA should be performed[291]. False positive results occur, however,[292] and a positive test result, particularly if the values are low, should be confirmed by another nucleic acid amplification test such as the detection of HIV-1 DNA in peripheral blood mononuclear cells. The fourth generation EIAs incorporating p24 antigen detection can also be useful in this context, reducing the risk of missing early, unsuspected infections[293].

HIV-1 PROVIRAL DNA DETECTION IN PERIPHERAL BLOOD MONONUCLEAR CELLS

A qualitative PCR for the detection of HIV-1 proviral DNA in peripheral blood mononuclear cells is not available commercially but is offered by specialist laboratories using in-house PCR. The sample to be submitted is the same as that required for viral load (in EDTA), but the laboratory should be given advance warning and the request clearly marked 'for proviral DNA' so that the white cells are harvested and stored appropriately. In a meta-analysis of ninety-six studies amongst adults, sensitivities ranged from 10% to 100% and specificities from 40% to 100%[294]. The authors concluded that the PCR assay is not sufficiently accurate for diagnosis without confirmation. However, the test may be useful in confirming a positive result for HIV RNA in early infection before antibodies become detectable (see pp. 171–172). This is the preferred test for the early detection of HIV infection in infancy, when maternal antibodies confuse the picture. In a meta analysis involving 271 infected infants of 271 infected mothers, HIV-1 DNA was detected in an estimated 38% of neonates on the day of birth or on the subsequent day[326]. By 14 days of birth, the sensitivity of the test was 93% (90% CI, 76–97%). Steketee and colleagues, however, have presented data to sugges that the detection of HIV-1 RNA is a more sensitive tests for neonatal infection.[327] They noted that HIV-1 RNA and HIV-1 DNA were detected in 56% and 33% of samples from 36 infants under the age of 28 days. In 81 samples from 49 infants over the age of 14 days, HIV-1 RNA was detected in 98%. The specificity of this test, however, has been questioned.[431]

HIV p24 ANTIGEN

Serum HIV p24 antigen is detected by an antigen capture EIA. Confirmation of the reactive result with a neutralization assay is recommended. Dissociation of immune complexes before antigen assay increases the sensitivity of the test[295]. Before the introduction into clinical practice of the nucleic acid amplification methods, the determination of serum p24 antigen was used in the diagnosis of primary HIV infection before antibodies became detectable, and in the monitoring of patients. It is now clear that the detection of viral RNA is more sensitive than antigen detection in the diagnosis of this primary illness. Viral RNA is detectable up to 5 days before antigen is found in the blood[296, 297]. Recently, as mentioned above, fourth generation antibody assays incorporating p24 antigen detection have been introduced for screening with a view to identification of more early HIV infections without resorting to nucleic acid tests.

HIV-2 INFECTION

The majority of the available anti-HIV assays detect between 55% and 91% of HIV-2 infections[268]. It is recommended that a repeatedly reactive serum in a combined HIV-1/HIV-2 EIA should be tested by HIV-1 immunoblot; a positive result by HIV-1 immunblot confirms HIV-1 infection, and testing for HIV-2 is recommended only if risk factors are present. If the HIV-1 immunoblot is negative or indeterminate an HIV-2 EIA should be performed, and positive sera should then be submitted to an HIV-2 specific Western blot[298].

Polymerase chain reaction can also be used to discriminate between HIV-1 and HIV-2. Using primers derived from the *vif* and *pol* regions of HIV-1, and from the *gag* and LTR regions of HIV-2, Walther-Jallow et al.[97] found that there was a high concordance between HIV type-specific tests and PCR in individuals from Guinea-Bissau, West Africa, who had dual infection.

Routine assessment of the HIV-infected patient

In the case of the *newly diagnosed* individual, a complete medical history should be taken, and a comprehensive physical examination performed as soon as the patient's psychological state allows it. Certain further investigations, summarized in Table 7.2, should be completed.

It is the authors' practice to assess *previously diagnosed* patients who are clinically well, either *untreated* or *stable on therapy*, at 3-monthly intervals. At this time, medical, social, and sexual histories are taken to identify areas of concern, such as adherence to therapy if on ART (see pp. 192–193), the development of symptoms suggestive of increasing immunodeficiency, loss of employment, or a recent change of sexual partner. A physical examination should be undertaken to identify minor or major opportunistic infections or neoplasms such as Kaposi's sarcoma. Blood should be sent to the laboratory for hematological examination; abnormalities are not uncommon and in some instances, such as thrombocytopenia, antiretroviral treatment may be indicated irrespective of CD4+ cell count. Plasma enzyme tests of liver function should be performed routinely, and at each 3-monthly attendance, the CD4+ T-cell count and plasma viral load is measured.

LYMPHOCYTE SUBSET ESTIMATION

T lymphocytes broadly subdivide into two subsets – CD4+ and CD8+ – determined by the surface expression of specific antigens. In an HIV-negative individual the CD4+ T-cell count is usually between 500 and 1500 cells/mm³, and the ratio of CD4+ to

Table 7.2 Investigations that are undertaken in the investigation of the newly diagnosed HIV-infected individual

Investigation	Comment
Full blood count	Unsuspected anemia or thrombocytopenia may be identified. Pancytopenia is common in late-stage HIV infection.
Peripheral blood lymphocyte subset determination	See text.
Plasma viral load	Prognostic significance, see text.
Plasma enzyme tests of liver function	Partly to assess effects of co-infections such as HCV, but also as a baseline if antiretroviral therapy is considered.
Serological tests for	
Syphilis	Natural history of untreated syphilis may be different from the HIV-non-infected patient (Chapter 15).
Toxoplasma gondii infection	For evidence of past infection. Reactivation may lead to disease; see text.
Cytomegalovirus infection	For evidence of past infection. Reactivation may lead to disease, see text.
Hepatitis A virus infection	Vaccinate the non-immune individual.
Hepatitis B virus infection	Identify the carrier, see Chapter 8.
Hepatitis C virus infection	Co-infection with HIV may alter natural history, for treatment considerations see text and Chapter 8.
Chest radiograph	Baseline.
Tuberculin skin test	Establish prior exposure.

CD8+ is greater than 1. Intercurrent illness may lead to a temporary fall in CD4+ T-cell count to less than 500/mm³, but the CD4+ to CD8+ ratio is usually preserved. Patients with HIV infection may have a CD4+ T-cell count that is low or within the normal range, but the CD4+ to CD8+ ratio is less than 1.

As a general rule the CD4+ T-cell count in the peripheral blood reflects the damage that has already been done to immune function, and is an indicator of the likelihood of clinical disease within the short term. Patients who have CD4+ T-cell counts repeatedly greater than 300/mm³ are unlikely to develop HIV-related symptoms or opportunistic infections. At counts of between 200 and 300/mm³, minor opportunistic infections may develop. As the CD4+ T-cell count falls to less than 200 cells/mm³, there is an increasing risk of major opportunistic infections such as PCP, and prophylaxis should be considered.

These figures should not be regarded as absolute since serious illnesses may present in those with CD4+ T-cell counts greater than 200/mm³, and occasional patients may present with CD4+ T-cell counts of less than 10/mm³ and have no symptoms at all.

VIRAL LOAD

Estimation of plasma RNA viral load can predict the rate and risk of disease progression (Figure 7.32), and the combination of CD4+ T-cell count and viral load estimation allows a calculation of the probability for the development of opportunistic infections or neoplasms (AIDS) (Table 7.3). This information helps to inform decisions about the benefits of introducing ART.

Serial testing has shown the relative stability of plasma HIV-1 RNA levels over the short term (weeks to months), with a biological variation of approximately 0.3 $\log_{10}$ copies/mL. Given these factors, changes of greater than 0.5 to 0.7 $\log_{10}$ copies/mL (three- to fivefold) are likely to reflect significant changes in HIV-1 replication.

Viral load also plays a central role in assessing the response to ART (see pp. 186–188).

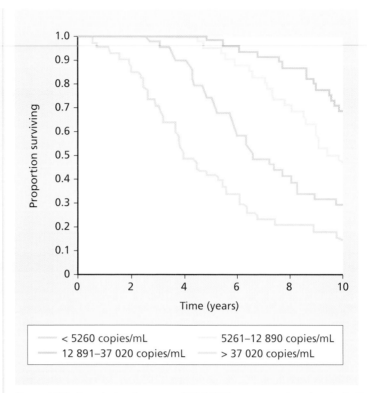

Figure 7.32 Association between HIV-1 RNA concentrations (copies/mL) obtained between 6 and 12 months after the initial infection and the subsequent risk of disease progression (reproduced with permission from Mellors *et al.* 1996[80])

SCREENING FOR OTHER INFECTIONS AND CONDITIONS

All sexually active individuals should be offered tests for other STIs, even if HIV was acquired by a non-sexual route. Untreated gonococcal or chlamydial infections may facilitate transmission of HIV to a sexual partner, and untreated syphilis may follow an aggressive natural history in HIV infection (Chapter 15).

Serological tests for previous infection with *T. gondii* and CMV should be undertaken particularly in patients with low CD4+ T-cell counts. For example, the results of toxoplasma serology will influence the management of a patient presenting with signs or symptoms of an intracranial space-occupying lesion. A negative result would favor an alternative etiology. Similarly, negative CMV serology influences the management of patients who have CD4+ T-cell counts of less than 100/mm³ and a complaint of visual disturbance or other syndrome in which CMV may be implicated.

In addition, if blood transfusion becomes necessary, it is unwise to transfuse the patient with anti-CMV positive blood.

Serological tests for current or past infection with hepatitis A and B viruses should be undertaken, and if there is no evidence of immunity, vaccination should be offered to those considered to be at risk of this infection (Chapter 8). As there may be therapeutic implications in those found to be infected with hepatitis C virus (HCV), screening for antibody against HCV should be undertaken routinely at the patient's initial visit. If the test is negative but the individual continues to undertake unsafe injecting practices, the test should be repeated at regular intervals thereafter.

A chest radiograph should also be carried out at, or as close as practicable to, the initial clinic attendance, especially in intravenous drug users and/or patients from countries where tuberculosis is common.

Because of the increased prevalence of squamous intraepithelial abnormalities

Table 7.3 Risk of progression to AIDS defining illness in a cohort of homosexual men predicted by baseline CD4+ T cell count and viral load (after Mellors *et al*[82])

	Plasma viral load (copies/ml)[a]		% AIDS (AIDS-defining complication)[b]			
	bDNA	RT-PCR	n	3 years	6 years	9 years
CD4 ≤ 200	≤500	≤1500	0[c]	–	–	–
	501–3000	1501–7000	3[c]	–	–	–
	3001–10 000	7001–20 000	7	14.3	28.6	64.3
	10 001–30 000	20 001–55 000	20	50.0	75.0	90.0
	>30 000	>55 000	70	85.5	97.9	100.0
CD4 201–350						
	≤500	≤1500	3[c]	–	–	–
	501–3000	1501–7000	27	0	20.0	32.2
	3001–10 000	7001–20 000	44	6.9	44.4	66.2
	10 001–30 000	20 001–55 000	53	36.4	72.2	84.5
	>30 000	>55 000	104	64.4	89.3	92.9
CD4 >350						
	≤500	≤1500	119	1.7	5.5	12.7
	501–3000	1501–7000	227	2.2	16.4	30.0
	3001–10 000	7001–20 000	342	6.8	30.1	53.5
	10 001–30 000	20 001–55 000	323	14.8	51.2	73.5
	>30 000	>55 000	262	39.6	71.8	85.0

[a] MACs numbers reflect plasma HIV RNA values obtained by bDNA testing. RT-PCR values are consistently 2 to 2.5 fold higher than bDNA values, as indicated.
[b] in this study AIDS was defined according to the 1987 CDC definitions and does not include asymptomatic individuals with CD4+ T cells <200 mm³.
[c] Too few subjects were in the category to provide a reliable estimate of AIDS risk.

(SILs) amongst HIV-infected women (Chapter 5), annual cervical cytological examination or colposcopy should be offered. Infected men who have had sex with other men are also at risk of SILs of the anal canal (Chapter 5), and cytological screening for such lesions should be considered.

PSYCHOLOGICAL ISSUES

Psychological issues may remain important throughout the patient's life, but they are particularly important in the initial period after the patient has learned of his/her infection. Patients may experience a range of emotions on discovering they are HIV-positive including shock, fear, grief, anger, numbness, and disbelief. They may feel confused and disorientated and find it difficult to concentrate. Considerable support is often required in the early weeks after diagnosis and regular clinic appointments should be offered.

Support may also be obtained from partners, friends, and/or family. However, patients should be advised to exercise caution in choosing their confidants. In many instances disclosure of status may lead to anger, hostility, rejection, and even violence or eviction from home. Patients who have told their employer have been demoted or lost their jobs. Except for healthcare workers carrying out exposure-prone procedures, HIV-positive people are under no obligation to disclose their status to an employer.

Written information should be given to the patient, and he or she should be encouraged to seek help from voluntary organizations that have often been established by individuals who are themselves HIV-infected. National organizations in the UK include the Terence Higgins Trust, NAT, and NAM. Websites such as www.aidsmap.com are also helpful sources of information and support.

PARTNER NOTIFICATION

Current partners

If there has been a risk of transmission to or from a current partner, either through unprotected sex or via needle sharing, it is recommended that partners be tested for HIV. There are two main reasons for this. If the partner is also HIV-infected then diagnosis allows the opportunity for measurement of CD4+ cell count and viral load and assessment of the need for ART. If the partner is HIV-negative, the couple should be encouraged to adopt practices which minimize the risk of transmission of infection.

Partners usually ask to be tested immediately, and for many couples this is appropriate. Some prefer to allow for a period of adjustment to the first diagnosis of HIV infection before having to cope with the possibility of a second diagnosis.

Previous partners

There has been a reluctance to undertake notification of previous partners because of the potential upset. In addition, the relatively ineffective treatments available for HIV left health professionals reluctant to apply pressure on contacts to be tested.

However, in the light of advances in ART, these arguments are less easy to defend. Indeed, failure to contact potentially infected ex-partners may lead to extended chains of infection to other sexual partners or via materno-fetal transmission in heterosexual networks.

Clearly there may be practical constraints. There may be insufficient information regarding the whereabouts of ex-partners. The relationship may not have ended in an amicable fashion. It may be difficult to assess the degree of risk to ex-partners if there is uncertainty about the duration of infection in the index case. The risk of transmission in a single sexual encounter is much less than in a long-term relationship.

Much will depend upon the question as to whether the contact sought is thought to be the source of the index patient's infection, or whether the index patient could have infected the contact.

It is the authors' practice to attempt to trace all regular partners with whom the index case had unprotected sex during the likely period of infection. The patient is encouraged to make the contact, but clinic staff, for example health advisers, will undertake the task if the patient requests this. Ideally this would be face-to-face at a time when the contact is alone, but it is often impossible to predict domestic circumstances. The main alternative is making contact by telephone. Writing to the patient is not recommended if at all possible, even if the letter does not explicitly mention HIV.

In the case of patients who have a young family, the question of serological testing of the children for HIV may be an issue. When the duration of infection of the mother is unknown, testing may be indicated.

Infected patients should be counseled about the need to practice safer sex (Chapter 3).

PREGNANCY

If pregnant at the time of diagnosis, the woman should be managed as detailed below.

Patients may ask about the advisability of a planned pregnancy in an HIV-infected woman. The potential hazards should be explained carefully and supported by written information.

The technique of 'sperm washing' is now practised in several centers in industrialized countries to reduce the risk of transmission of HIV from an HIV-infected man to an HIV-non-infected woman. At the time of writing more than 300 healthy children have been born after more than 3000 cycles of sperm washing and intrauterine insemination treatment or *in vitro* fertilization[299]. There have been no HIV seroconversions amongst the sperm recipients. In the case of prevention of transmission from an infected woman to a non-infected man, self-insemination using quills is advocated[299].

In addition to the general advice given to pregnant women about issues such as nutrition and screening for genetic disorders, HIV-infected women should be counseled about

- the selection of effective contraception to reduce the risk of an unintended pregnancy
- the risks of perinatal transmission and the strategies to reduce these risks
- potential effects of HIV or treatment on the course and outcomes of pregnancy
- initiation or modification of an antiretroviral treatment regimen to achieve a maximally suppressed viral load and reduce the risk of perinatal transmission.

CONTRACEPTION

Contraception should be discussed with HIV-infected women who do not want to become pregnant. In reaching a decision on the choice of method it is important to consider

- the efficacy of the contraceptive method
- its ability to reduce the risk of transmission of HIV to a partner
- its ability to protect against acquisition of other STIs
- in the case of oral contraception, possible interactions with antiretroviral therapy.

The male latex condom is highly effective in reducing the risk of pregnancy and the transmission of HIV and other STIs (Chapter 2), and of course, there is no risk of drug–drug interactions. This is the preferred method of contraception. Fewer data are available on the efficacy of the female condom in reducing the risk of transmission or acquisition of infections, and there have been concerns about possible transfer of viruses through the polyurethane barrier (Chapter 2). In addition, the use of female condoms has not proved universally popular amongst women.

Hormonal methods of contraception, although effective as contraceptive agents, do not prevent HIV transmission, and may indeed lead to increased shedding of virus from the cervix. In a cross-sectional study, Mostad et al.[112] found that the shedding of HIV-1 infected cells from the cervix was independently associated with the use of depot medroxyprogesterone acetate (odds ratio 2.9, 95% confidence interval 1.5–5.7), and with the use of low-dose (odds ratio 3.8, 95% confidence interval 1.4–9.9) and high-dose (odds ratio 12.3,

95% confidence interval 1.5–101) oral contraceptive pills. It has been postulated that the suppression of endogenous hormones by synthetic estrogens and progestins may result in a loss of control of viral replication[112]. In addition, steroids bind to regulatory sequences of HIV[300] and up regulate expression of the virus. Oral contraceptives may interact with antiretroviral agents, particularly the protease inhibitors that may inhibit or induce the enzymes of the cytochrome P450 system. Individuals receiving such therapy should use alternative methods of contraception.

Modern intrauterine devices (IUDs) are more than 99% effective in preventing pregnancy over 1 year of use. In addition, it has been shown that the incidence of IUD-related complications, including pelvic inflammatory disease, is no greater amongst HIV-infected women than amongst non-infected women[301]. In addition, the insertion of an IUD does not appear to alter the prevalence of shedding of HIV-1 infected cells from the cervix: 50% and 43% of 98 HIV-infected women had viral shedding before and about 4 months after IUD insertion respectively[302]. The IUD offers little protection against STIs, and the heavier and more prolonged menstrual periods associated with the use of copper-bearing IUDs may increase the risk of HIV infection to a sexual partner. Use of the levonorgestrel-releasing intrauterine system, however, is associated with less menstrual blood loss and, although more expensive than other IUDs, this may be the intrauterine device of choice in the HIV-infected woman who opts for this form of contraception.

The use of occlusive pessaries (diaphragm, cervical cap, vault cap, and the vimule) can be less efficacious than the above methods. Although they may provide some protection against STIs, the spermicides that are recommended for use in conjunction with these barriers may result in genital inflammation, possibly increasing the risk of HIV transmission (Chapter 2).

Sterilization may be an option for those women whose families are complete, but, of course, protection against transmission of HIV or protection against other STIs is not afforded.

Antiretroviral therapy

The principles underpinning the use of ART have changed frequently in the past and are likely to do so in the future, therefore evidence-based guidelines such as those issued by the British HIV Association (BHIVA) should be consulted. These are available at www.aidsmap.com and they are updated regularly in accordance with new developments. The March 2001 draft of the guidelines forms the template for this section.

The ideal antiretroviral drug would have the following properties,

- it would be sufficiently powerful to inhibit fully HIV replication
- it would require several mutations in the viral genome before resistance developed
- it would have no short-term side-effects such as rash, nausea, or diarrhea
- it would have no long-term side-effects such as lipodystrophy
- it could be taken once or twice daily with no food restrictions.

Indeed it could be argued that a removable depot preparation to be replaced every few months would be optimal. Unfortunately, no such agent is available at present. Currently, a minimum of two or more antiretroviral drugs are required to inhibit HIV replication. Resistance, short and long-term side-effects are problematic, and inconvenient dosing schedules may interfere with activities of daily living.

TARGETS IN THE HIV LIFE CYCLE

Several targets for drug therapy have been identified

1. reverse transcriptase – nucleoside analog reverse transcriptase inhibitors (NRTIs), non-nucleoside analog reverse transcriptase inhibitors (NNRTIs) and nucleotide analog reverse transcriptase inhibitors
2. protease – protease inhibitors (PIs)
3. integrase*
4. fusion with target cell*

* these drugs are currently in development.

MODE OF ACTION OF ANTIRETROVIRAL DRUGS

Reverse transcriptase has a three-dimensional structure that approximates the human right hand. Nucleoside-analog reverse transcriptase inhibitors are phosphorylated intracellularly before being incorporated by reverse transcriptase into the growing DNA strand in place of one of the naturally available nucleosides; NRTIs lack a 3′ hydroxyl group for the next nucleotide to attach, and thus the DNA chain terminates, for example stavudine and zidovudine are thymidine analogs.

Non-nucleoside reverse transcriptase inhibitors do not require intracellular phosphorylation but bind directly to the enzyme, primarily through hydrophobic interactions. In the case of nevirapine, the position of critical amino acids within the enzyme's catalytic site is altered, with significant slowing of the reaction catalyzed by reverse transcriptase[303].

Most of the protease inhibitors (PIs) contain a synthetic analog of the phenylalanine–proline sequence at positions 167 and 168 of the gag–pol polyprotein that is cleaved by the protease. They prevent cleavage of gag and gag–pol precursor proteins during virion assembly, thereby resulting in the production of immature and non-infectious virus.

Nucleotide analog reverse transcriptase inhibitors are being evaluated for use in HIV infection. Tenofovir is a monophosphorylated derivative of adenine that, after phosphorylation to the active triphosphate, replaces deoxyadenosine monophosphate, resulting in DNA chain termination.

ANTIRETROVIRAL DRUGS

Nucleoside analog reverse transcriptase inhibitors

Zidovudine

This was the first antiretroviral agent introduced for the treatment of HIV infection.

Pharmacokinetics (mostly from the Glaxo Wellcome Data Sheet 2000)

When given orally the drug is well absorbed with a bioavailability of between 60% and 70%. Following oral administration of 200 mg of zidovudine every 4 hours, the C_{max} was 1.2 µg/mL, and the C_{min} was 0.1 µg/mL. The mean terminal plasma half-life after intravenous administration of zidovudine is 1.1 hours. The drug is excreted by the kidney and, as the renal clearance of zidovudine exceeds that of creatinine, tubular secretion occurs. The major metabolite found in both plasma and urine is the 5′ glucuronide. Plasma protein binding is low (33% to 38%). Zidovudine penetrates the CSF, the average CSF:plasma concentration ratio being about 0.5. In rabbits diffusion of zidovudine from the CSF to brain tissue is considerable[304]. Pregnancy does not appear to alter the pharmacokinetics of zidovudine. The drug crosses the placenta by passive transfer and plasma levels in the neonate at birth are similar to those in the mother. In placental infusion studies, zidovudine is metabolized in the placenta into the triphosphate, and therefore may give additional protection against materno-fetal transmission. Zidovudine can also be detected in breast milk. Zidovudine is found in semen at concentrations that are higher than simultaneous plasma concentrations, the semen AUC to plasma AUC ratio being 3.31[305].

As the glucuronidation enzyme system is immature, the zidovudine half-life (3.1 hours) and clearance (10.9 mL min^{-1} kg^{-1} body weight) are prolonged in neonates[306]. These parameters are further prolonged in immature infants.

Mutagenicity and carcinogenicity

In mouse lymphoma cell studies, zidovudine has been shown to be mildly mutagenic at the highest concentrations tested, in the absence of metabolic activation (4000 to 5000 µg/mL), and again to be weakly mutagenic at lower concentrations in the presence of metabolic activation (1000 µg/mL)[307]. Dose-related chromosomal alterations have been noted in human lymphocytes exposed to high concentrations of zidovudine *in vitro*, and BALB/c-3T3 cells can be transformed with high doses of the drug[307]. In mice and rats given large oral doses of zidovudine, vaginal squamous cell carcinoma can be induced in some animals. When the drug is given to pregnant mice from day 10 of gestation, the incidence (2 of 11 animals given 20 or 40 mg kg^{-1} day^{-1} for 24 months) and the time of onset of vaginal epithelial cell tumors was similar to that of animals given zidovudine only after birth[308]. The authors concluded that zidovudine was not a transplacental carcinogen. Although long-term follow-up of uninfected children exposed to zidovudine *in utero* or in the neonatal period have yet to be completed, current data do not show an increased incidence of cancers amongst such children. No malignancies were noted amongst 727 infants from the Pediatric AIDS Clinical Trials Group Protocol 076[308a] who had been monitored for up to 6 years.

Adverse events

Nausea, vomiting, abdominal pain, diarrhea, headache, malaise, and insomnia are all common side effects of zidovudine during the first few weeks of therapy. Anemia and neutropenia are recognized adverse events that do not usually occur before 4 to 6 weeks of therapy. Pancytopenia has also been reported. Myalgia, myopathy, and peripheral neuropathy may (occasionally) occur and, probably as a result of mitochondrial dysfunction, lactic acidosis may also develop (see page 192). Nail and skin pigmentation may complicate the use of zidovudine.

Preparations available

Capsules containing 100 mg, 250 mg, or 300 mg zidovudine are available. A syrup containing 50 mg zidovudine/5 mL is also marketed. The drug may be taken with or without food. A formulation for intravenous infusion is also available: the solution contains 10 mg zidovudine/mL and must be diluted prior to administration. The desired dose of zidovudine is added to and mixed with Glucose Intravenous Infusion (5% w/v) to give a concentration of either 2 mg/mL or 4 mg/mL, the infusion should be given over 1 hour.

Zidovudine is a component of Combivir® (Glaxo Wellcome), each film-coated tablet containing 300 mg zidovudine and 150 mg lamivudine. It is also a component of Trizivir® (Glaxo Wellcome), each film-coated tablet containing 300 mg zidovudine, 150 mg lamivudine, and 300 mg abacavir (as abacavir sulfate). The pharmacokinetic properties of each drug are not altered in these combinations.

Lamivudine

Pharmacokinetics (mostly from the Glaxo Wellcome Data Sheet 2000)

Lamivudine is well absorbed after oral administration, the bioavailability being between 80% and 85%. The mean time to C_{max} is 1 hour, the C_{max} being 1.5 to 1.9 μg/mL. The elimination half-life is 5 to 7 hours, most of the drug being excreted unchanged in the urine; about 5% to 10% of the drug is metabolized in the liver. Dosage adjustment is necessary in patients with renal dysfunction and a creatinine clearance below 50 mL/min. Plasma protein binding is low (less than 16% to 36%). Lamivudine penetrates the CSF, and during chronic oral dosing the CSF concentration of the drug 4.5 to 7 hours after an oral dose has been reported as being 0.36 ± 0.19 μmol/L[309]. Lamivudine is found in semen at semen to plasma ratios of between 4.6 and 8.7 when samples are obtained 2 to 4 hours and 8 to 12 hours after dosing respectively[310].

The pharmacokinetics of lamivudine are not affected by pregnancy. The drug crosses the placenta by simple diffusion and it is secreted in breast milk.

Mutagenicity, carcinogenicity, and teratogenicity tests

In bacterial tests, lamivudine is not mutagenic but it showed activity in the mouse lymphoma assay and in an *in vitro* cytogenetic assay; the mutagenic activity of the drug could not be shown *in vivo* (Glaxo Wellcome Data Sheet 2000). Early embryolethality can be induced in pregnant rats, and administration of the drug during the first trimester of pregnancy is not recommended (Glaxo Wellcome Data Sheet 2000).

Adverse events

Headache, insomnia, nausea, vomiting, abdominal pain, diarrhea, malaise, and myalgia are reported side effects of lamivudine therapy. Peripheral neuropathy and pancreatitis have been described rarely during therapy, and lactic acidosis may be a complication (see page 192). In patients with chronic hepatitis B who have received lamivudine, recurrence of hepatitis with hepatic decompensation may result if therapy is discontinued. Whenever possible it may be wise to continue lamivudine, even when it may not be active against HIV in that particular patient.

Preparations available

Lamivudine is available as tablets, each containing 150 mg of the drug. An oral solution containing 10 mg/mL lamivudine is also available.

Lamivudine is a component of Combivir® (Glaxo Wellcome), each film-coated tablet containing 300 mg zidovudine and 150 mg lamivudine. It is also a component of Trizivir® (Glaxo Wellcome), each film-coated tablet containing 300 mg zidovudine, 150 mg lamivudine, and 300 mg abacavir (as abacavir sulfate). The pharmacokinetic properties of each drug are not altered in these combinations.

Didanosine

Pharmacokinetics[316]

Following oral administration of the tablet, didanosine is rapidly absorbed from the intestinal tract, the bioavailability being 42 ± 12%. The pharmacokinetics of didanosine are dose-linear. After dosing with 200 mg didanosine tablets twice daily, the C_{max} mean is 1.05 μg/mL, and is observed 0.25 to 1.50 hours after administration. As the C_{max} and the AUC are decreased by about 55% when didanosine tablets are taken within 2 hours of a meal, the tablets should be taken on an empty stomach, at least 30 minutes before a meal or 2 hours after eating. The rate of absorption of didanosine from the gastro-resistant capsules is significantly slower than from the tablets; the time to attain C_{max} is about 2 hours. In addition the C_{max} is about 60% of that obtained with the tablet. Didanosine is distributed into total body fluid, and crosses the blood–brain barrier, although concentrations in the CSF are low after a single oral dose of 250 mg. Didanosine crosses the placenta by passive diffusion; concentrations of the drug in the placenta and fetal circulation are 20% to 50% that of the maternal plasma concentrations because of metabolism in the placenta. There are no data on secretion of didanosine in human breast milk. Plasma protein binding is less than 5%. Didanosine is metabolized to the triphosphate, to uric acid, or it enters the purine metabolic pool. About 30% to 60% is excreted unchanged in the urine within 8 hours of an oral dose. Dose adjustment is necessary in individuals with renal impairment. The mean plasma half-life is 1.4 hours, but the intracellular concentration of the active moiety (didanosine triphosphate) ranges from 8 to 24 hours, making once daily dosing feasible.

Mutagenicity, carcinogenicity, and teratogenicity tests

As observed with other NRTIs, didanosine gives positive results in the bacterial mutagenicity assay, and the mouse lymphoma gene mutation assay. There is activity in the *in vitro* chromosomal aberration assays in cultured human lymphocytes and in Chinese hamster lung cells, and in the *in vitro* BALBc/c 3T3 transformation assay. Mutagenicity was not observed in rat or mouse *in vivo* micronucleus assays. In rats and rabbits given doses up to 12 and 14.2 times the estimated human exposure, there is no evidence of harm to the fetus.

Adverse events

One of the most common side effects of didanosine tablets is diarrhea, attributable to the buffer component of the tablet. The incidence of diarrhea is lower in patients treated with enteric-coated tablets. Nausea and vomiting occur in fewer than 5% of patients. Pancreatitis is a well-recognized complication of didanosine, occurring in 5% of treated individuals, and developing particularly in those receiving high doses of the drug. If possible it is prudent to avoid the use of didanosine in individuals who have other risk factors for pancreatitis such as alcoholism or hypertriglyceridemia. Dry mouth and dry eyes have also been reported during drug therapy. Peripheral sensory neuropathy develops in about 16% of patients, but is reversible on discontinuation of the drug. Retinal toxicity and optic neuritis are less common adverse events. Reversible hyperglycemia has also been noted in patients treated with didanosine, and diabetes mellitus has developed during treatment. Lactic acidosis and hepatic steatosis have been reported (see page 192).

Preparations available

Didanosine is available as chewable/dispersible buffered tablets, each containing either 25 mg, 100 mg, or 150 mg of didanosine. This preparation should be taken at least 30 minutes before a meal. Gastro-resistant hard capsules, containing 125 mg, 200 mg, 250 mg, or 400 mg didanosine have recently become available.

These capsules should be taken at least 2 hours before a meal.

Zalcitabine

Pharmacokinetics (mostly from Roche Products Data Sheet 2000)

The mean absolute bioavailability of zalcitabine is over 80%. After administration of an oral dose of 1.5 mg of zalcitabine, the mean plasma C_{max} is 25.2 ng/mL (range 11.6 to 37.5 ng/mL), and is achieved after a mean of 0.8 hours. Food reduces the absorption rate resulting in a 39% decrease in the mean plasma C_{max} and in a twofold increase in the time to reach plasma C_{max}; in addition, the area under the curve is reduced by 14%. There is little (less than 4%) plasma protein binding. There have been few studies on zalcitabine metabolism in humans, but there appears to be little hepatic metabolism, the majority of the drug being excreted in the urine (about 70%). The mean elimination half-life is 2 hours (range 1 to 3 hours), but is prolonged in patients with renal impairment who may require dose adjustment (Roche Products Ltd Data Sheet 2000). Little zalcitabine appears in the CSF; in animal studies the ratio of CSF: plasma concentration is 0.03[311].

Zalcitabine crosses the placenta by passive diffusion, it is not known if the drug is secreted in breast milk.

Mutagenicity, carcinogenicity, and teratogenicity tests

There is no evidence of mutagenicity in the Ames tests, but dose-related increases in chromosomal aberration is seen in human lymphocytes exposed to the drug (Roche Products Ltd Data Sheet 2000). Zalcitabine given in high doses has the potential to cause thymic and other lymphomas in different mouse models systems. It has also been shown that zalcitabine can produce developmental toxicity in mice, i.e. malformations, reduced body weight, and resorptions.

Adverse events

Gastrointestinal symptoms, including nausea, vomiting, abdominal pain, diarrhea, and dry mouth are not uncommon side effects. The most serious complication of therapy, however, is a sensorimotor peripheral neuropathy that is potentially irreversible. Pancreatitis has also been reported as an adverse event, and abnormalities of plasma enzyme tests of liver function may occur. Cardiac arrythmias and heart failure have been reported, but as in the case of other apparent side effects with any of the antiretroviral drugs, it is sometimes difficult to differentiate toxicity from underlying disease. Anemia, neutropenia, thrombocytopenia, and eosinophilia are noted uncommonly.

Preparations available

Zalcitabine is available as tablets, each containing 0.375 mg or 0.750 mg of the drug. The drug can be taken with or without food.

Abacavir

Pharmacokinetics

Abacavir is well absorbed when given by mouth, the oral bioavailability being about 83%, absorption is not affected by food. After oral administration, the mean time to C_{max} is about 1.5 hours for the tablet formulation, and 1 hour for the oral solution. In steady state studies the C_{max} is about 3 µg/mL. There is good penetration into body tissues and fluids including the CSF, the CSF concentration being 30% to 44% of the plasma AUC. Probably because it is more lipophilic than the other currently available NRTIs, it penetrates brain tissue better[312]. Although data are not currently available for humans, abacavir is secreted into the breast milk of lactating rats. Protein binding is low or moderate (about 49%), indicating a low likelihood of drug interactions through plasma protein binding displacement. The mean half-life of abacavir is about 1.5 hours. Abacavir is metabolized in the liver, the primary pathways are by alcohol dehydrogenase and glucuronidation. Abacavir is contraindicated in severe hepatic impairment. About two-thirds of the dose is excreted in urine as the 5'-carboxylic acid and the 5'-glucuronide; only about 2% of the dose is excreted unchanged in the urine.

The remainder of the dose is excreted in the feces. No dosage adjustment is necessary in patients with renal impairment. There is no clinically significant interaction between ethanol use and abacavir.

Mutagenicity, carcinogenicity, and teratogenicity tests

Abacavir is not mutagenic in bacterial tests, but as with other nucleoside analogs, there is activity *in vitro* in the human lymphocyte chromosome aberration assay, the mouse lymphoma assay, and the *in vivo* micronucleus test. Data on carcinogenicity are not currently available. Abacavir crosses the placenta, and although there is no evidence of toxicity in rabbits, decreased body weight, fetal edema, and an increased incidence of skeletal malformations have been observed in rats. The use of abacavir in pregnancy should therefore be avoided.

Adverse events

Nausea, vomiting, and malaise are the most common side effects; these are genrally mild and transient. There may be abnormalities in plasma enzyme tests of liver function. The most serious adverse event, that may be fatal, is hypersensitivity; this reaction occurs in about 3% of patients treated with abacavir.

As the risk of life-threatening reactions or death are greater when the patient is re-challenged with the drug, it is imperative that when a diagnosis of abacavir hypersensitivity has been made, or is thought possible, that that patient is never re-challenged with abacavir.

Symptoms of hypersensitivity usually develop within the first 6 weeks of initiation of therapy with a median onset of 11 days. Most patients present with fever (80% of cases) and gastrointestinal symptoms (about half of cases), including nausea, vomiting, and abdominal pain. Dyspnea is a less common feature. A maculopapular or urticarial skin rash is present in about 70% of cases, and sometimes conjunctival injection, oral mucosal lesions, or facial edema may be found. Symptoms tend to evolve over a few days, and characteristically, the severity of the symptoms increases after each dose of abacavir. Discontinuation of the drug leads to rapid resolution of the symptoms.

Preparations available

Abacavir is available as tablets, each containing 300 mg of the drug as sulfate, and as an oral solution containing 20 mg/mL of abacavir as sulfate. Abacavir can be taken with or without food.

Abacavir is a component of Trizivir® (Glaxo Wellcome), each film-coated tablet containing 300 mg zidovudine, 150 mg lamivudine, and 300 mg abacavir (as abacavir sulfate). The pharmacokinetic properties of each drug are not altered in these combinations.

Stavudine

Pharmacokinetics (Bristol-Myers-Squibb Pharmaceuticals Ltd Data Sheet 2000)

Stavudine is well absorbed when given by mouth, the oral bioavailability being 86 ± 18%. After multiple oral dosing with 0.5 to 0.67 mg/kg, the C_{max} is 810 ± 175 ng/mL. The terminal elimination half-life is 1.3 ± 0.2 hours when a single oral dose is given, and 1.4 ± 0.2 hours after multiple doses. The intracellular half-life of stavudine triphosphate is 3.5 hours in T cells, supporting twice daily dosing (Bristol-Myers-Squibb Pharmaceuticals Ltd Data Sheet 2000). About 40% of the dose of stavudine is excreted unchanged in the urine by glomerular filtration and by tubular secretion; the remainder is metabolized. In patients with renal impairment, dosage adjustment may be necessary. Stavudine crosses the placenta by simple diffusion[313], and is present in the fetus as parent compound or its inactive metabolites[314]. It is also found in breast milk (Bristol-Myers-Squibb Pharmaceuticals Ltd Data Sheet 2000). Stavudine is found in the CSF, the concentration being 0.28 ± 0.08 μmol/L in patients receiving the drug in an oral dosage of 40 mg every 12 hours[309]. Although stavudine is sometimes not detected in semen, concentrations approach those in plasma when it is detected[310].

Mutagenicity, carcinogenicity, and teratogenicity tests

Although stavudine, when given in very large doses, is carcinogenic in mice and rats, carcinogenicity is not found when these animals are administered the drug in doses that are up to 168 times the expected human exposure (Bristol-Myers-Squibb Pharmaceuticals Ltd Data Sheet 2000). As with the other nucleoside analog agents, stavudine is genotoxic in *in vitro* tests, and in an *in vivo* test for chromosomal aberrations.

Adverse events

Sensory peripheral neuropathy has been reported in patients receiving stavudine, particularly those with advanced HIV disease and in combination with other neurotoxic drugs such as didanosine. Headache, insomnia, nausea, vomiting, diarrhea, and skin rash have all been reported in patients receiving stavudine. Lactic acidosis has also been recorded (see page 192).

Preparations available

Stavudine is available as capsules, each containing 15 mg, 20 mg, 30 mg, or 40 mg of the drug. A powder for oral solution is also marketed, the reconstituted solution containing 1 mg of stavudine/mL. Stavudine should be taken at least 30 minutes before a meal.

Non-nucleoside reverse transcriptase inhibitors

Nevirapine

Pharmacokinetics[303]

Nevirapine is well absorbed when given orally, the bioavailability being 93.7 ± 9% after a 50 mg tablet. The rate of absorption is decreased with both food and antacids, but the extent of absorption is unaffected. A C_{max} of 7.5 μM is achieved about 4 hours after a single 200 mg dose of nevirapine. After multiple doses C_{max} increases linearly in the dose range 200 to 400 mg/day. Steady-state peak and trough concentrations on 400 mg daily dosing are 7.2 and 4 mg/L respectively. Nevirapine is widely distributed in tissues, including the CSF where the concentration is about 45% of that in plasma.

The isoenzyme CYP3A (including CYP4A) is the family of cytochrome P450 responsible for the oxidative metabolism of nevirapine to its major metabolites. CYP2B6 is also important in the formation of the 3-hydroxy-nevirapine. Nevirapine induces its own rate of metabolism. As treatment continues from a single dose to 2 to 4 weeks of 200 to 400 mg/day dosing, there is up to a twofold increase in systemic clearance. There is a corresponding decrease in the terminal half-life in plasma from 45 hours (after a single dose) to 25 to 30 hours with multiple dosing. Following induction, the pharmacokinetics remain linear in the dose-range 200 to 400 mg/day. The principal route of excretion of the hydroxylated glucuronides (about 80%) is in the urine, with the remainder in the feces. Less than 3% of drug is excreted unchanged in the urine. About 60% of the drug is plasma protein bound.

After a single oral dose given to pregnant women, the median half-life is 61 to 66 hours. Nevirapine crosses the placenta and the half-life of the drug in neonates born to mothers given a single 200 mg dose during labor is 45 to 54 hours[315]. The breast milk concentration of nevirapine is about 75% of that in the maternal serum. Nevirapine penetrates into semen, with a semen to plasma concentration ratio that varies between 0.6 and 1[310].

Mutagenicity, carcinogenicity, and teratogenicity tests

Teratogenicity was not detected in studies performed on rats and rabbits (Boehringer Ingelheim Hospital Division Data Sheet 2000). There do not appear to be any published reports of mutagenesis or carcinogenesis.

Adverse events

Nausea, fatigue, fever, headache, and somnolence may be side effects of nevirapine therapy. One of the most common adverse events is skin rash, developing in about 17% of individuals, usually within 6 weeks of initiation of therapy. Although most rashes are maculopapular and of mild to moderate severity, severe and sometimes life-threatening rashes, including erythema multiforme exudativum and toxic epidermal necrolysis, that require discontinuation of treatment occur in about 7% of cases. When nevirapine is introduced as part of an antiretroviral regimen, it is recommended that the dose should be 200 mg once daily for the first 14 days and, if a rash does not develop within that time, the dose should be increased to 200 mg every 12 hours. The use of steroids to reduce the incidence of rash is ineffective. Abnormalities of plasma glutamyl aminotransferase occur in just under 20% of patients during treatment with nevirapine, and are indicative of enzyme induction. As acute hepatitis and hepatic failure have been described most commonly during the first 2 to 8 weeks of treatment[317], estimation of plasma enzyme tests of liver function should be performed at regular intervals during the initial 8 weeks of therapy, say at 2, 4 and 8 weeks. Occasionally, hepatitis may develop months after the start of treatment[318].

Preparations available

Nevirapine is available as tablets, each containing 200 mg nevirapine anhydrate. The drug may be given with or without food.

Efavirenz

Pharmcokinetics (from DuPont Pharma Data Sheet 2000)

Efavirenz is well absorbed when given orally, the peak plasma concentrations of between 1.6 and 9.1 µM being reached within 5 hours of a single dose of 100 mg to 1600 mg. After multiple dosing, steady-state plasma concentrations are reached in 6 to 7 days. In patients receiving 600 mg daily, the steady-state C_{max} was 12.9 µM and the C_{min} was 5.6 µM, the area under the curve being 184 µM/h. More than 99.5% of absorbed drug is bound to plasma protein, particularly albumin. Efavirenz is metabolized principally by the cytochrome P450 system, the isoenzymes CYP3A4 and CYP2B6 being involved. The principal metabolite is 8-hydroxy efavirenz which subsequently undergoes glucuronidation to form the glucuronide conjugate of 8-hydroxy efavirenz. The metabolites are inactive against HIV-1. Efavirenz induces its own metabolism by inducing the synthesis of the cytochrome P450 enzymes, especially CYP3A. This accounts for the observation that multiple dosing with the drug results in a shorter terminal half-life (40 to 55 hours) compared with the administration of a single dose (52 to 76 hours). Efavirenz can be used in patients with mild to moderate hepatic impairment, but regular monitoring of plasma enzyme tests of liver function is recommended. Individuals with severe liver disease should not be treated with efavirenz. The metabolites of efavirenz are excreted in the urine with less than 1% of unchanged drug being eliminated by the kidneys.

Efavirenz penetrates into the CSF, with levels in that fluid some three times higher than that of the non-bound drug in the plasma. Although it is unknown if efavirenz is secreted in human breast milk, the drug can be found in the milk of lactating rats at concentrations higher than those in the plasma.

Mutagenicity, carcinogenicity, and teratogenicity tests

In conventional genotoxicity studies, efavirenz is not mutagenic or clastogenic.

As malformations have been observed in fetuses or the newborn of cynomolgus monkeys given efavirenz, the drug should not be administered to pregnant women.

Carcinogenicity studies have not yet been completed.

Adverse events

Nausea is common during the first few weeks of initiation of therapy. Central nervous system symptoms are also common, more than half of patients complaining of dizziness, impaired concentration, drowsiness, abnormal dreams, and insomnia. In about 3% of patients, these side effects are sufficiently severe as to necessitate withdrawal of the drug. In general symptoms begin within a few days of initiating therapy and resolve within about 4 weeks. Administration of the drug at bedtime lessens the impact of these features. Skin rash is another adverse event that can be disturbing to patients. Up to about 17% of individuals develop a diffuse maculopapular rash that is noticed a median of 11 days from start of therapy. Treatment discontinuation is not usually necessary, the rash resolving spontaneously in about 14 days. The use of antihistamines and/or corticosteroids may hasten resolution of the rash. In a few patients, there may be vesiculation and desquamation, sometimes with fever; these patients should discontinue treatment with efavirenz.

Elevations of plasma alanine aminotransferase are found in about 2% of patients treated with efavirenz, and in those with dual infection with HIV and hepatitis B or C virus infections, 13% have been noted to have greater than fivefold in the alanine aminotransferase. Abnormal levels of gammaglutamyl transferase are found in 6% of patients treated with efavirenz, and in 11% of those with hepatitis B or C infections.

Preparations available

Efavirenz is available as capsules, each containing 50 mg, 100 mg, or 200 mg of the drug. The drug can be given with or without food.

Delavirdine

This non-nucleoside reverse transcriptase inhibitor is not licensed for use in the UK. It is well absorbed when given orally. It is metabolized through desalkylation catalyzed by CYP3A4 and CYP2D6, and by pyridine hydroxylation by CYP3A4. It is an irreversible inhibitor of CYP3A4, and can partially inhibit other cytochrome P450 isoenzymes[319]. The most common side effect is skin rash, occurring in about 25% of treated patients, the rash may necessitate discontinuation of the drug. Rash often recurs when the patient is re-challenged with delavirdine and about 70% of individuals have cross reactivity with nevirapine[320]. Fatigue, nausea, headache, and diarrhea may also occur.

Protease inhibitors

The characteristics of drugs of this class when administered alone (with the exception of lopinavir) are presented below.

However, advantage can be taken of the drug interactions associated with these drugs. Treatment regimens can include two protease inhibitors, one as an antiviral agent and the other, usually ritonavir, as an inhibitor of the cytochrome P450 isoenzymes involved in the metabolism of these agents. Drug interactions are discussed further on pp. 193–194.

Nelfinavir

Pharmacokinetics (mostly from Roche Products Ltd Data Sheet 2000).

Nelfinavir is well absorbed when given by mouth, the oral bioavailability exceeding 78%. The peak plasma concentrations and AUC are some two to threefold higher when nelfinavir is given with food compared with when given in the fasting state. The C_{max} values after multiple dosing of 750 mg every 8 hours with food average between 3 to 4 μg/mL, and are achieved 2 to 4 hours after the dose. The steady state C_{min} before the next dose of nelfinavir varies between 1 to 3 μg/mL. In serum, nelfinavir is highly protein bound (over 98%). There is extensive tissue penetration but data on CNS penetration are unavailable. It is unknown if nelfinavir crosses the human placenta. Although there are no available human data, nelfinavir is secreted in the milk of lactating rats. The cytochrome P450 enzyme system, including the isoenzymes CYP3A4 and CYP2C19, is involved in the metabolism of nelfinavir into one major metabolite (M8) that has antiviral activity equal to that of the parent drug, and into several minor metabolites. In steady-state studies, the terminal half-life is between 3.5 and 5 hours. Excretion of the drug and its metabolites is chiefly in the feces, with only 1% to 2% of the unchanged drug being excreted in the urine. In moderate to severe liver disease, there may be acquired CYP2C19 deficiency, resulting in decreased M8 formation; as a consequence, low dose nelfinavir dosage may be effective in such patients[321].

Mutagenicity, carcinogenicity, and teratogenicity tests

In vitro and in vivo tests have shown that nelfinavir, with or without metabolic activation, is not associated with mutagenicity or genotoxicity. Data on carcinogenicity are currently unavailable. Teratogenicity has not been observed.

Adverse events

Diarrhea is the most common side effect, affecting about one-quarter of patients treated with nelfinavir. The metabolic effects of the protease inhibitors are discussed on page 192.

Preparations available

Nelfinavir is available as tablets, each containing 292.25 mg nelfinavir mesylate corresponding to 250 mg nelfinavir as free base. The tablets are given orally and should be ingested with food. An oral powder, containing 58.45 mg/g of the mesylate, corresponding to 50 mg/g of nelfinavir as free base, is also available. The powder is mixed with water or milk, but not with acidic food or juice as this causes a bad taste.

Indinavir

Pharmacokinetics (mostly from Merck Sharp & Dome Data Sheet 2000)

When given by mouth, indinavir is well absorbed, the oral bioavailability of an 800 mg dose being in the order of 65%. Administration with a meal high in fat, calories, and protein reduces absorption, resulting in an 80% reduction in the AUC and an 86% reduction in the C_{max}. After a single 800 mg dose given in the fasting state, the C_{max} is 7.7 μg/mL, this concentration being reached after 0.8 ± 0.3 hours. Protein binding is in the order of 60% to 65%. During multiple dosing, the CSF concentration of indinavir 2 to 4 hours after a dose varies between 0.1 and 0.14 μM/L[322]. Co-administration of a small dose of ritonavir results in an increased CSF concentration of indinavir, possibly through inhibition of P-glycoprotein[323]. The concentration of indinavir in semen is high, and similar to that in plasma[310]; as with its effect on CSF concentrations, the addition of ritonavir to the treatment regimen increases the concentration of indinavir in the semen[323].

Indinavir is metabolized by the cytochrome P450 enzyme system, particularly the CYP3A4 isoenzyme, and is an inhibitor of this system. The metabolites are not active against HIV-1. Indinavir is mostly cleared by hepatic metabolism, less than 20% of the dose is excreted in the urine; about 10% to 12% is excreted as unchanged drug. The terminal half-life is short (1.8 ± 0.4 hours). In the presence of moderate hepatic insufficiency, there is an increase of up to 60% in the AUC, and the mean half-life is increased to about 2.8 hours. Dose reduction to 600 mg every 8 hours is therefore necessary. It is not known if indinavir crosses the human placenta or if it is found in breast milk. In lactating rats, however, the drug is found in the milk.

Mutagenicity, carcinogenicity, and teratogenicity tests

In standard tests indinavir does not have mutagenic or genotoxic effects. Carcinogenicity has not been noticed in mice, although an increased incidence of thyroid adenomas has been observed in rats given similar doses. There is also no evidence of teratogenicity.

Adverse events

Nausea, diarrhea, abdominal pain, and taste perversion have been described. Dry skin, skin rash, and pruritus may also occur. Nephrolithiasis, resulting from crystallization of indinavir in the urine, occurs in about 4% of individuals. The symptoms are loin pain with or without hematuria; occasionally acute renal failure, reversible on discontinuation of the drug, has been reported. Discontinuation of indinavir and adequate hydration usually results in resolution of nephrolithiasis. A fluid intake of at least 1.5 L/day is recommended for patients receiving indinavir to reduce the risk of nephrolithiasis. Anaphylactoid reactions are rare, and hemolytic anemia is an unusual complication of indinavir therapy. Hyperbilirubinemia is a not infrequent finding in routine laboratory tests. The metabolic complications of protease inhibitor therapy and drug interactions are discussed on pp. 192 and 194.

Preparations available

Indinavir is available as capsules, each containing 200 mg or 400 mg of the drug

as indinavir sulfate. The drug should be taken without food or 2 hours after a meal. Alternatively, indinavir can be taken with a light, low-fat meal. These dietary restrictions are unnecessary when indinavir is given with ritonavir.

Ritonavir

Pharmacokinetics (mostly from Abbott Laboratories Ltd Data Sheet 2000)

The oral bioavailability of ritonavir has been estimated at between 66% and 75%. Administration of food with ritonavir capsules increases absorption by about 15%, but there is a 7% reduction in absorption when the liquid formulation is given with a meal. In individuals who have been given ritonavir 600 mg twice daily for several weeks, the steady-state C_{max} and C_{min} are 11.2 ± 3.6, and 3.7 ± 2.6 µg/mL respectively; C_{max} is reached between 2 and 4 hours. The terminal half-life is 3 to 5 hours. Plasma protein-binding to α_1-acid glycoprotein is high (98% to 99%). There is little penetration into the CSF or into semen. It is unknown if ritonavir is secreted in breast milk. The drug is metabolized by oxidative metabolism primarily by the CYP3A4 isoenzyme of cytochrome P450 in the liver. There are four metabolites, one of which has antiviral activity similar to that of the parent drug, although the AUC is less than 3% of the latter. Over 85% of the dose is excreted in the feces as metabolites or unchanged ritonavir. Ritonavir is a substrate of the cytochrome P450 enzyme system and also acts as an inhibitor. It can also induce CYP3A4, and indeed can induce its own metabolism. This is shown by the reduction by some two to threefold in steady-state trough plasma concentrations during the first 2 weeks of initiation of therapy. As the drug is metabolized in the liver, caution should be exercised in its administration to individuals with mild to moderate hepatic impairment, and should be avoided in those with severe disease.

Mutagenicity, carcinogenicity, and teratogenicity tests

In the standard tests, ritonavir has not been found to be mutagenic or genotoxic. Long-term carcinogenicity studies are not yet complete. High doses of ritonavir given to pregnant rats has led to embryo death,

decreased litter size, decreased fetal weight, and visceral abnormalities such as delayed testicular descent. Similar changes were noted in treated rabbits. Ritonavir should only be used in pregnancy if the advantages of treatment outweigh any likely adverse effect on the fetus.

Adverse events

Nausea, diarrhea, vomiting, dyspepsia, abdominal pain, and taste perversion are the most common side effects. Circumoral paraesthesiae occur in about one-quarter of patients given standard doses of ritonavir, and peripheral paraesthesiae is also common. Skin rash is frequent but generally mild. Elevation of plasma levels of alanine aminotransferase and gamma glutamyl transferase may occur, and some patients develop clinical hepatitis. The association of protease inhibitors with lipodystrophy, and their drug–drug interactions are discussed on pp. 192 and 194.

Preparations available

Ritonavir is available as capsules, each containing 100 mg of the drug. An oral solution, containing 80 mg/mL is also available. It should be ingested with food.

Saquinavir

Saquinavir was originally available as a hard capsule, the bioavailability was low and a gel-filled capsule that had better pharmacodynamic properties was introduced.

Pharmacokinetics (Roche Products Ltd Data Sheet 2000[324])

Absorption of saquinavir, when given orally as the hard capsule preparation, is poor, the oral bioavailability being less than 4%. Administration of hard capsule saquinavir with a meal, however, increases absorption by almost 700%. The soft capsule preparation of saquinavir is better absorbed, although the oral bioavailability is presently unknown. After the administration of soft capsule saquinavir to individuals who had received the drug in an oral dosage of 1200 mg every 8 hours for 3 weeks, the mean C_{max} (21.8 µg/mL), the C_{min} (2.2 µg/mL) and the AUC (72.5 µg h^{-1} mL^{-1}) are significantly higher than those obtained with hard capsule saquinavir (2 μg/mL, 0.8 μg/mL, and 8.7 μg/mL respectively). There is extensive protein binding in the plasma (more than 98%), and saquinavir does not penetrate well into the CSF. The effects of saquinavir in pregnant women are unknown, and there are no data on the secretion of the drug into breast milk. Saquinavir does not appear to penetrate well into semen[325]. Saquinavir is metabolized by the cytochrome P450 CYP3A4 isoenzyme into a variety of mono- and dihydroxylated metabolites that have little antiviral activity. Less than 1% of the dose is excreted in the urine. After administration of the hard capsule preparation, the plasma half-life is 1.1 to 1.9 hours.

Mutagenicity, carcinogenicity, and teratogenicity tests

In standard tests, saquinavir does not have mutagenic or genotoxic effects. Results of carcinogenicity experiments are awaited. Teratogenic effects have not been observed when saquinavir has been given to pregnant rats or rabbits.

Adverse events

The most common side effects are diarrhea, nausea, and abdominal discomfort. Peripheral neuropathy has been described in patients who have received hard capsule saquinavir, and the occurrence of headache and dizziness have been reported. Skin rashes occur occasionally, but serious dermatological adverse events such as erythema multiforme exudativum are rare. Buccal and mucosal ulceration have also been reported in the absence of skin rash. Increased plasma alanine aminotransferase levels and/or gammaglutamyl transferase concentrations have been reported in about 5% of patients.

Preparations available

Saquinavir gel-filled capsules (Fortovase®, Roche Products Ltd) are available, each capsule containing 200 mg saquinavir as free base. The drug is also available as hard capsules (Invirase®, Roche Products Ltd), each containing saquinavir mesylate equivalent to 200 mg saquinavir. When given as the only protease inhibitor in a regimen, each preparation should be taken within 2 hours of a meal.

Amprenavir

Pharmacokinetics (Glaxo Wellcome Data Sheet 2000)

Amprenavir is well absorbed when given orally, and has an estimated oral bioavailability of more than 90%. The mean time to C_{max} is between 1 and 2 hours after administration of the capsule, and 0.5 to 1 hour for the oral solution. After multiple dosing, the mean steady-state C_{max} is 5.36 μg/mL and the C_{min} is 0.28 μg/mL. Although the AUC is reduced by about 25% when the drug is given with food, the C_{min} is unaffected. Amprenavir penetrates well into tissues, although the CSF concentration is less than 1% of that in the plasma. Although amprenavir is secreted in breast milk of lactating rats, it is unknown if it is secreted into human milk. Plasma protein binding primarily to α_1-acid glycoprotein and albumin is about 90%, drug interactions from plasma-binding protein displacement have not been observed. Amprenavir is metabolized principally in the liver by the CYP3A4 isoenzyme of cytochrome P450, of which the drug is an inhibitor. Unchanged amprenavir and its metabolites in feces account for about 75% of the dose, and in urine for about 14%. As the liver is the principal site of metabolism, dose modification is necessary in those with moderate to severe hepatic impairment.

Mutagenicity, carcinogenicity, and teratogenicity tests

Amprenavir has not been found to be mutagenic or hepatotoxic in standard tests. Carcinogenicity studies have not yet been completed. When amprenavir has been given to pregnant mice and rats, minor skeletal abnormalities and thymic elongation has been noted; treatment of pregnant women, therefore, is not recommended.

Adverse events

Most side effects are mild or moderate in severity. The most common are nausea, vomiting, diarrhea, and abdominal discomfort. Erythematous or maculopapular rashes occur in just under 20% of patients, and usually appear within 2 weeks of initiation of therapy. The rash usually resolves spontaneously within 2 weeks. Erythema multiforme exudativum is a rare complication. Headache may occur, and oral or perioral parasthesiae develop in up to 2% of patients. Elevated levels of alanine aminotransferase has been reported in about 5% individuals with concurrent hepatitis B or C virus infections.

Preparations available

Amprenavir is available as soft capsules, each containing 150 mg amprenavir. The dose can be taken with or without food. Antacids, however, may impair absorption. It is also available as an oral solution.

Lopinavir with ritonavir

Lopinavir is a protease inhibitor that has recently been introduced into clinical practice. It is given in a preparation that contains a small dose of ritonavir that by its inhibition of CYP3A, responsible for most of the metabolism of lopinavir, leads to high C_{max} and AUC.

Pharmacokinetics (Abbott Laboratories Ltd Data Sheet 2001)

After the oral administration of lopinavir/ritonavir (400 mg/100 mg) to individuals who have had twice daily doses of the drug for 3 to 4 weeks, the C_{max} of 9.6 ± 4.4 μg/mL is achieved about 4 hours after dosing. The mean steady-state C_{min} just before the morning dose of drug is 5.5 ± 4.0 μg/mL. The absolute oral bioavailability of lopinavir/ritonavir is currently unknown. Administration of lopinavir/ritonavir capsules with a moderate fat meal increases the C_{max} and the AUC by 23% and 48% respectively, the corresponding increases after administration of lopinavir/ritonavir oral solution being 54% and 80% respectively. Therefore, it is recommended that liponavir/ritonavir is taken with a meal. Lopinavir is highly protein bound (98% to 99%) to plasma proteins, primarily α_1-acid glycoprotein. Although lopinavir is secreted in the milk of lactating rats, data in humans are unavailable. Lopinavir undergoes oxidative metabolism in the liver to at least thirteen metabolites, two of which have antiviral activity, although they are present in small concentrations in the plasma. Lopinavir is metabolized almost exclusively by the CYP3A isoenzyme of the cytochrome P450 system. Because the liver is the main site of metabolism lopinavir/

ritonavir should be used cautiously in those with mild to moderate hepatic insufficiency, and should be avoided in patients with severe hepatic impairment. More than 80% of the dose of lopinavir is excreted in the feces, and about 10% in urine; after multiple dosing only 3% of lopinavir is found unchanged in the urine. Dose adjustment is unnecessary in patients with renal impairment.

Mutagenicity, carcinogenicity, and teratogenicity tests

Lopinavir/ritonavir has not been found to be mutagenic or clastogenic in *in vitro* or *in vivo* tests, including the Ames bacterial reverse mutation assay, the mouse lymphoma assay, the mouse micronucleus test and chromosomal aberration assays in human lymphocytes. Carcinogenicity tests have not been completed. In rats, pregnancy loss, decreased fetal body weights, and skeletal abnormalities have been observed. Use of the drug should therefore be avoided in pregnancy unless there is no alternative therapy.

Adverse events

Diarrhea, of mild to moderate severity, is the most common side effect, affecting just under 15% of patients. Less common unwanted effects include nausea, vomiting, abdominal pain, and headache. Pancreatitis has been reported rarely. Lipodystrophy as a complication of protease inhibitor therapy, and drug interactions with this class of drug are considered on pp. 192 and 194.

Preparations available

Lopinavir/ritonavir is available as soft capsules, each containing 133.3 mg of lopinavir and 33.3 mg of ritonavir. An oral solution is also available. The drug is given with food.

Nucleotide reverse transcriptase inhibitor

Tenofovir disoproxil fumarate

Tenofovir disoproxil fumarate is the prodrug of tenofovir, a nucleotide analog reverse transcriptase inhibitor. The terminal half-life of intravenous tenofovir varies between 4

and 8 hours, and the prodrug can be given by mouth in a single daily dose. Unlike adefovir, another nucleotide analog reverse transcriptase inhibitor, the risk of nephrotoxicity appears to be low. In combination with other antiretroviral agents, it has proved effective by producing significant and sustained decreases in plasma viral RNA compared with placebo[328]. Tenofovir is active against strains of HIV that have the more common resistance patterns for zidovudine and lamivudine, and, uniquely, against multinucleoside resistant HIV expressing Q151M mutation. There is, however, cross-resistance to T69S insertions[329]. Further studies on its efficacy and safety are awaited.

Other drugs

Hydroxyurea

Hydroxyurea has been used as a supplement to antiretroviral therapy. The drug inhibits ribonucleotide reductase, a cellular enzyme that is the rate-limiting step in the production of deoxynucleoside triphosphates (dNTPs)[330]. HIV can only replicate in replicating cells, and by diminishing the pool of dNTPs through the action of hydroxyurea, viral replication is inhibited. The antiviral action adenosine analogs such as didanosine is potentiated because the reduction in intracellular concentrations of dNTPs increases the chances of incorporation of nucleoside analog reverse transcriptase inhibitors into the growing viral DNA. Hydroxyurea also compensates for resistance to didanosine because, as the endogenous dNTP is depleted, NRTIs will still be incorporated into viruses that harbor mutations.

Hydroxyurea is well absorbed from the gastrointestinal tract, peak concentrations being achieved in 2 hours. More than 80% of the administered dose is excreted in the urine. As the drug is mutagenic, and teratogenicity has been observed, hydroxyurea should not be used in pregnancy. It is also secreted in breast milk and should not be administered to lactating women.

There are dose-related adverse effects on the bone marrow, with the possible development of leukopenia, thrombocytopenia, and anemia. These effects are

reversible on discontinuing therapy. Peripheral neuropathy as a side effect has been reported, most commonly in patients receiving combination therapy that has included didanosine.

Hydroxyurea is available as capsules, each containing 500 mg of the drug.

Mycophenolic acid

By selectively inhibiting inosine monophosphate dehydrogenase that converts inosine monophosphate to guanosine monophosphate, mycophenolic acid inhibits the *de novo* synthesis of guanine nucleotides in lymphocytes. The depletion of the intracellular pool of guanine nucleotides results in apoptosis of a large proportion of activated CD4+ T cells[331]. *In vitro*, the combination of abacavir and mycophenolic acid inhibits synergistically HIV-1 replication in stimulated peripheral mononuclear cells[332]. Strains of HIV-1 that encode the M184V mutation appear to be sensitive to this combination of drugs. Mycophenolic acid and didanosine also act synergistically, but stavudine and zidovudine are antagonistic. The ester derivative of mycophenolic acid, mycophenolate mophetil, can be given orally, and preliminary studies have shown that treatment of patients already receiving antiretroviral therapy with this drug results in a reduction in the number of dividing CD4+ and CD8+ T cells, and in the inhibition of virus isolation from CD4+ T cells[331]. The place of this agent as an adjuvant to combination antiretroviral therapy remains to be established.

Tables 7.4 to 7.6 show the most commonly used dosage regimens for available antiretroviral drugs. Tenofovir disoproxil is given in a single daily dose of 300 mg by mouth with food.

EFFICACY OF ANTIRETROVIRAL REGIMENS

In the initial years of the epidemic, death was an almost invariable outcome for patients with HIV disease. The early trials of antiretroviral drugs such as zidovudine concentrated on patients with the most advanced disease, in whom development of clinical endpoints such as death and/or new opportunistic infections could be

Table 7.4 Nucleoside analog reverse transcriptase inhibitors

Drug	Dose
Zidovudine (AZT)[a]	250–300 mg every 12 hours by mouth
Stavudine (D4T)	40 mg every 12 hours by mouth if weight is > 60 kg, or 30 mg every 12 hours if weight is < 60 kg
Didanosine (DDI)	400 mg capsule as a single oral dose once daily on an empty stomach if weight is > 60 kg or 250 mg once daily if weight is < 60 kg
Lamivudine (3TC)[a]	150 mg every 12 hours by mouth
Zalcitabine	0.75 mg every 8 hours by mouth
Abacavir[a]	300 mg every 12 hours by mouth

[a] Also available in combinations of zidovudine/lamivudine and zidovudine/lamivudine/abacavir – both one tablet every 12 hours by mouth.

compared quickly between the active and placebo arms[333].

Although these endpoints remain valid for patients with low CD4+ T-cell counts, trials involving patients with relatively well-preserved immune function will take many years to demonstrate significant differences in clinical endpoints when comparing two antiretroviral regimens. For that reason, surrogate markers in the form of decline in plasma HIV RNA (viral load) and rise in CD4+ T-cell count are regarded as favorable outcomes in determining the efficacy of specific antiretroviral drugs or regimens. It is anticipated that clinical benefits including longer life expectancy will follow for regimens introduced within the last few years[334].

Goals of therapy

Benefit from a drop in viral load was demonstrated in the Delta study[335], but it was soon recognized that partial reduction in the viral load was temporary in most patients as resistant mutants of HIV emerged. Since then increasingly rigorous falls in viral load have been sought. Studies show that for patients whose viral load fell to below 400 copies/mL but remained detectable, viral rebound was much more likely than if the viral load was less than 20 to 50 copies/mL[336, 337]. As assays with a lower limit of detection of 20 copies/mL are not available in routine clinical practice, the main goal has been to achieve a viral load of less than 50 copies/mL. This is usually achieved by 12 weeks after the introduction of HAART, although occasionally it may take up to 24 weeks.

A second goal of therapy is to achieve an increase in the CD4+ T-lymphocyte count. This is more likely to be achieved in patients with a pre-treatment CD4+ T-cell nadir of more than 200 cells/mm3[338] than in patients with severe depletion of CD4+ T cells (less than 50 cells/mL), in whom a rise in CD4+ T-cell count is less predictable. A significant reduction in the incidence of opportunistic infections is seen if the CD4+ T-cell count rises above 50/mm3[339, 340].

The increase in CD4+ T-cell count after introduction of HAART is biphasic[341]. The first phase, which is observed within the first 8 weeks of treatment, may represent release and redistribution of CD4+ memory T cells from lymphoid follicles. The second phase is characterized by a slower increase in CD4+ T cells, and probably represents thymic production of naïve CD4+ T cells. During this period, there is an increase in the numbers of CD4+ naïve and CD8+ naïve T cells, memory CD4+ T cells stabilize, and CD8+ T cells decrease in numbers in the peripheral blood[341].

Table 7.5 Non-nucleoside reverse transcriptase inhibitors

Drug	Dose
Efavirenz	600 mg once daily by mouth as a single dose (usually at bedtime)
Nevirapine	200 mg every 12 hours by mouth (once daily for the first 14 days)
Delavirdine	400 mg every 8 hours by mouth

Table 7.6 Protease inhibitors

Drug	Dose
Indinavir	800 mg every 8 hours by mouth on an empty stomach. Fluid intake should exceed 1.5 liters of fluid/day
Nelfinavir	750 mg every 8 hours, or 1250 mg every 12 hours, by mouth
Ritonavir	600 mg every 12 hours by mouth
Saquinavir soft gel capsule (SGC)	1200 mg every 8 hours by mouth
Amprenavir	1200 mg every 12 hours by mouth
Lopinavir/ritonavir	Three capsules (total dose lopinavir 400 mg and ritonavir 100 mg) every 12 hours

There is considerable variation in the CD4[+] T-cell response to antiretroviral therapy. In patients who have a high baseline viral load, and a rapid decline in the CD4[+] T-cell count before treatment, there is likely to be a higher rate of increase in the CD4[+] T-cell count in the peripheral blood than amongst those with a lower pre-treatment viral load and slower decline in cell numbers[341]. The biphasic increase in circulating CD4[+] T cells may not be observed. In some patients there may be no, or only a modest, increase in these cells, despite viral suppression[341]. The place of IL-2 in the treatment of such patients is currently being explored (see page 195).

Although there may be sufficient immune function to protect against opportunistic infections in patients treated during the late stages of HIV infection, the CD4[+] T-cell count and function of these cells is often abnormal[341]. It is as yet uncertain if continued antiretroviral therapy will eventually restore T-cell function in these patients. Notwithstanding, there is growing evidence of improvement in immune function after the introduction of effective antiretroviral therapy. Spontaneous improvement may be seen in previously poorly controlled infections such as molluscum contagiosum, cryptosporidiosis, *M. avium intracellulare* infection, and progressive multifocal leukoencephalopathy. Spontaneous regression of Kaposi's sarcoma has also been described.

It is therefore possible to discontinue prophylaxis against

1. *P. carinii* in patients who maintain CD4[+] T-cell counts above 200/mm[3] for at least 3 months[342]
2. *M. avium* complex in patients who maintain the CD4[+] T-cell count above 100/mm[3] for 3 to 6 months
3. CMV in patients who maintain the CD4[+] T-cell count above 100/mm[3] for 3 months[343].

Unfortunately, HIV-specific immunity does not appear to regenerate in response to viral suppression in those whose therapy is commenced in established HIV infection. However, treatment of primary HIV infection may allow preservation of HIV cytotoxic T-cell activity, with control of viral replication even after antiretroviral therapy is discontinued.

TREATMENT REGIMENS

The options for combining the various antiretroviral drugs in such a way as to reduce viral load to undetectable levels are shown in Table 7.7 (BHIVA draft guidelines at www.aidsmap.com).

Indications for starting antiretroviral therapy

Acute seroconversion illness

Antiretroviral therapy should be considered in the treatment of ASI. The early use of HAART during primary infection preserves HIV-specific CD8[+] T cells physically and functionally while HIV-specific T-cell help is sustained; such effects are not seen when

Table 7.7 Antiretroviral treatment regimens (British HIV Association 2001[427])

Regimen	Advantages	Disadvantages
2NRTIs + PI[a]	1. randomized clinical trial evidence with clinical endpoints 2. evidence of efficacy in late disease 3. long-term follow-up	1. toxicity common 2. high pill burden 3. drug interactions
2NRTIs + 2PIs[b]	1. easier adherence 2. better PK 3. evidence of improved efficacy for lopinavir/ritonavir when compared to nelfinavir	1. no clinical endpoint data 2. possible increased toxicity and drug interactions
2NRTIs + NNRTI	1. equivalent in surrogate marker trials when compared to PI based regimens 2. easier adherence	1. no clinical endpoint data 2. shorter follow up 3. single mutations may lead to cross-class resistance
3NRTIs	1. useful if there are concerns about adherence 2. fewer drug interactions 3. low pill burden	1. no clinical endpoint data 2. short-term surrogate only marker data 3. may be less effective at high viral load

[a] Hard-gel saquinavir should not be used as the sole PI. There are fewer data concerning use of saquinavir soft-gel in this context than for other PIs.

[b] Combinations of PIs in clinical use are ritonavir/saquinavir, ritonavir/indinavir, and ritonavir/lopinavir. These have advantages over agents used alone in terms of improved pharmacokinetics (PK), with higher trough levels and reduced fluctuations in plasma concentration over time. This allows lower doses to be taken at longer intervals, i.e. twice instead of three times a day, and without dietary restrictions, this should assist adherence. The additive or synergistic antiviral effects of PIs in combination may improve potency compared with regimens including a single PI. Possible disadvantages of combining PIs are an increased risk of lipodystrophy and severe lipid abnormalities. Unfavorable PK interactions between the PIs or with other drugs may necessitate drug dosage modification. In addition, the interation between PIs and other agents may result in toxic concentrations of the latter; an example is the combination of ritonavir and rifabutin.

therapy is delayed[344]. The successful control of HIV by the immune system has been shown in a recent study[345]: 8 patients who were treated with HAART during acute infection had complete suppression of plasma viremia, and developed HIV-1-specific T-helper cell responses. After one or two interruptions of HAART, 5 of 8 patients remained off therapy with viral loads that were less than 500 copies/mL after a median 6.5 months (range 5 to 8.7 months). Virus-specific cytotoxic T-cell responses increased significantly both quantitatively and qualitatively with respect to broadening of the repertoire of targeted epitopes.

The role of drugs that are known to inhibit CD4+ activation, such as hydroxy-urea[346] and cyclosporin A[347], in the suppression of viral replication and boosting of CD4+ lymphocyte responses in this setting is unclear, and requires further evaluation. Interleukin-2 therapy has also been used and has resulted in higher CD4+ cell counts than in those who did not receive IL-2[348].

As the optimal antiretroviral regimen for primary HIV infection has not been elucidated, patients should be entered into a clinical trial if possible.

Chronic infection

Asymptomatic patients

Once HIV infection is established, the possibility of restoring HIV-specific immune control by ART alone appears to be lost. The timing of introduction of ART is therefore based on a careful consideration of the advantages and disadvantages for each individual patient. Arguments in favor of early introduction of ART generally relate to the prevention of loss of the full immune repertoire, and an inability to restore any gaps following therapy. Control of viral replication by ART may also decrease the risk of evolution of drug-resistant virus. From a broader public health perspective there may be a decreased risk of transmission of infection to others.

Arguments against early introduction of ART highlight the toxicity of currently available drugs, the interference with daily living in taking regular medication, unknown duration of efficacy of current antiretroviral therapy, and the risk of limited future choices of antiretroviral agents if resistance occurs. Of greatest relevance may be the paucity of evidence to indicate any benefit of starting ART before the CD4+ T-cell count falls to 200 cells/mm³ [349, 350]. As there is evidence of adverse clinical outcome and impaired response to ART if the CD4+ cell count falls to below 200 cells/mm³ [338, 351], the optimal time to start ART is likely to be at a CD4+ T-cell count of approximately 250 to 300 cells/mm³.

Table 7.8 indicates the BHIVA recommendations[427] for the management of HIV-infected symptomless patients. Broadly similar guidelines have been produced in the USA by the Panel on Clinical Practices for the Treatment of HIV Infection (2001) (www.hivatis.org).

Symptomatic patients

The onset of symptoms is a clear indicator of the need for introduction of ART. Minor opportunistic infections tend to be followed by more severe infections, and treatment is therefore indicated to alleviate early symptoms and to prevent the development of more serious infections or cancers

Management strategy

Before starting ART, all patients should receive education about the importance of adherence to therapy, and literature relating to the specific drugs they will be taking.

Ongoing support with adherence is essential for patients, within clinics and in the community, as wastage of antiretroviral regimens is costly both in terms of patients' health and financially to health care systems. Patients should be reviewed 2 weeks after initiation of therapy to check for adverse effects of drugs in the regimen. Peripheral blood CD4+ cell count and viral load measurement are usually carried out 4 weeks after commencing ART. If viral load has fallen as expected (about 1 log$_{10}$/10 days) and there are no adverse effects, the regimen should be left unchanged. If the viral load has not fallen appropriately adherence should be checked. A resistance assay for possible pre-existing resistance mutations should be considered, with modification of ART accordingly.

Twelve to 16 weeks after initiation of ART, the CD4+ T-cell count and viral load should be repeated using an ultra-sensitive assay with a cut off of less than 50 copies/mL. If the viral load is undetectable, and there are no side effects, the regimen should be continued. If the viral load remains detectable but less than 2000 copies/mL, the ART should be modified, either by intensification (addition of a fourth drug) or substitution of one or more drugs depending upon the initial regimen. For a viral load greater than 2000 copies/mL, a resistance test should be performed

VIRAL RESISTANCE TESTING

HIV reverse transcriptase lacks a 39 to 59 exonuclease activity or 'proofreading' ability. As a result, spontaneous mutations that occur regularly are not corrected[352]. An average of one mutation occurs during each replication cycle, creating a huge pool of variants called quasispecies. Most of these mutations result in defective or non-functional virions, but some retain enough replicative capacity to be able to survive. The dominant (wild-type) virus will be the strain that has the most efficient replicative capacity, a concept referred to as 'viral

Table 7.8 Recommendations for management of symptomless HIV-infected patients (British HIV Association 2001[427])

CD4+ T-cell count (cells/mm³ or/mL)	Plasma viral load (copies/mL)	Recommendation
500	Any	Defer treatment
350–500	< 30 000	Defer treatment
350–500	> 30 000	Consider treatment or defer and monitor at least 3 monthly
0–350	Any	Offer treatment

Table 7.9 Mutations associated with resistance to nucleoside analog reverse transcriptase inhibitors

	41	65	67	69*	70	74	75	115	151	184	210	215	219
AZT	41		67	69*	70				151		210	215	219
3TC				69*					151	184			
DDI		65		69*		74			151	184			
DDC		65		69*		74			151	184			
D4T	41		67	69*	70		75		151		210	215	219
ABC		65		69*		74		115	151	184			

AZT = zidovudine; 3TC = lamivudine; DDI = didanosine; DDC = zalcitabine;
D4T = stavudine; ABC = abacavir.
Multiple AZT mutations predict ABC failure.
69* = 69SS insertion, which along with other RT-mutations leads to cross resistance for the class and is difficult to identify in genotypic testing.
151 = leads to cross-resistance to NRTI class when present along with 3 or more mutations.

fitness'. By chance, some mutations will confer resistance to antiretroviral drugs. When these drugs are prescribed, selection pressure will render the resistant strains 'more fit' than wild-type virus and the dominant strain will change.

The principal mutations associated with resistance to antiretroviral drugs are shown in Tables 7.9 to 7.11.

There are two methods of testing for drug resistance

1. *genotypic* tests that look for specific mutations in the reverse transcriptase or protease genes that have been linked to resistance to anti-HIV drugs

2. *phenotypic* tests that measure the concentration of a drug required to reduce viral replication by either 50% or 90% (IC$_{50}$ or IC$_{90}$).

Both methods have the disadvantage of only reliably identifying major quasispecies, that is, those that account for approximately 20% or more of the specimen. Archived mutants selected by any previous antiretroviral therapies are likely to go unrecognized.

Genotypic tests are quicker and cheaper than phenotypic tests but only provide an indirect measure of resistance. They require complex interpretation, may be insensitive to some HIV subtypes, for example non-clade B, and are unreliable at viral load levels below 2000 copies/mL or difficult to perform.

Phenotypic tests directly measure the sensitivity of the virus to a drug and they are relatively easy to interpret. The disadvantages are that they take 2 to 3 weeks to perform and they are more expensive. None the less, a number of prospective clinical trials have shown improved treatment outcomes following genotypic[353, 354] or phenotypic[355, 356] assays.

Indications for resistance studies[357]

Acute seroconversion illness, because of the narrow repertoire of HIV quasispecies at ASI, any resistant mutant transmitted is likely to be detected easily by genotypic testing. Therefore resistance testing is advised. In chronic, untreated infection, resistant mutants are likely to be submerged by wild-type virus. These mutants only become dominant, and therefore detectable on testing, when there is the selection pressure of ART. Any patient with a viral load in excess of 2000 copies/mL, in whom treatment modification is planned, should have a resistance test. This is particularly important in situations where others are affected, for example pregnancy, where optimal control reduces risk of transmission to the child, or following percutaneous exposure in a health care worker to whom post-exposure prophylaxis is to be administered.

Table 7.10 Mutations associated with resistance to non-nucleoside analog reverse transcriptase inhibitors

	100	103	106	108	179	181	188	190	225	236
EFV	100	103		108	179	181	188	190	225	
NVP	100	103	106	108		181	188	190		
DLV		103				181			225	236

EFV = efavirenz; NVP = nevirapine; DLV = delavirdine.

Table 7.11 Mutations associated with resistance to protease inhibitors

	10	20	24	30	32	33	46	47	48	50	54	73	77	82	84	88	90	150*
IDV	10	20	24		32		46				54	73		82	84		90	
RTV	10	20			32	33	46				54			82	84		90	
SQV	10	20							48		54	73		82	84		90	
NFV	10			30			46						77	82	84	88	90	
APV	10						46	47		50	54			82	84			150*
LPV	10	20	24				46			50	54			82	84		90	

IDV = indinavir; RTV = ritonavir; SQV = saquinavir; NFV = nelfinavir; APV = amprenavir; LPV = lopinavir.
Primary mutations are 30, 48, 54, 82, 84, 90. Resistance to all PIs is likely if two or more of these mutations are present.
*Primary mutation for amprenavir is 150.

'BLIPPERS'

Once the plasma viral load has fallen to less than 50 copies/mL, it will usually remain undetectable as long as there is good adherence to the antiretroviral regime. Some patients experience transient rises, 'blips', in viral load of several hundred copies/mL. In one study[358] viral load blips to more than 50 copies/mL occurred in 40% of 241 patients on triple antiretroviral therapy, and 10% experienced more than one episode. It is not clear if these blips reflect temporary non-adherence to the antiretroviral regime, or a failure of that particular regimen to suppress viral replication completely. Havlir *et al.*[358] noted that baseline viral load and the time taken to achieve a viral load of less than 200 copies/mL were predictors of blips. Ongoing viral replication can be recognized by finding unintegrated copies of DNA forming circles with two copies of the long terminal repeat (2-LTR circles). These are unstable structures that are lost from cells within days; thus their detection indicates recent viral turnover[359]. The detection of multiply spliced HIV-1 mRNA is also indicative of ongoing viral replication. Treatment should not be altered on the basis of a single blip, as in the majority of cases viral load will return to undetectable levels. For example, in the study reported by Havlir *et al.*[358], only nine of 96 blippers experienced viral load rebound (more than 200 copies/mL). Repeatedly detectable viral load (more than 50 copies/mL), however, should lead to consideration of ART modification.

CHANGING ANTIRETROVIRAL TREATMENT

The new combination will depend on previous drug history and the current test results, especially if a resistance study has been performed. Ideally the whole regimen should be changed if there is treatment failure, although this may be difficult in heavily pre-treated patients. A single drug change or addition should not normally be made to a failing regimen.

Because of cross-resistance within NNRTIs in particular, and to a lesser extent within PIs, it is probably safer to switch this part of the combination, even if there is no evidence of resistance. Therefore, if an NNRTI-based triple combination was prescribed, any new regimen is likely to include three (or possibly four) new drugs including one or two PIs. If a protease-based combination has been used, then a change to three new drugs including an NNRTI is likely.

Sometimes, if a protease-based combination is changed early enough, the regimen can be changed to include two new protease inhibitors (one of which will probably be ritonavir as pharmacokinetic enhancer – see page 193) in a four-drug combination. Drugs such as hydroxyurea and mycophenolate may have a role in boosting the antiretroviral effect of some NRTIs (although they are not licensed for this purpose).

Salvage of heavily pre-treated patients

Complex patterns of resistance mutations in heavily pre-treated patients make the interpretation of genotypic resistant assays particularly difficult. If possible, a phenotypic assay should be performed. Antiretroviral regimens including six or more agents have been prescribed (mega-HAART), but toxicity is often prohibitive. It is the authors' opinion that patients who have been heavily pre-treated and have a detectable viral load with multiple drug resistance mutations should continue that regimen of therapy until newer and perhaps more effective drugs become available. The rationale for this approach is the observation that when antiretroviral therapy is discontinued in such patients, there is emergence of drug-sensitive (wild-type) virus with an increase in the plasma viral load and a rapid decline in the numbers of CD4+ cells in the peripheral blood[360].

Changing therapy because of toxicity

Switch studies indicate that changing one drug is safe as long as the plasma viral load is undetectable[361].

TOXICITY OF ANTIRETROVIRAL TREATMENT

Drug hypersensitivity is extremely common in HIV-infected patients and occurs with agents such as cotrimoxazole, as well as with many of the antiretroviral drugs. Abacavir, the NNRTIs nevirapine, delavirdine, and efavirenz, and amprenavir are the drugs most commonly implicated. About half of patients with hypersensitivity may continue on the drug with spontaneous resolution. The exception to this is abacavir hypersensitivity in which immediate and permanent discontinuation is mandatory. The adverse events with the individual agents are described above, and class-specific toxicity is discussed here.

Class specific toxicities

Nucleoside analog reverse transcriptase inhibitors

Nucleoside analog reverse transcriptase inhibitors may inhibit mitochondrial DNA polymerase gamma, resulting in impaired synthesis of mitochondrial enzymes that generate ATP by oxidative phosphorylation. As a result there is depletion of mitochondrial DNA and mitochondrial dysfunction. The pathogenesis of mitochondrial dyfunction has been reviewed by Rustin[362]. The two tissues most sensitive to the resultant reduction in intracellular energy production are muscle and nerves. This in turn may explain why myopathy (zidovudine) and neuropathy (stavudine, didanosine, zalcitabine) have been prominent side-effects. Other side-effects of related etiology include hepatic steatosis and lactic acidemia (didanosine, stavudine, zidovudine), peripheral lipoatrophy (predominantly with stavudine) and pancreatitis (didanosine). Severe neurological disease (two cases), and less severe symptoms (three cases) or laboratory abnormalities (three cases), all possibly indicating mitochondrial dysfunction, have been reported amongst infants who had been exposed to zidovudine with or without lamivudine *in utero*[363]. Such neurological abnormalities, however, were not found in other studies that have used zidovudine or zidovudine and lamivudine as prophylaxis against mother-to-child transmission[364, 365]. In addition, there is no evidence of cardiac dysfunction amongst children who have been exposed to zidovudine *in utero*[366].

Some of the toxicity of the NRTIs may reflect additional insult upon pre-existing organ damage such as chronic liver disease from Hepatitis B or C virus infections, or prior neuropathy commonly seen in long-standing HIV infection.

Lactic acidosis and lactic acidemia

The above terms are not interchangeable. Blood pH is not often measured in conjunction with serum lactate, and without this measurement the term lactic acidosis is incorrect. Lactic acidosis: arterial pH < 7.35, venous lactate > 2 mmol/L.

Lactic acidemia occurs predominantly amongst women, and particularly those of high body weight[367]. Although cases of severe and fatal lactic acidosis have been reported in women receiving stavudine and didanosine in combination with a NNRTI or PI (Bristol-Myers-Squibb Data Sheet 2001), it is unclear if pregnancy increases the incidence of lactic acidosis. There is no rationale for performing routine serum lactate measurements, as they are not predictive of the development of lactic acidosis. Serum lactate should only be measured if there are symptoms such as nausea, malaise, weight loss, or hepatic enzyme abnormalities; or in potentially related syndromes such as peripheral neuropathy, lipoatrophy, and osteopenia. At serum concentrations of 2 to 5 mmol/L with related symptoms, either stopping the ART or frequent observation and monitoring is indicated. If there are no symptoms, the patient should be observed and the serum lactate level measured 1 to 2 weeks later. Moderately high levels of serum lactate (between 5 to 10 mmol/L) are usually accompanied by clinical features and the drugs should be stopped until other causes are found and the features resolve. If there are no symptoms at this level, then it is likely that the measurement reflects marked dehydration or even artefact. A serum concentration above 10 mmol/L is usually accompanied by marked symptoms and significant mortality (about 80%). All drugs should be stopped and the patient should be admitted to hospital.

Protease inhibitors

Lipid abnormalities

Increased levels of plasma cholesterol and triglycerides are commonly found in individuals after initiation of PI-containing regimens. The cause is uncertain but there may be homology with lipid receptors and carrier protiens[16]. These increased blood lipid concentrations may be important in individuals with other cardiovascular risk factors, such as cigarette smoking and a family history. Coronary artery disease has been reporterd in patients receiving protease inhibitors[368]. Very high levels of triglycerides may also be complicated by acute pancreatitis.

Lipodystrophy

Lipodystrophy affecting HIV-1-infected patients was first described in 1999[369]. The main clinical features are peripheral fat loss (lipoatrophy in the face, limbs, and buttocks) and central fat accumulation (within the abdomen, breasts, and over the dorsocervical spine, the 'buffalo hump'). Metabolic features significantly associated with lipodystrophy and protease-inhibitor therapy include hypertriglyceridemia, hypercholesterolemia, insulin resistance (raised C-peptide and insulin concentrations), and type 2 diabetes mellitus. The prevalence of diabetes mellitus is about 8% to 10%; most cases are identified after oral glucose loading[370]. Few individuals present with symptoms such as polyuria, blurred vision, or weight loss, and ketoacidosis is rare. A further 15% of patients have impaired glucose tolerance. Most cases of diabetes have been identified in recipients of protease inhibitors but a causal relation has not been established.

The pathogenesis of the syndrome is unknown. One hypothesis suggests that it might be caused by inhibition of lipid and adipocyte regulatory proteins that have partial homology to the catalytic site of HIV-1 protease, to which protease inhibitors all bind[16]. *In-vitro* studies have shown that protease inhibitors can inhibit lipogenesis, and that indinavir may do this via altered retinoid acid signaling[371, 372]. More recently, some features of this syndrome have been suggested to represent mitochondrial toxicity of NRTIs, since lipoatrophy and buffalo hump have been reported in patients who have received only NRTIs in association with lactic acidemia, and both can occur in HIV-uninfected patients with mitochondrial defects[373].

The management of lipodystrophy is unclear. Switching from a protease inhibitor-containing regimen may be helpful in some cases, but the condition seldom appears to be reversible.

Osteopenia and osteoporosis

Recent reports suggest that osteopenia (thinning of bone) in HIV-infected patients is significantly higher amongst those receiving protease inhibitor therapy (40% to 50%) compared with those who are untreated or who are receiving a protease-sparing regimen (20% to 23%)[190]. In addition a sizeable proportion (9% to 20%) of protease inhibitor recipients have osteoporosis (severe loss of bone mass and disruption of the bone microarchitecture). Symptomatic osteoporosis, however, is rare. The pathogenesis of these conditions is uncertain, although lactic acidemia may be associated with osteopenia[374].

ADHERENCE TO ANTIRETROVIRAL THERAPY

With increasing experience with HAART, it has become apparent that adherence to medication is crucial in maintaining treatment efficacy. The subject has been reviewed by Cinti[375]. Factors that contribute to lack of adherence include toxicity of the treatment regimens such as diarrhea and lipodystrophy, and pill burden, particularly with some of the protease inhibitors. Measuring adherence can difficult, but several methods have been described.

1. The use of *Medication Event Monitoring System* (MEMS) caps have provided useful data on adherence to drug therapy, and one study showed a good correlation between the MEMS readings and virological failure[376]. These devices, however, are cumbersome and may not be entirely reliable in patients who remove multiple doses at one time.

2. *Self-reporting* using questionnaires. In theory this is a simple method but unfortunately a standardized questionnaire does not exist. Although questionnaires suitable for use in the clinic may give some useful information, self-reporting overestimates adherence by up to 20% when compared with MEMS[375].

3. *Pill counts.* Unannounced pill counts are difficult to manage and announced counts may lead to deception by the patient.

4. *Pharmacy records.* When patients collect their prescriptions from only one pharmacy, consideration of these records may identify gaps in having drugs dispensed. Gaps have been shown to correlate with virological failure[375].

5. *Clinician or nurse assessment.* This method of measuring adherence has been shown to be inaccurate in several studies[375].

6. *Antiretroviral drug levels.* This method is unreliable as variable absorption of drugs may lead to overestimation of lack of adherence.

7. *Directly observed therapy.* Although such a means of improving adherence can be effective[377], it is expensive in terms of time and staff, and is therefore impracticable for routine use.

8. *Genotypic resistance testing.* The presence of a high viral load in an individual whose virus has no genotypic mutations to the drugs in the treatment regimen, may give a clue about non-adherence. Such a conclusion can only be tentative, as variability of absorption may be responsible for that observation.

There appear to be many reasons for non-adherence. Although age, sex, race, socioeconomic status, and level of education do not predict adherence to treatment[378], psychosocial factors are important. Depression strongly correlates with lack of adherence[375], and heavy alcohol and drug use are factors in contributing to lack of adherence. In an attempt to improve adherence, depression should therefore be treated[379], and illicit substance users should be offered a place in a rehabilitation program. It has been shown that a belief that a particular treatment is beneficial aids adherence[380], and if patients have confidence in their health care providers, they are more likely to be adherent to their treatment regimen than if they do not[375].

Drug toxicity clearly affects adherence, but several studies have shown that adherence is not adversely affected by the number of drugs in a regimen[375]. The major reason for missing medication appears to be forgetfulness[375].

It is the authors' belief that to reduce the risk of non-adherence the patient who requires antiretroviral therapy should be fully prepared psychologically. The various treatment regimens and options should be carefully explained, with a full discussion about possible adverse effects. This counseling should be supported by written information on the drugs, and how treatment efficacy is assessed. Decisions should not be taken at the first consultation, and adequate time should be given to consider the treatment options. It is sometimes helpful to give the individual the opportunity of discussing treatment options with a patient who is well established on a therapeutic regimen. The ultimate choice of drug therapy should be tailored to the patient's lifestyle.

Ideally, the same health care provider should assess the patient at each follow-up attendance, particularly during the first few months after initiation of therapy.

ANTIRETROVIRAL TREATMENT AND DRUG INTERACTIONS

This important topic has been reviewed by Piscitelli & Gallicano[381], and a detailed discussion of drug interactions is outwith the scope of this text.

There are a variety of methods by which other drugs, including those used in the treatment and prophylaxis of opportunist infections, may interact with antiretroviral agents. In addition, antiretroviral drugs may interact with each other. For example antacids, by increasing the gastric pH, may decrease the absorption of indinavir, resulting in low plasma concentrations of that drug, thereby increasing the risk of selection of drug resistance. As the NRTIs are not highly plasma protein bound, interactions with other drugs through plasma protein binding displacement are unlikely.

Many of the drug interactions are the consequence of the mechanisms by which antiretroviral agents are metabolized. The protease inhibitors and the NNRTIs are metabolized by the cytochrome P450 enzyme system*. The liver is the primary site of drug metabolism by the P450 enzyme system, but enterocytes in the small intestine also contain CYP3A4, and drugs that inhibit this isoenzyme may alter the intestinal and hepatic metabolism of other drugs. Some drugs are substrates for the P450 cytochrome system, whilst others are inhibitors or inducers. The plasma concentration of substrates is increased when a drug that inhibits the enzyme system is co-administered. Although some drugs may result in irreversible inhibition of the enzymes, most inhibitors are competitive and reversible. Advantage can be taken of such interactions. For example, when a small dose of ritonavir is given with indinavir, the C_{min} and AUC of the latter drug increases, but the C_{max} decreases, permitting twice daily dosing (instead of three times daily) of indinavir. In addition, there is no need for the dietary restrictions that are necessary when indinavir is used without ritonavir. Through the avoidance of large swings in plasma concentration of indinavir, the incidence of nephrolithiasis appears to be reduced, compared with treatment with indinavir as sole protease inhibitor. Inhibition of the P450 cytochrome enzyme system, however, can have unfavorable effects. The concurrent administration of rifabutin with the protease inhibitors may raise the plasma concentration of that drug by some threefold, and increase the risk of uveitis. In contrast, inducers of the P450 cytochrome system, such as nevirapine, may reduce the plasma concentrations and AUC of protease inhibitors.

---

* In humans, there are three important families of enzymes of the cytochrome P450 system: CYP1, CYP2 and CYP3. These families of proteins are subdivided into subfamilies, designated by a letter, and these are further subdivided into isoenzymes, designated by a number (for example CYP2B6).

Drugs may also act on the P-glycoprotein, one of several membrane-bound proteins that increase the efflux of drugs from cells by pumping out large lipid-soluble compounds. This protein is found on enterocytes, hepatocytes, renal tubular cells, and endothelial cells. The inhibition or induction of P-glycoprotein on the enterocyte can influence the rate of absorption of drugs but, because of the overlap in substrate specificity between CYP3A and P-glycoprotein, it is often difficult to predict the effect on plasma concentrations[381]. In the CNS endothelial cells express P-glycoprotein. As protease inhibitors are a substrate for P-glycoprotein, this protein limits the penetration of ritonavir and saquinavir into brain tissue. Co-administration of ketoconazole, a potent inhibitor of P-glycoprotein, however, produces large increases in CSF concentrations of these drugs compared with increases in unbound plasma concentrations[381].

Drug interactions with different classes of antiretroviral agents

Nucleoside analog reverse transcriptase inhibitors

As these are not metabolized by the cytochrome P450 enzyme system, there are no significant interactions with the other classes of antiretroviral agents. Zidovudine and stavudine compete for the same phosphorylation pathway and should not be administered concurrently. Similarly, lamivudine inhibits phosphorylation of zalcitabine.

Non-nucleoside analog reverse transcriptase inhibitors

Nevirapine and efavirenz are inducers of CYP3A4, and nevirapine can decrease plasma concentrations of saquinavir and indinavir when co-administered. Although efavirenz increases the plasma concentration of ritonavir and nelfinavir, possibly by inhibiting CYP2C9 or CYP2C19 pathways, it reduces the plasma concentrations of lopinavir, amprenavir, indinavir, and saquinavir[381]. Plasma levels of saquinavir, however, are not affected when ritonavir is co-administered[381]. Delavirdine is a potent inhibitor of cytochrome P450, and can therefore cause serious interactions with hypnotics, antiarrythmic drugs, and etoposide[381].

Protease inhibitors

As inhibitors of the CYP3A4 enzymes, this is the class of antiretroviral agents that is most often associated with drug interactions. Ritonavir is the most potent inhibitor of the cytochrome system but, in addition, can be an enzyme inducer, as evidenced by its autoinduction during the first 14 days of therapy. As a result of an increase in glucuronosyltransferase activity, there may be reductions in the plasma concentrations of ethinylestradiol when given with ritonavir and nelfinavir. Concurrent use of other potent enzyme inducers, such as phenytoin and carbamazepine, can reduce the plasma levels of the protease inhibitors. Patients should be aware of the potentially lethal interaction between protease inhibitors, particularly ritonavir, and 'Ecstasy' (3,4-methylenedioxymethamphetamine – MDMA). 'Ecstasy' is metabolized by demethylenation, the reaction being catalyzed by CYP2D6, and toxic concentrations of the drug can accumulate when this isoenzyme is inhibited[382]. Drug interactions with herbal therapies have also been shown: St John's Wort (Hypericum) induces CYP3A4 or P-glycoprotein, and can result in a decreased AUC for indinavir[383].

It is quite impossible for the clinician to be familiar with all possible antiretroviral drug interactions, and several web sites that are constantly updated should be consulted for details of possible interactions. The following have proved most useful in the authors' clinical practice.

- www.hiv-druginteractions.org
- www.hopkins.aids.edu

THERAPEUTIC DRUG MONITORING

Several studies have shown an association between plasma concentrations of protease inhibitors and anitviral effects. For example, treatment failure has been associated with low plasma concentrations of indinavir[384]. Inter-individual variability in pharmacokinetics may result in significant differences in plasma and tissue concentrations of antiviral drugs, as shown by the differences in plasma concentrations of indinavir in patients treated with the same dose of the drug[385]. A study that showed

that the appearance of resistance mutations was delayed in patients who had high plasma concentrations of ritonavir when this drug was used as monotherapy, illustrates the potential deleterious effect of low plasma drug levels[386]. Monitoring of plasma concentrations of protease inhibitors during therapy therefore may help to identify those individuals who are likely to develop treatment failure. A recent study on HIV-infected patients treated with zidovudine, lamivudine, and indinavir, 13 of whom received standard therapy and 11 received plasma concentration-controlled treatment, showed possible benefit from the latter approach. Compared with those who received standard therapy, plasma drug concentration monitoring significantly reduced inter-patient variability in zidovudine concentrations and significantly increased indinavir concentrations[387]. The usefulness of therapeutic drug monitoring, however, was questioned in the study reported by Clevenbergh et al.[388] who found that there was no difference in virological response between patients who had therapeutic drug monitoring and those who had not.

The place of therapeutic drug monitoring, therefore, has not been fully established. It may be helpful under certain circumstances.

1. In severe liver impairment metabolism of the protease inhibitors by the cytochrome P450 system may be greatly delayed, and standard dosing may result in toxicity.
2. It may be helpful to identify the effects of drug interactions, for example, in patients receiving a single PI and an NNRTI, or a PI and an inducer/inhibitor of CYP3A4. There are, however, some limitations in the use of therapeutic drug monitoring in this context
   - there is considerable variability in pharmacokinetics
   - there are few data on specific therapeutic ranges and target concentrations
   - there are variations in binding to α_1-acid glycoprotein and albumin
   - there are slow viral responses to changes in plasma drug concentrations
   - the results are difficult to interpret[381].

3. To reduce the incidence of dose-related toxicity. A high plasma concentration of drug may allow dosage reduction in patients who are unlikely to have a drug resistant virus.

4. In the assessment of failure of anti-retroviral therapy. There is probably little advantage in undertaking therapeutic drug monitoring when high-level antiviral resistance has developed. It may be considered, however, when treatment intensification is an option, for example

- when the reduction in plasma viral load following a new treatment regimen is sub-optimal
- where viral resistance testing suggests that resistance is unlikely
- to overcome a low-level virological rebound.

IMMUNE RECONSTITUTION DISEASE

In patients with CD4+ T-cell counts in the peripheral blood of less than 50 cells/mm³, the institution of antiretroviral therapy can precipitate a marked inflammatory response to subclinical infections, with dramatic results. For example, within the first few weeks of initiation of therapy in an individual with untreated *M. avium* complex infection, there may be a severe illness with fever, leukocytosis, and lymphadenitis; granulomatous inflammation is found in lymph node biopsies[389]. It is postulated that antiviral therapy results in the recruitment of immune competent T cells to infected tissues, resulting in inflammation. Similarly, an inflammatory response to antiretroviral therapy may occur in patients with symptomless or subclinical CMV retinitis[390]. The authors have also observed acute inflammatory pulmonary reactions within a few weeks of initiation of antiretroviral therapy in individuals with unsuspected *P. carinii* infection. Apart from specific antimicrobial therapy, steroids may have a role to play in limiting this inflammatory reaction.

Following initiation of antiretroviral and anti-tuberculous treatment, there may be transient worsening of the symptoms of tuberculous disease (paradoxical response). This paradoxical response is related to the initiation of ART rather than to

that of anti-tuberculous chemotherapy. The reaction tends to occur at a mean of 15 days (standard deviation 11 days) after initiation of the ARV regimen[391]. This phenomenon results from immune reconstitution and, in the majority of patients, is associated with tuberculin skin test conversion from negative to positive.

IMMUNE MANIPULATION

After initiation of antiretroviral therapy, CD8+ cytotoxic T-cell activity declines as the plasma viral load and HIV antigen expression are reduced[70]. In addition, CD4+ T-cell proliferative responses, previously undetectable, may become detectable in up to one third of treated patients[392]. Efforts have been made to re-establish HIV-specific T help and CTL by active immunization; studies, however, have failed to show durable clinical benefit.

Interleukin-2 is a polypeptide hormone derived from activated T cells that can induce the activation, proliferation, and differentiation of T- and B-lymphocytes, thereby forestalling the development of immune deficiency. *In vitro* it has been shown that exogenous IL-2 increases natural killer cell activity and CMV-specific cytotoxic effects in peripheral blood mononuclear cells from patients with advanced HIV infection[393]. Highly significant increases in the CD4+ cell count in the peripheral blood have been found in patients on antiretroviral therapy with a CD4+ T-cell count between 200 and 500 cells/mm³ who have been treated with intermittent subcutaneous IL-2 compared with those who only received antiviral drugs[394]. Although it had been noted previously that IL-2 infusion did not result in an increase in the number of peripheral blood CD4+ T cells in patients on antiviral treatment with a CD4+ T-cell count of less than 200 cells/mm³, Arno et al.[395] found that intermittent low-dose subcutaneous doses of IL-2 significantly increased the number of CD4+ T cells in the peripheral blood compared with those who received antiviral therapy alone. It is still uncertain if these increases in CD4+ cell counts confer clinical advantage. However, in an analysis of three published studies that had been commenced before 1995, Emery et al.[396] showed a non-significant trend

towards improved clinical outcome. Treatment does not appear to increase plasma or tissue levels of HIV or to result in sustained expression of previously latent quasi species[397]. As viral rebound occurs after discontinuation of antiretroviral therapy even in patients who have also received IL-2, it appears that IL-2 does not eradicate latent HIV infection[398].

A novel approach to the treatment of primary HIV infection, using cyclosporin A, was reported by Rizzardi et al.[347]. Cyclosporin A reduces T-cell activation, and as HIV requires T-cell activation for replication, use of the drug should reduce the pool of activated cells. They treated 9 patients with zidovudine, lamivudine, saquinavir, ritonavir, and cyclosporin A, and compared their outcome with 29 patients given the antiviral agents only. There was a highly significant and sustained increase in the CD4+ T-cell count in the peripheral blood in those given cyclosporin A compared with those who were not. The results of further studies will be of interest.

MANAGEMENT OF THE HIV-INFECTED PREGNANT WOMAN

There should be a team-work approach to the management of the pregnant HIV-infected woman, involving the HIV specialist, obstetrician, pediatrician, and general practitioner.

At the initial assessment note should be made of the gestational age, and whether the patient has been treated previously with, or is currently receiving, antiretroviral drugs. A social history should also be elicited. Blood should be obtained for the determination of the CD4+ T-cell count and the plasma viral load. It should be noted that physiological changes during pregnancy may result in changes in the absolute CD4+ T-cell count in the peripheral blood; the percentage of these cells, however, is more stable, and is a more accurate reflection of her immune status[399].

When these results are available they, and the options available to reduce transmission of the virus to her child, should be discussed with the woman. The various treatment regimens should be discussed and known or uncertain risks of particular drugs should be carefully explained.

Strategies to reduce the risk of mother-to-child transmission of HIV

Risk factors for the transmission of HIV from an HIV-infected woman to her child have been considered above. The efficacy of zidovudine given to both the pregnant woman before and during birth, and to her new-born child was shown clearly in the Pediatric AIDS Clinical Trials Group study (Protocol 076) whose results were published in 1994[400]. In this placebo-controlled trial, women were treated with zidovudine (100 mg five times/day) or placebo, given by mouth, at varying intervals from 14 to 34 weeks gestation, and with intravenous zidovudine during parturition (2.0 mg/kg infusion over 1 hour, followed by a continuous infusion of 1.0 mg kg^{-1} h^{-1}). The child was treated with a 6-week course of either oral zidovudine (2 mg/kg orally every 6 hours) or placebo. Of the children whose infection status was known, the proportions infected at 18 months of age were 8.3% (95% confidence interval 3.9–12.8%) of the zidovudine group (180 children), and 25.5% (95% confidence interval 18.4–32.5%) in the placebo group (183 children). The use of zidovudine then resulted in a 67.5% (95% confidence interval 40.7–82.1%) relative reduction in the risk of HIV transmission. Analysis of the 402 mother–infant pairs enrolled in this study confirmed the protection afforded by zidovudine treatment: the rate of transmission of HIV was 7.6% (95% confidence interval 4.3–12.3%) and 22.6% (95% confidence interval 17.0–29.0%) in zidovudine and placebo recipients respectively[401]. A reduction in the materno-fetal transmission rate by the use of zidovudine has also been found amongst women with advanced HIV infection[402]. The mechanisms by which zidovudine reduces materno-fetal transmission are unknown. With the subsequent adoption of this regimen, perinatal transmission rates in Europe and the USA declined to less than 6%[403].

Reduction in risk of materno-fetal transmission of HIV with a shorter course of zidovudine was shown in a placebo-controlled trial in Thailand[404]. Pregnant HIV-infected women were given either zidovudine, 300 mg by mouth twice daily from 36 weeks' gestation, and every 3 hours from the onset of labor until delivery, or placebo. None of these women breast fed their infants. Based on the proportion of infected children aged 6 months, the estimated transmission rates were 9.4% (95% confidence interval 5.2–13.5%) on zidovudine and 18.9% (95% confidence interval 13.2–24.2%) on placebo. These data suggested a relative efficacy of short course zidovudine therapy of about 50%. This is higher than the 37% efficacy with the same treatment regimen reported from the Cote d'Ivoire[405]. In the latter study, however, women breast fed their infants.

The importance of giving zidovudine to the pregnant woman for a sufficient length of time was shown in a complex trial that compared four regimens of zidovudine in the prevention of materno-fetal transmission amongst non-breast-feeding HIV-infected women in Thailand[406]. Women were given zidovudine (300 mg twice daily) from either 28 weeks or 35 weeks gestation and during delivery (300 mg by mouth every 3 hours), and their infants were given the drug in an oral dose of 2 mg/kg every 6 hours for either 3 days or 6 weeks. It was found that the rate of *in utero* transmission was significantly higher with regimens with short-term treatment of the mother (from 35 weeks gestation) than with longer treatment (from 28 weeks gestation) (5.1% compared with 1.6%). It was also noted that longer treatment of the infant did not substitute for longer treatment of the mother.

The value of using zidovudine post-partum as the only prophylaxis against mother-to-child transmission is controversial. Wade *et al.*[407], however, found that when zidovudine was given to the child within 48 hours of birth, the rate of transmission by 6 months was 9.3% (95% confidence interval 4.1–17.5%), compared with 18.4% (95% confidence interval 7.7–34.3%) when it was given on day 3 of life or later.

Even amongst women receiving zidovudine, materno-fetal transmission of HIV is still possible, and Mofenson *et al.*[408] demonstrated that amongst such women, the maternal plasma viral load was the best predictor of the risk of perinatal transmission.

Amongst women who have been treated previously with the drug, zidovudine has been reported as giving protection against mother-to-child transmission at a level similar to that seen in zidovudine-naïve patients[402]. It is uncertain if genotypic resistance mutations for zidovudine increase the risk of perinatal transmission. A recent study of 142 isolates of HIV from women who had received zidovudine monotherapy before their pregnancy, however, showed that having at least one zidovudine-associated mutation was independently associated with perinatal transmission[409]. Different results were obtained in a Swiss study of 62 HIV-infected women, 10% of whom were infected with virus that had high-level resistance to zidovudine; none of these women transmitted virus to their children, despite receiving only zidovudine prophylaxis[410].

A combination of zidovudine and lamivudine, given orally from 36 weeks gestation, intrapartum, and for 1 week after birth, has been shown to reduce by about 50% the risk of HIV transmission amongst a cohort of breast-feeding African women[411]. In this placebo-controlled trial, at age 6 weeks, transmission had occurred in the infants of 9% of active drug recipients, compared with 17% who had been given placebo.

In many countries where mother-to-child transmission of HIV plays an important role in the spread of the virus, the expense of zidovudine treatment is outwith the means of the majority of the infected population. For this reason, and because the drug has a long half-life in pregnant women and their babies (see page 178), nevirapine has been assessed as a possible agent for use in preventing materno-fetal transmission. A study from Kampala, Uganda, compared the efficacy of nevirapine with zidovudine in reducing the risk of materno-fetal transmission of HIV[412]. Nevirapine was given to the mother in a single oral dose of 200 mg at the onset of labor and, 48 hours after birth, to the neonate in a single oral dose of

2 mg/kg. A comparison group of women received zidovudine, given orally to the mother in a dose of 600 mg at the onset of labor and 300 mg every 3 hours thereafter until delivery; their babies were treated with zidovudine in an oral dose of 4 mg/kg twice daily for 7 days. Almost all the babies were breast fed. At birth the estimated risk of HIV transmission in the zidovudine and nevirapine groups were 10.4% and 8.2% respectively. By age 14 to 16 weeks these estimates were 25.1% and 13.1% respectively. At 14 to 16 weeks the relative efficacy of this nevirapine regimen was 47%.

Although zidovudine or nevirapine monotherapy significantly reduces the risk of materno-fetal transmission of HIV, this is sub-optimal therapy for the mother, and in industrialized countries is not recommended.

There is an association between the risk of mother-to-child transmission and the plasma viral load (see pp. 152–153), but it is unknown if lowering the viral load to undetectable levels (less than 50 copies/mL) reduces the risk of materno-fetal transmission. A recent retrospective study, however, has shown that none of 24 women who had a satisfactory viral load response on combination therapy transmitted the virus[413].

Little is known about the effect of antiretroviral therapy on the HIV viral load in the genital secretions. Amongst a group of 310 pregnant, HIV-infected, Thai women who participated in a trial of zidovudine prophylaxis in the prevention of HIV transmission, HIV RNA was detected in cervicovaginal secretions significantly more often in placebo recipients (52%) than in those given zidovudine (23%)[414]. It was further shown that the risk of infection was more likely in the babies of those women who had detectable HIV RNA in the genital tract and a high plasma viral load (28.7%) than in the babies of those who had undetectable viral RNA and a low plasma viral load (1%).

In studies undertaken before viral load testing and HAART, cesarean section before labor and ruptured membranes has been shown to reduce the rate of mother-to-child transmission by about 50%[133, 415]. In the meta-analysis reported by The International Perinatal HIV Group[133] it was further shown that the likelihood of transmission was reduced by about 87% with both elective cesarean section and the use of antiretroviral treatment (mainly zidovudine monotherapy) given during the prenatal, intrapartum, and neonatal periods, compared with those women who had had other modes of delivery and no antiviral treatment. Cesarean section, however, is not without risk, and 6.7% of 225 women delivered by this means developed post-partum fever, compared with 1.1% of 183 women delivered vaginally[415].

Currently there are no published data on the cost-effectiveness of elective cesarean section in the prevention of mother-to-child transmission of HIV amongst women receiving potent antiretroviral therapy, but as the risk of transmission when the viral load is below the limit of detection (less than 50 copies/mL), it is unlikely that cesarean section will reduce the transmission rate further.

An interesting recent finding is that women on combination therapy from before pregnancy or during the first trimester were twice as likely to deliver prematurely as those starting therapy in the third trimester[416]. The authors of that report suggested that elective cesarean section to reduce the risk of vertical transmission of HIV should be undertaken at 36 weeks rather than 38 weeks gestation in women on combination therapy.

Recommendations for the treatment of HIV-1 infected pregnant women (Public Health Service Task Force Recommendations for the Use of Antiretroviral Drugs in Pregnant HIV-1 Infected Women for Maternal Health and Interventions to Reduce Perinatal Transmission in the United States. May2001, www.hivatis.org)

The following discussion is based on the recommendations of the expert panel. It should be emphasized, however, that these are guidelines and it is often necessary to tailor treatment to the individual patient.

Treatment of the naïve woman

Recommendations for initiation and choice of antiretroviral regimen should be based on the same parameters used for non-pregnant patients. As the safety of some drugs in early pregnancy is uncertain, some women may wish to postpone initiation of therapy until the start of the second trimester.

Zidovudine should be considered as a component of the regimen, and it is recommended that the drug should also be given to the mother during labor and delivery, and to the infant. As it has also been shown that the administration of zidovudine three times per day maintains intracellular triphosphate at levels comparable to those found with more frequent dosing, the maternal dose during the pregnancy can be either 200 mg every 8 hours or 300 mg every 12 hours. If the woman does not have zidovudine as part of her antiretroviral regimen, this drug should be given intrapartum and to the neonate (2 mg/kg body weight every 6 hours) who should be treated for 6 weeks.

When it is necessary to use zidovudine at the time of elective cesarean section, the drug should be given by intravenous infusion (in 5% glucose) of 2 mg/kg body weight over 1 hour, followed by 1 mg kg^{-1} h^{-1} until the umbilical cord is clamped. The infusion should be initiated 4 hours before the operation.

Because there are uncertainties about the risk of lactic acidosis or hepatic steatosis in pregnancy (see page 192), women receiving NRTIs should have plasma electrolytes and plasma enzyme tests of liver function estimated every 2 weeks during the last trimester. The combination of stavudine and didanosine should only be used in pregnant women when they are intolerant of other regimens or if other treatments have failed.

When women are treated with antiretroviral drugs principally to reduce mother-to-child transmission, it may be appropriate to stop such treatment after delivery, and reintroduce therapy when necessary (see section on initiation of therapy in the non-pregnant individual, pp. 188–189). The regimen based on the PACTG 076 study may be considered in such women.

Treatment of the experienced patient

When a woman who is receiving antiretroviral therapy becomes pregnant, the treatment regimen should be reviewed and drugs, such as hydroxyurea and efavirenz, that are known to be harmful to the fetus should be replaced by other less toxic agents. If the viral load is undetectable (less than 50 copies/mL) on a drug regimen that is as safe as possible, that regimen should be continued. Ideally, zidovudine should be a component of the regimen after the first trimester. Irrespective of the drug regimen used, zidovudine should be given intrapartum, and to the neonate. An exception, however, may be the woman who is receiving stavudine as part of the combination therapy. As these drugs compete for phosphorylation, stavudine should be discontinued during the intrapartum zidovudine treatment, or the stavudine should be continued during labor, and the administration of zidovudine to the mother withheld. If treatment is interrupted during the first trimester, the drugs should be stopped and re-introduced simultaneously to reduce the risk of development of drug resistance.

Treatment of the HIV-infected woman in labor who has not received antiretroviral drug during pregnancy

A single 200 mg oral dose of nevirapine can be given to HIV-infected women who have not been treated antenatally. The significance of genotypic nevirapine resistance mutations that have been identified in women given single dose therapy[417] is uncertain. The neonate can be treated with nevirapine, given in an oral dose of 2 mg/kg, 48 hours after delivery. Alternatively, zidovudine by intravenous infusion may be given intrapartum (dosage as above) and to the neonate as above. Zidovudine given in an oral dose of 600 mg at the onset of labor, followed by 300 mg every 3 hours until delivery, *with* lamivudine given in a dose of 150 mg by mouth at the onset of labor followed by 150 mg every 12 hours until delivery. The infant is treated with zidovudine 4 mg/kg orally every 12 hours, *with* lamivudine 2 mg/kg every 12 hours for 7 days. Studies comparing directly the efficacy of each of these regimens have not been undertaken.

Treatment of infants born to mothers who have had no antiretroviral therapy during pregnancy or at delivery

Zidovudine should be given in the above dosage, treatment beginning as soon as possible, and preferably, within 8 to 12 hours of birth.

Mode of delivery

When the maternal viral load is less than 50 copies/mL, cesarean section is unlikely to reduce further the risk of perinatal transmission, and is considered unnecessary by most obstetricians. As an adjunct to antiretroviral therapy, the American College of Obstetricians and Gynecologists, however, recommend delivery by cesarean section if the viral load is more than 1000 copies/mL. The College recommends that when cesarean section is indicated to reduce the risk of HIV transmission, it should be undertaken at 38 weeks gestation[418].

Guidance on breast feeding

There is now much evidence that HIV can be transmitted by breast milk (see pp. 152–153). Ideally, HIV-infected women should not breast feed their infants. In developing nations, however, this approach may not be practicable. Although formula feeding results in a lower rate of transmission of HIV from mother to child, this mode of feeding may not be acceptable. At present it is difficult to offer guidance to mothers in resource-poor countries on how best to reduce the risk of mother-to-child transmission of HIV through breast feeding. From the data discussed above, however, it may be prudent to advise women not to undertake mixed feeding. Clearly more research is needed in this difficult area.

Prevention

Aspects of the prevention of acquisition of HIV and other blood-borne viral infections and STIs are discussed in Chapters 2 and 8. Although there are several candidate vaccines undergoing clinical trials, it is premature to consider these here.

POST-EXPOSURE PROPHYLAXIS
Health care workers

In the early 1980s a number of reports described cases where a health care worker had become HIV-infected following percutaneous exposure to HIV-contaminated blood or other fluid, usually as a result of a 'needle-stick' injury. It was felt justified to offer post-exposure prophylaxis, initially with zidovudine monotherapy, to a health care worker suffering such exposure to potentially infected material. An observational study published in 1997 estimated an 80% reduction in infection if post-exposure prophylaxis were taken within 2 hours of exposure[419]. As combination antiretroviral therapy became available, further guidelines advocated prophylaxis with dual therapy of zidovudine and lamivudine, and most recent practice advocates the use of triple therapy[420]. Given the potential toxicity of these regimens, careful triage of percutaneous and mucous membrane exposures is required in order to limit unnecessary risk to health care workers. Guidance has been produced in the USA by the Centers for Disease Control and Prevention[421] and in the UK by the Department of Health[420].

There are two components to risk assessment, the source patient and the nature of the injury.

Source patient

This is clear when the status of the source is known to be HIV-infected. In such situations an assessment should be made of the patient's clinical condition, as blood and other body fluids tend to be more infectious in late-stage disease, almost certainly reflecting a higher viral load. Recent results of CD4+ cell estimation and viral load should be scrutinized if available. If the source patient is taking ART, the viral load may be low or undetectable, indicating less risk of transmission. If recent results are unavailable, the source patient should be asked about adherence to the regimen. If poor adherence is admitted, and/or viral load is detectable, it is prudent to assume that any transmitted virus will be resistant to those particular drugs, which in turn should not be prescribed to the health care worker involved if at all possible.

The nature of the injury

In the case-control study that demonstrated the benefit of post-exposure zidovudine[419], three factors pertaining to the injury were found to increase the risk of transmission

1. a deep injury
2. the presence of visible blood on the device causing the injury
3. an injury with a needle that had been placed in the source patient's artery or vein.

Wearing latex (or similar) gloves reduces the risk of transmission as blood on the outside of the needle will be 'washed off' during penetration. A hollow-bore needle containing blood remains a significant source of risk especially if the injury is deep, preventing easy expression of injected material by squeezing. Injuries involving blood tend to carry greater risk than other bodily fluids in which the concentration of virus is likely to be less. After any injury, the site of exposure should be washed with soap and water, and wounds should be encouraged to bleed. Exposed mucous membranes should be irrigated with water.

Source whose HIV-infection status is unknown

Inevitably, each case must be judged on an individual basis. The nature of the injury, and the epidemiological likelihood of infection should be considered.

Post-exposure prophylaxis should be offered to an individual who has sustained a significant exposure (Box 7.2) to blood or another high-risk body fluid (Box 7.3) from a patient known to be HIV-infected or at high risk of infection.

Drugs for use in post-exposure prophylaxis

Non-nucleoside reverse transcriptase inhibitors such as nevirapine have been prescribed as part of post-exposure prophylaxis regimens because of the theoretical advantage of a quicker onset of action since no phosphorylation is required for activation. However, reports of fulminant hepatitis in health care workers given

---

Box 7.2 Injuries associated with high risk of HIV infection (Departments of Health 2000[420])

Percutaneous injury from, for example, needles or bites that break the skin

Exposure of broken skin, including eczema

Exposure of mucous membranes, including the conjunctivae

Box 7.3 Body fluids that may pose risk of HIV transmission if significant occupational exposure has occurred (Departments of Health 2000[420])

Amniotic fluid

Cerebrospinal fluid

Human breast milk

Pericardial, peritoneal, or pleural fluid

Saliva when the injury has been associated with dentistry

Synovial fluid

Unfixed human organs and tissues

Any other blood-stained fluid

Exudate from burns or skin lesions

Box 7.4 Drugs regimens for occupational post-exposure prophylaxis (Centers for Disease Control and Prevention 1998[421]; Departments of Health 2000[420])

Zidovudine in an oral dose of 500 mg initially, followed by 500 mg 2 hours later, and then 250 mg every 6 hours for 3 days, the dose then being reduced to
either
200 mg every 8 hours
or
250 mg every 12 hours for 28 days

PLUS

Lamivudine 150 mg by mouth immediately, and then in a dose of 150 mg every 12 hours for 28 days

PLUS

Nelfinavir 750 mg by mouth immediately, and then
either
750 mg every 8 hours
or
1200 mg every 12 hours

OR

Indinavir 800 mg by mouth immediately, and then 800 mg every 8 hours before food or with a light fat meal

---

nevirapine suggest that this drug should not be used in such a scenario[422, 423]. The most recent guideline advocates zidovudine/lamivudine and either indinavir or nelfinavir taken for a total of 4 weeks. Box 7.4 indicates the drug regimens. Post-exposure prophylaxis should be initiated as soon as possible after the injury, but some reports suggest that it might be worth considering starting the regimen even if up to 2 weeks has elapsed since the event[420]. The individual should be followed-up at regular intervals during treatment to identify adverse events from the therapy, and to assess adherence to the regimen.

The injured worker should receive counseling about the risks of HIV infection from the injury, and safer sexual practices should be discussed and practised, and blood donation should be avoided until there is clear serological evidence that HIV infection has not occurred. There is no need to limit the individual's working practice during the time before freedom from infection is confirmed. A blood sample should be obtained from the health care worker as soon as possible after the incident, and the serum should be stored. HIV antibody testing should be offered 6 months after the incident. Should this test yield positive results, the initial serum specimen should be tested for anti-HIV; demonstration of seroconversion will influence compensation. Clearly every reported injury must be carefully documented by the physician.

The possibility of transmission of other blood-borne viruses such as hepatitis B and C should also be considered.

Prevention remains crucial and the guidelines produced by the UK Health Departments[420] should be followed.

Post-exposure prophylaxis after sexual exposure

The place of post-exposure prophylaxis against HIV infection is unknown. Although there is no definitive evidence that it is efficacious, analogy with post-exposure prophylaxis and prevention of perinatal transmission suggest that it is biologically plausible[424] and increasing numbers of individuals are seeking such intervention. Post-exposure prophylaxis may be considered if there has been high-risk exposure (see Epidemiology, page 153) to a partner who is known to be HIV-infected, or is at high risk of infection. In the former case

1. the clinical status of the individual should be ascertained
2. has he or she received antiretroviral treatment within the preceding 30 days?
3. if so, is the plasma viral load known?

This information is helpful in deciding on a prophylaxis regimen. Treatment should be initiated as soon as possible after the event, and probably not later than 72 hours[424]. In macaques infected with SIV by the intravenous route, zidovudine therapy, particularly when given within 24 hours, suppressed or delayed infection but rarely prevented it[425]. In post-sexual exposure prophylaxis, the treatment regimens described above may be used, but these may need to be modified if the source of possible infection is known or is suspected to harbor resistant virus. Treatment is usually given for 28 days, and serological testing should be offered 6, 12, and 24 weeks later[424]. Individuals should be counseled about future risk reduction.

References

1 Barre-Sinoussi, F, Chermann, Rey F, *et al.* Isolation of a T-lymphotropic retrovirus from a patient at risk for the acquired immune deficiency syndrome (AIDS). *Science* 1983; **220**: 868–871.

2 Gallo RC, Salahuddin SZ, Popovic M, *et al.* Frequent detection and isolation of cytopathic retroviruses (HTLV-III) from patients with AIDS and at risk of AIDS. *Science* 1984; **224**: 500–503.

3 Levy JA, Hoffman AD, Kramer SM, *et al.* Isolation of lymphocytopathic retroviruses from San Francisco patients with AIDS. *Science* 1984; **220**: 840–842.

4 Coffin J, Haase A, Levy JA, *et al.* Human immunodeficiency viruses. *Science* 1986: **232**: 697.

5 Kornfield H, Van de Stouwe RA, Lange M, *et al.* T-lymphocyte subpopulations in homosexual men. *N Engl J Med* 1982; **307**: 729–731.

6 Dalgleish AG, Beverley PCL, Clapham P, *et al.* The CD4 (T4) antigen is an essential component of the receptor for the AIDS retrovirus. *Nature* 1984; **312**: 763–767.

7 Klatzman D, Hampagne E, Chamaret S, *et al.* T-lymphocyte T4 molecule behaves as the receptor for human retrovirus. *Nature* 1984; **312**: 767–768.

8 Clavel F, Guetard D, Brun-Vezinet F, *et al.* Isolation of a new human retrovirus from West African patients with AIDS. *Science* 1986; **233**: 343–346.

9 Fischl MA, Dickinson GM, La Voie L. Safety and efficacy of sulfamethoxazole and trimethoprim chemoprophylaxis for *Pneumocystis carinii* pneumonia in AIDS. *JAMA* 1988; **259**: 1185–1189.

10 Anonymous. Concorde: MRC/ANRS randomised double-blind controlled trial of immediate and deferred zidovudine in symptom-free HIV infection. Concorde Coordinating Committee. *Lancet* 1994; **343**: 871–881.

11 Delta: a randomised double-blind controlled trial comparing combinations of zidovudine plus didanosine or zalcitabine with zidovudine alone in HIV-infected individuals. Delta Coordinating Committee. *Lancet* 1996; **348**: 283–291.

12 Hammer S, Katzenstein DA, Hughes MD, *et al.* A trial comparing nucleoside monotherapy with combination therapy in HIV-infected adults with CD4 counts from 200 to 500 per cubic millimetre. *N Engl J Med* 1996; **335**: 1081–1090.

13 Ho DD, Neumann AU, Perelson AS, Chen W, Leonard JM, Markowitz M. Rapid turnover of plasma virions and CD4 lymphocytes in HIV-1 infection. *Nature* 1995; **373**: 123–126.

14 Perelson AS, Neumann AU, Markowitz M, Leonard JM, Ho DD. HIV-1 dynamics in vivo: virion clearance rate, infected cell life-span and viral generation time. *Science* 1996; **271**: 1582–1586.

15 Cameron DW, Heath-Chiozzi M, Danner S, *et al.* Randomised placebo-controlled trial of ritonavir in advanced HIV-1 disease. The Advanced HIV Disease Ritonavir Study Group. *Lancet* 1998; **351**: 543–549.

16 Carr A, Samaras K, Burton S, *et al.* A syndrome of peripheral lipodystrophy, hyperlipidaemia, and insulin resistance in patients receiving HIV protease inhibitors. *AIDS* 1998; **12**: F51–F58.

17 Schrager LK, D'Souza MP. Cellular and anatomical reservoirs of HIV-1 in patients receiving potent antiretroviral combination therapy. *JAMA* 1998; **280**: 67–71.

18 Gao F, Bailes E, Robertson DL, *et al.* Origin of HIV-1 in the chimpanzee *Pan troglodytes troglodytes*. *Nature* 1999; **397**: 436–441.

19 Chen Z, Telfier P, Gettie A, *et al.* Genetic characterization of new West African simian immunodeficiency virus SIVsm: geographic clustering of household-derived SIV strains with human immunodeficiency virus type 2 subtypes and genetically diverse viruses from a single feral sooty mangabey troop. *J Virol* 1996; **70**: 3617–3627.

20 UNAIDS. Report on the global HIV/AIDS epidemic. June 2000.

21 Pizzo PA, Wilfert CM (eds) *Pediatric AIDS. The Challenge of HIV Infection in Infants, Children and Adolescents* 3rd edition. Baltimore; Williams & Wilkins: 1998.

22 Rous P. A sarcoma of the fowl transmissible by an agent separable from the tumour cells. *J Exp Med* 1911; **13**: 397–411.

23 Poiesz BJ, Ruscetti FW, Gadzar AF, *et al.* Detection and isolation of type C retrovirus particles from fresh and cultured lymphocytes of a patient with cutaneous T-cell lymphoma. *Proc Natl Acad Sci USA* 1980; **77**: 7415–7419.

24 Sigurdsson B. Observations on three slow infections of sheep. *Br Vet J* 1954; **110**: 255–270.

25 Haase AT. Pathogenesis of lentivirus infections. *Nature* 1986; **332**: 130–136.

26 Robertson DL, Sharp PM, McCutchan FE, Hahn BH. Recombination in HIV-1. *Nature* 1995; **374**: 124–126.

27 Robertson DL, Anderson J, Bradac J, *et al.* HIV-1 subtype and recombinant nomenclature proposal. *Science* 2000; **288**: 55–56.

28 UNAIDS. HIV-1 subtypes: implications for epidemiology, pathogenicity, vaccines and diagnostics. *AIDS* 1997; **11**: 17–36.

29 Pope M, Frankel SS, Mascola JR, *et al.* Human immunodeficiency virus type 1

strains of subtypes B and E replicate in cutaneous dendritic cell–T-cell mixtures without displaying subtype-specific tropism. *J Virol* 1997; **71**: 8001–8007.

30 Peeters M, Sharp PM. Genetic diversity of HIV-1: the moving target. *AIDS* 2000; **14**: S129–S140.

31 Nelson K, Rungruengthanakit K, Margolick J, *et al.* High rates of transmission of subtype E human immunodeficiency virus type 1 among heterosexual couples in Northern Thailand: role of sexually transmitted diseases and immune compromise. *J Infect Dis* 1999; **180**: 337–343.

32 Alaeus A, Lidman K, Sonnerborg A, Albert J. Subtype specific problems with quantification of plasma HIV-1 RNA. *AIDS* 1997; **11**: 859–865.

33 Debyser Z, Van Wijngaerden E, Van Laethem K, *et al.* Failure to quantify viral load with two of the three commercial methods in a pregnant woman harboring an HIV type 1 subtype G strain. *AIDS Res Hum Retroviruses* 1998; **15**: 889–894.

34 Descamps D, Collin G, Letourner F, *et al.* Susceptibility of human immunodeficiency virus type 1 group O isolates to antiretroviral agents: in vitro phenotypic and genotypic analysis. *J Virol* 1997; **71**: 8893–8898.

35 Feng Y, Broder C, Kennedy PE, Berger EA. Functional cDNA cloning of a seven-transmembrane, G protein-coupled receptor. *Science* 1996; **278**: 872–877.

36 D'Souza P, Harden VA. Chemokines and HIV-1 second receptors: confluence of two fields generates optimism in AIDS research. *Nat Med* 1996; **2**: 1293–1300.

37 Kostirkis LG, Huang Y, Moore JP, *et al.* A chemokine receptor CCR2 allele delays HIV-1 disease progression and is associated with a CCR5 promoter mutation. *Nat Med* 1998; **4**: 350–353.

38 Ghoparde A, Xia MQ, Hyman BT *et al.* Role of beta-chemokine receptors CCR3 and CCR5 in human immunodeficiency virus type 1 infection of monocytes and microglia. *J Virol* 1998; **72**: 3351–3361.

39 Samson M, Libert F, Doranz BJ, *et al.* Resistance to HIV-1 infection in caucasian individuals bearing mutant alleles of the CCR-5 chemokine receptor gene. *Nature* 1996 ; **382**: 722–725.

40 Dean M, Carrington M, Winkler C, *et al.* Genetic restriction of HIV-1 infection and progression to AIDS by a deletion allele of the *CKR*5 structural gene. *Science* 1996; **273**: 1856–1862.

41 McDermott DH, Zimmerman PA, Guignard F, Kleeberger CA, Leitman SF, Murphy PM. CCR5 promoter polymorphism and HIV-1 disease progression. Multicenter AIDS Cohort Study (MACS). *Lancet* 1998; **352**: 866–870.

42 Guerin S, Meyer L, Theodorou I, *et al.* CCR5 Δ32 deletion and response to highly active antiretroviral therapy in HIV-1-infected patients. *AIDS* 2000; **14**: 2788–2789.

43 Tang J, Makhatadze N, Y Zhang, *et al.* CCR5 genotypes determine progression of HIV-1 by regulating early viral load. *Seventh Conference on Retroviruses and Opportunistic Infections*; San Francisco: 2000, Abstract 651A.

44 Winkler C, Modi W, Smith MW, *et al.* Genetic restriction of AIDS pathogenesis by an SDF-1 chemokine gene variant. *Science* 1998; **279**: 389–393.

45 De Jong JJ, Goudsmit J, Keulen W, *et al.* Human immunodeficiency virus type 1 clones chimeric for the envelope V3 domain differ in syncytium formation and replication capacity. *J Virol* 1992; **66**: 757–765.

46 Koot M, Keet IPM, Vos AHV, *et al.* Prognostic value of HIV-1 syncitium-inducing phenotype for rate of CD4⁺ cell depletion and progression to AIDS. *Ann Intern Med* 1993; **118**: 681–688.

47 Richman DD, Bozzette SA. The impact of the syncitium-inducing phenotype of human immunodeficiency virus on disease progression. *J Infect Dis* 1994; **169**: 968–674.

48 Whittle HC, Ariyoshi K, Rowland-Jones S. HIV-2 and T cell recognition. *Curr Op Immunol* 1998; **10**: 382–387.

49 McKnight A, Dittmar MT, Moniz-Periera J, *et al.* A broad range of chemokine receptors are used by primary isolates of human immunodeficiency virus type 2 as co-receptors with CD4. *J Virol* 1998; **72**: 4065–4071.

50 Trono, D. HIV accessory proteins: leading roles for the supporting cast. *Cell* 1995; **82**: 189–192.

51 Strebel K, Bour S. Molecular interactions of HIV with host factors. *AIDS* 1999; **13**: S13–24.

52 Kotler M, Simm M, Zhao YS, *et al.* Human immunodeficiency virus type 1 (HIV-1) protein vif inhibits the activity of HIV-1 protease in bacteria and in vivo. *J Virol* 1997; **71**: 5774–5781.

53 Selig L, Pages J-C, Tanchou V, *et al.* Interaction with p6 domain of the gag precursor mediates incorporation into virions of vpr and vpx proteins from primate lentiviruses. *J Virol* 1999; **73**: 592–600.

54 Kerkau T, Bacik I, Bennink JR, *et al.* The human immunodeficiency virus type 1 (HIV-1) Vpu protein interferes with an early step in the biosynthesis of major histocompatibility complex (MHC) class molecules. *J Exp Med* 1997; **185**: 1295–1305.

55 Collins KL, Chen BK, Kalams SA, Walker BD, Baltimore D. HIV-1 nef protein protects infected primary cells against killing by cytotoxic T lymphocytes. *Nature* 1998; **391**: 397–401.

56 Casella CR, Rapaport EL, Finkel TH. Vpu increases susceptibility of human immunodeficiency virus type 1-infected cells to fas killing. *J Virol* 1999; **73**: 92–100.

57 Collette Y, Dutartre H, Benziane A, Olive D. The role of HIV1 Nef in T-cell activation: Nef impairs induction of Th1 cytokines and interacts with the Src family tyrosine kinase Lck. *Res Virol* 1997; **148**: 52–58.

58 Kirchhoff F, Greenough TC, Brettler DB, Sullivan JL, Desroisiers RC. Brief report: absence of intact nef sequences in a long-term survivor with non-progressive HIV-1 infection. *N Engl J Med* 1995; **332**: 228–232.

59 Martin-Serrano J, Li K, Bieniasz PD. Regulation of Cyclin T1 expression. *Eighth Conference on Retroviruses and Opportunistic Infections*; Chicago: 2001, Abstract 121.

60 Jeang KT, Xiao H, Rich EA. Multifaceted activities of the HIV transactivator of transcription, Tat. *J Biol Chem* 1999; **274**: 28837–28840.

61 Saphire AC, Bobardt MD, Gallay PA. Human immunodeficiency virus type 1 hijacks host cell cyclophilin A for its attachment to target cells. *Immunol Res* 2000; **21**: 211–217.

62 Switzer WM, Wiktor S, Soriano V, *et al.* Evidence of nef truncation in human immunodeficiency virus type 2 infection. *J Infect Dis* 1998; **177**: 65–71

63 Markowitz DM, Hannibal M, Perez VL, *et al.* Differential regulation of human immunodeficiency viruses (HIVs): a specific regulatory element in HIV-2 responds to stimulation of the T-cell antigen receptor. *Proc Natl Acad Sci* 1990; **87**: 9098–9102.

64 Baldwin A. The NF-kappa B and I kappa B proteins: new discoveries and insights. *Ann Rev Immunol* 1996; **14**: 649–683.

65 Geijtenbeek TB, Kwon DS, Torensma R, *et al.* DC-SIGN, a dendritic-cell specific HIV-1 binding protein that enhances trans-infection of T cells. *Cell* 2000; **100**: 587–597.

66 Mascola JR, Frankel SS, Broliden K. HIV-1 entry at the mucosal surface: role of antibodies in protection. *AIDS* 2000; **14**: S167–174.

67 Clark SJ, Saag MS, Decker WD, *et al.* High titers of cytopathic virus in plasma of patients with symptomatic primary HIV-1 infection. *N Engl J Med* 1991; **324**: 954–960.

68 Daar ES, Moudgil T, Meyer RD, Ho DD. Transient high levels of viremia in patients with primary human immunodeficiency virus type 1 infection. *N Engl J Med* 1991; **324**: 961–964.

69 Rosenberg ES, Billingsley JM, Caliendo AM, et al. Vigorous HIV-1-specific CD4+ T cell responses associated with control of viremia. Science 1997; 278: 1447–1450.

70 Ogg GS, Jin X, Bonhoeffer S, et al. Quantitation of HIV-1-specific cytotoxic T lymphocytes and plasma load of viral RNA. Science 1998; 279: 2103–2106.

71 Cao Y, Qin L, Zhang L, Safrit J, Ho DD. Virologic and immunologic characterization of long-term survivors of human immunodeficiency virus type 1 infection. N Engl J Med 1995; 332: 201–208.

72 Migueles S, Sabbhagian MS, Shupert WL, et al. HLA B*5701 is highly associated with restriction of viral replication in a subgroup of HIV-infected long term progressors. Proc Natl Acad Sci USA 2000; 97: 2709–2714.

73 Johnson RP. The dynamics of T-lymphocyte turnover in AIDS. AIDS 2000; 14: S3–S9.

74 Zhang Z, Notermans DW, Sedgewick G, et al. Kinetics of CD4+ T cell repopulation of lymphoid tissues after treatment of HIV-1 infection. Proc Natl Acad Sci USA 1998; 95: 1154–1159.

75 Chun T-W, Carruth L, Finzi D, et al. Quantification of latent tissue reservoirs and total body viral load in HIV-infection. Nature 1997; 387: 183–188.

76 Rosok BI, Bostad L, Voltersvik P, et al. Reduced CD4 cell counts in blood do not reflect CD4 cell depletion in tonsillar tissue in asymptomatic HIV-1 infection. AIDS 1996; 10: F35–F38.

77 Pantaleo G, Graziosi C, Demarest JF, et al. HIV infection is active and progressive in lymphoid tissue during the clinically latent stage of disease. Nature 1993; 362: 355–358.

78 Embretson J, Zupancic M, Ribas JL, et al. Massive covert infection of helper T lymphocytes and macrophages by HIV during the incubation period of AIDS. Nature 1993; 362: 359–362.

79 Finkel TH, Tudor-Williams G, Banda NK, et al. Apoptosis occurs predominantly in bystander cells and not in productively infected cells of HIV- and SIV-infected lymph nodes. Nat Med 1995; 1: 129–134.

80 Mellors JW, Rinaldo CR, Gupta P, White RM, Todd JA, Kingsley LA. Prognosis of HIV-1 infection predicted by quantity of virus in plasma. Science 1996; 272: 1167–1170.

81 Coombs RW, Welles SL, Hooper C, et al. Association of plasma human immunodeficiency virus type 1 RNA level with risk of clinical progression in patients with advanced infection. J Infect Dis 1996; 174: 704–712.

82 Mellors JW, Munoz A, Giorgi J, et al. Plasma viral load and CD4+ lymphocytes as prognostic markers of HIV-1 infection. Ann Intern Med 1997; 126: 946–954.

83 Saag MS, Holodnity M, Kuritzkes DR, et al. HIV viral load markers in clinical practice. Nat Med 1996; 2: 625–629.

84 Multicohort Analysis Project Workshop. Immunologic markers of AIDS progression: consistency across five HIV-infected cohorts. AIDS 1994; 8: 911–921.

85 Pezzotti P, Phillips AN, Dorrucci M, et al. Category of exposure to HIV and age in the progression to AIDS: longitudinal study of 1199 people with known dates of seroconversion. HIV Italian Seroconversion Study Group. Br Med J 1996; 313: 583–586.

86 Sterling TR, Vlahov D, Astemborski J, Hoover DR, Margolick JB, Quinn TC. Initial plasma HIV-1 RNA levels in progression to AIDS in women and men. N Engl J Med 2001; 344: 720–725.

87 Marlink R, Kanki P, Thior I, et al. Reduced rate of disease development after HIV-2 infection as compared to HIV-1. Science. 1994; 8: 1587–1590.

88 Whittle H, Morris J, Todd J, et al. HIV-2-infected patients survive longer than HIV-1-infected patients. AIDS 1994; 8: 1617–1620.

89 Ariyoshi K, Jaffar S, Alabi AS, et al. Plasma viral load predicts the rate of CD4 T cell decline and death in HIV-2-infected patients in West Africa. AIDS 2000; 14: 339–344.

90 Berry N, Ariyoshi K, Jaffar S, et al. Low peripheral blood viral HIV-2 RNA in individuals with high CD4 percentage differentiates HIV-2 from HIV-1 infection. J Hum Virol 1998; 1: 457–468.

91 Cohen J. Can one type of HIV protect against another type? Science 1995; 268: 1566.

92 Travers K, Mboup S, Marlink R, et al. Natural protection against HIV-1 infection provided by HIV-2. Science 1995; 268: 1612–1615.

93 Ariyoshi K, Schim van der Loeff M, Sabally S, Cham F, Corrah T, Whittle H. Does HIV-2 infection provide cross-protection against HIV-1 infection? AIDS 1997; 11: 1053–1054.

94 Norrgren H, Andersson S, Biague AJ, et al. Trends and interaction of HIV-1 and HIV-2 in Guinea-Bissau, west Africa: no protection of HIV-2 against HIV-1 infection. AIDS 1999; 13: 701–707.

95 Wiktor SZ, Ekpini ER, Karon JM, et al. Short-course oral zidovudine for prevention of mother-to-child transmission of HIV-1 in Abidjan, Cote d'Ivoire: a randomised trial. Lancet 1999; 353: 781–785.

96 Ishikawa K, Fransen K, Ariyoshi K, et al. Improved detection of HIV-2 proviral DNA in dually seroreactive individuals by PCR. AIDS 1998; 12: 1419–1425.

97 Walther-Jallow L, Andersson S, da Silva Z, Biberfeld G. High concordance between polymerase chain reaction and antibody testing of specimens from individuals dually infected with HIV types 1 and 2 in Guinea-Bissau, West Africa. AIDS Res Hum Retroviruses 1999; 15: 957–962.

98 Nkengasong JN, Kestens L, Ghys PD, et al. Dual infection with human immunodeficiency virus type 1 and type 2: impact on HIV type 1 viral load and immune activation markers in HIV-seropositive female sex workers in Abidjan, Ivory Coast. AIDS Res Hum Retroviruses 2000; 16: 1371–1378.

99 Andersson S, Norrgren H, da Silva Z, et al. Plasma viral load in HIV-1 and HIV-2 singly and dually infected individuals in Guinea-Bissau, West Africa: significantly lower plasma virus set point in HIV-2 infection than in HIV-1 infection. Arch Intern Med 2000; 160: 3286–3293.

100 Royce RA, Sena A, Cates W, Cohen MS. Sexual transmission of HIV. N Engl J Med 1997; 336: 1072–1078.

101 Quinn TC, Wawer MJ, Sewankambo N, et al. Viral load and heterosexual transmission of human immunodeficiency virus type 1. N Engl J Med 2000; 342: 921–929.

102 Gray RH, Wawer MJ, Brookmeyer R, et al. Probability of HIV-1 transmission per coital act in monogamous, heterosexual, HIV-1-discordant couples in Rakai, Uganda. Lancet 2001; 357: 1149–1153.

103 Quinn T, Gray R, Sewankambo N, et al. Therapeutic reductions of HIV viral load to prevent HIV transmission: data from HIV discordant couples; Rakai, Uganda. Thirteenth International AIDS Conference; Durban: 2000, Abstract TuPeC3391.

104 Vernazza PL, Gilliam B, Dyer JR, et al. Quantification of HIV in semen: correlation with antiviral treatment and immune status. AIDS 1997; 11: 987–995.

105 Coombs RW, Speck CE, Hughes JF, et al. Association between culturable human immunodeficiency virus type 1 (HIV-1) in semen and HIV-1 RNA levels in semen and blood: evidence for compartmentalization of HIV-1 between semen and blood. J Infect Dis 1998; 177: 320–330.

106 Chakraborty H, Sen PK, Helms RW, et al. Viral burden in genital secretions determines male-to-female sexual transmission of HIV-1: A probabilistic empiric model. Eighth Conference on Retroviruses and Opportunistic Infections; Chicago: 2001, Abstract 223.

107 Dyer J, Gilliam B, Eron JJ, Cohen MS, Fiscus S, Vernazza P. Shedding of HIV in semen during primary infection. AIDS 1997; 11: 543–545.

108 Sewankambo N, Gray RH, Wawer MJ, et al. HIV-1 infection associated with abnormal vaginal flora morphology and bacterial vaginosis. Lancet 1997; 350: 546–550.

109 Clemetson DB, Moss GB, Willerford DM, et al. Detection of HIV DNA in cervical and vaginal secretions. Prevalence and correlates among women in Nairobi, Kenya. JAMA 1993; 269: 2860–2864.

110 Lazzarin A, Saracco A, Musicco M, Nicolosi A. Man-to-woman sexual transmission of the human immunodeficiency virus. Risk factors related to sexual behaviour, man's infectiousness and woman's susceptibility. Italian study group on HIV heterosexual transmission. *Arch Int Med* 1991; **151**: 2411–2416.

111 European Study Group on Heterosexual Transmission of HIV. Comparison of female to male and male to female transmission of HIV in 563 stable couples. *Br Med J* 1992; **304**: 809–813.

112 Mostad SB, Overbaugh J, De Vange DM, *et al.* Hormonal contraception, vitamin A deficiency, and other risk factors for shedding of HIV-1 infected cells from the cervix and vagina. *Lancet* 1997; **350**: 922–927.

113 Martin HL, Nyange PM, Richardson BA, *et al.* Hormonal contraception, sexually transmitted diseases, and heterosexual transmission of human immunodeficiency virus. *J Infect Dis* 1998; **178**: 1053–1059.

114 Downs AM, De Vincenzi I. Probability of heterosexual transmission of HIV: relationship with number of unprotected sexual contacts. European study group on heterosexual transmission of HIV. *J Acquir Immune Defic Syndr Hum Retrovirol* 1996; **11**: 388–395.

115 Musicco M, Lazzarin A, Nicolosi A, *et al.* Antiretroviral treatment of men infected with human immunodeficiency virus type 1 reduces the incidence of heterosexual transmission. *Arch Intern Med* 1994; **154**: 1971–1976.

116 Vernazza P, Troiani L, Flepp M, *et al.* Potent antiretroviral treatment of HIV-infection results in suppression of the seminal shedding of HIV. *AIDS* 2000; **14**: 117–121.

117 Imrie A, Beveridge A, Genn W, Vizzard J, Cooper DA. Transmission of human immunodeficiency virus type 1 resistant to nevirapine and zidovudine. Sydney Primary HIV Infection Study Group. *J Infect Dis* 1997; **175**: 1502–1505.

118 Hecht FM, Grant RM, Petropoulos CJ, *et al.* Sexual transmission of an HIV-1 variant resistant to multiple reverse transcriptase and protease inhibitors. *N Engl J Med* 1998; **339**: 307–311.

119 Yerly S, Kaiser L, Race E, Bru J-P, Clavel F, Perrin L. Transmission of antiretroviral-drug-resistant HIV-1 variants. *Lancet* 1999; **354**: 729–733.

120 Caceres CF, van Griensven GJP. Male homosexual transmission of HIV-1. *AIDS* 1994; **8**: 1051–1061.

121 DeGruttola V, Seage GR, Mayer KH, Horsburgh CR. Infectiousness of HIV between male homosexual partners. *J Clin Epidemiol* 1989; **42**: 849–856.

122 Lampinen TM, Critchlow CW, Kuypers JM, *et al.* Association of antiretroviral therapy with detection of HIV-1 RNA in the anorectal mucosa of homosexual men. *AIDS* 2000; **14**: F69–F75.

123 Vittinghoff E, Douglas J, Judson F, *et al.* Per-contact risk of human immunodeficiency virus transmission between male sexual partners. *Am J Epidemiol* 1999; **150**: 306–311.

124 Des Jarlais DC, Friedman SR, Choopanya K, Vanichseni S, Ward TP. International epidemiology of HIV and AIDS among injecting drug users. *AIDS* 1992; **6**: 1053–1068.

125 Krai AH, Bluthenthal RN, Lorvick J, Gee L, Bacchetti P, Edin BR. Sexual transmission of HIV-1 among injecting drug users in San Francisco: risk factor analysis. *Lancet* 2001; **357**: 1397–1401.

126 Newell M-L. Mechanisms and timing of mother-to-child transmission of HIV-1. *AIDS* 1998; **12**: 831–837.

127 Nicholl A, Newell M-L, Peckham C, Luo C, Savage F. Infant feeding and HIV-1 infection. *AIDS* 2000: **14**: S57–S74.

128 Cao Y, Krogstad P, Korber BT, *et al.* Maternal HIV-1 viral load and vertical transmission of infection: the Ariel Project for the prevention of HIV transmission from mother to infant. *Nature Med* 1997; **3**: 549–552.

129 Mayaux M-J, Teglas J-P, Mandelbrot L, *et al.* Acceptability and impact of zidovudine for prevention of mother-to-child human immunodeficiency virus-1 transmission in France. *J Pediatr* 1997; **131**: 857–862.

130 Thea DM, Steketee RW, Pliner V, *et al.* The effect of maternal viral load on the risk of perinatal transmission of HIV-1. *J Infect Dis* 1997; **175**: 707–711.

131 Mock PA, Shaffer N, Bhadrakom C, *et al* Maternal viral load and timing of vertical transmission of HIV-1, Bangkok, Thailand. *AIDS* 1999; **13**: 407–414.

132 Landesman SH, Kalish LA, Burns DN, *et al.* Obstetrical factors and the transmission of human immunodeficiency virus type 1 from mother to child. *N Engl J Med* 1996; **334**: 1617–1623.

133 The International Perinatal HIV Group. The mode of delivery and the risk of vertical transmission of human immunodeficiency virus type 1 – a meta analysis of 15 prospective cohort studies. *N Engl J Med* 1999; **340**: 977–987.

134 European Collaborative Study. Risk factors for mother-to-child transmission of HIV-1. *Lancet* 1992; **329**: 1007–1012.

135 Dunn DT, Newell ML, Ades AE, Peckham CS. Risk of human immunodeficiency virus type 1 transmission through breastfeeding. *Lancet* 1992; **340**: 585–588.

136 Nduati R, John G, Mbori-Ngacha D, *et al.* Effect of breastfeeding and formula feeding on transmission of HIV-1: a randomized clinical trial. *JAMA* 2000; **284**: 956–957.

137 Coutsoudis A, Pillay K, Spooner E, Kuhn L, Coovadia HM, for the South African Vitamin A Study Group. Influence of infant-feeding patterns on early mother-to-child transmission of HIV-1 in Durban, South Africa: a prospective cohort study. *Lancet* 1999; **354**: 471–476.

138 Van de Perre P, Simonon A, Msellati P, *et al.* Postnatal transmission of human immunodeficiency virus type 1 from mother to infant. *N Engl J Med* 1991; **325**: 593–598.

139 Leroy V, Newell ML, Dabis F, *et al.* International multicentre pooled analysis of late postnatal mother-to-child transmission of HIV-1 infection. Ghent International Working Group on Mother-to-Child Transmission of HIV. *Lancet* 1998; **352**: 597–600.

140 Semba RD, Kumwenda N, Hoover DR, *et al.* Human immunodeficiency virus load in breast milk, mastitis, and mother-to-child transmission of human immunodeficiency virus type 1. *J Infect Dis* 2000; **181**: 800–801.

141 Simonsen L, Kane A, Lloyd J, Zaffran M, Kane M. Unsafe injections in the developing world and transmission of bloodborne pathogens: a review. *Bull WHO* 1999; **77**: 789–800.

142 Kane A, Lloyd J, Zaffran M, Simonsen L, Kane M. Transmission of hepatitis B, hepatitis C and human immunodeficiency viruses through unsafe injections in the developing world: model-based regional estimates. *Bull WHO* 1999; **77**: 801–807.

143 Ghys PD, Fransen K, Diallo MO, *et al.* The associations between cervicovaginal HIV shedding, sexually transmitted diseases and immunosuppression in female sex workers in Abidjan, Cote d'Ivoire. *AIDS* 1997; **11**: F85–F93.

144 Schim van der Loeff MFS, Aaby P. Towards a better understanding of the epidemiology of HIV-2. *AIDS* 1999; **13**: S69–S84.

145 O'Donovan D, Ariyoshi K, Milligan P, *et al.* Maternal plasma viral RNA levels determine marked differences in mother-to-child transmission rates of HIV-1 and HIV-2 in the Gambia. *AIDS* 2000; **14**: 441–448.

146 Cooper DA, Gold J, Maclean P, *et al.* Acute AIDS retrovirus infection. Definition of a clinical illness associated with seroconversion. *Lancet* 1985; **i**: 537–540.

147 Brew BJ, Perdices M, Darveniza P, *et al.* The neurological features of early and 'latent' human immunodeficiency virus infection. *Aust N Z J Med* 1989; **19**: 700–705.

148 Pena JM, Martinez-Lopez MA, Arnalich F, Barbado FJ, Vazquez JJ. Esophageal candidiasis associated with acute infection due to human immunodeficiency virus: case report and review. *Rev Infect Dis* 1991; **13**: 872–875.

149 Kahn JO, Walker BD. Acute human immunodeficiency virus type 1 infection. *N Engl J Med* 1998; **339**: 33–39.

150 Boag F, Dean K, Hawkins DA, *et al.* Abnormalities of liver function during HIV

seroconversion illness. *Int J STD AIDS* 1992; **2**: 46–48.

151 Sinicco A, Fora R, Sciandra M, *et al*. Risk of developing AIDS after primary acute HIV-1 infection. *J AIDS*. 1993; **6**: 575–581.

152 Vanhems P, Lambert J, Cooper DA, *et al*. Severity and prognosis of acute human immunodeficiency virus type 1 illness: a dose–response relationship. *Clin Infect Dis* 1998; **26**: 323–329.

153 Soeprono FF, Schinella RA, Cockerell CJ, Comite SL. Seborrheic-like dermatitis of acquired immunodeficiency syndrome. A clinicopathologic study. *J Am Acad Dermatol* 1986; **14**: 242–248.

154 Soeprono FF, Schinella RA. Eosinophilic pustular folliculitis in patients with acquired immunodeficiency syndrome. Report of three cases. *J Am Acad Dermatol* 1986; **14**: 1020–1022.

155 Friedman-Kien A, Laubenstein L, Marmor M, *et al*. Kaposi's sarcoma and *Pneumocystis* pneumonia among homosexual men – New York and California. *MMWR* 1981; **30**: 305–308.

156 Antman K, Chang Y. Kaposi's sarcoma. *N Engl J Med* 2000; **342**: 1027–1038.

157 Francis ND, Parkin JM, Weber J, Boylston AW. Kaposi's sarcoma in acquired immune deficiency syndrome (AIDS). *J Clin Pathol* 1986; **39**: 469–474.

158 Cockerell CJ, Whitlow MA, Webster GF, Friedman-Kien AE. Epithelioid angiomatosis: a distinct vascular disorder in patients with the acquired immunodeficiency syndrome or AIDS-related complex. *Lancet* 1987; **ii**: 654–656.

159 Koehler JE, Sanchez MA, Garrido CS, *et al*. Molecular epidemiology of Bartonella infections in patients with bacillary angiomatosis-peliosis. *N Engl J Med* 1997; **337**: 1876–1883.

160 Adal KA, Cockerell CJ, Petri WA. Cat scratch disease, bacillary angiomatosis, and other infections due to rochalimea. *N Engl J Med* 1994; **330**: 1509–1515.

161 Greenspan D, Greenspan JS. HIV-related oral disease. *Lancet* 1996; **348**: 729–733.

162 Jacobson JM, Greenspan JS, Spritzler J, *et al*. Thalidomide for the treatment of oral aphthous ulcers in patients with human immunodeficiency virus infection. *N Engl J Med* 1997; **336**: 1487–1493.

163 Phair J, Munoz A, Detels R, *et al*. The risk of *Pneumocystis carinii* pneumonia among men infected with human immunodeficiency virus type 1. *N Engl J Med* 1990; **322**: 161–165.

164 Antonucci G, Girardi E, Raviglione MC, Ippolito G. Risk factors for tuberculosis in HIV-infected persons. A prospective cohort study. The Gruppo Italiano di Studio Tuberculosi e AIDS (GISTA). *JAMA* 1995; **274**: 143–148.

165 Havlir DV, Barnes PF. Tuberculosis in patients with human immunodeficiency

virus infection. *N Engl J Med* 1999; **340**: 367–373.

166 Rieder HL, Cauthen GM, Bloch AB, *et al*. Tuberculosis and acquired immunodeficiency syndrome – Florida. *Arch Intern Med* 1989; **149**: 1268–1273.

167 Klein NC, Duncanson FP, Lenox TH III, Pitta A, Cohen SC, Wormeser GP. Use of mycobacterial smears in the diagnosis of pulmonary tuberculosis in AIDS/ARC patients. *Chest* 1989; **95**: 1190–1192.

168 Brown TJ, Power EG, French GL. Evaluation of three commercial detection systems for *Mycobacterium tuberculosis* where clinical diagnosis is difficult. *J Clin Pathol* 1999; **52**: 193–197.

169 Hirschtick RE, Glassroth J, Jordan MC, *et al*. Bacterial pneumonia in persons infected with the human immunodeficiency virus. *N Engl J Med* 1995; **333**: 845–851.

170 Sharpstone D, Gazzard B. Gastrointestinal manifestations of HIV infection. *Lancet* 1996; **348**: 379–383.

171 Stockman M, Fromm M, Schmitz H, Schmidt W, Riecken E-O, Schulzke J-D. Duodenal biopsies of HIV-infected patients with diarrhoea exhibit epithelial barrier defects but no active secretion. *AIDS* 1998; **12**: 43–51.

172 Chen Y, Brennessel D, Walters J, Johnson M, Risner F, Raza M. Human immunodeficiency virus-associated pericardial effusion: report of 40 cases and review of the literature. *Am Heart J* 1999; **137**: 516–521.

173 Anderson DW, Virmani R. Cardiac pathology of HIV disease. In: Joshi V (ed.) *Pathology of AIDS and Other Manifestations of HIV Infection*. New York; Igaku-Shoin: 1992.

174 Barbaro G, Di Lorenzo G, Grisorio B, Barbarini G. Incidence of dilated cardiomyopathy and detection of HIV in myocardial cells of HIV-positive patients. Gruppo Italiano per lo Studio Cardiologico dei Pazienti Affetti da AIDS Investigators. *N Engl J Med* 1998; **339**: 1093–1099.

175 Currie PF, Jacob AJ, Foreman AR, Elton RA, Brettle RP, Boon NA. Heart muscle disease related to HIV infection: prognostic implications. *Br Med J* 1994; **309**: 1605–1607.

176 Mehta NJ, Khan IA, Mehta RN, Sepkowitz DA. HIV-related pulmonary hypertension: analytical review of 131 cases. *Chest* 2000; **118**: 1133–1141.

177 Dalakas MC, Illa I, Pezeshkpour GH, Laukatis JP, Cohen B, Griffin JL. Mitochondrial myopathy caused by long-term zidovudine therapy. *N Engl J Med* 1990; **322**: 1098–1105.

178 Hambleton J. Hematologic complications of HIV infection. *Oncology* 1996; **10**: 671–680.

179 Harris CE, Biggs JC, Concannon AJ, Dodds AJ. Peripheral blood and bone marrow

findings in patients with acquired immune deficiency syndrome. *Pathology* 1990; **22**: 206–211.

180 Aboulafia DM. Use of hematopoietic hormones for bone marrow defects in AIDS. *Oncology* 1997; **11**: 1827–1844.

181 Calenda V, Chermann JC. The effects of HIV on haematopoiesis. *Eur J Haematol* 1992; **48**: 181–186.

182 Fauci AS, Lane HC. Human immunodeficiency virus (HIV) disease: AIDS and related disorders. In: Isselbacher KJ, Braunwald E, Wilson JD, Martin JB, Fauci AS, Kasper DL (eds) *Harrison's Principles of Internal Medicine* 13th edition. New York; McGraw-Hill: 1994, pp. 1566–1618.

183 Mitsuyasu R. Oncological complications of human immunodeficiency virus disease and hematologic consequences of their treatment. *Clin Infect Dis* 1999; **29**: 35–43.

184 Moore RD, Keruly JC, Chaisson RE. Neutropenia and bacterial infection in acquired immunodeficiency syndrome. *Arch Intern Med* 1995; **155**: 1965–1970.

185 Walsh CM, Nardi MA, Karpatkin S. On the mechanism of thrombocytopenic purpura in sexually active homosexual men. *N Engl J Med* 1984; **311**: 635–639.

186 Savona S, Nardi MA, Lennette ET, Karpatkin S. Thrombocytopenic purpura in narcotic addicts. *Ann Intern Med* 1985; **102**: 737–741.

187 Ballem PJ, Belzberg A, Devine DV, *et al*. Kinetic studies of the mechanism of thrombocytopenia in patients with human immunodeficiency virus infection. *N Engl J Med* 1992; **327**: 1779–1784.

188 Toulon P. Hemostasis and human immunodeficiency virus (HIV) infection. *Annales de Biologie Clinique* 1998; **56**: 153–160.

189 Witz M, Lehman J, Korzets Z. Acute brachial artery thrombosis as the initial manifestation of human immunodeficiency virus infection. *Am J Hematol* 2000; **4**: 137–139.

190 Powderly WG. Bone disorders in HIV-infected patients. Expert Column. *Medscape HIV/AIDS* 2001; **7**(1).

191 Wong D, Cheung A, O'Rourke K, *et al*. Effect of alpha-interferon treatment in patients with hepatitis Be antigen-positive chronic hepatitis B: a meta-analysis. *Ann Intern Med* 1993; **119**: 312–323.

192 Wong D, Colina Y, Naylor C. Interferon alfa treatment of chronic hepatitis B: Randomized trial in a predominantly homosexual male population. *Gastroenterology* 1996; **108**: 165–171.

193 Carne C, Weller I, Waite J. Impaired responsiveness of homosexual men with HIV antibodies to plasma-derived hepatitis B vaccine. *Br J Med* 1987; **294**: 866–868.

194 Collier A, Corey L, Murphy V. Antibody to human immunodeficiency virus and

suboptimal response to hepatitis B vaccination. *Ann Intern Med* 1988; **109**: 101–105.

195 Manucci M, Zanetti A, Gringeri A. Long-term immunogenicity of a plasma-derived hepatitis B vaccine in HIV-seropositive and HIV-negative hemophiliacs. *Arch Intern Med* 1989; **149**: 1333–1337.

196 Bonacini M, Nussbaum J, Ahluwalia C. Gastrointestinal, hepatic, and pancreatic involvement with *Cryptococcus neoformans* in AIDS. *J Clin Gastroenterol* 1990; **12**: 295–297.

197 Bonacini M. Hepatobiliary complications in patients with human immunodeficiency virus infection. *Am J Med* 1992; **92**: 404–411.

198 Knowles DM, Chamulak G, Subar M, *et al.* Clinicopathologic, immunophenotypic, and molecular genetic analysis of AIDS-associated lymphoid neoplasia. Clinical and biologic implications. *Pathology Annual.* 1988; **23** Pt 2: 33–67.

199 Furrer H. Prevalence and clinical significance of splenomegaly in asymptomatic human immunodeficiency virus type 1-infected adults. *Clin Infect Dis* 2000; **30**: 943–945.

200 Laguna F, Adrados M, Alvar J, *et al.* Visceral leishmaniasis in patients infected with the human immunodeficiency virus. *Eur J Clin Microbiol Infect Dis* 1997; **16**: 898–903.

201 Puoti M, Spinetti A, Ghezzi A, *et al.* Mortality for liver disease in patients with HIV infection: a cohort study. *J AIDS* 2000; **24**: 211–217.

202 Blumberg R, Kelsey P, Perron T. Cytomegalovirus and cryptosporidium-associated acalculour cholecystitis. *Am J Med* 1984; **76**: 1118–1123.

203 Kavin H, Jonas R, Chowdhury L, *et al.* A calculous cholecystitis and cytomegalovirus infection in the acquired immunodeficiency syndrome. *Ann Intern Med* 1986; **104**: 53–54.

204 Cello J. Acquired immunodeficiency syndrome cholangiopathy: spectrum of disease. *Am J Med* 1989; **86**: 539–546.

205 Benhamou Y, Caumes E, Gerosa Y, *et al.* AIDS-related cholangiopathy. Critical analysis of a prospective series of 26 patients. *Dig Dis Sci* 1993; **38**: 1113–1118.

206 Pol S, Romana CA, Richard S, *et al.* Microsporidia infection in patients with the human immunodeficiency virus and unexplained cholangitis. *N Engl J Med* 1993; **328**: 95–99.

207 Ducreaux M, Buffet C, Beaugerie L. Diagnosis and prognosis of AIDS-related cholangitis. *AIDS* 1995; **9**: 875–880.

208 Rao TKS, Filippone EJ, Nicastri AD, *et al.* Associated focal and segmental glomerulosclerosis in the acquired immunodeficiency syndrome. *N Engl J Med* 1984; **310**: 669–673.

209 Brook MG, Miller RF. HIV associated nephropathy: a treatable condition. *Sex Transm Inf* 2001; **77**: 97–100.

210 Sharer LR. Pathology of HIV infection of the central nervous system: a review. *J Neuropathol Exp Pathol* 1992; **51**: 3–11.

211 McArthur JC, Hoover DR, Bacellar H, *et al.* Dementia in AIDS patients: incidence and risk factors. *Neurology* 1993; **43**: 2245–2252.

212 Koralnik IJ, Beaumanoir A, Hausler R, *et al.* A controlled study of early neurologic abnormalities in men with asymptomatic human immunodeficiency virus infection. *N Engl J Med* 1990; **323**: 864–870.

213 Navia BA, Price RW. Clinical and biologic features of the AIDS dementia complex. In: Gendelman HE, Lipton SA, Epstein L, Swindells S (eds) *The Neurology of AIDS.* New York; Chapman & Hall: 1998.

214 Budka H. HIV-associated neuropathology. In: Gendelman HE, Lipton SA, Epstein L, Swindells S (eds) *The Neurology of AIDS.* New York; Chapman & Hall: 1998.

215 Pohl P, Vogl G, Fill H, Rossler H, Zangerle R, Gerstenbrand F. Single photon emission computed tomography in AIDS dementia complex. *J Nucl Med* 1988; **29**: 1382–1386.

216 Gonzales RG, Ruiz A, Tracey I, McConnell J. Structural, functional, and molecular neuroimaging in AIDS. In: Gendelman HE, Lipton SA, Epstein L, Swindells S (eds) *The Neurology of AIDS.* New York; Chapman & Hall: 1998.

217 Brew BJ, Dunbar N, Pemberton L, Kaldor J. Predictive markers of AIDS dementia complex: CD4 cell count, and cerebrospinal fluid concentrations of β_2-microglobulin. *J Infect Dis* 1996; **174**: 294–298.

218 Ho D, Rota TR, Schooley RT, *et al.* Isolation of HTLV-III from cerebrospinal fluid and neural tissues of patients with neurologic symptoms related to the acquired immunodeficiency syndrome. *N Engl J Med* 1985; **313**: 1493–1497.

219 Goudsmit J, Wolters EC, Bakker M, *et al.* Intrathecal synthesis of antibodies to HTLV-III in patients without AIDS or AIDS related complex. *Br Med J* 1986; **292**: 1231–1234.

220 Shuanak S, Albright RE, Klotman ME, Henry SC, Bartlett JA, Hamilton JD. Amplification of HIV-1 provirus from cerebrospinal fluid and its correlation with neurologic disease. *J Infect Dis* 1990; **161**: 1068–1072.

221 Brew JB, Pemberton L, Cunningham P, Law MG. Levels of human immunodeficiency virus type 1 RNA in cerebrospinal fluid correlate with AIDS dementia stage. *J Infect Dis* 1997; **175**: 963–966.

222 Cinque P, Vago L, Ceresa D, *et al.* Cerebrospinal fluid HIV-1 RNA levels: correlation with HIV encephalitis. *AIDS* 1998; **12**: 389–394.

223 Petito CK, Navia BA, Cho E-S, Jordan BD, George DC, Price RW. Vacuolar myelopathy pathologically resembling subacute combined degeneration in patients with the acquired immunodeficiency syndrome. *N Engl J Med* 1985; **312**: 874–879.

224 Harrison LH, Vaz B, Quinn TC, *et al.* Myelopathy among Brazilians coinfected with human T-cell lymphotropic virus type I and HIV. *Neurology* 1997; **48**: 13–18.

225 Oksenhendler E, Charreau I, Tournerie C, Azihary M, Carbon C, Aboulker J-P. *Toxoplasma gondii* infection in advanced HIV infection. *AIDS* 1994; **8**: 483–487.

226 Remington JS, Desmont G. Toxoplasmosis. In: Remington JS, Klein JO (eds) *Infectious Diseases of the Fetus and Newborn Infant.* Philadelphia; WB Saunders: 1990, pp. 84–179.

227 Porter SB, Sande MA. Toxoplasmosis of the central nervous sytem in the acquired immunodeficiency syndrome. *N Engl J Med* 1992; **327**: 1643–1648.

228 Ruiz A, Ganz WI, Post JD, *et al.* Use of thallium-201 SPECT to differentiate cerebral lymphoma from toxoplasma encephalitis in AIDS patients. *Am J Neuroradiol* 1994; **15**: 1885–1894.

229 Raffi F, Aboulker JP, Michelet C, *et al.* A prospective study of criteria for the diagnosis of toxoplasmic encephalitis in 186 AIDS patients. The BIOTOXO Study Group. *AIDS* 1997; **11**: 1529–1530.

230 Cinque P, Scarpellini P, Vago L, Linde A, Lazzarin A. Diagnosis of central nervous system complications in HIV-infected patients: cerebrospinal fluid analysis by the polymerase chain reaction. *AIDS* 1997; **11**: 1–17.

231 Leading article. Cryptococcosis and AIDS. *Lancet* 1988; **i**: 1434–1435.

232 Chuck SL, Sande MA. Infections with *Cryptococcus neoformans* in the acquired immunodeficiency syndrome. *N Engl J Med* 1989; **321**: 794–799.

233 Van der Horst CM, Saag MS, Cloud GA, *et al.* Treatment of cryptococcal meningitis associated with the acquired immunodeficiency syndrome. *N Engl J Med* 1997; **337**: 15–21.

234 Quagliarello VJ, Viscoli C, Horwitz RI. Primary prevention of cryptococcal meningitis by fluconazole in HIV-infected patients. *Lancet* 1995; **345**: 548–552.

235 Cohen BA, Berger JR. Neurologic opportunistic infections in AIDS. In: Gendelman HE, Lipton SA, Epstein L, Swindells S (eds) *The Neurology of AIDS.* New York; Chapman & Hall: 1998.

236 Whiteman ML, Post MJ, Berger JR, Tate LG, Bell MD, Limonte LP. Progressive multifocal leucoencephalopathy in 47 HIV-seropositive patients: neuroimaging with clinical and pathologic correlation. *Radiology* 1993; **187**: 233–240.

237 Krachmarov CP, Chepenik LG, Barr-Vagell S, Khalili K, Johnson EM. Activation of the JC virus Tat-responsive transcriptional control element by association of the Tat protein of human immunodeficiency virus 1 with cellular protein Pur alpha. *Proc Natl Acad Sci USA* 1996; **93**: 14112–14117.

238 Albrecht H, Hoffmann C, Degen O, *et al.* Highly active antiretroviral therapy significantly improves the prognosis of patients with HIV-associated progressive multifocal leukoencephalopathy. *AIDS* 1998; **12**: 1149–1154.

239 De Luca A, Giancola ML, Ammassari A, *et al.* The effect of potent antiretroviral therapy and JC virus load in cerebrospinal fluid on clinical outcome of patients with AIDS-associated progressive multifocal leukoencephalopathy. *J Infect Dis* 2000; **182**: 1077–1083.

240 Bishburg E, Sunderham G, Reichman LB, *et al.* Central nervous system tuberculosis with the acquired immunodeficiency syndrome and its related complex. *Ann Intern Med* 1986; **105**: 210–213.

241 Villoria MF, De La Torre J, Fortea F, Munoz L, Hernandez T, Alarcon JJ. Intracranial tuberculosis in AIDS: CT and MRI findings. *Neuroradiology* 1992; **34**: 11–14.

242 De Angelis LM. Primary brain tumours in the acquired immunodeficiency syndrome. *Curr Opin Neurol* 1995; **8**; 419–423.

243 MacMahon EM, Glass JD, Hayward SD, *et al.* Epstein–Barr virus in AIDS-related primary central nervous system lymphoma. *Lancet* 1991; **338**; 969–973.

244 Berger JR, Harris JO, Gregorios J, Norenberg M. Cerebrovascular disease in AIDS: a case-control study. *AIDS* 1990; **4**: 239–244.

245 Griffin JW, Crawford TO, McArthur JC. Peripheral neuropathies associated with HIV infection. In: Gendelman HE, Lipton SA, Epstein L, Swindells S (eds) *The Neurology of AIDS*. New York; Chapman & Hall: 1998.

246 Cornblath DR, McArthur JC, Kennedy PGE, Witte AS, Griffin JW. Inflammatory demyelinating peripheral neuropathies associated with human T-lymphotropic virus type III infection. *Ann Neurol* 1987; **21**: 32–40.

247 Gherardi RK, Chretien F, Delfau-Larue M-H, *et al.* Neuropathy in diffuse infiltrative lymphocytosis syndrome. An HIV neuropathy, not a lymphoma. *Neurology* 1998; **50**: 1041–1044.

248 Craddock C, Pasvol G, Bull R, Protheroe A, Hopkins J. Cardiorespiratory arrest and autonomic neuropathy in AIDS. *Lancet* 1987; **ii**: 16–18.

249 Tagliati M, Morgello S, Simpson DM. Myopathy in HIV infection. In: Gendelman HE, Lipton SA, Epstein L, Swindells S (eds) *The Neurology of AIDS*. New York; Chapman & Hall: 1998.

250 Simpson DM, Citak KA, Godfrey E, Gobold J, Wolfe D. Myopathies associated with human immunodeficiency virus and zidovudine: can their effects be distinguished? *Neurology* 1993; **43**: 971–976.

251 Till M, MacDonnell KB. Myopathy with human immunodeficiency virus type 1 (HIV-1) infection: HIV-1 or zidovudine. *Ann Intern Med* 1990; **113**: 492–494.

252 Lowder CY, McMahon JT, Meisler DM, *et al.* Microsporidial keratoconjunctivitis caused by *Septata intestinalis* in a patient with acquired immunodeficiency syndrome. *Am J Ophthalmol* 1996; **121**: 715–717.

253 Glasgow BJ, Weisberger AK. A quantitative and cartographic study of retinal microvasculopathy in acquired immunodeficiency syndrome. *Am J Ophthalmol* 1994; **118**; 46–56.

254 Jabs DA, Bartlett JG. AIDS and ophthalmology: a period of transition. *Am J Ophthalmol* 1997; **124**; 227–233.

255 Whitcup SM, Fortin E, Lindblad AS, *et al.* Discontinuation of anticytomegalovirus therapy in patients with HIV infection and cytomegalovirus retinitis. *JAMA* 1999; **282**: 1633–1637.

256 Torriani FJ, Freeman WR, Macdonald JC, *et al.* CMV retinitis recurs after stopping treatment in virological and immunological failures of potent antiretroviral therapy. *AIDS* 2000; **14**: 173–180.

257 Zegans ME, Walton RC, Holland GN, O'Donnell JJ, Jacobson MA, Margolis TP. Transient vitreous inflammatory reactions associated with combination antiretroviral therapy in patients with AIDS and cytomegalovirus retinitis. *Am J Ophthalmol* 1998; **125**: 292–300.

258 Cunningham ET, Margolis TP. Ocular manifestations of HIV infection. *N Engl J Med* 1998; **339**: 236–244.

259 Poretsky L, Can S, Zumoff B. Testicular dysfunction in human immunodeficiency virus-infected men. *Metabolism* 1995; **44**; 946–953.

260 Lambert M. Thyroid dysfunction in HIV infection. *Baillières Clinical Endocrinology and Metabolism.* 1994; **8**: 825–835.

261 Marks JB. Endocrine manifestations of human immunodeficiency virus (HIV) infection. *Am J Med Sci* 1991; **302**: 110–117.

262 Gurtler L. Difficulties and strategies of HIV diagnosis. *Lancet* 1996; **348**; 176–179.

263 McAlpine L, Parry JV, Shanson D, Mortimer PP. False negative results in enzyme linked immunosorbent assays using synthetic HIV antigens. *J Clin Pathol* 1995; **48**: 490–493.

264 Zaaijer HL, Exel-Oehlers PV, Kraaijeveld T, Altena E, Lelie PN. Early detection of antibodies to HIV-1 by third generation assays. *Lancet* 1992; **340**: 770–772.

265 Constantine NT, van der Groen G, Belsey EM, Tamashiro H. Sensitivity of HIV-antibody assays determined by seroconversion panels. *AIDS* 1994; **8**: 1715–1720.

266 Gurtler L, Muhlbacher A, Michl U, *et al.* Reduction of the diagnostic window with a new combined p24 antigen and human immunodeficiency virus antibody screening assay. *J Virol Methods* 1998; **75**: 27–38.

267 Van Binsbergen J, Siebelink A, Jacobs A, *et al.* Improved performance of seroconversion with a 4th generation HIV antigen/antibody assay. *J Virol Methods* 1999; **82**: 77–84.

268 Busch MP, Petersen L, Schable C, Perkins H. Monitoring blood donors for HIV-2 infection by testing anti-HIV-1 reactive sera. *Transfusion* 1990; **30**: 184–187.

269 Sullivan PS, Schable C, Koch W, *et al.* Persistently negative HIV-1 antibody enzyme immunoassay screening results for patients with HIV-1 infection and AIDS: serologic, clinical, and virologic results. *AIDS* 1999; **13**: 89–96.

270 Ellenberger DL, Sullivan PS, Dorn J, *et al.* Viral and immunologic examination of human immunodeficiency virus type 1-infected, persistently seronegative persons. *J Infect Dis* 1999; **180**: 1033–1042.

271 Kassler WJ, Haley C, Jones WK, Gerber AR, Kennedy EJ, George JR. Performance of a rapid, on-site human immunodeficiency virus antibody assay in a public health setting. *J Clin Microbiol* 1995; **33**: 2899–2902.

272 Kelen GD, Bennecoff TA, Kline R, Green GB, Quinn TC. Evaluation of two rapid screening assays for the detection of human immunodeficiency virus-1 infection in emergency department patients. *Am J Emerg Med* 1991; **9**: 416–420.

273 Lyons SF. Evaluation of rapid enzyme binding assays for the detection of antibodies to HIV-1. *S Afr Med J* 1993; **83**: 115–117.

274 Van Kerckhoven I, Vercauteren G, Piot P, van der Groen G. Comparative evaluation of 36 commercial assays for detecting antibodies to HIV. *Bull WHO* 1991; **69**: 753–760.

275 Emmons WW, Paparello SF, Decker SF, Sheffield JM, Lowe-Bey FH. A modified ELISA and western blot accurately determine anti-human immunodeficiency virus type 1 antibodies in oral fluids obtained with a special collecting device. *J Infect Dis* 1995; **171**: 1406–1410.

276 Gallo D, George JR, Fitchen JH, Goldstein AS, Hindhal MS. Evaluation of a system using oral mucosal transudate for HIV-1 antibody screening and confirmatory testing. OraSure HIV Clinical Trials Group. *JAMA* 1997; **277**: 254–258.

277 King SD, Wynter SH, Bain BC, Brown WA, Johnston JN, Delk AS. Comparison of testing saliva and serum for detection of antibody to human immunodeficiency virus in Jamaica, West Indies. *J Clin Virol* 2000; **19**: 157–161.

278 Centers for Disease Control and Prevention. Interpretive criteria used to report western blot results for HIV-1 antibody testing – United States. *MMWR* 1991; **40**: 692–695.

279 MacDonald KL, Jackson JB, Bowman RJ, et al. Performance characteristics of serologic tests for human immunodeficiency virus type 1 (HIV-1) antibody among Minnesota blood donors. Public health and clinical implications. *Ann Intern Med* 1989; **110**: 617–621.

280 Jackson JB, MacDonald KL, Cadwell J, et al. Absence of HIV infection in blood donors with indeterminate western blot tests for antibody to HIV-1. *N Engl J Med* 1990; **322**: 217–222.

281 Celum CL, Coombs RW, Lafferty W, et al. Indeterminate human immunodeficiency virus type 1 Western blots: seroconversion risk, specificity of supplemental tests, and an algorithm for evaluation. *J Infect Dis* 1991; **164**: 656–664.

282 Celum CL, Coombs RW, Jones M, et al. Risk factors for repeatedly reactive HIV-1 EIA and indeterminate western blots. A population-based case-control study. *Arch Intern Med* 1994; **154**: 1129–1137.

283 Sullivan MT, Mucke H, Kadey SD, Fang CT, Williams AE. Evaluation of an indirect immunofluorescence assay for confirmation of human immunodeficiency virus type 1 antibody in US blood donors. *J Clin Microbiol* 1992; **30**: 2509–2510.

284 Ho DD, Moudgil T, Alam M. Quantitation of human immunodeficiency virus type 1 in the blood of infected persons. *N Engl J Med* 1989; **321**: 1621–1625.

285 Taylor-Robinson D, Thomas B, Ison C. Diagnostic procedures in genitourinary medicine: practical laboratory aspects. In: Barton SE, Hay PE (eds) *Handbook of Genitourinary Medicine*. London: Arnold; 1999.

286 Ariyoshi K, Bloor S, Bieniasz PD, Bourrelly M, Foxall R, Weber JN. Development of a rapid quantitative assay for HIV-1 plasma infectious viraemia-culture-PCR (CPID). *J Med Virol* 1994; **43**: 28–32.

287 Sninsky JJ, Kwok S. The application of quantitiative polymerase chain reaction to therapeutic monitoring. *AIDS* 1993; **7** (Suppl. 2): S29–S34.

288 Mulder J, Resnick R, Saget B, et al. A rapid and simple method for extracting human immunodeficiency virus type 1 RNA from plasma: enhanced sensitivity. *J Clin Microbiol* 1997; **35**: 1278–1280.

289 Volderbing PA. HIV quantification: clinical applications. *Lancet* 1996; **347**: 71–74.

290 Collins ML, Irvine B, Tyner D, et al. A branched DNA signal amplification assay for quantification of nucleic acid targets below 100 molecules /ml. *Nuc Acid Res* 1997; **25**: 2979–2984.

291 Daar ES, Little S, Pitt J, et al. Diagnosis of primary HIV infection. *Ann Intern Med* 2001; **134**: 25–29.

292 Rich JD, Merriman NA, Mylonakis E, et al. Misdiagnosis of HIV infection by HIV-1 plasma viral load testing: a case series. *Ann Intern Med* 1999; **130**: 37–39.

293 Ly TD, Edlinger C, Vabret A. Contribution of combined detection assays of p24 antigen and anti-human immunodeficiency virus (HIV) antibodies in diagnosis of primary HIV infection by routine testing. *J Clin Microbiol* 2000; **38**: 2459–1461.

294 Owens DK, Holodniy M, Garber A, et al. Polymerase chain reaction for the diagnosis of HIV infection in adults: a meta-analysis with recommendations for clinical practice and study design. *Ann Intern Med* 1996; **124**: 803–815.

295 Miles SA, Balden E, Magpantay L, et al. Rapid serologic testing with immune-complex-dissociated HIV p24 antigen for early detection of HIV infection in neonates. Southern California Pediatric AIDS Consortium. *N Engl J Med* 1993; **328**: 297–302.

296 Henrard DR, Phillips J, Windsor I, et al. Detection of human immunodeficiency virus type 1 p24 antigen and plasma RNA: relevance to indeterminate serologic tests. *Transfusion* 1994; **34**: 376–380.

297 Busch MP, Lee LL, Satten GA, et al. Time course of detection of viral and serologic markers preceding human immunodeficiency virus type 1 seroconversion; implications for screening of blood and tissue donors. *Transfusion* 1995; **35**: 91–7.

298 O'Brien TR, George JR, Epstein JS, Holmberg SD, Schochetman G. Testing for antibodies to human immunodeficiency virus type 2 in the United States. *MMWR* 1992; **41** (No. RR-12): 1–9.

299 Gilling-Smith C, Smith JR, Semprini AE. HIV and infertility: time to treat. *Br Med J* 2001; **322**: 566–567.

300 Kolesnitchenko V, Snart RS. Regulatory elements in the human immunodeficiency virus type 1 long terminal repeat LTR (HIV-1) responsive to steroid hormone stimulation. *AIDS Res Hum Retroviruses* 1992; **8**: 1977–1980.

301 Sinei SK, Morrison CS, Sekadde-Kigondu C, Allen M, Kokonya D. Complications of use of intrauterine devices among HIV-1-infected women. *Lancet* 1998; **351**: 1238–1241.

302 Richardson B, Morrison CS, Sekadde-Kigondu C, et al. Effect of intrauterine device use on cervical shedding of HIV-1 DNA. *AIDS* 1999; **13**: 2091–2097.

303 Murphy RL, Montaner J. Nevirapine: a review of its development, pharmacological profile and potential for clinical use. *Exp Opin Invest Drugs* 1996; **5**: 1183–1199.

304 Wang Y, Sawchuk RJ. Zidovudine transport in the rabbit brain during intravenous and intracerebroventricular infusion. *J Pharm Sci* 1995; **84**: 871–876.

305 Anderson PL, Noormohamed SE, Henry K, et al. Semen and serum pharmacokinetics of zidovudine and zidovudine-glucuronide in men with HIV-1 infection. *Pharmacotherapy* 2000; **8**: 917–922.

306 Boucher FD, Modlin JF, Weller S, et al. Phase I evaluation of zidovudine administered to infants exposed at birth to the human immunodeficiency virus. *J Pediatr* 1993; **122**: 137–144.

307 Ayers KM, Tucker WE, Hajan G, De Miranda P. Nonclinical toxicology studies with zidovudine: acute, subacute and chronic toxicity in rodents, dogs, and monkeys. *Fund Appl Toxicol* 1996; **32**: 129–139.

308 Ayers KM, Torrey CE, Reynolds DJ. A transplacental carcinogenicity bioassay in CD-1 mice with zidovudine. *Fund Appl Toxicol* 1997; **38**: 195–198.

308a Hanson IC, Antonelli TA, Sperling RS, et al. Lack of tumors in infants with perinatal HIV-1 exposure and fetal/neonatal exposure to zidovudine. *J Acquir Immune Defic Syndr Hum Retrovirol* 1999; **20**: 463–467.

309 Foudraine N, Hoetelmans R, Lange JMA, et al. Cerebrospinal fluid (CSF) HIV-RNA and drug concentrations during treatment with lamivudine (3TC) in combination with zidovudine (AZT) or stavudine (d4T). *Lancet* 1998; **351**: 1547–1551.

310 Taylor S, Van Heeswijk R, Hoetelmans RMW, et al. Concentrations of nevirapine, lamivudine and stavudine in semen of HIV-1 infected men. *AIDS* 2000; **14**: 1979–1984.

311 Kelley JA, Litterst CL, Roth VS, et al. The disposition and metabolism of 2′,3′-dideoxycytidine, an in vitro inhibitor of HTLV-III infectivity, in mice and monkeys. *Drug Metab Dispos* 1987; **15**: 595–601.

312 Daluge SM, Good SS, Faletto MB, et al. 1592U89, a novel carbocyclic nucleoside analog with potent, selective anti-human immunodeficiency virus activity. *Antimicrob Agents Chemother* 1997; **41**: 1082–1093.

313 Tuntland T, Odinecs A, Pereira CM, Nosbisch C, Unadkat JD. In vitro models to predict the in vivo mechanism, rate, and extent of placental transfer of dideoxyribonucleoside drugs against human immunodeficiency virus. *Am J Obstet Gynecol* 1999; **180**: 198–206.

314 Patterson TA, Binienda ZK, Newport GD, et al. Transplacental pharmacokinetics and fetal distribution of 2′,

3'-didehydro-3'-deoxythymidine (d4T) and its metabolites in late-term rhesus macaques. *Teratology* 2000; **62**: 93–99.

315 Musoke P, Guay LA, Bagenda D, *et al.* A phase I/II study of the safety and pharmacokinetics of nevirapine in HIV-1-infected pregnant Ugandan women and their neonates (HIVNET 006). *AIDS* 1999; **13**: 479–486.

316 Perry CMJ, Balfour JA. Didanosine. An update on its antiviral activity, pharmacokinetic properties and therapeutic efficacy in the management of HIV disease. *Drugs* 1996; **52**: 928–962.

317 Havlir D, Cheesman SH, McLaughlin M, *et al.* High dose nevirapine: safety, pharmacokinetics, and antiviral effect in patients with HIV infection. *J Infect Dis* 1995; **171**: 537–544.

318 Clarke S, Harrington P, Condon C, Kelleher D, Smith OP, Mulcahy F. Late onset hepatitis and prolonged deterioration in hepatic function associated with nevirapine therapy. *Int J STD AIDS* 2000; **11**: 336–337.

319 Voorman RL, Payne NA, Wienkers LC, Hauer MJ, Sanders PE. Interaction of delavirdine with human liver microsomal cytochrome P450: inhibition of CYP2C9, CYP2C19, and CYP2D6. *Drug Metabolism Disposition* 2001; **29**; 41–47.

320 Gangar M, Arias G, O'Brien JG, Kemper CA. Frequency of cutaneous reactions on rechallenge with nevirapine and delavirdine. *Ann Pharmacother* 2000; **34**: 839–842.

321 Khaliq Y, Gallicano K, Seguin I, *et al.* Single and multiple pharmacokinetics of nelfinavir and CYP2C19 activity in human immunodeficiency virus-infected patients with chronic liver disease. *Br J Clin Pharmacol* 2000; **50**: 108–115.

322 Brinkman K, Kroon F, Hugen PWH, Burger DM. Therapeutic concentrations of indinavir in cerebrospinal fluid of HIV-1-infected patients. *AIDS* 1998; **12**: 537.

323 Van Praag R, Wavering G, Portegies P, *et al.* Enhanced penetration of indinavir in cerebrospinal fluid after addition of low dose ritonavir. *AIDS* 2000; **14**: 1187–1194.

324 Moyle G. Saquinavir: a review of its development, pharmacological properties and its clinical use. *Exp Opin Invest Drugs* 1996; **5**: 155–167.

325 Reijers M, Van Heeswijk P, Jurrianns S, *et al.* The concentrations of D4T, 3TC, nelfinavir, and saquinavir in plasma, cerebrospinal fluid, and semen. *Seventh International Conference on Retroviruses and Opportunistic Infections*. San Francisco: 2000: Abstract 316.

326 Dunn DT, Brandt CD, Krivine A, *et al.* The sensitivity of HIV-1 DNA polymerase chain reaction in the neonatal period and the relative contributions of intra-uterine and intra-partum transmission. *AIDS* 1995; **9**: F7–11.

327 Steketee RW, Abrams EJ, Thea DM, *et al.* Early detection of perinatal human immunodeficiency virus (HIV) type 1 infection using HIV RNA amplification and detection. New York City Perinatal HIV Transmission Collaborative Study. *J Infect Dis* 1997; **175**: 707–711.

328 Schooley R, Myers R, Runae P, Beall G, Lampiris H, McGowan I. A double-blind, placebo-controlled study of tenofovir disoproxil fumarate (TDF) for the treatment of HIV infection. *Thiry-ninth Interscience Conference on Antimicrobial Agents and Chemotherapy*; San Francisco: 1999, Abstract LB-19.

329 Miller MD, Margot NA, Hertogs K, Larder B, Miller V. Antiviral activity of tenofovir (PMPA) against nucleoside-resistant HIV samples. *Fortieth Interscience Conference on Antimicrobial Agents and Chemotherapy*; Toronto: 2000, Abstract 2115.

330 Foli A, Lori F. Hyroxyurea combination therapy. *J HIV Therapy* 1999; **4**: 45–48.

331 Chapuis AG, Paolo Rizzardi G, D'Agostino C, *et al.* Effects of mycophenolic acid on human immunodeficiency virus infection in vitro and in vivo. *Nat Med* 2000; **6**: 762–768.

332 Margolis D, Heredia A, Gaywee J, Oldach D, Drusano G, Redfield R. Abacavir and mycophenolic acid, an inhibitor of inosine monophosphate dehydrogenase, have profound and synergistic anti-HIV activity. *J AIDS* 1999; **21**: 362–370.

333 Fischl MA, Richman DD, Grieco MH, *et al.* The efficacy of azidothymidine in the treatment of patients with AIDS and AIDS-related complex. *N Engl J Med* 1987; **317**: 185–191.

334 Mocroft A, Katlama C, Johnson AM, *et al.* AIDS across Europe, 1994–98: the EuroSIDA study. *Lancet* 2000; **356**: 291–296.

335 Brun-Vezinet F, Boucher C, Loveday C, *et al.* HIV-1 viral load, phenotype, and resistance in a subset of drug-naïve participants from the Delta trial. The National Virology Groups. Delta Virology Working Group and Co-ordinating Committee. *Lancet* 1997; **350**: 983–990.

336 Pilcher CD, Miller WC, Beatty ZA, Eron JJ. Detectable HIV-1 RNA at levels below quantifiable limits by amplicor HIV-1 monitor is associated with virologic relapse on antiretroviral therapy. *AIDS* 1999; **13**: 1337–1342.

337 Raboud JM, Rae S, Vella S, *et al.* Meta-analysis of two randomized controlled trials comparing combined zidovudine and didanosine therapy with combined zidovudine, didanosine, and nevirapine therapy in patients with HUV. INCAS study team. *J AIDS* 1999; **22**: 260–266.

338 Hogg RS, Yip B, Wood E, *et al.* Diminished effectiveness of antiretroviral therapy among patients initiating therapy with CD4+ cell counts below 200/mm³. *Eighth Conference on Retroviruses and Opportunistic Infections*; Chicago: 2001, Abstract 342.

339 Lederberger B, Egger M, Erard V, *et al.* AIDS-related opportunistic illness occurring after initiation of potent antiretroviral therapy. *JAMA* 1999; **282**: 2220–2226.

340 Miller V, Staszewski S, Nisius G, Cozzi Lepri A, Sabin CA, Phillips AN. Risk of new AIDS diseases in people on triple therapy. *Lancet* 1999; **353**: 463.

341 Lederman M, Valdez H. Immune restoration with antiretroviral therapies: implications for clinical management. *JAMA* 2000; **284**: 223–228.

342 Kovacs JA, Masur H. Prophylaxis against opportunistic infections in patients with human immunodeficiency virus infection. *N Engl J Med* 2000; **342**: 1416–1429.

343 Whitcup SM. Cytomegalovirus retinitis in the era of highly active antiretroviral therapy. *JAMA* 2000; **283**: 653–657.

344 Oxenius A, Price DA, Easterbrook PJ, *et al.* Early highly active antiretroviral therapy for acute HIUV-1 infection preserves immune function of CD8+ and CD4+ T lymphocytes. *Proc Natl Acad Sci USA* 2000; **97**: 3382–3387.

345 Rosenberg ES, Altfield M, Poon SH, *et al.* Immune control of HIV-1 after early treatment of acute infection. *Nature* 2000; **407**: 523–526.

346 Ravot E, Tambussi G, Jessen H, *et al.* Effects of hydroxyurea on T cell count changes during primary HIV infection. *AIDS* 2000; **14**: 619–622.

347 Rizzardi GP, Capiluppi B, Tambussi *et al.* Effect of cyclosporin A in combination with highly active antiretroviral therapy in primary HIV-1 infection. *Eighth Conference on Retroviruses and Opportunistic Infections*; Chicago: 2001, Abstract 759.

348 Hecht FM, Levy JA, Martinez-Marino B, *et al.* A randomized trial of interleukin-2 (IL-2) added to HAART for primary HIV. *Eighth Conference on Retroviruses and Opportunistic Infections*; Chicago: 2001, Abstract 407.

349 Phillips A, Staszewski S, Weber R, *et al.* Viral load changes in response to antiretroviral therapy according to the baseline CD4 lymphocyte count and viral load. *Fifth International Congress on Drug Therapy in HIV Infection*; Glasgow: 2000, Abstract PL3.4.

350 Sterling TR, Chaisson RE, Bartlett JG, Moore RD. CD4+ lymphocyte level is better than HIV-1 plasma viral load in determining when to initiate HAART. *Eighth Conference on Retroviruses and Opportunistic Infections*; Chicago: 2001, Abstract 519.

351 Kaplan J, Hanson D, Karon J, *et al.* Late initiation of antiretroviral therapy (at CD4+ lymphocyte count < 200 cells/µl) is associated with increased risk of death. *Eighth Conference on Retroviruses and Opportunistic Infections*; Chicago: 2001, Abstract 520.

352 Havlir DV, Richman DD. Viral dynamics of HIV: implications for drug development and therapeutic strategies. *Ann Intern Med* 1996; **124**: 984–994.

353 Durant J, Clevenbergh P, Halfon F *et al.* Drug resistance genotyping in HIV-1 therapy: the VIRADAPT randomised controlled trial. *Lancet* 1999; **353**: 2195–2199.

354 Baxter JD, Mayers DL, Wentworth DN *et al.* A randomised study of antiretroviral management based on plasma genotypic resistance testing in patients failing therapy. CPCRA 046 study team for the Terry Beirn Community Programs for Clinical Research on AIDS. *AIDS* 2000; **14**: F83–F93.

355 Cohen C, Kessler H, Hunt S *et al.* Phenotypic resistance testing significantly improves response to therapy: final analysis of a randomized controlled trial (VIRA 3001). *Antiviral Ther* 2000, **5** (Suppl. 3): 67.

356 Meynard JL, Wray M, Mourand-Joubert L *et al.* Impact of treatment guided by phenotypic and genotypic resistance tests on the response to antiretroviral therapy: a randomized controlled trial (NARVAL, ANRS 088). *Antiviral Ther* 2000, **5** (Suppl. 3): 67–68.

357 Hirsch MS, Brun-Vezinet F, D'Aquila R, *et al.* Antiretroviral drug resistance testing in adult HIV-1 infection. *JAMA* 2000; **283**: 2417–2426.

358 Havlir D, Hirsch MS, Richman DD, *et al.* Prevalence and predictive value of intermittent viremia in patients with viral suppression. *Thirteenth International AIDS Conference*; Durban: 2000, Abstract TuPeB3195.

359 Sharkey ME, Teo I, Greenough T, *et al.* Persistence of episomal HIV-1 infection intermediates in patients on highly active antiretroviral therapy. *Nat Med* 2000; **6**: 76–81.

360 Deeks SG, Barbour JD, Martin JN, Swanson MS, Grant RM. Sustained CD4+ T cell response after virologic failure of protease inhibitor-based regimens in patients with human immunodeficiency virus infection. *J Infect Dis* 2000; **181**: 946–953.

361 Paredes R, Ruiz L. Changing from a protease inhibitor to a non-nucleoside reverse transcriptase inhibitor. *J HIV Ther* 2000; **5**: 64–66.

362 Rustin P. Mitochondrial dysfunction in HIV infection: an overview of pathogenesis. *J HIV Ther* 2001; **6**: 4–12.

363 Blanche S, Tardieu M, Rustin P, *et al.* Persistent mitochondrial dysfunction and perinatal exposure to antiretroviral nucleoside analogues. *Lancet* 1999; **354**: 1084–1089.

364 Lange J, Stellato R, Brinkman K, *et al.* Review of neurological adverse events in relation to mitochondrial dysfunction in the prevention of mother to child transmission of HIV: PETRA study. *Second Conference on Global Strategies for the Prevention of HIV Transmission from Mothers to Infants*; Montreal: 1999, Abstract 250.

365 The Perinatal Safety Review Working Group. Nucleoside exposure in the children of HIV-infected women receiving antiretroviral drugs: absence of clear evidence for mitochondrial disease in children who died before 5 years of age in five United States cohorts. *J Acquir Immune Defic Syndr Hum Retrovirol* 2000; **15**: 261–268.

366 Lipshultz SE, Easley KA, Orav EJ, *et al.* Absence of cardiac toxicity of zidovudine in infants. *N Engl J Med* 2000; **343**: 759–766.

367 Boxwell DE, Styrt BA. Lactic acidosis (LA) in patients receiving nucleoside reverse transcriptase inhibitors (NRTIs). *Thirty-ninth Interscience Conference on Antimicrobial Agents and Chemotherapy*; San Francisco: 1999, Abstract 1284.

368 Henry K, Melroe H, Huebsch J, *et al.* Severe premature coronary artery disease with protease inhibitors. *Lancet* 1998; **351**: 1328.

369 Carr A, Samaras K, Thorisdottir A, Kaufmann GR, Chisholm DJ, Cooper DA. Diagnosis, prediction, and natural course of HIV-I protease inhibitor-associated lipodystrophy, hyperlipidaemia, and diabetes mellitus: a cohort study. *Lancet* 1999; **353**: 2093–2099.

370 Walli R, Goebel FD, Demant T. Impaired glucose tolerance and protease inhibitors. *Ann Intern Med* 1998; **129**: 837–838.

371 Zhang B, MacNaul K, Szalkowski D, Li Z, Berger J, Moller DE. Inhibition of adipocyte differentiation by HIV protease inhibitors. *J Clin Endocrinol Metab* 1999; **84**: 4274–4277.

372 Lenhard J, Weiel JE, Paulki MA, Furfine ES. Stimulation of vitamin A1 acid signaling by the HIV protease inhibitor indinavir. *Biochem Pharmacol* 2000; **59**: 1063–1068.

373 Brinkman K, Smeitink JA, Romijn JA, Reiss P. Mitochondrial toxicity induced by nucleoside-analogue reverse-transcriptase inhibitors is a key factor in the pathogenesis of antiretroviral-therapy-related lipodystrophy. *Lancet* 1999; **354**: 1112–1115.

374 Carr A, Miller J, Cooper D. Osteopenia in HIV-infected men: association with lactic acidemia and lower weight pre-antiretroviral therapy. *Antiviral Ther* 2000; **5** (Suppl. 5): 20–21, Abstract O32.

375 Cinti SK. Adherence to antiretrovirals in HIV disease. *AIDS Reader* 2000; **10**: 709–717.

376 Paterson D, Swindells S, Mohr J, *et al.* How much adherence is enough? A prospective study of adherence to protease inhibitor therapy using MEMS caps. *Sixth Conference on Retroviruses and Opportunistic Infections*. Chicago; 1999: Abstract 92.

377 Fischl M, Rodriguez A, Scerpella E, *et al.* Impact of directly observed therapy on outcomes in HIV clinical trials. *Seventh Conference on Retroviruses and Opportunistic Infections*; San Francisco: 2000, Abstract 71.

378 Besch CL. Compliance in clinical trials. *AIDS* 1995; **9**: 1–10.

379 Markowitz JC, Kocsis JH, Fishman B, *et al.* Treatment of depressive symptoms in human immunodeficiency virus-positive patients. *Arch Gen Psychiatry* 1998; **55**: 452–457.

380 Geletko SM, Ballard CR, Matthews WC. Health beliefs and discontinuation of zidovudine therapy. *Am J Health System Pharm* 1995; **52**: 505–507.

381 Piscitelli SC, Gallicano KD. Drug therapy: interactions among drugs for HIV and opportunistic infections. *N Engl J Med* 2001; **344**: 984–996.

382 Henry JA, Hill IR. Fatal interaction between ritonavir and MDMA. *Lancet* 1998; **352**: 1751–1752.

383 Piscitelli SC, Burstein AH, Chaitt D, Alfaro RM, Falloon J. Indinavir concentrations and St John's wort. *Lancet* 2000; **355**: 547–548.

384 Burger DM, Hoetelmans RM, Hugen PW, *et al.* Low plasma concentrations of indinavir are related to virological treatment failure in HIV-1-infected patients on indinavir-containing triple therapy. *Antiviral Ther* 1998; **3**: 215–220.

385 Acosta EP, Kakuda TN, Brundage RC, Anderson PL, Fletcher CV. Pharmacodynamics of human immunodeficiency virus type 1 protease inhibitors. *Clin Infect Dis* 2000; **30** (Suppl. 2): S151–S159.

386 Molla A, Korneyeva M, Gao Q, *et al.* Ordered accumulation of mutations in HIV protease confers resistance to ritonavir. *Nat Med* 1996; **2**: 760–766.

387 Kakuda TN, Page LM, Anderson PL, *et al.* Pharmacological basis for concentration-controlled therapy with zidovudine, lamivudine, and indinavir. *Antimicrob Agents Chemother* 2001; **45**: 236–242.

388 Clevenbergh P, Durant J, Garaffo R, Kirstetter M, Daures JP, Dellamonica P, and Infectio-SUD Group. Usefulness of protease inhibitor therapeutic drug monitoring? PharmAdapt: a prospective multicentric randomized controlled trial: 12 weeks results. *Eighth Conference on Retroviruses*

and Opportunistic Infections; Chicago: 2001, Abstract 260B.

389 Race EM, Adelson-Mitty J, Kriegel GR, *et al.* Focal mycobacterial lymphadenitis following initiation of protease-inhibitor therapy in patients with advanced HIV-1 disease. *Lancet* 1998; **351**: 252–255.

390 Jacobson MA, Zegans M, Pavan PR, *et al.* Cytomegalovirus retinitis after initiation of highly active antiretroviral therapy. *Lancet* 1997; **349**: 1443–1445.

391 Narita M, Ashkin D, Hollender ES, Pitchenik AE. Paradoxical worsening of tuberculosis following antiretroviral therapy in patients with AIDS. *Am J Respir Crit Care Med* 1998; **158**: 157–161.

392 Deeks SG, Hoh R, Troiano J, *et al.* Virologic and immunologic evaluation of structured treatment interruption (STI) in patients experiencing long-term virologic failure. *Seventh Conference on Retroviruses and Opportunistic Infections*; San Francisco: 2000.

393 Rook AH, Masur H, Lane HC, *et al.* Interleukin-2 enhances the depressed natural killer and cytomegalovirus-specific cytotoxic activities of lymphocytes from patients with the acquired immune deficiency syndrome. *J Clin Invest* 1983; **72**: 398–403.

394 Davey RT, Murphy RL, Graziano FM, *et al.* Immunologic and virologic effects of subcutaneous interleukin 2 in combination with antiretroviral therapy: a randomized controlled trial. *JAMA* 2000; **284**: 183–189.

395 Arno A, Ruiz L, Juan M, *et al.* Efficacy of low-dose subcutaneous interleukin-2 to treat advanced human immunodeficiency virus type 1. *J Infect Dis* 1999; **180**: 56–60.

396 Emery S, Capra WB, Cooper DA, *et al.* Pooled analysis of 3 randomized, controlled trials of interleukin-2 therapy in adult human immunodeficiency virus type 1 disease. *J Infect Dis* 2000; **182**: 428–434.

397 Kovacs JA, Imamichi H, Vogel S, *et al.* Effects of intermittent interleukin-2 therapy on plasma and tissue human immunodeficiency virus levels and quasi-species expression. *J Infect Dis* 2000; **182**: 1063–1069.

398 Davey RT, Chaitt DG, Albert JM, *et al.* A randomized trial of high versus low-dose subcutaneous interleukin-2 outpatient therapy for human immunodeficiency virus type 1 infection. *J Infect Dis* 1999; **179**: 849–858.

399 Tuomala RE. Prevention of transmission. Pharmaceutical and obstetric approaches. *Obstet Gynecol Clin NA* 1997; **24**: 785–795.

400 Connor EM, Sperling RS, Gelber R, *et al.* Reduction of maternal–infant transmission of human immunodeficiency virus type 1 with zidovudine treatment. *N Engl J Med* 1994; **331**: 1173–1180.

401 Sperling RS, Shapiro DE, Coombs RW, *et al.* Maternal viral load, zidovudine treatment, and the risk of transmission of human immunodeficiency virus type 1 from mother to infant. *N Engl J Med* 1996; **335**: 1621–1629.

402 Stiehm ER, Lambert JS, Mofenson LM, *et al.* Efficacy of zidovudine and hyperimmune HIV immunoglobulin for reducing perinatal HIV transmission from HIV-infected women with advanced disease: results of Pediatric AIDS Clinical Trials Group Protocol 185. *J Infect Dis* 1999; **179**: 567–575.

403 Mofenson LM, McIntyre JA. Advances and research directions in the prevention of mother-to-child HIV-1 transmission. *Lancet* 2000; **355**: 2237–2244.

404 Shaffer N, Chuachoowong R, Mock PA, *et al.* Short-course zidovudine for perinatal HIV-1 transmission in Bangkok, Thailand: a randomised controlled trial. *Lancet* 1999; **353**: 773–780.

405 Wiktor SZ, Nkengasong JN, Ekpini ER, *et al.* Lack of protection against HIV-1 infection among women with HIV-2 infection. *AIDS* 1999; **13**: 695–699.

406 Lallemant M, Jourdain G, Le Coeur S, *et al.* A trial of shortened zidovudine regimens to prevent mother-to-child transmission of human immunodeficiency virus type 1. *N Engl J Med* 2000; **343**: 982–991.

407 Wade NA, Birkhead GS, Warren BL, *et al.* Abbreviated regimens of zidovudine prophylaxis and perinatal transmission of the human immunodeficiency virus. *N Engl J Med* 1998; **339**: 1409–1414.

408 Mofenson LM, Lambert JS, Stiehm ER, *et al.* Risk factors for perinatal transmission of human immunodeficiency virus type 1 in women treated with zidovudine. *N Engl J Med* 1999; **341**: 385–393.

409 Welles SL, Pitt J, Colgrove R, *et al.* HIV-1 genotypic zidovudine drug resistance and the risk of maternal–infant transmission in the Women and Infants Transmission Study. *AIDS* 2000; **14**: 263–271.

410 Kully C, Yerly S, Erb P, *et al.* Codon 215 mutations in human immunodeficiency virus-infected pregnant women. *J Infect Dis* 1999; **179**: 705–708.

411 Saba J on behalf of the PETRA Trial Study Team. Interim analysis of early efficacy of three short ZDV/3TC combination regimens to prevent mother-to-child transmission: the PETRA trial. *Sixth Conference on Retroviruses and Opportunistic Infections*; Chicago: 1999, Abstract S-7.

412 Guay LA, Musoke P, Fleming T, *et al.* Intrapartum and neonatal single-dose nevirapine compared with zidovudine for prevention of mother-to-child transmission of HIV-1 in Kampala, Uganda: HIVNET 012 randomised trial. *Lancet* 1999; **354**: 795–802.

413 McGowan JP, Crane M, Wiznia AA, Blum S. Combination antiretroviral therapy in human immunodeficiency virus-infected pregnant women. *Obstet Gynecol* 1999; **94**: 641–646.

414 Chuachoowong R, Shaffer N, Siriwasin W, *et al.* Short-course antenatal zidovudine reduces both cervicovaginal human immunodeficiency virus type 1 RNA levels and the risk of perinatal transmission. Bangkok Collaborative Perinatal HIV Transmission Study Group. *J Infect Dis* 2000; **181**: 99–106.

415 The European Mode of Delivery Collaboration. Elective Caesarean-section versus vaginal delivery in prevention of HIV-1 transmission: a randomised clinical trial. *Lancet* 1999; **353**: 1035–1039.

416 The European Collaborative Study and the Swiss Mother + Child Cohort Study. Combination antiretroviral therapy and duration of pregnancy. *AIDS* 2000; **14**: 2913–2920.

417 Jackson JB, Becker-Pergola G, Guay L, *et al.* Identification of the K103N resistance mutation in Ugandan women receiving nevirapine to prevent HIV-1 vertical transmission. *AIDS* 2000; **14**: F111–F115.

418 American College of Obstetricians and Gynecologists Committee Opinion. Scheduled cesarean delivery and the prevention of vertical transmission of HIV infection. Number 234. May 2000.

419 Cardo DM, Culver DH, Ciesielski CA, *et al.* A case-control study of HIV seroconversion in health care workers after percutaneous exposure. Centers for Disease Control and Prevention Needlestick Surveillance Group. *N Engl J Med* 1997; **337**: 1485–1490.

420 United Kingdom Health Departments. HIV post-exposure prophylaxis: guidance from the UK Chief Medical Officers' Expert Advisory Group on AIDS. 2000.

421 Centers for Disease Control and Prevention. Public Health Service guidelines for the management of health-care worker exposures to HIV and recommendations for postexposure prophylaxis. *MMWR* 1998; **47** (RR-7): 1–28.

422 Centers for Disease Control and Prevention. Serious adverse events attributed to nevirapine regimens for postexposure prophylaxis after HIV exposures. *MMWR* 2001; **49**: 1153–1156.

423 Benn PD, Mercey DE, Brink N, Scott G, Williams IG. Prophylaxis with a nevirapine-containing triple regimen after exposure to HIV-1. *Lancet* 2001; **357**: 687–688.

424 Katz MH, Gerberding JL. Post-exposure prophylaxis after sexual exposure to HIV. *J HIV Ther* 2000; **5**: 5–9.

425 Martin LN, Murphey-Corb M, Soike KF, *et al.* Effects of initiation of 3'-azido, 3'-deoxythymidine (zidovudine) treatment at different times after infection of

rhesus monkeys with simian immunodeficiency virus. *J Infect Dis* 1993; **168**: 825–835.

426 Blattner W, Cooper E, Charurat M, *et al.* Effectiveness of potent antiretroviral therapies on reducing perinatal transmission of HIV-1. *Program and Abstracts of the XIII International AIDS Conference*; July 9–14 2000: Durban, South Africa, Abstract LbOr4.

427 British HIV Association, 2001. www.aidsmap.com

428 Mandell GL, Dolin R. *Mandell, Douglas, and Bennett's Principles and Practice of Infectious Diseases* 5th edition. Churchill Livingstone; Edinburgh: 1999.

429 UNAIDS 2001. www.unaids.org

430 McMillan A, Scott GR. *Sexually Transmitted Infections, Colour Guide.* Churchill Livingstone; Edinburgh: 2000.

431 Yeung SM, Gibb DM. Paediatric HIV infection – diagnostic and epidemiological aspects. *Int J STD AIDS* 2001; **12**: 549–554.

Chapter 8

Sexually transmissible viral hepatitis
A McMillan, M M Ogilvie

Viral hepatitis is a notifiable infection caused by one of the hepatotropic viruses spread principally enterically, via feces (hepatitis A) or fecally contaminated water (hepatitis E), or acquired parenterally as with hepatitis B, hepatitis D, and hepatitis C. The clinical features of acute hepatitis and results of biochemical investigations are presented later in this chapter. The epidemiology and diagnostic virological investigations are described individually for hepatitis A to D, the infections of concern in the context of sexual health medicine. Milder abnormalities of liver function are found in symptomatic primary infections with herpesviruses, particularly cytomegalovirus and Epstein–Barr virus infections. It is also convenient to consider hepatitis G virus infection here.

Hepatitis A virus infection

Hepatitis A virus (HAV), classified in genus *Hepatovirus*, family Picornaviridae, is a very small non-enveloped virus (25–28 nm) possessing cubic symmetry. The small RNA genome, a positive-sense single-stranded linear molecule, contains one large ORF that acts as messenger RNA for synthesis of a single polyprotein that is processed by a virus-encoded proteinase (3C) to produce structural and non-structural proteins[1]. After the usual mode of entry by ingestion, the virus is transported across the intestinal epithelium and reaches the liver where replication takes place within the cytoplasm of hepatocytes. There is a short viremic phase in the 2 to 3 weeks before onset of symptoms. New virions are also secreted through the biliary tree to the intestine and are shed in feces. Maximum shedding of infectious virus occurs in the week before the onset of jaundice[2], and the virus particles are remarkably stable. There is little infectivity in fecal extracts by the time most patients are seen by a physician (Figure 8.1).

EPIDEMIOLOGY

The virus of hepatitis A is transmitted by the fecal–oral route and undetected

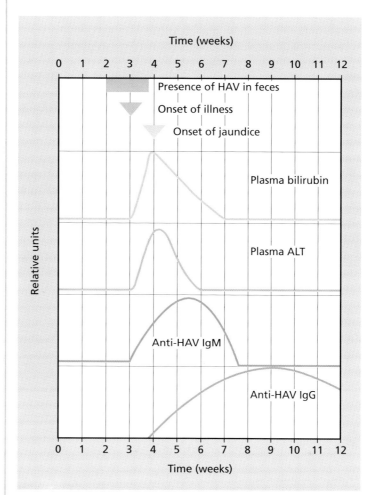

Figure 8.1 Diagrammatic representation of clinical, plasma enzyme, and virological features in symptomatic hepatitis A infection (adapted from Robertson *et al.*[261])

asymptomatic cases may be an important source of infection. Feces of infected persons become infective 2 to 4 weeks after exposure and remain so for about 3 weeks (Figure 8.1). Patients are not infective when jaundice appears. In developed countries infections occur at all ages, with about 50% of clinical cases being seen in children less than 15 years old. In tropical and subtropical areas most infections are probably acquired in childhood and the majority are subclinical. The virus is excreted in the feces and infection is acquired orally under conditions of poor hygiene and sanitation and overcrowding, as in childrens' homes and camps. The incubation period can be 15 to 50 days.

The prevalence of antibody (anti-HAV) in the serum can be used to give information about previous exposure to the virus in various populations. In developed countries its prevalence increases with age. In people under 50 years of age the prevalence of anti-HAV is higher in the lower socioeconomic groups than in the higher socioeconomic groups. In individuals aged 50 years or over, however, these differences are not significant statistically; this finding suggests that all groups were exposed during their youth at a time when hygienic conditions were generally inferior to those of the present day[2]. In some countries the incidence of hepatitis A has declined with increased susceptibility in adults under 40 years of age: this was confirmed in a survey of over 7000 sera submitted to Public Health Laboratories in 1986/87 from people across all age groups in England[3].

Although the sexual transmission of HAV probably plays a small part in the global epidemiology of hepatitis A, the finding, in Halifax, Nova Scotia, of a higher prevalence of serum anti-HAV among patients (both male and female) who attended a STI clinic than amongst volunteer blood donors[4], suggested that possibility.

It has been known for about two decades that the prevalence of enteric infections, such as giardiasis, is higher in men who attend STI clinics and who give a history of homosexual contact, than in heterosexual male attendees. As most of these infections are acquired by oral–anal

sexual contact ('rimming'), it is perhaps not surprising that outbreaks of hepatitis A described amongst homosexual men in Europe, the USA, and in Australia were attributed to sexual practices. In some of these reports, however, the spread of infection was significantly related to occupational factors such as food handling, or to travel to areas of the world where HAV is prevalent. Early studies which showed that the prevalence of antibody against HAV was significantly higher in the sera of homosexual men than in heterosexual men who attended STI clinics, however, appeared to support the conclusion that men who had sex with other men were at increased risk of hepatitis A infection[5, 6]; this increased prevalence of specific antibody was independent of age. The annual incidence of infection was also reported to be higher in homosexual men than in heterosexual men in Amsterdam and in Seattle. These studies also showed that the acquisition of hepatitis A was correlated with a high number of sexual partners and frequent oral–anal sexual contact.

More recent studies, however, have yielded conflicting data on the importance of homosexual contact in the epidemiology of HAV infection. Some reports have confirmed the results of the earlier seroprevalence studies[7], but others have shown that the prevalence of anti-HAV in the sera of homosexual men does not differ from that in heterosexual men. In addition, oral–anal sex has not consistently been associated with an increased prevalence of specific antibody[8]. Although a recent study from San Francisco also failed to show a correlation between oral–anal sexual contact and recent infection, insertive anal intercourse and sharing contaminated needles were significant risk factors[9]. In a report on an outbreak of hepatitis A in New York City, digital–rectal intercourse was also found to be associated with infection[7].

Notwithstanding the conflicting data that have been discussed above, men who have sex with other men, particularly with multiple partners, can be at risk of HAV infection, as exemplified by recent reports of outbreaks of the infection in London that were apparently unrelated to occupational risk or travel[10, 11].

CLINICAL AND LABORATORY FEATURES

It is likely that in the majority of individuals infection with HAV is asymptomatic or produces mild transient and non-specific clinical features. Szmuness *et al.*[12] found that less than 5% of individuals whose sera contained anti-HAV gave a history of icteric hepatitis.

The clinical and biochemical features of hepatitis A are similar to those of any other viral hepatitis (see pp. 220–221). In general the course of the illness is shorter and less severe than that of hepatitis B, with resolution of both clinical and biochemical abnormalities within 1 month of the onset of the illness.

DIAGNOSIS

The diagnosis of hepatitis is made by finding elevated levels of plasma enzymes and bilirubin in tests of liver function (see page 221). As the clinical features in individual cases are not sufficiently specific, the diagnosis of hepatitis A is made by the finding of specific anti-HAV IgM in the patient's serum (Figure 8.1). The most widely used method for the detection of this antibody is an enzyme immunoassay. The specific IgM antibody is usually only detectable for 3 to 4 months after the onset of the illness.

PREVENTION

Simple preventative measures should be discussed such as showering soon after anal sex, washing the hands after digital anal intercourse, and the use of 'clingfilm', a dental dam, or a square of latex cut from a condom for oral–anal sex. Such advice is particularly important for young men who have sex with men and who, with the declining incidence of HAV in the industrialized world, are reaching sexual maturity without immunity.

Hepatitis A vaccine

The vaccines in general use in Europe and the USA are derived from HAV propagated in cell culture and inactivated by formalin before use. As the cell culture-adapted strains of HAV are antigenically indistinguishable from the wild-type virus, and, as there is no evidence of antigenic variation between different strains of HAV, it is likely that the vaccines will confer protection against all wild-type strains. The inactivated vaccines contain both viral particles and immunogenic empty capsids, adsorbed to aluminum hydroxide for adjuvant effect.

Within 2 weeks of a single injection of vaccine, antibody against HAV is detectable by modified solid-phase immunoassay or virus neutralization tests in the sera of 80% of individuals; by 4 weeks, 95% of vaccinees have seroconverted (Havrix Data Sheet 2000). As these antibody levels are significantly higher than those achieved after passive immunization with serum immunoglobulin, it is likely that they are protective.

Evidence for efficacy of formalin-inactivated vaccines comes from two studies in children. In the placebo-controlled, double-blind, randomized trial of the Vaqta vaccine[13] in 1037 children living in a community around Monroe, New York State, USA, that had a high incidence of hepatitis A, complete protection against disease was noted within 3 weeks of a single dose of the vaccine. Seven of the 519 vaccinated children developed hepatitis A within 18 days of vaccination, but there was no evidence that the severity of the illness was greater than in children who had not received vaccine. Similar findings were reported by Innis and colleagues[14] in a randomized, double-blind study amongst children in Thailand. These investigators used the Havrix vaccine in 20 000 children and assessed efficacy after the second of two injections given at an interval of 1 month. This study also showed convincingly that vaccination reduced the risk of inapparent infection. A recent study comparing the immunogenicity of the two vaccines in young adults confirmed the excellent responses to a single dose of either vaccine[15].

Unwanted effects

The most common unwanted effect of a vaccine is discomfort at the injection site, sometimes with erythema. Systemic features that are generally mild and that may be unrelated to the vaccine have been described, they include nausea, fever, malaise, and skin rash. Anaphylaxis has rarely been described.

Use in pregnancy and lactation

Although the effects of vaccination on fetal development are unknown, it is unlikely that there is a risk to the fetus. Similarly, there are no data to guide the physician on the use of hepatitis A vaccine in mothers who are breast feeding. It is therefore recommended that the vaccine should only be used in pregnant or breast-feeding mothers when clearly needed.

Use of inactivated hepatitis A vaccines

Vaccination should be offered to certain individuals, namely

1. Those traveling to countries where hepatitis A is endemic and sanitation is poor.
2. Men who have sex with men. Hepatitis A vaccination of homosexual men has recently been recommended[16]. Two strategies for hepatitis A vaccination have been proposed
   - universal vaccination, in which all individuals are vaccinated without previously serological testing for immunity
   - serology-based vaccination, when vaccine is given only to those without serological evidence of immunity.

In the determination of the least costly strategy, account should be taken of the prevalence of immunity to hepatitis A, the costs of serological testing and of vaccination, and adherence to the vaccination regimen[17]. When these variables are entered into a mathematical model, it is apparent that universal vaccination is the preferred strategy, except amongst populations with a high seroprevalence of specific antibody against hepatitis A (more than 50%), such as people over the age of 50 years. It should be noted that the serological response to vaccination of HIV-infected individuals may be impaired, particularly in those with a low CD4+ cell count in the peripheral blood. It is recommended that susceptible patients should be vaccinated early in HIV infection[18].

3. Injecting drug users.
4. Individuals with chronic HCV infection who acquire HAV are at risk of fulminant hepatitis, and it is recommended that these individuals should be immunized[19]. Although there are conflicting data on the risk of fulminant hepatitis in those with chronic HBV infection who become infected with HAV, vaccination is recommended in these patients.

Vaccination schedule

Each vial of Havrix vaccine that is intended for use in adults, contains 1440 ELISA units of HAV antigen (the viral protein content established by the manufacturer according to an 'in-house' reference standard) per 1 mL dose. A preparation of Havrix, containing 720 ELISA units per 0.5 mL dose, for use in children over the age of 2 years* and adolescents up to the age of 15 years is also available. The vaccine is given by intramuscular injection, with a booster dose 6 to 12 months after the initial dose. As there may be an impaired immune response if the injection is made into adipose tissue, it is important that the dose of vaccine is given into muscle, the deltoid is the preferred site in adults. The length of protection by vaccination is unknown. Antibody levels induced by vaccination tend to be lower than those elicited by natural infection, and are often below the limit of detection by standard assay systems. It is not current practice to estimate anti-HAV levels after vaccination.

A recent advance has been the introduction into clinical practice of a combined hepatitis A and B vaccine (Twinrix, SmithKlineBeecham) that has the same dosing schedule as hepatitis B vaccine (Engerix B, SmithKlineBeecham) (see page 228).

---

* Infants respond well to the vaccine, provided that there is no maternal antibody. Maternal antibody will largely have gone by 12 months in those whose mothers are seropositive.

Passive immunization

It is well recognized that human immunoglobulin, given in a dose of 0.02 mL/kg by intramuscular injection, is effective in preventing hepatitis A when given during epidemics or to household contacts of cases. It is, however, only effective when given within 2 weeks of exposure. Human immunoglobulin may prevent HAV infection or modify its clinical features. The variables that influence the outcome of exposure to HAV probably include the size of the inoculum of virus, the timing of administration of immunoglobulin in relation to exposure, and the level of plasma anti-HAV[20]. Passive immunization of travelers, and of children or adults in day-care facilities or institutions and their household contacts, has largely been replaced by active immunization. It should, however, be offered to sexual or household contacts of individuals with acute hepatitis A if exposure had occurred within the preceding 14 days. They should also be offered active immunization, but the vaccine must be given at a different injection site to that of the immunoglobulin. There is some evidence that the antibody response to vaccination is less in those who are given simultaneous vaccine and immunoglobulin[21]; the clinical significance of this, however, is uncertain.

Hepatitis B virus infection

Hepatitis B virus belongs to a family of closely related DNA viruses called the hepadnaviruses, all of which have similar tropism for the liver and similar life cycles in their hosts. Blumberg[22] described an antigen in blood, that reacted with serum from patients who had been given many blood transfusions. This antigen was found most commonly in Australian aborigines and Asians, and was termed 'Australia' antigen. The same antigen was subsequently discovered in the serum of patients with serum hepatitis. It is now known as the hepatitis B surface antigen (HBsAg).

The antigen in the serum consists of three morphologically distinct particles (Figure 8.2)

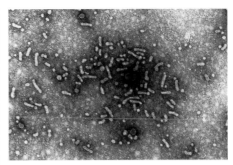

Figure 8.2 Electronmicrograph of hepatitis B virus particles (tungstophosphoric acid stain, × 100 000) (reproduced from McMillan and Scott 2000[260])

1. hepatitis B virus itself (HBV), a large (42 nm) double-shelled spheroidal particle with an inner core particle or capsid, approximately 34 nm in diameter, composed of core protein (HBc) and enclosing viral DNA

2. small spherical particles with an average diameter of 22 nm that do not contain DNA and are not infective, they are always the predominant form and can reach concentrations of 10^{13}/mL of serum, these structures are composed of excess viral surface (HBs) antigen.

3. tubular or filamentous particles with a diameter of 22 nm, but varying in length, also composed of HBs antigen.

The molecular virology of hepatitis B virus has recently been reviewed by Kann and Gerlich[23] and much of the following discussion is taken from that review.

THE GENOME

The genome of HBV is small (3.2 kb), circular and partially double-stranded. One of the DNA strands is incomplete (Figure 8.3), and so endogenous DNA polymerase reaction is possible. The 3′ end of this plus-strand is connected with the HBV polymerase that is able to complete the strand when supplied with deoxynucleotide triphosphates. The 5′ end is formed by an 18-base-long oligoribonucleotide which is capped like mRNA. The minus strand of DNA that encodes the viral proteins is of full length but it is not covalently closed. It has a redundancy of some 9 to 10 bases at the ends, and carries at its 5′ terminus a covalently bound part of the viral polymerase known as primase because it is necessary for priming synthesis of the minus strand.

All the nucleotides encode for protein and about half are in regions where two open reading frames (ORFs) overlap (Figure 8.3). There are four ORFs localized on one viral strand in the same transcriptional orientation (Figure 8.3). The C and S regions specify structural proteins of the virion core and surface, respectively; these genes have upstream genes known as pre-C and pre-S respectively. The longest ORF, P, encodes a polyprotein, which contains primase and replicase activities necessary for viral replication. The smallest ORF, X, encodes a transcriptional transactivator and may be an early gene product that upregulates the viral promoters.

THE SURFACE PROTEINS

The viral surface antigen is comprised of small, middle-sized and large proteins, which appear in glycosylated forms. The ORF S is completely located in the ORF P: the pre-S/S ORF contains three start codons and a common stop codon that divide this gene into pre-S1, pre-S2, and S regions encoding the large, middle-sized and small envelope proteins respectively. The small molecular weight surface protein (SHBs) occurs in stable subtypes. There is a common antigenic determinant *a* with other subtype-specific antigens. These are mutually exclusive pairs, named *d* and *y*, and *w* and *r*. Thus the HBsAg can be typed as *adw*, *adr*, *ayw*, and *ayr*: these findings are of epidemiological significance and have broad geographical associations. In Europe, the Americas and Australia, *adw* predominates, while in northern and western Africa, the eastern Mediterranean and the Indian subcontinent *ayw* predominates. At least six genotypes (A–F) have now been identified by sequencing the SHBs gene, and these loosely correlate with antigenic subtypes. Much of the polypeptide chain of the HBs sphere is folded to α-helices, formed by 4 or 5 hydrophobic stretches of SHBs. The helices (I–V) are inserted cotranslationally into the endoplasmic reticulum (ER) membrane. The hydrophobic sequence between helix I and II remains cytosolic, and after budding into the ER

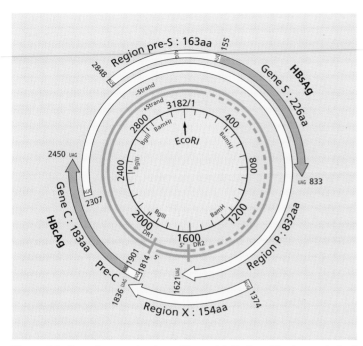

Figure 8.3 Genetic organization of hepatitis B virus. The inner circle shows a restriction map of the *ayw* genome. The partially double-stranded genome is represented as a thick line. Four open reading frames encoding seven peptides are indicated by large arrows. DR1 and DR2 are two directly repeated sequences located at the extremities of the viral DNA strands (adapted from Zuckerman and Thomas 1998[109])

lumen, is within the particle. A sequence of amino acids is exposed at the particles' surface and forms the HBs antigenic region.

The largest HBs protein (LHBs) contains two domains: pre-S (composed of the pre-S1 and pre-S2 sequence) and S. In mature virions or HBs particles, the S domain and part of the pre-S2 sequence are hidden by the pre-S1 sequence. Although the entire pre-S domain of LHBs is synthesized in the cytosol, during maturation of the virion or HBs particle about half of the pre-S domain reconfigures and translocates to the surface of the particle. The other half of the pre-S domain remains on the cytosolic side. The external pre-S region is necessary for binding to the host cell receptor, and the internal pre-S sequence is required for the envelopment of the core particles. The pre-S domain is one of the most variable regions of the HBV genome, and pre-S1 and pre-S2 represent two of the most immunogenic portions of HBsAg.

Mutations in the HBV S gene have been reported. A mutation in the S gene resulting in an amino acid substitution of arginine for glycine at codon 145 (G145R), and a conformational change affecting several epitopes in the region of the *a* determinant, has been described in infants immunized after birth to carrier mothers[24]. Because vaccines induce a predominantly anti-HBs/*a* response, there was therefore loss of reactivity for the HBsAg/*a* epitope.

THE CORE PROTEINS

The precore/core ORF contains two start codons. Translation from the precore start codon produces a precore polypeptide that is post-translationally modified to hepatitis B e antigen (HBeAg). The pre-C sequence at the 5′ terminal part of the ORF C encodes a hydrophobic α-helix that is a secretion signal and allows for translocation of the HBe protein into the lumen of the ER. The HBe protein is not essential for the viral life cycle, but in some way it may suppress the immune elimination of HBV-producing hepatocytes. Precore stop mutants are sometimes found in HBeAg-negative patients who nevertheless have detectable HBV DNA in the serum. A

mutation in the precore region of the viral genome has been associated with a failure to generate HBeAg. A one base-pair change (guanosine to arginine) at position 1896 (A1896) converts the codon at the site into a 'stop' codon, so that during synthesis of the viral proteins, HBeAg is not synthesized[25]. This mutant is only found in patients infected with HBV genotypes, B, C, D and E, that have a thiamine at nucleotide 1858 (T1858)[26]. The G–A mutation increases stability of the secondary structure of the pregenome encapsidation sequence (e) in HBV genotypes that have T1858, suggesting that the A1896 mutant may replicate better than the wild-type virus[26].

HBc protein is a product of ORF C from the second start codon of the pre-C/C ORF and is synthesized in the cytosol of the infected cell. It packages its own mRNA and the viral polymerase after formation of the RNA–polymerase complex and assembles into core particles. These core particles are then enveloped by segments of the ER which contain the three HBs proteins, and the HBV particles are formed. Some regions within the HBc seem to be essential for genome maturation.

ORF P

ORF P (coding for viral polymerase) has four domains

1. the amino-terminal domain that encodes the part of the protein linked to the 5′ end of the minus-strand of virion DNA – the primase
2. a spacer or tether
3. a reverse transcriptase/DNA polymerase
4. an RNaseH which cleaves RNA if it is present in hybrids of RNA and DNA.

THE LIFE CYCLE OF HEPATITIS B VIRUS

The life cycle of HBV is shown schematically in Figure 8.4. As attachment of serum-derived HBs particles to HepG2 cells (a human hepatoma cell line) can be blocked by antibodies to preS1 sequence 21–47, the preS1 sequence appears to be important in initiating infection of hepatocytes. The receptor for human HBV, however, has not yet been identified, and

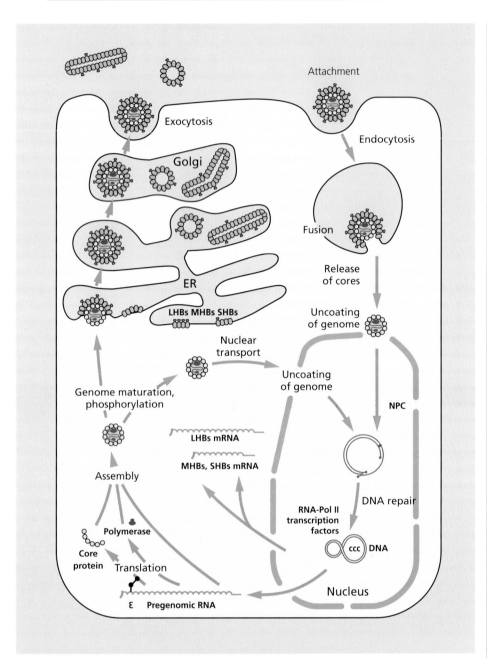

Figure 8.4 Schematic view of the life cycle of hepatitis B virus. In many details this model is still speculative. It is assumed that the virus is endocytosed after attachment, the nucleocapsid is released to the cytosol and binds to the nuclear pore. The genome is transported into the nucleus, converted to cccDNA, and transcribed to three essential classes of mRNA. The non-essential HBe and HBx synthesis is omitted for the sake of simplicity. Translation of the core/pol transcript in the cytosol allows for assembly of core particles that contain the pregenome. The transcripts for LHBs and M/SHBs are translated at the rough endoplasmic reticulum and the MBs proteins are inserted in that membrane. The HBs particles bud to the lumen of the intermediate compartment, and at least a part of LHBS-rich endoplasmic reticulum-membrane areas envelops core particles. The HBV and HBs particles are secreted thereafter by the constitutive pathway (adapted from Zuckerman and Thomas 1998[109])

the mechanism of entry into hepatocytes is not well understood. It is likely, however, that the virus enters by receptor-mediated endocytosis into endosomal vesicles. The viral membrane then fuses with the cell membrane, thereby releasing viral nucleocapsid into the cytoplasm. The core particle mediates the transport of the viral genome to the nuclear pore complex. Replication requires firstly completion of the single-stranded gap and the conversion of the virion DNA into a double-stranded covalently closed circle (an episome), possible through the action of cellular polymerases.

Replication of HBV requires RNA intermediates. The episomal DNA is transcribed by cell RNA polymerase to various RNAs

1. pregenomic mRNA, larger than genome length, for replication of HBV genome
2. shorter (subgenomic) mRNA, including those encoding for the surface proteins, HBc protein and polymerase.

The latter two proteins assemble together with their mRNA to the replication complex. The encapsidation signal e at the 5′ end governs the packaging of the RNA and the priming of the minus strand DNA synthesis. The redundant part of the 3′ end acts as a signal for reverse transcription after priming. The primase domain of the viral polymerase serves as a primer for the reverse transcriptase, and the growing minus DNA strand is linked at its 5′ end to the primase. The RNase H activity associated with the reverse transcriptase degrades the RNA template but leaves an 18-base-long capped RNA fragment at its 5′ end. This functions as a primer for plus strand DNA synthesis. One episomal HBV genome can be transcribed to many pregenome molecules by the cellular RNA polymerase II. Newly-synthesized HBV DNA can enter the nucleus from the cytoplasm and become a further source of covalently closed circular DNA. It is this replication of the HBV genome via the reverse transcription of an RNA intermediate that makes it prone to mutations.

After assembly and genome maturation, HBc protein exhibits an affinity for intracellular membranes that contain inserted LHBs molecules, and core particles bind to these. For secretion of enveloped virions an excess of SHBs is necessary. The envelope is formed by mixed aggregates of LHBs, middle-sized proteins and SHBs. For secretion, virions move from the ER via the Golgi apparatus to the cell surface. During this migration the HBs is modified in a manner similar to that of normal cellular secreted proteins.

EPIDEMIOLOGY

The carrier state

The persistent carrier state has been defined as the presence of HBsAg in the serum of the individual for more than 6 months. It is estimated that, worldwide, there are about 400 million carriers of HBV[27]. In the UK less than 1% of the population are found to have HBsAg in the serum. The prevalence in apparently healthy adults varies from 0.1% in parts of Europe, North America, and Australia to 20% in several tropical countries. Within each country considerable differences in prevalence may exist between different ethnic and socioeconomic groups. In the pre-AIDS era and before the widespread introduction of vaccination against hepatitis B, the prevalence of HBsAg amongst homosexual men who attended clinics for STIs was some 50 times higher than that in unpaid blood donors in the UK[28].

The major determinant of chronic carriage of hepatitis B is age at the time of exposure to the virus. Without immunization, about 90% of infants born to HBeAg-positive mothers become carriers[29]. When exposed to infection between the ages of 1 and 5 years, 25% to 50% of children become chronically infected, but the probability of chronic carriage falls to about 5% to 10% among older children, and 1% to 6% of adults. The carrier state is also more common in individuals with natural or acquired immune deficiencies.

Modes of spread

In areas of low prevalence one mode of spread continues to be the inoculation of blood. Hepatitis B virus may be transmitted as a result of inoculation of minute quantities of blood, for example during intravenous drug use, tattooing, and acupuncture if care is not taken to sterilize the needles or other equipment. In industrialized countries health-care professionals and medical laboratory personnel are immunized against the virus, thereby reducing the risk of transmission during either surgical procedures or the handling of infected material. Donated blood for transfusion is also screened for HBsAg, and the risks of transfusion-associated hepatitis B have been

completely eliminated in developed nations. The sharing of razors and toothbrushes has been implicated as an occasional cause of hepatitis B.

Experimental studies in non-human primates have shown that inoculation of HBV-containing blood, semen, or saliva, but not the oral ingestion of HBV-containing saliva, results in infection[30, 31]. Kissing, therefore is an unlikely means of transmission of the virus, although a human bite could result in infection. Although HBsAg can be found in tears, breast milk, urine, feces, bile, and pancreatic secretions, these fluids have not been described as sources of infection.

Spread of HBV from carrier mothers to babies is a very significant factor in some regions, as well as the spread from those with an acute infection. In Taiwan, for example, where the prevalence of HBsAg is 5% to 20% it was found that, in about 40% of cases, babies born to asymptomatic mothers became antigen positive within the first 6 months of life[32]. If an acute infection occurs in the second or third trimester or within 2 months after delivery there is a substantial risk that the baby will be infected. Women whose serum contains HBeAg will pass on hepatitis B virus to their babies, whereas those with anti-HBe generally do not[33]. This probably reflects the active viral replication that occurs in e-antigen-positive individuals. The infection of the baby is usually anicteric and most children infected (about 85%) will become persistent carriers. Intra-uterine infection seems to be rare. Goudeau et al.[34] failed to identify anti-HBc IgM in the serum of neonates born to HBsAg carriers, a finding that argued against the *in utero* acquisition of HBV.

The prevalence of serological markers of HBV infection in African communities has been shown to increase throughout childhood. Although only 25% of children aged 3 years in a rural area of Senegal, West Africa, had evidence of current or past infection with HBV, by the age of 7 years 50% of children were seropositive for the virus, and by 15 years of age 80% of the population had been infected[35]. The mode of spread of HBV in this community was unknown. In another study from West Africa (the Gambia), among children who

were e-antigen positive persistent carriers of HBsAg, there was a significant relationship with the presence of bed bugs in their beds[36]. Elimination of bed bugs by insecticides, however, failed to reduce the risk of HBV infection in Gambian children[37].

Jeffries et al.[38] observed that the prevalence of HBsAg in the sera of patients who attended a STI clinic in London was some ten times higher than that in blood donors. They noted that high rates were found in homosexual and non-European patients. Results of other studies, summarized in Table 8.1, have shown clearly an association between homosexual activity and the acquisition of hepatitis B virus; the prevalence of HBV in men who have sex with men will vary geographically and will be particularly high in countries with high prevalence in the general population. Several studies have shown that the sera of more than 70% of homosexual men who are persistent carriers of HBsAg contain e antigen[39], suggesting that their sexual contacts would be likely to be at particular risk of infection.

Measures to reduce the transmission of HIV amongst men who have sex with men, and vaccination against hepatitis B virus would be expected to reduce the incidence of hepatitis B amongst this population. Studies from England in the early 1990s, however, showed that, although the prevalence of serological markers of hepatitis B virus infection was lower than previously, a significant number of young homosexual men were seropositive for anti-HBc[40, 41]. Sera from 288 (14.6%) of 1977 homosexual men who attended the STI clinic in Edinburgh, UK, between 1989 and 1998 gave positive results for anti-HBc and/or anti-HBs. None of these men had been vaccinated previously against hepatitis B. The median age of seropositive men (34.0 years) was significantly higher than that of seronegative men (27.0 years), but there was no significant difference between each year in the median ages of the seropositive men. These results suggest that hepatitis B virus continues to be transmitted amongst young homosexual and bisexual men in this population, and this is exemplified by finding that 7% of men under the age of 30 years had anti-HBc in

Table 8.1 Prevalence of hepatitis B surface antigen (HBsAg) and antibody (anti-HBs or anti-HBc) in the sera of homosexual and heterosexual men in various cities

Geographical area	HBsAg		Anti-HBs or anti-HBc	
	Homosexual	Heterosexual	Homosexual	Heterosexual
	No. (%) positive/ No. tested	No. (%) positive/ No. tested	No. (%) positive/ No. tested	No. (%) positive/ No. tested
UK				
London[a]	3 (4.2)/71	0 (0)/129	21 (29.6)/71	7 (5.4)/129
London[b]	11 (6.2)/177	nt	89 (53.6)/166	nt
Glasgow[c]	4 (1.9)/208	0 (0)/124	65 (31.3)/208	9 (7.3)/124
Edinburgh[d]	32 (1.6)/1977	nt	288 (14.6)/1977	nt
Bristol[e]	18 (3.0)/599	nt	nt	nt
USA				
New York City[f]	29 (4.3)/674	8 (1.3)/597	295 (45.3)/645	99 (16.8)/589
Chicago, Los Angeles, San Francisco, Denver, St Louis[g]	234 (6.1)/3816	nt	1999 (52.4)/3582	nt
The Netherlands				
Amsterdam[h]	140 (4.8)/2946	nt	1596 (56.9)/2806	nt

nt = not tested
[a] Lim et al. 1976[105]
[b] Coleman et al. 1979[106]
[c] Follett and McMillan 1980[107]
[d] McMillan, unpublished
[e] Lacey et al. 1983[39]
[f] Szmuness et al. 1975[47]
[g] Schreeder et al. 1982[43]
[h] Coutinho et al. 1981[108]

their serum, and 50% of the 32 men with hepatitis B surface antigenemia were less than 30 years old. Data supporting the continued transmission of the virus amongst young men in the USA have been presented by Seage et al.[42] in Boston who found that 12.9% of 508 homo- or bisexual men aged 18 to 29 years had serological evidence of prior exposure to hepatitis B.

Schreeder et al.[43] noted that seropositivity for HBV was related to the duration of regular homosexual activity and to the number of different sexual partners. Practices likely to result in mucosal trauma, including genital–anal and oral–anal intercourse and rectal douching, correlated with the presence of HBV serological markers. Reiner et al.[44] studied 22 homosexual men whose serum contained HBsAg (17 sera were HBeAg positive) and found asymp-tomatic rectal mucosal lesions, in the form of multiple punctate bleeding points in 13 men. HBsAg was detected in specimens taken from the rectal lesions in 10 of these 13 patients and less frequently from the normal mucosa and feces. Such specimens were more likely to give positive results if the serum contained large quantities of HBsAg. Gingival swabs from 20 patients contained HBsAg.

HBsAg-positive individuals of either sex may transmit HBV to their sexual con-tacts[45, 46]. Szmuness et al.[47] found that 26% of spouses of HBsAg carriers were seropositive for anti-HBs.

In a sample of 293 female sex-industry workers in Athens, there was evidence of hepatitis B infection in 61% compared with 28% of 379 controls. When the prevalence of HBsAg and anti-HBs were related to years in prostitution a substantially higher rate of HBsAg was noted in women in their first 5 years of prostitution (9%), decreasing substantially in those who had been in prostitution for 5 years or more[48]. De Hoop et al.[49] also noted an increased prevalence of anti-HBs in the sera of female sex-industry workers who attended an STI clinic in Rotterdam. Sexually promiscuous persons clearly have a higher incidence of seropositivity than the general population in areas of low prevalence.

ACUTE HEPATITIS

Clinical features and course in acute hepatitis infections

In many cases of hepatitis, whether type A or B, the disease is asymptomatic and detectable only by biochemical tests for hepatocellular damage. In those who develop clinical manifestations of the disease, following an incubation period of 30 to 50 days in the case of hepatitis A, and 40 to 160 days in hepatitis B, there is a pre-icteric stage (prodrome) during which the symptoms of the disease develop. The patient complains of nausea, malaise, anorexia, and discomfort in the upper right abdomen. Tender enlargement of the liver is found in most cases, and in about 20% of patients the spleen is also enlarged. In less than 5% of symptomatic cases, manifestations of immune-complex disease appear, consisting of erythematous, maculopapular, or urticarial skin rashes, and arthralgia.

Jaundice usually develops within a week of the development of the symptoms, and is preceded by the onset of dark urine and pale stools. The onset of jaundice in hepatitis B may not always be associated with prodromal illness. With the development of jaundice, the patient's condition improves, and within 2 to 4 weeks most infections have resolved. Uncommonly (less than 1% of cases), acute liver failure with encephalopathy, cerebral edema, and coagulopathy, develops within 4 weeks of the onset of symptoms (the majority of these patients having hepatitis B infection). This complication may be related to

- an enhanced immune response with rapid clearing of the virus
- super-infection with another virus such as hepatitis C or hepatitis D viruses
- restoration of immunity after iatrogenic immunosuppression.

The role of HBV variants in the pathogenesis of fulminant hepatitis B is controversial[50].

The mortality rate of acute hepatitis B is less than 1%.

Plasma enzyme tests in viral hepatitis and its sequelae

In hepatocellular damage there is a release, particularly, of soluble cytoplasmic enzymes such as alanine aminotransferase (ALT) and aspartate aminotransferase (AST). Increases of ALT are usually greater than those of AST in early hepatitis. AST has both cytoplasmic and mitochondrial isoenzymes and tends to be released more than ALT in chronic hepatocellular disease.

Gamma-glutamyl transferase (GGT) and alkaline phosphatase are enzymes located close to the biliary canaliculi. These tend to be released in small amounts in hepatocellular damage but in much greater amounts when there is cholestasis, providing a sensitive marker for detecting mild cirrhosis.

In the pre-icteric phase of viral hepatitis, plasma ALT and AST activities are increased. Urobilinogen is present in the urine, and later bilirubin will be found. By the time jaundice appears aminotransferase activities are usually more than five times reference values and sometimes more than 100 times reference values. Alkaline phosphatase activity is usually only slightly increased (twice the upper reference value) unless there is a marked cholestatic element.

In chronic disease, which is more likely to follow anicteric hepatitis B than the acute icteric hepatitis B, plasma ALT and AST activities may remain high for many months. Plasma enzyme tests and tests for hepatitis B antigens and antibodies are important in the follow-up of HBsAg-positive asymptomatic patients.

Other chemical tests in viral hepatitis and its sequelae

Plasma contains two forms of bilirubin

1. the unconjugated lipid-soluble form which is transported bound to albumin from the lymphoreticular system to the liver
2. the conjugated water-soluble form which has been regurgitated from the liver to the plasma.

Normally most of the bilirubin in the plasma is unconjugated. For most purposes measurement of the total bilirubin is sufficient for clinical purposes when interpreted in relation to the laboratory tests and other clinical investigations (e.g. plasma enzyme tests and tests for hepatitis B antigens and antibodies).

In hepatitis and cirrhosis hepatocellular damage may interfere with the conjugation of bilirubin, or with the excretion of conjugated bilirubin into the bile, or with both. This and other abnormalities lead to cholestasis and bring about an increase in plasma bilirubin and bilirubinuria.

Urobilinogen is water-soluble and is formed from degraded bilirubin glucuronide

in the colon and is normally excreted in the feces. Some is reabsorbed and excreted in the urine where it spontaneously oxidizes into a brown pigment called urobilin. In hepatitis urobilinogen excess is found in the urine in the pre-icteric stage, but as the stools become pale, because of impairment of excretion of bilirubin, urobilinogen disappears from the urine.

Since gross increases in alpha-fetoprotein (AFP) occur in the serum of 50% to 90% of patients with hepatocellular carcinoma (HCC) this investigation may help in the longer term follow-up of patients who are chronic HBsAg carriers.

Infectivity of hepatitis B virus in acute hepatitis B

The patient is infectious for about 2 weeks before the onset of jaundice until he or she becomes HBsAg negative.

Pregnancy and acute hepatitis B

Acute hepatitis B infection in the first trimester of pregnancy is associated with transmission to the infant in about 10% of cases. In later pregnancy, the risk is significantly higher and up to 90% of infants are infected[51]. Complications of pregnancy, most commonly premature delivery, and less frequently, spontaneous abortion or stillbirth, are found in about 25% of women with acute hepatitis B[52].

Immune response in acute hepatitis B

The humoral immune response to acute hepatitis B virus infection and its relation to clinical features and plasma enzyme tests of liver function are shown in Figure 8.5.

Hepatitis B surface antigen and its antibody (HBsAg and anti-HBs)

Hepatitis B surface antigen is found 14 to 120 days following exposure to infection, the interval between exposure and appearance of detectable serum HBsAg is related to the infectivity of the inoculum. A rise in the serum titer of HBsAg occurs gradually and, after reaching a peak, falls rapidly. The serum ALT level rises after the HBsAg peak, and by the time symptoms develop in

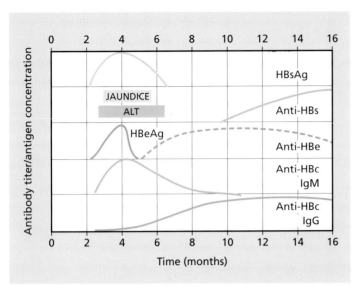

Figure 8.5 Diagrammatic representation of clinical, plasma enzyme, and virological features in symptomatic hepatitis B infection (adapted from Robertson et al.[261])

uncomplicated cases, the transaminase levels are falling. In most cases, the disappearance of HBsAg and subsequent appearance of anti-HBs signal recovery from infection and the development of immunity to re-infection. Anti-HBs can appear at the time HBsAg disappears or may not appear for several months. The persistence of HBsAg for more than 3 months, in some 5% to 10% of cases, suggests the development of the carrier state. In fulminant hepatitis there is some evidence to suggest that an unusually strong and rapid immune clearance of HBsAg, associated with the early appearance of anti-HBs during the peak of liver damage, may be involved in the pathogenesis of this severe form of infection.

Enzyme immunoassays have largely replaced the radioimmunoassays that were used formerly for the detection of HBsAg. Anti-HBs is bound to a solid phase to capture HBsAg from the serum specimen and a second labeled anti-HBs probe is used to identify bound antigen. Modified enzyme immunoassays that use microparticles and computerized instrumentation produce rapid and automated assays[53].

Anti-HBs can be estimated by radioimmunoassay, enzyme immunoassay, or microparticle enzyme immunoassay in which HBsAg is affixed to a solid phase and is labeled with ^{125}I or enzyme. As anti-HBs/a is the predominant antibody in the convalescent serum of most patients or in the serum of vaccinated patients, the choice of HBV strain for the reagent antigen is not too important. Semi-quantitative values of anti-HBs have been determined with the immunoassays, and are expressed in milli-international units per milliliter (mIU/mL). These are pertinent to assessing immune response to vaccination.

The detection of HBsAg is the main approach in the diagnosis of acute and chronic cases. Other antigen and antibody tests are available for some individual cases, especially during the recovery from acute illness and to assess the carrier state.

Hepatitis B core antigen and its antibody (HBcAg and anti-HBc)

Although HBcAg has been obtained from HBV-rich plasma and from infected liver tissue, free core antigen has not been detected in circulating blood because of the HBsAg envelope that surrounds it. However, anti-HBc is found in the serum 2 to 10 weeks after the appearance of HBsAg and before the appearance of anti-HBs (Figure 8.5). It often appears during the acute infection while HBsAg is still present and remains detectable for a considerable period after recovery. The anti-HBc is detected by either a competitive or direct assay. Hepatitis B core antigen is fixed to a solid phase and used to capture anti-HBc from the serum specimen. In the competitive test, this captured antibody inhibits the binding of labeled anti-HBc antibody.

Antibodies of the IgM class against HBcAg can be detected by an IgM capture method. Anti-human IgM, attached to a solid phase, is incubated with the patient's serum. Captured IgM antibodies are then incubated with HBcAg particles and then with labeled anti-HBc. These IgM antibodies can be found in the sera of almost all patients with acute hepatitis B; they appear about 2 weeks before the onset of jaundice and generally become undetectable by commercially available assays within 6 months. Although this antibody can be found in the sera of patients with chronic hepatitis B and carriers, it is present in very low titer and, therefore, the presence of serum anti-HBc IgM can be taken as an indication of recent infection[54,55]. As HBsAg becomes undetectable, anti-HBc IgM may be the only serological evidence of fulminant hepatitis B.

Hepatitis B e antigen and its antibody (HBeAg and anti-HBe)

Hepatitis B e antigen can be detected in serum by a sandwich immunoassay similar to that for HBsAg. A competitive assay is used to detect anti-HBe. Hepatitis B e antigen is found in the sera of almost all patients with acute hepatitis B, becoming detectable at about the same time as HBsAg. The presence of this antigen and specific DNA polymerase reflects viral replication. When this ceases, levels of HBeAg in the serum fall and anti-HBe becomes detectable, usually a short time after disappearance of HBeAg from the serum.

Cell-mediated immunity

The observation that carriers of hepatitis B with high-level viral replication do not always have liver damage suggests that HBV itself is not directly cytopathic. However, small epitopes of viral proteins, especially HBcAg are present on the surface of the hepatocyte. It is probable that these, in association with major histocompat-ibility complex (MHC) class I molecules whose expression may be increased by the production of interferon-α in response to viral infection, make the cell a target for cytotoxic CD8⁺ T-cell lysis. During acute HBV infection, there is a marked MHC class I restricted cytotoxic T-cell response to the nucleocapsid and envelope antigens of HBV[56]. T-lymphocyte reactivity is main-tained for years after apparent resolution of acute infection[57], suggesting that HBV is not eliminated entirely.

CHRONIC HEPATITIS B

Chronic hepatitis B may be defined as a primary inflammatory condition of the liver that has persisted without improve-ment for more than 6 months. There are four main consequences of hepatitis B infection.

1. *Chronic carrier state*. In this state of the virus there is a normal or minimally abnormal histological appearance[58]. Randomly distributed ground-glass hepatocytes are found in varying numbers in histological sections. These are enlarged liver cells with finely granular cytoplasm that contains HBsAg as shown by immunoper-oxidase methods (Figure 8.6).
2. *Chronic persistent hepatitis*. This is a histological diagnosis as neither clini-cal features nor biochemical tests differentiate this type of chronic hepatitis from chronic active hepatitis. Histologically the lobular architecture is intact, but the portal tracts are enlarged with a dense infiltration of lymphocytes, sometimes forming folli-

cles. 'Piecemeal' necrosis (interface hepatitis) is *not* a feature. The prog-nosis is generally good, but there can be progression to chronic active hepatitis. Progressive changes, how-ever, cannot be predicted based on a specimen taken at a single time.
3. *Chronic active hepatitis*. This is again a histological diagnosis. The hallmark of this type of chronic hepatitis is 'piece-meal' necrosis which is defined as necrosis of liver cells at the junction of the interface between the liver paren-chyma and the connective tissue of the portal tracts or septa of a fibrotic or cirrhotic liver. There is a predomi-nantly lymphocytic infiltration of the portal tracts extending into the hepatic parenchyma. Fibrous tissue septa of varying size surround groups of liver cells. Ground-glass hepatocytes are seen in both chronic active and chronic persistent hepatitis. Although this form of chronic hepatitis may progress to cirrhosis, the prognosis in individual cases is difficult to predict.
4. *Hepatocellular carcinoma* (see pp. 225–226).

Immune response in chronic hepatitis B

Humoral antibody response

In almost all cases of chronic hepatitis B serum HBsAg and anti-HBc are detectable, generally anti-HBs is not produced. Although serum anti-HBc IgM can be detected by sensitive tests, this antibody is present in low titer.

Hepatitis B e antigen and high levels of HBV DNA (detectable by direct hybridiza-tion, branched chain (b-DNA) or PCR methods) persist for a variable period after infection is established. Patients in the replicative state are defined as those with high-level HBV DNA and ALT, and usually HBeAg, whereas patients in the non-replicative state have low levels of HBV DNA (undetectable by direct hybridization tests that are less sensitive than b-DNA or PCR methods), have normal plasma ALT levels, and are negative for HBeAg. In the latter patients, only HBV DNA integrated into the cell genome is found in hepatic

tissue. Individuals in the replicative state are much more likely to transmit infection through sexual contact than those in the non-replicative state. After an indefinite period, many patients show seroconversion from HBeAg to anti-HBe. Such a transition is preceded by an increase in serum transaminase levels that are significantly lower than those recorded when the patient's serum was HBeAg positive[59]. However, seroconversion is not associated with improvement in hepatic histology, and, indeed, progression to cirrhosis is known to occur in HbsAg-positive patients with serum anti-HBe. Some of these individuals with anti-HBe have moderate to high serum levels of HBV DNA, and it is likely that many are infected with HBV mutants that are incapable of making HBeAg. A mutation in the precore region of the nucleocapsid ORF creates a termina-tion codon that prevents production of the HBeAg. Seroconversion to anti-HBe is not always permanent. Perillo et al.[59] showed spontaneous transient reactivation in three patients who had had documented seroconversion from HBeAg positive to anti-HBe several months previously. Reactivation was associated with a sharp increase in serum transaminase levels.

Anti-idiotype antibodies may play an important role in viral persistence. These antibodies are directed against the variable region of immunoglobulin, and may limit the immune response. Between 70% and 80% of patients with persistent HBV infection have anti-idiotype antibodies in the sera, and subsequent clearance of infection is more likely to occur if these antibodies are absent or present in low titer.

Cellular immunity

As discussed above, cytotoxic T cells recog-nize and kill hepatocytes that bear nucleo-capsid proteins on their surface. In chronic HBV infection, cytotoxic T lymphocyte res-ponses are almost undetectable. A possible mechanism for interference with cytotoxic T-cell responses and viral persistence may involve anti-HBc. This antibody is produced early in infection, and both it and anti-HBe have been shown to inhibit cytotoxic T-cell lysis of HBV-infected cells.

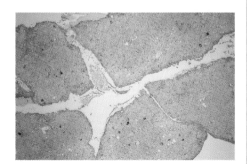

Figure 8.6 Expression of HBsAg in hepatocytes (immunoperoxidase stain × 40)

This blocking effect may be the result of steric hindrance if the B and T-cell epitopes are displayed close to each other on the cell membrane.

Factors leading to viral persistence

This issue has been reviewed by Thomas and Thursz[60].

Viral factors

Induction of tolerance

Hepatitis B e antigen crosses the human placenta, and it has been shown in a transgenic mouse model that exposure *in utero* to HBeAg induces T-cell tolerance to HBeAg and HBcAg in non-transgenic offspring of HBeAg-expressing transgenic female mice. This immunological tolerance may be an important factor in the chronicity of infection in neonates born to HBeAg-positive mothers.

Another mechanism for viral persistence may be the secretion of surplus HBs into the serum where it is seen as 22 nm particles (see page 216). This protein may compete with intact virions for neutralizing antibody (anti-HBs), reducing the chances of neutralization of the latter.

Inhibition of cytotoxic T lymphocyte lysis of infected hepatocytes

Because the viral replication cycle involves a reverse transcriptase mechanism similar to that of retroviruses, the HBV genome has a high mutation rate, resulting in the generation of genetic heterogeneity. Theoretically, there could be inhibition of cytotoxic T-cell recognition and lysis of infected hepatocytes.

Emergence of HBeAg-negative variant of HBV

See humoral responses, page 223.

Hepatitis B virus integration

HBV becomes covalently integrated into the host cell genome at some time during chronic infection. Some of the viral genes are transcribed with those of the hepatocyte DNA, with the production of viral surface proteins (HBsAg). As the preferred integration site is in the promoter region of the HBV core gene and this is destroyed during integration, no core antigens are produced. Unless the infected cell is recognized by cytotoxic T cells, integration of the virus will lead to viral persistence.

Host factors

In addition to antibody to nucleocapsid antigens, and anti-idiotype antibody formation, HBV persistence may be determined by other host factors.

Genetic susceptibility

The outcome of infection may be partly determined by the host genotype. Certain MHC class II alleles – DRB1*1302, DRB1*02, and DRB1*04 – are associated with resistance to persistent HBV infection, whereas DRB1*07 is associated with increased susceptibility to persistent infection.

Gender

Men are much more likely to become persistently infected than women, significant liver disease is more likely to develop in men. The reasons are uncertain, but hormonal factors may be important.

Clinical features and course in chronic hepatitis B infections

Although chronic disease can follow acute icteric hepatitis B, it seems more likely to be a consequence of anicteric hepatitis. Most patients with chronic disease do not give a past history of jaundice.

The clinical features of chronic hepatitis B vary considerably and often there are no symptoms or signs of the disease, the diagnosis being made after routine testing of the patient's serum for HBsAg. Some patients with chronic active hepatitis and cirrhosis present with clinical evidence of hepatic decompensation with edema, ascites, or bleeding varices. From time to time patients with chronic hepatitis B develop episodes of acute hepatitis caused by other viruses, including cytomegalovirus. In an individual with acute hepatitis whose serum is found to be HBsAg positive but anti-HBc IgM negative, it is likely that he has chronic hepatitis B with some other super-added viral infection.

Plasma enzyme tests of liver function are abnormal in chronic hepatitis but there is such a wide variation in levels of ALT and AST that it is not possible to differentiate between chronic persistent and chronic active hepatitis. Based on a study that compared the results of plasma enzyme tests of liver function, hepatic histology, and HBV DNA assay, Ter Borg *et al.*[61] found that AST and not ALT was the best predictor of chronic active hepatitis in patients with HBsAg and anti-HBe. They also reported that the estimation of HBV DNA did not improve the predictive accuracy of the AST estimation. Alkaline phosphatase levels are only slightly elevated. Although the presence of HBeAg in the sera of patients with chronic hepatitis was considered to indicate progression to cirrhosis, this is no longer considered to be so. During the phase of active viral replication, HBe antigenemia occurs early in the course of chronic hepatitis; seroconversion from HBeAg to anti-HBe is frequent, 5% to 10% of adults spontaneously clearing the virus per year[62]. When the patient becomes anti-HBe positive, disease activity decreases, but chronic active hepatitis continues in up to 10% of HBV carriers with anti-HBe[63], each year just over 1% of this group of patients develop cirrhosis[64].

Rates of progression to cirrhosis and HCC vary according to the state of the immune system, age of the patient, serological findings, and geographical and genetic factors[65]. The relative risk of death due to cirrhosis in HBsAg carriers, as compared with non-infected individuals, ranges from 12 to 79, and the relative risk of HCC ranges from 148 in Alaska to 30 to 98 in the Far East.

HEPATITIS B VIRUS INFECTION AND HIV INFECTION

The risk of chronic carriage of HBV in HIV-infected individuals is significantly higher than that in HIV-seronegative patients. In a large study of unvaccinated homosexual men, 21% of HIV-seropositive men who were subsequently exposed to HBV became persistent carriers of the virus, compared with 7% of HIV-seronegative men[66]. HIV-infected individuals with a high CD4+ cell count in the peripheral blood are more likely to clear HBsAg than those with low counts[67]. Although there is greater expression of HBeAg and HBV polymerase in HIV-infected patients, hepatic necrosis and fibrosis is significantly less than that seen in HIV-seronegative patients[68].

Reactivation of HBV in HIV-infected patients has been described[69], although the pathogenic mechanism is uncertain. A sudden increase in the levels of ALT in a HIV-positive patient should alert the physician to the possibility of reactivation of HBV. However, HBeAg may not be detectable in the peripheral blood, and the diagnosis may only be apparent when HBV DNA is found in the serum.

Management of hepatitis B virus infection

Acute hepatitis B

In most cases, acute hepatitis B virus infection is a self-limiting condition, and there is no specific therapy. Vomiting, dehydration, or the development of hepatic decompensation (somnolence or change of personality) necessitates admission to hospital and referral to a hepatologist for specialist management. Other than the avoidance of alcohol during the acute illness and convalescence, dietary restrictions are unnecessary. Individuals should be advised about the risks of sexual transmission, and they should avoid unprotected sexual intercourse, and both oral–anal and oral–genital contact until they have become HBsAg negative or their sexual partners have been successfully vaccinated.

Chronic hepatitis B

A detailed discussion of the therapy of chronic hepatitis B is outwith the scope of this textbook. Patients should be referred to a hepatologist for expert management. The aim of therapy is to suppress HBV replication before there is irreversible liver damage. Current therapies for chronic hepatitis B infection are interferon-α and lamivudine.

Interferon-α

The efficacy of interferon-α in the treatment of HBeAg-positive patients was shown in a meta-analysis of randomized controlled trials[70]: there was a significant difference between treated patients and controls with respect to clearance of HBeAg (33% versus 12%), serum HBV DNA (37% versus 17%), and HBsAg (7.8% versus 1.8%). Those who lose HBeAg commonly become HBsAg negative during the next 5 to 7 years[71]. Fewer than 10% of HBeAg-positive individuals with high levels of serum HBV DNA but normal plasma enzyme tests of liver function, however, respond to interferon therapy[72]. Although interferon-α treatment can suppress viral replication and induce remission in patients with chronic hepatitis B who are HBeAg negative, relapse is common[73]. The most important factor predictive of a good response to interferon therapy is a high ALT level, and low serum HBV DNA levels. The treatment response of children who are HBeAg positive is as good as that in adults.

The recommended dose of interferon-α is 5 million units given once daily or 10 million units, given three times per week by subcutaneous injection, for 4 months. Plasma enzyme tests of liver function are measured at 2 to 4-week intervals, and serological markers of HBV infection are examined at the end of therapy and 6 months later. Transient increases in the ALT levels are seen during therapy particularly in those who become HBeAg negative. Loss of HBeAg may not be apparent for several months after discontinuation of treatment.

Treatment with interferons is associated with unwanted effects such as fever and chills, and later malaise, depression, and myelosuppression may necessitate dosage reduction or, in up to 10% of cases, discontinuation of therapy.

Lamivudine

Lamivudine is a nucleoside analog reverse transcriptase inhibitor that is used widely in the treatment of HIV infection (Chapter 7). In a group of Chinese patients with chronic hepatitis B, Lai et al.[74] found that 16% of 143 patients given 100 mg lamivudine by mouth once daily for 1 year had loss of HBeAg and undetectable serum HBV DNA at the end of therapy. The plasma enzyme tests of liver function returned to normal in more than 70% of the treated individuals. Lai et al.[74] also noted that there was a reduced rate of progression of hepatic fibrosis in these treated patients compared with placebo recipients. Viral replication, however, commonly returns when treatment is stopped, and the emergence of drug resistance may be problematic. Substitutions at codons in the YMDD motif or in the HBV polymerase gene are common, genotypic resistance being found in up to 25% of patients who had been given lamivudine for 1 year, and almost 50% of those treated for 3 years. Although break-through infection may be the consequence of such mutations, the long-term clinical significance is uncertain[75]. A combination of interferon and lamivudine treatments confers no added advantage over the use of the agents singly[75].

There are many uncertainties about the treatment of chronic hepatitis B[75]. Treatment of patients with viral replication but normal ALT levels, and individuals with cirrhosis were previously excluded from interferon therapy because of the poor response, or, in the case of cirrhosis, life-threatening adverse reactions. Lamivudine, however, can be used for such individuals, and, although relapse is common after cessation of therapy, the clinical and histological benefits warrant its use in patients with HBeAg-negative chronic hepatitis[75].

HEPATOCELLULAR CARCINOMA

Several lines of evidence suggest a causative role for HBV in hepatocellular carcinoma (HCC). In geographical areas, especially Southeast Asia, where HBsAg carriers are common, HCC is also frequently found; the converse is also true in that the tumor is rare where the HBsAg carriage rate is low. Case control studies have shown that the serum of patients with HCC is much more likely to be positive for HBsAg. In Taiwan, the association between HCC and HBV is stronger in children than in adults[76]. Beasley et al.[77] showed that HBV infection preceded the development of HCC. The incidence of HCC is highest in patients with cirrhosis, although it may also occur in those with chronic hepatitis and asymptomatic carriers. Further evidence for the association between HCC and HBV comes from DNA hybridization studies. Hepatitis B virus DNA sequences have been found by PCR in tumor tissue in 17 of 28 patients with HCC, including 8 of 10 with serological evidence of HBV infection and 6 of 13 individuals without such markers of infection[78]. Circumstantial evidence of a role for HBV in HCC comes from the observation that the incidence of HCC amongst children declined significantly in Taiwan after the introduction of universal vaccination against HBV[79]. Between 1981 and 1986, before the introduction of mass vaccination, the average annual incidence of HCC in children aged 6 to 14 years was 0.70 per 100 000 children. However, after institution of universal vaccination of children in 1984, the incidence between 1990 and 1994 had fallen to 0.36 per 100 000.

Although the mechanism of carcinogenesis is unknown, integration of HBV DNA into the host cell genome appears to be essential, resulting in activation of cellular proto-oncogenes or suppression of growth regulatory genes[80].

Patients with HCC may present with features of hepatic cirrhosis or with right hypochondrial pain in association with fever, weight loss, and a palpable mass. In some cases the diagnosis is made during routine examination or from the results of liver scanning of patients with chronic liver disease.

Although fluctuating levels of AFP are common in non-malignant liver disease, sustained or high values are strongly suggestive of HCC in non-pregnant patients.

SCREENING FOR VIRUS MARKERS IN THE SERUM OF ASYMPTOMATIC PATIENTS

Routine screening of serum for HBV markers (anti-HBc and, ideally, HBsAg) from

- men who have had homosexual contact
- intravenous drug users
- HIV seropositive individuals
- female sex-industry workers
- the sexual partners of positive or high-risk individuals

is recommended so that appropriate advice with respect to infectivity and the individual's future health can be given. Vaccination of at-risk individuals with hepatitis B vaccine deserves active consideration. If the initial tests give negative results in those who decline vaccination, the authors recommend repeat serological screening at an interval that should be determined by either the sexual activity or injecting drug use pattern of the individual.

Figure 8.7 gives, in outline, recommendations on the management of asymptomatic patients whose sera are found to be HBsAg positive. Box 8.1 indicates the advice that is given to a patient with chronic HBV infection.

Other serological findings in hepatitis B virus infection

When the pattern of serological markers of HBV at different times from infection are considered (Figure 8.5), interpretation of the results of tests is generally straightforward. Sometimes, however, unusual patterns are found.

HBsAg without anti-HBc

This may occur in the very early stages of infection before symptoms develop or before the production of detectable anti-HBc. This may also be a finding in immunosuppressed patients[81].

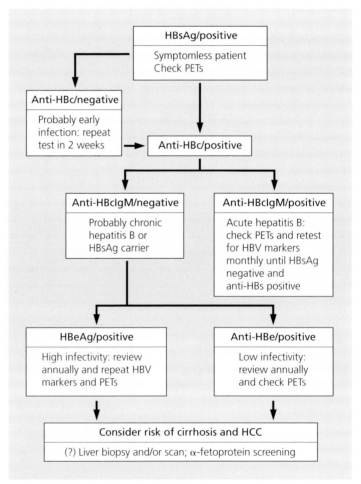

Figure 8.7 A scheme of management of asymptomatic individuals found to be HBsAg positive on routine testing. The abbreviation 'PETs' is used for 'plasma enzyme tests in liver disease'; plasma alanine and aspartate aminotransferase (ALT and AST) activities are most often measured but ALT is more liver specific (adapted from Robertson *et al.*[261])

HBsAg and anti-HBs

This pattern is occasionally found in patients who are recovering from acute hepatitis B. It is, however, a common finding in chronic infection, particularly in those with chronic active hepatitis in whom it may be indicative of a greater inflammatory reaction in the liver. Occasionally the presence of both HBsAg and anti-HBs is evidence of an HBV escape mutant (see page 217).

Anti-HBc alone

Some of these reactions, particularly when the titers are low, are false positive results, possibly resulting from an IgM-like component in the serum sample. In other cases, there has been exposure to HBV in the past but HBsAg and serological markers have become undetectable. A few patients have high titered anti-HBc, and HBV DNA can be detected by PCR. Some of these patients have concurrent infection with hepatitis C virus, HIV, or both[82].

Anti-HBs alone

This antibody alone is found in those who have been vaccinated against HBV, and is occasionally found in patients who give no history of vaccination. The latter finding may reflect previous infection but the other serological markers are below the limits of detection of the assay systems, or exposure without infection. As false positive reactions sometimes occur in the tests, it is recommended that, when there is no clear history of previous acute infection or vaccination, these individuals should be vaccinated.

VACCINATION FOR HEPATITIS B

Vaccination should be offered to certain groups of individuals who lack immunity to HBV (Box 8.2). Compared with other population groups, the prevalence of serological markers of previous HBV infection (anti-HBc) amongst men who have sex with men, and injecting drug users, is high, and it may be cost effective to undertake screening for such markers. It is generally recommended, however, that to increase patient adherence to the vaccination program, the initial dose of vaccine should be given at the time of testing[83]. Immune individuals, of course, do not receive further doses.

Efficacy of hepatitis B vaccine

Both the effectiveness and safety of the hepatitis B vaccine were shown in a placebo-controlled, randomized, and double-blind trial in 1083 homosexual men known to be at high risk for hepatitis B. The vaccine prepared by the Merck Institute for Therapeutic Research, consisted of a 1 mL, 40 μg dose of HBsAg, subunit *ad*, formulated in an alum adjuvant, administered intramuscularly at 0, 1, and 6 months. Within 1 month of the first vaccination 31.4% of recipients acquired anti-HBs, within 2 months this rate had increased to 77%, within 3 months to 87%, and within 6 months, but before the third injection, to 90%. The final booster injection increased the antibody response to 96%. For the first 18 months of follow-up hepatitis B or subclinical infection developed only in 1.4% to 3.4% of the vaccinated recipients, compared with 18.1% to 21.7% of placebo recipients, a difference that was highly significant (log-rank summary chi-square test, $P > 0.0001$). The study provided evidence also that the presence of anti-HBs is synonymous with protection[84]. No HBsAg-positive events, with or without hepatitis, occurred among subjects who received all three vaccinations and developed an immune response. Although protection is correlated with anti-HBs titers above 10 mIU/mL, low anti-HBs levels may mask significant infection and some countries, including the UK, adopt a higher reference point such as 100 mIU/mL[85].

The occasional appearance (8 cases) of anti-HBc conversion without surface antigen, anti-HBs or biochemical evidence of liver damage probably occurred when incompletely immunized subjects were exposed to HBV, since this anti-HBc seroconversion declined sharply after the booster injection was given and immunity firmly established, whereas it increased during the same period in the placebo recipients[84].

The effectiveness of the vaccine was firmly established by this trial, and it has been shown that, in adults, a dose of 20 µg of HBsAg is as effective as the earlier 40 µg and is now standard[86]. A dose of 10 µg is sufficient for young children. Recombinant DNA techniques have been used for expressing HBsAg in eukaryotic cells, particularly in yeast cells, and modern vaccines, prepared in this manner, have replaced the earlier, plasma-derived vaccines. There is no significant difference in the quantity or specificity of the anti-HBs response induced by the recombinant hepatitis B vaccines and the plasma-derived hepatitis B vaccine[87].

The anti-HBs response to vaccination is reduced in those over 40 years of age, and in immunocompromised individuals, including those with HIV infection. Collier et al.[88] found that after vaccination with plasma-derived vaccine, a low or absent anti-HBs response was found in 7 of 16 HIV-infected homosexual men, compared with 6 of 68 HIV seronegative men. An additional observation is that immunocompromised HIV-infected individuals have an accelerated loss of serum anti-HBs after vaccination[89]. Smoking tobacco may also result in impaired responses to hepatitis B vaccine[90].

Hepatitis B vaccine

The most widely used vaccine (Engerix B, SmithKline Beecham Pharmaceuticals) is a suspension of hepatitis B surface antigen produced by yeast cells using a recombinant DNA method. It is available as a 1 mL suspension, each mL containing 20 µg protein, adsorbed on aluminum hydroxide adjuvant.

Adverse reactions

These are generally mild, the most common being discomfort at the injection site with erythema and/or induration. Less frequent side effects include malaise, low-grade fever, arthralgia, headache, thrombocytopenic purpura, and, rarely, rashes, including urticaria. Neurological features that have been reported include neuropathy, including the Guillain–Barré syndrome; no causal relationship to the vaccine has been established (Data Sheet 1999/2000). Anaphylactic reactions are rare but have been reported.

Use in pregnancy

The safety of hepatitis B vaccine in pregnancy has not been established and its use is not recommended unless there is a serious risk if infection.

Vaccination schedules

In *adults* 1 mL of vaccine is given by *intramuscular* injection into the deltoid muscle. Injection into the buttock or into adipose tissue results in an impairment of the immune response[91]. The second dose is given at 1 month and the third at 6 months after the initial dose. The subcutaneous route may be used in those with severe coagulation defects. The combined hepatitis A and B vaccine is given in an identical manner.

Another vaccination schedule that is sometimes used, is one in which 20 µg doses of vaccine are given at 0, 1, and 2 months, with a booster at 12 months. It is stated that 1 month after the first dose, 15% of recipients have protective levels of antibody and 89% have protective antibody levels after the third dose. One month after the booster, 95% of vaccinees have protective levels.

An alternative accelerated course is used when it is necessary to induce protective antibodies as quickly as possible. The 20 µg vaccine is given at days 0, 7, and 21, plus a booster at 12 months. One week and 5 weeks after completion of the primary vaccination course, 65% and 76% of vaccinees respectively have protective antibodies, and 1 month after the booster dose, 98% of vaccinees have protective antibody levels. This is the regimen that the authors favour in the management of victims of sexual assault.

In *neonates and children less than 12 years of age*, 0.5 mL of vaccine is given intramuscularly through the anterolateral thigh in infants and into the deltoid muscle in older children. The dosing schedule is that used for adults.

Monitoring the response to hepatitis B vaccine

It is the authors' policy to measure the anti-HBs levels in the serum 6 to 8 weeks after the third dose of vaccine. If the plasma level of anti-HBs is greater than 100 mIU/mL, the individual is likely to have life-long immunity to hepatitis B, and further vaccination is not required[92]. It is postulated that proliferation of memory B cells is likely to occur within a few days of exposure to HBV, even when vaccine has been given years previously[93]. Even when anti-HBs was no longer detectable, immunological priming of peripheral blood B cells was shown in each of over 150 individuals who had received hepatitis B primary vaccination years previously[94]. Further evidence for long-term protection comes from the observation in a community with a high prevalence of infection: in a 10-year follow-up only 0.8% of 1630 vaccinated people developed anti-HBc and none had clinical disease[95].

Further booster doses of hepatitis B vaccine, however, should be given to those individuals who show poor or absent responses to the standard three-dose vaccine course. Support for this approach comes from a study conducted by SmithKline Beecham[96]: after a single booster 65% of 162 persons developed anti-HBs levels greater than 100 mIU/mL, 18% were low-responders (anti-HBs 10 to 99 mIU/mL), and 17% were non-responders (anti-HBs less than 10 mIU/mL). After a second booster, given 2 months after the first, all low-responders achieved a level of anti-HBs greater than 100 mIU/mL, and after a third dose given 2 months later, all non-responders had such protective serum levels of antibody. HIV-infected individuals with a CD4+ cell count in the peripheral blood less than 500/mm³ often respond poorly to hepatitis B vaccination (see page 228). In the case of non-responders, three additional monthly doses of vaccine (20 μg) have been shown to increase the response rate significantly[97]. Because antibody is likely to persist for less time in immunocompromised patients, including those with chronic renal failure and HIV infection, it is recommended that post-vaccination testing for anti-HBs is undertaken every 6 to 12 months, and if plasma levels are less than 10 mIU/mL, booster doses should be given[92].

Prevention of infection in infants

HBV can be transmitted at birth from a HBsAg-positive mother to her child, particularly if she carries HBeAg. The aim of immunization of neonates is to prevent the establishment of the carrier state. As judged by the development of anti-HBc and anti-HBs months after the immediate postnatal administration of hepatitis B immunoglobulin (HBIG), infection with the virus is not prevented. However, studies have shown a striking reduction in the carrier rate of neonates given HBIG immediately after delivery or within 48 hours of birth. Beasley *et al.*[98] noted that 32 (91%) of 35 placebo-treated infants, but only 19 (45%) of 42 infants given a single injection

of HBIG, became HBsAg carriers. The carrier rate was further reduced to 23% when multiple doses (at birth, and 3 and 6 months later) of HBIG were given. It is likely that infants are protected against perinatal infection when HBIG is administered after birth but later acquire the virus from their mothers when levels of anti-HBs become ineffective. The results of Beasley's study[98] seem to indicate that the older the infant is when it is infected, the less likely it is that he will become a chronic carrier.

When given just after delivery and 1 month later, a serological response to hepatitis B vaccine develops within 3 to 6 months[99]. Such an observation prompted studies into active immunization of infants born to mothers who were chronic HBsAg carriers or who developed acute hepatitis B during their second or third trimesters. However, Maupas *et al.*[99] found that the protective efficacy rate* was only in the order of 75% which is similar to that for HBIG alone.

In Taipei, Taiwan, where the carrier rate for hepatitis B in the general population is 15% to 20% a well-controlled trial of immunization was carried out in infants born to HBsAg carrier mothers who were also HBeAg-positive[100]. When 0.5 mL hepatitis B immune globulin was given immediately after birth and followed by various vaccination schedules with the Merck HBV vaccine, the combined efficacy was 94%, compared with that of HBIG alone (71%) or of vaccination alone (75%). In Hong Kong, Wong *et al.*[101] obtained similarly good results with HBIG and a heat-inactivated vaccine in somewhat different schedules.

In the prevention of infection in infants born to HBsAg-positive mothers, 200 units of hepatitis B immunoglobulin should be given by intramuscular injection as soon as possible after birth, and preferably within 12 hours of delivery. Simultaneously, hepatitis B vaccine (10 μg) is given, but at a different anatomical site. The active

$$*\text{Protective efficacy rate} = \frac{100 \times \text{attack rate in placebo group} - \text{attack rate in treatment group}}{\text{attack rate in placebo group}}$$

immunization is continued with further doses of hepatitis B vaccine (10 μg) at 1 and 6 months after birth.

Post-exposure prophylaxis

Individuals who are not known to be immune to the infection and who have had sexual contact with a patient with acute hepatitis B or an infectious carrier, should be given 500 units of hepatitis B immunoglobulin by intramuscular injection as soon as possible after the most recent sexual exposure, and certainly within 7 days. The effectiveness of HBIG in preventing infection was shown in a study amongst the spouses of individuals with acute hepatitis B[102]. It was shown that only 1 of 25 spouses who had received HBIG developed symptomatic disease, compared with 9 of 33 who had received placebo. A further individual developed subclinical infection, compared with five placebo recipients. In addition to receiving passive immunization, sexual contacts should be given hepatitis B vaccine, preferably as an accelerated course at 0, 1, and 2 months, followed by a booster at 12 months (see page 228). A similar passive/active immunization regimen is recommended after parenteral exposure to the virus.

New hepatitis B vaccine and escape mutants

Up to 10% of immunocompetent individuals either fail to mount an antibody response or have an impaired response to vaccination with plasma-derived or recombinant vaccines[103]. A new vaccine, containing pre-S1, pre-S2, and S antigenic components of both viral surface antigen subtypes *adw* and *ayw* has shown promise in the vaccination of health-care workers who have failed to respond to licensed vaccine[104]. Seventy per cent of 100 individuals seroconverted after a single dose of vaccine. The results of larger studies on efficacy and safety are awaited.

Vaccines such as this may overcome concerns about vaccine escape mutants (see page 217). Although the G145R mutant has now been described in several countries, the prevalence of such mutants is still low.

Hepatitis C virus infection

VIROLOGY

Hepatitis C virus (HCV) was the first virus to be isolated using molecular cloning. Large volumes of plasma from a chronically infected chimpanzee were centrifuged to pellet the virus particles. All the nucleic acids were extracted from the pellet and transcribed into cDNA. About a million colonies in a lambda gt11 expression system were screened with serum from a patient with chronic non-A, non-B hepatitis. A single positive clone that expressed a virus-specific immunogenic peptide was finally identified[110]. By using overlapping clones, the entire sequence of the HCV genome was obtained. As HCV cannot be grown in tissue culture or propagated in small animal models, theories on the pathogenesis of the disease and the replication of the virus have been inferred from studies of other positive-strand viruses, particularly the flaviviruses and the pestiviruses.

Hepatitis C virus is a member of the family Flaviviridae, which includes flaviviruses and pestiviruses. There has been a proposal for HCV to become a separate genus – hepacivirus. There are at least six genotypes and over fifty subtypes of HCV. The virion, which is thought to contain a nucleoprotein and an outer envelope composed of a lipid membrane and envelope proteins, contains a positive, single-stranded RNA genome about 9.6 kilobases (kb) in length. It contains a single open reading frame (ORF) of about 9 kb that encodes a polyprotein of about 3000 amino acids. At both ends the ORF is flanked by untranslated regions (UTR), which are the most conserved regions of the genome. The polyprotein is cleaved during and after translation by viral and cellular proteases. Figure 8.8 shows diagramatically the HCV genome and the cleavage products. The structural (virion) proteins (C, E1, and E2) are encoded by the 5' quarter of the ORF, and the non-structural proteins (NS2, NS3, NS4A/B, and NS5A/B) by the 3' three-quarters of the ORF. The latter proteins are involved in polyprotein processing and replicative functions of the virus.

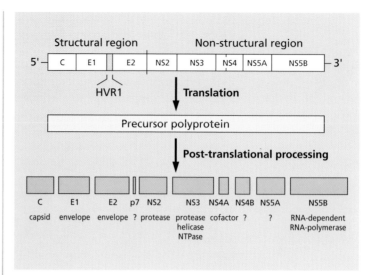

Figure 8.8 Hepatitis C virus genome, open reading frame translation, and post-transitional processing of viral proteins (adapted from Pawlotsky 2000[118])

HCV replication cycle

HCV is produced mainly in the liver. It is postulated that HCV enters susceptible cells through attachment to a cell surface receptor. The identity of the receptor is uncertain, although CD81 that is expressed on various cell lines, including hepatocytes, may be important. Following endocytosis, it is probable that the envelope proteins fuse with the endosomal membrane, with subsequent release of nucleocapsid into the cytoplasm[111]. The nucleocapsid associates with ribosomes resulting in release of the capsid protein, and the genomic RNA serves as a template for protein translation. Non-structural proteins, cleaved from the polyprotein encoded by the genomic RNA, the HCV RNA template and cellular factors are thought to form a ribonucleoprotein complex. Within this complex, a negative-strand copy of viral RNA genome is produced that serves as a template for the production of positive-strand RNA.

A nucleocapsid is produced by an interaction between capsid proteins and, specifically, positive-strand, genomic RNA. The positive-strand RNA is thought to possess an encapsidation signal, resulting in specific binding affinity for the capsid protein[111]. It is postulated that nucleocapsids bud into the endoplasmic reticulum or similar structures and acquire envelopes. It is not known how the envelope is added.

The assembled virions are released from cells via the exocytic pathway.

Genotypes and quasispecies

The HCV genome displays considerable heterogeneity. Hepatitis C virus isolates, collected from different parts of the world, have been sequenced, and can be classified into six genotypes[112]. A large number of subtypes have been recognized within five of the six main genotypes. Genotypes differ by around 30% sequence, and within any genotype the subtypes differ by 21% to 23%.

HCV circulates as a heterogeneous population of genetically distinct but closely related variants in various proportions, and known collectively as a quasispecies. The quasispecies composition of HCV results from the accumulation of mutants during viral replication in the host (see above).

PATHOGENESIS

The mechanisms by which HCV evades the immune system and establishes persistent infection are uncertain. The high incidence of chronic hepatitis C implies that most individuals are unable to mount an effective immune response that will clear the virus. CD4+ T cells and their cytokines appear to play an important role in determining outcome of infection with HCV. In individuals who have *acute*, self-limiting, HCV infection, there is a marked HCV-specific T_h-cell response. The NS3 protein appears to be an important antigen in this respect because CD4+ T-cell responses against its helicase domain are significantly stronger in patients who have self-limiting hepatitis compared with those who have persistent infection. Within this protein is a short immunodominant region that is well-conserved within most genotypes, and that binds to several HLA class II alleles with high affinity[113]. The T cells mediating the NS3-specific immune response produce cytokines of the T_{h1} or T_{h0} profile[114]. These cytokines (interleukin-2, interferon-γ and tumor necrosis factor-α) may have direct antiviral effects by stimulating nitric oxide production by macrophages and hepatocytes. Tsai *et al.*[114] found that peripheral blood mononuclear cells from patients who developed *chronic hepatitis*, however, were characterized by T_{h2} profiles, and had significantly weaker proliferative responses than cells from patients with self-limiting disease. The cytokines produced by T_{h2} cells downregulate the T_{h1} response, and it is this imbalance between T_{h1} and T_{h2} responses that may result in persistence of infection and disease progression. Little is known about HCV-specific cytotoxic T-cell (CTL) responses in acute HCV infection. It has been shown, however, that termination of infection correlates with the onset of an *intrahepatic* CTL response[115]. Although the frequency of HCV-specific CTL is about one hundred times higher in the liver than in the peripheral blood[116], it is too weak to clear the virus from chronically infected individuals. In addition, infected hepatocytes lack the co-stimulatory molecules that promote contact between the T-cell receptor and peptide–MHC complex via CD28-B7 interaction, or engagement of CD4 and CD8 co-receptors.

Neutralizing antibodies are produced during the course of chronic hepatitis C[117], but are clearly unable to terminate infection. Although specific antibodies may interfere with entry of HCV into cells (binding of HCV E2 protein to the major extracellular loop of CD81 is inhibited by HCV neutralizing antibodies), they cannot eliminate the virus from infected cells. Rapid viral mutation may also be partly responsible for HCV persistence. Viral heterogeneity arises from a high error rate of RNA-dependent RNA polymerase, encoded by the NS5B gene (Figure 8.8). The majority of mutant virus particles are replication deficient but others propagate efficiently, the 'fittest' viruses being selected continuously by the pressure resulting from immune responses[118]. This confers a survival advantage on HCV. This is suggested by the finding that patients with persistent viremia have higher early quasispecies complexity than those with spontaneous clearance[119]. During chronic HCV infection, viral quasispecies are in a state of equilibrium at any given time, but their composition may alter. The E1 and E2 regions of the genome have the highest mutation rate at the nucleotide and (predicted) amino acid levels, suggesting that this region is under selective pressure by the immune system. The hypervariable region 1 (HVR 1) is located at the 5′ end of E2, and is one of the main targets of neutralizing antibodies[120]. Viral persistence is associated with the continuous generation of new HVR1 mutants, and the continuous selection of mutants escaping recognition by neutralizing antibodies[118].

Some HCV-seronegative individuals who are exposed repeatedly to HCV mount HCV-specific Th and CTL responses in the absence of viremia or a humoral immune response[121], suggesting that such responses are protective.

Although the mechanism of damage to the liver is uncertain, HCV is not thought to be cytopathic. The damage most probably results from the low-grade immune response that is, albeit, insufficient to clear the virus.

EPIDEMIOLOGY

Hepatitis C virus is a blood-borne virus that is endemic throughout the world. As the virus has only recently been identified, data on the incidence and prevalence of infection are incomplete. It has been estimated, however, that 170 million people are infected worldwide, representing 3% of the population[122].

Geographical distribution of hepatitis C virus genotypes

Although some genotypes of HCV, such as 1a, 2a, 2b, and 3a, are of world wide distribution, their relative frequencies vary from one geographical area to another[123]. For example, in the USA and in western Europe, types 1a and 1b predominate, but type 1b is more prevalent in southern and eastern Europe than in northern Europe or the USA. Almost three-quarters of cases of HCV in Japan are associated with type 1b. In northern Africa and in the Middle East, type 4 predominates, and types 5 and 6 appear to be confined to South Africa and Hong Kong respectively[123].

Risk factors for transmission of hepatitis C virus

Injecting drug use

In the USA, injecting drug use accounts for most HCV transmission. Although the prevalence of HCV infection was low in the late 1960s, the incidence of infection increased during the 1980s, an average of 230 000 new infections occurring each year. Since 1989, the incidence of infection has declined by more than 80% so that by 1996 the annual number of new infections was about 36 000[124]. Infection mostly occurred amongst young adults, and was principally the result of injecting drug use with sharing of contaminated syringes and needles. A similar incidence pattern has been reported from Australia[125].

Several studies have shown a high prevalence of HCV infection amongst injecting drug users in both industrialized and developing countries. In the USA, it has been estimated that the average prevalence of infection amongst such individuals is 79%[124]. About one-third of injecting users attending specialist agencies for the management of drug misuse in England and Wales during 1998 to 1999 had markers of infection, and in Scotland, 62% of 1905 specimens from injecting users tested between 1995 and 1996 gave positive results[126]. Within countries, however, there are regional differences in prevalence. In Scotland, for example, 74% of injecting drug users in Glasgow and 37% in Aberdeen were anti-HCV positive[126].

Similarly, the prevalence of HCV was significantly higher amongst injecters in Ho Chi Minh City (87% of 67 users) than in Hanoi (31% of 200 users)[127].

HCV is acquired more rapidly after initiation of injecting than other blood-borne viral infections. For example, amongst injecting drug users in Sydney, Australia, the incidence of HCV among 152 initially negative users was 20.9 per 100 person years; this compared with an incidence of HIV-1 among 426 initially negative individuals of 0.17 per 100 person years[128]. The incidence of HCV amongst injecting drug users under the age of 20 years was particularly high – 75.6 per 100 person years – and the propensity for spread of the virus amongst new, young users is clear. For example, in a prospective study, it was shown that seroconversion for HCV was significantly associated both with injecting for less than 2 years and continuing to inject[129]. These observations probably reflect the high prevalence of HCV infection in the injecting drug user population and hence the greater likelihood of exposure to the virus in young injecters. After 5 years of injecting, up to 90% of individuals have been found to be HCV seropositive[124].

Sexual transmission

Although HCV can be transmitted sexually there are still unanswered questions regarding some aspects of its transmission by this route.

Tests for anti-HCV in the sera of 21 241 people who participated in the third National Health and Nutrition Examination Survey conducted in the USA between 1988 and 1994 showed an overall prevalence of HCV infection of 1.8%[130]. Factors with the strongest associations with HCV infection were illicit drug use, and high-risk sexual behaviour (an early age at first intercourse or more than 50 lifetime sexual partners) in the absence of drug use.

Alter et al.[131] were the first to suggest that heterosexual intercourse may play a role in the transmission of HCV. In the comparison of 52 individuals with non-A, non-B hepatitis, who had no recognized risk factors for the infection, with 104 non-infected controls, these authors found that the former group were eleven times more likely to have had multiple sexual partners.

Several studies in the early 1990s, however, suggested that sexual transmission of HCV was uncommon. Bresters et al.[132] reported that none of 50 heterosexual partners of anti-HCV positive individuals had become infected after a median duration of sexual relationship of 13 years. Similarly, specific antibodies against HCV were not found in the serum of any sexual partner of 40 patients with hemophilia who were anti-HCV positive, 35 having detectable plasma HCV RNA[133].

Amongst individuals who have attended STI clinics in the USA but who had not been injecting drug users, the prevalence of anti-HCV has been high. For example, in a Baltimore clinic, 7% of 555 men and 4% of 484 women were seropositive for HCV[134]. As in the study referred to above, there was a significant relationship between a high number of sexual partners and seropositivity. In addition, anti-HCV was associated with a history of other STIs, namely Trichomonas vaginalis and HIV infection. It was also shown that women whose sexual partner was anti-HCV positive were 3.7 times more likely to be seropositive than women who were contacts of anti-HCV negative men[134]. In the same study, nucleotide sequencing was undertaken, and the similarities of the nucleic acid sequences of these women and their sexual partners suggested a common source of HCV, as would be expected with sexual transmission. These data seem to corroborate earlier reports on sexual transmission of HCV. Peano et al.[135] detected anti-HCV in the serum of 13% of 100 sexual partners of HCV-infected individuals. The disparity between the findings in these studies and those that showed little evidence of sexual transmission of HCV may be that other factors, such as genital ulceration, may facilitate the transmission of the virus. Amongst female sex-industry workers with HCV infection in Brazil, it was shown that there was a significant relationship between the time spent in prostitution and positive serological tests for syphilis (FTA-ABS), suggesting a significant role for sexual transmission of the virus in those who have multiple sexual partners[136]. Plasma viral load of HCV may also be an important factor in determining sexual transmission. Although earlier studies failed to detect HCV RNA in semen, HCV RNA has now been found in semen, but viral loads in this fluid are low[137]. As the plasma HCV load is higher in individuals who have co-infection with HIV than in those who have HCV infection alone[138], HIV co-infection may also facilitate transmission of HCV. Eyster et al.[139] found that the frequency of HCV transmission to sexual partners was five times higher when HIV was also transmitted: 5 (3%) of 164 female sexual partners of HIV-positive/ HCV-positive men were infected compared with none of 30 partners of anti-HIV-negative/anti-HCV-positive men. In a multicenter study to investigate the risk of sexual transmission of HIV and HCV from infected hemophiliac men, it was found that a higher viral load was associated with an increased risk of HIV transmission, but that a higher HCV viral load was not associated significantly with increased risk of transmission of HCV[140].

Although HCV can be detected in cervicovaginal secretions[141], the risk of female-to-male transmission appears to be low. In the study reported by Thomas et al.[134], there was no apparent increased risk for men who had sexual intercourse with HCV-infected women.

Amongst homosexual men attending STI clinics, higher prevalence rates of anti-HCV have been reported than amongst control subjects. In San Francisco, for example, during 1983 to 1984 at a time when unprotected anal intercourse was prevalent in the community, 9.2% of 435 men were seropositive for HCV[142]. Over one-fifth of these men gave a history of injecting drug use, the prevalence of HCV infection in this group being 25%. Amongst men who gave no history of intravenous drug use, sera from 5% contained anti-HCV, a prevalence rate that was significantly higher than amongst blood donors (odds ratio 3.4, 95% confidence interval 2.8–4.2). Several risk factors for HCV, including receptive anal intercourse and 'fisting', were identified, but on multivariate analysis only intravenous drug use was significantly associated with anti-HCV positivity. Similar results from a large cohort of homo-sexually active men were reported from Sydney[143] where 7.6% of 1038 men were seropositive for HCV. In multiple logistic regression analyses, only HIV co-infection and a history of injecting drug use cor-related with HCV infection.

In conclusion, although sexual trans-mission of HCV undoubtedly occurs, the risk of transmission from an infected individual appears to be low.

Perinatal transmission

The prevalence of HCV in pregnant women varies geographically, reflecting the prevalence of the infection in the general population. Hepatitis C virus can be trans-mitted from an infected mother to her child, the most probable time of infection being in the peripartum period. In a systematic review of 976 infants from 28 studies, Thomas *et al*.[144] reported that the rate of transmission of HCV from mother to child averaged 6%. The risk of maternal transmission of the virus is very low in those who are not viremic, but appears to increase as the plasma viral load increases[144]. Higher rates of transmission, however, have been observed in women who are co-infected with HIV: an average of 14% and 17% of infants born to mothers with HIV and HCV infection had detectable anti-HCV and HCV RNA respectively[145]. This finding probably reflects the higher levels of HCV RNA in immune-suppressed patients. Although Granovsky *et al*.[146] noted an increased risk of HCV infection amongst children born vaginally to HCV-infected mothers compared with those delivered by cesarean section, larger studies have failed to confirm this finding[147]. Des-pite the fact that the virus can be present in breast milk[141], there is little epidemiological evidence that HCV is transmitted by breast feeding[144].

Acquisition of hepatitis C virus from receipt of blood or blood products, and organs

Although the transfusion of blood or blood products was an important risk factor for HCV infection in industrialized countries before 1990, serological screening of donated blood, and inactivation of blood products has all but eliminated this mode

of transmission of HCV. Similarly, the risk of acquisition of the virus from organ transplants is now negligible. Although there is much geographical variation in the prevalence of HCV infection amongst hemodialysis patients, about 20% may be infected[148]. This high prevalence is the result of receipt of blood before screening procedures were in place, and patient-to-patient spread because of a breakdown in infection-control practices.

Occupational risk

Blood-borne viruses pose a hazard to health-care professionals who have exposure to blood. Although the prevalence of HCV infection amongst health-care workers in areas of the UK is low (2.05 to 2.8 per 1000 persons), it is almost three times higher than in the general popula-tion, as judged by the prevalence of anti-HCV in blood donors[149]. A history of needle-stick injury is the only occupational risk factor associated with HCV infec-tion[150]. Although the average incidence of anti-HCV seroconversion after such injury from an HCV-infected patient is reported as 1.8% (range 0% to 7%)[124], researchers from Japan detected HCV infection by HCV reverse transcriptase PCR, in 10% of injured individuals[151]. One report sug-gested that only contaminated hollow-bore needles posed a risk[152]. This risk is significantly higher than for HIV sero-conversion after a needle-stick injury involving an HIV-infected individual (on average 0.3%). Although the degree of risk is unknown, transmission of HCV from blood splashes to the conjunctivae has occurred[153].

The risk of transmission of HCV from an infected health-care worker to a patient is very low. There has been a report on such an occurrence, a cardiac surgeon having infected five patients[154].

Body piercing, tattooing, acupuncture, and ritual practices

The undertaking of these procedures with inadequately sterilized equipment has the potential to transmit HCV in addition to other blood-borne viruses. In the indus-trialized world, however, there are few data to show that they are a significant risk[124].

Procedures related to health care

There have been instances of patient-to-patient transmission of HCV through the use of contaminated phlebotomy needles, multi-dose vials, and inadequately dis-infected endoscopes[155]. In a recent report, genotype and molecular characterization of HCV isolates proved useful in providing evidence for patient-to-patient transmission of HCV during colonoscopy[156].

In Japan, geographical clustering of anti-HCV positive individuals over the age of 40 years has suggested that, in addition to surgical operations, certain folk remedies, including acupuncture and cutting of the skin with unsterilized knives, are a risk factor for infection[157]. The low prevalence of anti-HCV amongst children and younger people, however, suggest that these pro-cedures are no longer the most important means of transmission of HCV in these localities.

In some countries, such as Egypt, the prevalence of HCV infection is high in all age groups and increases steadily with age, indicating high risk in the past with an ongoing high risk for acquisition of HCV[155]. Mass treatment for schistosomia-sis with potassium antimony tartrate has been implicated as a cause for the high prevalence of infection in rural areas of Egypt[158]. Until oral treatment for schisto-somiasis became available, the drug was administered by the parenteral route, often using inadequately sterilized syringes. Unsafe injecting practices appear to be responsible for the sustained transmission of HCV in Egypt[159].

Household contacts

Although there are inadequate data to draw conclusions, the risk of infection to non-sexual household contacts of indivi-duals with HCV infection is probably low. In one study, however, more patients with non-A, non-B hepatitis compared with control subjects had had household contact with a person who had a history of hepatitis[131].

No recognized source of infection

In the USA about 10% of individuals with HCV have no apparent source of infection[124].

NATURAL HISTORY

There are several possible outcomes of HCV infection

- complete recovery
- persistent viremia without abnormalities of plasma enzyme tests of liver function
- chronic hepatitis with abnormal liver enzyme tests but without signs of disease progression
- progression to hepatic fibrosis and cirrhosis
- cirrhosis without evidence of hepatic decompensation
- progressive cirrhosis culminating in hepatic failure
- development of hepatocellular carcinoma.

The natural history of hepatitis C virus infection with respect to the frequency and rates of development of serious liver disease, however, is incompletely understood for the following reasons[160]

- the onset of acute infection is rarely identified
- many affected individuals are asymptomatic
- disease progression may take decades to become apparent, thereby making prospective studies difficult
- the risk of infection is highest amongst individuals whose underlying condition is itself associated with considerable morbidity and mortality
- many studies have included patients referred to tertiary treatment centers, hence introducing bias, these studies representing 'worst-case' scenarios
- most studies have omitted from analysis those who have recovered from acute hepatitis C and those with mild disease who have not sought medical attention.

Notwithstanding these difficulties some conclusions can be reached regarding the natural history of HCV infection[160].

Conclusions from prospective studies regarding the natural history of HCV infection

Several prospective studies of transfusion-associated disease have shown that progression from acute to chronic hepatitis is common[161–163]. Cirrhosis developed in 7% to 16% of cases during a follow-up period that averaged 16 years and liver-related mortality ranged from 1.3% to 3.7%. Unfortunately, longer-term data (20 to 40 years) were not available from these cohorts, and none contained a control group.

Several studies have investigated the natural history of hepatitis C beginning with patients who had established chronic hepatitis. A follow-up study from Germany of 838 patients with chronic hepatitis C yielded useful information[164]. One hundred and forty-one patients had cirrhosis at study entry. During the follow-up period, median 50.2 months, 62 patients died, 18 from cirrhosis, 13 from hepatocellular carcinoma, and 31 from other causes. Overall mortality was higher in those infected with HCV than in the general population, and mortality was strongly related to the presence of cirrhosis and duration of infection. Among the 696 patients without cirrhosis, however, the mortality rate did not differ from that of the general population. All individuals who had hepatocellular carcinoma had had cirrhosis at study entry. Cirrhosis, long disease duration, chronic alcoholism, injecting drug use, and older age were identified as factors resulting in decreased survival.

In a follow-up study of 384 European patients with compensated cirrhosis, Fattovich et al.[165] found that hepatocellular carcinoma developed in 29 (8%) patients, and hepatic decompensation developed in 65 (18%) of the remaining 355 patients. In total 9% of the cohort died from liver-related causes, 9 to 124 months after enrolment into the study.

It appears that, provided decompensation does not occur, early stage cirrhosis seems compatible with survival.

Conclusions from retrospective studies regarding the natural history of HCV infection

Retrospective studies that have assessed patients with established chronic hepatitis C have shown a high frequency of cirrhosis, hepatic decompensation, and hepatocellular carcinoma. For example, in a highly selected group of 70 Japanese patients with chronic hepatitis, Yano et al.[166] reported the development of cirrhosis in 50% of individuals who were followed-up for between 2 and 26 years, and who had had serial liver biopsies. In a retrospective evaluation of 213 patients with chronic hepatitis C and short-term follow-up (mean duration 3.9 years) of 131 patients, Tong et al.[167], working in a tertiary referral center in Los Angeles, found chronic hepatitis in 21%, chronic active hepatitis in 23%, cirrhosis in 51%, and hepatocellular carcinoma in 5.3% of initial biopsy specimens. The average intervals between infection and the development of chronic hepatitis, chronic active hepatitis, cirrhosis, and hepatocellular carcinoma were 14 years, 18 years, 21 years, and 28 years respectively. In their follow-up study, a further 5.3% of patients developed hepatocellular carcinoma. Similarly, Gordon et al.[168] found a high frequency of cirrhosis amongst a group of patients from the USA, and noted that cirrhosis was much more likely to occur in individuals who had acquired HCV through blood transfusion than through other routes (55% of 215 versus 21% of 195 patients). They also noted that hepatocellular carcinoma was more likely to develop in the former group of patients than in the latter (4% versus 1%).

Conclusions from non-concurrent prospective studies regarding the natural history of HCV infection

These studies involve the identification and follow-up of a cohort of patients who had a clearly recognized initial infection. One such study involved a group of Irish women who had received contaminated anti-D immune globulin at the time of delivery for Rh incompatibility[169]. Three hundred and seventy-six women who were seropositive for HCV and had HCV RNA in the plasma were evaluated. The mean interval from infection to enrolment in the study was 17 years. Serum alanine aminotransferase levels were normal in 45%, mildly elevated (40–99 IU/mL) in 47%, and moderately elevated (> 100 IU/mL) in 8% of women. Liver biopsies were available from 363 women. Mild inflammatory or necrotic changes were found in 41% of cases, moderate inflammatory changes in 51%, and marked inflammation in 4%, there was no evidence of inflammation or necrosis in 2% of biopsies. There was no evidence of fibrosis in 49% of biopsies, 34% had portal or periportal fibrosis only, 15% had bridging fibrosis, and 2% had cirrhosis. These findings suggested a more benign natural history than had been previously reported, and the authors suggested that this may reflect the small size of inoculum, the sex of the patients (women have a higher frequency of spontaneous clearance of HCV[170]), young age at the time of infection, and possibly viral strain.

An analysis of five prospective studies of post-transfusion hepatitis C was published by the National Heart, Lung, and Blood Hepatitis Working Group[171]: 568 patients had non-A, non-B hepatitis and mortality rates in this group were compared with those of 984 matched control subjects who had been transfusion recipients but who did not have hepatitis. At the initiation of follow-up, an average of 18 years from transfusion, the overall mortality was 51% for those with non-A, non-B hepatitis and 51% for the control subjects. Liver-related deaths occurred in 3.3% of those with hepatitis, and in 1.5% of the controls, a difference that was statistically significant. In a follow-up report[172], 5 years of evaluation were added. Overall mortality was similar in both hepatitis and control groups (69.1% and 69.4% respectively), but higher than in the general population. Liver-related death was 4.0% for those with hepatitis and 1.7% for controls, a significant difference. A third report from the same group[173] examined morbidity amongst 103 HCV-related cases 18 to 20 years from transfusion. In this group 74% had detectable serum HCV RNA, 16% were anti-HCV positive but HCV RNA negative, and 10% had no markers of HCV infection. About 50% of subjects had abnormal ALT levels: liver biopsy showed cirrhosis in one-third and chronic hepatitis in two-thirds of these patients. Thus, cirrhosis developed in 15% of the original cases of acute hepatitis C.

Another study[174] examined the natural history of HCV infection acquired in younger individuals (US Air Force recruits, average age 23 years). The authors found that, although the overall morbidity amongst anti-HCV-positive individuals over a 45-year period was similar to that of seronegative individuals, liver-related events were more common in the HCV seropositive group than in the HCV seronegative group (2 of 17 versus 115 of 3566). Seven of the 17 HCV-infected individuals had died, but only one from liver disease. It was concluded therefore that only 20% of the original cohort had continuing infection or liver disease.

Evidence that chronic hepatitis C in childhood is more benign or slowly progressive than in adults was suggested by Vogt et al.[175]. This study involved 458 children who had had a blood transfusion during their childhood, at a mean of 17 years previously, and age- and sex-matched controls from the general population. Anti-HCV was detected in 67 patients, 37 (55%) of whom were HCV RNA positive; 36 of the 37 had normal ALT levels. Liver biopsies from 17 patients were available, two showed portal fibrosis and one had cirrhosis.

Spontaneous loss of hepatitis C virus

It appears that a sizeable proportion of individuals who become infected with HCV recover from their infection. For example, in the National Health and Nutrition Examination Survey (NHANES III)[176], 1.8% of 21 241 individuals were seropositive for HCV. Plasma specimens from 74% of these people were positive for HCV RNA, indicating that 26% of infected individuals recover. It is uncertain, however, when recovery occurs, but it is suspected that spontaneous viral loss occurs relatively early after infection, probably within 6 months, or perhaps in the first 2 years[160].

Persistent infection may be more likely with some genotypes than others. Amoroso et al.[177] found that amongst 42 patients in whom a diagnosis of acute hepatitis C had been made, chronicity was associated with genotype 1b, persistent infection was found in 92% of individuals infected with this genotype compared with 30% to 50% of patients exposed to other genotypes.

Association of hepatitis C virus genotypes and persistence of infection

The role of HCV genotypes in the progression of liver disease is controversial[178].

In patients with chronic HCV infection, infection with genotype 1b has been reported to be associated with more severe liver disease and more rapid disease progression than infection with other genotypes[179]. This genotype is also found more frequently among patients with cirrhosis and those with decompensated liver disease than amongst those with chronic active hepatitis[180, 181]. Genotype 1b may carry a higher risk for the development of hepatocellular carcinoma than other genotypes. In the study reported by Zein et al.[182] genotype 1b was found in 5 of 18 patients with this cancer, only 1 of 30 patients infected with other genotypes had this tumor. Patients infected with genotype 1b tend to be older than those infected with other types, and it is possible that it is a marker for more severe disease, reflecting a longer duration of infection[178].

HIV AND HEPATITIS C VIRUS DISEASE PROGRESSION

HIV infection does not appear to influence the severity of acute hepatitis C virus infection, and fulminant disease is rare. Simultaneous HIV infection, however, seems to be an important cofactor in chronic HCV disease progression. Darby et al.[183] found that amongst 4865 men with hemophilia who were exposed to HCV the cumulative risk of liver disease-related death was 1.4% (range 0.7% to 3%) in those who were anti-HIV negative, compared with 6.5% (range 4.5% to 9.5%) in men infected with HIV. HIV infection results in an unusually rapid progression to cirrhosis. Soto et al.[184] compared disease progression in 547 patients with chronic HCV infection, 116 of whom were co-infected with HIV. In the first 10 years, cirrhosis had developed in 13 (15%) of 87 HIV-infected patients, but in only 7 (3%) of 272 persons who were not infected with HIV. The mean interval from estimated time of HCV infection to cirrhosis was significantly shorter in the HIV-infected than in the uninfected patients (6.9 years versus 23.2 years). Other workers, however, have failed to show a more rapid progression of disease in HIV-infected individuals[185, 186]. The reasons for the differences between these studies is not immediately obvious, but factors such as selection bias, duration of infection, and differences in the timing of the two infections may play a part.

PATHOLOGY

The pattern of injury in acute hepatitis C is similar to that found in acute hepatitis caused by other hepatotropic viruses such as hepatitis A and B. In chronic hepatitis C, the pattern of injury is similar to that of chronic hepatitis B or D and to autoimmune hepatitis[187]. There is inflammatory destruction of hepatocytes accompanied by progressive fibrosis. The most distinct histological finding is 'piecemeal' necrosis (interface hepatitis) that may be focal or involve the entire circumference of the portal area. The inflammatory infiltrate is predominantly CD4+ T cells. Periportal collagen deposition eventually replaces the destroyed hepatocytes. Portal inflammation is also common, particularly in the early stages of the disease, and dense lymphoid aggregates are seen more frequently in chronic hepatitis C virus infection than in chronic hepatitis B. Another histological finding that is more common in hepatitis C than in hepatitis B is the presence of reactive epithelial changes in the bile ducts within the lymphoid aggregates or at their edges (Poulsen lesions). Small foci of inflammatory cells associated with hepatocyte apoptosis may be found in the liver parenchyma. Fatty change (steatosis) is also common. Fibrosis begins in the portal areas and with the passage of time, continuing inflammation and fibrosis with destruction of acini and regenerative changes (cirrhosis) may develop. The histology of the chronic hepatitis C in HIV co-infected patients is similar to that of HIV-non-infected individuals[188].

Grading and staging of liver biopsies can provide useful information to the clinician when planning therapy.

CLINICAL FEATURES

Acute hepatitis C

The incubation period of acute hepatitis C ranges from 2 to 12 weeks, with an average of 7 weeks[189]. The symptoms and signs resemble those of other forms of acute viral hepatitis (see pp. 220–221). Figure 8.9 shows the clinical, biochemical, and serological course of a typical case of acute hepatitis C with recovery.

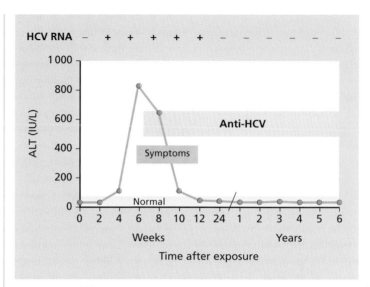

Figure 8.9 Self-limited acute hepatitis C (adapted from Hoofnagle 2000[189])

Chronic hepatitis C

The majority of patients with chronic HCV infection are asymptomatic until complications such as cirrhosis or hepatocellular carcinoma develop; most patients with chronic hepatitis C do not have a past history of icteric hepatitis. Of those who are symptomatic, fatigue is the most common complaint. There may be no abnormal clinical signs, but in more severe hepatitis, hepatic and splenic enlargement, and spider nevi may be found. In some patients extrahepatic manifestations are encountered.

1. There is a strong association between HCV infection and *mixed cryoglobulinemia*. Cryoglobulins are proteins that reversibly precipitate from serum on cooling. Three types of cryoglobulins are recognized
   - Type I, composed entirely of monoclonal immunoglobulins
   - Type II composed of a mixture of monoclonal IgM with rheumatoid factor activity, and polyclonal IgG
   - Type III composed of polyclonal IgG and polyclonal IgM rheumatoid factor.

It is difficult to determine the prevalence of mixed cryoglobulinemia in patients with chronic HCV infection because of lack of standardization of the measurements of cryoglobulins, and patient selection. In one study from France, 20% of patients with chronic hepatitis C had Type II cryoglobulinemia[190]. The pathogenesis of mixed cryoglobulinemia in association with HCV infection is unknown. The mechanisms involved in the proliferation of B cells that results in the production of both polyclonal rheumatoid factor and monoclonal rheumatoid factor are speculative[191]. The most prominent clinical feature of mixed cryoglobulinemia is *palpable purpura*, but the vasculitis that affects small and medium-sized blood vessels may involve viscera resulting in life-threatening disease. Hepatitis C virus antigens, HCV RNA and IgM and IgG have been detected in the cutaneous lesions[191]. Membranoproliferative glomerulonephritis occurs in about one-third of patients with cryoglobulinemia secondary to HCV infection (predominantly Type II)[191]. Arthralgia, weakness, peripheral neuropathy, and Raynaud's phenomenon are also described in association with mixed cryoglobulinemia.

2. Several studies have shown an increased prevalence of HCV infection

amongst patients with *porphyria cutanea tarda*. In one study from the USA, for example, 56% of 70 patients with this condition were infected with HCV[192]. The pathogenesis of porphyria cutanea tarda in relation to HCV infection, however, remains unexplained. Hepatitis C virus is certainly neither necessary nor sufficient for its development, and it has been postulated that alcoholism, a condition common to both HCV and porphyria may be the link between the two[192].

3. There is a high incidence of salivary gland lesions in patients with chronic hepatitis C. Lymphocytic capillaritis and lymphocytic adenitis have been reported in about 50% and up to 80% of infected patients respectively. The condition differs from Sjögren's syndrome in that fewer females are affected, antinuclear antibodies are absent, there is less of an association with HLA DR 3, fewer individuals have xerostomia, and none have xerophthalmia[191].

4. A variety of autoantibodies occur in HCV infection, including rheumatoid factor, anti-smooth muscle antibody, and, less frequently, antinuclear antibody[191]. Clinical features related to the presence of these antibodies, however, are unusual.

Although serum ALT levels decline from the peak levels found in acute infection, they usually remain persistently elevated some two- to eightfold. Serum ALT levels, however, can fluctuate over time and intermittently may be normal. The serum of most patients with chronic hepatitis C who have elevated ALT levels contains detectable HCV RNA. When elevated ALT levels then are found in a patient who is seropositive for HCV, a test for HCV RNA should be undertaken to confirm that HCV is the cause of the abnormality and not some other liver disease. With the development of cirrhosis, the serum aspartate aminotransferase level usually becomes higher than the ALT, the serum albumin concentration is reduced, and the prothrombin time is prolonged. However, there is a poor correlation between symptoms and biochemical markers and liver histology[193].

DIAGNOSIS

Diagnostic tests

Serological tests

The detection in plasma or serum of antibodies against HCV protein antigens, encoded by the viral RNA, is based on the use of enzyme immunoassays (EIAs). The first two proteins, 5-1-1 and c100-3, are derived from non-structural regions of the HCV genome, NS3 and NS4 regions (Figure 8.8). Using 5-1-1 as a hybridization probe, c100 was expressed in yeast and used as antigen in the so-called first-generation enzyme immunoassays for HCV infection. The false positive rate, however, was high, particularly amongst low prevalence populations such as blood donors, and, as anti-c100-3 was not present in the sera of all individuals with past or current infection, sensitivity was low.

Second generation EIAs incorporated two extra HCV-derived recombinant proteins, thereby increasing the sensitivity of the test. One of these proteins, c22-3 antigen, representing the majority of a 22 kDa nucleoprotein whose amino-terminus encoded an immunodominant epitope, was derived from the core region of the HCV genome. Using this antigen in enzyme immunoassays, antibodies against HCV were detected earlier and more frequently than in assays with c100-3 as antigen. The c33c antigen derived from the non-structural region NS3 (Figure 8.8) was also included in the second-generation tests. Although the sensitivity of these tests was improved over the first-generation assays, specificity was little altered.

In the third generation tests, a recombinant NS5 antigen has been added to the four other antigens used in the second-generation tests. In high-prevalence, immunocompetent populations, the sensitivity of these tests has ranged from 98.8% to 100%[194, 195]. However, amongst immunocompromised individuals, including those with HIV infection, the sensitivity of the enzyme immunoassays is lower, ranging from 50% to 95%, depending on the degree of immunodeficiency[196–198]. The specificity of third-generation enzyme immunoassays in low prevalence popula-

tions lies between 99.3% and 100%[194, 195]. Cross-reactivity with other viral antigens may result in false positive results.

For the confirmation of positive results in the EIAs, recombinant immunoblot assays (RIBA) are used. In these assays, the patient's serum is incubated with recombinant HCV antigens coated as parallel bands on a nitrocellulose strip, and enzyme-labeled anti-human IgG is used to detect bound antibody. The first-generation RIBA used c100-3 and 5-1-1 as antigens, and the second-generation RIBA added bands coated with c22-3 and c33c. Peptides replaced c100-3, 5-1-1 and c22-3 in the third-generation RIBA, and another modified c33c antigen and a recombinant NS5 protein were added. RIBA have been successful in excluding false positive results[199]. Indeterminate results (i.e. samples that react with only one antigen in the immunoblot assay) however, do occur, and with respect to the second-generation immunoblot assays, the HCV genotype appears to affect the interpretation of the results. Zein *et al.*[200] who examined serum specimens from the USA, noted that the HCV genotype distribution in patients with indeterminate results was different from that on those with clearly positive results. Genotypes that were less common in the USA were over-represented in the indeterminate results group.

The identification of antibodies against genotype-specific HCV epitopes located in the NS4 and/or core proteins has been used as an indirect marker for the infecting HCV genotype. Two tests are currently available: a RIBA and a competitive EIA. In immunocompetent individuals, the sensitivity range is about 85% to 90%, relative to the molecular methods for genotyping, and their concordance with genotypic assays is about 95%[201].

Molecular methods for diagnosis

A standardized reverse-transcription PCR assay is the most common method used for the detection of HCV RNA in serum. During chronic infection it has been shown that the viral load (amount of circulating genome equivalents per volume of plasma) is stable over periods of months to years[202]. The first-generation tests appeared to be somewhat less sensitive for HCV genotypes 2 and 3 than for genotype 1, but a second generation test, in addition to being more sensitive (stated detection cut-off 100 copies/mL) has a sensitivity that is the same for all genotypes. The specificity of this test is 97% to 99%[203].

Two quantitative assays for HCV RNA that are helpful in clinical management are available: a signal amplification-based 'branched DNA' assay and a competitive reverse-transcription PCR-based assay.

The most definitive method for HCV genotyping is sequencing of a specific PCR-amplified portion of the HCV genome (NS5, core, E1 and 5′ UTRs) obtained from the patient, followed by phylogenetic analysis[123]. For routine use, however, this method is impracticable. Most techniques for HCV genotyping are based on amplification of HCV RNA by PCR, followed by either reamplification with type-specific primers, hybridization with type-specific probes, or digestion of PCR products with restriction endonucleases that recognize genotype-specific cleavage sites[123]. These methods are useful in identifying the major genotypic groups, but only direct sequencing can discriminate between subtypes.

Hepatitis C virus markers in acute hepatitis C

Anti-HCV usually becomes detectable during the icteric phase of the illness, or, occasionally, during the late pre-icteric stage. In about one-third of patients, the test is negative at the onset of symptoms or jaundice[204]. The presence of anti-HCV in an individual with acute hepatitis does not necessarily indicate that HCV is the cause of the hepatitis, for example acute infection with another virus in an individual who already has HCV may be responsible. Acute symptomatic exacerbations of chronic hepatitis C may also be the cause of the patient's symptoms and signs. In a series of 194 patients with chronic hepatitis C, 151 episodes of acute exacerbations occurred in 98 patients, 45% of the episodes were symptomatic[205]. Seroconversion to anti-HCV positivity is the most reliable means of reaching a diagnosis of acute hepatitis C virus infection. In addition, testing for antibodies to specific HCV proteins may help to identify seroconversion[206]. On the other hand, the detection of anti-HCV IgM is not helpful in making a diagnosis of acute hepatitis C. Although this antibody can be detected in the serum of up to 90% of individuals with acute hepatitis C virus infection, it is also found in 50% to 70% of patients with chronic hepatitis C[207]. In the course of acute HCV infection, HCV RNA is detectable in the serum during the incubation period, in the anicteric and in the icteric phases of the disease, and its detection precedes seroconversion (Figure 8.9). Although the detection of HCV RNA suggests the diagnosis of acute hepatitis C in the correct clinical setting, this test fails to differentiate between acute and chronic infection. As the laboratory diagnosis of acute hepatitis C virus infection can therefore be difficult, diagnostic tests for other causes of acute hepatitis may be necessary (Table 8.2).

Diagnosis of chronic hepatitis C virus infection

As the majority of individuals with chronic HCV infection do not have a history of a clinically apparent icteric hepatitis, the diagnosis is made by the detection of specific antibody against HCV in the serum by EIA. In screening of low-risk populations such as blood donors, false positive results in the EIAs occur, and confirmation by RIBA is recommended[208]. However, in individuals with elevated ALT levels or in high-risk patients, these confirmatory tests are unnecessary, and the detection of HCV RNA in serum by PCR is the preferred confirmatory test[208]. Currently, serological tests cannot differentiate between those who have recovered from acute hepatitis C, false positive result, and those with chronic hepatitis but with viral RNA below the limit of detection.

In at least 80% of patients with chronic hepatitis C and normal ALT levels, the liver histology is normal or shows mild hepati-

Table 8.2 Differential diagnosis of acute hepatitis

Condition	Diagnostic tests
Hepatitis A virus infection	Anti-HAV IgM
Hepatitis B virus infection	HBsAg, anti-HBc IgM, HBV DNA
Hepatitis C virus infection	Anti-HCV, HCV RNA
Hepatitis D virus infection (in association with hepatitis B virus infection)	Anti-HDV
Hepatitis E virus infection	Anti-HEV IgG
Infectious mononucleosis	Anti-EBV VCA IgM
Cytomegalovirus	Anti-HCMV IgG seroconversion
Toxoplasmosis	Anti-Toxoplasma IgM
Drug-induced hepatitis	History of ingestion
Syphilis	Anti-treponemal antibodies
Autoimmune hepatitis	Antinuclear antibodies, anti-smooth muscle antibodies, antineutrophil antibodies, histology
Wilson's disease	Serum copper and ceruloplasmin, slit-lamp examination
Hemochromatosis	Serum ferritin
Cholangitis	Abdominal ultrasound or CT scan

tis[209]. Liver biopsy in such patients has not been considered necessary[208]. As the histology shows moderate to severe hepatitis in more than 50% of patients with elevated ALT levels, liver biopsy is indicated in this group of individuals[208]. These guidelines, however, have been challenged recently[210], and a significant number of individuals (almost 20% in Nutt's series[211]) with chronic HCV infection but with normal ALT levels may have advanced histological liver damage[211]. It has therefore been suggested that all patients with HCV RNA in their plasma should be considered for liver biopsy irrespective of their ALT level.

In HIV-infected individuals, antibodies to one or several antigens may be lost, with false negative results in the earlier EIA tests. Indeterminate results for antibody against HCV in HCV viremic patients have also been noted more frequently in samples from HIV-infected than from HIV-non-infected persons: in one study 23% of 167 and 15% of 318 samples respectively[212]. The detection of HCV RNA by PCR should be undertaken if HCV infection is suspected but the serological tests are negative.

Diagnosis of perinatal hepatitis C virus infection

Children born to mothers who are HCV infected should be tested for infection. It is recommended that testing for anti-HCV should not be undertaken until the child is at least 1 year old, by which time maternally acquired antibodies will be undetectable. Alternatively, plasma can be tested for HCV RNA by PCR when the child is 1 to 2 months old[124]. Infected children should be referred to a pediatrician with a special interest in hepatology for further evaluation, and treatment if necessary.

MANAGEMENT OF HEPATITIS C VIRUS INFECTION

Individuals who have confirmed hepatitis C virus infection should be counseled with respect to the prevention of further liver damage, and prevention of transmission of infection (Box 8.3). All patients with chronic HCV infection with detectable HCV RNA should be referred to a hepatologist.

Box 8.3 Information to be given to a HCV-infected individual (after Centers for Disease Control and Prevention 1998[83])

To protect the liver from further harm

avoid alcohol

do not take any medication, including herbal remedies that may harm the liver (consult physician)

be vaccinated against hepatitis A.

To reduce risk of transmission to others

do not donate blood, organs, or semen

do not share toothbrushes, razors, or other personal care items that might be contaminated with blood

cover wounds on the skin

use condoms with a new partner, if in a long-term relationship discuss the small but possible risk of infection with partner and, if that person is uninfected, consider condom use.

TREATMENT OF CHRONIC HEPATITIS C

The aim of therapy is to inhibit viral replication to decrease the activity of the hepatitis, and thereby decrease the risk of subsequent cirrhosis and hepatocellular carcinoma. Although only a proportion of infected individuals eventually develop cirrhosis (see pp. 234–235), it is not usually possible to predict the likelihood of cirrhosis in an individual patient. Box 8.4 indicates the minimal criteria for the treatment of patients with chronic hepatitis C, as proposed (with modifications) by the panel of the 1997 National Institutes of Health Consensus Development Conference on 'Management of Hepatitis C'[213] and the EASL International Consensus Conference on Hepatitis C[208]. Liver biopsy before therapy is recommended, inapparent cirrhosis can be diagnosed and other forms of liver disease can be excluded.

Box 8.4 Minimal criteria for treatment of chronic hepatitis C

Elevations in serum alanine aminotransferase levels for at least 6 months.

Presence of HCV RNA in serum.

Some degree of fibrosis or moderate inflammation on liver biopsy.

Compensated liver disease.

Compliance and acceptance of therapy.

Abstinence from alcohol and illicit drugs.

No contraindication to therapy.

Currently, combination therapy with interferon-α and tribavirin (ribavirin) is the preferred treatment regimen[208]. Interferon-α is usually given by subcutaneous injection, in a dose of 3 million units three times per week, and tribavirin is administered orally in a daily dose of 1.0 to 1.2 g, depending on body weight. Monotherapy with interferon is reserved for those with contraindications to tribavirin. Tribavirin is a synthetic guanosine-like nucleoside analog that has, *in vitro*, a broad spectrum of activity against several viruses, including flaviviruses. In trials of monotherapy for HCV infection, it has resulted in significant decreases in ALT levels, but not in serum HCV RNA. In combination with interferon-α, however, studies have shown higher virological responses (undetectable HCV RNA at least 24 weeks after therapy) and biochemical responses (normal ALT levels at the end of treatment and for at least 24 weeks later) than with interferon monotherapy. Combination therapy for 24 or 48 weeks gave overall sustained virological response rates of 33% and 41% respectively, compared with 6% and 16% with interferon alone[214, 215]. Improvement in liver histology was also more likely in those given combination therapy than in those given monotherapy. As measured at six and 12 months after cessation of treatment, 48 weeks of therapy resulted in a higher sustained virological response rate than 24 weeks of treatment. Virological relapse, that is, HCV RNA becoming detectable again, was noted in 45% of patients given the shorter course of therapy, compared with 20% treated for the longer period[214, 215].

In patients who have a sustained virological response to combination therapy, serum ALT levels and HCV RNA levels fall rapidly and become normal or undetectable within 2 months[216].

Factors predictive of a response to combination therapy include the following.

1. *Genotype*: in the two studies referred to above, patients infected with genotype 1a or 1b were much less likely than those infected with other types to have a sustained response (overall in these studies only 17% of individuals infected with genotype 1a or 1b had a sustained response to 24 weeks of therapy, compared with 62% of those with other infecting genotypes)[216]. In those with HCV genotype 1 infection, continuing therapy for a further 24 weeks was associated with an increased response rate (29%); this effect was not seen in patients infected with other types. The inference is that individuals with type 1 HCV infection should be treated for 48 weeks, whereas those with other infecting types need only be given 24 weeks.

2. *Initial HCV viral load*: in patients infected with HCV genotype 1a or 1b and given treatment for 24 weeks, a sustained virological response has been shown to be less likely in those whose initial plasma viral load was high ($> 2 \times 10^6$ copies/mL)[214, 215]. The response rate amongst individuals infected with these types and given 48 weeks of treatment, however, increased significantly even amongst those with a high viral load. An effect of initial viral load in patients infected with other HCV genotypes was not found, irrespective of duration of treatment.

3. *Other factors*: other predictive factors include young age (less than 45 years), being female, and having lesser degrees of bridging fibrosis[215]. African-Americans appear to be less likely to respond, but the reasons for this observation are speculative[216].

In the management of patients given combination therapy, it is recommended that patients who have detectable HCV RNA after 24 weeks should discontinue treatment. Persistence of HCV RNA at 24 weeks predicts a lack of sustained response in almost every case[214, 215].

In patients who have responded but relapsed, that is, had an undetectable viral load at the end of treatment but with subsequent reappearance of HCV RNA, retreatment with combination therapy for 24 weeks has been shown to produce a sustained response in about 50% of cases[217]. It is recommended, however, that patients infected with HCV genotype 1 who have relapsed should be treated for 48 weeks[216].

The treatment of those who fail to respond to interferon-α or to combination therapy is problematic with few other options[216].

Adverse events with combination therapy with interferon-α and tribavirin

Fatigue, malaise, depression, emotional lability, forgetfulness, and bone marrow suppression with thrombocytopenia and neutropenia are amongst the common side effects of interferon treatment. Dose-related hemolytic anemia, pruritus, nasal congestion, dyspnea, and cough are noted with tribavirin therapy. In general most side effects are mild to moderate and reversible. As tribavirin can cause fetal abnormalities, women and men who cannot use contraception during and for 6 months after therapy should not be treated with this drug.

Contraindications to combination therapy

These include: decompensated liver disease, hemolysis, anemia, bone marrow suppression, active autoimmune disease, alcohol or illicit drug abuse, depression, coronary artery disease, cerebrovascular disease, and renal insufficiency.

TREATMENT OF ACUTE HEPATITIS C

The general measures outlined in the sections on acute hepatitis A and B are the mainstays of management. Although several studies have shown that interferon treatment given to patients with acute hepatitis C appears to reduce the risk of the development of chronicity[215, 218], the long-term outcome of treated individuals is unknown. In the treatment of acute hepatitis C, there are several unresolved issues, such as when to initiate treatment, the dose of interferon, and the duration of therapy[189].

TREATMENT OF HEPATITIS C VIRUS INFECTION IN PATIENTS WITH HIV CO-INFECTION

Studies have shown that treatment of HCV-HIV co-infected individuals with interferon-α for 1 year can produce biochemical and virological responses by the end of treatment that are similar to those seen in HIV-non-infected persons[219]. However, amongst those with HIV infection, the relapse rate within 12 months of stopping therapy is significantly higher than in those without HIV infection. One study has shown that the rate of improvement of histological features is poor among HIV-infected persons[220]. In consideration of the treatment of HCV infection in HIV-seropositive patients, most physicians use HAART to control the latter infection before initiating interferon therapy for HCV. There are few data on the use of combination therapy with tribavirin and interferon in the management of HCV and HIV co-infected patients. There are concerns about the possible toxicity of tribavirin in HIV-infected patients. For example, some individuals have bone marrow suppression, and others have depression. An additional concern is that tribavirin inhibits the intracellular phosphorylation of zidovudine, stavudine, and zalcitabine, and increases the intracellular conversion of didanosine to its active metabolite, thereby possibly increasing its toxicity[221].

PREVENTION

In the case of primary prevention of transmission of HCV by blood, blood products, organs, tissues, and semen, donors should be excluded if they give a history of risk for the virus. All potential donors should be screened by serological tests for anti-HCV, and those found to be positive should be excluded from donating blood, organs, tissues, or semen. Plasma derivatives should undergo procedures to inactivate the virus, but if this is impossible, the products must be screened for HCV RNA by PCR before release[124].

Counseling and education to prevent initiation of injecting drug use is important, but when an individual wishes to inject illicit drugs, several risk-reduction strategies should be explained (Box 8.5). Syringe and needle-exchange programs are effective in reducing the incidence of blood-borne virus infections[222], and methadone substitution programs also help in this regard[223].

Although the risk of sexual transmission of HCV appears to be low, individuals who have multiple partners should be encouraged to use condoms. Hepatitis C virus-infected persons with a long-term sexual partner do not need to change their sexual practices[124]. It is advisable, however, that they should discuss the small risk of HCV transmission with the partner, and the possible use of condoms to reduce the risk even further.

Health-care workers should be properly trained in infection-control measures, including the need to wear gloves when undertaking invasive procedures, to avoid re-sheathing used needles, and to dispose safely of used needles and sharp instruments. Strict attention to detail is particularly important in the setting of a hemodialysis unit. In resource-poor countries, every effort should be made to reduce the risk of transmission of HCV from inadequately sterilized or disinfected medical surgical or dental equipment.

An animal model has shown that the administration of immune globulin after exposure to HCV is not effective in prophylaxis[224]. A chimpanzee was infected with HCV and given hepatitis C immune globulin, containing high titers of anti-E2 antibodies, 1 hour later; hepatitis C virus-infection was detected a few days later. Compared with another two animals, one of whom had been given anti-HCV negative immune globulin, and the other untreated, the administration of anti-HCV positive immune globulin had the effect of prolonging the incubation period of acute hepatitis C. There are no data on the efficacy of interferons alone or in combination with tribavirin in post-exposure prophylaxis.

If a health-care worker sustains percutaneous or mucosal exposure to blood, the source of the blood should be tested if possible. If that person is anti-HCV positive, the worker should be offered testing for anti-HCV 6 months later (a baseline sample would be stored at the time of the incident for retrospective testing if necessary). A positive result should be confirmed by RIBA, and by PCR for HCV RNA. If it is considered important to identify the infection earlier, a test for HCV RNA can be performed four to six weeks after exposure. Confirmation of seroconversion may lead to claims for compensation. The infected health-care worker should be referred to a hepatologist for further management, including, possibly, early treatment with antiviral agents.

Practitioners who undertake tattooing, body piercing, acupuncture, and other ritual practices should be educated to use only sterilized equipment.

Prevention of vertical transmission of HCV by cesarean section is controversial, and is not currently recommended by the Centers for Disease Control and Prevention[124]. There is no evidence that an HCV-infected mother should avoid breast feeding, unless they have cracked or bleeding nipples.

Hepatitis D virus infection

Hepatitis D virus (HDV) is a small subviral agent (36 nm), or satellite, that depends on hepatitis B virus for surface proteins of its envelope[225]. Transmission of HDV requires co-infection with HBV or superinfection in individuals who are HBV carriers. The HDV RNA genome is very small and circular, quite unusual except in subviral particles found in plants, and has been placed in a new floating genus, *Deltavirus*. The spherical particles contain all three forms of HBs antigen on the surface, and internally have the nucleoprotein delta antigen (HDAg), the only known functional protein encoded by the HDV RNA. The virus only infects hepatocytes in life; the mode of entry into the cells is unknown but probably utilizes the same receptor as HBV. Replication of HDV RNA occurs in cell nuclei, by RNA-directed RNA synthesis using a rolling circle mechanism. Hepatitis D antigen is found in two forms (large and small) in both serum and liver from patients. Both forms are essential for replication, the small one for genome replication and the large delta antigen for assembly of HDV nucleoprotein into new enveloped viral particles.

The pathogenesis of HDV infection is not understood.

EPIDEMIOLOGY

Hepatitis D virus is transmitted by blood or blood products and is found amongst injecting drug users who share syringes and needles, and recipients of blood or blood products. It is also transmissible sexually and vertical transmission occurs.

The prevalence of HDV infection amongst chronic carriers of HBV varies geographically. For example, in Asia, 11% of 1651 carriers were seropositive for anti-HDV, but only 4% of 1556 carriers in Eastern Europe[235]. Three patterns of HDV infection can be identified

1. endemic, such as occurs in southern Italy and Greece, where the route of transmission is uncertain
2. epidemic
3. occurrence in high risk groups such as injecting drug users.

Transmission of HDV occurs through homosexual and heterosexual activity. The prevalence of HDV in homosexual men with chronic HBV infection has varied geographically, but in most countries, fewer than 10% are infected[226, 227]. The route of acquisition of HDV is unknown. In Taiwan, Wu et al.[228] found that sexual contact with female prostitutes and the use of non-disposable needles were associated with HDV infection. The prevalence of antibody to HDV amongst HBV carriers with a history of sexual contact with sex-industry workers was 10%, and 59% of prostitutes in that study were seropositive for HDV. Further evidence for the sexual transmission of the virus came from another study from Taiwan. Of 30 men with HDV infection, 27 (90%) had had sexual intercourse with a female prostitute within the preceding 3 months[229]. Hepatitis D virus genomes from HDV-antibody positive spouses of infected individuals have been found to be almost identical, but significantly different from other couples, further supporting the evidence for sexual transmission[230].

CLINICAL FEATURES

The clinical features of acute hepatitis D are indistinguishable from those of hepatitis caused by other agents. The illness, however, tends to be more severe, and more likely to result in fulminant hepatitis[231]. In the majority of individuals, the hepatitis of HDV co-infection* is self-limiting; plasma enzyme

---

* The term co-infection is used when both HDV and HBV are acquired simultaneously. Superinfection refers to HDV infection in an individual who is already chronically infected with HBV.

tests of liver function generally return to normal within 2 to 10 weeks. In less than 10% of patients, the infection becomes chronic and cirrhosis may develop within a relatively short time.

Superinfection of hepatitis B carriers with HDV is more likely to result in persistence of HDV, with the sequelae of chronic hepatitis and cirrhosis. In a study from Taiwan, 20% of 38 patients with HDV superinfection developed cirrhosis during a 4-year follow-up period[228]. Acute HDV superinfection may precipitate hepatic decompensation in those with cirrhosis secondary to chronic HBV infection.

DIAGNOSIS

The detection of antibody against HDV (anti-HDV) by enzyme immunoassay is reliable for the diagnosis of HDV infection. Antibodies become detectable within 1 to 2 months of infection. In HDV *co-infection* in which infection is transient, titers of anti-HDV are low, but total anti-HDV can remain detectable for a long period after the acute illness. Specific IgM antibodies appear transiently in more than 90% of patients with co-infection, and when found together with rising levels of total anti-HDV, confirms the diagnosis. In patients with HDV *superinfection* anti-HDV becomes detectable earlier than in co-infection, and high titers are often found. IgM antibodies may remain detectable into the chronic stage of the infection, and may remain detectable as long as there is viral replication.

Molecular hybridization methods permit the detection of HDV RNA in serum from patients. In acute infection, HDV RNA can be found within the first week of the illness in about two-thirds of cases. Its appearance is transient, but in those who develop chronic HDV hepatitis, the viremia persists[232].

The histology of the acute hepatitis is non-specific, and biopsy is not indicated as a diagnostic test in patients with acute hepatitis. The histological changes in the liver in chronic HDV hepatitis resemble those of chronic hepatitis B, but chronic active hepatitis and cirrhosis is more likely to be found. Immunochemical staining may reveal HDAg in a few cells.

TREATMENT

It is important to recognize HDV super-infection in the chronically infected HBV individual because the response to interferon treatment is less satisfactory and the dose of interferon-α is different. The subcutaneous injection of interferon-α in a dosage of 9 million units given three times per week for 12 months led to remission in about a third of patients[233]. Lower doses are ineffective.

PREVENTION

Immunization against hepatitis B protects against hepatitis D. Those individuals who are already chronic carriers of HBV should be given advice on avoiding superinfection with HDV from blood-contaminated needles or sexual partners.

Hepatitis E virus infection

Hepatitis E virus (HEV) is a small non-enveloped virus (27–32 nm) with the morphology of human caliciviruses. However its single-stranded positive-sense RNA genome seems to be closer to that of members of the superfamily of alpha-viruses, particularly rubella virus. Infection with HEV resembles that of hepatitis A virus in its pattern of transmission and because it can cause a self-limiting hepatitis without long-term sequelae.

The virological aspects of this infection, the clinical features and diagnosis have been reviewed recently [109]. Infection with HEV is endemic in Asia, Africa, the Middle East, and Central America, especially in underdeveloped areas where outbreaks are associated with drinking fecally contaminated water. Recurrent epidemics occur in certain areas while sporadic endemic cases are found in others. In non-endemic areas, HEV accounts for less than 1% of cases of acute viral hepatitis, mostly related to travel to an endemic region. There is an unusually high mortality rate associated with HEV infection, up to 2% in hospitalized patients in general, and 15% to 20% amongst women in the third trimester of pregnancy. Person-to-person transmission of HEV seems to be uncommon, unlike

HAV, and there is no clear evidence that it is sexually transmitted. Serological diagnosis of infection is now available, usually based on an enzyme immunoassay for IgG antibody to hepatitis E virus.

Hepatitis G virus infection

Hepatitis G virus (HGV) of GB virus C (GBV-C) is a member of the flavivirus family that was identified using molecular cloning techniques on the plasma from patients with non-A–E hepatitis[234]. It is a positive, single-stranded RNA virus whose genome contains about 9400 nucleotide sequences. The virus can be detected in serum or plasma by PCR[236] or by the branched DNA (bDNA) technique. Serological assays for antibody against the envelope E_2 protein are also available[237, 238]. Recent studies suggest that HGV is primarily a lymphotropic virus, negative and positive-strand RNA being detected in bone marrow and spleen, but seldom in other tissues[239].

The virus can establish persistent infection: 14 of 16 individuals whose plasma contained HGV RNA were still viremic more than 1 year later[240]. Most of these patients with persistent infection have normal plasma enzyme tests of liver function[241]. In other individuals, the virus is cleared from the serum and antibodies against E_2 become detectable[237]. Although these antibodies may persist for a long period, more than 50% of initially seropositive hemophiliac patients appear to become seronegative after 10 years of follow-up[252].

It appears that the majority of individuals who acquire HGV do not develop acute hepatitis[241], and, although some patients have persistent infection, there is little evidence that this results in chronic liver disease[242]. Recent studies on infection of macaques with HGV have shown that although part of the genome of HGV and antigen are expressed in hepatocytes, only a very mild hepatitis results[243].

The epidemiology of HGV infection is incompletely understood. Amongst blood donors with no known risk of other blood-borne virus infections, the prevalence of HGV RNA in the serum has varied geographically, but in most countries it is about 1% to 2%[244]. In comparison with other blood-borne virus infections, this is a high rate, and may reflect infection during birth, or during childhood or young adulthood. Hepatitis G virus infection appears to be common in children and young adults. For example, Handa et al.[245] detected HGV RNA or E_2 antibody in the blood of 160 American children, and showed that 13.6% had evidence of current or previous infection. Although the source of their infection was unknown, transmission during birth may play a role. HGV can be transmitted from an infected mother to her infant, at a much higher frequency than for HCV (see page 233). In an Italian study[246], the virus was transmitted to 6 of 9 infants born to HGV RNA-positive mothers, the RNA becoming detectable in the babies' serum by the third month of life. HCV was transmitted to the infant in only 9 of 71 anti-HCV positive mothers. The risk of transmission of HGV to an infant seems to depend on the viral RNA load[247], and infants born to infected mothers by cesarean section have a lower incidence of infection[247].

The virus can be transmitted by blood transfusion, but it has been shown that fewer than 50% of recipients of infected blood become HGV viremic[248]. HGV is also a common infection amongst hemophiliacs and patients who have had multiple blood transfusions[249].

A high prevalence of HGV has been noted amongst injecting drug users. In a study from Berlin, Germany[250], about 43 (33%) of 130 injecting drug users were HGV viremic, compared with 2% of blood donors.

In addition to the parenteral transmission of HGV, it is probable that it can be spread by sexual contact. Evidence for sexual transmission of the virus comes from the observation that HGV viremia is more prevalent amongst men who have sex with men, and amongst prostitutes than amongst blood donors[250–252]. For example, amongst homosexual men attending a STI clinic in Edinburgh, Scotland, HGV RNA was detected in the serum of 31% of 87 men, and 23% were seropositive for antibody against E_2[252]. Fiordalisi et al.[253] had shown previously that the seroprevalence of HGV amongst homosexual men was significantly greater amongst those who had had more than 100 lifetime partners compared with those who had fewer partners. From the results of sequential sampling of 22 homosexual men, Scallan et al.[252] estimated that the annual incidence of infection was 11%. Amongst female sex-industry workers, the seroprevalence of HGV is also higher than in the blood donor population: in one study, HGV RNA and anti-E_2 were found in the serum of 9 of 50, and 11 of 41 women respectively[252]. A relationship between the time in prostitution and the likelihood of HGV viremia has also been shown[253]. Further evidence for the sexual transmission of HGV comes from a study of the sexual partners of 161 hemophiliac men, 77 of whom were seropositive for HGV RNA and/or E_2 antibody. Hepatitis G virus infection of these women was significantly more likely if their partner was HGV-infected, rates of infection increasing by two- to threefold[254].

Other individuals at risk of HGV infection include liver transplant recipients[255], and, to a lesser extent than with hepatitis C virus infection, hemodialysis patients[256].

Not surprisingly, HGV infection can co-exist with other blood-borne viruses. For example, HGV RNA is found in the serum of up to 20% of patients with chronic HCV infection[257]. Co-infection with HGV, however, does not appear to affect the likelihood of response to interferon in patients with chronic hepatitis C[257]. HGV is also found commonly in individuals infected with HIV: in a study from France 66% of 80 HIV-seropositive patients were seropositive for HGV RNA and/or E_2 antibody[258]. The influence of HGV co-infection on the natural history of HIV infection is unknown, although a recent study found that, compared with individuals who had no evidence of HGV infection, patients with current or previous HGV infection had higher CD4+ lymphocyte counts and increased AIDS-free survival rates[259].

Treatment of individuals found to be HGV-infected is not necessary.

References

1 Koff RS. Hepatitis A. *Lancet* 1998; **351**: 1643–1649.

2 World Health Organization. *Advances in Viral Hepatitis*. World Health Organization Technical Report Series No 602; Geneva: 1977.

3 Gay NJ, Morgan-Capner P, Wright J, Farrington CP, Miller E. Age-specific antibody prevalence to hepatitis A in England: implications for disease control. *Epidemiol Infect* 1994; **113**: 113–120.

4 McFarlane ES, Embil JA, Manuel FR, Thiebaux HJ. Antibodies to hepatitis A antigen in relation to the number of lifetime sexual partners in patients attending a STD clinic. *Br J Vener Dis* 1981; **57**: 58–61.

5 Corey L, Holmes KK. Sexual transmission of hepatitis A in homosexual men. *N Engl J Med* 1980; **302**: 435–438.

6 Coutinho RA, Albrecht van Lent P, Lelie N, Nagelkerke N, Kuipers H, Rijsdijk T. Prevalence and incidence of hepatitis A among male homosexuals. *Br Med J* 1983; **287**: 1743–1745.

7 Henning KJ, Bell E, Braun J, Barker ND. A community-wide outbreak of hepatitis A: risk factors for infection among homosexual and bisexual men. *Am J Med* 1995; **99**: 132–136.

8 Nandwani R, Caswell S, Boag F, Lawrence AG, Coleman JC. Hepatitis A seroprevalence in homosexual and heterosexual men. *Genitourin Med* 1994; **70**: 325–328.

9 Katz MH, Hsu L, Wong E, Liska S, Anderson L, Janssen RS. Seroprevalence of and risk factors for hepatitis A infection among young homosexual and bisexual men. *J Infect Dis* 1997; **175**: 1225–1229.

10 Walsh B, Sundkvist T, MacGuire H, Young Y, Heathcock R, Iverson A. Rise in hepatitis A among gay men in the Thames regions 1995 and 1996. *Genitourin Med* 1996; **72**: 449–450.

11 Sundkvist T, Aitken C, Duckworth G, Jeffries D. Outbreak of acute hepatitis A among homosexual men in east London. *Scand J Infect Dis* 1997; **29**: 211–212.

12 Szmuness W, Dienstag JL, Purcell RH, Harley EJ, Stevens CE, Wong DC. Distribution of antibody to hepatitis A antigen in urban populations. *N Engl J Med* 1976; **295**: 755–759.

13 Werzberger A, Mensch B, Kuter B, *et al.* A controlled trial of a formalin-inactivated hepatitis A vaccine in healthy children. *N Engl J Med* 1992; **327**: 453–457.

14 Innis BL, Snitbhan R, Kunasol P, *et al.* Protection against hepatitis A by an inactivated vaccine. *JAMA* 1994; **271**: 1328–1334.

15 Ashur Y, Adler R, Rowe M, Shouval D. Comparison of immunogenicity of two hepatitis A vaccines – VAQTA and HAVRIX – in young adults. *Vaccine* 1999; **17**: 2290–2296.

16 Salisbury TM, Begg NT (eds). *Immunisation Against Infectious Diseases*. Edward Jeenner Bicentenary Edition. London; HMSO: 1996.

17 Saab S, Martin P, Yee HF. A simple cost-decision analysis model comparing two strategies for hepatitis A vaccination. *Am J Med* 2000; **109**: 241–243.

18 Neilsen GA, Bodsworth NJ, Watts N. Response to hepatitis A vaccination in human immunodeficiency virus-infected and uninfected homosexual men. *J Infect Dis* 1997; **176**: 1064–1067.

19 Leading Article. Are HCV-infected individuals candidates for hepatitis A vaccine? *Lancet* 1998; **351**: 924–925.

20 Lemon SM, Stapleton JT. Prevention. In: Zuckerman AJ, Thomas HC (eds) *Viral Hepatitis* 2nd edition. London; Churchill Livingstone: 1998.

21 Green MS, Cohen D, Lerman Y, *et al.* Depression of the immune response to an inactivated hepatitis A vaccine administered concomitantly with immune globulin. *J Infect Dis* 1993; **168**: 740–743.

22 Blumberg BS. Polymorphism of serum proteins and the development of isoprecipitins in transfused patients. *Bull N York Acad Med* 1964; **40**: 377–386.

23 Kann M, Gerlich W. Structure and molecular virology. In: Zuckerman AJ, Thomas HC (eds) *Viral Hepatitis*. 2nd edition. London; Churchill Livingstone: 1998.

24 Hsu HY, Chang MH, Ni YH, Lin HH, Wang SM, Chen DS. Surface gene mutants of hepatitis B virus in infants who develop acute or chronic infections despite immunoprophylaxis. *Hepatology* 1997; **26**: 786–791.

25 Carman WF, Zanetti AR, Karayiannis P, *et al.* Vaccine-induced escape mutant of hepatitis B virus. *Lancet* 1990; **336**: 325–329.

26 Lok AS, Akarca U, Greene S. Mutations in the pre-core region of hepatitis B virus serve to enhance the stability of the secondary structure of the pre-genome encapsidation signal. *Proc Natl Acad Sci USA* 1994; **91**: 4077–4081.

27 Kane M. Global programme for control of hepatitis B infection. *Vaccine* 1995; **13** (Suppl. 1): S47–S49.

28 Ellis WR, Murray-Lyon IM, Coleman JC, *et al.* Liver disease among homosexual males. *Lancet* 1979; **i**: 903–905.

29 Beasley RB, Hwang LY, Lin CC, *et al.* Hepatitis B immune globulin (HBIG) efficacy in the interruption of perinatal transmission of hepatitis B virus carrier state. *Lancet* 1981; **ii**: 388–393.

30 Bancroft WH, Snitbhan R, Scott RM, *et al.* Transmission of hepatitis B virus to gibbons by exposure to human saliva containing hepatitis B surface antigen. *J Infect Dis* 1977; **135**: 79–85.

31 Alter HJ, Purcell RH, Gerin JL, *et al.* Transmission of hepatitis B to chimpanzees by hepatitis B surface antigen-positive saliva and semen. *Infect Immun* 1997; **16**: 928–933.

32 Stevens CE, Beasley RP, Tsin J. Vertical transmission of hepatitis B antigen in Taiwan. *N Engl J Med* 1975; **292**: 771–774.

33 Okada K, Kamiyama I, Inomata M, Imai M, Miyakawa Y, Mayumi M. e antigen and anti-e in the serum of asymptomatic carrier mothers and indicators of positive and negative transmission of hepatitis B virus to their infants. *N Engl J Med* 1976; **294**: 746–749.

34 Goudeau A, Yvonnet B, Lesage G, *et al.* Lack of anti-HBcIgM in neonates with HbsAg carrier mothers argues against transplacental transmission of hepatitis B virus infection. *Lancet* 1983; **ii**: 1103–1104.

35 Feret E, Larouze B, Diop B, *et al.* Epidemiology of hepatitis B virus infection in the rural community of Tip, Senegal. *Am J Epidemiol* 1987; **125**: 140–149.

36 Mayans MV, Hall AJ, Inskip HM, *et al.* Risk factors for transmission of hepatitis B virus to Gambian children. *Lancet* 1990; **336**: 1107–1109.

37 Mayans MV, Hall AJ, Inskip HM, *et al.* Do bedbugs transmit hepatitis B? *Lancet* 1994; **343**: 761–763.

38 Jeffries DJ, James WH, Jefferiss FJG, MacLeod KG, Willcox RR. Australia (hepatitis-associated) antigen in patients attending a venereal disease clinic. *Br Med J* 1973; **i**: 455–456.

39 Lacey CJM, Meaden JD, Clarke SKA. Hepatitis B virus infection in homosexual men. *Br J Vener Dis* 1983; **59**: 277–278.

40 Hart GJ, Dawson J, Fitzpatrick RM, *et al.* Risk behaviour, anti-HIV and anti-hepatitis B core prevalence in clinic and non-clinic samples of gay men in England, 1991–1992. *AIDS* 1993; **7**: 863–869.

41 Gilson RJC, de Ruiter A, Waite J, *et al.* Hepatitis B virus infection in patients attending genitourinary medicine clinic: risk factors and vaccine coverage. *Sex Transm Inf* 1998; **74**: 110–115.

42 Seage GR, Mayer KH, Lendrking WR, *et al.* HIV and hepatitis B infection and risk behavior in young gay and bisexual men. *Public Health Rep* 1997; **112**: 158–167.

43 Schreeder MT, Thompson SE, Hadler SC, *et al.* Hepatitis B in homosexual men: prevalence of infection and factors related to transmission. *J Infect Dis* 1982; **146**: 7–15.

44 Reiner NE, Judson FN, Bod WW, Francis DP, Petersen NJ. Asymptomatic rectal mucosal lesions and hepatitis B surface antigen at sites of sexual contact in homosexual men with persistent hepatitis B virus infection. *Ann Int Med* 1984; **96**: 170–173.

45 Hersh T, Melnick JL, Goyal RK, Hollinger FB. Non-parenteral transmission of viral hepatitis type B Australia antigen-associated hepatitis. *N Engl J Med* 1971; **285**: 1363–1364.

46 Heathcote J, Sherlock S. Spread of acute type B hepatitis in London. *Lancet* 1973; **i**: 1468–1470.

47 Szmuness W, Much MI, Prince AM, *et al.* On the role of sexual behavior in the spread of hepatitis B infection. *Ann Int Med* 1975; **83**: 489–495.

48 Papaevangelou G, Trichopoulos D, Kremastinou T, Papoutsahis G. Prevalence of hepatitis B antigen and antibody in prostitutes. *Br Med J* 1984; **ii**: 256–258.

49 De Hoop D, Anker WJ, van Strik R, Masurel N, Stolz E. Hepatitis B antigen and antibody in the blood of prostitutes visiting an outpatient venereology department in Rotterdam. *Br J Vener Dis* 1984; **60**: 319–322.

50 Williams R. Treatment of fulminant hepatitis. In: Zuckerman AJ, Thomas HC (eds) *Viral Hepatitis*. 2nd edition. London; Churchill Livingstone: 1998, pp. 477–488.

51 Sweet RL. Hepatitis B infection in pregnancy. *Obstet Gynecol Rep* 1990; **2**: 128–139.

52 Medhat A, el-Sharkawy MM, Shaaban MM, Makhlouf MM, Ghaneima SE. Acute viral hepatitis in pregnancy. *Int J Gynaecol Obstet* 1993; **40**: 25–31.

53 Eble K, Clemens J, Krenc C, *et al.* Differential diagnosis of acute viral hepatitis using rapid, fully automated immunoassays. *J Med Virol* 1990; **33**: 240–247.

54 Gerlich WH, Luer W, Thomssen R, *et al.* Diagnosis of acute and inapparent hepatitis B virus infections by measurement of IgM antibody to hepatitis B core antigen. *J Infect Dis* 1980; **142**: 95–101.

55 Lemon SM, Gates NL, Simms TE, Bancroft WH. IgM antibody to hepatitis B core antigen as a diagnostic parameter of acute infection with hepatitis B virus. *J Infect Dis* 1981; **143**: 803–809.

56 Nayersina R, Fowler P, Guilhot S, *et al.* HLA A2 restricted cytotoxic T lymphocyte responses to multiple hepatitis B surface antigen epitopes during hepatitis B virus infection. *J Immunol* 1993; **150**: 4659–4671.

57 Penna A, Artini M, Cavalli A, *et al.* Long-lasting memory T cell responses following self-limited acute hepatitis B. *J Clin Invest* 1996; **98**: 1185–1194.

58 De Franchis R, Meucci G, Vecchi M. The natural history of asymptomatic hepatitis B surface antigen carriers. *Ann Int Med* 1993; **118**: 191–194.

59 Perillo RP, Campbell CR, Sanders GE, Regenstein FG, Bodicky CJ. Spontaneous clearance and reactivation of hepatitis B virus infection among male homosexuals with chronic type B hepatitis. *Ann Int Med* 1984; **100**: 43–46.

60 Thomas HC, Thursz MR. Pathogenesis of chronic hepatitis B. In: Zuckerman AJ, Thomas HC (eds) *Viral Hepatitis* 2nd edition. London; Churchill Livingstone: 1998.

61 Ter Borg F, ten Kate FJW, Cuypers HTM, *et al.* Relation between laboratory test results and histological hepatitis activity in individuals positive for hepatitis B surface antigen and antibodies to hepatitis e antigen. *Lancet* 1998; **351**: 1914–1918.

62 Fattovich G, Rugge M, Brollo L, *et al.* Clinical, virologic and histologic outcome following seroconversion from HBeAg to anti-HBe in chronic hepatitis type B. *Hepatology* 1986; **6**: 167–172.

63 De Franchis R, Meucci G, Vecchi M. The natural history of asymptomatic hepatitis B surface antigen carriers. *Ann Int Med* 1993; **118**: 191–194.

64 Liaw Y-F, Tai D-I, Chu C-M, Chen T-J. The development of cirrhosis in patients with chronic type B hepatitis: a prospective study. *Hepatology* 1988; **8**: 493–496.

65 Lee WM. Hepatitis B virus infection. *N Engl J Med* 1997; **337**: 1733–1745.

66 Hadler SC, Judson FN, O'Malley PM, *et al.* Outcome of hepatitis B virus infection in homosexual men and its relation to prior human immunodeficiency virus infection. *J Infect Dis* 1991; **163**: 454–459.

67 Bodsworth NJ, Cooper DA, Donovan B. The influence of human immunodeficiency virus type 1 on the development of the hepatitis B virus carrier state. *J Infect Dis* 1991; **163**: 1138–1140.

68 Goldin RD, Fish DE, Hay A, *et al.* Histological and immunohistochemical study of hepatitis B virus in human immunodeficiency virus infection. *J Clin Pathol* 1990; **40**: 203–205.

69 Levy P, Marcellin P, Martinot PM, *et al.* Clinical course of spontaneous reactivation of hepatitis B virus infection in patients with chronic hepatitis B. *Hepatology* 1990; **12**: 570–574.

70 Wong DK, Cheung AM, O'Rourke K, Naylor CD, Detsky AS, Heatcote J. Effect of alpha-interferon treatment in patients with hepatitis B e antigen-positive chronic hepatitis B. A meta-analysis. *Ann Int Med* 1993; **119**: 312–323.

71 Lau DTY, Everhart J, Kleiner DE, *et al.* Long-term follow-up of patients with chronic hepatitis B treated with interferon alfa. *Gastroenterology* 1997; **113**: 1660–1667.

72 Lok AS, Wu PC, Lai CL, *et al.* A controlled trial of interferon with or without prednisone priming for chronic hepatitis B. *Gastroenterology* 1992; **102**: 2091–2097.

73 Fattovich G, Farci P, Rugge M, *et al.* A randomised control trial of lymphoblastoid interferon-alpha in patients with chronic hepatitis B lacking HBeAg. *Hepatology* 1992; **15**: 584–589.

74 Lai CL, Chien RN, Leung N, *et al.* A one-year trial of lamivudine for chronic hepatitis B. *N Engl J Med* 1998; **339**: 61–68.

75 Lok AS. Hepatitis B infection: pathogenesis and management. *J Hepatol* 2000; **32** (Suppl. 1): 89–97.

76 Wu TC, Tong MJ, Hwang B, Lee SD, Hu MM. Primary hepatocellular carcinoma and hepatitis B infection during childhood. *Hepatology* 1987; **7**: 46–48.

77 Beasley RB, Hwang LY, Lin CC, *et al.* Hepatitis B immune globulin (HBIG) efficacy in the interruption of perinatal transmission of hepatitis B virus carrier state. *Lancet* 1981; **ii**: 388–393.

78 Paterlini P, Gerken G, Nakajima E, *et al.* Polymerase chain reaction to detect hepatitis B virus DNA and RNA sequences in primary liver cancers from patients negative for hepatitis B surface antigen. *N Engl J Med* 1990; **323**: 80–85.

79 Chang MH, Chen CJ, Lai MS, *et al.* Universal hepatitis B vaccination in Taiwan and the incidence of hepatocellular carcinoma in children. *N Engl J Med* 1997; **336**: 1855–1859.

80 Matsubara K, Tokino T. Integration of hepatitis B virus DNA and its implications for hepatocarcinogenesis. *Mol Biol Med* 1990; **7**: 243–260.

81 Brown JL, Carman WF, Thomas HC. The clinical significance of molecular variation within the hepatitis B virus genome. *Hepatology* 1992; **15**: 144–148.

82 Decker RH. Diagnosis of acute and chronic hepatitis B. In: Zuckerman AJ, Thomas HC (eds) *Viral Hepatitis* 2nd edition. London; Churchill Livingstone: 1998.

83 Centers for Disease Control and Prevention. 2002 Guidelines for treatment of sexually transmitted diseases. *MMWR* 2002; **51**: RR-6.

84 Szmuness W, Stenes CE, Harley EJ, *et al.* Hepatitis B vaccine: demonstration of efficacy in a controlled clinical trial in a high-risk population in the United States. *N Engl J Med* 1980; **303**: 833–841.

85 Salisbury TM, Begg NT (eds). *Immunisation Against Infectious Diseases*. Edward Jeenner Bicentenary Edition. London; HMSO: 1996.

86 Szmuness W, Stevens CE, Zang EA, Harley EJ, Kellner A. A controlled clinical trial of the efficacy of the hepatitis B vaccine (Heptavax B): a final report. *Hepatology* 1981; **1**: 377–385.

87 Brown SE, Stanley C, Howard CR, Zuckerman AJ, Stewart MW. Antibody responses to recombinant and plasma derived hepatitis B vaccines. *Br Med J* 1986; **292**: 159–162.

88 Collier AC, Corey L, Murphy VL, Handsfield HH. Antibody to human immunodeficiency virus (HIV) and suboptimal response to hepatitis B vaccination. *Ann Int Med* 1988; **109**: 101–105.

89 Biggar RJ, Goedert JJ, Hoofnagle J. Accelerated loss of antibody to hepatitis B surface antigen among immunodeficient homosexual men infected with HIV. *N Engl J Med* 1987; **316**: 630–631.

90 Winter AP, Follett EA, McIntyre J, Stewart J, Symington IS. Influence of smoking on immunological responses to hepatitis B vaccine. *Vaccine* 1994; **12**: 771–772.

91 Shaw FE, Guess IJA, Roets JM, *et al.* Effect of anatomic site, age and smoking on the immune response to hepatitis B vaccination. *Vaccine* 1989; **7**: 425–430.

92 European Consensus Group on Hepatitis B Immunity. Are booster immunisations needed for lifelong hepatitis B immunity? *Lancet* 2000; **355**: 561–565.

93 Jilg W, Schmidt M, Deinhardt F. Four-year experience with a recombinant hepatitis B vaccine. *Infection* 1989; **17**: 70–76.

94 Boland GJ, de Gast GC, Italiander E, van der Reijden J, van Huttum L. Long-term immunity to hepatitis B infection after vaccination with recombinant hepatitis B vaccine. *Hepatology* 1995; **22**: 325.

95 Wainwright RB, Bulkow LR, Parkinson AJ, Zanis C, McMahon BJ. Protection provided by hepatitis B vaccine in a Yupik Eskimo population: results of a 10-year study. *J Infect Dis* 1997; **175**: 674–677.

96 Clemens R, Sanger R, Kruppenbacher J, *et al.* Booster immunization of low- and non-responders after a standard three dose hepatitis B vaccine schedule – results of a post-marketing surveillance. *Vaccine* 1997; **15**: 349–352.

97 Rey D, Krantz V, Partisani M, *et al.* Increasing the number of hepatitis B vaccine injections augments anti-HBs response rate in HIV-infected patients. Effects on HIV-1 viral load. *Vaccine* 2000; **18**: 1161–1165.

98 Beasley RB, Hwang LY, Lin CC, Chien CS. Hepatocellular carcinoma and hepatitis B virus. A prospective study of 22,707 men in Taiwan. *Lancet* 1981; **ii**: 1129–1133.

99 Maupas P, Chiron JC, Barin F, *et al.* Efficiency of hepatitis B vaccine in prevention of early HBsAg carrier state in children. Controlled trial in an endemic area (Senegal). *Lancet* 1981; **i**: 289–292.

100 Beasley RP, Hwang LY, Lee GC, *et al.* Prevention of perinatally transmitted hepatitis B virus infections with hepatitis B immune globulin and hepatitis B vaccine. *Lancet* 1983; **ii**: 1099–1102.

101 Wong VCW, Ip HMH, Lelie PN, Reerink-Brongers EE, Young CY, Ma HK. Prevention of the HBsAg carrier state in newborn infants of mothers who are chronic carriers of HBsAg and HBeAg by administration of hepatitis B vaccine and hepatitis B immunoglobulin. Double blind randomised placebo-controlled study. *Lancet* 1984; **i**: 921–926.

102 Redeker AG, Mosley JW, Gocke DJ, McKee AP, Pollack W. Hepatitis B immune globulin as a prophylactic measure for spouses exposed to acute type B hepatitis. *N Engl J Med* 1975; **293**: 1055–1059.

103 Craven DE, Awdeh ZL, Kunches LM, Yunis EJ, Dienstag JL, Werner DG. Non-responsiveness to hepatitis B vaccine in healthcare workers. *Ann Int Med* 1986; **105**: 356–360.

104 Zuckerman JN, Sabin C, Craig FM, Williams A, Zuckerman AJ. Immune response to a new hepatitis B vaccine in healthcare workers who had not responded to standard vaccine: randomised double blind dose-response study. *Br Med J* 1997; **314**: 329–333.

105 Lim KS, Taam V, Fulford KWM, Catterall RD, Briggs M, Dane DS, Simpson P. Australia antigen-positive hepatitis as a sexually transmitted disease. In: Catterall RD, Nicol CS (eds) *Sexually Transmitted Diseases*. London; Academic Press: 1976, pp. 197–206.

106 Coleman JC, Evans BA, Thornton A, Zuckerman AJ. Homosexual hepatitis. *J Infect* 1979; **1**: 61–66.

107 Follett EAC, McMillan A. Homosexuals – a true 'high risk' group for hepatitis B infection. *Communicable Diseases in Scotland*. CDS Unit, Glasgow. 1980; **14**: vii–viii.

108 Coutinho RA, Schut BJTh, van-Lent WA, Reorink-Brongers EE, Jesdigk LS. Hepatitis B among homosexual men in the Netherlands. *Sex Transm Dis* 1981; **8**: 333–335.

109 Zuckerman AJ, Thomas HC. Viral hepatitis. 2nd ed. London. Churchill Livingstone. 1998.

110 Choo QL, Kuo G, Ralston R, *et al.* Isolation of a cDNA clone derived from a blood-borne non-A, non-B hepatitis genome. *Science* 1989; **244**: 359–362.

111 Thomson M, Liang TJ. Molecular biology of hepatitis C virus. In: Liang TJ, Hoofnagle JH (eds). *Hepatitis C.* San Diego; Academic Press: 2000, pp. 1–23.

112 Simmonds P. Hepatitis C virus genotypes. In: Liang TJ, Hoofnagle JH (eds) *Hepatitis C.* San Diego; Academic Press: 2000, pp. 53–70.

113 Diepolder HM, Gerlach J-t, Zachoval R, *et al.* Immunodominant CD4+ T-cell epitope within nonstructural protein 3 in acute hepatitis C virus infection. *J Virol* 1997; **71**: 6011–6019.

114 Tsai S-L, Liaw Y-L, Chen M-H, Huang C-Y, Kuo GC. Detection of type 2-like T-helper cells in hepatitis C virus infection: implications for hepatitis C virus chronicity. *Hepatology* 1997; **25**: 449–458.

115 Cooper S, Erickson AL, Adams EJ, *et al.* Analysis of a successful immune response against hepatitis C virus. *Immunity* 1999; **10**: 439–449.

116 Rehermann B. Immunopathogenesis of hepatitis C. In: Liang TJ, Hoofnagle JH (eds) *Hepatitis C.* San Diego; Academic Press: 2000.

117 Shimizu YK, Hijikata M, Iwamoto A, Alter HJ, Purcell RH, Yoshikura H. Neutralizing antibodies against hepatitis C virus and the emergence of neutralization escape mutant viruses. *J Virol* 1994; **68**: 1494–1500.

118 Pawlotsky J-M. Hepatitis C: viral markers and quasispecies. In: Liang TJ, Hoofnagle JH (eds) *Hepatitis C.* San Diego; Academic Press: 2000, pp. 25–52.

119 Ray SC, Wang YM, Laeyendecker O, Ticehurst JR, Villano SA, Thomas DL. Acute hepatitis C virus structural gene sequences as predictors of persistent viremia: hypervariable region 1 as a decoy. *J Virol* 1999; **73**: 2938–2946.

120 Weiner AJ, Geysen HM, Christopherson C, *et al.* Evidence for immune selection of hepatitis C virus (HCV) putative envelope glycoprotein variants: potential role in chronic HCV infections. *Proc Natl Acad Sci USA* 1992; **89**: 3468–3472.

121 Scognamiglio P, Accapezzato D, Casciani A, *et al.* Presence of effector CD8+ T cells in hepatitis C virus-exposed healthy seronegative donors. *J Immunol* 1999; **162**: 6681–6689.

122 World Health Organization. Global surveillance and control of hepatitis C. *J Viral Hepatitis* 1999; **6**: 35–47.

123 Zein NN. Clinical significance of hepatitis C virus genotypes. *Clin Microbiol Rev* 2000; **13**: 223–235.

124 Centers for Disease Control and Prevention. Recommendations for prevention and control of hepatitis C virus (HCV) infection and HCV-related chronic disease. *MMWR* 1998; **47** (No. RR-19): 1–39.

125 Lowe D, Cotton R. Hepatitis C: a review of Australia's response. Canberra: Publications Production Unit, Commonwealth Department of Health and Aged Care, Commonwealth of Australia. 1999.

126 Unlinked Anonymous Surveys Steering Group. *Prevalence of HIV and Hepatitis Infections in the United Kingdom 1999.* London; Department of Health, Public Health Laboratory Service, Institute of

Child Health (London), Scottish Centre for Infection and Environmental Health: 2000.

127 Nakata S, Song P, Duc DD, *et al*. Hepatitis C and B virus infections in populations at low and high risk in Ho Chi Minh and Hanoi, Vietnam. *J Gastroenterol Hepatol* 1994; **9**: 416–419.

128 Van Beek I, Dwyer R, Dore GJ, Luo K, Kaldor JM. Infection with HIV and hepatitis C virus among injecting drug users in a prevention setting: retrospective cohort study. *Br Med J* 1998; **317**: 433–437.

129 Garfein RS, Doherty MC, Monterroso ER, Thomas DL, Nelson KE, Vlahov D. Prevalence and incidence of hepatitis C virus infection among young adult injection drug users. *J Acqu Immun Def Syndrom* 1998; **18** (Suppl. 1): S11–S19.

130 Alter MJ, Kruszon-Moran D, Nainan OV, *et al*. The prevalence of hepatitis C virus infection in the United States. *N Engl J Med* 1999; **341**: 556–562.

131 Alter MJ, Coleman PJ, Alexander WJ, *et al*. Importance of heterosexual activity in the transmission of hepatitis B and non-A, non-B hepatitis. *JAMA* 1989; **262**; 1201–1205.

132 Bresters D, Mauser-Bunschoten EP, Reesink HW, *et al*. Sexual transmission of hepatitis C virus. *Lancet* 1993; **342**: 210–211.

133 Scaraggi FA, Lomuscio S, Perricci A, de Mitrio V, Napoli N, Schiraldi O. Intrafamilial and sexual transmission of hepatitis C virus. *Lancet* 1993; **342**: 1300–1301.

134 Thomas DL, Zenilman JM, Alter HJ, *et al*. Sexual transmission of hepatitis C virus among patients attending sexually transmitted diseases clinics in Baltimore – an analysis of 309 sex partnerships. *J Infect Dis* 1995; **171**: 768–775.

135 Peano GM, Fenoglio LM, Menardi G, Balbo R, Marenchino D, Fenoglio S. Heterosexual transmission of hepatitis C virus in family groups without risk factors. *Br Med J* 1992; **305**: 1473–1474.

136 Mesquita PE, Granato CF, Castelo A. Risk factors associated with hepatitis C virus (HCV) infection among prostitutes and their clients in the city of Santos, Sao Paulo State, Brazil. *J Med Virol* 1997; **51**: 338–343.

137 Leruez-Ville M, Kunstmann JM, De Almeida M, Rouzioux CH, Chaix ML. Detection of hepatitis C virus in the semen of infected men. *Lancet* 2000; **356**: 42–43.

138 Sanchez-Quijano A, Andreu J, Gavilan F, *et al*. Influence of human immuno-deficiency virus type 1 infection on the natural course of chronic parenterally acquired hepatitis C. *Eur J Clin Microbiol Infect Dis* 1995; **14**; 949–953.

139 Eyster ME, Alter HJ, Aledort LM, Quan S, Hatzakis A, Goedert JJ. Heterosexual co-transmission of hepatitis C virus (HCV)

140 Hisada M, O'Brian TR, Rosenberg PS, Goedert JJ. Virus load and risk of heterosexual transmission of human immunodeficiency virus and hepatitis C virus by men with hemophilia. The Multicenter Hemophilia Cohort Study. *J Infect Dis* 2000; **181**: 1475–1478.

141 Tang Z, Yang D, Hao L, Tang Z, Huang Y, Wang S. Detection and significance of HCV RNA in saliva, seminal fluid and vaginal discharge in patients with hepatitis C. *C J Tongji Med Univ* 1996; **16**; 11–13.

142 Buchbinder SP, Katz MH, Hessol NA, Liu J, O'Malley PM, Alter MJ. Hepatitis C virus infection in sexually active homosexual men. *J Infect* 1994; **29**: 263–269.

143 Bodsworth NJ, Cunningham P, Kaldor J, Donovan B. Hepatitis C virus infection in a large cohort of homosexually active men: independent associations with HIV-1 infection and injecting drug use but not sexual behaviour. *Genitourin Med* 1996; **72**: 118–122.

144 Thomas SL, Newell ML, Peckham CS, Ades AE, Hall AJ. A review of hepatitis C virus (HCV) vertical transmission: risks of transmission to infants born to mothers with and without HCV viraemia or human immunodeficiency virus infection. *Int J Epidemiol* 1998; **27**: 108–117.

145 Centers for Disease Control and Prevention. Recommendations for prevention and control of hepatitis C virus (HCV) infection and HCV-related chronic disease. *MMWR* 1998; 47 (No. RR-19): 1–39.

146 Granovsky MO, Minkoff HL, Tess BH, *et al*. Hepatitis C virus infection in the mothers and infants cohort study. *Pediatrics* 1998; **102**: 355–359.

147 Conte D, Fraquella M, Prati D, *et al*. Prevalence and clinical course of chronic hepatitis C virus (HCV) infection and rate of HCV vertical transmission in a cohort of 15,250 pregnant women. *Hepatology* 2000; **31**: 751–755.

148 Quer J, Esteban JI. Epidemiology. In: Zuckerman AJ, Thomas HC (eds) *Viral Hepatitis* 2nd edition. London; Churchill Livingstone: 1998, pp. 271–283.

149 Neal KR, Dornan J, Irving WL. Prevalence of hepatitis C antibodies among healthcare workers of two teaching hospitals. Who is at risk? *Br Med J* 1997; **314**: 179–180.

150 Polish LB, Tong MJ, Co RL, *et al*. Risk factors for hepatitis C virus infection among health care personnel in a community hospital. *Am J Infect Control* 1993; **21**: 196–200.

151 Mitsui T, Iwano K, Masuko K, *et al*. Hepatitis C virus infection in medical personnel after needlestick accident. *Hepatology* 1992; **16**: 1109–1114.

152 Puro V, Petrosillo N, Ippolito G, Italian Study Group on Occupational Risk of HIV

and Other Bloodborne Infections. Risk of hepatitis C seroconversion after occupational exposures in health care workers. *Am J Infect Control* 1995; **23**: 273–277.

153 Ippolito G, Puro V, Perosillo N, *et al*. Simultaneous infection with HIV and hepatitis C virus following occupational conjunctival blood exposure. *JAMA* 1998; **280**: 28.

154 Esteban JI, Gomez J, Martell G, *et al*. Transmission of hepatitis C virus by a cardiac surgeon. *N Engl J Med* 1996; **334**: 555–560.

155 Alter MJ, Hutin YJF, Armstrong GL. Epidemiology of hepatitis C. In: Liang TJ, Hoofnagle JH (eds) *Hepatitis C*. San Diego; Academic Press: 2000, pp. 169–183.

156 Bronowicki JP, Venard V, Botte C, *et al*. Patient-to-patient transmission of hepatitis C virus during colonoscopy. *N Engl J Med* 1997; **337**: 237–240.

157 Kiyosawa K, Tanaka E, Sodeyama T, *et al*. Transmission of hepatitis C in an isolated area in Japan: community-acquired infection. *Gastroenterol* 1994; **106**: 1596–1602.

158 Darwish MA, Raouf TA, Rushdy P, Constantine NT, Rao MR, Edelman R. Risk factors associated with a high seroprevalence of hepatitis C virus infection in Egyptian blood donors. *Am J Trop Med Hyg* 1993; **49**: 440–447.

159 Mohamed MK, Hussein MH, Massoud AA, *et al*. Study of the risk factors for viral hepatits C infection among Egyptians applying for work abroad. *J Egypt Public Health Assoc* 1996; **71**: 113–142.

160 Seeff LB. Natural history of hepatitis C. In: Liang TJ, Hoofnagle JH (eds) *Hepatitis C*. San Diego; Academic Press: 2000, pp. 85–105.

161 Di Bisceglie AM, Goodman ZD, Ishak KG, Hoofnagle JH, Melpolder JJ, Alter HJ. Long-term clinical and histopathological follow-up of chronic post-transfusion hepatitis. *Hepatology* 1991; **14**: 969–974.

162 Koretz RL, Abbey H, Coleman E, Gitnick G. Non-A, non-B post-transfusion hepatitis: looking back in the second decade. *Ann Int Med* 1993; **119**: 110–115.

163 Tremolada F, Casarin C, Alberti A, *et al*. Long-term follow-up of non-A, non-B (type C) post-transfusion hepatitis. *J Hepatol* 1992; **16**: 273–281.

164 Niederau C, Lange S, Heintges T, *et al*. Prognosis of chronic hepatitis C: results of a large, prospective cohort study. *J Hepatol* 1998; **28**: 1687–1695.

165 Fattovich G, Giustina G, Degos F, *et al*. Morbidity and mortality in compensated cirrhosis type C: a retrospective follow-up of 384 patients. *Gastroenterology* 1997; **112**: 463–472.

166 Yano M, Kumada H, Kage M, *et al*. The long-term pathological evolution of

chronic hepatitis C. *Hepatology* 1996; **23**: 1334–1340.

167 Tong MJ, El-Farra NS, Reikes AR, Co RL. Clinical outcomes after transfusion-associated hepatitis C. *N Engl J Med* 1995; **332**: 1463–1466.

168 Gordon S, Bayati N, Silerman AL. Clinical outcome of hepatitis C as a function of mode of transmission. *Hepatology* 1998; **28**: 562–567.

169 Kenny-Walsh E, for the Irish Hepatology Research Group. Clinical outcomes after hepatitis infection from contaminated anti-globulin. *N Engl J Med* 1999; **340**: 1228–1233.

170 Yamakawa Y, Sata M, Suzuki H, Noguchi S, Tanakiwa K. Higher elimination rate of hepatitis C virus among women. *J Viral Hepatitis* 1996; **3**: 317–321.

171 Seeff LB, Buskell-Bales Z, Wright EC, *et al.* Long-term mortality after transfusion-associated non-A, non-B hepatitis. *N Engl J Med* 1992; **327**: 1906–1911.

172 Wright EC, Seeff LB, Hollinger FB, *et al.* Updated long-term mortality of transfusion-associated hepatitis (TAH), non-A, non-B and C. *Hepatology* 1998; **28**: 272A.

173 Seeff LB, Hollinger FB, Alter HJ, Wright EC, Bales ZB, NHLBI Study Group. Long-term morbidity of transfusion-associated hepatitis (TAH) C. *Hepatology* 1998; **28**: 407A.

174 Seeff LB, Miller RN, Rabkin CS, *et al.* Forty-five year follow-up of hepatitis C virus infection among healthy young adults – a retrospective cohort study. *Ann Int Med* 2000; **132**: 105–111.

175 Vogt M, Lang T, Frosner G, *et al.* Prevalence and clinical outcome of hepatitis C infection in children who underwent cardiac surgery before the implementation of blood-donor screening. *N Engl J Med* 1999; **341**: 866–870.

176 Alter MJ, Kruszon-Moran D, Nainan OV, *et al.* The prevalence of hepatitis C virus infection in the United States. *N Engl J Med* 1999; **341**: 556–562.

177 Amoroso P, Rapicetta M, Tosti ME, *et al.* Correlation between virus genotype and chronicity rate in acute hepatitis C. *J Hepatol* 1998; **28**: 939–944.

178 Zein NN. Clinical significance of hepatitis C virus genotypes. *Clin Microbiol Rev* 2000; **13**: 223–235.

179 Nousbaum JB, Pol S, Nalpas B, *et al.* Hepatitis C virus type 1b (II) infection in France and Italy. *Ann Int Med* 1995; **122**: 161–168.

180 Zein NN, Rakela J, Poterucha JJ, Steers JL, Wiesner RH, Persing DH. Hepatitis C genotypes in liver transplant recipients: distribution and 1-year follow-up. *Liver Transplant Surg* 1995; **1**: 354–357.

181 Zein NN, Rakela J, Krawitt EL, *et al.* Hepatitis C virus genotypes in the United States: epidemiology, pathogenicity and response to interferon treatment therapy. *Ann Int Med* 1996; **125**: 634–639.

182 Zein NN, Poterucha JJ, Gross JB, *et al.* Increased risk of hepatocellular carcinoma in patients infected with hepatitis C genotype 1b. *Am J Gastroenterol* 1996; **91**: 2560–1562.

183 Darby SC, Ewart DW, Giangrande PL, *et al.* Mortality from liver cancer in haemophilic men and boys in UK given blood products contaminated with hepatitis C. UK Haemophilia Centre Directors' Organisation. *Lancet* 1997; **350**: 1425–1431.

184 Soto B, Sanchez-Quijano A, Rodrigo L, *et al.* Human immunodeficiency virus infection modifies the natural history of chronic parenterally-acquired hepatitis C with an unusually rapid progression to cirrhosis. *J Hepatol* 1997; **26**: 1–5.

185 Quan CM, Krajden M, Grigoriew GA, Salit IE. Hepatitis C virus infection in patients infected with the human immunodeficiency virus. *Clin Infect Dis* 1993; **17**: 117–119.

186 Wright TL, Hollander H, Pu X, *et al.* Hepatitis C in HIV-infected patients with and without AIDS: prevalence and relationship to patient survival. *Hepatology* 1994; **20**: 1152–1155.

187 Kleiner DE. Pathology of hepatitis C. In: Liang TJ, Hoofnagle JH (eds) *Hepatitis C.* San Diego; Academic Press: 2000, pp. 107–124.

188 Guido M, Rugge M, Fattovich G, *et al.* Human immunodeficiency virus infection and hepatitis C pathology. *Liver* 1994; **14**: 314–319.

189 Hoofnagle JH. Acute hepatitis C. In: Liang TJ, Hoofnagle JH (eds) *Hepatitis C.* San Diego; Academic Press: 2000, pp. 71–83.

190 Lunel F, Musset L, Cacoub P, *et al.* Cryoglobulinemia in chronic liver diseases: the role of hepatitis C virus and liver damage. *Gastroenterology* 1994; **106**: 1291–1300.

191 Agnello V. Mixed cryoglobulinemia and other extrahepatic manifestations of hepatitis C virus infection. In: Liang TJ, Hoofnagle JH (eds) *Hepatitis C.* San Diego; Academic Press: 2000, pp. 295–313.

192 Bonkovsky HL, Poh-Fitzpatrick M, Pimstone N, *et al.* Porphyria cutanea tarda, hepatitis C, and HFE gene mutations in North America in the USA. *Hepatology* 1998; **27**: 1661–1669.

193 Haber MM, West AB, Haber AD, Reuben A. Relationship of aminotransferases to liver histological status in chronic hepatitis C. *Ann Gastroenterol* 1995; **90**: 1250–1257.

194 Vrielink H, Zaaijer HL, Reesink HW, van der Poel CL, Cuypers HT, Lelie PN. Sensitivity and specificity of three third-generation anti-hepatitis C virus ELISAs. *Vox Sanguis* 1995; **69**: 14–17.

195 Lavanchy D, Steinmann J, Moritz A, Frei PC. Evaluation of a new automated third-generation anti-HCV enzyme immunoassay. *J Clin Lab* 1996; **10**: 269–276.

196 Ragni MV, N'Dimbie OK, Rice EO, Bontempo FA, Nedjar S. The presence of hepatitis C virus (HCV) antibody in human immunodeficiency virus-positive hemophilic men undergoing HCV 'seroreversion'. *Blood* 1993; **82**: 1010–1015.

197 Quaranta JF, Delaney SR, Alleman S, Cassuto JP, Dellamonica P, Allain JP. Prevalence of antibody to hepatitis C virus (HCV) in HIV-1-infected patients (Nice SEROCO Cohort). *J Med Virol* 1994; **42**: 29–32.

198 De Medina M, Hill M, Sullivan HO, *et al.* Detection of anti-hepatitis C virus antibodies in patients undergoing dialysis by utilizing a hepatitis C virus 3.0 assay: correlation with hepatitis C virus RNA. *J Lab Clin Med* 1998; **132**: 73–75.

199 Sayers MH, Gretch DR. Recombinant immunoblot and polymerase chain reaction testing in volunteer whole blood donors screened by a multi-antigen assay for hepatitis C virus antibodies. *Transfusion* 1993; **33**: 809–813.

200 Zein NN, Germer JJ, Wendt NK, *et al.* Indeterminate results of the second-generation hepatitis C virus (HCV) recombinant immunoblot assay: significance of high-level c22–3 reactivity and influence of HCV genotypes. *J Clin Microbiol* 1997; **35**: 311–312.

201 Lee JH, Roth WK, Zeuzem S. Evaluation and comparison of different hepatitis C virus genotyping and serotyping assays. *J Hepatol* 1997; **26**: 1001–1009.

202 N'guyen T, Sedghi-Vaziri A, Wilkes L, *et al.* Fluctuations in viral load (HCV RN) are relatively insignificant in untreated patients with chronic HCV infection. *J Viral Hepatitis* 1996; **3**: 75–78.

203 Damen M, Cuypers HT, Zaaijer HL, *et al.* International collaborative study on the second EUROHEP HCV-RNA reference panel. *J Virol Methods* 1996; **58**: 175–185.

204 Gretch D. Diagnostic tests for hepatitis C. *Hepatology* 1997; **26** (Suppl. 1): 43S–47S.

205 Sheen IS, Liaw TF, Lin DY, Chu CM. Acute exacerbations in chronic hepatitis C: a clinico-pathological and prognostic study. *J Hepatol* 1996; **24**: 525–531.

206 Fournillier-Jacob A, Lunel F, Cahour A, *et al.* Antibody responses to hepatitis C envelope proteins in patients with acute or chronic hepatitis C. *J Med Virol* 1996; **50**: 159–167.

207 Quiroga JA, Campillo M, Castillo I, Bartolome J, Porres JC, Carreno V. IgM antibody to hepatitis C virus in acute and chronic hepatitis C. *Hepatology* 1991; **14**: 38–43.

208 EASL International Consensus Conference on Hepatitis C. Consensus Statement. *J Hepatol* 1999; **30**: 956–961.

209 Marcellin P. Hepatitis C: clinical spectrum of the disease. *J Hepatol* 1999; **31** (Suppl. 1): 9–16.

210 Hirsch KR, Wright TL. The dilemma of disease progression in hepatitis C patients with normal aminotransferase levels. *Am J Med* 2000; **109**: 66–67.

211 Nutt AK, Hassan HA, Lindsey J, Lamps L, Raufman J-P. Liver biopsy in the evaluation of patients with chronic hepatitis C who have repeatedly normal or near-normal serum alanine aminotransferase levels. *Am J Med* 2000; **109**: 62–64.

212 Marcellin P, Martinot-Peignoux M, Elias A, *et al.* Hepatitis C virus (HCV) viraemia in human immunodeficiency virus-seronegative and -seropositive patients with indeterminate recombinant immunoblot assay. *J Infect Dis* 1994; **170**: 433–435.

213 National Institutes of Health Consensus Development Conference Panel. Statement: management of hepatitis C. *Hepatology* 1997; **26** (Suppl. 1): 2S–10S.

214 McHutchison JG, Gordon SC, Schiff ER, *et al.* Interferon alfa-2b alone or in combination with ribavirin as initial treatment for chronic hepatitis C. *N Engl J Med* 1998; **339**: 1485–1492.

215 Poynard T, Leroy V, Cohard M, Thevenot T, Mathurin P, Opolon P. Meta-analysis of interferon randomized trials in the treatment of viral hepatitis C: effects of dose and duration. *Hepatology* 1996; **24**: 778–189.

216 McHutchison JG, Hoofnagle JH. Therapy of chronic hepatitis C. In: Liang TJ, Hoofnagle JH (eds) *Hepatitis C*. San Diego; Academic Press: 2000, pp. 203–239.

217 Davis GL, Esteba-Mur R, Rustgi V, *et al.* Interferon alpha-2b alone or in combination with ribavirin for the treatment of relapse of chronic hepatitis C. *N Engl J Med* 1998; **339**: 1493–1499.

218 Vogel W. Treatment of acute hepatitis C virus infection. *J Hepatol* 1999; **31** (Suppl. 1): 189–192.

219 Soriano V, Garcia-Samaniego J, Bravo R, *et al.* Interferon alpha for the treatment of chronic hepatitis C in patients infected with human immunodeficiency virus. Hepatitis-HIV Spanish Study Group. *Clin Infect Dis* 1996; **223**: 585–591.

220 Boldorini R, Vigano P, Monga G, *et al.* Hepatic histology of patients with HIV infection and chronic hepatitis C treated with interferon. *J Clin Pathol* 1997; **50**: 735–740.

221 Sulkowski MS, Mast EE, Seeff LB, Thomas DL. Hepatitis C virus infection as an opportunistic disease in persons infected with human immunodeficiency virus. *Clin Infect Dis* 2000; **30**: S77–S84.

222 Hagan H, Des Jarlais DC, Friedman SR, Purchaase D, Alter MJ. Reduced risk of hepatitis B and hepatitis C among injection drug users in the Tacoma syringe exchange program. *Am J Public Health* 1995; **85**: 1531–1537.

223 Broers B, Junet C, Bourquin M, Deglon JJ, Perrin L, Hirshel B. Prevalence and incidence rate of HIV, hepatitis B and C among drug users on methadone maintenance treatment in Geneva between 1988 and 1995. *AIDS* 1998; **12**: 2059–2066.

224 Krawczynski K, Alter MJ, Tankersley DL, *et al.* Effect of immune globulin on the prevention of experimental hepatitis C virus transmission. *J Infect Dis* 1996; **173**: 822–828.

225 Monjardino J, Lai MMC. Structure and molecular virology. In: Zuckerman AJ, Thomas HC (eds) *Viral Hepatitis* 2nd edition. London; Churchill Livingstone: 1998.

226 Bodsworth NJ, Donovan B, Gold J, Cossart YE. Hepatitis delta virus in homosexual men in Sydney. *Genitourin Med* 1989; **65**: 235–238.

227 Weisfuse JB, Hadler SC, Field HA, *et al.* Delta hepatitis in homosexual men in the United States. *Hepatology* 1989; **9**: 872–874.

228 Wu JC, Lee SD, Govindarajan S, *et al.* Sexual transmission of hepatitis D virus infection in Taiwan. *Hepatology* 1990; **11**: 1057–1061.

229 Liaw YF, Chiu KW, Chu CM, Sheen IS, Huang MJ. Heterosexual transmission of hepatitis delta virus in the general population of an area endemic for hepatitis B virus infection: a prospective study. *I Infect Dis* 1990; **162**: 1170–1172.

230 Wu JC, Chen CM, Sheen IJ, Lee SD, Tzeng HM, Choo KB. Evidence of transmission of hepatitis D virus to spouses from sequence analysis of the viral genome. *Hepatology* 1995; **22**: 1656–1660.

231 Smedile A, Verne G, Cargnel A, *et al.* Influence of delta infection on severity of hepatitis B. *Lancet* 1982; **ii**: 945–947.

232 Buti M, Esteban R, Roggendorf M, *et al.* Hepatitis D virus RNA in acute delta infection: serological profile and correlation with other markers of hepatitis D virus infection. *Hepatology* 1988; **8**: 1125–1129.

233 Farci P, Mandas A, Coiana A, *et al.* Treatment of chronic hepatitis D with interferon alpha-2a. *N Engl J Med* 1994; **330**: 88–94.

234 Kim JP, Fry KE. Structure and molecular virology of HGV (GBV-C). In: Zuckerman AJ, Thomas HC (eds) *Viral Hepatitis* 2nd edition. London; Churchill Livingstone: 1998.

235 Di Bisceglie AM. Epidemiology and diagnosis. In: Zuckerman AJ, Thomas HC (eds) *Viral Hepatitis* 2nd edition. London; Churchill Livingstone: 1998.

236 Schlueter V, Schmolke S, Stark K, *et al.* Reverse transcription-PCR detection of hepatitis G virus. *J Clin Microbiol* 1996; **34**: 2660–2664.

237 Pilot-Matias TJ, Carrick RJ, Coleman PF, *et al.* Expression of the GB virus E_2 glycoprotein using the Semliki Forest Virus Vector System and its utility as a serologic marker. *Virology* 1996; **225**: 282–292.

238 Tacke M, Schlueter V, Ofenloch-Haehnle B, *et al.* Detection of antibodies to a putative hepatitis G virus envelope protein. *Lancet* 1997; **149**: 318–320.

239 Tucker TJ, Smuts HE, Eedes C, *et al.* Evidence that the GBV-C/hepatitis G virus is primarily a lymphotropic virus. *J Med Virol* 2000; **61**: 52–58.

240 Dawson GJ, Schlauder GG, Pilot-Matias TJ, *et al.* Prevalence studies of GB virus-C infection using reverse transcriptase-polymerase chain reaction. *J Med Virol* 1996; **50**: 97–103.

241 Alter MJ, Gallacher M, Morris TT, *et al.* Acute non-A–E hepatitis in the United States and the role of hepatitis G virus infection. *N Engl J Med* 1997; **336**: 741–746.

242 Alter HJ, Nakatsuji Y, Melpolder J, *et al.* The incidence of transfusion-associated hepatitis G virus infection and its relation to liver disease. *N Engl J Med* 1997; **336**: 747–754.

243 Cheng Y, Zhang W, Li J, *et al.* Serological and histological findings in infection and transmission of GBV-C/HGV to macaques. *J Med Virol* 2000; **60**: 28–33.

244 Hadziyannis S, Hess G. Epidemiology and natural history of HGV (GBV-C). In: Zuckerman AJ, Thomas HC (eds) *Viral Hepatitis* 2nd edition. London; Churchill Livingstone: 1998.

245 Handa A, Jubran RF, Dickstein B, *et al.* GB virus C/hepatitis G virus infection is frequent in American children and young adults. *Clin Infect Dis* 2000; **30**: 569–571.

246 Hess G, Papakonstantinou A, Fry K, *et al.* Coinfection of the hepatitis G and C viruses. In: Rizzetto M, Purcell RH, Gerin JL, Verma G (eds) *Viral Hepatitis and Liver Disease*. Turin; Edizioni Minerva Medica: 1997.

247 Ohto H, Ujiie N, Sato A, Okamoto H, Mayumi M. Mother-to-infant transmission of GB virus type C/HGV. *Transfusion* 2000; **40**: 725–730.

248 Roth WK, Waschk D, Marx S, *et al.* Prevalence of hepatitis G virus and its strain variant, the GB agent, in blood donations and their transmission to recipients. *Transfusion* 1997; **37**: 651–656.

249 Hadziyannis SJ, Dawson GJ, Vrettou E, *et al.* Infection with the novel GB-C virus in multiply transfused patients and in various forms of liver disease. *J Hepatol* 1995; **23** (Suppl. 1): 218A.

250 Stark K, Bienzle U, Hess G, Engel AM, Hegenscheid B, Schluter V. Detection of the hepatitis G virus genome among injecting drug users, homosexual and bisexual men, and blood donors. *J Infect Dis* 1996; **174**: 1320–1323.

251 KaoJH, Chen W, Chen PJ, Lai MY, Lin RY, Chen DS. GB virus C/hepatitis G virus infection in prostitutes: possible role of sexual transmission. *J Med Virol* 1997; **52**: 381–384.

252 Scallan MF, Clutterbuck D, Jarvis LM, Scott GR, Simmonds P. Sexual transmission of GB virus C/hepatitis G virus. *J Med Virol* 1998; **55**: 203–208.

253 Fiordalisi G, Bettinardi A, Zanella I, *et al.* Parenteral and sexual transmission of GB virus C and hepatitis C virus among human immunodeficiency virus-positive patients. *J Infect Dis* 1997; **175**: 1025–1026.

254 Yeo AET, Matsumoto A, Shih JW, Alter HJ, Goedert JJ. Prevalence of hepatitis G virus in patients with hemophilia and their steady female sexual partners. *Sex Transm Dis* 2000; **27**: 178–182.

255 Berenguer M, Terrault NA, Piatak M, *et al.* Hepatitis G virus (HGV) in hepatitis C virus (HCV) infection following liver transplantation (OLTx). *Hepatology* 1995; **22**: 151A.

256 Masuko K, Mitsui T, Iwano K, *et al.* Infection with hepatitis GB virus C in patients on maintenance hemodialysis. *N Engl J Med* 1996; **334**: 1485–1490.

257 Brandhagen DJ, Gross JB, Poterucha JJ, *et al.* The clinical significance of simultaneous infection with hepatitis G virus in patients with chronic hepatitis C. *Am J Gastroenterol* 1999; **94**: 1000–1005.

258 Bourlet T, Guglielminotti C, Evrard M, *et al.* Prevalence of HGV-C/hepatitis G virus RNA and E2 antibody among subjects with human immunodeficiency virus type 1 after parenteral or sexual exposure. *J Med Virol* 1999; **58**: 373–377.

259 Yeo AE, Matsumoto A, Hisada M, Shih JW, Alter HJ, Goedert JJ. Effect of hepatitis G virus infection on progression of HIV infection in patients with hemophilia. Multicenter Hemophilia Cohort Study. *Ann Int Med* 2000; **132**: 959–963.

260 McMillan A, Scott GR. *Sexually Transmitted Infections, Colour Guide*. Churchill Livingstone; Edinburgh: 2000.

261 Robertson DHH, McMillan A, Young H. *Clinical Practice in Sexually Transmissible Diseases* 2nd edition. Edinburgh; Churchill Livingstone: 1989.

Chapter 9

Other sexually transmissible viruses
A McMillan, M M Ogilvie

Molluscum contagiosum

The lesions of molluscum contagiosum, caused by a poxvirus, are benign tumors that affect the skin and, rarely, conjunctivae and mucosal surfaces, these tumors are self-limiting in the immunocompetent individual. The virus does not become latent, but it escapes the immune system through the action of various viral specific proteins that inhibit immune defenses and increase resistance of infected host cells to cell death.

ETIOLOGY

The virus of molluscum contagiosum (MCV) (Figure 9.1), although easily obtained in abundance from skin lesions, cannot be grown in culture outside the human host. From its size (300 × 200 × 100 nm), shape, fine structure, cytoplasmic site of replication, and characteristic inclusion body, the virus is classed as a member of the poxvirus family in a genus of its own: *Molluscipoxvirus*[1]. In contrast to other DNA viruses, poxviruses lack icosohedral symmetry and have a complex structure. The genome is a single linear molecule of double-stranded DNA and the virion contains a virus-specified DNA-dependent RNA polymerase[2]. The virus replicates entirely within the cytoplasm of the keratinocytes and the virion colony is isolated in a protective sac that, until recently, has been thought to prevent triggering of the host immune response (page 252). Although molluscum contagiosum virus cannot be propagated in cell culture, DNA can be extracted from single lesions in sufficient quantities for molecular analysis. Using restriction enzyme analysis and DNA-DNA hybridization patterns, the

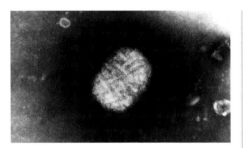

Figure 9.1 Electron micrograph of a molluscum contagiosum virus (× 200 000)

virus can be classified into three major subtypes: MCV I, MCV II, and the rarely identified MCV III[3, 4]. Minor variants, for example of MCV I (MCV Iv), have been described. There is no clear relationship between viral type and anatomical site, and lesions from different sites on the same patient are associated with the same MCV type[5]. It has also been shown that lesions on the same individual that appear at different times, are associated with the same viral type[5].

The receptor molecule for entry of MCV into host cells has not been identified. The rarity of molluscum contagiosum lesions on the mucous membranes* and their absence from the palms and soles, however, suggest that hair follicles may be the site of such receptor molecules. This hypothesis is supported by the finding that the bulk of the molluscum bodies are within the epithelium of the follicular infundibulum[6].

PATHOLOGY

The lesion consists of a localized mass of hypertrophied and hyperplastic epidermis

---

* It has been proposed that mucosal lesions develop only on aberrantly located follicular units[6].

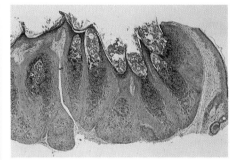

Figure 9.2 Histological section of a molluscum contagiosum lesion (hematoxylin and eosin, × 40) (reproduced from Rein 1996[115])

extending into the underlying dermis, without breaching the limiting basement membrane and projecting above the surface as a papule (Figure 9.2). Beginning in the lower cells of the stratum spinosum, the intracytoplasmic inclusion bodies (Henderson-Paterson or molluscum bodies), growing larger as the infected cells migrate through the stratum granulosum, ultimately enlarge the host cells, pushing aside their nuclei and assuming dimensions varying between 24–27 mm in width and 30–37 mm in length. The core of the lesion consists of degenerating epidermal cells with inclusion bodies and keratin.

PATHOGENESIS

As the infection cannot be transmitted to laboratory animals and an *in vitro* system for MCV replication is not available, much of the pathogenesis of the infection is unknown. However, something of the means by which the immune system is evaded can be deduced from a consideration of the function of the proteins of vaccinia and variola viruses that have been characterized.

The lesions of stable molluscum contagiosum contain few immunocompetent cells

- Langerhans cells are absent within the lesion but present in normal or increased numbers in the perilesional skin[7]
- natural killer (NK) cells are absent in the lesion[7]
- T lymphocytes are absent in the molluscum but are usually present in small numbers in the surrounding dermis[8]

In addition, molluscum bodies lack β_2-microglobulin reactivity[9], indicating lack of expression of HLA class I antigens on the cell surfaces.

DNA sequencing of the MCV genome has shown that about two-thirds of the predicted proteins encoded by the MCV DNA are homologous with proteins of variola and vaccinia viruses many of which have been characterized functionally. The predicted function of some of the specific genes of the molluscum contagiosum virus may explain the ability of the virus to evade an immune response without the development of latency[6].

- One gene codes for a homolog of the major histocompatibility complex (MHC) class I heavy chain that lacks the conserved amino acids important in peptide binding, and therefore cannot present peptides on the infected cell's surface.
- The viral MHC peptide gene product can compete with host MHC proteins for assembly, transport and function, thereby interfering with the presentation of molluscum contagiosum specific peptides.
- The homolog of MHC I interferes with cytotoxic T-cell killing of molluscum contagiosum virus infected cells.
- The genome of MCV encodes a CC chemokine homolog to macrophage inflammatory protein (MIP)-Ib. This homolog lacks the NH_2-terminal region, and, although binding the receptor, has no activity and therefore inhibits inflammation.
- A glutathione peroxidase is encoded by the MCV genome, thereby protecting cells from oxidative damage by peroxides that can lead to apoptosis.
- In the poxviruses, there are 13 caspases (cytoplasmic endoproteinases that

mediate the effector phase of apoptosis) which differ in their substrate specificities and MCV encodes a caspase 8 inhibitor. This decreases apoptosis secondary to FAS-FAS-Ligand and TNF-α-TNF-receptor I binding at the cell surface.

In lesions that are undergoing spontaneous regression or that have been traumatized, there is a dense lymphocytic infiltrate in the surrounding epidermis, but a more limited inflammatory response in the dermis[10,11]. Although it is often considered that epidermal injury releases viral antigen thereby initiating an immune response, the mechanism of this response remains unknown.

EPIDEMIOLOGY

Studies on the epidemiology of molluscum contagiosum virus have been hampered by the inability to culture the virus, and, until recently, the lack of suitable serological tests. Published work has principally relied on the results of clinical examination for the characteristic lesions, and, as a result, knowledge of the epidemiology of the virus is incomplete. There have been several small studies on the molecular epidemiology of molluscum contagiosum virus (see page 253).

The virus is worldwide in its distribution, and the disease can be sporadic or endemic, particularly in conditions of poor hygiene and overcrowding. There are two peaks in the incidence of molluscum contagiosum, one in childhood and the other in early adulthood (Figure 9.3). A recent seroepidemiological study from Sydney, Australia, showed that the prevalence of IgG antibody against MCV was strongly age related: 3% of 37 children aged 6 to 24 months and 39% of 44 adults aged 50 years or over were seropositive[12]. Although molluscum contagiosum is found more commonly in males than in females aged 3 years and over (Figure 9.3), there appears to be no significant difference in the prevalence of specific antibody between the sexes. As the overall seroprevalence of infection (23% of 357 individuals) in the Sydney study was much higher than would have been expected from estimates based on the number of clinically apparent infections, it is likely that subclinical or minor infections are more common than previously considered.

In children, molluscum contagiosum principally affects the face, trunk, and limbs, and is usually spread by direct contact with the skin of an infected individual and, much less commonly, from

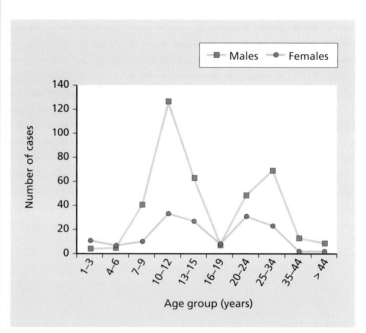

Figure 9.3 Age distribution of clinical cases of molluscum contagiosum in Scotland (data from Postlethwaite *et al.* 1967[14] and Information and Statistics Division, Scottish Health Service)

fomites[13]. The incidence and prevalence of infection amongst children in tropical countries is higher than in temperate climates. The peak incidence in the former countries tends to be at a younger age than in the latter. For example, in Fiji the peak incidence is between 2 and 3 years, but in Scotland it is between 10 and 12 years[14], the difference probably reflecting the difference in clothing between the two countries and the warm moist environment in Fiji that facilitates spread. Mechanical trauma may facilitate transmission of the virus. In temperate climates it has been associated with outbreaks amongst children using communal facilities such as swimming pools where the virus may have been transmitted by towels[14]. Transmission of MCV to siblings within families is common in the tropics.

Sometimes molluscum contagiosum may appear in endemic form. In 1977 it occurred in this way mainly among the young children of the Massai pastoralists of the Rift Valley (70 km west of Nairobi) at a time after famine when the relief diet was different from the normal milk diet. This endemic, it was suggested, was an example of a suppressed infection in patients being fed after a period of moderate famine. The molluscum attained an unusually large size (12 mm)[15].

Among adults, the infection is usually acquired during sexual contact. The evidence for sexual transmission of the virus is as follows

- the peak age incidence parallels that of other STIs such as chlamydia (Figure 9.4)
- lesions in adults are most commonly found in the genital area and on the thighs[16]
- lesions have been reported in sexual partners[16]
- genital molluscum contagiosum infection is often associated with concurrent STIs, over 30% of male and female patients with molluscum contagiosum, who attended a STI clinic in London had at least one concurrent STI[17].

Over the past three decades there has been an increase in the number of cases of molluscum contagiosum reported from STI clinics in England (Figure 9.5) and from

STI clinics and private practices in the USA[18]. The prevalence of infection in men attending English STI clinics is twice that in women.

Non-sexual transmission of infection has been associated with tattooing and wrestling[19, 20].

Small studies on the molecular epidemiology of MCV have been conducted in Europe, Australia, and Japan and have shown that MCV I is the predominant infecting type in children with only a small proportion of cases being associated with MCV II, the ratio of MCV I to MCV II being up to 56:1[21–23]. By contrast, a significantly higher proportion of adult infections are caused by MCV II, than MCV I[22]. Yamashita *et al.*[23], however, noted that 44% of lesions in men were associated with MCV II but only 8% of lesions in women. The viral types found in lesions in women whose children had molluscum contagiosum caused by MCV I were also MCV I, and it has been postulated that mothers and their offspring are infected from each other by casual contact mainly at home[23]. Molluscum contagiosum virus III is found much less commonly than the other types (1.1% of 261 patients[24]), and MCV Iv is mostly found in Japan[3]

Molluscum contagiosum infection that may be extensive and recalcitrant to conventional therapy has been described in a

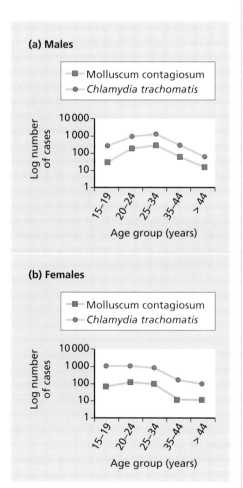

Figure 9.4 Number of cases of molluscum contagiosum and *Chlamydia trachomatis* infection in Scotland during 1996–1998 inclusive (data from Information and Statistics Division, Scotland)

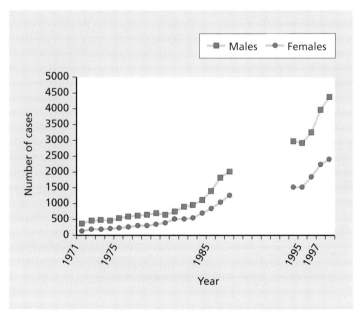

Figure 9.5 Number of new cases of molluscum contagiosum reported from STI clinics in England 1971–1997 (Public Health Laboratory Service)

variety of immunodeficiency conditions (see below), including HIV infection in which up to 20% of HIV-infected individuals with severe immunodeficiency may be affected[25]. Molluscum contagiosum virus II is more commonly associated with the lesions of molluscum contagiosum from HIV-seropositive individuals than MCV I. In a study from an STI clinic in Sydney, Australia, MCV II was the infecting type in 17 (59%) of 29 HIV-infected patients and in only 15 (31%) of 48 HIV-seronegative individuals[26]. This finding suggests that mollusca in HIV-infected persons are likely to have been acquired in adulthood. The same workers also showed that there was no correlation between either the viral type and stage of HIV infection or anatomical site of the lesions.

CLINICAL FEATURES

In the immunocompetent patient

Experimental studies involving the inoculation of volunteers with the virus have shown that the pre-patent period of molluscum contagiosum varies between 2 weeks and 6 months, with an average interval of 2 to 7 weeks after inoculation[20, 27]. In children lesions appear in a generalized distribution, or they may be localized to the face, forearms, or hands. The lesions are pearly, flesh-colored, raised, firm, umbilicated skin nodules, and usually about 2 to 5 mm in diameter (Figure 9.6). They may appear in most skin areas, singly or in groups, except for the palms and soles, where they are exceedingly rare. From the central pit, a white curdy material can be expressed. If the lesion is opened with a sterile needle the central core may not be easily detached. The core was described at the turn of the 18th century in Edward Jenner's notebook as a 'white body … equal in solidity but not so opaque as the boild crystalline humour of a fishes eye'[28]. Molluscum contagiosum can spread by autoinoculation, particularly in atopic patients, and may produce linear lesions (Koebner phenomenon).

Where transmission by sexual intercourse is the likely method of spread, lesions are seen on the inner aspect of the thigh and vulva in the case of the female (Figure 9.7), and on the penis (Figure 9.8), anterior aspect of the scrotum, and pubic area in the male. Spontaneous regression of molluscum contagiosum lesions usually occurs within 2 to 3 months often following trauma or bacterial infection, but new lesions may appear from autoinoculation so that the mean duration of the condition is 8 months[29,11]. The most common complications of molluscum contagiosum are inflammation and secondary infection. Inflammation of the lesions is common (just under 20% of cases)[10], and may precede spontaneous regression by about 7 days[11]. An itchy eczematous dermatitis surrounding the mollusca occurs in up to 10% of patients (molluscum dermatitis)[30]. Scarring may be found at the site of lesions that have undergone spontaneous regression, especially if they had been secondarily infected.

Molluscum contagiosum may develop during the second half of pregnancy, and lesions may be extensive. Spontaneous resolution after delivery is usual.

In the immunocompromised patient

In the immunocompromised patient molluscum contagiosum can be a distressing condition. Table 9.1 shows the immunosuppressive conditions that have been associated with extensive or aggressive disease. In addition, profuse lesions of molluscum contagiosum have been described in atopic individuals[31, 32], perhaps as a result of a pattern of immune dysregulation in the skin of atopic individuals that is

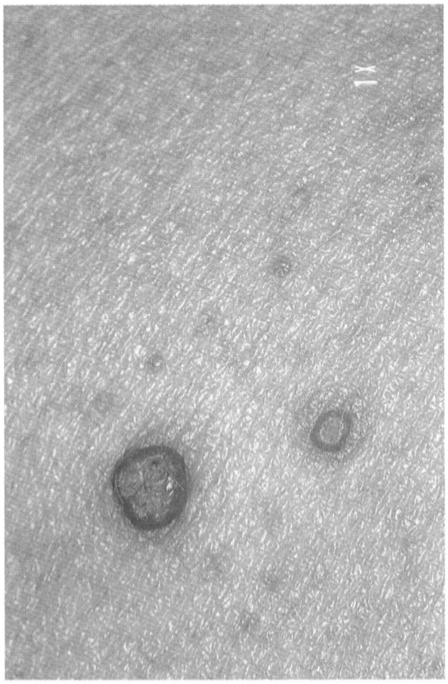

Figure 9.6 Molluscum contagiosum lesions

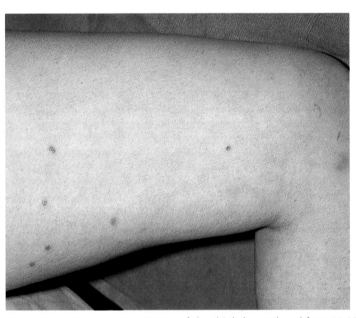

Figure 9.7 Molluscum contagiosum of the thigh (reproduced from McMillan and Scott 2000[166])

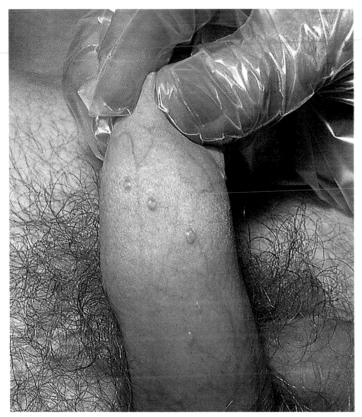

Figure 9.8 Molluscum contagiosum of the penis (reproduced from McMillan and Scott 2000[166])

Table 9.1 Conditions that may be associated with extensive or aggressive molluscum contagiosum virus infection

Condition that may be associated with extensive or aggressive molluscum contagiosum virus infection	Reference
HIV infection	Schwartz and Myskowski 1992[35]
Topical steroid use	Hellier 1971[49]
Systemic immunosuppressive drugs	Rosenberg and Yusk 1970[50]
Congenital immunodeficiency states	Mayuma *et al.* 1986[48]
Lymphoproliferative states	Cotton *et al.* 1987[47]

- multiple monomorphic papules without the usual umbilicated center[36]
- giant molluscum contagiosum lesions (> 1 cm in diameter)[35, 6]
- verrucous, warty lesions[37].

In such cases biopsy is often necessary to establish the diagnosis.

When immunosuppression continues, as, for example, in late-stage and untreated HIV infection, the infection is chronic and the clinical course is one of disease progression despite aggressive treatment with cryotherapy or curettage.

DIAGNOSIS

Diagnosis of molluscum contagiosum is usually made by the characteristic appearance of the lesion. To identify the virus the surface of the lesion may be opened with the point of a disposable needle and the core extracted with forceps. Fine-toothed ophthalmological forceps are ideal for this purpose. The core is placed on the inner wall of a dry specimen tube and ringed on the outside for ease of identification. In the laboratory, the core is teased out in a drop of water, virions are allowed to adsorb to a formvar-coated grid which is then floated on a drop of tungstophosphoric acid. This negatively stained preparation is examined by electron microscopy, and typical brick-shaped pox-virions are readily identified (see Figure 9.1).

Although characteristic lesions are often found in the *immunocompromised* patient and diagnosed as above, atypical mollusca are not unusual; the differential diagnosis of such lesions is shown in Box 9.1[38, 39]. Histological confirmation of the diagnosis is desirable, and is essential when there are additional clinical features such as fever that may be associated with systemic fungal infection.

TREATMENT

In children, regression usually occurs following trauma or abrasion, and treatment is usually not required. In the immunocompetent adult with genital lesions, treatment is often requested for cosmetic reasons. Although it is considered advisable to treat individuals with molluscum contagiosum lesions[40], there is no clear evidence that treatment either prevents the transmission of the virus to others or limits the spread of

similar to that seen in HIV-infected patients[33, 34]. Most recent reports of mollusca in immunocompromised patients have concerned the manifestations of the infection in late-stage HIV-infection. When the individual is not severely immunocompromised, mollusca may regress spontaneously after several months. Lesions with the characteristic morphology of molluscum contagiosum may be seen and they

may be localized or extensive (more than 12 in number) (Figure 9.9), often affecting the face and neck (Figure 9.10), a site that is unusual in immunocompetent adults[35, 26]. In the context of HIV infection, there is a good correlation between the degree of immunosuppression and the number of lesions[35]. The clinical appearance of the lesions may be atypical and the following have been described

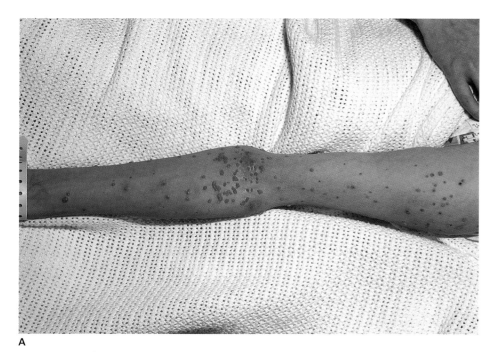

A

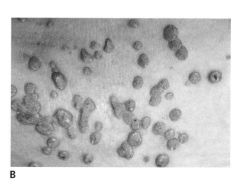

B

Figure 9.9A and 9.9B Multiple molluscum contagiosum lesions in a severely immunocompromised woman with HIV infection

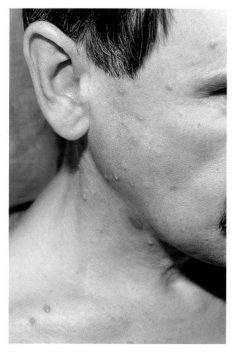

Figure 9.10 Molluscum contagiosum lesions of the face in a HIV-infected man

the virus by autoinoculation. If treatment is considered necessary, lesions can be treated by destruction by one of the following methods

- cryotherapy
- piercing the lesion with a sharpened wooden probe impregnated with liqui-

Box 9.1 Differential diagnosis of molluscum contagiosum in the immunocompromised patient

Basal cell carcinoma

Common warts

Giant condylomata acuminata

Keratoacanthoma

Ecthyma

Sebaceous nevus of Jadassohn

Atypical mycobacterial infection

Systemic fungal infections:

  Cryptococcus neoformans

  Histoplasma capsulatum

  Penicillium marneffei

fied phenol (80% w/w solution of phenol in water) or povidone iodine 10% in an alcoholic solution (Betadine, antiseptic paint, Seton Scholl), possibly using Emla cream (Astra) for analgesia.
- expressing the body of the lesion with forceps, possibly using Emla cream (Astra) for analgesia
- curettage after infiltration of the skin with local anesthetic

- electrocautery after infiltration of the skin with local anesthetic.

Evidence for the efficacy of any of these methods, however, is lacking. Although there is no significant difference in terms of resolution between physical expression of the core of the lesion and piercing with a phenol-impregnated wooden probe, the latter method results in more scarring[41].

The self application of podophyllotoxin cream (0.5% w/w) (see Chapter 5 for details about this agent) twice daily for three consecutive days per week for up to four weeks has been found to be satisfactory for the treatment of molluscum contagiosum. In the study reported by Syed *et al.*[171], 92% of 80 patients evaluated at the end of the treatment period were cured. A lower concentration (0.3%) of podophyllotoxin was found to be less efficacious.

In a recent, placebo-controlled trial[42], the application of imiquimod (see pp. 94–95) cream three times per day for 5 consecutive days per week for 4 weeks was found to have cured 82% of 50 male patients, whereas complete resolution of infection was found in only 16% of 50 placebo recipients. The place of this agent in the treatment of molluscum contagiosum, however, remains to be defined.

Treatment of molluscum contagiosum in HIV-infected patients

In late-stage HIV infection, the above treatments are very seldom successful. Recurrence is often seen after removal of lesions, and this may be explained by the presence of virus in the skin surrounding the lesions[43]. There have now been several case reports on the complete and maintained regression of molluscum contagiosum, including the verrucous variety, in individuals who have been treated with combination antiretroviral therapy that has included a protease inhibitor[37, 44, 45]. Regression of lesions has been reported to begin as early as 4 weeks and is generally complete within 3 to 4 months of initiation of treatment.

The antiviral agent cidofovir (a nucleoside analog of deoxycytidine monophosphate) shows activity against a range of DNA viruses, and clearing of MCV lesions has been noted in patients on intravenous cidofovir for CMV retinitis, and those who have had 3% cidofovir cream applied to molluscum lesions[46]. However, the outcome of any controlled trials is not yet known.

Epstein–Barr virus infection

The etiological role of the Epstein–Barr virus (EBV) as the causative agent of infectious mononucleosis is established, and its acquisition during adolescence or early adulthood as a result of intimate kissing, is an important facet of the epidemiology of this virus infection in the industrialized nations of the world. The classic triad of fever, sore throat, and generalized lymph node hyperplasia, and the typical blood picture occur in some 50% of primary infections in the 15 to 25 year age group, in contrast to the generally asymptomatic primary infection in childhood. In developed countries about 75% to 80% of the population ultimately become infected, whereas in developing countries nearly all children are already infected by about the age of 3 years. The delayed infection is more frequent in privileged classes of western societies, enjoying high standards of hygiene, than in the lower socioeconomic groups. The uniformly early age of EBV infection in developing countries, which leaves no adolescents or young adults susceptible, accounts for the virtual absence of infectious mononucleosis. The annual incidence of infectious mononucleosis in the United Kingdom is about 20–60 per 100 000. Whenever infection takes place the infected individual carries the virus for life.

In addition EBV can cause a rare fulminant infectious mononucleosis, first termed Duncan's disease, in individuals with predominantly an X-linked recessive genetically determined defect. The ubiquitous virus also has an etiological role, albeit with co-factors, in the induction of tumors, Burkitt's lymphoma and undifferentiated nasopharyngeal carcinoma. Epstein–Barr virus is a component in the induction of some malignant lymphomas in immunocompromised individuals, including those with HIV infection (Chapter 7).

THE EPSTEIN–BARR VIRUS

Epstein–Barr virus (EBV) is so named after two of the people who discovered the virus particles in cultured lymphoblastoid cells from the unusual malignant tumor, African endemic Burkitt's lymphoma. It is a herpesvirus, morphologically identical, but serologically distinct from the other herpesviruses that affect humans. By reason of its characteristic feature of latency in lymphoblastoid cells, EBV has been placed in the subfamily Gammaherpesvirinae with 'human herpesvirus 4' as its specific name. Two EBV types have been identified (EBV1 and EBV2), but they are much more closely related than herpes simplex virus types 1 and 2.

EBV antigens are classified as

1. *latent phase antigens*: EBV-nuclear antigens (EBNA) and latent membrane proteins (LMP) which are expressed in viral latency
2. *activated phase antigens*: early antigens (EA), viral capsid antigens (VCA), and membrane antigens (MA), and membrane antigens expressed in the viral productive cycle[51].

The EA components function during the lytic replicative cycle. The EA appears before the cycle of viral replication begins in productively infected cells, and therefore its expression does not require viral DNA replication. In viral replication, immediate early genes are expressed first and then early genes. Viral capsid antigens CA appear following the replication of viral DNA and this protein constitutes the protein coat (capsid) of the virus. Progeny virus particles are assembled in the cell nucleus, after which some pass into the cytoplasm and are released as enveloped virions through the cell membrane.

Shedding of virus into the buccal fluid occurs as early as 8 days after the onset of symptoms. Virus is regularly detectable in the saliva of infectious mononucleosis patients and seropositive healthy persons[52]. The site of virus production is thought to be the B lymphocytes of the oropharynx because only these cells are known to have EBV receptors. It was previously considered that EBV could infect and replicate in normal epithelial cells. More sensitive methods, however, have shown that all the infected cells in epithelial tissue are B lymphocytes[53].

IMMUNE RESPONSES

In primary infection the first antibody to become detectable is IgM specific for VCA, however IgG to VCA is also usually detectable at clinical presentation. During recovery from the acute phase of infectious mononucleosis, and usually within 4 months, IgM production ceases. Early in the disease IgM against MA is found, but IgG antibody production to MA occurs later than that to VCA and EBNA. At the time of onset of the illness, IgG against EA is detectable only for a short time. During convalescence, antibodies to EBNA-1 develop. The IgG antibodies to VCA and EBNA-1, but not to EA, persist for life in most cases. Antibodies to the virus envelope, whose titers peak later than those of anti-VCA and EBNA and persist for life, neutralize viral infectivity, kill lytically infected cells by antibody-dependent cell-mediated cytotoxicity, and protect against re-infection.

A virus-determined surface antigen on B lymphocytes is directly responsible for the disease and especially the hematological manifestations. It is recognized by helper and suppressor T cells and eventually by cytotoxic CD8[+] T cells that are produced in great quantities and are responsible for the clinical features of the disease, namely hepato-splenomegaly, jaundice, abnormal plasma enzyme tests of liver function, tonsillar and adenoidal changes and the typical blood picture. The characteristic mononucleosis and atypical cells have been shown to consist largely of NK cells and T lymphocytes which are specifically cyto-toxic *in vitro* for EBV genome-positive B-cell lines. Only a minority of the atypical cells in the blood are EBV-carrying B cells. In addition to the production of disease, these T-cell responses eliminate large numbers of infected cells from the body.

PATHOGENESIS

This is a complex subject that has been reviewed recently by Ward & Roizman[54] and Thorley-Lawson[55], and much of the following discussion summarizes these reviews that are highly referenced. It must be emphasized that some of the conclusions reached have yet to be established beyond doubt.

Viral entry and establishment of infection

The virus is thought initially to infect B cells (either naïve or memory cells) in the mucosal epithelium. B lymphocytes have the receptor for the virus, namely CD21, and can carry the viral genome *in vivo*. CD21 is the B-cell receptor for the C3d component of complement. The major viral surface glycoprotein gp350/220 recognizes and binds to the same motif on CD21 as C3da[55]. CD21 forms part of a multimeric signal transduction complex, and cross-linking of this complex with gp350/220 provides the necessary signal to move the resting B cells out of the resting phase, and, together with the earliest expressed latent proteins, to drive the cells on their way to entering the cell cycle. Immediately after the individual becomes infected with EBV there is likely to be binding of only a few virions to a small number of B cells, and it is unlikely that there is sufficient virus to cross-link enough of the CD21 receptor to push the resting cell into the cell cycle. It is postulated that the first infections are lytic until sufficient virions are produced to transform B cells. During

the viral productive cycle, the EBV BCRF1 gene encodes a homolog of IL-10 that inhibits interferon-γ production by T-helper cells and NK cells, thereby suppressing the local immune response to the virus and increasing the efficiency of viral trans-formation. Eventually there is sufficient virus to cross-link enough of the viral receptors of the newly infected cells to push them into the cell cycle and become lymphoblasts. These proliferating cells are initially localized to the site of original infection through the binding of adhesion molecules such as CD48 to heparin sulfate in the basal epithelium and lamina propria. Viral IL-10 also acts synergistically with heparan sulfate to increase the efficiency of transformation. Another factor that may play a part in establishing infection is the expression of a superantigen that stim-ulates T cells in an antigen-independent fashion. Lymphokines produced by these activated T cells may push infected B cells more efficiently into the lytic cycle. Another consequence may be the delay of a specific immune response, allowing the virus more time to establish infection. Proliferating infected lymphoblasts expand and migrate into the peripheral circulation. These infected cells express all six EBNA genes, LMP1, LMP2, and the EBV encoded RNA (EBERs) 1 and 2. T-cell responses develop quickly and destroy B cells express-ing the growth program genes, most of which are targets for cytotoxic T cells.

When EBV infects resting B cells they become activated B-cell blasts and express a variety of virally encoded latent proteins, including nuclear antigens (EBNAs) and membrane proteins (LMPs). These cells pro-liferate indefinitely and are called immor-talized or transformed lymphoblastoid cell lines (LCL).

Epstein–Barr virus only immortalizes resting B cells. A critical event in establish-ing latency is circularization of the linear viral genome to form an episome, so that it is replicated along with the cellular DNA in the proliferating LCL. Failure to achieve this results in loss of viral DNA and cell death. This is the consequence when the virus infects already activated B cells.

The virus encodes a set of latent pro-teins that are expressed as the cell traverses and exits the first G_1 before entry into the

cell cycle*. These proteins mimic those delivered by antigen-specific T-helper cells, and as a consequence, the B cell expresses an activated phenotype and starts to proliferate.

LMP1 is one of the virally encoded proteins expressed in latently infected B cells immortalized by EBV. It is expressed in newly infected B cells *in vitro* as they emerge from the first G_1 into the S phase of the growth cycle, and it is thought that the role of LMP1 is to drive the cell into S and through the cell cycle. In a normal prolif-erating B cell, the CD40 molecule (CD40 is a transmembrane receptor with large extra-cellular domains that bind ligands) on the surface of the B cell interacts with its ligand CD40L on the surface of an antigen-specific T-helper cell. This results in binding of cytoplasmic molecules called TNFR-associated factors (TRAFs) to the cyto-plasmic tail of CD40. This in turn leads to activation of the cytoplasmic transcription factor NFκB that then translocates to the nucleus resulting in survival and growth of the B cell. The amino-terminal sequence of LMP1 is tethered to the cytoskeleton and functions as a receptor–ligand complex. The carboxyl terminus associates with TRAF molecules and activates NFκB.

Unlike the normal B cell that when activated in response to antigen and T-cell signaling terminally differentiates into a plasma cell secreting specific antibody, B cells activated through infection with EBV proliferate indefinitely. The virus must then in some way block the terminal differen-tiation of the B cell. Proliferating cells arrest growth and begin to differentiate through a mechanism mediated by the Notch receptor and the DNA-binding pro-tein RBPJk. The Notch receptor interacts with its ligand and as a result there is a cleavage reaction that releases the cyto-plasmic domain of Notch which then

---

* The cell cycle is divided into four main stages: 1) the *M phase*, consisting of mitosis and cytoplasmic division, 2) the G_1 phase in which there is a considerable degree of biosynthesis and growth, 3) the *S phase* in which there is doubling of the cellular DNA and replication of the chromosomes, and 4) the G_2 *phase* that precedes cell division.

migrates to the nucleus to bind to RBPJk. This interaction leads to transcription of a gene which in turn represses expression of a master transcription factor which is required for the cell to arrest growth and differentiate. The first latent protein to be detected in newly infected cells is EBNA2, this binds to the same region of RBPJk as Notch, and as a result growth cannot be arrested and proliferation continues driven by LMP1.

Long-term latency and viral reactivation

The site of long-term latency is the resting, long-term memory B cell. The infection in these cells is tightly latent, as shown by the absence of linear EBV genomes in the peripheral blood, and the failure to detect growth-promoting viral latent genes such as LMP1 and EBNA2. The expression of the LMP2A gene, however, has been detected in the blood. It has been proposed that the gene product acts as a dominant negative inhibitor, preventing the B cell from responding to exogenous signals, and maintaining the viral infection in a tightly latent form.

In the first week of infectious mononucleosis up to 1 in 2000 blood lymphocytes carries the virus, as judged by the ability to infect other lymphocytes in tissue culture. Over ensuing weeks the proportion of infected lymphocytes falls to reach control levels – about 5 in 10^7 cells – 3 months after the onset. As the number of infected B cells in the peripheral blood is stable over several years, it is probable that they are being maintained as though they were normal B memory cells.

Although not proven beyond doubt, it is likely that EBV-infected B cells behave as uninfected activated B cells. The B cells circulate through lymphoid tissue and if no signals are encountered they exit back into the peripheral circulation. On the other hand, if they encounter antigen in the presence of T cells expressing the ligand for CD40 (CD40L), they become activated to express the EBNA1-only program that allows the episomal viral genome to replicate without being recognized by cytotoxic T cells. When the cells re-enter a quiescent phase, EBNA1 transcription again ceases.

Prolonged exposure to CD40L and lymphokines cause the B cell to cease growing and become a resting memory cell which can re-enter the circulation to maintain the levels of latently infected cells. If CD40L is no longer expressed but the presence of lymphokines is sustained, the B cells stop proliferating and undergo terminal differentiation into plasma cells. The cells that express a differentiated phenotype appear to home to the mucosal surface where infectious virus is shed. Apoptosis may also be a signal for reactivation. The pool of latently infected cells is therefore replenished and there is a continuous supply of cells that replicate and release infectious virus.

Avoidance of the immune system

To persist for the lifetime of the infected individual, EBV must evade the immune system. The virus has evolved several strategies to evade recognition by antigen-specific cells[54].

1. EBV inhibits antigen processing for presentation to effector T cells in the context of MHC class I molecules.
2. EBV down regulates the expression of intracellular adhesion molecule-1 (ICAM-1) and LFA-3 molecules that are necessary for interactions between effector cells and their targets.
3. The tropism of EBV for resting B cells precludes T-cell recognition because of the absence of certain cell surface molecules required for activating and differentiating effector T cells. Activation of naïve T cells requires both antigen recognition via the T-cell receptor/MHC molecules and also a secondary signal mediated by ligation of the C28 antigen on T cells with the co-stimulatory molecule B7 that is expressed on B cells. This interaction signals resting T cells to produce IL-2, to proliferate, and to differentiate into effector cells. Resting B cells do not express B7, and therefore viral antigens remain hidden from the immune system.
4. EBV can block signal transduction that could activate a switch from latent to productive infection. Signal transduction, mediated by the B-cell surface

receptor that leads to differentiation of the B cell and subsequent activation of the lytic phase of viral replication may be blocked by LMP2A produced by the virus.

The EBV gene, EBNA1, encodes a function that interferes with antigen presentation at an early stage by interfering with proteolytic processing of viral proteins. This gene is expressed not only in latent infection but also during lytic infection, and therefore the EBNA1 protein may be important for evasion of the immune system when infected B cells begin to differentiate.

The EBV BCRF1 gene encodes a homolog of IL-10 that inhibits interferon-γ production by T-helper cells and NK cells and suppresses certain T-cell and NK-cell responses.

The EBV BHRF1 gene encodes a homolog of the anti-apoptosis protein bcl-2, and the virus also up regulates the expression of cellular bcl-2 via another EBV-encoded protein, LMP1. As BHRF1 is not expressed during latent infection, it is unlikely to play a role in maintaining latency. However, it is an abundant early protein during the EBV lytic cycle, so its function may be to prolong cell life and maximize viral replication[54]. Protection against apoptosis has been attributed to three latency-associated proteins: LMP1, EBNA 2, and EBNA 4, all of which can up regulate bcl-2 expression. Inhibition of apoptosis would therefore allow the virus to persist in the memory B cell population.

INFECTIOUS MONONUCLEOSIS
Epidemiology

Inapparent primary infection with EBV generally occurs in childhood and is always accompanied by seroconversion and immunity to infectious mononucleosis. If the primary infection is delayed, however, until late adolescence or early adulthood then this event leads to infectious mononucleosis in about 50% of cases. As in herpes simplex virus (HSV) infections, EBV is most frequently acquired as a primary infection during childhood, particularly in the lower socioeconomic groups and, in developing countries, almost all children are infected before the age of 10, so that very few young adults can develop a primary infection and infectious mononucleosis is therefore virtually unknown. However or whenever infected, the individual will carry EBV for life.

In previously uninfected adolescents, often from privileged classes, large doses of EBV are ingested when kissing; this virus is shed in the saliva of seropositive healthy carriers who themselves have practically never shown signs of their original primary infection. In the case of young children indirect methods of spread probably operate and are responsible for the smaller infecting doses, which seem to play a part in determining inapparent infection without disease. Although infectious mononucleosis tends to occur within the 15 to 25-year age group, it may occasionally occur in those outside the group.

Genital lesions in infectious mononucleosis have rarely been described but the recovery of EBV from ulcerative lesions on the labia minora in a single case has raised interest in the sexual transmission of the virus[56].

EBV has now been detected in cervical secretions[57]. As the virus was found in cervical secretions from women with infectious mononucleosis and in individuals with serological evidence of past EBV infection, it is possible that the uterine cervix as well as the oropharynx may be a site of EBV replication and chronic viral shedding. This study suggests that EBV can be transmitted sexually, possibly by orogenital contact, but perhaps also from the male genital tract.

Clinical manifestations

Infectious mononucleosis consists of an acute illness characterized by certain clinical and hematological criteria. The incubation period is difficult to determine as evidence in case-to-case infection is rarely clear cut. Figures are frequently quoted within the range 6 to 60 days. The young adult presenting with malaise, fever with tachycardia, sore throat, and skin rash, who is found to have lymphadenopathy and splenomegaly, is the classic clinical picture. There may also be headache, dysphagia and anorexia, myalgia, nausea, neck stiffness, photophobia and

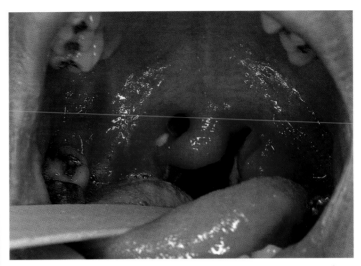

Figure 9.11 Pharyngitis of infectious mononucleosis (reproduced from McMillan and Scott 2000[166])

chest pain, and even a mild jaundice in a few patients. Hyperplasia of the pharyngeal lymphoid follicles is common and a pharyngeal exudate is seen in about half the patients (Figure 9.11). In up to one-third of cases there are petechial lesions 0.5 to 1.00 mm in diameter at the junction of the hard and soft palate near the midline. Discrete, slightly tender, lymph nodes are noted, especially in the posterior cervical region.

Skin rashes, when present, usually consist of a faint diffuse erythematous eruption, mostly on the trunk and proximal portions of the limbs. The rash is not diagnostic and may have been drug-induced as patients with infectious mononucleosis are particularly prone to hypersensitivity reactions of this kind. Ampicillin will precipitate a rash in about 8% of individuals, but in patients with infectious mononucleosis or lymphatic leukemia, a rash develops in more than 70% of cases[58]. This may be caused by alteration of the normal immune mechanisms resulting from the abnormal, but immunologically competent lymphocytes. Impurities of high molecular weight in ampicillin may also play a part.

Genital lesions have only rarely been described in infectious mononucleosis. In one such case, a 14-year-old girl developed buccal and labial ulceration following oral–genital contact[59]. In another case, a shallow single punched-out painless subpreputial erosion was found[60]. In the case where EBV was recovered from genital

ulcers, Portnoy et al.[56], describe how a 23-year-old patient first saw a bluish-black irregular lesion on the labia minora which was followed later by tender ulcers in this area which remained painful until healing occurred 32 days after the first appearance of the lesions.

Other objective signs sometimes found include also hepatomegaly, peri-orbital edema, arthropathy, cough, and diarrhea. Most of the unusual symptoms are associated with some rare complication and their undue emphasis tends to distort descriptions of the true clinical picture which, for the most part, is somewhat stereotyped. The most important and characteristic symptom is the sore throat that develops a few days after the onset of the illness.

Hematological manifestations

The hematological features of infectious mononucleosis are characterized by an absolute lymphocytosis, $4.5–5.0 \times 10^9$/L. A relative lymphocytosis of more than 60% of total leukocytes is seen in 95% of cases. The lymphocytosis tends to persist for 2 weeks unless bacterial infection supervenes. Twenty per cent or more of the lymphocytes are atypical and pleomorphic, varying in size, shape, and staining qualities of the cytoplasm and chromatin configurations of the nuclei (Figure 9.12). Many lymphocytes show a tendency to flow round adjacent erythrocytes. Rapid changes in this picture may occur from day to day.

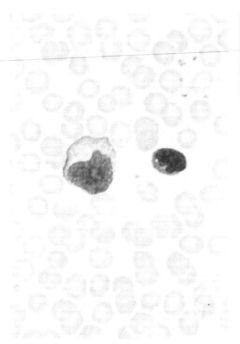

Figure 9.12 Blood film from a patient with infectious mononucleosis, showing an atypical lymphocyte (Leishman's stain, × 1000) (reproduced from McMillan and Scott 2000[166])

Plasma enzyme tests

Plasma enzyme tests for hepatocellular damage (alkaline phosphatase, alanine aminotransferase) show increased activity in 85% to 100% of patients with infectious mononucleosis. Abnormalities increase during the first week and are most pronounced by the middle or end of the second week. They almost invariably return to normal by the third to fifth week of the illness.

Prognosis

The usual pattern is one of mild fever lasting about 2 weeks. Complications are rare although a wide variety, including hemolytic anemia and thrombocytopenia due to auto-antibodies, occasionally develop. Fatalities are very rare (less than 1 per 1000 cases) and may be associated with ruptured spleen, neurological complications, asphyxia, and 'toxic' effects. A syndrome has been recognized in which an X-chromosome-linked immunological deficiency has led to deaths as a result of primary virus infection[61]. In this condition (often designated XLP or Duncan's disease) individuals die of fatal infectious mononucleosis in which a genetically determined failure of specific T-cell and other cellular immunological responses lead to a huge uncontrolled proliferation of B cells infected with EBV.

Some patients with infectious mononucleosis do not fully recover clinically for several months or even years and there are occasional reports of recrudescences. In patients who fail to make a complete recovery, high levels of T-suppressor cells may be found. Although remaining unwell for a year at least, recovery is the rule, when a return to normal of the lymphocyte subsets is seen[62].

Laboratory diagnosis

The presence of the hematological abnormalities described above in an individual with the classic clinical features of infectious mononucleosis suggests the diagnosis, and the detection of heterophil antibodies by a rapid and specific screening test, for example, the monospot slide test, is helpful in such cases. In infectious mononucleosis the heterophil antibodies agglutinate sheep red blood cells, but unlike those of the Forssman type, are not absorbed by guinea-pig kidney cells, although ox cells absorb the antibody. The test can also be made more specific by using horse erythrocytes. In the monospot test, serum is mixed thoroughly with guinea-pig kidney stroma (GPK) on one spot and with beef erythrocyte stroma on another, and unwashed preserved horse erythrocytes are added immediately to each spot. If agglutination of erythrocytes on the spot with GPK is stronger than on the spot with BES, the result of the test is positive. If the agglutination is stronger on the spot with BES, the result is negative. The test is also negative if no agglutination appears on either spot, or if agglutination is equal on both spots. The sera of up to 85% of patients with infectious mononucleosis contain heterophil antibodies, with negative results in the monospot test being reported more frequently in children under 4 years old. False positive tests for heterophil antibodies have been recorded in pregnancy and autoimmune disease.

The presence of IgM antibodies against VCA is regarded as the most reliable diagnostic test (page 257), and sero-conversion of anti-VCA from negative to positive in paired sera is also a useful test. Single high or paired IgG antibody titers are not helpful in diagnosing recent EBV infections, but a fourfold or greater increase in IgG antibody titer is regarded as suggestive evidence. IgG antibody to EBNA indicates past infection, but takes some weeks to appear in convalescence and may not be detectable in immunocompromised hosts. Tissue and cytology samples can be examined for EBERS and EBV antigens, and PCR may be applied to monitor viral DNA in blood samples post-transplant, for instance.

Differential diagnosis

In patients without antibodies to EBV, other conditions that may cause fever with lymph node enlargement should be considered in the differential diagnosis (Box 9.2). In addition, viral or streptococcal pharyngitis, diphtheria, Vincent's infection, or primary HSV stomatitis may cause sore throat of similar severity to infectious mononucleosis.

Treatment

Patients with uncomplicated infectious mononucleosis usually require rest in bed during the acute phase of the illness. Saline gargles and aspirin are useful for the relief of symptoms. As soon as the temperature is within normal range the patient may become ambulant, and full activity is commonly resumed after about a month from the onset. Violent exercise should be avoided for at least 3 weeks after the spleen is no longer palpable. Corticosteroids should

---

Box 9.2 Differential diagnosis of infectious mononucleosis

Primary HIV infection

Cytomegalovirus infection

Toxoplasmosis

Listeriosis

Tuberculosis

Secondary syphilis

Brucellosis

only be given for life-threatening pharyngeal edema, neurological complications, and thrombocytopenia or hemolytic anemia. Although aciclovir treatment has been shown to inhibit the virus replication cycle and does reduce oropharyngeal shedding of EBV, it has no effect on clinical infectious mononucleosis.

EPSTEIN–BARR VIRUS AND B-CELL LYMPHOMAS

In the transformed B cells of the three lymphomas associated with EBV, the virus establishes three patterns of latency[54]

1. latency I is found in latently infected Burkitt's lymphoma cells, and only the EBNA1 gene and the EBV encoded RNA (EBER) 1 and 2 are expressed
2. latency II is characteristic of Hodgkin's lymphoma (and nasopharyngeal carcinoma) and is characterized by the expression of EBERs, EBNA1, LMP1, and LMP2
3. latency III is found in immunoblastic lymphomas, and the full set of EBNAs and LMPs is expressed.

The pathogenesis of B-cell lymphomas in the context of EBV has been reviewed recently[63]. In individuals who are severely immunocompromised, for example those receiving post-transplant immunosuppressive therapy, there may be a fatal proliferation of EBV-transformed immunoblasts. Initially there is polyclonal B-cell proliferation, but later it becomes monoclonal. Additional genetic factors, however, are probably important.

Highly endemic Burkitt's lymphoma is almost always associated with EBV. Chronic infected B-cell proliferation, stimulated for example by malaria, increases the risk of genetic accidents, including translocation of c-myc gene to one of the three Ig loci. Because of the constitutive activation of c-myc in the B cell, there is a permanent signal for proliferation. Only some 20% of cases of the sporadic form of Burkitt's lymphoma are associated with EBV, but the Ig/c-myc translocation is found in almost 100% of individuals. Other secondary genetic changes, however, are probably necessary to produce the lymphoma.

Lymphomas associated with HIV infection

The etiology of these lymphomas is not clear. Only a subset of non-Hodgkin's lymphomas in HIV-infected individuals is associated with EBV: 30% of small non-cleaved cell lymphoma, 80% of large cell immunoblastic lymphoma, and almost 100% of primary central nervous system lymphoma. It is possible that the large cell immunoblastic lymphoma develops in a similar manner to the lymphomas seen in those who are iatrogenically immunocompromised: HIV infection results in a deficiency of the immune surveillance mechanisms that control EBV-infected B cells in the normal host. Some 30% of cases of small non-cleaved cell lymphomas contain EBV DNA sequences, the majority of which contain a Ig/c-myc translocation, and the pathogenesis may be similar to that of endemic Burkitt's lymphoma. Certainly chronic stimulation of B cells by HIV antigens is well recognized. Hodgkin's lymphoma has also been observed in HIV-infected patients, and unlike the neoplasms found in non-HIV-infected individuals, is almost always associated with EBV; the mechanism of induction of the tumor is unknown.

Cytomegalovirus infection

Cytomegaloviruses (CMVs) are ubiquitous agents widespread among many animals including man and non-human primates such as the owl monkey (Aotus spp.), spider monkey (Ateles spp.), marmoset (Callithrix spp.), capuchin monkey (Cebus spp.), and African green monkey (Cercopithecus spp.)[64]. These viruses are highly species-specific, and, as in the case of man, have been closely linked to their natural hosts over aeons of time, and over the generations, many, probably thousands, of genetically different strains have emerged to circulate continuously throughout the world. As with other herpesviruses, primary CMV infection is followed by persistence. Cells of the myeloid lineage have been identified as one site of CMV latency[65]. Reactivation of latent CMV may

occur subclinically, or present with disease in hosts with compromised cell-mediated immunity. Re-infection may also occur because of the antigenic diversity of CMV.

If transmission is expedited by poor environmental conditions, as in some tropical countries, the acquisition of HCMV in infancy or early childhood may confer a measure of protection. Primary infection, however, may be delayed until in adolescents or young adults, aged 15 to 35 years, the requirement of close physical contact such as kissing or sexual intercourse, enables the effective spread of the virus. Although generally asymptomatic the infection becomes important medically when it occurs as a primary infection during pregnancy, bringing with it a risk of placental passage of the virus to the fetus and brain damage. In the vast majority of cases, however, HCMV infections are subclinical including those acquired in utero and at, or shortly after, birth.

HUMAN CYTOMEGALOVIRUS

Human cytomegalovirus (HCMV) is one of the herpesviruses that is slow to produce a cytopathic effect in cell culture (family Herpesviridae, subfamily Betaherpesvirinae). On electron microscopy the virus particles, after negative staining, are indistinguishable from other members of the family. When inoculated in vitro into permissive human fibroblasts clinical specimens containing HCMV produce a characteristic cytopathic effect – striking cytomegaly with intranuclear inclusions – within days or weeks following infection. With inocula of high infectivity focal collections of swollen rounded refractile fibroblasts may be detectable in 24 to 72 hours, whereas with inocula of low infectivity it may take several weeks to produce sparse focal lesions[66].

Herpesvirions enter host cells directly by adsorption to cell receptors followed by fusion of the viral envelope with the cell plasma membrane. Within minutes of entry into the cytoplasm, the tegumented viral nucleocapsid is transported to the nuclear membrane where the core passes into the nucleus through a pore. Tegument protein has a role in initiating transcription of the immediate early genes.

Replicative cycle of human cytomegalovirus

HCMV has a very large genome (230 kbp), some 33% larger than that of HSV, and has a coding potential for over 200 proteins. The replication cycle, which is based on the appearance of different classes of viral proteins in an orderly sequence as the genome transcription is regulated, can be divided into three time periods (as with all herpesviruses).

1. *Immediate early period* (2 to 4 hours after infection, depending on cell transcription factors in association with stimuli from viral tegument protein) is characterized by DNA transcription in the absence of either protein synthesis or viral DNA replication. Restricted transcription of specific segments of the genome occurs with the production of what are referred to as '*regulatory immediate early proteins*' and which may control transcription of early messenger RNA.

2. *Early period* (follows (1) and persists through long eclipse phase of HCMV multiplication) characterized by DNA replication and the synthesis of a distinct class of non-structural proteins (e.g. viral DNA polymerase).

3. *Late period* (36 to 48 hours after infection) characterized by continued DNA replication, the formation of virion structural proteins referred to as '*late proteins*' and the release of infectious virus about 72 hours after infection. Quantitatively the production of *late proteins* is markedly increased as DNA replication reaches its maximum.

Studies *in vivo* of HCMV replication in compromised patients have recently shown that this is a very dynamic process, with a doubling time for CMV DNA of approximately 1 day[67].

A 'myriad' of proteins encoded by human cytomegalovirus

Among the 'myriad' of proteins encoded by HCMV there are an unknown number of non-structural proteins (*infected-cell proteins*); and about thirty-three *structural proteins*, mostly found in small amounts. Of the more abundant proteins there are a major and a minor capsid protein; two matrix proteins linking the capsid to the virion envelope; and at least six envelope glycoproteins, three of which (gB, gH, and gC) are involved in entry. Glycoprotein B (gB) appears to be immunodominant and does contain sites that are recognized by neutralizing antibodies. Other proteins, with as yet unknown functional and structural role in HCMV, have been found.

Heterogeneity of human cytomegalovirus

As can be shown by

- DNA–DNA re-association between strains
- the number and size of fragments produced by restriction enzyme analysis of DNA

HCMV isolates vary in base composition of their DNA. Restriction pattern polymorphisms caused by base substitutions and deletions are present and may be used to differentiate strains of HCMV[68]. At least four genotypes based on RFLP of the envelope glycoprotein gB are recognized, and may reflect differences in pathogenicity and cell tropism.

Immunology of human cytomegalovirus infection

The differences in the immunological responses of the body at different stages of infection are summarized in Table 9.2; it is convenient to discuss these separately.

Stages of human cytomegalovirus infection

During human cytomegalovirus mononucleosis – an event in a human cytomegalovirus primary infection

During the early acute phase of the illness which is seen almost always in young

Table 9.2 Immunological findings in individuals infected with cytomegalovirus (CMV) (from Robertson *et al.* 1989)

	CMV mononucleosis		Congenitally infected infant	Postnatally infected child	Pregnancy
	Acute	Convalescent			
Isolation of CMV from:					
Blood	+	−	?	?	−
Urine	+	+	?	?	+
Saliva	+	±	+	+	?
Serum immunoglobulin concentration	increased	normal	increased	normal	normal
Activated CD8+ cells	present	absent	?	?	?
Number of CD8+ cells	increased	increased	increased	normal	normal
Proliferative responses to mitogens	impaired	impaired	normal	normal	impaired*
Lymphokine production by leukocytes	impaired	?	normal	normal	impaired
Ability to produce cytotoxic effector cells	impaired	?	impaired	impaired	normal
Specific proliferative response of leukocytes to CMV	impaired	normal (late)	impaired	impaired	impaired

* With the exception of the proliferative response to phytohemagglutinin.

people after puberty, virus can be cultured from the buffy coat of blood samples and often, but not always, from urine, saliva, and semen. Human cytomegalovirus can only rarely be recovered from the peripheral blood leukocytes during convalescence, but viruria is common and may persist for weeks.

Figure 9.13 illustrates diagrammatically the humoral immune antibody response during HCMV mononucleosis. The IgM and IgG (usually IgG$_1$ and IgG$_3$) antibodies are directed against viral glycoproteins, and structural and non-structural viral antigens respectively. Neutralizing and complement-fixing antibodies are directed primarily against late structural antigens. The appearance of the former is often delayed with respect to the other antibodies, but neutralizing and complement-fixing antibodies persist indefinitely. Antibodies against immediate early and early antigen are present at high titer during active infection and often, but not always, decline in titer during convalescence.

During the acute phase of the illness various auto-antibodies are detectable, probably as the result of the polyclonal B-cell stimulation following exposure to HCMV.

In the peripheral blood there is an increased number of CD8$^+$ lymphocytes. The ability of mononuclear cells to proliferate and produce cytokines in response to *in vitro* exposure to various mitogens, including phytohemagglutinin, is impaired. The number of CD4$^+$ cells is normal. The CD8$^+$ cells have an increased spontaneous proliferation rate and their ability to produce effector cells may result from re-exposure to antigen that has previously produced memory CD8$^+$ cells. These abnormalities are maximal during the acute phase of the illness, and some resolve during convalescence. Specific delayed type hypersensitivity reaction develops as the mitogen-proliferative responses recover.

In congenitally infected infants

IgM against HCMV is detectable in the cord and neonatal blood of most congenitally infected infants. Complement-fixing antibodies are present in the serum at birth and remain detectable at high titer. Antibodies detected by immunofluorescence against early and late antigen are found at high titer in the neonate's serum. Antibodies against the late antigen persist for years, but those against the early antigen diminish and become undetectable generally within 3 to 4 years. Immune complexes, present in high concentrations in the blood of congenitally infected infants, may play a part in the disease process.

In contrast to HCMV mononucleosis, the proliferative responses of peripheral blood lymphocytes to mitogens other than HCMV is normal; specific responses are impaired for at least a year. Immunosuppression in congenital HCMV infection lasts much longer than in HCMV mononucleosis.

In postnatally infected infants

Although the humoral immune response is similar to that seen in HCMV mononucleosis, general cell-mediated immune responses are intact. Peripheral blood lymphocyte responses to HCMV antigen, however, are impaired and this impairment may persist for years.

During pregnancy

Human cytomegalovirus mononucleosis is rare in pregnancy. In seropositive pregnant women HCMV-specific peripheral blood lymphocyte responses become progressively depressed during pregnancy. Responses to other mitogens are also depressed. Within 4 months of delivery, however, the immune suppression has generally resolved. There is no correlation between the suppression of HCMV-specific proliferation and excretion of virus. During reactivation of HCMV infection there is usually no specific IgM response; however, low levels may be detected and cause difficulty in diagnosis.

Immune activation of HCMV from latently infected cells is clinically relevant. In the context of recipients of blood or bone marrow or solid organs, allogeneic stimulation is significant; in the HIV-infected individual viral activation following bacterial infection may be important. Cytokines are important mediators in these reactions.

Immune evasion by human cytomegalovirus during lytic infection

The means by which HCMV evades the human immune system are not entirely clear, but the following discussion, based on reviews by Ward & Roizman[69] and Hengel & Kosinowski[70] summarizes what mechanisms are currently thought to be important. Human cytomegalovirus carries several genes that function to interfere with

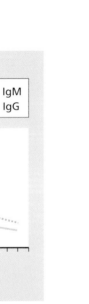

Figure 9.13 Diagrammatic illustration of the humoral antibody response during HCMV mononucleosis (adapted from Robertson *et al.* 1989[167])

antigen presentation by MHC class I molecules*.

The lack of MHC class I antigen expression diminishes the host's ability to recognize and kill HCMV-infected cells. However, it is known that the peripheral blood mononuclear cells of healthy seropositive individuals contain cytotoxic T cells that recognize HCMV-infected targets. It appears that certain HCMV proteins are not recognized by T lymphocytes, and it has been suggested that HCMV can selectively inhibit the presentation of certain viral antigens. The loss of T-cell cytotoxicity in immunocompromised hosts is associated with severe HCMV disease, indicating that this response is important in controlling infection.

The UL18 gene encodes a homolog to the human MHC class I heavy chain that binds to β_2-microglobulin. As virally infected cells may have completely lost MHC class I expression on the cell surface, it has been postulated that the homolog competes for binding to the light chain of the heterodimer, β-2 microglobulin. However, as cellular class I protein bound to β-2 microglobulin has been found in infected cells, and deletion of the UL18

gene does not restore surface expression of MHC class I molecules, this is not the main mechanism of interference with surface expression of these molecules. The expression of homolog protein on the cell surface, however, may protect against lysis by NK cells. It is known that MHC class I expression on the cell surface is necessary for protection of cell against destruction by NK cells, and in virus-infected cells that do not express this molecule on the cell surface, the expression of the homolog may be protective.

The US region of HCMV contains genes whose products interfere with the transport of peptides into the endoplasmic reticulum (ER) or with maturation or stability of newly synthesized MHC class I molecules. US2 and US11 act by reversing the normal process of translocation of the MHC class I heavy chains. US2 binds directly to heavy chains and, with US11, promotes retrograde transport of newly synthesized MHC I molecules from the ER to the cytosol where they are degraded. US3 in concert with US2 and US11 interfere with maturation and transport out of the ER of MHC class I molecules bound to β-2 microglobulin.

HCMV encodes molecules that interfere with the complement pathway. Human cytomegalovirus, HSV and VZV express Fc receptors, one a low-affinity receptor encoded by the viral glycoprotein E gene, and the other a high-affinity receptor formed as a complex of gE and gI. These receptors may function in immune escape by forming bipolar bridging of virus-specific antibody bound to a viral antigen via the Fab region of the immunoglobulin molecule while the Fc portion of the antibody binds the virally encoded Fc receptor. This would result in interference with antibody and complement-mediated killing of the infected cell and the virion, and with antibody-dependent cellular cytotoxicity.

Human cytomegalovirus also encodes two proteins, IE1 and IE2, that prevent apoptosis by an unknown mechanism.

Pathology

When there is widely disseminated infection, almost every organ can be involved. Human cytomegalovirus characteristically

infects ductal epithelial cells. Human cytomegalovirus-infected cells are large with prominent central nuclei that contain marginated chromatin and intranuclear inclusions surrounded by a clear halo (owl's-eye inclusions). In the kidneys the proximal tubules are most commonly affected, but the loop of Henle and collecting tubules are also affected. In HIV-infected or otherwise immunocompromised patients, the gastrointestinal tract is often the site of HCMV pathology. Ulceration, which may be superficial or deep, localized or diffuse, is the most common manifestation; the colon, esophagus, rectum, and jejunum are affected in decreasing order of frequency of involvement. The hepatitis of HCMV infection in children and adults is associated with mononuclear cell infiltrates of the portal triads; when present, cytomegalovirus changes are seen within duct epithelium, and in adults hepatocytes may contain inclusion-bearing cells. Cytomegalovirus infection has also been shown in vascular epithelium, and giant endothelial cells with multilobed nuclei become detached from these vessel walls.

In HIV infection, the most common pathological finding of HCMV infection is that of microglial nodules with central cytomegalic cells and surrounding gliosis throughout the subcortical gray matter and brainstem. Another histological finding is parenchymal necrosis with macrophages, cytomegalic cells, and axonal swelling in necrotic areas. The finding of cytomegalic cells in small vessel endothelial cells in necrotic foci suggests that hematogenous seeding of the vascular epithelium occurs[71]. The ependymal lining may be necrotic with fibrinous exudates and intraventricular hemorrhage. In some cases, the only evidence of CNS involvement by HCMV is the finding of isolated inclusion-bearing cells, particularly in the capillary epithelium of the brain.

Epidemiology

Human cytomegalovirus is an important cause of disease in HIV-infected individuals (Chapter 7), and is a major cause of disease in congenitally infected infants. In the USA, the estimated rates of congenital HCMV infection ranges between 2 and 40 per 1000

---

* Activated CD8+ T lymphocytes have cytolytic activity against virally infected cells and recognize peptides associated with MHC class I molecules. Cytoplasmic antigens are processed into peptides by an organelle known as the proteasome. Peptides are translocated across the membrane of the endoplasmic reticulum (ER) by the transporter associated with antigen processing (TAP). This transporter, encoded within the MHC, is a heterodimer composed of two homologous proteins, TAP1 and TAP2, and translocation occurs in an ATP-dependent manner. The MHC class I molecules are composed of a transmembrane heavy chain, a light chain, β-2 microglobulin, and a short peptide. MHC class I heterodimers assemble with the TAP via the TAP1 subunit. Binding of high-affinity peptides to the MHC class I molecules results in dissociation of the TAP–MHC class I complex and the exit of the heterotrimeric complex from the endoplasmic reticulum, and via the Golgi apparatus to the cell surface. Class I molecules lacking bound antigenic peptide are degraded within the cell (description modified from Hengel & Koszinowski et al.[70]).

births[72]. About 10% of these infected children have neurological sequelae, and it is estimated that 4000 to 7000 infants in the USA will suffer neurological damage as a result of congenital CMV infection[73]. In the UK, it is thought that about 2800 infants are congenitally infected with HCMV, and that 500 children develop severe brain damage[74].

Transmission

After a primary infection, HCMV persists in the body in latent form, probably for life. Although antibody is present in the serum, virus excretion because of reactivation occurs in pregnancy and in immunocompromised individuals. Human cytomegalovirus has been recovered, for example, from the cervix of 18% of pregnant Chinese women in Taiwan, 14% of Navajo women, 5% of Negro women, and 4% of Caucasian women in Pittsburgh. If recovery of HCMV from the cervix is the result of reactivation of a latent infection, then a measure of the reactivation rate within these infected groups is provided by dividing the number with positive cervical cultures for HCMV by the number with complement-fixing antibody to HCMV (i.e. latent infection) and, when these calculations are applied to the Pittsburgh and Navajo populations, the rates are about the same (about 14%). Reactivation occurs more often in the third trimester than in the first or second and more often in the younger and primiparous, than in the older and multiparous patient[75].

Young infants and children seem to be the major source of primary infection in pregnant women[76]. Maternal immunity is an important determinant of the frequency of transmission of HCMV to the fetus, and of the virulence of the ensuing infection. Congenital infection in babies is associated with primary HCMV infection in the pregnant mother, the rate of infection being about 40%. In contrast, the risk of transmission to the fetus from a woman who has recurrent infection, or re-infection, is only 0.2% to 2%[77, 78]. Maternal immunity can reduce significantly the transmission of HCMV to the fetus: Fowler et al.[79] showed that the incidence of congenital HCMV infection in babies born to mothers who had HCMV immunity before conception was 91% less than in those whose mothers did not have immunity. Viral neutralizing antibodies appear to be important in protecting the fetus. In a study of HCMV-specific antibody responses after primary infection in pregnancy, anti-glycoprotein B IgG antibodies were significantly higher at delivery in women who had transmitted the virus to the fetus than those who had not, indicating that the amount of antibody did not reflect protection[80]. However, it was shown in the same study that women who transmitted infection had lower levels of neutralizing antibody and reduced levels of high-affinity antibodies than non-transmitters. This suggested that a defect in affinity maturation may play a role in intrauterine transmission of HCMV.

The other main mode of transmission to the neonate is breast feeding. Amongst infants fed infected breast milk, 12% developed neonatal infection[81].

The prevalence of serum HCMV antibody increases with age, at a rate that varies from country to country and between communities. In developing countries most individuals are seropositive by the age of 5 years, whereas less than 5% of children in the developed countries are seropositive by that age. Living under crowded conditions is the most likely reason for this difference in antibody prevalence.

In clinics for STIs in Leicester, HCMV was isolated from the cervix in about 3% of women, and in Manchester antenatal clinics an isolation rate of 0.7% was obtained[82]. Handsfield et al.[83] showed that the prevalence of HCMV antibodies was greater amongst male contacts of seropositive women than those of seronegative females. They showed further, by DNA restriction enzyme typing, that isolates from partners were identical. Sexual intercourse, as a method for the spread of HCMV, is supported by the finding of the virus, as extracellular aggregates, in the semen of asymptomatic men convalescent from heterophil-antibody-negative HCMV mononucleosis[84, 85]. Sero-

Table 9.3 Prevalence of cytomegalovirus (CMV) antibody in homosexual and heterosexual men attending sexually transmitted infections clinics

Locality	Percentage (number tested) of seropositive individuals		Reference
	Homosexual men	Heterosexual men	
San Francisco	94 (139)	54 (70)	Drew et al. (1981)[90]
Copenhagen	87 (170)	50 (50)	Melbye et al. (1983)[168]
Aarhus	73 (89)	50 (50)	Melbye et al. (1983)[168]
Antwerp	71 (191)	57 (95)	Coester et al. (1984)[169]
London	93 (152)	56 (108)	Mindel and Sutherland (1984)[170]
Amsterdam	71 (710)	nt	Coutinho et al. (1984)[89]
Edinburgh	90 (207)	59 (183)	Edmond et al. (unpublished data 1984)

nt, not tested

positivity has also correlated with the number of lifetime sexual partners and young age at first intercourse[86].

The prevalence of HCMV antibodies amongst young homosexual men is higher than amongst heterosexual men (Table 9.3). Up to 15% of homosexual men who attended a STI clinic in Copenhagen excreted HCMV in the semen[87]. Reports on HCMV infection amongst homosexual men living in Amsterdam and San Francisco suggest attack rates of 71% and 27% over a 9 and 23 month period respectively[88, 89]. Among 501 seropositive homosexual men, Coutinho and his colleagues[89] found a recurrence rate (fourfold increase in titer-paired sera) of 6.2% within the 23-month follow-up period.

Re-infection of the genital tract is common in sexually active populations and co-infection with multiple strains of the HCMV has been detected in the semen of homosexual men and others attending STI clinics[90].

Persons acquiring a primary infection, perhaps those experiencing re-infection, and some with activation of an existing infection may excrete virus in urine or saliva for months. The urine may contain 10^6 infectious CMV plaque-forming units per mL. Infection rates in England, as determined serologically, rise appreciably in adolescents. Human cytomegalovirus, like infectious mononucleosis caused by EBV, may be a 'kissing disease'.

Viral excretion is markedly increased in the immunocompromised seropositive individual and HCMV is commonly shed from multiple sites in HIV-infected individuals, particularly when the CD4$^+$ cell count in the peripheral blood is low[91]. After organ transplantation, HCMV excretion is almost invariably found in seropositive recipients, the source of the virus, including reactivation of latent HCMV, transfused blood, and the transplanted tissue.

Clinical features

A primary HCMV infection in adolescents or young adults is almost invariably subclinical. A clinical syndrome may occasionally occur characterized by low-grade fever, diffuse lymphadenopathy, hepato-megaly, and pharyngitis; a lymphocytosis develops with atypical lymphocytes in the peripheral blood. Heterophil antibodies are not produced and the monospot test is therefore negative.

Similarly primary postnatal infections are usually asymptomatic, but hepatitis with hepatomegaly may occur with abnormalities of plasma enzyme tests of liver function. Serious ill effects in previously healthy adults, as for example, chorioretinitis or thrombocytopenia are exceedingly rare.

In the post-perfusion syndrome, named for its frequent association with the use of extracorporeal circulation and characterized by splenomegaly and heterophil-antibody-negative HCMV mononucleosis, the infection is primary and the virus may be transmitted with fresh blood in the fraction rich in leukocytes.

Those with immunological deficiencies, whether due to debilitating conditions or therapy with suppressive agents (particularly organ transplant recipients), are also susceptible to HCMV illness when the infection may be localized or confined to one organ. Interstitial pneumonitis, hepatitis, swinging pyrexia, and colitis are the common presentations in transplant recipients and in those with severe HIV infection (the latter may develop CMV retinitis in advanced immunodeficiency (Chapter 7)).

In the UK 40% to 60% of women enter pregnancy without complement-fixing antibodies to HCMV and about 3% of them suffer primary infection at some time during the course of the pregnancy. In about 50% of cases the fetus is affected. About 0.5% to 1% of all babies are congenitally infected and are excreting virus in the throat and urine[74]. The consequences of fetal infection may range from inapparent infection to the classic syndrome of neonatal cytomegalic inclusion disease (hepatosplenomegaly, purpura, chorioretinitis, uveitis, and microcephaly). The non-neurological manifestations of congenital HCMV disease are self-limiting, but intrauterine infection of the CNS invariably leads to permanent sequelae. Progressive bilateral sensorineural hearing loss, resulting from damage to the cochlea and, possibly, the eighth nerve, is the most common feature of CNS involve-ment. There is now good evidence that the severity of HCMV infection in the neonatal period is related to maternal immunity; symptomatic disease following recurrent infection or re-infection in women with pre-existing immunity is rare. In infected infants born to seropositive mothers, the incidence of sequelae is lower than if the mother had no previous exposure to the virus[73]. Neutralizing antibodies are thought to play a role in fetal protection. These antibodies are of the IgG$_1$ subclass and are transported to the fetal circulation by an active transport system specific for IgG$_1$ antibodies. Because these transport mechanisms are not fully developed until the early third trimester, fetuses infected in the first or early second trimesters may be more likely to have significant sequelae compared with those born to women infected in the third trimester (although serious disease can occur when infection has been acquired at this time)[72].

Laboratory diagnosis

Immunocompetent adult

The diagnosis of acute HCMV infection in normal adults is made by examination of paired sera, taken at an interval of 10 to 14 days apart, for HCMV IgG seroconversion. An enzyme immunoassay (EIA), using recombinant antigens, is the most widely used method for the detection of these antibodies[92]. When only a single specimen of serum is available an EIA to detect HCMV IgM antibodies is useful; the IgM antibody response persists for up to 16 to 20 weeks after infection[93]. The sensitivity of the assay in different populations has varied between 50% and 90%[94]. A particular difficulty arises in diagnosis of maternal infection during pregnancy if no earlier (antibody-negative) sample is available for comparison, and low levels of IgM antibody are found. An IgG avidity test has been found useful in such circumstances, as it may reveal low avidity (recently acquired primary antibody responses) or high avidity (long-standing antibody responses)[95].

Fetal and congenital infection

To investigate whether HCMV infection of the fetus has occurred it is important to look for the virus in amniotic fluid (by PCR) after 21 weeks gestation if cases are not to be missed[95]. The detection of virus by culture is the most widely used diagnostic test for congenital HCMV infection. Specimens of urine or pharyngeal secretion aspirate should be sent to the laboratory as soon as possible (as described for HSV, Chapter 6). If storage is required samples may be kept at 4°C, but should *not* be frozen prior to inoculation into cell cultures of human fibroblasts[96]. Whereas in postnatal HCMV standard tube culture may not yield a result for up to 28 days, in congenitally infected infants, high titers of virus are excreted for much of the first year and may be detected within a few days. A modification of culture, involving centrifugation enhancement of the inoculum and the immunological detection of the products of immediate early gene expression, the shell vial assay, can provide rapid results usually within 24 hours of receipt of the specimen. The sensitivity of the method is up to 95% when compared with routine culture (in the detection of virus in blood, however, the shell vial assay lacks sensitivity compared to conventional tube culture). For the purpose of establishing whether the infection was acquired *in utero*, samples must be submitted before the neonate is 3 weeks old.

Polymerase chain reactions for the detection of HCMV DNA have been used for the diagnosis of congenital HCMV infection[97], and when PCR is more widely available, it is likely to replace isolation in the detection of infection.

Patients with HIV infection

Serological methods are of limited value because of the inability to differentiate between infection and invasive disease. The most direct evidence of disease comes from the detection of the histological changes of HCMV[98]. Significant levels of viremia have been shown to predict disease[99].

Treatment

The treatment of CMV mononucleosis is symptomatic and similar to that of infectious mononucleosis (pp. 261–262). The management of HCMV disease in HIV-infected patients is outlined in Chapter 7.

Prevention

The prevention of HCMV infection in allograft recipients by a combination of strategies such as donor selection and ganciclovir prophylaxis is now well established, but a discussion of such antiviral prophylaxis lies outwith the scope of this text book. When transfusion of an immunocompromised individual is required, it is sensible to avoid use of HCMV seropositive blood. Since the use of leuko-depleted blood was introduced in the UK, the risk of acquiring HCMV from transfusion has decreased.

The prevention of congenital HCMV infection is much more complicated than the prevention of congenital rubella. Unlike the situation with maternal rubella diagnosed in the first trimester, where 90% of fetuses are at risk of serious disease, even primary CMV infection of the mother-to-be is usually asymptomatic, it is transmitted in less than 60% of cases, and results in serious disease in less than 20%. The fetus can, however, be severely damaged following maternal CMV later in the second trimester, when termination is impracticable.

A live attenuated vaccine for HCMV, the Towne vaccine, was developed early, but was not effective in the protection of pregnant women, although it did prove of benefit to renal transplant recipients. There has been little advance until recently when, in common with the development of other herpesvirus vaccines, subunit or recombinant vaccines based on viral glycoproteins have been produced. One of these, in a canarypox vector, was found to prime trial recipients to produce an improved neutralizing antibody response to subsequently administered Towne vaccine[100].

Work on adoptive transfer of HLA-compatible cytotoxic T-cell clones has progressed in recent years, to the benefit of patients with severe immunodeficiency states[101].

Human herpesvirus type 8

INTRODUCTION

Kaposi's sarcoma (KS) was first described by Kaposi in 1872 as an indolent tumor amongst elderly Europeans. In the 1950s, a slightly more aggressive variant of the condition was recognized in African populations, and in the 1970s KS was described in immunosuppressed patients, for example, following organ transplantation. The emergence of Kaposi's sarcoma as a feature of HIV infection in homosexual men was reported by Friedman-Kien and colleagues in 1981[102]. Four forms of KS are therefore recognized

1. classic 'Mediterranean'
2. endemic 'African'
3. post-transplant
4. HIV-associated.

All are caused by human herpesvirus type 8 (HHV-8) and all share common histological features (Figure 9.14), although the clinical course is variable.

The epidemiology of Kaposi's sarcoma (KS) in the 1980s suggested the likelihood of an infectious etiology with clustering of the infectious agent in specific groups such as men who had had sex with men, and inhabitants of eastern Africa.

Parts of a viral genome were identified in KS tissue in 1994[103]. Although initially referred to as Kaposi's sarcoma herpes virus (KSHV), the virus has been named human herpesvirus-8, a member of the Gamma herpesvirus family. This family is divided into γ1, represented in humans by the Epstein–Barr virus, and γ2, represented in humans by HHV-8. A family of similar viruses, referred to as Rhadinoviruses, has been described in primates[104, 105]. HHV-8 is also implicated in the etiology of primary effusion lymphoma[106] and Castleman's disease[107].

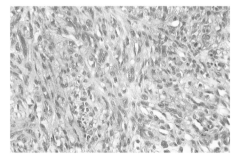

Figure 9.14 Kaposi's sarcoma of skin, showing spindle cell proliferation (hematoxylin and eosin, × 25).

VIROLOGY AND PATHOGENESIS

The size and shape of the virions of HHV-8 characterize them as members of the herpesvirus family. It is thought that the virus persists in a latent form in most spindle cells of KS lesions, in the perifollicular B cells of Castleman's disease, and in some infected blood mononuclear cells[108]. Lytic viral replication also occurs in some cells in these tissues and in blood. The virus appears to have incorporated human cell genes during its evolution, and their function can be compared with those of the host cell genes. A number of proteins encoded by the viral genome have been identified[109]

- a cyclin that inhibits the retinoblastoma protein, which controls the G1 to S phase of cell growth (page 73)
- a Bcl-like protein that inhibits apoptosis
- a G-protein-coupled receptor that is homologous to the cellular IL-8 receptor, IL-8 binds the HHV-8 G-protein-coupled receptor*
- an inhibitor of apoptosis mediated by FLICE (Fas-associated death domain-like interleukin-1β-converting enzyme) pathway*
- an immunoreceptor*
- an inhibitor of the interferon signaling pathway*, viral interferon regulatory factor prevents interferon from repressing the c-myc oncogene
- viral cytokines, including a homolog of interleukin-6 that induces B-cell proliferation, and others that may activate angiogenesis.

Latency-associated nuclear antigen (LANA) can interact with p53 (Chapter 5) and inhibit transcriptional activity mediated by p53. There appear to be differences in expression of the HHV-8 proteins, depending on the type of cell that the virus infects. For example, viral interleukin-6 is found only in B cells and has been shown to be capable of inducing B-cell and plasma cell proliferation.

In the early stages KS behaves as a reactive, inflammatory, angio-proliferative lesion, triggered by HHV-8, and probably

* These proteins may disrupt control of cellular proliferation.

driven by high levels of cytokines such as interferon-γ, tumor necrosis factor (TNF), and interleukin-1. In AIDS-associated KS, the Tat protein may enhance angiogenesis. Early lesions are polyclonal and may regress. In time, lesions tend to become monoclonal and can evolve into a true sarcoma. This may be because of increased expression of proto-oncogenes such as Bcl-2, which is expressed in endothelial and spindle cells in KS lesions, and which inhibits apoptosis.

EPIDEMIOLOGY

Human herpesvirus type 8 variants

K1 is a highly variable gene that is subject to evolutionary pressure. Five major variants have been described A–E; B predominates in Africa, and B and C in Europe and the USA. There is a large repertoire of HHV-8 genotypes, but, although dual infection with different viral genotypes can occur, the development of most KSs and primary effusion lymphomas is associated with a single viral genotype[110].

Seroprevalence studies and risk factors for human herpesvirus type 8 infection

Indirect immunofluorescence assays (IFA) for LANA, and enzyme immunoassays (EIA), using recombinant antigens from HHV-8 ORF proteins 65.2 and K8.1A are useful for diagnostic and screening purposes, the combined use of EIA and IFA having a sensitivity of 94%[111].

Serological studies have shown that HHV-8 infection is widespread in Africa. For example in Uganda, the seroprevalence of HHV-8 among 82 HIV-infected and HIV-non-infected individuals with and without cancers was 66% by immunoblot LANA, and 51% by IFA[112]. Amongst black South African blood donors, about 20% are seropositive for HHV-8, compared with 5% of whites. The reasons for this difference in prevalence are unknown, but as in the case of hepatitis B virus infection, poverty and poor hygienic conditions increase the risk of infection[113]. Sexual activity appears to be less important in the transmission of the

virus in endemic areas such as Africa, many infections occurring in childhood[113]. In a study from French Guiana, the seroprevalence increased from 1.2% of children under the age of 5 years, to plateau at about 15% between the ages of 15 and 40 years[114]. These authors also noted a strong familial aggregation in HHV-8 seroprevalence, with high mother–child and sibling–sibling correlations; there was, however, no significant correlation between spouses. These data suggested that routes of transmission other than sexual are important in endemic areas. The low prevalence in children aged less than 5 years would imply that pregnancy and breast-feeding are not significant routes of transmission. In these circumstances spread of HHV-8 through saliva may be important (page 270).

In Italy and Greece the prevalence of specific antibodies against HHV-8 parallels the incidence of KS. In southern Italy, where the incidence of KS is moderately high, the seroprevalence of HHV-8 is between 10% and 35%[115]. Although sexual transmission may play a part in transmission of HHV-8 in these Mediterranean countries, non-sexual means of transmission are also possible. Such a hypothesis is supported by the finding of HHV-8-specific antibody in the serum of young children in southern Italy[116]. It is unknown how these children become infected but, as in Africa, saliva may be a vehicle of transmission.

HHV-8 infection is less prevalent in the USA and in northern Europe where the incidence of KS is lower than in Italy: less than 3% of blood donors in the UK and in the USA are found to be seropositive[111].

Amongst men who have sex with men, the seroprevalence of HHV-8 infection is significantly higher than in the general population. For example, Martin et al.[117] reported that 223 (37.6%) of 593 men in San Francisco had anti-LANA antibodies in their serum; none of the 195 exclusively heterosexual men were seropositive for anti-LANA. Evidence of infection was particularly noted amongst the 396 HIV-seropositive men, 47.7% of whom had anti-LANA. These authors also reported that there was a linear relationship between the prevalence of specific antibody against HHV-8 and the number of sexual partners, a finding that was confirmed by others[118, 119]. Amongst homosexual men, independent risk factors for HHV-8 include a past history of syphilis and of HSV-2 infection[120], and Dukers *et al.*[121] found that orogenital insertive sex (odds ratio 5.95, 95% confidence interval 2.88–12.29) and orogenital receptive oral sex (odds ratio 4.29, 95% confidence interval 2.11–8.71) were independently related to HHV-8 infection. An intriguing association was found between a history of deep kissing with an HIV-infected partner (odds ratio 5.4, 95% confidence interval, 1.3–22.7) and HHV-8 seropositivity[119]. The latter authors also noted an association between HHV-8 infection and a history of having a partner with KS, and the use of inhaled nitrites (odds ratio 5.1, 95% confidence interval 1.5–17.7). One unconfirmed study has suggested that oral–anal sexual contact may be a risk factor for HHV-8 infection[122].

These epidemiological data suggest that HHV-8 can be transmitted sexually, and in industrialized countries it is probably more readily transmitted through homosexual than through heterosexual activity[120]. As HHV-8 DNA is found uncommonly in cervicovaginal secretions[123] and in semen[124, 125], it has been postulated that other body fluids are more likely to transmit infection: human herpesvirus type 8 DNA has been detected in saliva from 18 (75%) of 24 HIV-infected patients with KS, three (15%) of 20 HIV-infected patients without KS, and from none of 24 control subjects[125]. Pauk and colleagues[119] investigated further mucosal shedding of HHV-8, and, using a quantitative PCR (HHV-8 cannot yet be cultured from specimens), found HHV-8 DNA significantly more frequently in oral cavity secretions than in anal or genital samples from a cohort of homosexual men. Overall, they identified viral DNA in 34% of 1134 oropharyngeal specimens, in 1% of 1087 anal samples, in 0.3% of 848 urethral samples, and in 5% of semen samples. In addition, they showed that HHV-8 DNA was present at higher titers in saliva samples than in other specimens, and that virus could be excreted for extended periods at high titer, in the absence of viral shedding from other anatomical sites. Human herpesvirus type 8 DNA was identified in buccal epithelial cells by *in situ* hybridization[119].

These data suggest that HHV-8 may be acquired through oral–oral contact, especially if there is high titer virus and persistent shedding. The reason for the relative rarity of HHV-8 infection in the general populations of the USA and of most European countries remains unexplained. It is possible, however, that the virus is not highly infectious and that transmission depends on the degree of exposure to infected persons, especially to those who are immunocompromised[119].

Recent data from the USA have shown that HHV-8 is transmissible through heterosexual sex. Cannon *et al.*[126] found a significant association between the seroprevalence of HHV-8 in women, and correlates of sexual activity, namely commercial sex and seropositivity for syphilis.

Viral DNA can be detected by PCR in the blood from 20% of homosexual men who are HIV-infected[127], but until recently, blood-borne transmission had not been clearly defined. In the study of risk factors for HHV-8 infection in women, there was an independent association between injecting drug use and HHV-8 seropositivity (odds ratio 3.2, 95% confidence interval 1.4–7.6)[126]. It was shown further, however, that HHV-8 is transmitted less efficiently than hepatitis B virus, hepatitis C virus, and HIV. These data also suggest that HHV-8 may be transmissible by blood transfusion, but the degree of risk is unknown.

Transplant recipients in industrialized nations can also be at risk of HHV-8 infection, both through primary infection from a donor or through reactivation of latent infection[128].

Association of human herpesvirus type 8 with Kaposi's sarcoma

Chang *et al.*[103] identified DNA sequences in KS skin lesions from a patient with HIV infection. Regardless of the clinical subtype, more than 95% of KS lesions are associated with HHV-8 infection. Immunosuppression is an important co-factor in the development of KS in HHV-8 infected patients. In the study reported by Martin *et al.*[117], amongst the men who had HIV and HHV-8 infections, the 10-year probability of KS was 49.6%. None of the HHV-8 seropositive

men who were anti-HIV negative developed KS, emphasizing the importance of HIV as a cofactor in the development of this neoplasm. O'Brien *et al.*[129] found that the seroprevalence of HHV-8 amongst 245 homosexual men in New York and Washington DC was 20.4% in 1982, and that, although the seroincidence was 15% during 1982–1983, it fell sharply thereafter. Amongst men who were seropositive for HHV-8, the 10-year cumulative risk of KS was 39%, the time from co-infection to KS ranging from 15 to 154 months (median 63.5 months). In a study from The Netherlands, it was shown that those who acquire HHV-8 after they have been infected with HIV are more likely to develop KS more rapidly than those whose HHV-8 infection has antedated the HIV infection[130].

Between 0.1% and 1% of transplant recipients in geographical areas with a low prevalence of HHV-8, develop KS[131], and in areas of high prevalence up to 5% develop the neoplasm[132].

The clinical features of KS in relation to HIV infection are described on pp. 155–156.

Human lymphotropic viruses

The human lymphotropic virus type I (HTLV-I) is a sexually transmissible retrovirus infection which can result in adult T-cell leukemia/lymphoma (ATLL) and tropical spastic paraparesis or HTLV-I-associated myelopathy (HAM/TSP). In endemic areas HTLV-II appears to be transmitted from mother-to-child, but in industrialized countries, injecting drug use is associated with its spread. The association of HTLV-II with disease is uncertain.

VIROLOGY

HTLV-I was first identified in 1980 in a patient with a T-cell lymphoma[133]. It is a complex type C retrovirus and is closely related to the family of Simian T-cell lymphotropic viruses (STLV) that have been found in many species of primates. These viruses are now classified in the genus deltaretrovirus. Analysis of molecular phylogenetics has revealed evidence of repeated interspecies transmissions, including humans and twenty primate species[134]. Genetically HTLV-II is closely related to HTVL-I.

HTLV-I and II are single-stranded, RNA viruses. The viral genome, consisting of 9032 nucleotides, contains *gag*, *pol*, and *env* genes, flanked by two long terminal repeats in which are contained the transcription initiation sequences, as well as the genes for two regulatory proteins – TAX and REX. TAX upregulates transcription, and is essential for viral replication. It is also strongly implicated in oncogenesis via induction of expression of a large number of cellular genes in the target cell infected by HTLV-I – the CD4$^+$ lymphocyte[135]. Transactivation of cellular genes results in cell proliferation, and with the production of provirus at each cell division, the pool of infected cells increases.

The life cycle is similar to that of other retroviruses: the virus enters a susceptible cell and RNA is released and transported to the nucleus. Proviral DNA is produced by reverse transcription and becomes integrated in a random fashion into the host cell genome. Transcription and translation of spliced RNA follow with the production of nucleocapsid proteins, enzymes, and envelope glycoproteins. REX down regulates transcription by reducing splicing of RNA, with a consequent reduction in viral protein production, including TAX.

IMMUNE RESPONSE TO HUMAN LYMPHOTROPIC VIRUS TYPE I

The first antibodies to become detectable after infection with HTLV-I are against *gag* protein, principally p24. Over the ensuing 2 months, anti-*env* antibodies develop and about 50% of individuals subsequently produce antibodies to the TAX protein[136].

During the chronic stage of infection, there is a strong cell-mediated immune response to HTLV-I, the anti-HTLV-I CD8$^+$ T cells, recognizing the TAX protein[137].

EPIDEMIOLOGY

HTLV-I is distributed worldwide with 15 to 20 million infected individuals. Infection is endemic in Japan, parts of the Caribbean and South America, as well as parts of Sub-Saharan Africa. In Europe and the USA, the virus is found in immigrants from endemic areas and amongst injecting drug users. Major routes of transmission are through breast feeding, and by sexual intercourse. Evidence of mother-to-child transmission was presented by Hino *et al.*[138] who found that two babies born to 38 HTLV-I seropositive women seroconverted between the ages of 12 and 19 months, and that 3 of 20 elder siblings were found to be seropositive between the ages of 3 and 6 years. They noted further that 12 of 13 mothers of seropositive students were HTLV-I seropositive. In a prospective study of 34 children born to HTLV-I seropositive women in Gabon, West Africa, Nyambi *et al.*[139] found that the risk of seroconversion over a 4-year period was 17.5%. As HTLV-I proviral DNA could not be detected in cord blood or in amniotic fluid, and because seroconversion occurred relatively late in these children, it was postulated that the virus was transmitted from mother-to-child postnatally, probably through breast milk. It has been shown that mother-to-child transmission can be reduced by limiting the duration of breast feeding. Working in a highly endemic area in Japan, Takezaki *et al.*[140] showed a significantly lower seroconversion rate amongst infants who were breast fed for 6 months or less (2 of 51 infants) compared with those who were fed for longer (13 of 64 infants). Wiktor *et al.*[141] made a similar observation, but also noted benefit from limiting the duration of breast feeding to less than 12 months.

Sexual transmission was shown clearly in the study reported by Stuver and colleagues[142] amongst Japanese married couples. Amongst the couples who were serodiscordant at entry into the study, there were seven seroconversions; the rate of transmission was 3.9 times higher if the carrier spouse was male. There is also a correlation between the HTLV-viral load and risk of transmission from a male to his partner[143]. In a group of men who attended a STI clinic in Jamaica, seropositivity for HTLV-I was associated with being married, being 15 years or older at the time of first sexual intercourse, and having a positive test for hepatitis B surface antigen[144]. Risk factors for women included having two or more sexual partners in the month preceding examination, being aged less than 15 years at sexual debut, and being seropositive for either HIV-1 or *Treponema pallidum*, or both. A recent study has shown that the seroprevalence of HTLV-I infection is higher in individuals who have serological evidence of syphilis than in HTLV-I non-infected people, and that the prevalence of HTLV-I is higher amongst homosexual men than amongst heterosexual men[145].

It is probable that HTLV-I can be transmitted through injecting drug use. Schwebke *et al.*[146] identified HTLV infection in 16.5% of 213 intravenous drug users in Seattle, USA: 11% of infections were with HTLV-1, the others being infected with the closely related virus, HTLV-II. They also noted a strong association with hepatitis B virus infection, a marker for unsafe injecting behavior. In a cross-sectional study of 499 HIV-infected individuals in Santos, Brazil, 6% were seropositive for HTLV-I, and injecting drug use was found to be an independent risk factor for this infection (odds ratio 2.99, 95% confidence interval 1.09–8.20)[147].

Transmission of infection via blood products is also possible. In Jamaica, seroconversion occurred amongst 24 (44%) of 54 recipients of HTLV-I-positive cellular blood products, but not amongst any of 12 recipients of non-cellular donor units, or amongst any of 52 HTLV-I-negative donor units[148].

Less is known about the epidemiology of HTLV-II infection because it has been difficult to differentiate infection with this virus and HTLV-I by standard serological tests. It appears to be common among several Amer-indian tribes of North, Central, and South America[149], amongst Pygmies in central Africa, and in Melanesia. Mother-to-child transmission can be shown in these populations. Vitek *et al.*[150] found that 36 of 219 children aged 1 to 10 years had been born to HTLV-II seropositive mothers, compared with only 3 of 997 born to seronegative mothers. Sexual transmission in endemic areas also seems to play a part in the spread of the virus: infection rates increase with age, beginning in early adulthood, and there is a strong association between HTLV-II infection and infection in a sexual partner[150]. In non-endemic areas, the prevalence of HTLV infections depends on several factors, including the prevalence of injecting drug use, and the extent of immigration from countries where the viruses are endemic. For example, amongst 20 366 pregnant women in Spain, 11 (0.054%) were seropositive for HTLV-II, compared with only 2 (0.01%) who had HTLV-1 infection[151]. All 11 HTLV-II infected women were Spanish, and 10 women had injected drugs. In contrast, in the UK, antibody against HTLV-I predominated (59) in the blood of infants born to 126 010 women; only 2 had HTLV-II infection[152]. The prevalence of HTLV-I antibody was highest amongst infants born to mothers born in the Caribbean (17.0 per 1000). A high prevalence of HTLV-II infection has been found amongst injecting drug users in both the USA and in Europe. For example Egan et al.[153] from Dublin, found that 15 (14%) of 103 HIV-1-infected injecting drug users were seropositive for HTLV-II. Phylogenetic analysis of the nucleotides of the long terminal repeat showed that most subjects were infected with the HTLV-IIa subtype. This subtype predominates amongst injecting drug users in the USA, and is distinct from the HTLV-II β subtype that is prevalent in southern Europe, and in many areas in Central and South America. A recent study has shown that individuals infected with HIV are more likely to be infected with HTLV-II than HIV-seronegative individuals[145]. Unlike HTLV-I, these authors did not find an association between HTLV-II seropositivity and positive treponemal serology.

DIAGNOSIS

The diagnosis of HTLV infections is confirmed serologically. Antibodies can be detected by EIA or gelatin particle agglutination, using recombinant peptides as antigen. Various commercial kits for the detection of HTLV-I antibodies are available, and, compared with earlier assays, have high sensitivity for the detection of HTLV-II antibodies. Positive test results are confirmed by western blot that incorporates HTLV-I and HTLV-II antigens on a nitrocellulose strip. The patterns on western blotting can distinguish between these viral infections[154]. In HIV-infected individuals, EIAs may give false negative results[155].

A polymerase chain reaction can be used to confirm viral type (and subtype), and to measure plasma viral load[156, 157].

CLINICAL ASPECTS OF HUMAN LYMPHOTROPIC VIRUS TYPE I INFECTION

The two major sequelae are ATLL and HTLV-I associated myelopathy/tropical spastic paraparesis (HAM/TSP). The HTLV proviral load varies among those infected, with high levels carrying a greater likelihood of disease[158].

Adult T-cell leukemia/lymphoma

The lifetime risk of ATLL for an individual infected with HTLV-I before the age of 20 years is about 5%, with approximately 0.1% annual incidence[159]. Symptoms are those of a non-Hodgkin's lymphoma. About 40% of cases have widespread or localized skin lesions at diagnosis. Large nodules, plaques, ulcers, and a generalized papular rash are common lesions, and may appear on the limbs, trunk, or face. Lymphadenopathy, hepatosplenomegaly, and hypercalcemia are also common. Immunosuppression is well documented, manifesting as bacterial and opportunistic infections which contribute to a poor prognosis. The leukemic cells are CD4+, and are usually CD25+.

Treatment

Standard chemotherapy for non-Hodgkin lymphoma is ineffective in ATLL. The median survival for acute and lymphoma subtypes is less than a year; patients with chronic ATLL may survive longer. A combination of interferon-α and zidovudine has been found effective[160, 161], but randomized trials comparing this regimen with standard therapy for non-Hodgkin lymphoma have not been undertaken.

Human lymphotropic virus type I associated myelopathy/tropical spastic paraparesis

Human lymphotropic virus type I associated myelopathy/tropical spastic paraparesis presents as a progressive spastic paraparesis, incontinence, and paresthesiae. Examination may reveal weakness, hyperreflexia, clonus, and extensor plantar reflex. The rate of progression and degree of disability are variable. Women are more commonly affected than men, although the reason for this is not clear[162]. Co-infection with HIV may result in more rapid progression of HAM/TSP[163].

There are scattered lesions of demyelination throughout the cerebrum, and the lower cervical and upper thoracic spinal cord. There is an infiltration of predominantly CD8+ T cells into these areas[164]. The pathogenesis of HAM/TSP is uncertain. It has been postulated that the CNS is damaged by lymphocytes that are chronically activated by the HTLV-I TAX protein. These cells migrate to the CNS as a result of TAX-induced upregulation of adhesion molecules on their surface. Large amount of cytokines secreted from these activated lymphocytes may damage neural tissue[136].

Other conditions

Other diseases in which HTLV-1 is implicated include polymyositis, arthropathy, uveitis, and infective dermatitis[165].

HUMAN LYMPHOTROPIC VIRUS TYPE II INFECTIONS

The clinical manifestations of this virus infection have not been clearly defined, although rare cancers associated with HTLV-II have been described in which CD8+ cells predominate.

References

1 Thompson CH, Yager JA, Van Rensburg IB. Close relationship between equine and human molluscum contagiosum virus demonstrated by in situ hybridisation. *Res Vet Sci* 1998; **64**: 157–161.

2 Fenner F. Poxvirus. In: Fields BN (ed.) *Virology*. Raven Press; New York: 1985, pp. 661–684.

3 Nakamura J, Muraki Y, Yamada M, Hatano Y, Nii S. Analysis of moluscum contagiosum virus genomes isolated in Japan. *J Med Virol* 1995; **46**: 339–348.

4 Birthistle K, Carrington D. Molluscum contagiosum virus. *J Infect* 1997; **34**: 21–28.

5 Porter CD, Muhlmann MF, Cream JJ, Archard LC. Molluscum contagiosum: characterization of viral DNA and clinical features. *Epidemiol Infect* 1987; **99**: 563–567.

6 Smith KJ, Yeager J, Skelton H. Molluscum contagiosum: its clinical, histopathologic, and immunohistochemical spectrum. *Int J Dermatol* 1999; **38**: 664–672.

7 Bhawan J, Dayal Y, Bhan AK. Langerhans cells in molluscum contagiosum, verruca vulgaris, plantar wart, and condyloma acuminatum. *J Am Acad Dermatol* 1986; **15**: 645–649.

8 Heng MCY, Steuer ME, Levy A, *et al.* Lack of host cellular immune response in eruptive molluscum contagiosum. *Am J Dermatopathol* 1989; **11**: 248–254.

9 Viac J, Chardonnet Y. Immunocompetent cells and epithelial cell modifications in molluscum contagiosum. *J Cutan Pathol* 1990; **17**: 202–205.

10 Henao M, Freeman RG. Inflamatory molluscum contagiosum: clinicopathological study of seven cases. *Arch Dermatol* 1964; **90**: 479–482.

11 Steffen C, Markman J. Spontaneous disappearance of molluscum contagiosum. *Arch Dermatol* 1980; **116**: 923–924.

12 Konya J, Thompson CH. Molluscum contagiosum virus: antibody response in persons with clinical lesions and seroepidemiology in a representative Australian population. *J Infect Dis* 1999; **179**: 701–704.

13 Postlethwaite R. Molluscum contagiosum: a review. *Arch Environ Health* 1970; **21**: 432–452.

14 Postlethwaite R, Watt JA, Hawley TG, Simpson I, Adam H. Features of molluscum contagiosum in the north-east of Scotland and in Fijian village settlements. *J Hyg* 1967; **65**: 281–291.

15 Murray MJ, Murray AB, Murray NJ, Murray MB, Murray CJ. Molluscum contagiosum and herpes simplex in Massai pastoralists: refeeding activation of virus infection following famine? *Trans R Soc Trop Med Hyg* 1980; **74**: 371–374.

16 Wilkin JK. Molluscum contagiosum venereum in a woman's out-patient clinic: a venereally transmitted disease. *Am J Obstet Gynecol* 1977; **128**: 531–535.

17 Radcliffe KW, Daniels D, Evans BA. Molluscum contagiosum: a neglected sentinel infection. *Int J STD AIDS* 1991; **2**: 416–418.

18 Becker TM, Blount JH, Douglas J, Judson FN. Trends in molluscum contagiosum in the United States, 1966–1983. *Sex Transm Dis* 1986; **13**: 88–92.

19 Foulds IS. Molluscum contagiosum: an unusual complication of tattooing. *Br Med J* 1982; **285**: 607.

20 Low RC. Molluscum contagiosum. *Edinburgh Med J* 1946; **53**: 657–670.

21 Scholz J, Rosen-Wolff A, Bugert J, *et al.* Molecular epidemiology of molluscum contagiosum. *J Infect Dis* 1988; **158**: 898–900.

22 Thompson CH, de Zwart-Steffe RT, Biggs IA. Molecular epidemiology of Australian isolates of molluscum contagiosum. *J Med Virol* 1990; **32**: 1–9.

23 Yamashita H, Uemura T, Kawashima M. Molecular epidemiologic analysis of Japanese patients with molluscum contagiosum. *Int J Dermatol* 1996; **35**: 99–1105.

24 Porter CD, Blake MW, Cream JJ, Archard LC. Molluscum contagiosum virus. In: Wright D, Archard L, (eds) *Molecular and Cell Biology of Sexually Transmitted Diseases*. London: Chapman and Hall: 1992, pp. 233–257.

25 Matis WL, Triana A, Shapiro R, Eldred L, Polk BF, Hood AF. Dermatologic findings associated with human immunodeficiency virus infection. *J Am Acad Dermatol* 1987; **17**: 746–751.

26 Thompson CH, de Zwart-Steffe RT, Donovan B. Clinical and molecular aspects of molluscum contagiosum infection in HIV-1 positive patients. *Int J STD AIDS* 1992; **3**: 101–106.

27 Goldschmidt H, Kligman AM. Molluscum contagiosum. *J Invest Dermatol* 1958; **31**: 175–179.

28 Woods B. Edward Jenner and molluscum contagiosum. *Br J Dermatol* 1977; **96**: 91–93.

29 Field LM, Johnson ML. Questions and answers: molluscum contagiosum reaction. *JAMA* 1980; **243**: 2526.

30 De Oreo GA, Johnson HH, Binkley GW. An eczematous reaction associated with molluscum contagiosum. *Arch Dermatol* 1956; **74**: 344–348.

31 Blattner RJ. Molluscum contagiosum infection in atopic dermatitis. *J Pediatr* 1967; **10**: 997–999.

32 Pauly CR, Artis WM, Jones HE. Atopic dermatitis, impaired cellular immunity, and molluscum contagiosum. *Arch Dermatol* 1978; **114**: 391–393.

33 Romagnani S, Del Prete G, Ravina MA, *et al.* Role of Th$_1$/Th$_2$ cytokines in HIV infection. *Immunol Rev* 1994; **140**: 73–92.

34 Kristal L, Clark RAF. Atopic dermatitis. In: Arndt KA, LeBoit PE, Robinson JK, Wintroub BU (eds) *Cutaneous Medicine and Surgery*. Philadelphia; WB Saunders: 1996, pp. 195–204.

35 Schwartz JJ, Myskowski PL. Molluscum contagiosum in patients with human immunodeficiency virus infection. *J Am Acad Dermatol* 1992; **27**: 583–588.

36 Ogg GS, Coleman R, Rosbotham JC, MacDonald DM. Atypical molluscum contagiosum – a diagnostic problem. *Acta Dermatovenereol* 1997; **77**: 77–78.

37 Hurni MA, Bohlen L, Furrer H, Braathen LR. Complete regression of giant molluscum contagiosum lesions in an HIV-infected patient following combined antiretroviral therapy with saquinavir, zidovudine and lamivudine. *AIDS* 1997; **11**: 1784–1785.

38 Tschachler E, Bergstresser PR, Stingl G. HIV-related skin diseases. *Lancet* 1996; **348**: 659–663.

39 Itin PH, Gilli L. Molluscum contagiosum mimicking sebaceous nevus of Jadassohn, ecthyma and giant condylomata acuminata in HIV-infected patients. *Dermatology* 1994; **189**: 396–398.

40 Brown TJ, Yen-Moore A, Tyring SK. An overview of sexually transmitted diseases. Part II. *J Am Acad Dermatol* 1999; **41**: 661–677.

41 Weller R, O'Callaghan CJ, MacSween RM, White M. Scarring in molluscum contagiosum: comparison of physical expression and phenol ablation. *Br Med J* 1999; **391**: 1540.

42 Syed TA, Goswami J, Ahmadpour OA, Ahmad SA. Treatment of molluscum contagiosum in males with an analog of imiquimod 1% in cream: a placebo-controlled study. *J Dermatol* 1998; **25**: 309–313.

43 Smith KJ, Skelton HG, Yaeger J, James WD, Wagner KF. Molluscum contagiosum: ultrastructural evidence for its presence in skin adjacent to clinical lesions in patients infected with human immunodeficiency virus type 1. *Arch Dermatol* 1992; **128**: 223–227.

44 Horn CK, Scott GR, Benton EC. Resolution of severe molluscum contagiosum on

effective antiretroviral therapy. *Br J Dermatol* 1998; **138**: 715–717.

45 Cattelan AM, Sasset L, Corti L, Stiffan S, Meneghetti F, Cadrobbi P. A complete remission of recalcitrant molluscum contagiosum in an AIDS patient following highly active antiretroviral therapy (HAART). *J Infect* 1999; **38**: 58–60.

46 Meadows KP, Tyring SK, Pavia AT, Rallis TM. Resolution of recalcitrant molluscum contagiosum virus lesions in human immunodeficiency virus-infected patients treated with cidofovir. *Arch Dermatol* 1997; **133**: 987–990.

47 Cotton DWK, Cooper C, Barrett DF, Leppard BJ. Severe atypical molluscum contagiosum infection in an immunocompromised host. *Br J Dermatol* 1987; **116**: 871–876.

48 Mayuma H, Yamaoka K, Tsutsui T, *et al.* Selective immunoglobulin M deficiency associated with disseminated molluscum contagiosum. *Eur J Pediatr* 1986; **145**: 99–103.

49 Hellier FF. Profuse mollusca contagiosa of the face induced by corticosteroids. *Br J Dermatol* 1971; **85**: 398.

50 Rosenberg EW, Yusk JW. Molluscum contagiosum: eruption following treatment with prednisolone and methotrexate. *Arch Dermatol* 1970; **101**: 439–441.

51 Sairenji T, Kurata T. Immune responses to Epstein–Barr viral infection. In: Medveczky PG, Friedman H, Bendinelli M (ed.) *Herpesviruses and Immunity.* New York. Plenum Press. 1998.

52 Golden HD, Chang RS, Prescott W, Simpson E, Cooper TY. Leukocyte-transforming agent: prolonged excretion by patients with mononucleosis and excretion by normal individuals. *J Infect Dis* 1973; **127**: 471–473.

53 Anagnostopoulos I, Hummel M, Kreschel C, Stein H. Morphology, immunophenotype, and distribution of latently and/or productively Epstein–Barr virus-infected cells in acute infectious mononucleosis: implications for the interindividual infection route of Epstein–Barr virus. *Blood* 1995; **85**: 744–750.

54 Ward PL, Roizman B. Evasion and obstruction: the central strategy if the interaction of human herpesviruses with host defenses. In: Medveczky PG, Friedman H, Bendinelli M (ed.) *Herpesviruses and Immunity.* New York; Plenum Press: 1998.

55 Thorley-Lawson DA. EBV persistence *in vivo.* Invading and avoiding the immune response. In: Medveczky PG, Friedman H, Bendinelli M (ed.) *Herpesviruses and Immunity.* New York; Plenum Press: 1998.

56 Portnoy J, Ahronheim GA, Ghiba F, Clecner B, Joncas JH. Recovery of Epstein–Barr virus from genital ulcers. *N Engl J Med* 1984; **311**: 966.

57 Sixbey JW, Lemon SM, Pagano JS. A second site for Epstein–Barr virus shedding: the uterine cervix. *Lancet* 1986; **ii**: 1122–1124.

58 Cameron SJ, Richmond J. Ampicillin hypersensitivity in lymphatic leukaemia. *Scott Med J* 1971; **10**: 425–427.

59 Brown ZA, Stenchever MA. Genital ulceration and infectious mononucleosis: report of a case. *Am J Obstet Gynecol* 1977; **127**: 673–674.

60 Lawee D, Shaffir MS. Solitary penile ulcer associated with infectious mononucleosis. *Can Med Assoc J* 1983; **129**: 146–147.

61 Epstein MA, Achong BG. Pathogenesis of infectious mononucleosis. *Lancet* 1977; **ii**: 1270–1273.

62 Hamblin TJ, Hussain J, Akbar AN, Tang YC, Smith JL, Jones DB. Immunological reason for chronic ill health after infectious mononucleosis. *Br Med J* 1983; **287**: 85–88.

63 Klein G. EBV and B cell lymphomas. In: Medveczky PG, Friedman H, Bendinelli M (ed.) *Herpesviruses and Immunity.* New York; Plenum Press: 1998.

64 Roizman B, Carmichael LE, Deinhart F, *et al.* Herpesviridae: definition, provisional nomenclature, and taxonomy. *Intervirology* 1981; **16**: 201–217.

65 Soderberg-Naucler C, Fish KN, Nelson JA. Reactivation of latent human cytomegalovirus by allogeneic stimulation of blood cells from healthy donors. *Cell* 1997; **91**: 119–126.

66 Weller TH. The cytomegaloviruses: ubiquitous agents with protean clinical manifestations. *N Engl J Med* 1971; **285**: 203–214; 267–274.

67 Emery VC, Cope AV, Bowen EF, Gor D, Griffiths PD. The dynamics of human cytomegalovirus replication in vivo. *J Exp Med* 1999; **190**: 177–182.

68 Mocarski ES. Cytomegaloviruses and their replication. In: Fields BN, Knope DM, Howley PM (eds). Fields *Virology* 3rd edition. Philadelphia; Lippincott-Raven: 1996.

69 Ward PL, Roizman B. Evasion and obstruction. The central strategy of the interaction of herpesviruses with host defences. In: Medveczky PG, Friedman H, Bendinelli M (ed.) *Herpesviruses and Immunity.* New York; Plenum Press: 1998.

70 Hengel H, Koszinowski UL. Inhibition of MHC class I function by cytomegalovirus. In: Medveczky PG, Friedman H, Bendinelli M (ed.) *Herpesviruses and Immunity.* New York; Plenum Press: 1998.

71 Wiley CA, Nelson JA. Role of human immunodeficiency virus and cytomegalovirus in AIDS encephalitis. *Am J Pathol* 1988; **133**: 73–81.

72 Britt WJ. Congenital cytomegalovirus infection. In: Hitchcock PJ, MacKay HT, Wasserheit JN (eds). *Sexually Transmitted*

Diseases and Adverse Outcomes of Pregnancy. Washington DC; ASM Press: 1999.

73 Fowler KB, Stagno S, Pass RF, Britt WJ, Boll TJ, Alford CA. The outcome of congenital cytomegalovirus infection in relation to maternal antibody status. *N Engl J Med* 1992; **326**: 663–667.

74 Stern H. Cytomegalovirus vaccine. Justification and problems. In: Waterson AP (ed.) *Recent Advances in Clinical Virology.* Edinburgh; Churchill Livingstone: 1977.

75 Montgomery R, Youngblood L, Medearis DN. Recovery of cytomegalovirus from the cervix of pregnancy. *Pediatrics* 1972; **49**: 524–531.

76 Pass RF, Little EA, Stagno S, Britt WJ, Alford CA. Young children as a probable source of maternal and congenital cytomegalovirus infection. *N Engl J Med* 1987; **316**: 1366–1370.

77 Stagno S, Pass RF, Dworsky ME, *et al.* Congenital cytomegalovirus infection: the relative importance of primary and recurrent maternal infection. *N Engl J Med* 1982; **306**: 945–949.

78 Stagno S, Pass RF, Cloud G, *et al.* Primary cytomegalovirus infection in pregnancy. Incidence, transmission to fetus, and clinical outcome. *JAMA* 1986; **256**: 1904–1908.

79 Fowler KB, Pass RF, Stagno S. Congenital cytomegalovirus infection risk in future pregnancies and maternal CMV infection. Abstract 191. In 6th *International Cytomegalovirus Workshop*: 1997.

80 Boppana SB, Britt WJ. Antiviral antibody responses and intrauterine transmission following primary maternal cytomegalovirus infection. *J Infect Dis* 1995; **171**: 26–32.

81 Dworsky M, Yow M, Stagno S, Pass R, Alford CA. Cytomegalovirus in breast milk and transmission to the infant. *Pediatric Research* 1982; **16**: 239A.

82 Harris JRW. Cytomegalovirus. In: Morton RS, Harris JRW (eds) *Recent Advances in Sexually Transmitted Diseases.* Edinburgh; Churchill Livingstone: 1975.

83 Handsfield HH, Chandler SH, Caine VA, *et al.* Cytomegalovirus infection in sex partners: evidence for sexual transmission. *J Infect Dis* 1985; **151**: 344–364.

84 Lang DJ, Kummer JF, Hartley DP. Cytomegalovirus in semen. Persistence and demonstration in extracellular fluids. *N Engl J Med* 1974; **291**: 121–123.

85 Oill PA, Fiala M, Schofferman J, Byfield PE, Guze LB. Cytomegalovirus mononucleosis in a healthy adult. Association with hepatitis, secondary Epstein Barr virus antibody response and immunosuppression. *Am J Med* 1977; **62**: 413–417.

86 Chandler SH, Holmes KK, Wentworth BB, *et al.* The epidemiology of cytomegaloviral

infection in women attending a sexually transmitted diseases clinic. *J Infect Dis* 1985; **152**: 597–605.

87 Biggar RJ, Anderson HK, Ebbesen P, *et al.* Seminal fluid excretion of cytomegalovirus related to immunosuppression in homosexual men. *Br Med J* 1983; **286**: 2010–2012.

88 Mintz L, Drew WL, Minec RC, Braff EH. Cytomegalovirus infections in homosexual men. An epidemiological study. *Ann Int Med* 1983; **99**: 326–329.

89 Coutinho RA, Wertheim-van Dillen P, Albrecht van Lent P, *et al.* Infection with cytomegalovirus in homosexual men. *Br J Vener Dis* 1984; **60**: 249–252.

90 Drew ML, Mintz RC, Miner L, Sands M, Ketterer B. Prevalence of cytomegalovirus in homosexual men. *J Infect Dis* 1981; **143**: 188–192.

91 Gallant JE, Moore RD, Richman DD, Keruly J, Chaisson RE. Incidence and natural history of cytomegalovirus disease in patients with advanced human immunodeficiency virus disease treated with zidovudine. *J Infect Dis* 1992; **166**: 1223–1227.

92 Landini MP, Guan MX, Jahn G, *et al.* Large-scale screening of human sera with cytomegalovirus recombinant antigens. *J Clin Microbiol* 1990; **28**: 1375–1379.

93 Stagno S, Tinker MK, Elrod C, Fuccillo D, Cloud G, O'Beirne AJ. Immunoglobulin M antibodies detected by enzyme-linked immunosorbent assay and radioimmunoassay in the diagnosis of cytomegalovirus infections in pregnant women and newborn infants. *J Clin Microbiol* 1985; **21**: 930–935.

94 Lazzarotto T, dalla Case B, Campisi B, Landini MP. Enzyme-linked immunosorbent assay for the detection of cytomegalovirus-IgM: comparison between eight commercial kits, immunofluorescence and immunoblotting. *J Clin Anal* 1992; **6**: 216–218.

95 Lazzarotto T, Varani S, Guerra A, Nicolosi A, Lanari M, Landini MP. Prenatal predictors of congenital cytomegalovirus infection. *J Pediatr* 2000; **137**: 90–95.

96 Alford CA, Britt WJ. Cytomegalovirus. In: Fields BN (ed.) *Virology*. New York; Raven Press; 1985.

97 Warren WP, Balcarek K, Smith R, Pass RF. Comparison of rapid methods of detection of cytomegalovirus in saliva with virus isolation in tissue culture. *J Clin Microbiol* 1992; **30**: 786–789.

98 Cotte L, Drouet E, Bissuel F, Denoyel GA, Trepo C. Diagnostic value of amplification of cytomegalovirus DNA from gastrointestinal biopsies from human immunodeficiency virus-infected patients. *J Clin Microbiol* 1993; **31**: 2066–2069.

99 Bowen EF, Sabin CA, Wilson P, *et al.* Cytomegalovirus (CMV) viraemia detected by polymerase chain reaction identifies a group of HIV-positive patients at high risk of CMV disease. *AIDS* 1997; **11**: 889–893.

100 Adler SP, Plotkin SA, Gonezol T, *et al.* A canarypox vector expressing cytomegalovirus (CMV) glycoprotein B primes for antibody responses to a live attenuated CMV vaccine (Towne). *J Infect Dis* 1999; **180**: 843–846.

101 Walter EA, Greenberg PD, Gilbert MJ, *et al.* Reconstitution of cellular immunity against cytomegalovirus in recipients of allogeneic bone marrow by transfer of T-cell clones from donor. *N Engl J Med* 1995; **333**: 1038–1044.

102 Friedman-Kien AE, Lauabenstein L, Marmor M, *et al.* Kaposi's sarcoma and Pneumocystis pneumonia among homosexual men – New York City and California. *MMWR* 1981; **30**: 305–308.

103 Chang Y, Cesarman E, Pessin MS, *et al.* Identification of herpesvirus-like DNA sequences in AIDS-associated Kaposi's sarcoma. *Science* 1994; **266**: 1865–1869.

104 Lacoste V, Mauclere P, Dubreuil P, Lewis J, Georges-Courbot MC, Gessain A. KSHV-viruses in chimps and gorillas. *Nature* 2000; **407**: 151–152.

105 Greenshill J, Schulz TF. Rhadinoviruses (γ2-herpesviruses) of old world primates: models for KSHV/HHV8-associated disease? *AIDS* 2000; **14**: S11–19.

106 Cesarman E, Chang Y, Moore PS, Said JW, Knowles DM. Kaposi's sarcoma-associated herpesvirus-like DNA sequences in AIDS-related body-cavity-based lymphomas. *N Engl J Med* 1995; **332**: 1186–1191.

107 Soulier J, Grollet L, Oskenhendler E, *et al.* Kapsoi's sarcoma-associated herpesvirus-like DNA sequences in multicentric Castleman's disease. *Blood* 1995; **86**: 1276–1280.

108 Schulz TF. KSHV (HHV8) infection. *J Infect* 2000; **41**: 125–129.

109 Antman K, Chang Y. Kaposi's sarcoma. *N Engl J Med* 2000; **342**: 1027–1038.

110 Gao S-J, Zhang YJ, Deng JH, Rabkin CS, Flore O, Jenson HB. Molecular polymorphism of Kaposi's sarcoma-associated herpesvirus (human herpesvirus 8) latent nuclear antigen: evidence for a large repertoire of viral genotypes and dual infection with different viral genotypes. *J Infect Dis* 1999; **180**: 1466–1476.

111 Simpson GR, Schulz TF, Whitby D, *et al.* Prevalence of Kaposi's sarcoma-associated herpesvirus infection measured by antibodies to recombinant capsid protein and latent immunofluorescence antigen. *Lancet* 1996; **348**: 1133–1138.

112 Gao S-J, Kingsley L, Li M, *et al.* KSHV antibodies among Americans, Italians and Ugandans with and without Kaposi's sarcoma. *Nature Med* 1996; **2**: 925–928.

113 Moore PS. The emrgence of Kaposi's sarcoma-associated herpesvirus (human herpesvirus 8). *N Engl J Med* 2001; **343**: 1411–1413.

114 Plancoulaine S, Abel L, van Bevern M, *et al.* Human herpesvirus 8 transmission from mother to child and between siblings in an endemic population. *Lancet* 2000; **356**: 1062–1065.

115 Rein MF (ed.). *Atlas of Infectious Diseases, Volume V. Sexually Transmitted Diseases*. Churchill Livingstone; Philadelphia; 1996.

116 Whitby D, Luppi M, Sabin C, *et al.* Detection of antibodies to human herpesvirus 8 in Italian children: evidence for horizontal transmission. *Br J Cancer* 2000; **82**: 702–704.

117 Martin JN, Ganem DE, Osmond DH, Page-Shafer KA, Macrae D, Kedes DH. Sexual transmission and the natural history of human herpesvirus 8 infection. *N Engl J Med* 1998; **338**: 948–954.

118 Blackbourn DJ, Osmond D, Levy JA, Lennette ET. Increased human herpesvirus 8 seroprevalence in young homosexual men who have multiple sex contacts with different partners. *J Infect Dis* 1999; **179**: 237–239.

119 Pauk J, Huang M-L, Brodie SJ, *et al.* Mucosal shedding of human herpesvirus 8 in men. *N Engl J Med* 2000; **343**: 1369–1377.

120 Smith NA, Sabin CA, Gopal R. *et al.* Serologic evidence of human herpesvirus 8 transmission by homosexual but not heterosexual sex. *J Infect Dis* 1999; **180**: 600–606.

121 Dukers NH, Renwick N, Prins M, *et al.* Risk factors for human herpesvirus 8 seropositivity and seroconversion in a cohort of homosexual men. *Am J Epidemiol* 2000; **151**: 213–224.

122 Grulich AE, Olsen SJ, Luo K, *et al.* Kaposi's sarcoma-associated herpesvirus: a sexually transmissible infection? *J Acquir Immune Defic Syndr Hum Retrovirol* 1999; **20**: 387–393.

123 Calabro ML, Fiore JR, Facero A, *et al.* Detection of human herpesvirus 8 in cervicovaginal secretions and seroprevalence in human immunodeficiency virus type 1-seropositive and -seronegative women. *J Infect Dis* 1999; **179**: 1534–1537.

124 Diamond C, Huang ML, Kedes DH, *et al.* Absence of detectable human herpesvirus 8 in the semen of human immunodeficiency virus-infected men without Kaposi's sarcoma. *J Infect Dis* 1997; **176**: 775–777.

125 Koelle DM, Huang M-L, Chandran B, Vieira J, Piepkorn M, Corey L. Frequent detection of Kaposi's sarcoma-associated herpesvirus (human herpesvirus 8) DNA in saliva of human immunodeficiency virus-infected men: clinical and immunologic correlates. *J Infect Dis* 1997; **176**: 94–102.

126 Cannon MJ, Dollard SC, Smith DK, *et al*. Blood-borne and sexual transmission of human herpesvirus 8 in women with or without risk for human immunodeficiency virus infection. *N Engl J Med* 2001; **344**: 637–643.

127 Whitby D, Howard MR, Tennant-Flowers M, *et al*. Detection of Kaposi's sarcoma-associated herpesvirus in peripheral blood of HIV-infected individuals and progression to Kaposi's sarcoma. *Lancet* 1995; **346**: 799–802.

128 Luppi M, Barozzi P, Sculz TF, *et al*. Bone marrow failure associated with human herpesvirus 8 infection after transplantation. *N Engl J Med* 2000; **343**: 1378–1385.

129 O'Brien TR, Kedes D, Ganem D, *et al*. Evidence for concurrent epidemics of human herpesvirus 8 and human immunodeficiency virus type 1 in US homosexual men: rates, risk factors, and relationship to Kaposi's sarcoma. *J Infect Dis* 1999; **180**: 1010–1017.

130 Renwick N, Halaby T, Weverling GJ. Seroconversion for Kaposi's sarcoma-associated herpesvirus is highly predictive of KS development in HIV-1 infected individuals. *AIDS* 1998; **12**: 2481–2488.

131 Farge D. Kaposi's sarcoma in organ transplant recipients. *Eur J Med* 1993; **2**: 339–343.

132 Lesnoni La Parola I, Masini C, Nanni G, Diociaiuti A, Panocchia N, Cerimele D. Kaposi's sarcoma in renal-transplant recipients: experience at the Catholic University in Rome. *Dermatology* 1997; **194**: 229–233.

133 Poiesz BJ, Ruscetti FW, Gazdar AF, Bunn PA, Minna JD, Gallo RC. Detection and isolation of type C retrovirus particles from fresh and cultured lymphocytes of a patient with cutaneous T-cell lymphoma. *Proc Natl Acad Sci USA* 1980; **77**: 7415–7419.

134 Slattery JP, Franchini G, Gessain A. Genomic evolution, patterns of global dissemination, and interspecies transmission of human and simian T-cell leukaemia/lymphotropic viruses. *Genome Res* 1999; **9**: 525–540.

135 Franchini G. Molecular mechanisms of human T-cell leukaemia/lymphotropic virus type 1 infection. *Blood* 1995; **6**: 3619–3639.

136 Bangham CRM. HTLV-I infections. *J Clin Pathol* 2000; **53**: 581–586.

137 Bangham CRM, Hall SE, Jeffery KJM, *et al*. Genetic control and dynamics of the cellular immune response to the human T-cell leukaemia virus HTLV-I. *Philos Trans R Soc Lond Ser B Biol Sci* 1999; **354**: 691–700.

138 Hino S, Yamaguchi K, Katamine S, *et al*. Mother-to-child transmission of human T cell leukemia virus type-I. *Jpn J Cancer Res (Gann)* 1985; **76**: 474–480.

139 Nyambi PN, Ville Y, Louwagie J, *et al*. Mother-to-child transmission of human T-cell lymphotropic virus types I and II (HTLV-I/II) in Gabon: a prospective follow-up of 4 years. *J Acquir Immun Def Syndr* 1996; **12**: 187–192.

140 Takezaki T, Tajima K, Ito M, *et al*. Short-term breast-feeding may reduce the risk of vertical transmission of HTLV-1. The Tsushima Study Group. *Leukemia* 1997; **11** (Suppl. 3): 60–62.

141 Wiktor SZ, Pate EJ, Rosenbereg PS, *et al*. Mother-to-child transmission of human T-cell lymphotropic virus type I associated with prolonged breast feeding. *J Hum Virol* 1997; **1**: 37–44.

142 Stuver SO, Tachibana N, Okayama A, *et al*. Heterosexual transmission of human T cell leukemia/lymphoma virus type I among married couples in southwestern Japan: an initial report from the Miyazaki cohort study. *J Infect Dis* 1993; **167**: 57–65.

143 Kaplan JE, Khabbaz RF, Murphy EL, *et al*. Male-to-female transmission of human T-cell lymphotropic virus types I and II association with viral load. The Retrovirus Epidemiology Donor Study Group. *J Acquir Immune Defic Syndr* 1996; **12**: 193–201.

144 Figueroa JP, Morris J, Brathwate A, *et al*. Risk factors for HTLV-I among heterosexual STD clinic attenders. *J Acquir Immune Defic Syndr* 1995; **9**: 81–88.

145 Giuliani M, Rezza G, Lepri C, *et al*. Risk factors for HTLV-I and II in individuals attending a clinic for sexually transmitted diseases. *Sex Transm Dis* 2000; **27**: 87–92.

146 Schwebke J, Calsyn D, Shriver K, *et al*. Prevalence and epidemiologic correlates of human T cell lymphotropic virus infection among intravenous drug users. *J Infect Dis* 1994; **169**: 962–967.

147 Etzel A, Shibata GY, Rozman M, *et al*. HTLV-I and HTLV-II infections in HIV-infected individuals from Santos, Brazil: seroprevalence and risk factors. *J AIDS* 2001; **26**: 185–190.

148 Manns A, Wilks RJ, Murphy EL, *et al*. A prospective study of transmission by transfusion of HTLV-I and risk factors associated with seroconversion. *Int J Cancer* 1992; **51**: 886–891.

149 Maloney EM, Cleghorn FR, Morgan Os, *et al*. Incidence of HTLV-I-associated myelopathy/tropical spastic paraparesis (HAM/TSP) in Jamaica and Trinidad. *J Acquir Immune Defic Syndr Hum Retrovirol*. 1998; **17**: 167–170.

150 Vitek CR, Gracia FI, Giusti R, *et al*. Evidence for sexual and mother-to-child transmission of human lymphotropic virus type II among Guaymi Indians, Panama. *J Infect Dis* 1995; **171**: 1022–1026.

151 Machuca A, Tuset C, Soriano V, *et al*. Prevalence of HTLV infection in pregnant women in Spain. *Sex Transm Inf* 2000; **76**: 366–370.

152 Ades AE, Parker S, Walker J, Edington M, Taylor GP, Weber JN. Human T cell leukaemia/lymphoma virus infection in pregnant women in the United Kingdom: population study. *Br Med J* 2000; **320**: 1497–1501.

153 Egan JF, O'Leary B, Lewis MJ, *et al*. High rate of human lymphotropic virus type IIa infection in HIV type 1-infected intravenous drug abusers in Ireland. *AIDS Res Hum Retroviruses* 1999; **15**: 699–705.

154 HERN. Seroepidemiology of the HTLV viruses in Europe. *J AIDS Hum Retrovirol* 1996; **13**: 68–77.

155 Zehender G, De Maddalena C, Gianotto M, *et al*. High prevalence of false-negative anti-HTLV type I/II enzyme-linked immunosorbent assay results in HIV type 1-positive patients. *AIDS Res Hum Retroviruses* 1997; **13**: 1141–1146.

156 Heneine W, Khabbaz RF, Lal RB, Kaplan JE. Sensitive and specific polymerase chain reaction assays for diagnosis of human T-cell lymphotropic virus type I (HTLV-I) and HTLV-II infections in HTLV I/II-seropositive individuals. *J Clin Microbiol* 1992; **30**: 1605–1607.

157 Heredia A, Soraiano V, Weiss SH, *et al*. Development of a multiplex PCR assay for the simultaneous detection and discrimination of HIV-1, HIV-2, HTLV-I and HTLV-II. *Clin Diagn Virol* 1997; **7**: 85–92.

158 Hisada M, Okayama A, Shioiri S, *et al*. Risk factors for adult T-cell leukemia among carriers of human T-lymphotropic virus type I. *Blood* 1998; **92**: 3557–3561.

159 Cleghorn FR, Manns A, Falk R, *et al*. Effect of human T-lymphotropic virus type I infection on non-Hodgkin's lymphoma incidence. *J Natl Cancer Inst* 1995; **87**: 1009–1014.

160 Gill PS, Harrington W, Kaplan M, *et al*. Treatment of adult T-cell leukemia-lymphoma with a combination of interferon alfa and zidovudine. *N Engl J Med* 1995; **332**: 1744–1748.

161 Hermine O, Bouscary D, Gessain A, *et al*. Brief report: Treatment for adult T-cell leukemia-lymphoma with zidovudine and interferon alfa. *N Engl J Med* 1995; **332**: 1749–1751.

162 Maloney E, Biggar R, Neel J, *et al*. Endemic human T-cell lymphotropic virus type II infection among isolated Brazilian Amerindians. *J Infect Dis* 1992; **166**: 100–107.

163 Goorney BP, Young AC. HIV and HTLV-1 co-infection. *Int J STD AIDS* 2000; **11**: 205–206

164 Umehara F, Izumo S, Nakagawa M, *et al*. Immunocytochemical analysis of the cellular infiltrate in the spinal cord lesions in HTLV-I-associated myelopathy. *J Neuropathol Exp Neurol* 1993; **52**: 424–430.

165 Manns A, Hisada M, La Grenade L. Human T-lymphotropic virus type 1 infection. *Lancet* 1999; **353**: 1951–1958.

166 McMillan A, Scott GR. *Sexually Transmitted Infections, Colour Guide*. Churchill Livingstone; Edinburgh: 2000.

167 Robertson DHH, McMillan A, Young H. *Clinical Practice in Sexually Transmissible Diseases* 2nd edition. Edinburgh; Churchill Livingstone: 1989.

168 Melbye M, Biggar RJ, Ebbesen P, Andersen HK, Vestergaard BF. Lifestyle and antiviral antibody studies among homosexual men in Denmark. *Acta Pathol Microbiol Scand* 1983; **91B**: 357–364.

169 Coester C-H, Avonts D, Colaert J, Desmyter J, Piot P. Syphilis, hepatitis A, hepatitis B and cytomegalovirus infection in homosexual men in Antwerp. *Br J Vener Dis* 1984; **60**: 48–51.

170 Mindel A, Sutherland S. Antibodies to cytomegalovirus in homosexual and heterosexual men attending an STD clinic. *British Journal of Venereal Diseases* 1984; **60**: 189–192.

171 Syed TA, Lundin S, Ahmad M. Topical 0.3% and 0.5% podophyllotoxin cream for self-treatment of molluscum contagiosum in males. *Dermatology* 1994; **189**: 65–68.

Section 3
Bacterial, protozoal, and arthropod infections

Non-specific genital tract infection and chlamydial infection, including lymphogranuloma venereum
A McMillan, R C Ballard

Non-specific urethritis (NSU) is a convenient term to describe the very common condition in men which presents clinically as a purulent or mucopurulent urethral discharge, often associated with the symptom of dysuria, and which occurs a few days to a few weeks after intercourse. The urethral discharge in a patient with NSU contains pus cells but *Neisseria gonorrhoeae* cannot be detected by microscopy of Gram-stained smears or by culture. The term non-specific genital infection (NSGI) has been applied to the clinically less defined infection in the female who may have neither symptoms nor easily detected signs.

Clinically non-specific urethritis varies widely in severity, and symptomless infections are common. Most cases are associated with infection with *Chlamydia trachomatis*. Other genital conditions that share the same etiology include epididymo-orchitis, cervicitis, and pelvic inflammatory disease. In non-gonococcal ophthalmia neonatorum (conjunctivitis of the newborn), *Chlamydia trachomatis* is the infecting organism and is transmitted from the genital tract of the mother during parturition. Pneumonia may complicate chlamydial infection in the neonate. Chlamydial conjunctivitis is seen in all age groups, and chlamydial proctitis may occur in men and women who have had receptive anal intercourse. Chlamydial infection may occasionally cause a mild pharyngitis.

There is experimental evidence that *Ureaplasma urealyticum* and *Mycoplasma genitalium* have a role in the etiology of NSU. Other organisms such as herpes simplex virus, *Trichomonas vaginalis* and *Candida* spp. may be causative in a minority of cases (less than 1%).

Chlamydial genital tract infection

Studies in the 1970s showed that the isolation rates for *C. trachomatis* in men with NSU varied from 23% to 70%, and in patients with gonococcal urethritis from 10% to 30%, while in control groups it was usually less than 5%. Significantly more pairs of sexual partners were concordant for chlamydial infection than were discordant, and the chlamydial isolation rate was higher in men who had casual sexual contact than in men claiming to have regular partners. These findings provided evidence for the sexual transmission of *C. trachomatis* and its etiological role in NSU. Indirect evidence for the association of *C. trachomatis* with NSU was provided by serological studies. The microimmunofluorescence (micro-IF) test used to demonstrate the existence of serovars can also be used to detect serum antibody[1]. With this method, the seropositivity rates in patients with NSU, gonococcal urethritis, and no urethritis were 79%, 55%, and 38% respectively; the corresponding isolation rates for *C. trachomatis* were 42%, 19%, and 7% respectively. The serovar correlated with the specificity of the serum antibody.

An increase in serum antibody titer gave good correlation with the isolation of *C. trachomatis*. When paired sera were examined, seroconversion from negative to positive was found in 54% of cases and a fourfold rise in titer in 30% of patients from whom *C. trachomatis* was isolated, whereas only 4% of patients with negative culture demonstrated seroconversion or a fourfold rise in titer[1]. In *C. trachomatis* infection of the urethra the antigenic stimulus is weak and results in a modest antibody response, with some 10% to 20% of men developing no detectable specific antibodies at all, although many studies have reported antibodies more frequently at higher titers in men with urethritis than in those with no apparent disease. In men experiencing their first episode, a number develop an IgM response[2]; in subsequent episodes IgG may develop early in infection but IgM may not be demonstrated.

Chlamydia trachomatis is responsible for a large proportion of cases of NSGI in women. It can be cultured from the cervix in at least 40% of women who have gonorrhea or who have been contacts of men with NSU. In the case of female contacts of men with *C. trachomatis*-positive NSU, the organism has been recovered from the cervix in about 58% of cases, compared with only 23% of contacts of men with *C. trachomatis*-negative NSU[3].

ETIOLOGY

Family Chlamydiaceae: Genus *Chlamydia*

Organisms belonging to the genus *Chlamydia* are the cause of ocular, genital, and systemic diseases in humans. Once regarded as viruses because of their obligate intracellular growth, many of their fundamental properties, however, are those of bacteria. Three species are recognized, namely *C. trachomatis*, *C. psittaci*, and *C. pneumoniae*. *Chlamydia trachomatis* has been divided into three biovariants (biovars)

- trachoma
- lymphogranuloma venereum (LGV)
- murine (mouse pneumonitis (MoPn) agent).

DNA homology studies of genomic DNA have shown that the trachoma and LGV biovar are almost identical and that the murine biovar is more distantly related[4]. As determined by serological assays, the trachoma biovar consists of serovariants (serovars) designated by the letters A to K, including serovars Ba, Da, and Ia. The LGV biovar consists of four serovars: L1, L2, L2a, and L3.

Developmental cycle of *Chlamydia* species

All chlamydiae, unique among prokaryotic cells, undergo a developmental cycle in the cytoplasm of eukaryotic cells. Two main structures in the growth cycle are recognized

- the elementary bodies (EB) that are the infectious stage of the developmental cycle
- the reticulate bodies (RB) that are concerned solely with the multiplication of chlamydial populations within the eukaryotic cell.

The EB are spherical, rigid-walled structures 200 to 300 nm in diameter, rich with DNA, thus rendering the core electron dense when examined with the electron microscope. The dense DNA core is surrounded by a cytoplasmic membrane and an outer envelope.

Attachment

Infection of the host cell is initiated by close adhesion of an EB to the host cell surface and entry of the attached EB is by endocytosis, where the invading organisms lie within a vacuole formed by the host membrane. The host cell receptor, however, has not been identified. Electrostatic interactions play an important part in at least the early stages of infection. A number of EB surface components have been proposed as potential ligands mediating attachment to host cells. Heparan sulfate-like proteoglycans may be important, at least in mediating the initial electrostatic interaction, and heparin and heparan sulfate can inhibit attachment of L2 organisms to HeLa cells[5]. It has been proposed that a chlamydia-specific glycosaminoglycan, possibly synthesized in a series of reactions involving both host and bacterial enzymes, bridges receptors on the EB and host surface. The major outer membrane protein (MOMP) and the cysteine-rich protein (OmcB) have been postulated as the glycosaminoglycan-binding proteins. It is also likely that other, glycosaminoglycan-independent, means of attachment to eukaryotic cells are also involved. The differential effects of glycosaminoglycans on attachment of serovars E and L2 that have been shown *in vitro*[5] possibly reflect the natural history of the different infections: heparan sulfate is concentrated on the basolateral surface of epithelial cells where it is important in infection by LGV from the submucosa, whereas trachoma strains are exposed to the apical surface which is deficient in heparan sulfate.

There is some evidence that MOMP acts as an adhesin. Serovar-specific monoclonal antibodies to the surface-exposed variable sequence 'domains' I or II and IV of MOMP neutralize chlamydial infectivity by blocking attachment[5]. Other experiments have led to the hypothesis that MOMP functions as an adhesin by mediating electrostatic and hydrophobic interactions with the host cell surface. Intact MOMP is not necessarily required for attachment of EB to host cells, but it appears that the variable domains of MOMP are critical. The host cell ligand bound by MOMP is currently unknown.

The cysteine-rich protein, OmcB, which is found only on EBs and is a component of its cell wall, may have a role in the early stages of chlamydial interaction with host cells, as may the putative outer membrane proteins (POMP) that are present in the chlamydial outer membrane complex[5].

Entry

Elementary bodies are initially seen attached near the base of the microvilli, from which they are subsequently internalized into tight endocytic vesicles. It would appear that both phagocytic (microfilament-dependent) and pinocytic (microfilament-independent) mechanisms of uptake are used by *C. trachomatis*, but the underlying molecular mechanisms are uncertain. The surface of all species of chlamydiae have dome-shaped bulges through which spike-like projections protrude. It has recently been recognized that chlamydiae possess genes for a type III secretory system, and it has been suggested that the surface projections represent a type III apparatus. In other Gram-negative bacteria, type III secretion is activated by contact with a host cell into which specific proteins are injected. These injected proteins disrupt host cell transduction mechanisms and cytoskeletal arrangements, leading to endocytosis of the bacterium by the epithelial cell. In chlamydiae, however, the secreted effector molecule is unknown.

Intracellular development

The EB is internalized by an invagination of the host cell membrane that envelops it in a vesicle. Little, however, is known about the vesicle in the very early stages of infection. Endocytic vesicles rapidly mature from early endosomes to late endosomes and lysosomes, as shown by the acquisition or loss of specific markers. Vesicles containing EBs are very slow to fuse with lysosomes, and it is clear that chlamydial inclusions are not lysosomal in character. Elegant studies with labeled sphingolipid analogs have shown that they are metabolized at the *cis* Golgi apparatus and delivered to the plasma membrane by a vesicle-mediated pathway. The chlamydial inclusion intersects this pathway[5]. One of the early events in chlamydial infection is the expression of gene products that isolate the inclusion from the endosomal or lysosomal pathway, thereby protecting it from lysis. As the chlamydial inclusion becomes dissociated from the endocytic pathway and intercepts vesicles from the exocytic pathway, there is a rapid and marked increase in the size of the inclusion during chlamydial growth[4]. Within 6 to 9 hours of ingestion the EBs enlarge to form RBs with a diameter of about 200 to 300 nm. Electron microscopy shows the structure of the mature RB to be essentially that of a Gram-negative bacterium. Reticulate bodies multiply by binary fission. The cell wall complex appears to contain unidentified factors that cause the RB-containing endosome to be non-fusogenic with lysosomes. It is suggested that delayed maturation of the endocytic vesicle gives the EBs a survival advantage within the cell until chlamydiae modify the intracellular environment through early protein synthesis. Within 2 hours of becoming internalized, the EBs are committed to progression through the developmental cycle. One of the early functions of protein synthesis is to direct transportation of the endocytic vesicles to the region of the Golgi apparatus, where they aggregate, and to establish an interaction with an endocytic pathway; microtubules have been implicated in this translocation. The insertion of specific proteins into the inclusion membrane (Incs) may be the means of controlling intracellular movement of the endocytic vesicle and altering its fusogenic properties. When cells are infected with multiple EBs, there is a tendency for them to fuse into one large vesicle. Chlamydiae actively modify the response of the host cell to chlamydial infection that requires *de novo* chlamydial protein synthesis. Sphingomyelin (and probably other lipids also) appears to be delivered directly from the Golgi apparatus to the inclusion where it is subsequently incorporated into the cell walls of the chlamydiae.

Effects on the host cell

There is little disruption of host cell functions, with little requirement for host macromolecular synthesis to support chlamydial multiplication. Chlamydia-infected cells are resistant to apoptosis by a variety of pro-apoptotic stimuli, suggesting a possible communication with the host cell cytosol to interrupt cell-signaling pathways that lead to apoptosis.

Virtually nothing is currently known about the luminal contents of the chlamydial inclusion, and, although chlamydiae obtain amino acids, nucleotides, and lipids from host cells pools, the means of nutrient exchange are unknown. The inclusion membrane does not contain pores that permit passive diffusion of even small molecules. As RBs are found in association with the inner surface of the inclusion membrane, it is likely that they derive nutrients from the host cell cytosol.

Release

The chlamydiae complete their intracellular development in 36 hours or longer. Although the LGV serovars of *C. trachomatis* are released by lysis of the host cell, other serovars are released following fusion of the inclusion membrane with the plasma membrane.

Biovars and serovars of *Chlamydia trachomatis*

Chlamydiae contain genetic information for several hundred different proteins and as a result are antigenically complex. Sensitive immunoblotting and radioimmune precipitation methods have enabled the identification of some chlamydial antigens reactive both with patients' sera and monoclonal antibodies. A commonly used complement fixation test, for example, is genus-specific, and chemical characterization of the genus-reactive antigen indicates that it is a lipopolysaccharide (LPS) similar to that of Gram-negative bacteria.

On the basis of a micro-immuno-fluorescence (micro-IF) test *C. trachomatis* has been classified into serovars, and the type-specific antigens have been identified as trypsin-labile proteins at the surface of the EB. Clinically distinct infections are associated with different serovars of *C. trachomatis*.

Eighteen serovars have been identified. In hyperendemic trachoma, *C. trachomatis* bv. *trachoma* contains serovars A, B, Ba, and C; in ocular infections of sexually transmitted origin (paratrachoma) or genital tract infection, *C. trachomatis* bv. *trachoma* contains serovars D, Da, E, F, G, H, I, Ia, J, and K; and in lymphogranuloma venereum, isolates contain the LGV serovars L1, L2, L2a, and L3. Two broad complexes of serovars occur, with little cross reactivity between the serovars belonging to the different complexes. Cross-reactions of a lesser titer in the micro-IF test are found, with other serovars forming part of the antigenic complex being studied (for example C, J, H, I, and A are serologically related and form the so-called C complex).

Diseases due to Chlamydia trachomatis *bv.* trachoma *(tropical trachoma)* sv. A, B, Ba, C

In hyperendemic tropical trachoma, due to *C. trachomatis* bv. *trachoma* (serovars A, B, Ba, and C), the organisms are spread by eye-to-eye transmission particularly in unhygienic conditions, affecting approximately 500 million people and causing blindness in some two million. Hyperendemic trachoma occurs in conditions of 'ocular promiscuity', that is to say in conditions that favor the frequent, unrestricted, and indiscriminate mixing of ocular contacts or of ocular discharges[6].

Diseases due to Chlamydia trachomatis *bv.* trachoma *(ocular or genital tract infections)* sv. D, Da, E, F, G, H, I, Ia, J, and K

The genital infections or ocular infections associated with them of western countries, on the other hand, tend to occur when there is frequent mixing of genital contacts or discharges with occasional, accidental transfer to the eye. These chlamydial infections, due to serovars D to K, are predominantly genital and the incidence of both adult chlamydial conjunctivitis and conjunctivitis of the newborn, with or without involvement of other sites, for example the nasopharynx, are dependent upon the incidence of genital infections in the adult population and, in the case of infants, in their mothers.

Serovars D to K, either alone or with *N. gonorrhoeae*, are a cause of pelvic inflammatory disease and perihepatitis (Curtis–Fitz-Hugh syndrome) (Chapter 12).

There is evidence to suggests that chlamydiae may be a cause of peripheral and axial forms of arthritis as a reactive arthritis (Chapter 14).

Disease due to Chlamydia trachomatis bv. lymphogranuloma venereum sv. L1, L2, L2a, L3

Biovar *LGV* is sexually transmitted (serovars L1, L2, L2a, and L3) and in contrast to biovar *trachoma*, which is pathogenic to the squamocolumnar cells of mucous membranes, it causes primarily a disease of the lymphatic tissue, involving characteristically the lymph nodes of the anogenital region.

All chlamydial infections have a tendency to be persistent as chronic or clinically inapparent forms.

IMMUNOLOGY AND PATHOGENESIS

Immunity to infection

There is now good evidence that immunity to re-infection with chlamydiae can develop and this subject has been reviewed recently[7]. The following are some of the observations that have been proffered as evidence for immunity.

- Amongst individuals attending an STI clinic, the risk of infection with *C. trachomatis* is significantly lower in those individuals with a history of chlamydial infection within the preceding 6 months[8].
- Spontaneous healing of trachoma is well documented[9].
- In non-human primates, strain-specific immunity follows ocular chlamydial infection[10].
- Re-infection is usually associated with strains of *C. trachomatis* that differ from that of the initial infection[11].
- The diversity in MOMPs. MOMP is the serovariant protein among *C. trachomatis* strains, and antibodies to MOMP neutralize infectivity in animal models. Flanked by sequences that are relatively conserved, MOMP consists of four serovar-variable sequences to which neutralizing antibodies are uniquely

directed, and it is probable that these sequences are arrayed as surface-exposed loops. Allelic variation of the single-copy MOMP gene (*omp 1*) probably accounts for the antigenic variation noted in *C. trachomatis*. The diversity in MOMPs is selected for by environmental factors, and amongst these would be the presence of neutralizing antibodies, targeting the variable segments. If this is so, then immunity to *C. trachomatis* must occur[12].

Mechanisms of host resistance to *Chlamydia trachomatis*

Little is known about the mechanisms that initiate and sustain an inflammatory response to chlamydiae, but the following section outlines our current knowledge. For further details the reader is referred to the monograph edited by Stephens[4].

Innate defenses

The following innate defenses may contribute to resistance to chlamydial infection.

1. Chlamydiae activate complement and are inactivated by normal human serum[13].
2. Lysozyme, which is present in mucosal secretions, partially inactivates chlamydiae[14].
3. Chlamydia-infected cells produce interferon-γ (IFN-γ) and interferon-β (IFN-β)[15], and interferons are known to inhibit chlamydial growth.
4. A potent host defense mechanism may be mediated by cytokine production that is dependent on bacterial protein synthesis within the infected cell. Epithelial cell production of the pro-inflammatory cytokines – interleukin-8 (IL-8), GRO-a, granulocyte-macrophage colony-stimulating factor (GM-CSF), and interleukin-6 (IL-6) – is induced by *C. trachomatis* infection of cervical epithelial cells[16]. Interleukin-8 is a powerful inducer of neutrophil chemotaxis, and neutrophils that accumulate at sites of chlamydial infection are known to inactivate chlamydiae. Infected cells also produce interleukin-1a (IL-1a) and, as pro-inflammatory cytokine production is blocked by antibody against IL-1a, it is possible that release of IL-1a

after lysis of infected epithelial cells amplifies the inflammatory reaction by stimulating cytokine production by adjacent cells. The acute host response to *C. trachomatis* then might be initiated and maintained by the epithelial cells of the mucosal surface, the target of chlamydial infection[17].

Adaptive immune responses

In addition to the cytokine responses of infected epithelial cells, chlamydial infection can also generate a response through interaction with cells of the immune system. The central role of CD4+ T cells in immunity to chlamydiae is clearly shown by the increased susceptibility of HIV-infected women to chlamydial infection, and the increased risk of complications such as pelvic inflammatory disease as the CD4+ cell count in the peripheral blood decreases[11, 18].

Lymphoproliferative responses of class II-restricted CD4+ T cells to chlamydial antigen are found in individuals with current or past chlamydial infection, as reviewed by Brunham[7]. These responses are species but not serovar-specific which is readily explained by the finding that the T-cell epitopes of MOMP are located in regions that are conserved in amino-acid sequences among different *C. trachomatis* serovars. Lymphocyte responses are long lived and increase in magnitude with age, thereby possibly explaining the observed increased resistance to infection with age.

In individuals with ocular infection with *C. trachomatis* that resolves spontaneously, lymphocyte proliferative responses are enhanced compared with those who have persistent infection and who have depressed reactivity[19]. Lymphocyte proliferation is markedly depressed in patients with scarring trachoma compared with those who do not have this complication[20]. Individuals with scarring trachoma less frequently have chlamydial MOMP-antigen specific IFN-γ-secreting peripheral blood T cells than the latter group, but they are more likely to have heat shock protein 60 (Hsp60) antigen-specific IL-4-secreting cells[21]. These results suggest that MOMP-specific T_{H1}-type CD4+ T cells are important in immunity to *C. trachomatis*, and that Hsp60-specific T_{H2}-type CD4+ T cells are associated with the complications of infection.

Animal studies confirm the importance of T_{H1}-type responses and IFN-γ in eradication of chlamydial infection, but care is required in extrapolating the results of these experiments to human immunopathology. Wild-type mice and mice deficient for IL-4 (required for differentiation of T_{H2}-type cells), CD8$^+$ T cells, or B cells, eradicated human serovar D strain of *C. trachomatis* inoculated intravaginally; these mice were also resistant to reinfection[22]. In contrast, mice deficient in IFN-γ (required for differentiation of T_{H1}-type cells), IFN-γ receptor or CD4$^+$ T cells, had an impaired ability to eradicate infection. As shown in mice, IL-6 produced by chlamydia-infected epithelial cells might be important together with interleukin-12 (IL-12) in sustaining the T_{H1}-type protective response[23]. In animal studies, IFN-γ-induced up regulation of nitric oxide synthase with the production of nitric oxide appearing to be an important mechanism of killing of chlamydiae[22], and this may also be relevant to man. *In vitro* experiments with a virus-transformed human epithelial cell line showed that nitric oxide induction by IFN-γ accounted for about 20% of chlamydial growth inhibition[24]. A further 30% of chlamydial replication was accounted for by IFN-γ-induced tryptophan catabolism (tryptophan is an amino acid essential for chlamydial replication).

Professional antigen-presenting cells, dendritic cells, are found in mucosal tissue from chlamydia-infected patients, and may have been recruited to these sites by inflammatory cytokines released from infected cells. In addition, GM-CSF, another cytokine produced by chlamydia-infected epithelial cells[16], is important in maturing dendritic cell antigen presentation. In the mouse model, dendritic cells phagocytose chlamydiae that become enclosed in macropinosomes that then fuse with lysosomes bearing major histocompatability complex (MHC) class II molecules, resulting in chlamydial death[25]. Major histocompatability complex class II-based presentation of chlamydial antigen to CD4$^+$ T cells then follows.

The role of CD8$^+$ T cells in immunity to *C. trachomatis* is less clear. It is uncertain if infected epithelial cells can present antigen to CD8$^+$ T cells through MHC class I molecules. As the organism grows in a membrane-bound vacuole, chlamydial peptides may not be available to the cell for binding to MHC class I molecules. Cytotoxic T-cell responses to chlamydial peptides, however, have been shown in about 10% of individuals living in an area where trachoma is endemic, suggesting that CD8$^+$ cells are induced during chlamydial infection[26]. The mechanism for this is unknown, but it may be that chlamydial proteins enter the cytoplasm via a type III secretory system[27]. Although epithelial cells cannot present antigen to naïve T cells, activated CD8$^+$ T cells can recognize MHC-presented peptides on cells, and if chlamydial peptides are presented in the context of MHC class I molecules, infected cells may be lysed by them.

Although serum antibodies may afford some protection against ascending infection by *C. trachomatis*, as suggested by a reduced risk in women undergoing surgical termination of pregnancy[28], local antibody production may be more directly involved in immunity. Shedding of *C. trachomatis* from the human endocervix is inversely related to the presence of specific immunoglobulin A (IgA) in the secretions, but not to the presence of serum antibodies[29]. Circulating spontaneously secreting IgA B cells that home to epithelial surfaces, are found in patients with uncomplicated chlamydial infection of the urethra or cervix[30]. By contrast, individuals with complicated infection have a decreased number of circulating IgA but increased numbers of IgG-antibody-secreting cells, suggesting that IgA is important in human immunity against chlamydiae.

The ability of elementary bodies to evade these defense mechanisms has been explained by their rapid entry into cells after release from the parent cell[7].

Persistence of chlamydial infection

Several factors probably account for the ability of chlamydiae to evade the immune system in the host.

1. The organisms grow in a membrane-bound vacuole within the cytoplasm, and chlamydial peptides are not freely available for binding to MHC class I molecules for presentation to effector cells of the immune system (but see above). The chlamydial vacuole is sited on the exocytic vesicular pathway and, as this is distinct from the class II-containing endolysosome, infected epithelial cells appear to lack the ability to present chlamydial peptides to CD4$^+$ T cells through MHC class II molecules.
2. *Chlamydia*-infected cells are resistant to apoptosis by blocking mitochondrial cytochrome *c* release and caspase activation[31].
3. Reduced T_{H1}-type CD4$^+$ T-cell cytokine responses.

Although productive infection in which infectious elementary bodies are eventually released to infect other cells is the norm, persistent infection, possibly associated with incomplete chlamydial development, may occur with sporadic production of elementary bodies, and thus disease. Factors thought to favor persistent infection include the action of penicillin, interferon-γ, other products of cell-mediated immunity, and the deprivation of the amino acids tryptophan and cysteine that are required for bacterial replication[17].

Although some evidence for persistence of genital tract chlamydial infection in humans has been reported, each study has been flawed in some way and it is difficult to draw conclusions from the results[17]. More convincing evidence of persistent infection has come from the study of Bell *et al.*[32] who found that of 22 infants who had been infected at birth and who had either not been treated or who had failed treatment; 22% were still infected 1 year later.

Indirect evidence for covert infection comes from the observation that the culture of chlamydiae from the endocervix of female contacts of men with urethritis associated with both *N. gonorrhoeae* and *C. trachomatis* is more likely if the woman has concurrent infection with *N. gonorrhoeae*[3]. As chlamydial activity is thought to be greatest in actively growing and replicating cells, the hypothesis is that *N. gonorrhoeae* increases epithelial cell turnover and thereby activates deep-seated covert chlamydial infection[17].

Although there seems to be little doubt that persistent infection occurs, it has not been proven conclusively that this results from an incomplete life cycle. In most individuals who become infected with *C. trachomatis*, spontaneous resolution of infection eventually occurs, most likely through the action of cytokines produced in T_{H1}-type reactions and of neutralizing antibodies such as secretory IgA. Some people, however, fail to clear the infection and have persistent infections or are susceptible to re-infection. A recent study has shown evidence of chronic persistence of *C. trachomatis*[33]. Forty-five isolates from seven women with three to ten repeated, same serovar infections over 2 to 5 years were selected for *omp 1* genotyping, and it was shown that four women had identical genotypes at each recurrence; in two women there were one or two amino-acid changes following treatment, and in another woman, there was persistent infection with a unique genotype. The authors concluded that the data demonstrated that cervical infections with C-class serovars could persist for years.

It is individuals with persistent infection who are most likely to develop long-term sequelae of chlamydial disease[34]. Mechanisms of disease are discussed under Pelvic Inflammatory Disease (Chapter 12).

PATHOLOGY

Intracellular inclusion bodies were first described in trachoma by Halberstaeder and von Prowazek in 1907 and later, in 1910, in urethral discharge. In histological sections of cervical mucosa similar inclusions appear as cytoplasmic vacuoles when examined by light microscopy and are most easily seen in columnar epithelial cells. The vacuoles may occupy nearly the entire volume of the cell and, on electron microscopy, are seen to contain numerous small spherical bodies about 1 mm in diameter; these represent the infectious elementary bodies, non-infectious reticulate bodies, and transitional stages[35]. Several studies of chlamydial infection with the oculogenital serovars of *C. trachomatis* of the conjunctiva, uterine cervix, endometrium, and uterine tubes have shown that there is an exudation of neutrophils into the mucus layer overlying the epithelial cells. The lamina propria is infiltrated with

activated T and B lymphocytes (both CD4+ and CD8+ cells), macrophages, histiocytes, and dendritic cells[7]. The B cells and lymphoblasts may be found as organized lymphoid follicles or germinal centers either in the conjunctiva (in trachoma) or in the genital tract. This finding is more common in women with upper genital tract infection. In the later fibrotic stages of chlamydial infection of the uterine tubes, there is a diffuse plasma cell infiltrate of the lamina propria, but T cells are not conspicuous[7].

In rectal infection with the oculogenital serovars of *C. trachomatis*, the histology may be normal or there may be the changes of a non-specific proctitis with a mild increase in the number of chronic inflammatory cells and polymorphonuclear leukocytes in the lamina propria[36].

EPIDEMIOLOGY

Over the past 25 years there have been many studies on the prevalence of chlamydial infection in different populations, particularly amongst attendees at STI clinics. As isolation of the organism or antigen-detection methods were used for diagnosis in the majority of these investigations, and as these techniques lack sensitivity compared with the more modern molecular methods, the true prevalence of infection in these study populations has often been grossly underestimated. Nevertheless, interpretation of temporal changes in the incidence of infection is possible if the same diagnostic methods have been used throughout the study period.

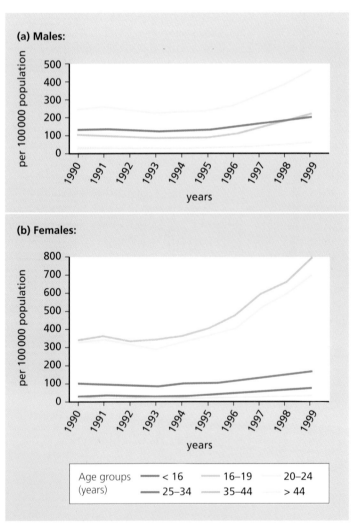

Figure 10.1 Rates of diagnoses of genital chlamydial infection made at genitourinary medicine clinics in the UK, by sex and age group[55]

Prevalence and risk factors

Genital chlamydial infection is worldwide in its distribution, and it has been estimated that more than 50 million individuals become infected annually[37].

In the US, during 1987 and 1995, the annual reported rate of infections increased 281% from 47.8 to 182.2 cases per 100 000 individuals[38]. The overall reported rate for women (290.3 per 100 000 population) was almost six times higher than that for men (52.1 per 100 000 population). A similar trend has occurred amongst men and women attending STI clinics in the UK (Figure 10.1), but the proportion of infected women was only 1.4 times greater than men[39]. However, selection bias may conceal the true prevalence rate in these populations.

In women

The prevalence of infection varies geographically and according to the population studied. For example, the prevalence was significantly higher amongst women attending a STI clinic in Jamaica (55% of 237 women)[40] where the diagnosis was made by culture and direct immunofluorescence than amongst those attending a clinic in Edinburgh (8% of 4431 women) where the diagnosis was made by ligase chain reaction. Irrespective of the geographical area, the majority of reported studies have shown that the majority of infected women are aged between 15 and 24 years: for example, the age distribution of women with chlamydial infection in Scotland is shown in Figure 10.2. Prevalence studies have been undertaken in other populations, including individuals attending family planning clinics, among whom, in the US, the rate of infection has decreased from 9.3% in 1988 to 3.3% in 1995[38]. A high prevalence and incidence of chlamydial infection has also been reported in a group of inner-city adolescent females who attended STI, family planning, or school-based clinics in Baltimore, US[41]. Infection was diagnosed at the first clinic attendance in 24.1% of 771 women, and 29.1% of adolescent females had at least one positive test over a 33-month period.

With the advent of chlamydial screening by ligase chain reaction (LCR) or polymerase chain reaction (PCR) on first-voided specimens of urine, opportunistic screening has become possible in settings in which genital examination might have been considered inappropriate. For example, at an anonymous and free HIV testing center in Paris, chlamydial infection was identified in 20 (3.9%) of 513 women who attended that facility[42]. Vuylsteke *et al.*[43] found that the prevalence of infection amongst 2784 sexually active adolescent female students, median age 17 years, was 1.4%. In a group of 890 women aged 18 to 35 who attended four general practices in London, the prevalence of infection as detected by LCR was 2.6% (95% confidence interval 1.6–3.9%)[44]. Using LCR for the detection of *C. trachomatis* in urine specimens, Gaydos *et al.*[45] found an overall prevalence of infection of 9.2% among 13 204 new female US army recruits, with a peak of 12.2% amongst those aged 17 years.

The prevalence of chlamydial infection in pregnant women has also been studied extensively. Amongst 1175 women who attended a clinic in Melbourne, Australia, for termination of pregnancy, the prevalence of infection was 2.8%[46]. It is important to identify these women, as post-abortal sepsis is commonly associated with untreated *C. trachomatis* infection[47]. In a study of pregnant teenage women from Jefferson County, Alabama, Oh *et al.*[48] identified chlamydial infection in 19% of 267 women at their first antenatal visit, and repeat infection was found in 8% of 218 women.

This finding suggested that high-risk sexual behavior continued during their pregnancy. Other population studies have shown a lower prevalence of infection.

Several risk factors for acquisition of *C. trachomatis* by women have been identified, but young age (less than 25 years) is the common factor in all reported studies. It has been suggested that this age effect is accounted for by eversion of the squamo-columnar junction in young women, exposing the columnar epithelium to infection. Intercourse with a new partner within the preceding 2 months, multiple sexual partners, and non-white race have all been identified as other risk factors for chlamydial infection[49-52].

In men

The prevalence of chlamydial infection in men has not been studied as closely as that in women. In a prospective study of 356 consecutive heterosexual men who attended a STI clinic in London in 1991, *C. trachomatis* was cultured from the urethras of 34 (9.5%) men[53]. Amongst a group of 480 young men who attended an HIV-testing center in Paris, *C. trachomatis* was detected in 11 individuals (2.3%, 95% confidence interval 1.0–3.6) using PCR on urine[43]. Young, 14 to 18-year-old, black prisoners in Birmingham, Alabama, had a high prevalence of chlamydial infection;

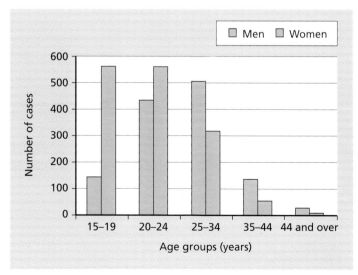

Figure 10.2 Prevalence of *C. trachomatis* infection amongst patients attending STI clinics in Scotland, 1998/99 (GUM Statistics Scotland 1998/99)

14.4% of 284 were infected, the majority being asymptomatic[54].

Although the incidence of chlamydial infection amongst men in the UK is highest in the 20 to 24-year age group (465 per 100 000 population)[55] the prevalence of infection is higher in those aged 25 to 34 years (data for Scotland are shown in Figure 10.2).

Earlier studies had shown that the rate of detection of *C. trachomatis* in the urethra of men who had sex with men and who had gonococcal or non-specific urethritis was significantly lower that than in heterosexual men[56]. However, more recent data, based on the detection of *C. trachomatis* by LCR on urine samples, indicate that the prevalence of chlamydial infection in homosexual or bisexual men with NSU or urethral gonorrhea is similar to that of heterosexual men[57]. Chlamydial infection was found more frequently in young men (less than 24 years of age) than in older either homo- or bisexual men. The frequency of chlamydial infection of the rectum amongst men who have had sex with men has not been investigated in detail in recent years. In the late 1970s, however, *C. trachomatis* was cultured from the rectums of 4% to 6% of homosexual men attending STI clinics[58].

Transmissibility of *Chlamydia trachomatis*

Data are not available on the risk of transmission of *C. trachomatis* from a single sexual exposure. However, it has been shown in a cross-sectional study, using PCR to detect *C. trachomatis* infection, that within sexual partnerships, and reflecting the cumulative result of multiple exposures, the frequency of male–female and female–male transmission is the same, i.e. 68%[59]. A broadly similar infection rate was reported by Lin et al.[60] who also showed that men and women were often infected with mixed serovars (6 of 12 men and 8 of 14 women).

Association of serovars with disease

Amongst women with cervical infection with *C. trachomatis*, the E, F, and D serovars predominated in a study conducted by Workowski et al.[61]. Serovars F and G were associated with fewer objective signs of infection and with fewer inclusion-forming units in cell culture. Workowski et al.[61] also noted that serovar F was found less often in rectal samples than in cervical specimens. The authors postulated that this finding reflected a lower level of cervical shedding of the organism with this serovar. Barnes et al.[62] had shown previously that the rectal isolates from women differed from those recovered from the cervix in respect of their serovar. Symptomatic rectal infection has been associated with serovars F and G[63].

However, genotyping has uncovered the heterogeneity of the serovars recognized by serological testing. Dean and colleagues, working in San Francisco[63a], examined cervical and endometrial isolates of *C. trachomatis* from women with lower genital tract infection or pelvic inflammatory disease, for *omp 1* gene (encoding the MOMP) polymorphism. They showed that the F variant genotypes were more frequently associated with upper genital tract pathology than the E genotypes. Dean and colleagues, and others, showed that mixed infections with several genotypes are possible. Class C serovars appear more likely to result in persistent infection than other serovars (see page 286).

Association of *Chlamydia trachomatis* infection and cervical carcinoma

Although it has been established that there is a causal relationship between certain types of human papillomavirus and cervical cancer, only a small proportion of women infected with these types progress to invasive disease (Chapter 5). Cofactors, including cigarette smoking, have been suggested as being important in the pathogenesis of cervical cancer. Recent studies that take into account the effect of human papillomavirus (HPV) infection and smoking strongly suggest that there is an independent relationship between lifetime exposure to chlamydial infection and cervical squamous cell carcinoma. The results of a prospective, nested case-control study from Finland, Norway, and Sweden were reported by Koskela and colleagues[64].

Serum samples that had been collected some years previously for research purposes were available for testing for specific IgG antibodies against *C. trachomatis* and HPV-16, HPV-18, and HPV-33, as well as for serum cotinine, a marker of tobacco smoking. Of the 530 000 women studied, 182 with invasive cervical carcinoma were identified. Baseline specimens had been collected an average of 56 months before the diagnosis of cervical carcinoma. The serological results were compared with those of well-matched subjects who did not have cervical cancer, and it was clear that serum IgG antibodies to *C. trachomatis*, indicating past infection, were associated with an increased risk for cervical squamous cell carcinoma (HPV and smoking-adjusted odds ratio 2.2, 95% confidence interval 1.3–3.5). There was no apparent increased risk for cervical adenocarcinoma, and there was no relationship between cervical carcinoma and seropositivity for *C. pneumoniae*. In an extension of this study it was shown that infection with *C. trachomatis* serovar G was most strongly associated with cervical squamous cell carcinoma (adjusted odds ratio 6.6, 95% confidence interval 1.6–27.0)[65]. Serovars I and D were also associated with the cancer, and exposure to more than one serovar increased the risk.

Although these data are intriguing the latter study does have limitations, particularly as the possibility of an additional unmeasured behavioral or biological variable cannot be excluded[66]. If *C. trachomatis* does indeed enhance progression of HPV to invasive cervical cancer, the mechanisms invloved remain to be determined.

HIV and chlamydia

Chlamydial infection as a risk factor for HIV infection was shown in a nested case-control study conducted amongst a group of female sex industry workers in Kinshasa, Zaire[67]. In those women exposed to HIV, the risk of infection was significantly associated with the presence of *C. trachomatis* infection (odds ratio 5.8, 95% confidence interval 2.3–15.0). Non-ulcerative STIs, including *C. trachomatis*, have been associated with an increase in the numbers of CD4+ cells in the endocervix[68], suggesting that HIV transmission could be increased as a result of such infection. Increased shedding of HIV has been shown in men with urethral chlamydial infection[69], and treatment of men with NSU has resulted in a reduction in HIV-1 in the semen[70]. Interestingly, Mostad *et al.*[71] found that *C. trachomatis* infection of the cervix did not correlate with significant increases in HIV-1 proviral DNA detection.

CLINICAL FEATURES

In men

Chlamydial infection of the urethra

A sizeable proportion (more than half) of men with urethral chlamydial infection are symptomless[53, 72]; men with *C. trachomatis* infection being more likely to be asymptomatic than those with non-chlamydial NSU[53]. In many cases, however, there may be objective signs of urethritis, and in this regard it is helpful to examine the urethra for discharge before the patient has passed urine in the morning. Gram-smear microscopy of a urethral smear can also be useful in symptomless men. For example, Swartz and Kraus[73] cultured *C. trachomatis* from the urethra of about 50% of symptomless men in whom microscopy had shown more than four polymorphonuclear leukocytes per high-power field. Men with symptoms complain of a urethral discharge associated with dysuria. The dysuria tends to be variable in severity with the discomfort localized to the shaft of the penis or to the region of the meatus. The onset may occur within a few days to a month or more after exposure. The urethral discharge may be small in quantity and mucoid

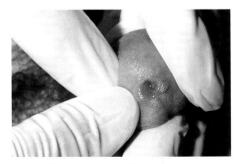

Figure 10.3 Mucoid urethral discharge in a young man with chlamydial urethritis

(Figure 10.3), or it may be copious and frankly purulent. Sometimes the discharge may dry at the urethral meatus to form a greyish crust and the discharge may appear to be more copious in the morning than at other times. Occasionally dysuria is very severe and the urethral discharge blood-stained. When there is a urethrocystitis, frank hematuria may occur with blood dispersed throughout the urinary stream.

In acute hemorrhagic cystitis the patient may complain of malaise and of passing blood after urinating, when dysuria may occur at the end of micturition (terminal dysuria). There may be frequency, urgency, and strangury.

Epididymitis, and, uncommonly, reactive arthritis may complicate chlamydial urethritis (Chapters 13 and 14).

Chlamydial infection of the rectum

Infection with the oculogenital serovars of *C. trachomatis* is usually symptomless, fewer than 40% of patients having symptoms of a distal proctitis[58]. Symptoms are usually mild and consist of a mucoid anal discharge, mucus, or pus streaking of the stool, anorectal bleeding, and perianal pain. At proctoscopy the rectal mucosa often appears normal, but in some patients there is loss of the normal vascular pattern with mucosal edema, friability, and small erosions.

In women

Cervical infection

More than two-thirds of women with uncomplicated genital chlamydial infection are symptomless and the cervix appears normal[74]. Infected women, however, may complain of increased vaginal discharge, post-coital or intermenstrual bleeding, and lower abdominal pain. Clinical findings, although not reliable criteria for diagnosis, do suggest that edema within an area of ectopy, congestion, friability of the endocervical epithelium, and a mucopurulent discharge (Figure 10.4) are associated with chlamydial infection of the cervix in a proportion of cases[75]. In chlamydial infection the cervix may occasionally have a follicular or 'cobblestone' appearance, because of the lymphoid follicle hyper-

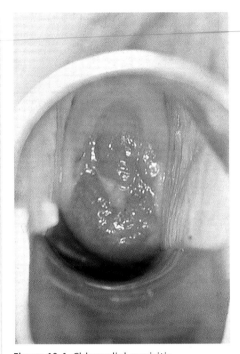

Figure 10.4 Chlamydial cervicitis

plasia. Although some degree of inflammatory reaction is induced by *C. trachomatis* it is unwise to imply that chlamydial infection can be diagnosed from this presentation. The differential diagnosis of chlamydial cervicitis includes gonococcal infection, endometritis, salpingitis, cervicitis associated with the use of an intrauterine device, trichomoniasis, and herpes simplex virus infection.

Urethral infection

Chlamydial infection of the genital tract is widespread and often induces subclinical infections. In a study of 99 chlamydia-infected women in Finland, *C. trachomatis* was cultured from the urethra and cervix of 46 women, from the urethra alone of 25 women, and from the cervix alone of 28 women[76]. In some cases, frequency and dysuria, in the absence of eubacterial infection of the urinary tract, may be caused by *C. trachomatis*. In the study reported by Stamm and colleagues[77], 10 of 16 women with sterile pyuria had chlamydial infection. Although there is objective evidence of urethritis – five or more polymorphonuclear leukocytes in a × 1000 microscope field – in more than 50% of women with cervical and/or urethral chlamydial infection, the majority of women, however, do not have frequency or dysuria[78].

Rectal infection

The rectum can also be infected and *C. trachomatis* has been cultured from that site in 5% of women attending an STI clinic[79]. As in the case of urethral infection, rectal chlamydial infection may be associated with microscopic signs of proctitis in the absence of clinical features[79]. When women have symptoms, they are those of a distal proctitis (see page 518).

Infection of the greater vestibular (Bartholin's) glands

Chlamydia trachomatis has been isolated from the duct exudate from women with Bartholinitis. In a series of 30 selected women, most of whom had gonorrhea, chlamydiae and *N. gonorrhoeae* were cultured from 7 women, and *C. trachomatis* alone from 2 women[80].

Complications of untreated infection include pelvic inflammatory disease, peri-hepatitis, and, uncommonly, reactive arthritis (Chapters 12 and 14).

In men and women

Pharyngeal infection

In most studies, the prevalence of pharyngeal infection with *C. trachomatis* amongst heterosexual men and women has been low. Using a commercially available PCR to detect chlamydial DNA, Ostergaard *et al.*[81] identified infection in only 1.7% of 179 women and none of 169 men, 80% of whom had had cunnilingus. The prevalence of infection amongst homosexual men is also low. McMillan *et al.*[82] isolated *C. trachomatis* from the pharynx of only 2 of 150 men. Although the small number of reported cases of chlamydial infection of the pharynx precludes detailed description of the clinical features, it is likely that the majority of infections are symptomless; a few patients complain of sore throat and there may be mild pharyngitis without specific features.

Ocular infections

In adults, chlamydial conjunctivitis usually results from accidental transfer of infected

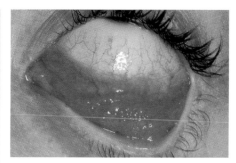

Figure 10.5 Chlamydial conjunctivitis

genital secretions to the eye[83]. About 90% of women and 50% of men who attended Moorfields Eye Hospital, London, with ocular chlamydial infection had concomitant genital infection with *C. trachomatis*. The infection presents as a chronic follicular conjunctivitis of acute or subacute onset, the incubation period varying between 2 and 21 days. The conjunctivitis is usually unilateral. There is a feeling of grittiness in the eye, lacrimation, a mucoid or mucopurulent discharge, redness, photophobia, and swelling of the lids[83]. The bulbar and palpebral conjunctiva are hyperemic (Figure 10.5) and occasionally there is edema. Follicular hypertrophy is found by the time most patients attend a clinic and is most pronounced in the upper and lower fornices. The pre-auricular node on the affected side is often affected. Persistent punctate keratitis, seen as a fine or coarse mottling of the epithelium, may follow several weeks after the onset of conjunctivitis.

CHLAMYDIAL INFECTION IN PREGNANCY

As endometritis, characterized by an infiltration of the endometrium with plasma cells, is a complication of chlamydial infection of the cervix[84], it has been suggested that this might predispose to failure of implantation or to spontaneous abortion in early pregnancy. Some evidence for this hypothesis comes from the studies of Witkin *et al.*[85], who examined the association between the presence of chlamydial DNA in cervical secretions from chlamydia-culture-negative women and the results of *in vitro* fertilization. They found a strong correlation between a positive test result and

1. failure to become pregnant after embryo transfer (10% of 135 women were chlamydia positive)

2. spontaneous abortion after embryo transfer (3 of 11 women who spontaneously aborted were chlamydia positive).

Chlamydia trachomatis was identified in 2 of 112 women who had term deliveries. An interesting observation on an association between the presence of IgA antibodies to the 57 kDa chlamydial heat shock protein (Hsp60) in endocervical secretions and failure to achieve pregnancy after embryo transfer, was made by the same group of investigators[86]. They detected antibodies to Hsp60 in 28% of 130 women, whose *in vitro* fertilization failed, but in only 7% of 68 women who had term births, a difference that is highly significant; 15 of these women had a positive test for chlamydial DNA. The authors concluded that unsuspected infection or reactivation of an immune response to the chlamydial heat shock protein might induce an inflammatory reaction in the endometrium that impairs embryo implantation or facilitates immune rejection after embryo transfer.

Despite these observations, however, the evidence that *C. trachomatis* is associated with spontaneous abortion remains inconclusive[87].

There is good correlation between the incidence of ectopic pregnancy and the prevalence of serum antibodies against chlamydiae[88], and Chow *et al.*[89] found that the matched-pair odds ratio for ectopic pregnancy and an anti-chlamydial IgG antibody titer of 64 or above was 3.0 (95% confidence interval 2.1–4.4). As shown by Hillis *et al.*[34] in a large retrospective cohort study amongst women living in Wisconsin, US, there is a significant trend between the number of chlamydial infections and the subsequent risks of ectopic pregnancy. Compared with those who had only one episode of chlamydial infection, women with two infections were four times more likely, and those with three or more infections were eleven times more likely to have an ectopic pregnancy. The mechanisms by which *C. trachomatis* damage the tubes are discussed on pp. 358–359.

Although the evidence is not entirely conclusive, *C. trachomatis* may be associated with premature rupture of the membranes, low birth weight, or both. As patients who have anti-chlamydial serum IgM antibody are at increased risk of perinatal complications, it appears that a recently acquired infection is responsible[90]. Successful treatment of chlamydial infection in pregnant women reduces the risk of premature delivery, premature rupture of the membranes and low birth weight, compared with those who have been untreated or in whom treatment has failed[91, 92]. Both of these studies showed that the incidence of premature delivery was significantly lower in treated than in uninfected and, hence, untreated women. It is tempting to speculate that the effect of treatment was not only on chlamydiae but also on other, less characterized infections susceptible to the antimicrobial agents used. In this regard it should be noted that Germain et al.[93] failed to show a relationship between intrauterine growth retardation (the only parameter recorded) and chlamydial infection.

LABORATORY DIAGNOSIS OF CHLAMYDIAL INFECTION

The laboratory diagnosis of *C. trachomatis* infections has been reviewed recently by Black[94]. Methods for the detection of nucleic acids have high sensitivity and specificity, and are the preferred diagnostic methods. Before discussing these methods, it is useful to consider the other methods that are, or have been, employed in diagnosis.

Detection of inclusion bodies by direct microscopy

In addition to Giemsa and immunofluorescence staining, iodine may also be used to detect the glycogen-containing inclusion bodies of *C. trachomatis* in smears made from urethral, cervical, and vaginal scrapings or swabs. Unfortunately, direct microscopy by any of these methods is too insensitive to be of any practical value.

Leukocyte esterase test

The basis of the leukocyte esterase test is the production of the enzyme by polymorphonuclear leukocytes, the principal cell type found in acute inflammation. Test strips for the detection of esterase in urine

are available, these have an absorbent pad containing indoxylester that turns a purple color when hydrolyzed by the enzyme. The test can detect urethritis, even when asymptomatic, but, of course, cannot identify the cause. It appears to be a sensitive indicator of urethritis. For example, Anestad et al.[95] found that 8 of 10 symptomless men with chlamydial urethral infection diagnosed by LCR had a positive leukocyte esterase test. It has been suggested that this is a useful screening test where resources are limited; a positive result would lead to testing for the cause of the urethritis[96].

Detection of chlamydial antigen by immunocytochemical methods

Although polyclonal antibodies against *C. trachomatis* have been developed and used successfully in the detection of chlamydial antigens in clinical specimens, the use of monoclonal antibodies in test systems has advantages because they react only with single antigenic determinants. Monoclonal antibodies were first produced by Stephens and colleagues[97]. Antibodies that reacted with genus-specific antigens reacted preferentially with reticulate body antigens whereas those that reacted to species, sub-species or type-specific antigens reacted with both reticulate body and elementary body antigens. Monoclonal antibodies have been used in fluorescent and enzyme immunoassay (EIA) methods for the detection of chlamydial antigens in conjunctival, urethral, and endocervical material and, in general, have shown a good correlation with those of conventional culture.

In the case of direct immunofluorescence tests using monoclonal antibodies against the MOMP of *C. trachomatis*, the sensitivity of the test on endocervical material is 80% to 90% relative to culture, but somewhat lower when male urethral specimens are tested[94]. As the staining characteristics of the elementary bodies or inclusions are visualized directly, the specificity of the test is high, but only when performed by an experienced microscopist. In addition, the adequacy of the specimen can be assessed. It is a somewhat laborious

test that does not lend itself to widespread screening. It is still used as a confirmatory test for positive results in other non-culture tests.

Enzyme immunoassays are used widely in the diagnosis of chlamydial infection. In both direct and indirect assays, antibodies against LPS are used because it is more abundant and more soluble than MOMP. Antibodies to LPS may cross react with the LPS of other species of bacteria and produce false positive results. In specimens yielding positive results in the EIA, confirmation of the result can be obtained by repeating the test in the presence of a monoclonal antibody specific for chlamydial LPS. This blocks the LPS epitope bound by the detector antibody, and a reduced signal confirms the initial result[94]. The sensitivities of commercially available EIAs compared with culture have varied but have been reported as being between 73% and 97% for male and female specimens; a sensitivity of only 83% has been reported with one EIA used on endocervical specimens[94]. The specificity of these assays is generally high (96% to 100%) provided blocking assays or direct immunofluorescence methods are used to confirm positive results. It should be noted that without confirmatory tests, the positive predictive value of a test in a population with a low prevalence of infection is low. The major advantages of immunocytochemical methods over culture are that they are simpler, quicker, and problems of transport are circumvented. The results with respect to sensitivity, however, do not compare favorably with those of molecular methods of diagnosis (see pp. 292–293). Enzyme immunoassays have been evaluated for the detection of chlamydial antigen in male urine. The sensitivity of these tests has varied from 53% to 86% compared with culture, being most reliable in symptomatic men, and the specificity ranges from 98% to 100%. As EIAs have low sensitivity and specificity when used on female urine samples, their use should be avoided in the diagnosis of chlamydial infection in women.

A solid-phase immunoassay (Clearview Chlamydia®, Unipath, UK) used in clinics in developing countries for the rapid diagnosis of cervical chlamydial infection has high specificity (from 95% to almost 100%) and, when compared with culture, of comparable sensitivity (79% to 90%) to EIA[98]. Other similar test systems are available commercially and include Surecell Chlamydia® (Kodak) and Testpack Chlamydia® (Abbott). When used for the detection of chlamydial antigen in first-voided specimens of urine from men, however, the sensitivities of these tests as compared with LCR are low, ranging from 62.9% to 70.9%, although their specificities remain high[99]. It is suggested, however, that the results of these methods should be considered presumptive, and a positive test should be confirmed by a laboratory test[94].

Culture

Isolation of C. trachomatis in McCoy cells, irradiated to stop their replication, was considered a sensitive method and, until the introduction into clinical practice of nucleic acid amplification methods, was considered the 'gold standard' diagnostic method.

As irradiation is inconvenient for many laboratories alternative methods of comparable sensitivity have been described, for example treatment with cycloheximide, 5-iodo-2-deoxyuridine or cytochlasin B. Treatment with these agents favors intracellular parasitism by preventing host cell replication and thus making more of the nutrients and precursors in the medium available to the chlamydiae. A simplified culture method uses cycloheximide, an inhibitor of protein synthesis in eukaryotic but not in prokaryotic cells, to favor the growth of chlamydiae. This method is suitable for routine isolation of C. trachomatis on a large scale as it does not involve pretreatment of the cells; cycloheximide is added after the chlamydiae have been taken up by the cells.

The clinical specimen is inoculated into flat-bottomed tubes containing the cell monolayers on cover-slips, and the tubes are then centrifuged for 1 hour at 3000 g at a temperature of 35°C to enhance the intracellular uptake of chlamydiae. The inoculated monolayers are then incubated for 48 to 72 hours, and the cells then stained by a direct immunofluorescence method using anti-MOMP monoclonal antibody. Inclusions may be demonstrated in positive cases.

Nucleic acid detection methods

Although isolation of chlamydiae in culture was long regarded as the 'gold standard' against which other diagnostic tests for chlamydial infection were compared, it is now clear that its sensitivity is significantly lower than that of the amplified molecular methods of diagnosis.

In the early 1990s the use of amplified DNA methods such as LCR and PCR that target nucleotide sequences on the plasmid, multiple copies of which are found within each elementary body, were evaluated as diagnostic methods for chlamydial infection in men and women. Early studies suggested that the sensitivity of PCR or LCR for the detection of C. trachomatis in the male urethra and in the uterine cervix was significantly higher than that of culture[100, 101]. The results from a multicenter study in which women who attended a variety of clinics were tested for C. trachomatis infection by culture and by LCR, the target sequence lying within the cryptic plasmid of the organism, are illustrative[101]. A total of 234 women were confirmed as being infected: 152 women were identified by culture and 221 by LCR. The corresponding sensitivities were 94% for LCR and 65% for culture. It was also shown that the sensitivity of LCR performed on urethral samples in the diagnosis of urethral infection in 542 men attending STI clinics in the US was about 98%, with a positive predictive value of 100%, and a negative predictive value of 99.5%[102].

The diagnosis of urethral chlamydial infection in men has traditionally relied upon the collection of urethral material for culture or antigen detection. Over the past decade, however, it has become clear that the detection of chlamydial DNA by either PCR or LCR in first-voided specimens of urine is a sensitive diagnostic method. Chernesky et al.[102] showed that the sensitivity of LCR assay on urine samples was 93.5%, compared with only 56.5% by culturing urethral swabs, and that there was no significant difference in the detection rate between those with or without symptoms; the specificity of the test was 100%.

As shown by isolation of C. trachomatis in culture, up to 60% of infected women have infection of both cervix and urethra,

30% have cervical infection only, and up to 30% have urethral infection only. With the high sensitivity of the amplified molecular diagnostic methods, it might be expected that chlamydial DNA will be found in the urine of the majority of infected women. This appears to be the case, as shown by the studies of Lee et al.[103]. From 1937 women, who attended a variety of clinics in the US and Canada, they obtained endocervical swabs for culture for C. trachomatis and first-voided urine samples for chlamydial DNA using a LCR test. The LCR test detected C. trachomatis in the urine of 150 (93.8%) of 160 infected women, but culture was positive in only 104 (65%). Broadly similar results were reported by Bassiri et al.[104] who studied a group of 447 women who attended a family planning clinic in Sweden, and Quinn et al.[59] who reported that 88% of 49 confirmed chlamydial infections in women attending STI clinics were identified by LCR on urine samples. In the studies referred to in this section, direct immunofluorescence tests or a second LCR assay, using a different target DNA for amplification resolved discordant results from matched patient samples assayed by culture and PCR or LCR. Clearly the detection of chlamydia-specific DNA sequences in a first-voided urine sample is a highly sensitive method for the diagnosis of chlamydial infection in men and women. It has the advantage of being non-invasive, thereby lending itself to use in population screening programs.

Other amplified molecular methods are also available. The transcription-mediated amplification assay (TMA), based on the amplification of chlamydial ribosomal RNA, has been shown to be highly sensitive for the detection of chlamydiae in endocervical specimens, and in urine from both men and women. When the assay was performed on 479 endocervical samples, the sensitivity and specificity were 100% and 99.5% respectively[105]. Although the specificity was 100%, the sensitivity of the test was shown to be somewhat lower when performed on 480 female urine specimens (93.8%). For 464 urine samples from men, the sensitivity and specificity were 95.6% and 98.7% respectively. However, experience with a second generation TMA test on cervical specimens has shown that the sensitivity is somewhat lower (92.1%), because some women are positive only in urine[106]. The latter authors also noted that the overall performance of this test was better than that of PCR or LCR.

An interesting observation by Moller et al.[107] was that the rate of detection of chlamydiae by either LCR or TMA decreased markedly in urine samples obtained during the third week after menstruation. As this phenomenon was not noted in vaginal-flush specimens, it was postulated that estrogen in urine may be an inhibitory factor in these tests. However, the percentage of positive women was significantly higher during the fourth week after menstruation than at other times.

Strand displacement amplification (SDA) is an isothermal *in vitro* method of amplifying a DNA sequence prior to its detection, and real-time SDA detection for the cryptic plasmid of *C. trachomatis* with high sensitivity has been shown. During SDA the probe is converted to a fully double-stranded form that specifically binds a genetically modified form of the endonuclease EcoRI which lacks cleavage activity but retains binding specificity. A fluorescein-labeled oligodeoxynucleotide detector probe hybridizes to the amplification product that rises in concentration during SDA and the single to double-strand conversion is monitored through an increase in fluorescence. When performed on urine samples from 825 men and 399 women, the sensitivity, specificity, and positive and negative predictive values of the test were 95.3%, 99.3%, 95.9%, and 99.2%[108]. Strand displacement amplification is therefore suitable for screening of urine specimens from both men and women.

The amplified molecular diagnostic methods have the additional advantage that there can be simultaneous detection of other STIs, including *N. gonorrhoeae* and *T. vaginalis*.

Serological methods

Serology is not generally useful in the diagnosis of genital tract infection due to *C. trachomatis*. Information on antibody responses during chlamydial infections is based largely on micro-IF tests in which reactions between antibodies and acetone-fixed organisms are detected by application of a fluorescein-labeled antiglobulin conjugate. In the micro-IF test[109], sera are screened against several antigens, either singly or in groups, representative of the many chlamydial serovars. Only a few laboratories offer this service. Although the test may yield useful epidemiological information on the extent to which a population has been exposed to genital chlamydial infections, it is of little value in the assessment of individual patients since the prescence of antibody could be a reflection of past infection.

A fourfold rise in titer or seroconversion from seronegative to seropositive has correlated well with the isolation of *C. trachomatis*, but this does not provide rapid diagnosis, since antibodies often take up to 1 month to become detectable. Tests for antichlamydial IgM are unreliable because specific IgM is not always present, often because the individual has been exposed previously to chlamydiae, and is generating an anamnestic response following the most recent exposure[94]. The detection of IgM antibody against *C. trachomatis* by the micro-IF test, however, may be helpful in the diagnosis of chlamydial pneumonia in the neonate (see pp. 299–300).

Collection of specimens for the detection of *Chlamydia trachomatis*

In the male

The following methods may be used for the detection of chlamydial infection in men.

Methods based on the detection of chlamydia-specific nucleic acid sequences

Where facilities exist for the detection of chlamydial DNA by PCR, LCR, TMA, or SDA, a first-voided 20 mL specimen of urine is obtained in a sterile universal container. Alternatively, urethral material can be collected for the detection of chlamydial nucleic acids by passing an endourethral swab into the anterior urethra for 5 cm, withdrawing, and placing in the buffer solution provided by the manufacturer of the test kit, before transporting to the laboratory. As the taking of an endourethral sample can cause considerable discomfort, tests based on urine are preferred.

Culture methods*‡

After moistening the swab with transport medium, an endourethral swab (Medical Wire and Equipment Company Ltd) is passed into the anterior urethra to a depth of 5 cm and withdrawn, and the tip of the swab is then agitated in a container of 2SP. Excess fluid is removed by rotating the swab while gently pressing against the inside of the container.

Antigen detection methods

In the enzyme immunoassay systems for which collection kits are available, urethral material is obtained as for PCR or LCR methods, and the swab is sent in the transport fluid provided. Alternatively, and when patient numbers are small, direct immunofluorescence for the detection of antigen is sometimes used (for example, the Microtrak® *C. trachomatis* direct specimen test (Syva, California, US)). In this test a urethral swab is rolled on to a slide and fixed in acetone. In some hands, examination by direct immunofluorescence of centrifuged urine sediment for antigen has been found to be almost as sensitive as that of a urethral smear in men with urethritis[110]. The sensitivity of EIA of urine sediment has also been shown to be high (89%)[110]. For antigen detection by these methods, a 20 mL first-voided urine sample collected in a sterile container that does not contain preservative should be obtained, and maintained at 4°C until transported to the laboratory.

---

* Specimens should be sent to the laboratory within 2 hours when possible; otherwise they should be taken in a cryoprotectant transport medium (e.g. 2SP) and stored at −70°C before inoculating monolayers. If this is not possible specimens should be transported in liquid nitrogen.
‡ Antibiotic treatment given to patients before specimens are taken adversely affects the chances of isolation. In patients treated with cephalosporins or penicillin the chances of negative results in primary isolation are increased.

In the female

For the detection of infection with *C. trachomatis*, specimens are obtained as follows.

Methods based on the detection of chlamydial nucleic acids

A cotton wool or rayon-tipped plastic swab is used. It is inserted about 1 cm into the endocervical canal, rotated several times, and, after withdrawal, it is cut off into a tube of the buffer fluid provided by the kit manufacturer. Alternatively, a first-voided specimen of urine may be obtained. Quinn *et al.*[111] compared the results of a PCR on matched endocervical and female urine specimens, and showed that urine PCR is as sensitive as endocervical PCR for the detection of *C. trachomatis*. Although the examination of urine by PCR or LCR for chlamydial DNA may conveniently replace the use of genital material for chlamydial detection, in the setting of a STI clinic, the authors consider it better to obtain cervical specimens directly. It should also be noted that a delay of more than 24 hours in the transport of urine specimens at room temperature to the laboratory may reduce the sensitivity of LCR[112]. Conversely, storage of urine specimens overnight, or thawing after freezing, may enhance sensitivity[113].

Several workers have examined the performance of amplified molecular methods when applied to self-collected specimens.

1. *Vaginal flush samples* have been obtained by introducing a pipette containing 5 mL sterile isotonic saline into the vagina, which is then flushed with the contents of the pipette after which the fluid is sucked back, and the pipette sealed before transport to the laboratory. In a series of 889 women, 45 of whom had chlamydial infection, vaginal flush material gave positive results in the TMA and LCR in 84% and 82% of the infected women[107]. These results were better than those obtained in the same tests performed on first-voided urine specimens (only 49% by LCR and 73% by TMA).

2. The detection of chlamydiae by PCR or LCR in self-collected *vaginal introital specimens* has been shown by several investigators to be a sensitive diagnostic method. The patient herself places a Dacron-tipped swab 2.5 cm into the distal vagina for 10 seconds, after which the swabs are placed by the patient into the appropriate transport media provided by the manufacturer. In a study of 2823 women, this diagnostic approach was reported to have a sensitivity of 87.5%[114]. Self-collected vaginal specimens have been shown to be acceptable to adolescent women[115].

3. *Tampons* can also be used for the detection of chlamydial infection. A tampon is introduced into the vagina and immediately withdrawn. Testing by PCR of tampon-collected specimens from 660 women was shown to be more sensitive than testing of a first-voided urine sample[116].

Culture methods*† (p. 293)

A cotton wool-tipped applicator stick is used as above, but after withdrawal it is agitated in the 2SP transport medium in which the specimen is transported to the laboratory.

Antigen detection methods

For the detection of chlamydial antigens by EIA, endocervical material is obtained as before with a swab similar to that used for the detection of nucleic acids. The swab is cut off into a tube of buffer provided by the manufacturer of the test kit. Endocervical specimens can also be examined by direct immunofluorescence, the material being rolled on a slide and fixed in acetone before transport to the laboratory. The detection of antigen in urine sediment by EIA is too insensitive for clinical use.

Chlamydia trachomatis has been recovered from the vaginas of women who have had hysterectomies[117], and it is recommended that specimens for the identification of infection should be taken from the vaginal vault of such patients attending STI clinics. In addition, urethral material for either antigen detection or for DNA detection should be obtained; alternatively, a first-voided specimen of urine should be collected for the latter test.

In both sexes

In the case of the conjunctiva, in the neonate particularly, the lower lid of each eye should be everted and a specimen taken by drawing a swab along its mucosal surface. Specimens should be taken from the upper lids also if possible.

Rectal specimens for the detection of chlamydial nucleic acids or for culture should be obtained, using either, in the case of the former, the swab provided by the manufacturer of the test kit, or, in the latter, a cotton wool-tipped applicator stick, the swab being inserted into the anal canal to a distance of about 5 cm and rotated several times before withdrawal. Pharyngeal specimens for amplified molecular methods or culture are obtained by passing the swab over the tonsils or tonsillar fossae, and then placing in the appropriate transport fluid. Enzyme immunoassays are not suitable for the detection of chlamydiae in either the pharynx or rectum.

NB In cases of sexual assault or abuse, culture methods alone are considered acceptable for medico-legal purposes.

Box 10.1 Circumstances in which screening for chlamydial infection should be considered (Scottish Intercollegiate Guidelines Network 2000[202])

All individuals attending STI clinics, irrespective of symptoms or signs of infection.

All patients with another STI such as genital warts.

Sexual partners of individuals with proven or suspected infection, including those with a condition for which *C. trachomatis* is a frequent (but undiagnosed) cause, such as epidiymo-orchitis and pelvic inflammatory disease.

Mothers of infants with chlamydial conjunctivitis.

All women undergoing termination of pregnancy.

All women undergoing uterine instrumentation, including the insertion of an intra-uterine contraceptive device, who have risk factors for chlamydial infection.

Semen and egg donors.

SCREENING FOR GENITAL CHLAMYDIAL INFECTION

Groups that should be offered screening for infection with *C. trachomatis* are listed in Box 10.1. The prevalence of infection amongst some of these patients, such as those attending STI clinics and women seeking termination of pregnancy, is high. Pelvic inflammatory disease is a complication in about 25% of untreated women undergoing termination of pregnancy[118]. As the semen of sperm donors may contain *C. trachomatis*[119], it is appropriate to screen potential donors for infection.

From consideration of the epidemiology of chlamydial infection, opportunistic screening should be considered in women who are under the age of 25 years and who are sexually active. In addition, screening may also be offered to older women with two or more partners or a partner change within the preceding year.

The value of screening for infection using non-cultural diagnostic methods is outlined in Chapter 2. The strategy of identifying, testing, and treating those women who are at increased risk of chlamydial infection is associated with a reduced incidence of pelvic inflammatory disease.[120]. In a randomized, controlled trial to determine if selective screening prevented pelvic inflammatory disease, this complication developed in 33 of 1598 women who had not been screened, but in only 9 of 645 women who had been screened at entry into the study and who, if infected, had been treated (relative risk 0.44, 95% confidence interval 0.2–0.9)[120].

TREATMENT

General considerations

In vitro studies have shown that *C. trachomatis* isolated from patients is sensitive to a variety of antimicrobial agents, but particularly to tetracyclines, macrolides, azithromycin, and some 4-fluoroquinolones. Generally there is a good correlation between the *in vitro* susceptibility of *C. trachomatis* and the treatment response. A notable exception, however, is that of ciprofloxacin that has a minimum inhibitory concentration (MIC_{90}) of 1.6 mg/L. Clinical trials, however, have shown that the failure rate is high: 11 of 21

men who had been given ciprofloxacin in an oral dosage of 750 mg twice daily for 7 days had a positive culture result when assessed 28 days after treatment[121].

The results of some clinical trials have been difficult to interpret because

1. small numbers of patients were enrolled or completed treatment
2. the follow-up period was inadequate
3. there was uncertainty whether the sexual partners had been treated
4. persistence and re-infection had not been clearly distinguished
5. only cultures had been used to ascertain cure[122].

However, it is clear that some agents are very effective and Table 10.1 indicates the treatment regimens that are currently recommended by the Centers for Disease Control and Prevention in the US[123], and by the Clinical Effectiveness Group in the UK[124]. With the exception of azithromycin, which can be given as a single oral dose, these drugs must be given for at least 7 days to ensure maximum efficacy. Patient adherence, however, is often unsatisfactory and medication may be inadvisably shared with a partner. For these reasons, a single dose of azithromycin, given under supervision, is the authors' preferred treatment. This drug is more expensive than the others, and this factor may have to be considered when designing clinic treatment protocols. Single-dose therapy with azithromycin, however, appears to be more cost-effective than multiple-dose regimens[125]. Unwanted side effects may also be a factor in adherence to treatment; for example 26% of patients treated with erythromycin in a daily dose of 2 g discontinued therapy because of gastrointestinal side effects[126]. It is therefore important to employ a drug

Table 10.1 Treatment regimens for uncomplicated anogenital chlamydial infection (Clinical Effectiveness Group 2001[124]; Centers for Disease Control and Prevention 2001[123])

Drug	Dosage
Azithromycin[a] *or*	1 g as single oral dose
Doxycycline[a] *or*	100 mg by mouth every 12 hours for 7 days
Erythromycin base[b] *or*	500 mg by mouth every 6 hours for 7 days
Erythromycin base[c] *or*	500 mg by mouth every 12 hours for 14 days
Erythromycin ethylsuccinate[d] *or*	800 mg by mouth every 6 hours for 7 days
Deteclo[c] *or*	300 mg every 12 hours for 7 days
Ofloxacin[b]	200 mg every 12 hours[c] *or* 300 mg every 12 hours[d] *or* 400 mg as single daily dose[c] given orally for 7 days
or Levofloxacin[d] *or*	500 mg once daily for 7 days
Tetracycline[c]	500 mg every 6 hours for 7 days

[a] Treatments recommended by Centers for Disease Control and Prevention 2002[123] and the Clinical Effectiveness Group 2002[124].
[b] Alternative regimens recommended by Centers for Disease Control and Prevention 2002[123] and Clinical Effectiveness Group 2001[124].
[c] Alternative regimen recommended by Clinical Effectiveness Group 2001[124].
[d] Alternative regimens recommended by Centers for Disease Control and Prevention 2002[123].

regimen that, in addition to potency, has minimal side effects.

Oral treatment is necessary to eradicate chlamydial eye infection; topical therapy may suppress the ocular symptoms but, of course, the underlying genital tract infection will not be cured.

Patients should be given oral and written information about chlamydial infection, and the issues to be discussed include[124]

- the sexually transmitted nature of the infection
- the fact that infection is often symptomless, particularly in women, and may not be apparent for many months if not years
- the complications of untreated infection
- the importance of adherence to the antimicrobial treatment regimen
- the unwanted side effects of treatment
- the need to investigate and treat the sexual partner(s)
- the need to abstain from sexual intercourse until a cure is effected
- the interaction between oral contraceptive pills and antimicrobial therapy.

Antimicrobial drugs for the treatment of anogenital chlamydial infection

Tetracyclines

In vitro *susceptibility of* Chlamydia trachomatis *to tetracyclines**

The MICs of doxycycline have mostly ranged from 0.016 to 0.5 mg/L, the MIC_{90}

---

* Drug susceptibility can be determined by methods similar to those described by Kuo et al.[127] . An inoculum of 10^3 to 10^5 inclusion forming units is centrifuged on to McCoy or HeLA cells grown in monolayers in the absence of antibiotics and pre-treated with diethylaminoethyl dextran. The supernate is replaced with minimal essential medium containing serial dilutions of the antibiotics. After incubation for 72 hours, the cells are fixed and stained, and the inclusions counted. The MICs are taken as the lowest dilutions that completely inhibit the formation of inclusion bodies. The minimum bactericidal concentration (MBC) is determined by incubation for 48 hours of infected cells with dilutions of antibiotics as described for MIC determination, followed by incubation for a further 48 hours in antibiotic-free medium, and one passage on to cell monolayers grown in antibiotic-free medium. The MBC is the lowest antibiotic concentration required to inhibit the development of a single inclusion.

being 0.064[128]; predictably, the minimum bactericidal concentrations (MBCs) have been higher, ranging from 0.5 to 8 mg/L, the MBC_{90} being 8 mg/L. The MIC range of minocycline is similar to that of doxycycline. The MIC of oxytetracycline ranges from 0.03 to 1.0 mg/L with a MIC_{90} of 0.06 mg/L; the MBC_{90} is 0.25 mg/L.

Efficacy of tetracyclines in the treatment of anogenital infections with Chlamydia trachomatis

Cure rates in men treated with doxycycline, oxytetracycline or tetracycline range from 97% to 100%[122], and in women from 92% to 100%[122, 129]. Deteclo® appears to be as effective as doxycycline; Munday et al.[130] detected C. trachomatis in endocervical material from 3 of 43 women who had been treated with Deteclo® for 7 days, and followed up for about 2 years. Minocycline in an oral dosage of 100 mg once daily has been shown to be as effective as doxycycline in the treatment of chlamydial genital infections[131].

Erythromycin

In vitro *susceptibility of* Chlamydia trachomatis *to erythromycin*

The MICs of erythromycin range from 0.064 to 0.128 mg/L, the MIC_{90} being 0.128 mg/L. The MBCs are in the range 4 to 64 mg/L and the MBC_{90} is 64 mg/L[128].

Efficacy of erythromycin in the treatment of anogenital infections with Chlamydia trachomatis

In the treatment of chlamydial infection in men given 500 mg every 12 hours for 14 to 15 days, cure rates have ranged from 90% to 100%[132], and in women from 86% to 100%[129, 133]. Although cure rates in excess of 95% have been reported in the use of erythromycin in an oral dosage of 500 mg twice daily for 7 days[134], this has not been the experience of others. Linnemann et al.[126] have shown that the cure rate with a dosage of 2 g per day is significantly higher than that with 1 g per day for 7 days: 27% of 45 patients who received the latter regimen were culture positive after treatment, compared with 10% of 37 patients who were given the

higher dose of erythromycin. These results suggest that erythromycin is not as effective as doxycycline or azithromycin in the treatment of oculogenital chlamydial infections.

Azithromycin

Azithromycin is the first of a class of antibiotics designated as azalides which are related to the macrolides. It differs structurally from erythromycin by the insertion of a methyl-substituted nitrogen at position 9a in the lactone ring, to create a 15-membered macrolide[135].

In vitro *susceptibility of* Chlamydia trachomatis *to azithromycin*

In vitro studies have shown that azithromycin is active against C. trachomatis.

In an early study[128], the MIC of azithromycin for eight clinical isolates, including an L2 isolate, and two laboratory strains, ranged from 0.064 to 0.025 mg/L, the MIC_{90} being 0.25 mg/L. The MBC for these strains was 2 to 8 mg/L, and the MBC_{90} was 8 mg/L. Welsh et al.[136] reported the MIC and MBC of azithromycin as ranging from 0.125 to 0.5 mg/L and 0.125 to 4.0 mg/L respectively. In both studies, the MICs and MBCs exceeded those of tetracycline or doxycycline. There appears to be some interstrain variation in susceptibility to antimicrobial agents, and Welsh et al.[136] noted that serovars F and K were most resistant to tetracyclines, azithromycin, and erythromycin.

Efficacy of azithromycin in the treatment of anogenital infection with the oculogenital serovars of Chlamydia trachomatis

Several studies have examined the use of azithromycin in the treatment of chlamydial infection, and most have compared the results with those of doxycycline. Cure can be achieved in 88% to 100% of men, and in 91% to 100% of women, as judged by a negative culture result after treatment of culture-proven urethral or cervical infection. An interesting recent study examined the treatment of women with either single-dose azithromycin or a course of doxycycline[137]. The outcome measure was a positive test for chlamydial DNA 1 month after treatment. A positive chlamydial test at 1 month was found in 5% of 98 women given azithromycin, and in 4% of 98 women treated with doxycycline; almost 95% of 73 women taking the doxycycline course adhered to the regimen. Hillis *et al.*[137] noted that all women who had a positive test result 1 month after treatment had had behavioral risk factors for re-infection.

Ofloxacin

Ofloxacin is a synthetic, fluorinated carboxyquinolone that is active against *C. trachomatis*, Enterobactericeae and Gram-positive organisms.

In vitro susceptibility of Chlamydia trachomatis *to ofloxacin*

The published MICs and the MBCs of ofloxacin for *C. trachomatis* range from 0.5 to 1.0 mg/L and 0.5 to 1.0 mg/L respectively, the MIC$_{90}$ being 0.8 mg/L[138].

Efficacy of ofloxacin in the treatment of anogenital infections with Chlamydia trachomatis

Different studies have used different treatment regimens, making direct comparisons difficult. However, when the drug has been compared with doxycycline, both drugs being given for 7 days, cure rates, as judged by negative cultures for *C. trachomatis* at least 1 week after completion of therapy, have ranged from 97% to 100%[122].

Levofloxacin

Levofloxacin for the treatment of chlamydial infection has not been studied in clinical trials, but as its pharmacology and antimicrobial activity are similar to ofloxacin, it is recommended for use[123].

Amoxicillin

The penicillins have an incomplete inhibitory effect on *C. trachomatis*, and for amoxicillin the reported MIC has varied widely, between 2.0 and over 4 mg/L[139]. *In vitro*, the rate of replication of *C. trachomatis* can be reduced, and a few clinical studies have shown apparent eradication of the organism. Csango *et al.*[140] reported clearance of chlamydiae from 10 men with urethral chlamydial and gonococcal infection after treatment with amoxicillin in a dosage of 750 mg three times per day for 7 days. Amoxicillin is used in pregnant women in whom other antimicrobial agents are contra-indicated.

Antimicrobial resistance of chlamydiae

Recently multiple drug-resistant strains of *C. trachomatis* have been isolated from 3 patients[141], 2 of whom failed to respond to antimicrobial treatment, and relapsing disease occurred in 1 man. In each case, both the MIC and MCC (minimum chlamydicidal concentration) of doxycycline was over 4.0 mg/L; the MIC of azithromycin was 0.5 mg/L in 2 cases, and over 4.0 mg/L in the other, and the MCC in each case was over 4.0 mg/L. In each case the MIC of ofloxacin was 4.0 mg/L or above, and the MCC exceeded 4.0 mg/L. The finding that in 2 instances, the MIC$_{90}$ of doxycycline was 0.03 mg/L, but the MIC was over 4.0 mg/L suggested that only a small proportion of organisms expressed resistance. The mechanism of this heterotypic resistance is unknown, and the most appropriate treatment of such infections has not been established. A suggestion has been made that longer courses of doxycycline or azithromycin may be effective, as has been the case in relapsing *C. pneumoniae* infection[141].

Treatment of chlamydial infections in pregnancy

The tetracyclines and the quinolones are contraindicated in the treatment of pregnant women. Erythromycin stearate, erythromycin ethyl succinate, or erythromycin base are safe, but treatment efficacy is not as good as with the other commonly used antimicrobial agents, and gastrointestinal side effects may influence adherence to the treatment regimen. The estolate is contraindicated in pregnancy because of possible hepatotoxicity. In a systematic review of interventions for treating genital chlamydial infection in pregnancy[142], eleven trials were included, and it was shown that amoxicillin, given in an oral dosage of 500 mg every 8 hours for 7 days, was as effective as erythromycin in achieving microbiological cure. In addition, it was noted that amoxicillin was better tolerated than erythromycin. The authors of the review, however, emphasize that there is a lack of suitable data on the long-term effectiveness of amoxicillin in terms of the risk of neonatal infection. It is not known, for example, if microbiological cure equates with eradication of the organism, and there is *in vitro* evidence that exposure of chlamydiae to penicillins can induce latency[143].

The issue of the efficacy and acceptability of azithromycin in the treatment of chlamydial infection in pregnant women has only recently been addressed. Adair and colleagues[144] undertook a randomized trial comparing treatment with single dose azithromycin (1 g) and erythromycin given in a dosage of 500 mg every 6 hours for 7 days. They noted cure, as defined as a negative test for specific DNA sequences at follow-up, in 37 (88%) of 42 women treated with azithromycin and 40 (93%) of 43 women given erythromycin. Four of the five women treated with azithromycin who had persistent infection at follow-up were considered to have been re-infected from an untreated partner, and the other woman vomited within 4 hours of administration of the drug. Although there was no significant difference in efficacy between the two treatment regimens, 58% of the women given erythromycin had gastrointestinal side effects leading to discontinuation of therapy in 19% of cases. In contrast, only 12% of those treated with azithromycin had gastrointestinal symptoms.

In the treatment of a pregnant woman with *C. trachomatis* infection, the following regimens have been recommended[123, 124]

1. erythromycin base, given in an oral dose of 500 mg every 6 hours for 7 days, *or* 500 mg every 12 hours for 14 days, *or*, if the woman is intolerant of this regimen,
2. amoxicillin, given orally in a dosage of 500 mg every 8 hours for 7 days.

Alternative regimens that have been proposed by the Centers for Disease Control[123] include:

1. erythromycin base, given orally in a dose of 250 mg every 6 hours for 14 days, *or*,

2. erythromycin ethyl succinate, in an oral dose of 800 mg every 6 hours for 7 days, *or*,

3. eythromycin ethyl succinate, 400 mg orally every 6 hours for 14 days, *or*,

4. azithromycin, in a single oral dose of 1 g, although there are insufficient data to recommend its routine use in pregnancy.

In all cases, a test of cure should be undertaken either 14 to 21 days after completion of treatment if culture is the diagnostic method, or 21 days post-treatment if molecular methods are used for diagnosis.

Management of sexual partners

In all cases, of course, partner notification (contact tracing) is mandatory. If the male has symptoms of urethritis, an arbitrary cut-off of 4 to 8 weeks is often used to identify sexual partners who have been at risk of infection[145]. It is often difficult to identify the source and the secondary contacts of infected but symptomless individuals, and there are no evidence-based guidelines. The most recent sexual partners, and those who have been at risk in the preceding 6 months, should be encouraged to attend for screening. It is the authors' practice to offer treatment to partners at risk, even before the results of the laboratory tests are available and even if negative results are obtained. Treatment on epidemiological grounds is justified in that laboratory tests are not always reliable, treatment is safe, and the risk of re-infecting the index patient is reduced. The identification of infection in a partner, of course, should be followed by contact tracing of that infected individual. Patients should be advised to abstain from sexual intercourse for at least 7 days after single-dose treatment, and until completion of a multiple-dosing regimen; they should also abstain from sexual intercourse until their partners are cured.

Follow-up of treated patients

The need for a test of cure in patients who have been treated for chlamydial infection is controversial. Although several studies have shown high recurrence rates after treatment (up to almost 40%), the populations studied have been at high risk for re-infection, and the results have been based on a limited number of tests. In a small study from general practice, 42 patients were invited to send a first-voided urine specimen and/or a self-collected vaginal fluid specimen at intervals after treatment for the detection of chlamydial DNA[146]. An incidence of recurrent infection of 29% during a 24-week follow-up period was found, and the authors proposed that retesting should be undertaken but not sooner than 12 to 24 weeks after treatment. However, in the authors' clinical practice, patients who have been treated are invited to attend about 3 weeks after completion of treatment. At this visit it is ascertained if they had adhered to the treatment regimen, if they had problems with adherence, for example the development of unwanted side effects, or if they had had sexual contact with an untreated sexual partner in the intervening period. If adherence had been less than optimal, if there has been a risk of re-infection, or if treatment has been with erythromycin (cure with this antimicrobial agent is less certain than with azithromycin or doxy-cycline) a test of cure is undertaken (either by a PCR or LCR). At the follow-up visit the opportunity should be taken to reinforce sexual health advice.

INFECTIONS IN THE NEWBORN DUE TO *CHLAMYDIA TRACHOMATIS*

Conjunctivitis is the most obvious clinical presentation of chlamydial neonatal infection. About 75% of infants delivered vaginally to infected mothers, and just over 20% born by cesarean section to infected women with intact membranes, become infected[147]. The latter finding suggests that infection *in utero* is possible. Infection is not confined to the conjunctiva, and the respiratory tract, the middle ear, the gut, and the vagina can also become infected[148].

Conjunctivitis

There are difficulties in assessing the true incidence of chlamydial neonatal conjunctivitis because babies are rarely in hospital

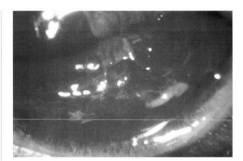

Figure 10.6 Chlamydial conjunctivitis in a neonate

for the full incubation period of 3 to 13 days, or longer when the inoculum is small. In the case of gonococcal conjunctivitis diagnosis is usually made 24 to 48 hours after birth.

Clinical features

The infection usually presents as a muco-purulent conjunctivitis, which may vary from mild to severe, within the incubation period already stated. The discharge may be only scanty and not obviously purulent, but it is sometimes more copious and frankly purulent, or on occasions bloodstained[75]. On examination the palpebral conjunctiva exhibits mild to severe inflammation and papillary hyperplasia (Figure 10.6). In its more severe form there is also edema of the eyelids and the palpebral conjunctiva, particularly of the lower lid, may also be involved. Signs may be minimal and the inflammatory reaction apparently is transitory but in some cases conjunctival scarring develops.

In the absence of specific treatment the course is usually benign, but it may be protracted. The sight is not compromised, although micropannus and conjunctival scarring may be found on long-term follow-up[149].

Diagnosis

In the investigation of neonatal conjunctivitis the following steps are essential.

1. Microscopy of a Gram-stained smear from the palpebral conjunctiva for Gram-negative diplococci (*N. gonorrhoeae*). Use a plastic inoculating loop to collect material for microscopy and culture.

2. Direct inoculation of selective medium with material from the palpebral conjunctiva to detect or exclude *N. gonorrhoeae*.

3. A swab from the palpebral conjunctiva should be placed in 2SP, or other chlamydial transport medium, for the isolation of *C. trachomatis*. Alternatively a swab may be taken for detection of chlamydial antigen by direct immuno-fluorescence or enzyme immunoassay. Although isolation of the organism is the accepted diagnostic method for neonatal chlamydial conjunctivitis, the latter tests have sensitivity (≥ 99%) and specificity (≥ 95%) compared with culture[150, 151]. It has recently been shown that a commercially available PCR has high sensitivity and specificity in the diagnosis of infection at this site. In a study of 75 infants with conjunctivitis, Hammerschlag *et al.*[152] observed that, compared with culture, the sensitivity and specificity of the PCR were 92.3% and 100% respectively.

4. Swabs should be taken and placed in Amies' or other transport medium for later isolation of other bacterial pathogens.

5. In the case of children in whom *C. trachomatis* infection has been identified, pelvic examination of the mother to exclude *N. gonorrhoeae*, *C. trachomatis*, or other pathogens, and examination of the mother's sexual partner.

Treatment of neonatal conjunctivitis

Once gonococcal conjunctivitis has been excluded, a mild neonatal conjunctivitis should be treated with a 0.5% (w/v) solution of neomycin as prescribed, as single-dose sterile eye drops, instilled into the eye every 4 hours. Neomycin is effective against most isolates of staphylococci and some strains of *Proteus vulgaris* and *Pseudomonas aeruginosa*. It has no action against fungi, viruses, or chlamydiae. If the conjunctivitis is marked and does not respond to neomycin then culture or antigen detection tests for chlamydiae should be undertaken. If the organism is discovered or suspected, the child should be treated with erythromycin base or ethylsuccinate

12.5 mg/kg by mouth every 6 hours for 10 to 14 days[123]. As nasopharyngeal infection is found in at least 50% of infants with chlamydial conjunctivitis, topical treatment alone is inadequate; there is no advantage in giving both systemic and topical treatment. As efficacy of erythromycin treatment is about 80%, follow-up of infants to ensure resolution of infection is recommended[123]. It should be noted that the use of oral erythromycin in neonates has been associated with an increased risk of infantile hypertrophic pyloric stenosis (IHPS). In February 1999 about 200 neonates born at a hospital in the US were given oral erythromycin as post-exposure prophylaxis against pertussis. The rate of IHPS during the 4 to 6 weeks following therapy was 32.3 per 1000 live infants, representing a sevenfold increase over the rate recorded during 1997 to 1998[153]. It is therefore recommended that infants treated with erythromycin for chlamydial ophthalmia should be monitored for signs of IHPS*.

Data on the use of azithromycin in the treatment of chlamydial ophthalmia are limited, but a 3-day course of the drug, given orally in a once daily dose of 20 mg/kg, has proved effective in a small number of infants[154].

Infection of the nasopharynx by *Chlamydia trachomatis* in the newborn

Although conjunctivitis is the most common clinical manifestation of neonatal chlamydial infection, the nasopharynx is the most commonly infected site. About three-quarters of infected infants have colonization of the nasopharynx, and about 50% of neonates with chlamydial conjunctivitis have nasopharyngeal involvement[155]. Most infants have no clinical signs of infection at this site, and infection

---

* In hypertrophic pyloric stenosis there is vomiting that becomes frequent and projectile. The vomitus is of gastric content (milk) and is not bile stained, although it may become bloodstained from gastritis. The baby becomes constipated and dehydrated, and fails to thrive. There may be visible gastric peristalsis.

has been shown to persist for up to 28.5 months after birth[32].

Pneumonia

Spread of the organism from the nasopharynx to the lower respiratory tract can result in pneumonitis, with an estimated incidence of 11% to 20% of babies born to infected mothers. Onset of the pneumonitis occurs later than that of conjunctivitis, usually between 3 and 11 weeks, with gradual development of a 'staccato' cough, partial nasal obstruction, and tachypnea. Typically the child is afebrile and not systemically unwell. Chest signs may be minimal when compared with the diffuse bilateral interstitial opacities and hyperinflation seen on chest X-ray (Figure 10.7). Crepitations are more commonly heard than ronchi. There may be an eosinophilia in the peripheral blood and serum immunoglobulins may be elevated.

Culture of the organism from the conjunctivae in concurrent conjunctivitis, or from the nasopharynx, supports the diagnosis of chlamydial pneumonitis. As enzyme immunoassays use group-specific antibodies and *C. pneumoniae* can also be detected by EIA in nasopharyngeal

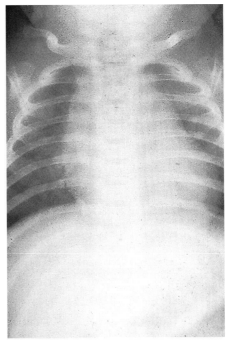

Figure 10.7 Chlamydial pneumonia in an infant

secretions, the value of these tests in the diagnosis of pneumonia caused by *C. trachomatis* is limited. Compared with culture, however, a commercially available PCR has been shown to have sensitivity, specificity, and positive and negative predictive values of 100%, 97.2%, 60%, and 100% respectively[152]. When available, the micro-IF test for antichlamydial IgM can be useful in that a titer of 32 or over is suggestive of *C. trachomatis* pneumonia. The presence of other respiratory pathogens (for example respiratory syncytial virus) must be excluded.

The infection is generally mild and self-limiting, but treatment in the form of erythromycin ethylsuccinate in an oral dose of 12.5 mg/kg every 6 hours for 14 days has been advocated. Most infants clear chlamydiae from the respiratory tract[156], but symptoms may persist for longer. There is, however, no clear evidence that permanent damage results.

Infection at other anatomical sites

Symptomless vaginal and rectal infection with *C. trachomatis* has been detected in about 14% of infants born to infected mothers[157]. Infection was found later (between 70 and 154 days after birth) than in the conjunctiva, and persisted at these anatomical sites for at least a year[32].

CHLAMYDIA TRACHOMATIS INFECTION IN OLDER CHILDREN

In contrast to the situation found in older women, *C. trachomatis* causes a true vaginitis in prepubertal girls. This is a direct consequence of the vagina being lined by columnar epithelial cells in this age group. As a result, vaginal and rectal infection with *C. trachomatis* has been reported in girls who have been sexually abused. Ingram *et al.*[158] found good correlation between vaginal infection and a history of sexual abuse; these authors, however, did not find a significant relationship with pharyngeal infection. As there may be difficulty in differentiating infection with *C. pneumoniae* and *C. trachomatis*, and as perinatally acquired pharyngeal infection

can persist for a long time[32], the Centers for Disease Control and Prevention[123] no longer advocate the examination of pharyngeal material for *C. trachomatis* in children who have been sexually abused. The majority of girls with vaginal or rectal infection are symptomless.

As a diagnosis of chlamydial infection in children has clear medico-legal implications, culture confirmation of the diagnosis is essential; this method of diagnosis is the most specific of those available.

Treatment of infected children who weigh less than 45 kg is with erythromycin base or ethylsuccinate, given in an oral dose of 50 mg^{-1} kg^{-1} day in four divided doses, for 14 days. In the case of children who weigh over 45 kg, but who are under the age of 8 years old, azithromycin in a single oral dose of 1 g can be given. A similar dose of azithromycin is appropriate for children who are over the age of 8 years, but an alternative treatment is with doxycycline, given in a dosage of 100 mg every 12 hours for 7 days[123].

Other possible causes of non-specific genital tract infection

ETIOLOGY

Family Mycoplasmataceae: Genus I *Mycoplasma*, Genus II *Ureaplasma*

The two genera within this family, *Mycoplasma* and *Ureaplasma*, are characterized by a lack of bacterial cell walls and being bounded by a plasma membrane only[159]. They stain poorly with aniline dyes and are best observed in Giemsa-stained smears. Both genera can grow in cell-free media, requiring cholesterol or a related sterol for growth. The basic medium required is a peptone-enriched beef heart infusion broth containing also horse serum and yeast extract as well as penicillin to inhibit bacterial growth. In broth, colonies grow best under aerobic conditions, but solid media are best incubated in a carbon dioxide-enriched atmosphere. Mycoplasmas

penetrate the surface of the agar and grow in the underlying medium, producing the characteristic 'fried-egg' appearance of colonies. The metabolic activity of mycoplasmas can be used to detect their growth in broth. Mycoplasmas metabolize arginine to form ammonia, while ureaplasmas produce urease that breaks down urea to form ammonia.

Mycoplasma species

Mycoplasmas and ureaplasmas have been found to be associated with human infection or disease, and in the case of urogenital infection, interest has concentrated largely on *M. hominis*, *M. genitalium*, and *U. urealyticum*.

The discovery of *M. genitalium* in urethral secretions was reported in 1981 by Tully *et al.*[160]. It is a bottle shaped organism with a terminal rod-like structure that contains an electron-dense core. The genome size is small, 580 kbp, compared with other mycoplasmas, and it has been estimated that it codes for less than 500 genes. It is fastidious in its growth requirements. The organism grows slowly, and produces 'fried-egg-like' colonies in an atmosphere of nitrogen and carbon dioxide, but not in air and carbon dioxide. It metabolizes glucose but not arginine or urea (c.f. *M. hominis* and *U. urealyticum*), and growth is inhibited by thallous acetate (c.f. other mycoplasmas) and a variety of antimicrobial agents[161]. *Mycoplasma genitalium* is motile and can adhere to glass and to other surfaces including epithelial cells, which it can invade[162]. The protein adhesin is 140 kDa in size and clusters on the terminal part of the organism. This mycoplasma, in common with *M. pneumoniae*, is susceptible to tetracyclines, and macrolide antibiotics including azithromycin[163].

Ureaplasma species

Members of the genus *Ureaplasma* are distinguished by their ability to hydrolyze urea and this is the minimum requirement for assigning a new isolate to the genus. The name *U. urealyticum* has been given to the single human species so far identified in this genus. Fourteen serologically distinct serovars have been recognized, and PCR has confirmed the differentiation into two biovars

- the parvo-biovar includes serovars 1, 3, 6, and 14
- the T960-biovar includes the other ten serovars[164].

Differentiation of strains of the organism using PCR is easy to perform and this method may be useful for epidemiological studies. The species occurs predominantly in the mouth, and respiratory, and urogenital tracts.

Both *M. hominis* and *U. urealyticum* are present on the genital mucosa of over half of sexually experienced adults[165], and it is against this background that their role, and particularly that of *U. urealyticum* in nonspecific urethritis should be considered. Colonization of the newborn is detected more often in infants delivered vaginally than in those delivered by cesarean section. Colonization does not persist and there is a progressive decrease with age in the proportion of infants colonized. Both mycoplasmas and ureaplasmas are seldom found in the genitourinary tract in prepubertal boys (for example in 2% of individuals) but more often in prepubertal girls (11%)[166].

Colonization, however, increases as a result of sexual contact. Thus, in a study of 156 young American women who had never had sexual contact, about 6% yielded ureaplasmas, compared with about 27% who had experienced genital apposition without vaginal penetration. In the case of those who had experienced sexual intercourse with only one partner, the colonization rate was about 38%; two partners about 55%; and three or more partners 75%[167]. Male Boston college students, those who had not experienced sexual intercourse were found to be virtually free of genital mycoplasmas. However, among those who had experienced sexual intercourse, colonization with ureaplasmas was significantly more prevalent and rose in relation to the number of sexual partners, ranging from about 19% in those who had one lifetime partner to about 56% in those who had experienced intercourse with fourteen or more women[168]. Subsequent work suggests that the prevalence of both

M. hominis and *U. urealyticum* diminish after the menopause[165].

Mycoplasmas are also associated with bacterial vaginosis (Chapter 17).

Ureaplasma urealyticum is susceptible to tetracyclines, the macrolides erythromycin, and clarithromycin, but is only partially susceptible to azithromycin[163]. Ureaplasmas may become resistant to tetracyclines by acquisition of a streptococcal *tetM* gene. This gene encodes a protein that binds to ribosomes and is associated on the chromosome with *Tn916*, a conjugative transposon. In the early 1980s, about 10% of isolates of *U. urealyticum* were tetracycline resistant[169], and a similar proportion was erythromycin resistant. Strains resistant to both antibiotics were rare.

Clinical and microbiological studies on the etiology of non-gonococcal, non-chlamydial urethritis

Mycoplasma hominis does not seem to play an important pathogenic role in NSU.

Studies on the isolation of *U. urealyticum* have yielded rates ranging from approximately 20% to 80% in patients with NSU, and about 10% to 50% in comparison groups[168]. Antibody against *U. urealyticum* has not been shown to develop with any regularity in cases of NSU.

The failure to provide unequivocal evidence about the role of *U. urealyticum* in the etiology of NSU results, in part, from the impossibility of finding control groups whose sexual behavior can be matched with that of the group of patients with urethritis being tested. Also variations in the efficiency of sampling and isolation methods, and the tendency of organisms to become latent, are likely to be important considerations. For these reasons attempts have been made to come to a firmer conclusion about the role of the organism by studying the effect of antibiotics in alleviating the clinical manifestations of the disease, and to determine whether there is a relationship between improvement and clearance of organisms from the urogenital tract.

In one clinical trial there was statistically significant evidence that sulfona-

mides (that have some activity against *C. trachomatis* but not *U. urealyticum*), were effective in treating chlamydia-positive cases, whereas spectinomycin, active against *U. urealyticum* but relatively inactive against *C. trachomatis*, was successful in treating ureaplasma-positive cases but not those associated with chlamydia. These results[170] support the theory that, although *C. trachomatis* is the principal pathogen in NSU, *U. urealyticum* is also implicated. In later quantitative culture studies also, response to treatment suggested that *U. urealyticum* may be the cause of some cases of chlamydia-negative NSU[171].

As ureaplasmas persist in some men despite complete clinical recovery, they are unlikely to be a major cause of NSU. Notwithstanding this situation, Coufalik *et al.*[172] were able to show by the use of differential antibiotics that ureaplasmas might be the cause of NSU in at least 10% of their patients. Basing their study on the fact that minocycline inhibits the multiplication of both *C. trachomatis* and *U. urealyticum* whereas rifampicin inhibits only chlamydiae, it was observed *inter alia* that patients in whom ureaplasmas disappeared recovered more frequently than those in whom the organisms persisted. Although the observation might be used as evidence for a causative role of ureaplasmas it is not, as the authors explain, possible to know whether the patients improved because the organisms disappeared or whether the organisms were not recoverable because the disease subsided spontaneously, isolation being less easily achieved in the absence of discharge.

Taylor-Robinson and McCormack's analytical discourse[165] on the etiology of NSU refers to the occurrence of naturally occurring tetracycline-resistant ureaplasmas and of a case of non-specific urethritis associated with these resistant organisms[173], and also to the probability that more observations of this kind might be possible and useful.

Further support for the role of *U. urealyticum* in the etiology of NSU was obtained from human inoculation experiments. Two medical men inoculated themselves with two strains of *U. urealyticum*. In this experiment, special precautions were taken to be sure that the inoculum contained *U. urealyticum* only, and that these were not in numbers in excess of what might be introduced during sexual intercourse. In one subject, the ureaplasma multiplied in the urethra and dysuria developed. Pus cells were detected in the urine and an immunological reaction of short duration was detected serologically. Tetracycline given 6 days after inoculation brought about rapid clearance of the organisms from the urine and a more gradual disappearance of symptoms and signs. In the second subject another ureaplasma 'strain' was inoculated and similar effects followed although there was evidence that prostatic involvement had occurred. Although treatment with tetracycline 1 month after inoculation eliminated the organisms, urinary threads containing epithelial cells and polymorphonuclear leukocytes persisted for at least 6 months[174]. As a result of their experiments it can be concluded that *U. urealyticum* is able to cause urethritis and may initiate chronic disease, but whether it is responsible for a major or only an insignificant part of the naturally occurring NSU remains unanswered. Nevertheless, regarding causes of NSU other than *C. trachomatis*, the results of early studies favored *U. urealyticum* as the most frequent alternative agent[165].

However, more recently evidence has accumulated to show that *M. genitalium* may play a part in the etiology of some cases of NSU. Early experiments on isolation of the organisms from clinical specimens were hampered by difficulties in culture[161]. The development of PCRs[175, 176] to detect specific DNA sequences, however, permitted more detailed investigation. Jensen *et al.*[177] detected *M. genitalium* DNA in urethral material from 13 (25%) of 52 men with acute urethritis, in 1 (7%) of 14 men with chlamydial urethritis, and in 12 (35%) of 34 men with non-gonococcal, non-chlamydial urethritis; they found the organism in only 4 (9%) of 47 men without urethritis. Similarly, Horner and colleagues[178] detected *M. genitalium* in urethral specimens from 23% of 103 men with acute NSU, but from only 6% of 53 men without urethritis; they also noted that 28% of men with non-gonococcal,

non-chlamydial urethritis were infected with *M. genitalium*. A remarkably similar prevalence amongst Japanese men was noted by Maeda *et al.*[179]. Studies on the effect of treatment, which might give valuable information on the true role of *M. genitalium* in the etiology of NSU, are incomplete, with small numbers of patients having been followed for only short periods.

Animal experiments, however, support the hypothesis that *M. genitalium* can cause urethritis. Two of four young male chimpanzees who were inoculated intra-urethrally with *M. genitalium* that had been recovered from a man with NSU became infected as shown by persistent recovery of organisms from the urethra for 13 weeks, and by the development of antibodies about 5 weeks after inoculation[180]. Infected animals developed an increase in the number of polymorphonuclear leukocytes in urethral secretions, and, in a subsequent study, *M. genitalium* was cultured from the blood of 2 chimpanzees, usually when there were large numbers of organisms in the urethra[181].

The role of *M. genitalium* as a cause of persistent or recurrent urethritis is uncertain. Using a DNA probe Hooton *et al.*[182] detected *M. genitalium* in the urethral secretions of 10 (27%) of 37 men with persistent or recurrent urethritis, and Taylor-Robinson *et al.*[183], using a PCR, demonstrated the organism in about 20% of men with chronic NSU. In a small number of cases the organism has become undetectable and the urethritis has resolved after a course of erythromycin.

Urethritis caused by organisms other than those discussed is very uncommon (less than 1%) in relation to the mass of patients with NSU. Herpes simplex virus, *Candida* spp. and *T. vaginalis* have been considered as causes. Although earlier studies had suggested a role for *Bacteroides ureolyticus* in the etiology of some cases of NSU, more recent work, in which the organism was isolated with equal frequency from symptomatic and symptomless men, has shown that *B. ureolyticus* is a commensal of the lower genital tract in men and women[184]. Cystitis due to *Mycobacterium tuberculosis* is now a very rare cause of urethritis in the UK, but in urinary tract infections due to other bacteria a urethrocystitis is not uncommon. Both trauma and

foreign bodies are occasional factors, and hypersensitivity may be involved.

The etiology of a proportion of cases of NSU is still far from clear as culture or molecular methods cannot detect organisms.

POST-GONOCOCCAL URETHRITIS

After treatment for gonorrhea with the penicillins or aminoglycosides up to 50% of men can be expected to develop postgonococcal urethritis (PGU), their urethral discharge persists or recurs and an excess of polymorphonuclear leukocytes is seen on microscopy but *N. gonorrhoeae* cannot be found on microscopy or on culture.

The sexually transmissible serovars of *C. trachomatis* have been implicated in the etiology of approximately 50% of cases of PGU while the organism could not be demonstrated in the control group of patients who did not develop PGU[185]. Others[186] have noted that men with gonococcal urethritis who also have a chlamydial infection are more liable to develop PGU. It may be that *N. gonorrhoeae* and *C. trachomatis* are sexually transmitted at the same time. It is presumed that both *U. urealyticum* or *M. genitalium* also play a significant role in the etiology of PGU, but few studies to determine the association have been undertaken.

ISOLATION OF *MYCOPLASMA* SPECIES AND *UREAPLASMA UREALYTICUM*

For optimal isolation of mycoplasmas specimens must not be allowed to become dry and should therefore be inoculated directly into medium, kept at 4°C, and transported to the laboratory as soon as possible. Urine samples should also be kept cool and, for best isolation, centrifuged to deposit epithelial and other cells.

In men, mycoplasmas may be found to colonize the urethra and the subpreputial sac. In the case of women, 'vaginal specimens' are more likely to contain these organisms than the urethra, endocervix, or posterior fornix. The method of obtaining 'vaginal' specimens involves simply spreading the labia with the gloved hand to expose the introitus and inserting a swab

2.5 to 5 cm into the vagina with the other hand and rubbing the swab against the vaginal wall[186a]. First-voided urine samples (40 mL) are an indirect and less sensitive method of sampling genital mucosa in both sexes.

In the laboratory the liquid-to-agar method is based on the fact that *U. urealyticum* metabolizes urea to ammonia, and *M. hominis* metabolizes arginine to ammonia. Aliquots of medium showing raised pH are then added to an agar medium containing urea and a sensitive indicator of ammonia, namely manganese II sulfate. After incubation, the colonies of *U. urealyticum* are dark brown. Colony morphology is not reliable.

Liquid cultures are normally incubated anaerobically at 37°C, while solid media are incubated in an atmosphere containing 95% nitrogen and 5% carbon dioxide. Results are usually available within 1 to 5 days. In the identification of the numerous subtypes of *U. urealyticum*, primers prepared against a nucleotide sequence of serovar 8 react with all fourteen reference strains and can detect about ten colony-forming units[187].

Mycoplasma genitalium can be isolated in SP-4 medium[160]. The medium contains a mycoplasma broth base, tryptone, peptone, yeast extract, fetal calf serum, glutamine, buffer, penicillin and an indicator (phenol red). This may be used in the liquid form without agar, or as a diphasic medium, or in the form of plates. Culture is undertaken at 37°C, in an atmosphere of nitrogen enriched with carbon dioxide (5%). As growth is very slow, culture does not lend itself to routine use, and amplified molecular methods (PCR) are most commonly employed for the detection of *M. genitalium*[161].

DIAGNOSIS OF NON-SPECIFIC URETHRITIS IN MEN AND NON-SPECIFIC GENITAL INFECTION IN WOMEN

The clinical features of NSU are identical to those of chlamydial urethritis. *Chlamydia trachomatis* is implicated in the etiology of many cases of NSU in the male and related infections in the female, and it can be detected by the microbiological tests as outlined below (see pp. 290–293). This service is often much less widely available

than is desirable, particularly in developing nations. Diagnosis in men presenting with a non-specific urethritis with urethral discharge will lead to the prescription of the appropriate effective antibiotic (for example, a tetracycline), whereas diagnosis in women on the grounds of clinical signs is quite unreliable and appropriate therapy will often not be given. Clearly an organismal diagnosis in the case of women at risk of chlamydial infection is an essential service. In the case of *M. hominis* and *U. urealyticum*, half of genital specimens will contain these ubiquitous organisms. With the interpretation of positive findings being difficult to assess in the individual patient, routine isolation is difficult to justify although quantitative cultures may give some help to the clinician.

Non-specific urethritis in men

In the case of urethritis in the male it is the clinician's prime duty to exclude the presence of the gonococcus, initially by careful microscopy of the Gram-stained smear, and also by inoculation of a culture plate at the same time. If the laboratory is distant then a swab may be sent in transport medium (Chapter 11).

An attempt should be made to milk any discharge from the penile urethra. If a discharge is present, the urethral meatus should be cleansed with a saline-soaked gauze swab and the discharge obtained by means of a disposable plastic inoculating loop. A 10 μL loop is inserted past the everted lips of the meatus and gently passed for 2 to 3 cm within the urethra. Where even minor urethral symptoms are present in the male a scraping should be taken and smeared on a microscope slide for Gram-staining. If the initial examination shows five or fewer polymorphonuclear leukocytes per × 1000 microscope field, averaged over five fields, but no Gram-negative diplococci are seen then a presumptive diagnosis of non-specific urethritis is made. The diagnosis of NSU of the anterior urethra is strengthened by finding haziness with or without urethral threads in a first-voided specimen of urine. A haze in urine due to precipitated phosphates may be differentiated from the haze due to pus by adding 10% v/v acetic acid to dissolve the phosphates. An alternative test for NSU is

the microscopical examination of urinary sediment. A 10 to 20 mL specimen of first-voided urine is centrifuged at 400 *g* for 10 minutes, after which most of the supernate is discarded, leaving 0.5 mL. An aliquot of the sediment is pipetted on to a microscope slide, covered with a cover-slip, and examined at a magnification of × 400. The number of polymorphonuclear leukocytes in each of five fields is recorded. Urethritis is diagnosed if there are more than fifteen cells in any of the five fields[188]. When patients have symptoms of urethritis, but microscopical findings are unhelpful, particularly when the man has recently passed urine, it is a useful procedure in such cases to ask patients to return the following morning after retaining urine overnight. The patient should empty his bladder late at night before retiring and come to the clinic in the early morning. Such early morning urethral smears, examined by microscopy and culture, are useful in the detection of minimal degrees of urethritis, whether non-gonococcal or gonococcal.

Routine tests need not be taken to exclude *T. vaginalis* and *Candida* spp. in the male, as cultures are frequently negative and the role of these organisms is probably not important. In the case of cystitis in the male, however, a mid-stream specimen should be taken for bacteriological investigation.

In men with recurrent or persistent urethritis, however, consideration should be given to culturing urethral material for herpes simplex virus, and undertaking the appropriate tests for trichomonal infection (Chapter 17). In such cases and where facilities exist, it may be helpful to test for *M. genitalium*, but testing for *U. urealyticum* usually contributes little to the diagnosis.

Epididymo-orchitis may complicate untreated NSU, and sexually acquired reactive arthritis is an uncommon complication developing in less than 1% of cases.

Non-specific genital infection in women

Non-specific genital infection is a term that extends to the theoretically expected involvement of the female, although it is a less precise clinical entity than NSU in the male. The diagnosis may be unsatisfactorily based on the existence of a non-specific urethritis in the partner, symptoms of increased vaginal discharge or dysuria and the evidence of inflammation of the cervix, vagina, urethra, or greater vestibular gland (Bartholinitis).

TREATMENT OF NON-SPECIFIC URETHRITIS

Acute non-specific urethritis

As the criteria are not well-defined, it is difficult to assess efficacy of treatment of non-gonococcal, non-chlamydial urethritis. The antimicrobial agents that have been detailed above for the treatment of chlamydial infection have all been used in NSU, and are the drugs of choice. Persistence or recurrence of urethritis, however, occurs more often after treatment of non-chlamydial NSU than after treatment for chlamydial urethritis[189], and at least 50% of men with acute NSU have recurrence. The reasons for relapse are speculative but persistence of organisms other than chlamydiae may be responsible. In a double-blind randomized trial of azithromycin (1 g as a single oral dose) and doxycycline (100 mg twice daily for 7 days) clinical cure rates were similar in both groups, irrespective of presence or absence of *C. trachomatis* or *U. urealyticum*[190]. It was noted, however, that the cure rate of urethritis associated with *U. urealyticum* was lower than for chlamydial urethritis at both 2 and 5 weeks follow-up (71% cure rate at 2 weeks and 53% cure rate at 5 weeks).

Although there are conflicting data on the influence of concurrent treatment of the sexual partners of men with acute non-chlamydial NSU on the relapse rate, treatment of partners is recommended, even when tests for chlamydiae yield negative results[124].

Follow-up of men who have been treated for acute non-specific urethritis

In the case of follow-up of men who have been treated for non-chlamydial NSU, it is good practice to invite these men to reattend about 1 week after completion of therapy. At this time, the results of the microbiological tests taken at the initial attendance will be available. The patient should be asked about

- his adherence to therapy, including difficulties associated with side effects
- possible re-infection from an untreated partner.

He should be examined for signs of persistent urethritis by taking a smear of urethral material for Gram-smear microscopy.

Persistent or recurrent non-specific urethritis

There is no consensus on the management of recurrent or persistent NSU. The diagnosis is made by finding a significant number of polymorphonuclear leukocytes in a × 1000 microscopic field of a Gram-stained smear of urethral material in a man who has been treated for acute NSU. At follow-up 2 weeks after treatment, if there are five or more polymorphonuclear leukocytes in the × 1000 microscope field one of the following procedures should be followed.

1. If the patient is asymptomatic without clinical signs of urethritis, reassurance may be all that is necessary, provided that he completed treatment and that his partner(s) has (have) been treated. When there has been difficulty with adherence to a particular drug, the initial drug may be prescribed again, but if problems have been caused by side effects a different antimicrobial should be given.
2. When there are symptoms or clinical signs of urethritis, consideration should be given to the use of erythromycin 500 mg every 6 hours for 2 weeks with metronidazole 400 mg by mouth every 12 hours for 5 days. One study showed the effectiveness of a 3-week regimen of erythromycin[191].

There is no evidence that retreatment of a sexual partner who has already received adequate treatment is necessary[124].

TREATMENT OF NON-SPECIFIC GENITAL TRACT INFECTION IN WOMEN

A diagnosis of NSGI in women implies that *N. gonorrhoeae* has been excluded as a cause. Although attempts must be made to eradicate *C. trachomatis* it must be emphasized that other organisms, including anaerobic bacteria, may be pathogenic on

occasions, such as after surgical procedures, and treatment with metronidazole may be necessary. Streptococci, staphylococci, Gram-negative bacilli, anaerobes, or facultative anaerobes, can be pathogens in the genital tract and antibiotic or chemotherapeutic treatment may be required, depending on the sensitivity of these organisms.

UREAPLASMA UREALYTICUM INFECTION IN PREGNANCY

Even when the membranes are intact, *U. urealyticum* can be cultured from the amniotic fluid, and ureaplasmas can be shown in the inflammatory infiltrates in the fetal membranes[192]. These results, together with those from cultures from endometrium and the results from several studies, has led to the proposal that *U. urealyticum* may be causative in some cases of spontaneous abortion[192]. Three studies have shown an association between isolation of the organism and premature birth[192]. Although other studies have failed to confirm these results, their design was such that they may have been unable to identify a role for *U. urealyticum*.

Lymphogranuloma venereum

Lymphogranuloma venereum is a sexually transmissible chlamydial infection and is found mainly in warm countries. In the cases seen in temperate climates the individual has acquired the infection when in the tropics. The incubation period is short (3 to 12 days) after which an evanescent primary lesion develops on the external genitalia or in the rectum, vagina or urethra, or, rarely, elsewhere on the body. Two or three weeks after infection the draining lymph nodes enlarge, become matted together, fluctuant, and eventually break down and discharge pus. If the disease is untreated the anogenital region may become scarred and edematous, and fistulae and strictures may develop. When pelvic nodes, which drain the cervix, upper vagina, and rectum, are involved, exudate may be discharged into the pelvic viscera and cause scarring; strictures may develop subsequently.

ETIOLOGY

Lymphogranuloma venereum is caused by *C. trachomatis* bv. *lymphogranuloma venereum*. The characteristics of chlamydiae have been discussed above (see pp. 282–283). Inclusion bodies composed of aggregates of the organisms may be identified in scrapings taken from primary lesions, in pus aspirated from buboes, and in histological sections of affected lymph nodes. Using micro-IF techniques, three serovars of *C. trachomatis* bv. *lymphogranuloma*, namely L1, L2, and L3, and one variant, L2a, have been identified.

Lymphogranuloma venereum is mostly acquired during sexual intercourse with an infected partner. Accidental infections, for example in doctors, are rare. Exudate from the primary lesions, discharging sinuses and the anus are infectious, as may be material from lesions which have persisted for years untreated.

EPIDEMIOLOGY

Lymphogranuloma venereum (LGV) has a worldwide distribution; it is common in tropical and subtropical areas, but rare in temperate climates. Infections diagnosed in the UK have almost always been acquired abroad; seamen and other travelers are most frequently affected. In tropical countries, sex workers serve as an important source of infection. It seems that the global incidence of the disease is falling. Lymphogranuloma venereum may be associated with other STIs in the same patient. Severe proctocolitis in men who have sex with men may be caused by LGV (Chapter 18).

PATHOLOGY AND PATHOGENESIS

The histological appearance of the primary genital lesion, a flat base of granulation tissue surrounded by a narrow zone of necrosis, is not specific. The margins of the ulcer are undermined and the adjacent epithelium may show pseudo-epitheliomatous hyperplasia. Lymphocytes and plasma cells infiltrate the underlying corium where there may be necrotic foci.

The micro-organisms spread from the site of the initial lesion to the regional lymph nodes. Multiple necrotic foci appear within the parenchyma of the gland, followed by infiltration – initially with polymorphonuclear leukocytes and later with plasma cells. Marked hyperplasia of the germinal centers occurs.

With the enlargement and coalescence of necrotic areas, abscesses develop. The gland capsule becomes inflamed early in the disease and perinodal tissues, including skin, become involved in this inflammatory process. Penetration of the abscess through the skin results in the formation of multiple sinuses.

In women, inguinal lymphadenitis is less common than in men. This is probably because lymphatic fluid from the upper vagina and cervix drains to the external and internal iliac nodes. The disease in females usually presents at a later stage characterized by chronic vulvar ulceration and edema of the labia, the latter resulting from obstruction of lymphatic vessels by fibrous tissue in the vulva and in the lymph nodes. Evidence of continuing inflammation is manifest as areas of granulomatous tissue in the genitalia[193, 194]. The name esthiomène, from the Greek meaning 'eaten away', has been applied to the disease at the stages when there has been marked destruction of tissue.

Rectal involvement, consisting essentially of ulceration of the mucosa with penetration of the muscular layer by inflammatory cells and subsequent stricture formation, although seen mainly in women, occurs also in gay men who have had anal intercourse. In LGV proctitis there is a diffuse infiltration of the lamina propria with neutrophils, plasma cells, and lymphocytes. Crypt abscesses and the formation of granulomas with multinucleated giant cells are common[195].

CLINICAL FEATURES

The interval between exposure to infection and the appearance of the primary lesion, if this develops, is usually 3 to 12 days; longer intervals of up to 5 weeks have been described. A further interval of 1 to 6 weeks usually elapses before regional lymph node enlargement is detected.

Untreated, the disease usually runs a course of between 6 and 8 weeks and may resolve completely. In many cases (at least 70%) there remain changes due to lymphatic obstruction and intermittent recrudescence of the disease can occur. In the early stages, LGV may conveniently be divided from the clinical point of view into two syndromes, namely the inguinal and the genito-anorectal[196].

Inguinal syndrome

This is the most frequent manifestation in men, it is uncommon in women as the primary lesion is not often found in the lower vagina or on the vulva. There are primary genital lesions, regional lymph node enlargement, and constitutional disturbances.

A history of a primary genital lesion, rare in women, is obtained in 20% to 50% of men. The lesion, usually a painless papulovesicle, tends to occur anywhere on the penis and heals within a few days. A lesion within the urethra may mimic an NSU. Extragenital lesions are rare, although oral infections are known to occur.

There is regional lymph node enlargement within 1 to 4 weeks of the appearance of the primary lesion. In most cases (at least 75%), there is unilateral involvement of the inguinal and/or femoral lymph nodes (Figure 10.8). The nodes are painful, tender, and although initially discrete, become matted together as a result of periadenitis.

Occasionally, multilocular abscesses develop and coalesce within the lymph nodes, which become fluctuant (bubo formation). Although untreated buboes may resolve spontaneously within a few weeks, abscesses may rupture through the overlying adherent skin, producing multiple sinuses. Enlargement of lymph nodes, above and below the inguinal ligament, produces a grooved appearance in the groin, 'sign of the groove', a sign almost pathognomonic of LGV. Healing with scarring eventually occurs, although there may be recurrent sinus formation.

In women the inguinal syndrome is uncommon unless the primary lesion is on the vulva or in the lower vagina, since lymphatic drainage from these sites is to the

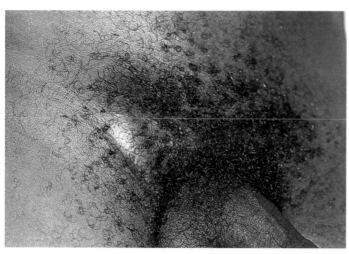

Figure 10.8 Lymphogranuloma venereum: unilateral inguinal lymph node enlargement

inguinal nodes which may show the changes already described. Lymphatic drainage from lesions in the middle and upper vagina and the cervix is to the external and internal iliac and the sacral lymph nodes; inflammation of these glands may produce backache or symptoms of peritonitis. More commonly, there may be few symptoms in the early stage of the disease, which shows itself with later manifestations such as esthiomène. Although symptoms and signs of iliac lymph node involvement are rare, the effects of inflammatory reaction in the lumbar glands can be shown by lymphography[197].

Constitutional symptoms occur more commonly in the inguinal syndrome than in the genito-anorectal syndrome. Pyrexia, malaise, nausea, arthralgia, and headache are frequent. Less commonly (about 10% in women and 2% in men) erythema nodosum or erythema multiforme may be seen.

Genito-anorectal syndrome

The clinical features of this syndrome are seen predominantly in women and in homosexual men. Extension of the inflammatory process by the lymphatic vessels of the rectovaginal septum to the submucous tissues of the rectum is thought to be the principal factor involved in the production of the syndrome in women when the primary lesion has been in the vagina[198].

The patient usually complains of bleeding from the anus and later a purulent anal discharge. On proctoscopy, the rectal mucosa is found to be inflamed with multiple punctate hemorrhages and there is a mucopurulent discharge. There may be superficial ulceration and polypoid growths. Histological examination of rectal biopsy material shows a non-specific granulomatous inflammatory reaction[36]. Although the rectum is most severely affected, a more generalized colitis often co-exists and can be demonstrated radiologically following administration of a barium enema[199].

In the later stages of both syndromes, if the disease is untreated, lymphedema may affect the genitalia of both sexes. The interval between the appearance of the early manifestations of the disease and the development of the later features varies between 1 and 20 years. Women may develop considerable edema (elephantiasis) of the vulva with the formation of polypoid growths, fistulae, ulceration, and scarring (esthiomène). Elephantiasis less frequently affects males, but obstruction of the lymphatic drainage of the external genitalia may lead to edema of the penis or scrotum and later to distortion of the penis. Strictures of the male and female urethra, with the formation of fistulae, are rare late complications.

In the genito-anorectal syndrome late complications include tubular rectal stricture, with or without proctitis and colitis, perianal abscesses, and perineal and rectovaginal fistulae. Intestinal obstruction may result from stricture formation, and carcinoma may develop on a chronic rectal stricture[200].

DIAGNOSIS

Diagnosis is based on the history and clinical features of the disease backed by bacteriological and serological tests; intradermal tests such as the Frei test are obsolete.

Culture of the organism

Attempts should be made to isolate *C. trachomatis* in tissue culture. Material, sent to the laboratory as quickly as possible on suitable transport medium, should be cultured in cycloheximide-treated McCoy or other susceptible cell lines. After incubation, cell cultures are stained by an immunofluorescence method and examined microscopically for inclusions. Chlamydiae are isolated only in about 30% of cases.

Demonstration of chlamydial antigen in tissue biopsies

Using immunofluorescence and immunoperoxidase methods Alacoque *et al.*[201] have detected chlamydial antigens within the macrophages of biopsy specimens of the granulation tissue from a patient with long-standing LGV and have suggested that such immunological methods may be useful in diagnosis.

Serological tests

Lymphogranuloma venereum complement fixation test (LGVCFT)

The chlamydial group LPS antigen used in this test is produced in embryonated hen eggs infected with *C. psittaci*. This test generally becomes positive during the initial 4 weeks of infection and the titer rises during this period in the untreated patient. Titers of 64 and over support the diagnosis of LGV, and a titer of 32 or less excludes the diagnosis.

In early LGV the LGVCFT titers fall after treatment and the test usually becomes negative after a variable period of months to several years. Treatment of chronic LGV rarely results in any change in the titer, which may remain high for the rest of the patient's life. If untreated, complement-fixing antibodies may persist for years at high titer; there is a tendency, however, for these titers to diminish, and the results of the test sometimes become negative spontaneously.

Micro-immunofluorescence typing

Using the micro-IF technique, which is far more sensitive than the LGVCFT, anti-chlamydial type-specific antibody can be detected in the serum and the particular infecting serovar (L1, L2, L2a, or L3) may be identified. Unfortunately, these anti-bodies tend to be highly cross-reactive, but occur at high titer (256 and above). Although this is the serological method of choice, it is available in only a few specialist centers.

Other laboratory tests

During the course of untreated LGV, the erythrocyte sedimentation rate is usually elevated, particularly in chronic cases. This presumably reflects changes in the levels of plasma proteins. The gamma globulin fraction of the serum is usually elevated, the albumin being normal or low. The total white cell count in the blood is often increased, with a relative lymphocytosis or monocytosis.

DIFFERENTIAL DIAGNOSIS

Genital ulceration due to LGV must be carefully differentiated from syphilis, chancroid, or genital herpes by appropriate tests (Chapters 6, 7, and 16).

Lymph node enlargement may occur in syphilis, genital herpes, granuloma inguinale, HIV, infectious mononucleosis, and in the reticuloses. Usually the onset of the glandular swelling in these cases is less acute and less painful, except in herpes genitalis.

Pyogenic infection, cat-scratch disease, and tuberculosis may produce painful swollen inguinal lymph nodes, with or without a history of a preceding lesion on the genitals.

TREATMENT

The aim of treatment is to eradicate the infecting organism as far as possible to prevent further damage and to correct any deformities caused by the disease. It is important to examine, if possible, sexual contacts of people with LGV.

The treatment of choice is doxycycline, given on an oral dosage of 100 mg every 12 hours for 21 days. Erythromycin base, given orally in a dose of 500 mg every 6 hours is an alternative regimen. Therapy is guided by resolution of suppurating lymph nodes, reduction in size of the nodes, healing of sinuses, and improvement in the patient's general condition.

Response to antibiotic treatment is better in LGV in the early stage than in the late stage when repeated prolonged courses may be required. At this stage improvement may not occur.

Buboes should be aspirated with aseptic precautions through a wide-bore needle (No. 19 SWG). Repeat aspiration may be required, even after initiation of appropriate antimicrobial chemotherapy, to prevent spontaneous rupture. Fluctuant glands should not be incised as this delays healing. Clean surgical removal of the affected glands appears to be an effective treatment.

Surgical treatment, with simultaneous antibiotic therapy, is often required in the management of late LGV. Polypoid growths on the vulva require excision, and fistulae need surgical repair. Rectal strictures will require regular dilatation, or excision and a colostomy. Stricture may cause acute intestinal obstruction.

References

1 Holmes KK, Handsfield HH, Wang S-P, *et al.* Etiology of non-gonococcal urethritis. *N Engl J Med* 1975; **292**: 1199–1205.

2 Wang S-P, Grayston JT, Kuo C-C, Alexander ER, Holmes KK. Serodiagnosis of *Chlamydia trachomatis* infection with the micro-immunofluorescence test. In: Hobson D, Holmes KK (eds) *Non-gonococcal Urethritis and Related Infections.* Washington DC: ASM: 1977.

3 Oriel JD, Ridgway GL. Studies of the epidemiology of chlamydial infection of the human genital tract. In: Mardh PA (ed.) *Chlamydial Infections.* Proceedings of the fifth international symposium on human chlamydial infections. Amsterdam: Elsevier Biomedical Press: 1982.

4 Stephens RS. *Chlamydia. Intracellular Biology, Pathogenesis, and Immunity.* Washington DC: ASM Press: 1999.

5 Hackstadt T. Cell biology. In: Stephens RS (ed.) *Chlamydia. Intracellular Biology,*

Pathogenesis, and Immunity. Washington DC: ASM Press: 1999.

6 Jones BR. The prevention of blindness from trachoma. The Bowman Lecture. *Trans Ophthalmol Soc UK* 1975; **95**: 16–33.

7 Brunham RC. Human immunity to chlamydiae. In: Stephens RS (ed.) *Chlamydia. Intracellular Biology, Pathogenesis, and Immunity.* Washington DC: ASM Press: 1999.

8 Katz BP, Batteiger BE, Jones RB. Effect of prior sexually transmitted disease on the isolation of *Chlamydia trachomatis. Sex Transm Dis* 1987; **14**: 160–164.

9 Grayston JT, Wang SP, Yeh LJ, Kuo CC. Importance of reinfection in the pathogenesis of trachoma. *Rev Infect Dis* 1985; **7**: 717–725.

10 Taylor HR. Development of immunity to ocular chlamydial infection. *Am J Trop Med Hyg* 1990; **42**: 358–364.

11 Brunham RC, Kimani J, Bwayo J, *et al.* The epidemiology of *Chlamydia trachomatis*

within a sexually transmitted diseases core group. *J Infect Dis* 1996; **173**: 950–956.

12 Brunham RC, Plummer FA, Stephens RS. Bacterial antigenic variation, host immune response, and pathogen–host coevolution. *Infect Immun* 1993; **61**: 2273–2276.

13 Johnson AP, Osborn MF, Rowntree S, Thomas BJ, Taylor-Robinson D. A study of inactivation of *Chlamydia trachomatis* by normal human serum. *Br J Vener Dis* 1983; **59**: 369–372.

14 Kondo L, Hanna L, Keshishyan H. Reduction in chlamydial infectivity by lysozyme. *Proc Soc Exp Biol Med* 1973; **142**: 131–132.

15 Hess CB, Jerrells TR, Haacktadt T, Klimpel GR, Niesel DW. Obligate intracellular bacteria induce interferon α/β production in fibroblasts. *Immunol Infect Dis* 1992; **2**: 13–16.

16 Rasmussen SJ, Eckmann L, Quayle AJ, *et al.* Secretion of proinflammatory cytokines by epithelial cells in response to chlamydial infection suggests a central role for

epithelial cells in chlamydial pathogenesis. *J Clin Invest* 1997; **99**: 77–87.

17 Ward ME. Mechanisms of chlamydia-induced disease. In: Stephens RS (ed.) *Chlamydia. Intracellular Biology, Pathogenesis and Immunity*. Washington DC; ASM Press:1999, pp. 171–210.

18 Kimani J, Maclean IW, Bwayo JJ, *et al.* Risk factors for *Chlamydia trachomatis* pelvic inflammatory disease among sex workers in Nairobi, Kenya. *J Infect Dis* 1996; **173**: 1437–1444.

19 Bailey RL. Holland MJ, Whittle HC, Mabey DC. Subjects recovering from human ocular chlamydial infection have enhanced lymphoproliferative responses to chlamydial antigens compared with those of persistently diseased controls. *Infect Immun* 1995; **63**: 389–392.

20 Holland MJ, Bailey RL, Hayes LJ, Whittle HC, Mabey DC. Conjunctival scarring in trachoma is associated with depressed cell-mediated immune responses to chlamydial antigens. *J Infect Dis* 1993; **168**: 1528–1531.

21 Holland MJ, Bailey RL, Conway DJ, *et al.* T helper type-1 Th1/Th2 profiles of peripheral blood mononuclear cells (PBMC); responses to antigens of *Chlamydia trachomatis* in subjects with severe trachomatous scarring. *Clin Exp Immunol* 1996; **105**: 429–435.

22 Johansson M, Schon K, Ward M, Lycke N. Genital tract infection with *Chlamydia trachomatis* fails to induce protective immunity in gamma interferon receptor-deficient mice despite a strong local immunoglobulin A response. *Infect Immun* 1997; **65**: 1032–1044.

23 Williams DB, Grubbs B, Darville T, Kelly K, Rank R. A role for interleukin 6 in host defense against *Chlamydia trachomatis*. In: Stephens RS, Byrne GI, Christiansen G *et al.* (eds) *Chlamydial infections*. Proceedings of the ninth international symposium on human chlamydial infection. San Francisco; International Chlamydia Symposium: 1998.

24 Igietseme JU, Perry LL, Ananaba GA, *et al.* Chlamydia infection in inducible nitric oxide synthase knockout mice. *Infect Immun* 1998; **66**: 1282–1286.

25 Ojcius DM, de Alba YB, Kannellopoulos JM, *et al.* Internalization of *Chlamydia* by dendritic cells and stimulation of *Chlamydia*-specific T cells. *J Immunol* 1998; **160**: 1297–1303.

26 Holland MJ, Conway DJ, Blanchard TJ, *et al.* Synthetic peptides based on *C. trachomatis* antigens identify cytotoxic T lymphocyte responses in subjects from a trachoma endemic population. *Clin Exp Immunol* 1997; **107**: 44–49.

27 Stephens RS, Kalman S, Lammel C, *et al.* Genome sequence of an obligate intracellular pathogen of humans. *Science* 1998; **282**: 754–759.

28 Osser S, Persson K. Postabortal pelvic infection associated with *Chlamydia trachomatis* and the influence of humoral immunity. *Am J Obstet Gynecol* 1984; **150**: 699–703.

29 Brunham RC, Kuo C-C, Cles L, Holmes KK. Correlation of host immune response with quantitative recovery of *Chlamydia trachomatis* from the human endocervix. *Infect Immun* 1983; **39**: 1491–1494.

30 Ghae-Maghami S, Hay PE, Lewis DJM. Antigen and isotype specificity of human B cell responses in immunopathogenesis of genital *Chlamydia trachomatis* infection. *Infect Dis Obstet Gynecol* 1996; **4**: 179–180.

31 Fan T, Lu H, Lu H, *et al.* Inhibition of apoptosis in *Chlamydia*-infected cells: blockade of mitochondrial cytochrome *c* release and caspase activation. *J Exp Med* 1998; **187**: 487–496.

32 Bell TA, Stamm WE, Wang SP, Kuo CC, Holmes KK, Grayston JT. Chronic *C trachomatis* infections in infants. *JAMA* 1992; **267**: 400–402.

33 Dean D, Suchland RJ, Stamm WE. Evidence for long-term cervical persistence of *Chlamydia trachomatis* by *omp 1* genotyping. *J Infect Dis* 2000; **182**: 909–916.

34 Hillis SD, Owens LM, Marchbanks PA, Amstredam LE, Mackenzie WR. Recurrent chlamydial infections increase the risk of hospitalization for ectopic pregnancy and pelvic inflammatory disease. *Am J Obstet Gynecol* 1997; **176**: 103–107.

35 Swanson J, Eschenbach DA, Alexander ER, Holmes KK. Light and electron microscopic study of *Chlamydia trachomatis* infection of the uterine cervix. *J Infect Dis* 1975; **131**: 678–687.

36 Quinn TC, Goodell SE, Mkrtichian E, *et al.* *Chlamydia trachomatis* proctitis. *N Engl J Med* 1981; **305**: 195–200.

37 Krul KG. Closing in on Chlamydia. *CAP Today* 1995; **9**: 1–20.

38 Centers for Disease Control and Prevention. *Chlamydia trachomatis* genital infections – United States, 1995. *MMWR* 1997; **46**: 193–198.

39 Lamagni TL, Hughes G, Rogers PA, Paine T, Catchpole M. New cases seen at genitourinary medicine clinics: England 1998. *Comm Dis Rep* 1999; **9** (Suppl. 6):S1–S12.

40 Dowe G, Smikle M, King SD, Wynter H, Frederick J, Hylton-Kong T. High prevalence of genital *Chlamydia trachomatis* infection in women presenting in different clinical settings in Jamaica: implications for control strategies. *Sex Transm Inf* 1999; **76**: 412–416.

41 Burstein GR, Gaydos CA, Diener West M, Howell MR, Zenilman JM, Quinn TC. Incident *Chlamydia trachomatis* infections among inner-city adolescent females. *JAMA* 1998; **280**: 521–526.

42 Malkin JE, Prazuck T, Bogar M, *et al.* Screening of *Chlamydia trachomatis* genital infection in a young Parisian population. *Sex Transm Inf* 1999; **75**: 188–189.

43 Vuylsteke B, Vandenbruaene M, Vandenbulcke P, Van Dyck E, Laga M. *Chlamydia trachomatis* prevalence and sexual behaviour among female adolescents in Belgium. *Sex Transm Inf* 1999; **75**: 152–155.

44 Grun L, Tassano Smith J, Carder C, *et al.* Comparison of two methods of screening for genital chlamydial infection in women attending in general practice: cross sectional survey. *Br Med J* 1997; **315**: 226–230.

45 Gaydos CA, Howell MR, Pare B, *et al.* *Chlamydia trachomatis* infections in female military recruits. *N Engl J Med* 1998; **339**: 739–744.

46 Garland SM, Tabrizi S, Hallo J, Chen S. Assessment of *Chlamydia trachomatis* prevalence by PCR and LCR in women presenting for termination of pregnancy. *Sex Transm Inf* 2000; **76**: 173–176.

47 Stevenson MM, Radcliffe KW. Preventing pelvic infection after abortion. *Int J STD AIDS* 1995; **6**: 305–312.

48 Oh MK, Cloud GA, Baker SL, Pass MA, Mulchahey K, Pass RF. Chlamydial infection and sexual behavior in young pregnant teenagers. *Sex Transm Dis* 1993; **20**: 45–50.

49 Handsfield HH, Jasman LL, Roberts PL, Hanson VW, Kothenbeutel RL, Stamm WE. Criteria for selective screening for *Chlamydia trachomatis* infection in women attending family planning clinics. *JAMA* 1986; **255**: 1730–1734.

50 Humphreys JT, Henneberry JF, Rickard RS, Beebe JL. Cost-benefit analysis of selective screening criteria for *Chlamydia trachomatis* infection in women attending Colorado family planning clinics. *Sex Transm Dis* 1992; **19**: 47–53.

51 Van Duynhoven YT, van de Laar MJ, Schop WA, Mouton JW, van der Meijden WI, Sprenger MJ. Different demographic and sexual correlates for chlamydial infection and gonorrhoea in Rotterdam. *Int J Epidemiol* 1997; **6**: 1373–1385.

52 Winter AJ, Sriskandabalan P, Wade AAH, Cummins C, Barker P. Sociodemography of genital *Chlamydia trachomatis* in Coventry, UK, 1992–6. *Sex Transm Inf* 2000; **76**: 103–109.

53 Zelin JM, Robinson AJ, Ridgway GL, Allason-Jones E, Williams P. Chlamydial urethritis in heterosexual men attending a genitourinary medicine clinic: prevalence, symptoms, condom usage and partner change. *Int J STD AIDS* 1995; **6**: 27–30.

54 Pack RP, DiClemente RJ, Hook EW, Oh MK. High prevalence of asymptomatic STDs in

incarcerated minority male youth: a case for screening. *Sex Transm Dis* 2000; **27**: 175–177.

55 PHLS, DHSS&PS and the Scottish ISD(D)5 Collaborative Group. *Trends in Sexually Transmitted Infections in the United Kingdom, 1990–1999*. London; Public Health Laboratory Service; 2000

56 Bowie WR, Alexander ER, Holmes KK. Etiologies of post-gonococcal urethritis in homosexual and heterosexual men; roles for *Chlamydia trachomatis* and *Ureaplasma urealyticum*. *Sex Transm Dis* 1978; **5**: 151–154.

57 Ciemens EL, Flood J, Kent CK, *et al.* Re-examining the prevalence of *Chlamydia trachomatis* infection among gay men with urethritis. *Sex Transm Dis* 2000; **27**: 249–251.

58 McMillan A. Bacterial infections. In: Adler MW (ed.) *Diseases in the Homosexual Male*. London; Springer-Verlag; 1988.

59 Quinn TC, Gaydos C, Shepherd M, *et al.* Epidemiologic and microbiologic correlates of *Chlamydia trachomatis* infection in sexual partnerships. *JAMA* 1996; **276**: 1737–1742.

60 Lin JS, Donegan SP, Heeren TC, *et al.* Transmission of *Chlamydia trachomatis* and *Neisseria gonorrhoeae* among men with urethritis and their female sex partners. *J Infect Dis* 1998; **178**: 1707–1712.

61 Workowski KA, Stevens CE, Suchland RJ, *et al.* Clinical manifestations of genital infection due to *Chlamydia trachomatis* in women: differences related to serotype. *Clin Inf Dis* 1994; **19**: 756–760.

62 Barnes RC, Rompalo AM, Stamm WE. Comparison of *Chlamydia trachomatis* serovars causing rectal and cervical infections. *J Infect Dis* 1987; **156**: 953–958.

63 Boisvert JF, Koutsky LA, Suchland RJ, Stamm WE. Clinical features of *Chlamydia trachomatis* rectal infection by serovar among homosexually active men. *Sex Transm Dis* 1999; **26**: 392–398.

63a Dean D, Oudens E, Bolan G, Padian N, Schachter J. Major outer membrane protein variants of *Chlamydia trachomatis* are associated with severe upper genital tract infections and histopathology in San Francisco. *J Infect Dis* 1995; **172**: 1013–1022.

64 Koskela P, Anttila T, Bjorge T, *et al. Chlamydia trachomatis* infection as a risk factor for invasive cervical cancer. *Int J Cancer* 2000; **85**: 35–39.

65 Anttila T, Saikku P, Koskela P, *et al.* Serotypes of *Chlamydia trachomatis* and risk of development of cervical squamous cell carcinoma. *JAMA* 2001; **85**: 47–51.

66 Zenilman JM. Chlamydia and cervical cancer. A real association? *JAMA* 2001; **285**: 81–83.

67 Laga M, Manoka A, Kivuvu M, *et al.* Non-ulcerative sexually transmitted diseases as risk factors for HIV-1 transmission in women: results from a cohort study. *AIDS* 1993; **7**: 95–102.

68 Levine WC, Pope V, Bhoomkar A, *et al.* Increase in endocervical CD4 lymphocytes among women with non-ulcerative sexually transmitted diseases. *J Infect Dis* 1998; **177**: 167–174.

69 Eron JJ, Gilliam B, Fiscus S, Dyer J, Cohen MS. HIV-1 shedding and chlamydia urethritis. *JAMA* 1996; **276**: 36.

70 Cohen MS, Hoffman IF, Royce RA, *et al.* Reduction of concentration of HIV-1 in semen after treatment of urethritis: implications for prevention of sexual transmission of HIV-1. *Lancet* 1997; **349**: 1868–1873.

71 Mostad SB, Overbaugh J, DeVange DM, *et al.* Hormonal contraception, vitamin A deficiency, and other risk factors for shedding of HIV-1 infected cells from the cervix and vagina. *Lancet* 1997; **350**: 922–927.

72 Hunter JM, Smith IW, Peutherer JF, MacAulay A, Tuach S, Young H. *Chlamydia trachomatis* and *Ureaplasma urealyticum* in men attending a sexually transmitted diseases clinic. *Br J Vener Dis* 1981; **57**: 130–133.

73 Swarz SL, Kraus SJ. Persistent urethral leukocytosis and asymptomatic chlamydial urethritis. *J Infect Dis* 1979; **140**: 614–617.

74 Harrison HR, Costin M, Meder JB, *et al.* Cervical *Chlamydia trachomatis* infection in university women: relationship to history, contraception, ectopy and cervicitis. *Am J Obstet Gynecol* 1985; **153**: 244–251.

75 Rees E, Tait A, Hobson D, Byng RE, Johnson FWA. Neonatal conjunctivitis caused by *Neisseria gonorrhoeae* and *Chlamydia trachomatis*. *Br J Vener Dis* 1977; **53**: 173–177.

76 Paavonen J. *Chlamydia trachomatis*-induced urethritis in female partners of men with nongonococcal urethritis. *Sex Transm Dis* 1979; **6**: 69–71.

77 Stamm WE, Wagner KF, Amsel R, *et al.* Causes of the acute urethral syndrome in women. *N Engl J Med* 1980; **303**: 409–415.

78 Horner PJ, May PE, Thomas T, Benton AM, Taylor-Robinson D. The role of *Chlamydia trachomatis* in urethritis and urethral symptoms in women. *Int J STD AIDS* 1995; **6**: 31–34.

79 Thompson CI, MacAulay AJ, Smith IW. *Chlamydia trachomatis* infections in the female rectum. *Genitourin Med* 1989; **65**: 269–273.

80 Davies JA, Rees E, Hobson D, Karayiannis P. Isolation of *Chlamydia trachomatis* from Bartholin's ducts. *Br J Vener Dis* 1978; **54**: 409–413.

81 Ostergaard L, Agner T, Krarup E, Johansen UB, Weisman K, Gutschik E. PCR for detection of *Chlamydia trachomatis* in endocervical, urethral, rectal, and pharyngeal swab samples obtained from patients attending an STD clinic. *Genitourin Med* 1997; **73**: 493–497.

82 McMillan A, Sommerville RG, McKie PMK. Chlamydial infection in homosexual men: frequency of isolation of *Chlamydia trachomatis* from the urethra, anorectum and pharynx. *Br J Vener Dis* 1981; **57**: 47–49.

83 Viswalingam ND, Wishart MS, Woodland RM. Adult chlamydial ophthalmia. *Br Med Bull* 1983; **39**: 123–127.

84 Paavonen J, Kiviat N, Brunham RC, *et al.* Prevalence and manifestations of endometritis among women with cervicitis. *Am J Obstet Gynecol* 1985; **152**: 280–286.

85 Witkin SS, Kligman I, Grifo JA, Rosenwaks Z. *Chlamydia trachomatis* detected by polymerase chain reaction in cervices of culture-negative women correlates with adverse *in vitro* fertilization outcome. *J Infect Dis* 1995; **171**: 1657–1659.

86 Witkin SS, Sultan KM, Neal GS, Jeremias J, Grifo JA, Rosenwaks Z. Unsuspected *Chlamydia* infection and *in vitro* fertilization outcome. *Am J Obstet Gynecol* 1994; **171**: 1208–1214.

87 Jones RB. Chlamydial infection. In: Hitchcock PJ, MacKay HT, Wasserheit JN (eds) *Sexually transmitted Diseases and Adverse Outcomes of Pregnancy*. Washington DC; ASM Press; 1999.

88 Osser S, Persson K. Chlamydial antibodies and deoxyribonucleic acid in patients with ectopic pregnancy. *Fert Steril* 1992; **57**: 578–582.

89 Chow JM, Yonekura ML, Richwald GA, Greenland S, Sweet RL, Schachter J. The association between *Chlamydia trachomatis* and ectopic pregnancy. A matched-pair, case-control study. *JAMA* 1990; **263**: 3164–3167.

90 Sweet RL, Landers DV, Walker C, Schachter J. *Chlamydia trachomatis* infection and pregnancy outcome. *Am J Obstet Gynecol* 1987; **156**: 824–833.

91 Cohen I, Veille JC, Calkins BM. Improved pregnancy outcome following successful treatment of chlamydial infection. *JAMA* 1990; **263**: 3160–3163.

92 Ryan GM, Abdella TN, McNeeley SG, Baselski VS, Drummond DE. *Chlamydia trachomatis* infection in pregnancy and effect of treatment on outcome. *Am J Obstet Gynecol* 1990; **162**: 34–39.

93 Germain M, Krohn MA, Hillier SL, Eschnebach DA. Genital flora in pregnancy and its association with intrauterine growth retardation. *J Clin Microbiol* 1994; **32**: 2162–2168.

94 Black CM. Current methods of laboratory diagnosis of *Chlamydia trachomatis*

infections. *Clin Microbiol Rev* 1997; **10**: 160–184.

95 Anestad G, Berdal BP, Scheel O, *et al.* Screening urine samples by leukocyte esterase test and ligase chain reaction for chlamydial infections among asymptomatic men. *J Clin Microbiol* 1995; **33**: 2483–2484.

96 Genc M, Ruusuvaara L, Mardh PA. An economic evaluation of screening for *Chlamydia trachomatis* in adolescent males. *JAMA* 1993; **270**: 2057–2064.

97 Stephens RS, Tam MR, Kuo CC, Nowinski RC. Monoclonal antibodies to *Chlamydia trachomatis* antibody specificities and antigen characterization. *J Immunol* 1982; **128**: 1083–1089.

98 Skulnick M, Small GW, Simor AE, *et al.* Comparison of the Clearview test, Chlamydiazyme, and cell culture for detection of *Chlamydia trachomatis* in women with a low prevalence of infection. *J Clin Microbiol* 1991; **29**: 2086–2088.

99 Chernesky M, Lang D, Krepel J, Sellors J, Mahony J. Impact of reference standard sensitivity on accuracy of rapid antigen detection assays and a leukocyte esterase dipstick for diagnosis of *Chlamydia trachomatis* infection in first-voided urine specimens from men. *J Clin Microbiol* 1999; **37**: 2777–2780.

100 Ratti G, Moroni A, Cevenni R. Detection of *Chlamydia trachomatis* DNA in patients with non-gonococcal urethritis using the polymerase chain reaction. *J Clin Pathol* 1991; **44**: 564–568.

101 Schachter J, Stamm WE, Quinn TC, Andrews WW, Burczak JD, Lee H. Ligase chain reaction to detect *Chlamydia trachomatis* infection of the cervix. *J Clin Microbiol* 1994; **32**: 2540–2543.

102 Chernesky MA, Lee H, Schachter J, *et al.* Diagnosis of *Chlamydia trachomatis* urethral infection in symptomatic and asymptomatic men by testing first-void urine in a ligase chain reaction assay. *J Infect Dis* 1994; **170**: 1308–1311.

103 Lee HH, Chernesky MA, Schachter J, *et al.* Diagnosis of *Chlamydia trachomatis* genitourinary infection in women by ligase chain reaction assay of urine. *Lancet* 1995; **345**: 213–216.

104 Bassiri M, Hu HY, Domeika MA, *et al.* Detection of *Chlamydia trachomatis* in urine specimens from women by ligase chain reaction. *J Clin Microbiol* 1995; **33**: 898–900.

105 Crotchfelt KA, Pare B, Gaydos C, Quinn TC. Detection of *Chlamydia trachomatis* by the Gen–Probe AMPLIFIED *Chlamydia trachomatis* Assay (AMP CT) in urine specimens from men and women and endocervical specimens from women. *J Clin Microbiol* 1998; **36**: 391–394.

106 Moncada J, Schachter J, Hook EW, *et al.* The effect of urine testing in evaluation of

the sensitivity of Gen-Probe APTIMA on cervical swabs for *Chlamydia trachomatis.* The infected patient standard reduces sensitivity of single site evaluation. Abstract. International Congress of Sexually Transmitted Infections. Berlin. June 2001. In: *Int J STD AIDS* 2001; **12** (Suppl. 2): 117.

107 Moller JK, Andresen B, Olesen F, Lignell T, Ostergaard L. Impact of menstrual cycle on the diagnostic performance of LCR, TMA, and PCE for detection of *Chlamydia trachomatis* in home obtained and mailed vaginal flush and urine samples. *Sex Transm Inf* 1999; **75**: 228–230.

108 Chan EL, Brandt K, Olienus K, Antonishyn N, Horsman GB. Performance characteristics of the Becton Dickinson ProbeTec System for direct detection of *Chlamydia trachomatis* and *Neisseria gonorrhoeae* in male and female urine specimens in comparison with the Roche COBAS System. *Arch Pathol Lab Med* 2000; **124**: 1649–1652.

109 Grayston JT, Wang SP. New knowledge of chlamydiae and the diseases they may cause. *J Infect Dis* 1975; **132**: 87–105.

110 Hay PE, Thomas BJ, Gilchrist C, Palmer HM, Gilroy CB, Taylor-Robinson D. The value of urine samples from men with non-gonococcal urethritis for the detection of *Chlamydia trachomatis. Genitourin Med* 1991; **67**: 124–128.

111 Quinn TC, Welsh L, Lentz A, *et al.* Diagnosis by AMPLICOR PCR of *Chlamydia trachomatis* infection in urine samples from women and men attending sexually transmitted disease clinics. *J Clin Microbiol* 1996; **34**: 1401–1406.

112 Caul PO, Horner PJ, Leech J, Crowley T, Paul I, Davey-Smith G. Population-based screening programmes for *Chlamydia trachomatis. Lancet* 1997; **349**: 1070–1071.

113 Mahony J, Chong S, Jang D, *et al.* Amplification inhibitors and detection of *Chlamydia trachomatis* in female urines by PCR, LCR and TMA. In: Stephens RS, Byrne GI, Christiansen G, *et al.* (eds) *Chlamydial Infections.* Proceedings of the ninth international symposium on human chlamydial infection. San Francisco; University of California: 1998, pp. 599–602.

114 Domeika M, Bassiri M, Butrimiene I, Venaalis A, Ranceva J, Vasjanova V. Evaluation of vaginal introital sampling as an alternative approach for the detection of genital *Chlamydia trachomatis* infection in women. *Acta Obstet Gynecol Scand* 1999; **78**: 131–136.

115 Smith K, Harrington K, Wingood G, Oh MK, Hook EW, DiClemente RJ. Self-obtained vaginal swabs for diagnosis of treatable sexually transmitted diseases in adolescent

girls. *Arch Pediatr Adolesc Med* 2001; **155**: 676–679.

116 Tabrizi SN, Paterson BA, Fairley CK, Bowden FJ, Garland SM. Comparison of tampon and urine as self-administered methods of specimen collection in the detection of *Chlamydia trachomatis, Neisseria gonorrhoeae* and *Trichomonas vaginalis* in women. *Int J STD AIDS* 1998; **9**: 347–349.

117 Barton SE, Thomas BJ, Taylor-Robinson D, Goldmeier D. Detection of *Chlamydia trachomatis* in the vaginal vault of women who have had hysterectomies. *Br Med J* 1985; **291**: 250.

118 Qvigstad E, Skaug K, Jerve F, Vik ISS, Ulstrup JC. Therapeutic abortion and *Chlamydia trachomatis* infection. *Br J Vener Dis* 1982; **58**: 182–183.

119 Tjiam KH, van Heijst BYM, Polak-Vogelzang AA, *et al.* Sexually communicable micro-organisms in human semen samples to be used for artificial insemination by donor. *Genitourin Med* 1987; **63**: 116–118.

120 Scholes D, Stergachis A, Heidrich FE, Andrilla H, Holmes KK, Stamm WE. Prevention of pelvic inflammatory disease by screening for cervical chlamydial infection. *N Engl J Med* 1996; **334**: 1362–1366.

121 Hooton TM, Rogers ME, Medina TG, *et al.* Ciprofloxacin compared with doxycycline for nongonococcal urethritis. Ineffectiveness against *Chlamydia trachomatis* due to relapsing infection. *JAMA* 1990; **264**: 1418–1421.

122 Weber JT, Johnson RE. New treatments for *Chlamydia trachomatis* genital infection. *Clin Infect Dis* 1995; **20** (Suppl. 1): S66–S71.

123 Centers for Diseases Control and Prevention 2002. Guidelines for treatment of sexually transmitted diseases. *MMWR* 2002; **51**: RR-6.

124 Clinical Effectiveness Group (Association of Genitourinary Medicine and the Medical Society for the Study of Venereal Diseases). *National Guideline for the Management of* Chlamydia trachomatis. *Genital Tract Infection.* 2001; www.mssvd.org.uk/ceg.htm.

125 Magid D, Douglas JM, Schwartz JS. Doxycycline compared with azithromycin for treating women with genital *Chlamydia trachomatis* infections: an incremental cost-effectiveness analysis. *Ann Int Med* 1996; **124**: 389–399.

126 Linnemann CC, Heaton CL, Ritchey M. Treatment of *Chlamydia trachomatis* infections: comparison of 1 and 2-g doses of erythromycin daily for seven days. *Sex Transm Dis* 1987; **14**: 102–106.

127 Kuo C-C, Wang S-P, Grayston JT. Antimicrobial activity of several antibiotics and a sulfonamide against *Chlamydia trachomatis* organisms in cell culture.

Antimicrob Agents Chemother 1977; **12**: 80–83.

128 Scieux C, Bianchi A, Chappey B, Vassias I, Perol Y. In-vitro activity of azithromycin against *Chlamydia trachomatis*. *J Antimicrob Chemother* 1990; **25** (Suppl A): 7–10.

129 Oriel JD, Ridgway GL. Comparison of erythromycin and oxytetracycline in the treatment of cervical infection by *Chlamydia trachomatis*. *J Infect* 1980; **2**: 96–97.

130 Munday PE. Thomas BJ, Gilroy CB, Gilchrist C, Taylor-Robinson D. Infrequent detection of *Chlamydia trachomatis* in a longitudinal study of women with treated cervical infection. *Genitourin Med* 1995; **71**: 24–26.

131 Romanowski B, Talbot H, Stadynk M, Kowalchik P, Bowie WR. Minocycline compared with doxycycline in the treatment of NGU and MPC. *Ann Int Med* 1993; **119**: 16–22.

132 Oriel JD, Ridgway GL, Tchamouroff S. Comparison of erythromycin stearate and oxytetracycline in the treatment of non-gonococcal urethritis: their efficacy against *Chlamydia trachomatis*. *Scott Med J* 1977; **22**: 375–379.

133 Hunter JM, Sommerville RG. Erythromycin stearate in treating chlamydial infection of the cervix. *Br J Vener Dis* 1984; **60**: 387–389.

134 Ross JDC, Crean A, McMillan A. Efficacy of anti-chlamydial therapy with oxytetracycline and erythromycin. *Int J STD AIDS* 1996; **7**: 373–374.

135 Bright GM, Nagel AA, Bordner J, *et al.* Synthesis, in-vitro and in-vivo activity of novel 9-deoxy-9a-aza-9a-homoerythromycin A derivatives; a new class of macrolide antibiotics, the azalides. *J Antibiotics* 1988; **41**: 1029–1047.

136 Welsh LE, Gaydos CA, Quinn TC. In vitro evaluation of activities of azithromycin, erythromycin, and tetracycline against *Chlamydia trachomatis* and *Chlamydia pneumoniae*. *Antimicrob Agents Chemother* 1992; **36**: 291–294.

137 Hillis SD, Coles FB, Litchfield B, *et al.* Doxycycline and azithromycin for prevention of chlamydial persistence or recurrence one month after treatment in women. A use-effectiveness study in public health settings. *Sex Transm Dis* 1998; **25**: 5–11.

138 Hooper DC, Wolfson JS. Fluoroquinolone antimicrobial agents. *N Engl J Med* 1991; **324**: 384–394.

139 Taylor-Robinson D. Genital chlamydial infections. In: Harris JRW, Forster SM (eds). *Recent Advances in Sexually Transmitted Diseases and AIDS*. Edinburgh: Churchill Livingstone: 1991, pp. 219–262.

140 Csango PA, Gundersen T, Martinsen I-M. Effect of amoxicillin on simultaneous *Chlamydia trachomatis* infection in men

with gonococcal urethritis: comparison of three dosage regimens. *Sex Transm Dis* 1985; **12**: 93–96.

141 Somani J, Bhullar VB, Workowski KA, Farshy CE, Black CM. Multiple drug-resistant *Chlamydia trachomatis* associated with clinical treatment failure. *J Infect Dis* 2000; **181**: 1421–1427.

142 Brocklehurst P, Rooney G. Interventions for treating genital *Chlamydia trachomatis* infection in pregnancy. *Cochrane Database of Systematic Reviews* Issue 1, 2000.

143 Bowie WR. *In vitro* activity of clavulanic acid, amoxicillin, and ticarcillin against *Chlamydia trachomatis*. *Antimicrob Agents Chemother* 1986; **29**: 713–715.

144 Adair CD, Gunter M, Stovall TG, McElroy G, Veille J-C, Ernest JM. Chlamydia in pregnancy: a randomized trial of azithromycin and erythromycin. *Obstet Gynecol* 1998; **91**: 165–168.

145 Fitzgerald MR, Welch J, Robinson AJ, Ahmed-Jushuf IH. Clinical guidelines and standards for the management of uncomplicated genital chlamydial infection. *Int J STD AIDS* 1998; **9**: 253–262.

146 Kjaer HO, Dimcsevski G, Hoff G, Olesen F, Ostergaard L. Recurrence of urogenital *Chlamydia trachomatis* infection evaluated by mailed samples obtained at home: 24 weeks' prospective follow-up study. *Sex Transm Inf* 2000; **76**: 169–172.

147 Bell TA, Stamm WE, Kuo CC, Wang SP, Holmes KK, Grayston JT. Risk of perinatal transmission of *Chlamydia trachomatis* by mode of delivery. *J Infect* 1994; **29**: 165–169.

148 Schachter J, Grossman M, Holt J, Sweet R, Spector S. Infection with *Chlamydia trachomatis*: involvement of multiple anatomic sites in neonates. *J Infect Dis* 1979; **139**: 232–234.

149 Hobson D, Rees E, Viswalingam ND. Chlamydial infections in neonates and older children. *Br Med Bull* 1983; **39**: 128–132.

150 Hammerschlag MR, Roblin PM, Gelling M, Worku M. Comparison of two enzyme immunoassays to culture for the diagnosis of chlamydial conjunctivitis and respiratory infections in infants. *J Clin Microbiol* 1990; **28**: 1725–1727.

151 Rapoza PA, Quinn TC, Kiessling LA, Green WR, Taylor HR. Assessment of neonatal conjunctivitis with a direct immunofluorescent monoclonal antibody stain for *Chlamydia*. *JAMA* 1986; **255**: 3369–3373.

152 Hammerschlag MR, Roblin PM, Gelling M, Tsumura N, Jule JE, Kutlin A. Use of polymerase chain reaction for the detection of *Chlamydia trachomatis* in ocular and nasopharyngeal specimens from infants with conjunctivitis. *Ped Infect Dis J* 1997; **16**: 293–297.

153 Honein MA, Paulozzi LJ, Himelright IM, *et al.* Infantile hypertrophic pyloric stenosis after pertussis prophylaxis with erythromycin: a case review and cohort study. *Lancet* 1999; **355**: 758.

154 Hammerschlag M, Gelling M, Roblin PM, Kutlin A, Jule JE. Treatment of neonatal chlamydial conjunctivitis with azithromycin. *Pediatr Infect Dis J* 1998; **11**: 1049–1050.

155 Hammerschlag MR, Chandler JW, Alexander ER, English M, Koutsky L. Longitudinal studies on chlamydial infections in the first year of life. *Pediatr Infect Dis* 1982; **1**: 395–401.

156 Beem MO, Saxon EM. Respiratory tract colonization and a distinctive pneumonia syndrome in infants infected with *Chlamydia trachomatis*. *N Engl J Med* 1977; **296**: 306–310.

157 Schachter J, Grossman M, Sweet RL, Holt J, Jordan C, Bishop E. Prospective study of perinatal transmission of *Chlamydia trachomatis*. *JAMA* 1986; **255**: 3374–3377.

158 Ingram DL, White ST, Occhiuti AR, Lynna PQ. Childhood vaginal infections: association of *Chlamydia trachomatis* with sexual contact. *Pediatr Infect Dis* 1986; **5**: 226–229.

159 Razin S, Freundt EA. Mycoplasmataceae etc. In: Krieg NR, Holt JC (eds) *Bergey's Manual of Systemic Bacteriology*. Baltimore and London; Williams & Wilkins: 1984.

160 Tully JG, Taylor-Robinson D, Cole RM, Rose DL. A newly discovered mycoplasma in the human urogenital tract. *Lancet* 1981; **i**: 1288–1291.

161 Taylor-Robinson D. The history and role of *Mycoplasma genitalium* in sexually transmitted diseases. *Genitourin Med* 1995; **71**: 1–8.

162 Jensen JS, Blom J, Lind K. Intracellular location of *Mycoplasma genitalium* in cultured Vero cells as demonstrated by electron microscopy. *Int J Exp Pathol* 1994; **75**: 91–98.

163 Taylor-Robinson D, Bebear C. Antibiotic susceptibilities of mycoplasmas and treatment of mycoplasmal infections. *J Antimicrob Chemother* 1997; **40**: 622–630.

164 Grattard F, Pozzetto B, de Barbeyrac B, *et al.* Arbitrarily-primed PCR confirms the differentiation of strains of *Ureaplasma urealyticum* into two biovars. *Mol Cell Probes* 1995; **9**: 383–389.

165 Taylor-Robinson D, McCormack WM. Medical progress: the genital mycoplasmas. *N Engl J Med* 1980; **302**: 1003–1010, 1063–1067.

166 Lee Y-H, McCormack WM, Maarcy SM, Klein JO. The genital mycoplasmas. Their role in disorders of reproduction and in pediatric infections. *Pediatr Clin N Amer* 1974; **21**: 457–466.

167 McCormack WM, Almeida PC, Bailey PE, Grady EM, Lee Y-H. Sexual activity and vaginal colonization with genital mycoplasmas. *JAMA* 1975; **221**: 1375–1377.

168 McCormack WM, Braun P, Lee YH, Klein JO, Kass EH. The genital mycoplasmas. *N Engl J Med* 1973; **288**: 78–89.

169 Taylor-Robinson D, Furr PM. Clinical antibiotic resistance of *Ureaplasma urealyticum*. *Pediatr Infect Dis* 1986; **5** (Suppl): S335–S337.

170 Bowie WR, Floyd JF, Millere Y, Alexander ER, Holmes J, Holmes KK. Differential response of chlamydial and ureaplasma associated urethritis to sulfafurazole. *Lancet* 1976; **ii**: 1276–1278.

171 Bowie WR, Wang S-P, Alexander ER, *et al.* Etiology of non-gonococal urethritis. Evidence for *Chlamydia trachomatis* and ureaplasma. *J Clin Invest* 1977; **59**: 735–742.

172 Coufalik ED, Taylor-Robinson D, Csonka GW. Treatment of non-gonococcal urethritis with rifampicin as a means of defining the role of *Ureaplasma urealyticum*. *Br J Vener Dis* 1979; **55**: 36–43.

173 Ford DK, Smith JR. Non-specific urethritis associated with a tetracycline-resistant T-mycoplasma. *Br J Vener Dis* 1974; **50**: 373–374.

174 Taylor-Robinson D, Csonka GW, Prentice MJ. Human intra-urethral inoculation of ureaplasmas. *Q J Med* 1977; **46**: 309–326.

175 Palmer HM, Gilroy CB, Furr PM, Taylor-Robinson D. Development and evaluation of the polymerase chain reaction to detect *Mycoplasma genitalium*. *FEMS Microbiol Lett* 1991; **77**: 199–204.

176 Jensen JS, Uldum SA, Sondergard-Andersen J, Vuust J, Lind K. Polymerase chain reaction for detection of *Mycoplasma genitalium* in clinical samples. *J Clin Microbiol* 1991; **29**: 46–50.

177 Jensen JS, Orsum R, Dohn B, Uldum S, Worm A-M, Lind K. *Mycoplasma genitalium*: a cause of male urethritis? *Genitourin Med* 1993; **69**: 265–269.

178 Horner PJ, Gilroy CB, Thomas BJ, Naidoo ROM, Taylor-Robinson D. Association of *Mycoplasma genitalium* with acute non-gonococcal urethritis. *Lancet* 1993; **342**: 582–585.

179 Maeda S, Tamaki M, Nakano M, Uno M, Deguchi T, Kawada Y. Detection of *Mycoplasma genitalium* in patients with urethritis. *J Urol* 1998; **159**: 405–407.

180 Taylor-Robinson D, Tully JG, Barile MF. Urethral infection in male chimpanzees produced experimentally by *Mycoplasma genitalium*. *Br J Exp Pathol* 1985; **66**: 95–101.

181 Tully JG, Taylor-Robinson D, Rose DL, Furr PM, Graham CE, Barile MF. Urogenital challenge of primate species with *Mycoplasma genitalium* and characteristics of infection induced in chimpanzees. *J Infect Dis* 1986; **153**: 1046–1054.

182 Hooton TM, Roberts MC, Roberts PL, Holmes KK, Stamm WE, Kenny GE. Prevalence of *Mycoplasma genitalium* determined by DNA probe in men with urethritis. *Lancet* 1988; **i**: 266–268.

183 Taylor-Robinson D, Gilroy CB Hay PE. Occurrence of *Mycoplasma genitalium* in different populations and its clinical significance. *Clin Infect Dis* 1993; **17** (Suppl 1): 66–68.

184 Woolley PD, Kinghorn GR, Bennett KW, Eley A. Significance of *Bacteroides ureolyticus* in the lower genital tract. *Int J STD AIDS* 1992; **3**: 107–110.

185 Vaughan-Jackson JD, Dunlop EMC, Darougar S, Treharne JD, Taylor-Robinson D. Urethritis due to *Chlamydia trachomatis*. *Br J Vener Dis* 1977; **53**: 180–183.

186 Oriel JD, Reeve P, Thomas BJ, Noicol CS. Infection with *Chlamydia* group A in men with urethritis due to *Neisseria gonorrhoeae*. *J Infect Dis* 1975; **131**: 376–382.

186a McCormack WM, Rankin JS, Lee Y-H. Localization of genital mycoplasmas in women. *Am J Obstet Gynecol* 1972; **112**: 920–923.

187 Blanchard A, Hentshel J, Duffy L, Baldus K, Cassell G. Detection of *Ureaplasma urealyticum* by polymerase chain reaction in the urogenital tract of adults, in amniotic fluid and in the respiratory tract of newborn. *Clin Infect Dis* 1993; **17** (Suppl. 1): S148–S153.

188 Bowie WR. Comparison of Gram stain and first-voided urine sediment in the diagnosis of urethritis. *Sex Transm Dis* 1978; **5**: 39–42.

189 Handsfield HH, Alexander ER, Pin Wang S, Pedersen AH, Holmes KK. Differences in the therapeutic response of chlamydia-positive and chlamydia-negative forms of nongonococcal urethritis. *J Am Vener Dis Assoc* 1976; **2**: 5–9.

190 Stamm WE, Hicks CB, Martin DH, *et al.* Azithromycin for empirical treatment of the nongonococcal urethritis syndrome in men. A randomised double-blind study. *JAMA* 1995; **274**: 545–549.

191 Hooton TM, Wong ES, Barnes RC, *et al.* Erythromycin for persistent or recurrent nongonococcal urethritis: a randomized, placebo controlled trial. *Ann Int Med* 1990; **113**: 9021–9026.

192 Cassell GH. Ureaplasma infection. In: Hitchcock PJ, MacKay HT, Wasserheit JN (eds) *Sexually Transmitted Diseases and Adverse Outcomes of Pregnancy*. Washington DC; ASM Press: 1999.

193 Koteen H. 'Lymphogranuloma venereum'. *Medicine* 1945; **24**: 1–69.

194 Smith EB, Custer P. The histopathology of lymphogranuloma venereum. *J Urol* 1950; **63**: 546–563.

195 Mindel A. Lymphogranuloma venereum of the rectum in a homosexual man. *Br J Vener Dis* 1983; **59**: 196–197.

196 Abrams A. Lymphogranuloma venereum. *JAMA* 1968; **205**: 199–202.

197 Osoba AO, Beetlestone CA. Lymphographic studies in acute lymphogranuloma venereum infection. *Br J Vener Dis* 1976; **52**: 399–403.

198 King AJ. Lymphogranuloma venereum. In: *Recent Advances in Venereology*. London; J & A Churchill Ltd: 1964, pp. 304–333.

199 Annamunthodod H, Marryatt J. Barium studies in intestinal lymphogranuloma venereum. *Br J Radiol* 1961; **34**: 53–57.

200 Morson BC. Anorectal venereal disease. *Proc R Soc Med* 1964; **57**: 179–180.

201 Alacoque B, Cloppet H, Dumontel C, Moulin G. Histological, immunofluorescent and ultrastructural features of lymphogranuloma venereum. *Br J Vener Dis* 1984; **60**: 390–395.

202 Scottish Intercollegiate Guidelines Network. *Management of Genital Chlamydia trachomatis Infection. A National Clinical Guideline*. Edinburgh; Royal College of Physicians: 2000.

203 Genitourinary Medicine Statistics Scotland 1998/99. Information and Statistics Division, National Health Service in Scotland; Edinburgh: 1999.

Chapter 11

Gonorrhea
H Young, A McMillan

Gonorrhea, an infection of the mucosal surfaces of the genitourinary tract with the bacterium *Neisseria gonorrhoeae*, is mainly transmitted by sexual intercourse. In men the infection is associated with acute purulent urethritis in approximately 90% of cases, but the organism may spread also to the epididymis and the prostate. In women the urethra and cervix are infected in 65% to 75% and in 85% to 90% of cases respectively, and the rectal mucosa in 25% to 50%. Occasionally (about 10% of cases) infection extends from the cervix to the endometrium and uterine tubes. Infection of the fauces may occur in both sexes (about 5%). Eye infections are rarely seen in adults. In men who have had receptive anal sex with other men, rectal infections also occur. In a small percentage of untreated cases, systemic spread gives rise to an entity known as disseminated gonococcal infection, characterized by arthritis with or without skin lesions.

The causative organism, *Neisseria gonorrhoeae*, commonly referred to as the gonococcus, derives its generic name from Albert Neisser who described it in 1879. The bacteria are small Gram-negative cocci, kidney shaped and arranged in pairs (diplococci) with the long axes in parallel and the opposed surfaces slightly concave; the organisms are typically intracellular.

By microscopy, it is impossible to differentiate the gonococcus from *Neisseria meningitidis* or other potentially pathogenic neisseriae, or from *Branhamella* (*Moraxella*) *catarrhalis*, commonly found in the upper respiratory tract. *N. meningitidis* and commensal neisseriae can also be found on the mucous surfaces of the genitourinary tract and anal canal, particularly in women and homosexual men respectively. The differentiation of the gonococcus from other neisseriae and *B. catarrhalis* is discussed below (see pp. 331–333).

The gonococcus is a delicate organism with exacting nutritional and environmental requirements. Media containing blood or serum, a temperature of 36°C to 37°C and a moist atmosphere enriched with 10% carbon dioxide, must be provided to ensure growth. The organism is liable to die if separated from its host and is easily killed by drying, soap and water, and by other cleansing or antiseptic agents.

In nature *N. gonorrhoeae* is a strictly human pathogen, although infections have been induced experimentally in the urethra of the chimpanzee.

Pathogenesis

Primary infection commonly occurs in the columnar epithelium of the urethra and paraurethral ducts and glands of both sexes, the greater vestibular glands (Bartholin's glands), the cervix, the conjunctiva, and the rectum. Primary infection may also occur in the soft stratified squamous epithelium of the vagina of young girls: involvement of this type of epithelium in other parts of the body such as the skin of the glans penis, cornea, and mouth is extremely rare. Mucosal infections are usually characterized by a marked local neutrophilic response that in uncomplicated gonorrhea results in a purulent discharge that is the hallmark of the disease[1].

During acute gonococcal urethritis, by the third day of infection, gonococci have penetrated the mucosal lining of the urethra and have become established in the subepithelial connective tissue[2]. The capillaries are dilated and there is an exudation of cells and serum. Dense cellular infiltrations, consisting of polymorphonuclear leukocytes, plasma cells, and mast cells, soon make their appearance beneath the columnar epithelium, being particularly numerous in the region of Littre's glands and ducts. The inflammatory reaction involves the deep tissue of the corpus spongiosum and may extend into the corpora cavernosa. Gonococci are thought to penetrate the intact mucosal surface by invasion through the cells rather than by passing between cell junctions.

Much of our knowledge of gonococcal invasion comes from studies with tissue culture cells such as Chang conjunctival cells and human oviduct organ culture cells. After gonococci attach to the non-ciliated epithelium, they are surrounded by microvilli that then draw them to the surface of the mucosal cell. Some of the ciliated cells are then damaged, probably by gonococcal lipo-oligosaccharide (LOS) and slough, but others are invaded by gonococci. The gonococci appear to enter the epithelial cells through a process called parasite-directed endocytosis. This process seems to be initialized by microbial factors because it does not occur unless the gonococci are viable and because it involves host cells that are not normally phagocytic. Gonococcal invasion depends on actin polymerization in order to trigger microfilament-dependent engulfment of the bound bacteria directly[3]. An unidentified factor in serum enhances the engulfment of the gonococci. The invasion and signal transduction in epithelial cells is reviewed in considerable detail elsewhere[4].

During endocytosis, the membrane of the mucosal cell retracts, pinching off a membrane-bound vesicle that contains gonococci. The gonococci may multiply within the phagocytic vesicle, which is then transported to the basal surface of the cell[5]. Enzymes, LOS, and other components are liberated from gonococci and contribute to the destruction of cell boundaries and the killing of the cell.

Gonococci at the base of the cell penetrate the sub-mucosal tissue, the epithelial cell is shed and the gonococci are exocytosed into the lumen of the mucosa, ready to infect other epithelial cells. Gonococci may also be discharged into deeper tissues through exfoliation and lysis of infected cells: exfoliation results in thinning of the mucosa[6]. An inflammatory reaction with the influx of polymorphonuclear leukocytes is evoked and gives rise to the typical symptoms of gonorrhea. Host responses usually localize the infection, but occasionally gonococci evade host defenses resulting in localized spread (to the accessory organs of the genitourinary tract such as the prostate, epididymis, endometrium, and oviducts) or disseminated infection. Although the vast majority of phagocytosed organisms are killed some may survive. It is possible that phagocytes, such as granulocytes, may facilitate the spread and transfer of gonococci while monocytes may serve as an intracellular niche and transportation vehicle for gonococci during systemic infections[4].

According to one concept, gonococcal pathogenicity may be based primarily on internal disorganization of human macrophages[7]. Gonococci in pus appear in specific clusters in which they are surrounded by organelles and granules derived from the host cells in which they multiplied. These clusters are called infectious units because

- the cocci multiply within them
- the whole complex makes contact with epithelial cells

- the cocci in units are not recognized by polymorphs as long as the coating of granules is dense enough
- the cocci are probably protected against humoral defense mechanisms.

Gonococci phagocytosed by polymorphonuclear leukocytes are killed. Those phagocytosed by macrophages, however, interfere with the cells' regulatory processes, survive and form a cluster of multiplying gonococci surrounded by granules and remnants of macrophages, i.e. the infectious units, the host cell remnants are utilized, the gonococci become less and less coated and are re-phagocytosed, and the cycle is repeated. Depending on the nature of the phagocytic cells involved, an abortive infection or a self-cure of gonorrhea may occur. Although this is an attractive model more recent work on gonococcal virulence and pathogenicity has focused on the development of gonococcal infection in terms of the interaction between the outer membrane of the gonococcal cell envelope, the host mucosal surfaces, and the immune system. The gonococcus is highly efficient in its ability to turn on or off the expression of cell surface components (phase variation) or to vary them (antigenic variation). Antigenic variation of surface proteins is thought to be the means of escape from host-specific antibody directed against the initial antigen that is expressed when the gonococcal infection starts. The role of the various gonococcal surface components involved in virulence and pathogenicity are reviewed briefly below.

GONOCOCCAL SURFACE STRUCTURES AND PATHOGENICITY

The cell envelope of Gram-negative bacteria including *N. gonorrhoeae*, is composed of three macromolecular components

- the outer membrane
- the rigid peptidoglycan layer.
- the cytoplasmic membrane

It is the components of the outer membrane that are important in the initial stages of adherence and invasion. Adherence of gonococci to the mucosal epithelium is a prerequisite for establishing infection. Attachment to mucosal cells is rapid as micturition after intercourse will not remove them[8].

Pili

Pili are important during initial attachment. They overcome the electrostatic forces of repulsion between the negatively charged bacterial surface and the sialic acid on the surface of the host cell and bind the organism loosely to the mucosal surface[9]. The gonococcus uses pili to recognize a receptor specific for human cells: the CD46 molecule, which is also a virus receptor, has recently been proposed to function as a *Neisseria* pilus receptor[10].

Pili are the hair-like appendages that extend up to several micrometers from the gonococcal surface. Pili are composed of stacked repeating peptide subunits called pilin proteins (molecular weight 17–21 kDa). Most strains of gonococci contain one copy of the expressed pilus subunit gene, *pilE*, and multiple copies of *pilS*, which are transcriptionally silent, incomplete pilin loci carrying variant sequences. PilC protein previously described as a pilus assembly factor is found on the bacterial surface and the tip of pili where it expresses an adherence function[4]. The amino-terminal of the pilus molecule, which contains a high percentage of hydrophobic amino acids is conserved. The amino acid sequence near the mid-portion of the molecule serves in the attachment to host cells and is less prominent in the immune response. The amino acid sequence near the carboxy terminal is highly variable; this portion of the molecule is most prominent in the immune response[11].

Gonococcal pili from different strains are antigenically diverse and a single gonococcal strain is capable of expressing multiple antigenically distinct types of pili. Antigenic variation results from recombination events between silent and expressed loci, which result in the formation of diverse pilins either by transformation with DNA released from lysed gonococci or by recombination between a silent and an expressed locus on the same chromosome.

There are several mechanisms of phase variation that switch between the presence (Pil+) and absence (Pil−) of pili on the cell surface: switching occurs at a frequency of about 1×10^{-4}. *PilA* and *PilB* are genes that form a two-component regulatory system that controls whether pili are assembled or secreted into the surrounding medium leading to the Pil+ or Pil- phenotype. This occurs by proteolytic cleavage at different sites of the *PilE* protein leading to the two possible phenotypes. Homologous recombination with uneven DNA exchanges between *pilE* and *pilS* genes can result in larger versions of PilE protein that are not assembled and lead to the Pil- phenotype. Slipped-strand DNA synthesis in the *pilC* gene leads to frame-shift mutations and determines whether or not PilC protein is expressed.

Phase and antigenic variation are important in evading the immune system and adaptation to new cell types. Clinical isolates from the genital tract are usually highly piliated and continue to express a strong Pil+ phenotype when initially cultured *in vitro*[3]. Shifts in the pilin antigens that are expressed occur during the course of an infection[12] and such variation in pili can endow the gonococci with specific cell tropism allowing it to spread from the cervix to the oviduct for example[13]. Apart from enhancing attachment to host cells piliated gonococci have increased resistance to phagocytosis[11]. There is evidence to suggest that a non-piliated phase is selected for during passage across a layer of epithelial cells[14]. The released bacteria contain a pool of clones that carry structurally altered pili that may have different antigenic and binding properties.

Non-piliated strains of GC are more susceptible to phagocytosis and are unable to infect human volunteers[15] but loss of pili may be an advantage to GC once within the host.

Protein II (PII) or opacity associated protein (Opa)

Once gonococci are loosely attached factors such as protein II, also known as opacity protein (Opa) because its presence is associated with opaque colonial (Opa+) forms, come into play. Protein II has a molecular weight of 24 to 32 kDa with one portion of the PII molecule in the outer membrane, and the rest exposed on the surface. Protein II functions in the attachment of gonococci to host cells and also promotes the adhesion of gonococci to each other to form microcolonies[16]. Microcolony formation

may aid the initial colonization of mucosal cells[1].

A strain of GC can express none, one, two, or occasionally three types of PII although each strain has eleven genes for different PIIs[8]. Each PII gene is complete with a functional promoter[17] and although all the PII genes are apparently transcribed, not all are translated. Thus, gonococci can fail to express, or can express different PIIs, through phase and antigenic variation. Antigenic variation of PII results from recombination amongst the eleven PII genes. Phase variation occurs more frequently and is caused by slipped-strand DNA synthesis during replication of a pentameric repeat (CTCTT) region of the *opa* gene. The result is that any number of genes may be expressed at a given time depending on whether they have shifted into or out of frame so that a gonococcus may produce several different Opa proteins at the same time, or none at all[1].

The variable expression of these proteins by gonococci represents important cell tropism determinants and aids the gonococcus to evade the host's immune response and to colonize different sites within the host. Antigenic variation of PII has been seen over the course of an infection within the host[18] and during the menstrual cycle[19] demonstrating the ability of PII to evade the host defenses. Different PII proteins allow the attachment of gonococci to epithelial cells and neutrophils. Variant Opa proteins bind to different receptors: proteins of the Opa^{50} class recognize heparin sulfate proteoglycan (HSPG), interact with epithelial cells and promote invasion while proteins of the Opa^{52} class recognize members of the CD66 receptor family and mediate binding to phagocytes[4]. Opa proteins are also thought to be important in cell invasion, although the most important surface component involved in invasion is thought to be the porin protein (PI).

Protein I (PI)

Protein I is a porin that extends through the gonococcal cell membrane. It occurs in trimers to form pores in the surface through which some nutrients enter the cell and waste products leave it. The molecular weight of PI varies from 34 to

37 kDa. Gonococci express one of two structurally related forms of PI termed IA or IB[20]. A single copy of the structural gene exists in the chromosome[21] which suggests that the PIA and PIB genes are alleles of the same gene. Each gonococcal strain expresses only one type of PI, but the PI of different strains is antigenically different[11]. Antigenic heterogeneity in PI is the basis of a serotyping scheme (see pp. 339–340). It is generally accepted that all strains of gonococci possess either PIA or PIB but not both. However, there are rare examples of PIA/IB hybrids in nature but little is known about them at present[22].

The actual role of PI in pathogenesis is unclear. Studies with lipid bilayers and erythrocytes have shown that gonococci transfer their porin molecules in an inverted manner into these membranes[23]. PIA-expressing strains of gonococci are more efficient at porin transfer than PIB-expressing strains; interestingly PIA strains are more often associated with disseminated gonococcal infection than are IB strains. Antibody to PI acquired during infection is bactericidal and prevents repeated attacks of salpingitis caused by strains with the same type of PI[24]. Protein I has also been shown to directionally insert into the membranes of neutrophils *in vitro*, collapsing their membrane potentials in the process. Degranulation of their cytoplasmic granules containing antimicrobial agents is then inhibited. It is not clear whether or not this occurs *in vivo* however[23].

Protein III (PIII)

This protein (molecular weight about 33 kDa) is antigenically conserved in all gonococci and is coded for by a single copy of the PIII gene. It is a reduction-modifiable protein (Rmp) that changes its apparent molecular weight when in a reduced state. It associates with PI in a ratio of 1:3 in the formation of pores in the cell surface[11]. Its actual function in the pathogenesis is not clear but a similar protein appears to be absent among non-pathogenic *Neisseria* species[25]. Mutants lacking PIII have been obtained indicating that PIII is not essential for gonococcal growth[26]. Antibodies to PIII are thought to increase susceptibility to gonococcal infection. Antibodies directed against PIII interfere with the bactericidal activity of antibodies directed against other surface antigens such as PI and LOS, probably by steric hindrance. The carboxy terminal of PIII shows a sequence homology with the carboxy terminal of the enterobacterial OmpA protein[27]. Therefore it is likely that these blocking antibodies arise naturally from cross-reactive Enterobacteriaceae in the body[28].

Lipo-oligosaccharide (LOS)

Lipopolysaccharide (LPS) is the major glycolipid of the outer membrane of Gram-negative bacteria. High molecular weight LPS from enteric bacteria such as *Escherichia coli* is composed of a lipid A moiety, a core oligosaccharide, and a repeating O-antigen polysaccharide. In comparison, gonococcal LPS is much smaller and lacks the repeating O-antigen polysaccharide[29]. It is thus called lipo-oligosaccharide (LOS) and has a molecular weight of 3 to 7 kDa.

Lipo-oligosaccharide possesses potent endotoxic activity and serves as the target antigen for much of the bactericidal antibody present in normal or convalescent sera[30]. Lipo-oligosaccharide contributes a great deal to the inflammatory response and tissue damage in gonorrhea by eliciting the release of tumor necrosis factor alpha (TNF-α)[1].

However, gonococci can modify their LOS to mimic host cells thus avoiding immune attack. It does this by an endogenous sialyltransferase enzyme which takes N-acetylneuraminic acid (NANA) from the human nucleotide sugar cytidine 5′ monophospho-N-acetylneuraminic acid (CMP-NANA) and adds it to the terminal galactose of a gonococcal acceptor LOS[11]. Sialylation of gonococcal LOS is associated with an increased resistance to killing by normal human serum. The addition of the sialic acid may down regulate the alternative complement pathway or mask protective epitopes. Gonococcal strains that cause uncomplicated gonorrhea are usually killed by normal human serum and are termed serum sensitive. Immunoglobulin M and immunoglobulin G antibodies mediate the

recognition of specific sites on the LOS and deposition of the C5b→9 membrane attack complex (MAC) on serum-sensitive strains destroys them. Strains that cause disseminated gonococcal infection are not killed by human serum and are referred to as serum resistant (these tend to be PIA strains). Sialylated strains are also less chemo-attractive to phagocytes and may explain why there is a lack of genital symptoms in disseminated gonococcal infection[1].

Recent work by Parsons *et al.*[31] has shown that lactic acid is a co-factor in blood that enhances the ability of CMP-NANA to sialylate gonococcal LOS and induce serum resistance. It does this by up regulating the activity of the sialyltransferase and also by providing more LOS sialyl acceptors. Lipo-oligosaccharide also undergoes antigenic variation at a frequency of 10^{-2} to 10^{-3}[32]. The antigenic variants have different molecular weights that may alter the spatial arrangements of other surface components thus altering exposed molecules and susceptibilities. Unlike pili and PII, the actual mechanism of this is unknown but it has been suggested that slippage in the poly-G tracts of certain genes involved in the biosynthesis of LOS may be involved[33]. Gonococcal strains appear to be sialylated *in vivo* but sialylated LOS is lost after growth *in vitro*[33a].

IgA protease

Many mucosal pathogens including *N. gonorrhoeae* produce IgA proteases. These proteases split antibodies of the IgA1 subclass of IgA at specific amino acid sites in the hinge region of the molecule. Once split, the IgA loses its antibody activity; the F$_{ab}$ fragments attach to the bacterial surface and mask the antigenic epitopes from further immune attack. The role of IgA protease in gonococcal pathogenesis is not clear. Although the enzyme presumably inactivates secretory IgA1 on the mucosal surface, antibody of the IgA2 subclass is unaffected. Recently it has been shown that *N. gonorrhoeae* does not require IgA1 protease activity to produce experimental urethritis in men[34].

IRON REGULATED PROTEINS

Iron is essential for bacterial growth. Unlike other bacteria that produce siderophores to utilize iron in the body, gonococci rely on scavenging host iron complexes through expression of transferrin and lactoferrin receptors[35]. These receptors are involved in the acquisition of iron from the host iron binding proteins and in this respect they can be considered virulence factors.

HOST RESPONSE

Not everyone who is exposed to the gonococcus develops infection. Non-specific factors have been implicated in natural resistance to gonorrhea. In women, changes in the genital pH and hormone levels may increase resistance to infection at certain times of the menstrual cycle. The osmolarity, pH, and high concentration of urea in urine are thought to protect some men from becoming infected. Invasion of the genital tract mucosal surfaces early in infection brings the gonococcus into contact with plasma. Immunoglobulin G and complement components are also found in cervical secretions and they may provide a primary defense system that will prevent some infections. The acute inflammatory response induced in localized gonococcal infection is in part mediated by the interaction of invading gonococci with natural antibody and complement[36]. These interactions generate chemotoxins that attract phagocytes to the site of infection. The majority of phagocytosed gonococci will be killed but some will survive[37]. Complement and natural non-specific antibodies have an important role in preventing dissemination. Individuals with deficiencies of the terminal components of the complement pathway are significantly more likely to develop bacteremia and disseminated gonococcal infection.

Most uninfected individuals have serum antibodies that react with gonococcal antigens. These antibodies probably result from colonization or infection with various Gram-negative bacteria that possess cross-reactive antigens, for example Enterobacteriaceae, and pharyngeal carriage of non-gonococcal neisseriae. Natural antibody of IgG, IgM, and IgA classes were detected by an indirect immunofluorescence test[38].

Natural IgM reacting with LPS in conjunction with complement is responsible for the bactericidal activity of normal human serum[39]. Antibody against PIII protects gonococci from killing by natural and anti-PI bactericidal antibody and complement by preventing bactericidal antibody binding to the gonococcal cells, presumably by steric hindrance.

Natural IgG can also function as a heat-stable opsonin promoting phagocytosis of gonococci by human PMNs. In this way it may constitute a part of the host's early defense mechanisms prior to the development of a specific antibody response.

MUCOSAL AND HUMORAL RESPONSE

Repeated gonococcal infections are common suggesting that the host does not mount a protective immune response. Mucosal antibodies are primarily IgA and IgG. In genital secretions, antibodies have been identified which react with PI, PII, and LOS. Complement is present in endocervical secretions but in much lower concentration than in the blood. There is, however, little evidence to suggest that there is a complement-mediated bactericidal defense mechanism on the genital mucosa. The IgA response is generally brief and declines rapidly after treatment. IgG levels decline more slowly.

Serum antibody to gonococci can be detected within a few days of infection but such antibodies are, in general, not protective with regard to mucosal re-infection. The majority of patients have increased levels of serum IgG, IgM, and secretory IgA reactive with the gonococcus. The main humoral antibody responses are to PI, LOS, and PIII[40, 41]. Although a study in a sex-worker cohort found some evidence for immunity derived from antibodies to PI (serovar-specific immunity)[42] others have found no evidence for such immunity[43]. Acquired specific antibody to PI prevented repeated attacks of salpingitis due to the same serovar but were unable to protect women from repeated local genital infection by homologous PI serovar strains[44].

Certain antibodies, such as those to PIII, may increase susceptibility to infection: IgG against PIII blocks the PI and LOS antibodies, presumably by steric hindrance.

A recent study of local and systemic antibody responses to uncomplicated gonococcal infection found that in addition to the potential ability of the gonococcus to avoid the effects of an immune response it does not elicit strong immune responses during uncomplicated genital infections[45].

CELL-MEDIATED IMMUNITY

There are few studies that examine T-cell responses to *N. gonorrhoeae* in humans and little evidence that cell-mediated immunity is important in protection from infection.

A recent study showed that T lymphocytes from a majority of patients with genital gonococcal infection proliferated on incubation with PI[46]. A significant increase in PI specific interleukin-4 producing CD4+ T helper lymphocytes occurred. The study concluded that mucosal gonococcal infection can induce PI specific circulating lymphocytes with a T_{h2} phenotype, and that a portion of these PI specific lymphocytes can potentially traffic to mucosal surfaces. Further studies are required to define antigonococcal T-cell responses and to elucidate their significance in the protection from disease and the ability to interrupt transmission.

Pathogenesis of disseminated gonococcal infection

Subtypes of *N. gonorrhoeae* that are associated with disseminated gonococcal infection may be more invasive than those confined to the mucosal surfaces. Gonococcal strains associated with disseminated gonococcal infection often belong to Protein IA serotype and auxotype AHU[47-49]. In areas such as Seattle, USA, where the prevalence of such strains has declined as a result of contact tracing and treatment of asymptomatic infected individuals, there has been a reduction in the number of cases of disseminated gonococcal infection[50]. Strains associated with disseminated gonococcal infection are usually resistant to the complement-dependent

bactericidal action of normal human serum[51, 52], and these strains, possibly by their inability to induce chemotaxis of neutrophils, are often associated with asymptomatic infection of mucosal surfaces. Although strains associated with disseminated gonococcal infection have been reported as being exquisitely sensitive to benzylpenicillin[53], isolates of *N. gonorrhoeae* with chromosomal or plasmid-mediated resistance to benzylpenicillin have been described in individuals with disseminated gonococcal infection. It is clear that the incidence of penicillin resistance in isolates from patients with disseminated gonococcal infection reflects the prevalence of resistant infection in the community[54].

As dissemination may occur from any site, but more often during or just after menstruation and in pregnancy, host factors may also be important in disseminated gonococcal infection. It has been suggested that, possibly influenced by changes in vaginal pH, cervicovaginal flora, or cervical mucus, gonococcal phenotype switching from opaque to transparent, which is more resistant to killing by normal human serum, may be a factor[55].

Recurrent bacteremia due to *N. gonorrhoeae* has been described in individuals with homozygous deficiency of the sixth, seventh, or eighth components of complement[56]. Screening for such deficiency, however, need only be undertaken in individuals who have had two or more episodes of bacteremia associated with *Neisseria* species.

Epidemiology

INCIDENCE AND PREVALENCE

Gonorrhea is a disease with a worldwide distribution. It has been estimated that in 1995, globally there were 62 million cases of gonorrhea[57]. Gonorrhea is common in developed as well as in developing countries, but differences and inadequacies in reporting systems make absolute comparisons of data between countries difficult. Nevertheless the data do give a reasonable guide as to trends.

In many countries, including the UK, the sharp increase in the incidence of gonorrhea noted in the 1960s and mid-1970s stabilized and declined thereafter until the mid-1990s. Within western Europe, the declining trend between 1991 and 1996 was particularly marked in the Scandinavian countries[58]. Since the mid-1990s, however, there has been a progressive increase in the number of reported cases in the UK (Figure 11.1) and elsewhere. In the UK between 1998 and 1999, diagnoses of gonorrhea rose by 25% (13 190 to 16 470), by 27% in men (8904 to 11 289) and 21% in women (4286 to 5181). Diagnoses in males outnumbered those in females by a ratio of more than 2:1[59]. In the UK in 1999, the diagnostic rates were highest in males aged 20 to 24 years (465 per 100 000 population), and in females aged 16 to 19 years (791 per 100 000 population) (Figure 11.1). In contrast, in the UK the rate for girls under the age of 16 years, however, is almost four times that of boys in the same age group.

In the USA, the incidence of gonorrhea decreased from the mid-1970s, and between 1985 and 1997, the reported rate of gonorrhea followed an overall decline of 64.2%[60]. This trend, however, was reversed in 1998, when an overall increase in incidence of 9% between 1997 and 1998 was reported (132.9 cases per 100 000 population in 1998 compared with 121.8 cases in 1997)[60]. During that period, the gonorrhea rate in women increased by 10.5% (from 119.2 to 131.7 per 100 000 population), and in men by 7.4% (from 124.5 to 133.7 per 100 000 population). Among women aged 15 to 19 years, the sex and age group with the highest incidence of gonorrhea, the rate increased by 11.4% (from 683.2 to 761.4 per 100 000 population). Amongst men aged 20 to 24 years, the rate increased by 11.3% (from 506.7 to 564.0 per 100 000 men). There were regional differences in the reported rates of infection in the USA, for example, the rate in the mid-west increased by 16.4%, but decreased by 0.8% in the north east.

Although changes in gonorrhea screening and surveillance practices, for example, the introduction of non-culture diagnostic methods that may have increased sensitivity under field conditions, may have contributed to the higher reported rates, data suggest that true increases in cases have occurred at least in some populations.

The incidence of gonorrhea in developing countries in Asia, Africa, and Central and South America is not known with certainty because of inadequacies in the reporting systems. The World Health Organization (WHO) in partnership with the Rockefeller Foundation, however, generated a set of estimates for the prevalence and incidence of gonorrhea in 1995 by region[57]. The data are shown in Table 11.1. These estimates highlight the public health importance of gonorrhea. In some developing countries public health campaigns targeted at reducing the incidence and prevalence of STIs have resulted in a steady decline in the number of reported cases of gonorrhea. For example in Thailand, although there was a modest decline in the number of cases since 1985, the institution of HIV-prevention programs in 1989 led to a marked drop in the incidence of infection (Figure 11.2).

Prostitution probably plays an important part in the spread of infection in developing countries. For example, in a cross-sectional study of 100 female sex-

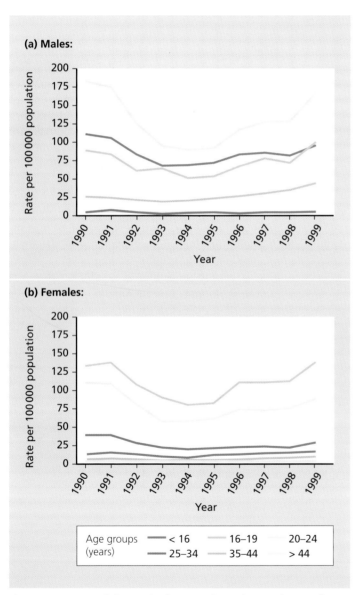

Figure 11.1 Rates of diagnosis of uncomplicated gonorrhea made at GUM clinics, by sex and age group, UK: 1990–1999 (adapted from PHLS, DHSS&PS and the Scottish ISD5 Collaborative Group 2000[59])

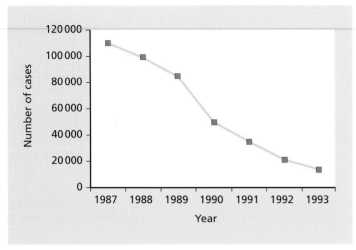

Figure 11.2 Number of reported cases of gonorrhea in men who attended STI clinics in Thailand (after Hanenberg *et al.* 1994[253])

industry workers in a port city in Peru, 14% had gonorrhea[61]. A similar high prevalence of gonorrhea was noted in female prostitutes in Dakar, Senegal, where 16% of 374 women were infected by *N. gonorrhoeae*[62].

In the UK there was a marked decrease in the incidence of homosexually acquired gonorrhea in the early to late 1980s, most probably reflecting concern about HIV infection. Since 1995, however, the incid-ence of infection has increased steadily (Figure 11.3). About 50% of men who had acquired gonorrhea through homosexual contact were aged 25 to 34 years, but between 1998 and 1999 the number of reported cases amongst this age group fell by 6%. The number of diagnoses in that period, in the 16 to 19, and in the 20 to 24 year age groups, however, increased by 51% and 25% respectively. In Amsterdam, between 1998 and 1999, there was a 46%

increase in the number of cases of gonor-rhea reported from the STI clinic[63]. The largest increase was noted amongst men who had sex with men, the number of cases of rectal gonorrhea in 1999 being double that of the previous year (186 versus 94 cases). Increased rates of rectal gonorrhea amongst men who had sex with men have also been reported from the USA[64]. Although the incidence of rectal gonorrhea declined between 1990 and 1993 (42, 33, 23, and 20 cases per year per 100 000 population), from 1994 through 1997, the incidence increased from 21 to 38 per 100 000 men. The increase in incidence of infection was highest amongst men aged 25 to 34 years (from 41 to 83 cases per 100 000 men).

TRANSMISSION OF INFECTION

Owing to the poor viability of the gono-coccus away from the mucosal surfaces of the host, gonorrhea is ordinarily acquired by sexual intercourse with an infected person. There are so many variable factors that it is difficult to assess the risk of acquiring an infection from a single exposure. Gonorrhea is regarded, however, as being of high infectivity, the risk for a female having intercourse with an infected male being higher, 60% to 90%[65–67], than that for a male with an infected female, 20% to 50%[68, 69]. The risk of transmission per exposure with an infected partner was 0.19 for white American men and 0.53 for black American men. The higher risk of infection among Afro-Caribbean Americans may be related to the increase susceptibility to neisserial infection of patients with blood group B[70]. On repeated exposure with a single infected partner the majority of men are susceptible to gonococcal infection.

Human volunteer studies associated with vaccine trials in men suggest that inoculum size is important in establishing infection. In challenge studies, increasing the challenge dose from 10^3 to 10^5 piliated gonococcal colony forming units (cfu) over-came the efficacy of a parenteral gonococ-cal pilus vaccine[71]. Similar numbers of organisms are readily acquired during sexual intercourse, as the number of gono-cocci recovered from cervical aspirates ranges from 5×10^3 to 8×10^6 cfu/mL

Table 11.1 Estimated prevalence and incidence of gonorrhea in 1995 in adults between the ages of 15 and 49 (modified from Gerbase *et al.* 1998[57])

	Prevalence of infection (%)		Annual incidence rate (per 100 000 population)	
	Males	Females	Males	Females
North America	0.1	0.4	1085	1204
Western Europe	0.07	0.2	559	601
Australasia	0.1	0.4	1085	1204
Latin America and the Caribbean	0.6	1.1	2756	2923
Sub-Saharan Africa	2.0	2.8	5771	6547
North Africa and the Middle East	0.2	0.4	915	976
Eastern Europe and Central Asia	0.3	0.5	1483	1467
East Asia and Pacific	0.1	0.1	435	379
South and Southeast Asia	1.0	1.4	3003	3180

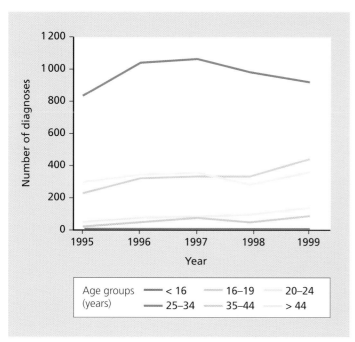

Figure 11.3 New diagnoses of uncomplicated gonorrhea in men who have sex with men by age group, UK: 1995–1999 (adapted from PHLS, DHSS&PS and the Scottish ISD5 Collaborative Group 2000[59])

(mean 1.0×10^6 cfu/mL); the corresponding figures for vaginal aspirates are 1.0×10^2 to 1.0×10^6 (mean 8.4×10^4 cfu/mL)[72].

There have been no studies on the inocula required to cause endocervical infection because of the risk of pelvic inflammatory disease and subsequent infertility. The observation, however, that the first 20 to 30 mL of urine from infected men contains 4.0×10^3 to 1.0×10^6 cfu/mL (mean 1.1×10^5 cfu/mL) (Young, unpublished observations) gives some idea of the numbers of gonococci likely to be transmitted.

The median pre-patent period of urethral gonorrhea in men is 5.8 days, with a range of 1 to 57 days[73]. In the female a precise incubation period is difficult to determine since approximately 70% or more of infections cause no symptoms. Such asymptomatic infections make it possible for individuals to remain as sources of infection within the community whilst at risk themselves of developing pelvic inflammatory disease or disseminated infection; the risk of developing these complications is generally given as 10% and 1% respectively. Patients infected with certain strains of gonococci are at greater risk of developing disseminated infection.

In those women who are symptomatic, 50% develop symptoms within 9 to 10 days of infection[74].

The gonococcus can be transmitted to the pharynx by orogenital contact. Infection is usually without symptoms. Pharyngeal transfer of gonococci by kissing is exceedingly rare. Oral to genital transmission is said to be uncommon, although it has been reported in relation to a subset of prostitutes in South East Asia who specialize in oral sex[75], and McMillan and Young (unpublished observations) noted that the pharynx was the only site of infection in the presumed source contacts of 6 of 62 homosexual men with urethral gonorrhea.

In males, rectal infection is usually the result of receptive anal intercourse with an infected partner. McMillan et al.[76], however, found that in 9 of 46 men with rectal gonorrhea the probable source of infection was the pharynx of the partner. Gonococci can be transmitted from the oropharynx to the rectum during receptive oral–anal sex or digital–anal contact. Colonization of the rectal mucosa in the female is common (25% to 50%)[77], and although long considered to be the result of backward extension of the infection because of contamination by infected vaginal secre-

tions, may more often result from receptive anal intercourse.

Vulvovaginitis in young children under the age of puberty is caused more commonly by organisms other than *N. gonorrhoeae*, but such infections can result from sexual abuse.

During birth a baby passing through an infected cervix may acquire gonococcal conjunctivitis of the newborn (ophthalmia neonatorum). This condition is uncommon nowadays in the UK because of general improvements in antenatal care and in the detection and treatment of gonococcal infection. In Nairobi, Kenya[77a], 42% of 67 babies born to mothers with untreated gonorrhea and who did not receive prophylaxis against infection, developed ophthalmia. Gonococcal conjunctivitis in older children and in adults is usually acquired by contact with fingers and/or moist towels contaminated with fresh pus.

ASSOCIATION OF GONORRHEA AND HIV INFECTION

Several studies have shown that the presence of ulcerative and non-ulcerative STIs, including gonorrhea, is a risk factor for acquisition of HIV-1[78]. For example, one such study reported by Laga et al.[79] identified 68 HIV-1 seroconverters amongst a group of 431 initially HIV-1 seronegative female sex-industry workers in Kinshasa, Zaire, who were followed prospectively for a mean duration of 2 years; these 68 seroconverters were with 126 women who did not seroconvert. Multivariate analysis on all variables that were associated with seroconversion on univariate analysis showed that gonorrhea was independently associated with seroconversion for HIV-1 with an odds ratio of 4.8 (95% confidence interval 2.4–9.8). Similar conclusions were reached by Beck et al.[80] in a case-control study from London, UK, in which about 80% of the patients were men who had had sex with men. They showed that a past history of STIs, including gonorrhea, was significantly associated with HIV-1 seropositivity. Craib et al.[81] working in Vancouver, Canada, conducted a case-control study amongst men who had sex with men and also found that gonorrhea was a risk factor for acquisition of HIV-1: 17% of 125 cases and 6% of 250 controls had had gonococcal infection during the seroconversion period. They showed further that rectal, but not urethral or pharyngeal, gonorrhea was independently associated with HIV-1 infection.

The impact of treatment of STIs, including gonorrhea, in reducing the incidence of HIV-1 was shown clearly in the Mwanza, Tanzania, study[82]. This was a randomized trial to evaluate the impact of improved STI case management on the incidence of HIV-1. The incidence of this infection was compared in six intervention communities and six pair-matched comparison communities. The study focused on enhanced syndromic diagnosis of symptomatic STI, including gonorrhea. Of those individuals who were initially HIV-1 seronegative, 1.2% of 4149 in the intervention communities and 1.9% of the 4400 in the comparison communities seroconverted, a reduction of 40%. HIV-1 has been detected in cervicovaginal secretions, as both cell-associated and cell-free virus (Chapter 7), and recent studies have shown that HIV-1 DNA is significantly more likely to be detected in endocervical material from women who have gonococcal infection than those who do not (odds ratio 3.1, 95% confidence interval 1.1–9.8)[83]. The same workers noted that the number of polymorphonuclear leukocytes in cervical mucus is a strong predictor of cervical HIV-1 DNA shedding. The increased shedding of cell-free virus and viral-infected cells in the cervicovaginal fluid of women with gonorrhea may increase their infectiousness to their sexual partners. If there are no other risk factors, HIV is easier to transmit from male to female, however, in the presence of a STI, female-to-male transmission is as likely as male-to-female[84]. In addition, the micro-ulcerations that are sometimes seen in women with gonococcal cervicitis, may be the portal of entry of HIV-1.

HIV-1 DNA can be detected in urethral secretions from HIV-seropositive men[85], and there is a good correlation between its detection and the CD4+ cell count in the peripheral blood. HIV-1 DNA is also more likely to be detected in urethral material from men with urethritis and gonorrhea, and successful treatment reduces its concentration. The presence of HIV-1 in semen is well documented (Chapter 7). Atkins et al.[86] showed high levels of HIV-1 proviral DNA in the semen of three men with gonococcal urethritis, and showed that these levels fell

rapidly after treatment; there was no significant change in plasma viral load. A larger study from Malawi[87] confirmed this finding. Cohen and colleagues showed that the median concentration HIV-1 RNA in cell-free seminal plasma from men with urethritis was eight times higher than that in HIV-seropositive men without urethritis (12.4 versus 1.51×10^4 copies/mL). Gonococcal urethritis was associated with the highest concentration of HIV-1 RNA in seminal plasma (15.8×10^4 copies/mL). As in Atkin's study, the concentration of HIV-1 RNA decreased significantly within 1 week of successful treatment, but the decline of HIV-1 RNA concentration in the seminal plasma was slower than the disappearance of leukocytes from the urethra, suggesting that increased viral shedding associated with urethritis is not simply a product of granulocytic inflammation. The increased level of shedding of HIV in genital secretions may lead to increased infectiousness and a greater possibility of HIV-1 transmission.

Clinical features

The clinical features of gonorrhea reflect the inflammatory changes induced by infection of mucosal surfaces by *Neisseria gonorrhoeae*: in some cases the inflammation may be so mild that the patient may be unaware of being infected. A chronic inflammatory process of mucous membranes may have serious sequelae, however, particularly in women in whom infertility or an increased risk of ectopic pregnancy may result. An infrequent but serious complication is systemic dissemination of the organism.

CLINICAL FEATURES IN THE ADULT MALE (UNCOMPLICATED GONOCOCCAL INFECTION)

Urethral infection

Urethral discharge and dysuria are the most common symptoms (47% of men), but some patients (34%) only complain of urethral discharge, and a few (5%) have dysuria as the sole symptom[73]. If infection has spread proximally to the posterior urethra there may be symptoms of frequency of micturition, urgency, and painful erec-

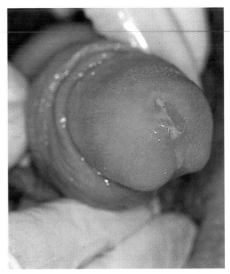

Figure 11.4 Gonococcal urethritis (reproduced from McMillan and Scott 2000[255])

tions. Clinical examination may reveal a reddened urethral meatus with a purulent or mucopurulent discharge (Figure 11.4). Inguinal lymph nodes may be enlarged on both sides. Examination of the urine by the two-glass test will show pus in the first glass if the anterior urethra is mainly affected, or in both glasses if the posterior urethra or bladder is involved (as the extent of the inflammatory process in the urethra does not influence management, however, this test has been abandoned by many physicians). If there is less severe inflammation in the urethra, 'threads' may be found in the urine. These threads are casts of mucus-secreting urethral glands, located in the submucosa and called Littre's glands. Invariably inflamed in urethral gonorrhea, the ducts of Littre's glands shed casts, composed of pus cells and desquamated tubular cells in the urine.

Although up to 10% of men with urethral gonorrhea who attend STI clinics are asymptomatic, many are in the pre-patent period of infection at the time of examination, and if untreated would become symptomatic[73].

Post-gonococcal urethritis may occur in at least 20% of men adequately treated with penicillins (Chapter 10).

Oropharyngeal infection

Infection of the pharynx results from transfer of organisms from the genitalia during fellatio or, less commonly, cunnilingus. Although there is a significant relationship between symptoms of pharyngitis and the practice of fellatio, the isolation of *N. gonorrhoeae* from the pharynx does not correlate with symptoms of pharyngitis[53]. Symptoms may be present in only about 20% of cases[88], when there may be sore throat, perhaps with referred pain in the area. Clinical examination may reveal no abnormalities, or a mild pharyngitis or tonsillitis.

Anorectal infection

Infection in this site in the male is usually the result of a homosexual act. More than half of men with uncomplicated rectal gonorrhea are asymptomatic[89]. In others there may be symptoms of a distal proctitis namely constipation, a mucopurulent anal discharge, anal bleeding, perianal discomfort or pruritus ani, and, in severe cases, pain and tenesmus. Proctoscopic examination may show a normal appearance, or there may be either patchy or generalized erythema of the rectal mucosa with mucopus in the lumen of the rectum and anal canal. The histology is that of a non-specific proctitis[89]. The inflammatory reaction does not extend into the sigmoid colon. In some cases the mucous membrane is friable and bleeding to the touch, in others it may have a granular appearance. The anal canal, constructed of stratified cuboid or squamous epithelium, is not affected by the gonococcus, although mucopus may be seen to exude from the orifices of the anal glands whose deeper parts are lined by columnar epithelium.

The differential diagnosis of anorectal gonorrhea includes ulcerative colitis, Crohn's disease, chlamydial infection caused by either oculogenital or lymphogranuloma venereum serovars of *Chlamydia trachomatis*, herpes simplex virus infection, cytomegalovirus proctocolitis in the immunocompromised patient, traumatic proctitis, chemical-induced proctitis, ischemic colitis, radiation or drug-induced colitis, amebiasis, and neoplasia.

Local complications of untreated anorectal infection include perianal and ischiorectal abscesses and anal fistulae.

Local complications of gonorrhea in the male

Inflammation and abscess formation in the parafrenal glands (Tyson's glands)

This is not common (less than 1%) but, when it occurs, it usually produces painful tender swellings on one or both sides of the frenum (Figure 11.5). Pus may be expressed from the duct.

Gonococcal balanitis

As the gonococcus tends not to attack the squamous epithelium of the penis this complication is uncommon.

Inflammation and abscess formation in the para-urethral glands on either side of the urethral meatus

This is rare now in areas where medical attention is easily available. A painful swelling develops on one or both sides of the urethral meatus. Pus may be expressed from the duct of the gland.

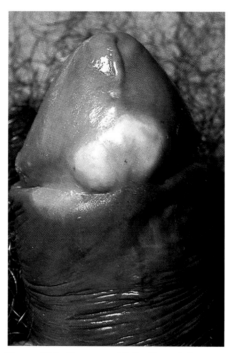

Figure 11.5 Gonococcal infection of the parafrenal glands (reproduced from McMillan and Scott 2000[255])

Periurethral cellulitis and abscess formation

This is rare except when medical help is delayed. The inflammatory reaction to the gonococcus in the subepithelial tissues of the urethra is particularly marked in the region of Littre's glands and ducts, which may become obstructed resulting in the formation of periurethral abscesses. These abscesses may rupture into the urethra or to the exterior, or may heal with scarring.

There is pain and swelling at the site of the abscess and there may be some restriction in urine flow if it bulges into the urethra. If the corpus spongiosum is affected, painful erections will be experienced, and there may be ventral angulation of the penis. On examination there is a tender fluctuant swelling, most commonly at the site of the fossa navicularis or bulb.

If untreated the abscess may point; the overlying skin becomes inflamed and edematous and the abscess may rupture, producing a fistula.

Urethral strictures

Although rare in developed countries, urethral strictures and fistulae as late complications are common in tropical countries. Fibrous strictures develop from healing of areas of periurethral cellulitis or abscesses. Further periurethral abscesses may develop proximal to the area of stricture and their rupture to the exterior results in the formation of urinary fistulae. Fistulae, either single or multiple, are most commonly found in the perineum or scrotum.

Strictures usually develop many years after infection, but may be found within 5 years of the initial infection[90]. Symptoms of urinary obstruction include straining at micturition, poor force of the urine stream, and prolonged micturition with dribbling. Increased frequency of micturition occurs from incomplete emptying of the bladder or from cystitis. Urinary retention eventually develops and death can result from ascending urinary infection and renal failure.

Inflammation and abscess formation of the bulbourethral glands (Cowper's glands)

This complication is uncommon in countries with good medical services. The patient complains of fever, throbbing pain in the perineum, painful defecation, and frequency of micturition. Reflex spasm of the sphincter urethrae may produce acute retention of urine. An abscess, which is usually unilateral, may point in the perineum. The inflamed glands are palpable on rectal examination and are exquisitely tender.

Prostatitis and seminal vesiculitis

Acute gonococcal prostatitis and seminal vesiculitis are rare. There are usually constitutional disturbances, fever, perineal discomfort, urgency of micturition, hematuria, and painful erections. Occasionally acute retention of urine results from reflex spasm of the external sphincter of the bladder. A tender swollen gland is detected on rectal examination. With abscess formation, symptoms become more severe with painful defecation and suprapubic pain. Pyrexia becomes more pronounced. Rectal examination shows a large, tense swelling bulging into the rectum. The abscess may rupture into the urethra or rectum.

Chronic prostatitis, inflammation of the bulbourethral glands (Cowperitis), and chronic inflammation of the seminal vesicles may be found in long-standing infections, and can produce vague symptoms of inflammation such as urethral discharge in the morning and perineal discomfort. Palpation of the glands may show irregular thickening.

Epididymitis

This is usually unilateral, when the patient complains of a painful swollen testis. On examination there may be erythema of the scrotum on the affected side, the epididymis is enlarged and tender, and there is often a secondary hydrocele. Inflammation of the testis itself is rare.

Infection of the median raphe of the penis

This is rare, but when it occurs a bead of pus may be expressed from a duct opening

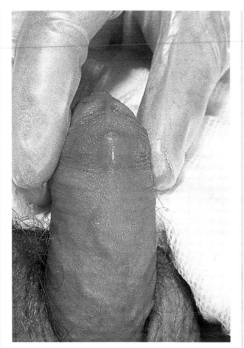

Figure 11.6 Gonococcal infection of the median raphe (reproduced from McMillan and Scott 2000[255])

on to the skin on the ventral surface of the penis (Figure 11.6).

CLINICAL FEATURES IN THE ADULT FEMALE (UNCOMPLICATED GONOCOCCAL INFECTION)

In most cases females with gonorrhea (70% or more) have few, if any symptoms. They may occasionally complain of increased

Table 11.2 Anatomical sites of infection by *Neisseria gonorrhoeae* in women with uncomplicated infection

Site affected	Frequency of infection at that site
Endocervix	85–90%
Urethra	65–75%
Anorectum	25–50%
Oropharynx	5–15%

vaginal discharge. Uncommonly, inflammation of the trigone of the bladder produces urinary frequency. The sites infected in the uncomplicated cases are shown in Table 11.2.

The affected cervix may appear normal on inspection, or there may be signs of inflammation with mucopus exuding from the cervical os (Figure 11.7). There may be no clinical evidence of urethritis but occasionally pus may be expressed from the orifice. Rectal gonorrhea in the female, as in the male, usually produces few symptoms. Oropharyngeal gonorrhea in the female results from fellatio and is usually asymptomatic.

Local complications in the female

Inflammation and abscess formation of the paraurethral glands, including those lying externally on either side of the external meatus (Skene's glands)

Abscess formation is not common, but involvement of these glands by the gonococcus is probably mostly present in urethral infection in the female.

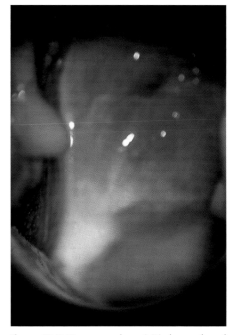

Figure 11.7 Gonococcal cervicitis (reproduced from McMillan and Scott 2000[255])

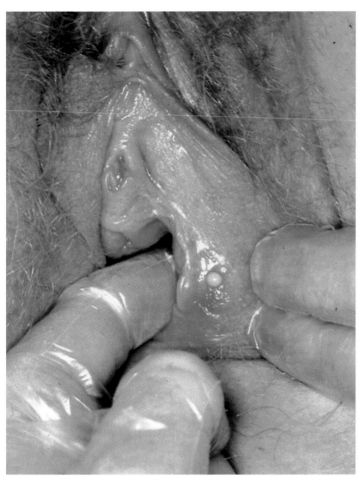

Figure 11.8 Gonococcal bartholinitis (reproduced with permission from Rein (ed.) 1996[254]).

Inflammation and abscess formation of the greater vestibular glands (Bartholinitis and Bartholin's abscess)

The glands may be involved on one or both sides. There may be few symptoms of Bartholinitis but, in the routine examination, on compressing the gland, pus may be expressed from the orifice of the duct (Figure 11.8). When an abscess forms, the patient may complain of pain in the vulva, and examination reveals a tender cystic swelling of the posterior half of the labium majus, the skin of which may be reddened (Figure 11.9). In less acute and partially treated cases, a chronic inflammation may result causing palpable thickening of the glands.

Pelvic inflammatory disease and salpingitis

These complications are considered in Chapter 12. The incidence of salpingitis in untreated cases is generally given as 10%.

DISSEMINATED GONOCOCCAL INFECTION AFFECTING BOTH SEXES

Disseminated gonococcal infection is an uncommon complication, occurring in less than 1% of cases, and is usually seen in women with asymptomatic anogenital infection. The female:male ratio of cases is about 1:4[91].

Arthritis and dermatitis

The clinical manifestations of disseminated gonococcal infection usually take the form of fever, rash, and arthralgia or arthritis. The spectrum of clinical features of this complication is fairly broad. It was considered previously that there was a bacteremic form of disseminated infection that, if untreated, progressed to septic joint. This is now discounted, as many individuals with gonococcal septic arthritis do not have a preceding illness suggestive of bacteremia,

spontaneous resolution of joint signs commonly occurs in those who present with fever, polyarthralgia, and dermatitis, and both modes of presentations can co-exist[92].

The clinical presentation in just under 50% of patients is that of a purulent arthritis, but in others, there is fever, rigors, joint pains with an asymmetrical, polyarticular arthritis involving usually the knees, wrists, small joints of the hands, ankles and elbows, without sufficient joint fluid to allow aspiration. If obtained, the fluid from joints from such patients is sterile on culture, but blood cultures are positive for *N. gonorrhoeae* in about one-third of patients[91] if taken within 2 days of onset of the illness. Nevertheless, *N. gonorrhoeae* DNA has been detected by PCR in synovial fluid from patients with disseminated infection[93] and it may be that the pathogenesis of this form of arthritis is similar to that associated with *Chlamydia trachomatis* (Chapter 14). There may be a tenosynovitis, affecting the hands and fingers, and, less commonly, tendons of the lower limbs.

About 90% of patients with non-suppurative arthritis have skin lesions, of which there are essentially two types[94]

1. hemorrhagic lesions
2. vesiculopapular lesions on an erythematous base.

Both types of lesion begin as erythematous macules, but in the hemorrhagic type the lesions become purpuric (Figure 11.10), especially on the palms and soles. In the second type lesions become papular and progress through vesicles to pustules. Generally resolution without scarring occurs in 4 to 5 days, but cropping may occur during febrile episodes. The lesions, often painful, have an asymmetrical distribution over the body, but generally sparing the head, and are particularly noticeable on the extremities and around affected joints. Histological examination of a skin lesion[95] shows a small vessel vasculitis in the dermis and subcutis and marked fibrinoid change. There is a perivascular infiltration of polymorphonuclear leukocytes and mononuclear cells. Degenerating polymorphs and evidence of hemorrhage are commonly seen. Although it can be difficult to culture *N. gonorrhoeae* from the skin lesions, organisms can be detected by direct immunofluorescence, for example Barr and Danielson[96] detected

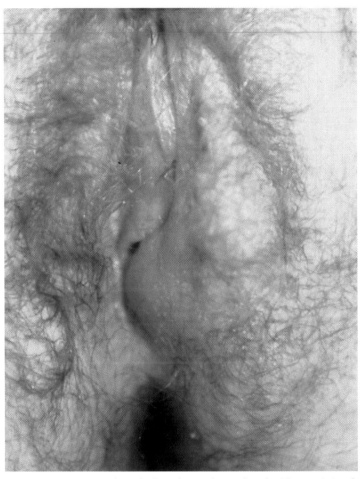

Figure 11.9 Gonococcal Bartholin's abscess (reproduced with permission from Rein (ed.) 1996[254])

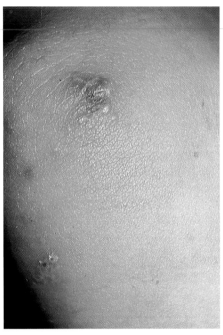

Figure 11.10 Disseminated gonococcal infection: purpuric lesions on elbow (reproduced from McMillan and Scott 2000[255])

gonococci in 14 of 16 cases of disseminated gonococcal infection. Erythema multiforme and erythema nodosum have also been described in patients with disseminated gonococcal infection.

Symptoms and signs of a septic joint may be the presenting feature in some patients (Figure 11.11). Usually a single large joint such as the knee is affected. Systemic features are usually milder than in patients who present as above, and skin lesions and tenosynovitis are less prevalent (about 40% and 20% of patients respectively). The affected joint is swollen, the overlying skin is red, and there is joint tenderness. The synovial fluid is turbid with a predominantly polymorphonuclear leukocyte exudate, and the glucose concentration is lower than normal. Culture of synovial fluid for *N. gonorrhoeae* yields positive results in less than 50% of cases and blood cultures are usually negative.

The differential diagnosis of arthritis caused by STIs is discussed in Chapter 14.

Meningitis, endocarditis, and pericarditis

Meningitis is an uncommon manifestation of disseminated gonococcal infection and is not usually found in association with arthritis and dermatitis[97].

Gonococcal endocarditis is also a rare but often fatal complication[98]. The degree of severity of the condition lies between the endocarditis due to *Staphylococcus aureus* and that due to oral streptococci. Most commonly the aortic valve is involved. Maculopapular skin lesions are common and appear in crops. Emboli to cerebral, renal, and peripheral arteries may occur[99].

Myocarditis and pericarditis may occur more commonly than hitherto recognized. Transient electrocardiographic abnormalities appear to be common in disseminated gonococcal infection[91]. Early referral in endocarditis for expert management by a cardiologist and cardiac surgeon is essential since deterioration may be rapid even when

there is an apparent response to antibiotic treatment.

Perihepatitis and hepatitis

Acute perihepatitis usually occurs in association with pelvic inflammatory disease in

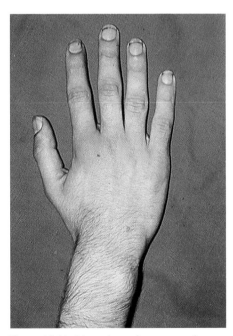

Figure 11.11 Disseminated gonococcal infection: septic joint (reproduced from McMillan and Scott 2000[255])

women, and a detailed account of the condition is found in Chapter 12. This complication is very rarely found in men. The patient complains of pain in the right hypochondrium and sometimes in the right shoulder from irritation of the right side of the diaphragm.

Hepatitis may occur following the bacteremia of disseminated gonococcal infection[91]. The hepatic histology is non-specific, there being scattered foci of mononuclear and polymorphonuclear leukocyte infiltrates in the parenchyma, with enlarged portal zones infiltrated with lymphocytes.

Diagnosis

As *N. gonorrhoeae* is not always isolated on culture of blood and synovial fluid, the diagnosis of disseminated gonococcal infection can be difficult. There may be non-specific abnormalities in the peripheral blood. Hematological tests may show an increase in the number of polymorphonuclear leukocytes: in one series 62% of 42 women had a white cell count that exceeded $10 \times 10^9/L$[91]. The erythrocyte sedimentation rate is elevated in most cases. Plasma enzyme tests of liver function are raised in about 50% of cases[91]. The diagnosis relies on the taking of a careful sexual history and obtaining material from the anogenital region and from the pharynx for microbiological examination for *N. gonorrhoeae* (see pp. 327–334).

GONOCOCCAL CONJUNCTIVITIS

This is rare except in the newborn and presents as a purulent conjunctivitis affecting one or both eyes. If untreated, keratitis or panophthalmitis with blindness may result.

GONORRHEA IN INFANTS AND CHILDREN UNDER THE AGE OF PUBERTY

Gonococcal ophthalmia neonatorum

This is a conjunctivitis with a purulent discharge in an infant, that appears within 21 days of birth and is a notifiable disease in the UK. Ophthalmia neonatorum was formerly caused chiefly by *N. gonorrhoeae*,

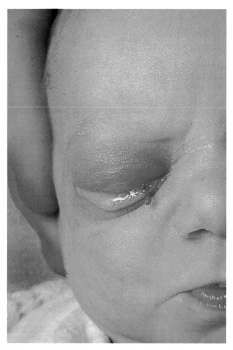

Figure 11.12 Gonococcal ophthalmia neonatorum (reproduced from McMillan and Scott 2000[255])

but is now more commonly caused by other organisms, including *C. trachomatis*. Gonococcal ophthalmia usually manifests itself within 48 hours of birth but it may be delayed for as long as a week and, if untreated, has dangerous consequences. The eyelids swell and pus collects in the conjunctival sac (Figure 11.12). Keratitis with corneal scarring may result if the condition is not treated.

Disseminated gonococcal infection

Septic arthritis is a rare complication of neonatal gonorrhea. It usually presents from 7 to 28 days after delivery. Multiple joints are affected, the infant refusing to move the involved limb[101]. Temperature instability and other features of neonatal sepsis* are common, and indeed these may

---

* Signs and symptoms of sepsis in the newborn are often non-specific. The most common symptoms are lethargy, poor feeding, and abdominal distention. There is prolonged capillary filling time resulting from hypotension, hepatic and splenic enlargement, abnormal neurological reflexes, petechiae or purpura, persistent acidosis, and glucose intolerance.

be the sole manifestations of disseminated gonococcal infection[101]. Meningitis may also be a complication.

Other features of gonorrhea in the neonate

Vaginitis, urethritis, and proctitis caused by *N. gonorrhoeae* have been reported in neonates born to infected mothers, and scalp abscesses complicating the use of scalp electrodes for fetal monitoring have been described[102].

Acute vulvovaginitis

This is uncommon in the UK nowadays. The parents usually notice discharge on the child's underwear and on examination a purulent vaginal discharge, with reddening and edema of the vulva, may be found (Figure 11.13). Other causes of vulvovaginitis include

1. hypersensitivity to detergents, bath foam, etc.
2. threadworm infestation
3. foreign body in the vagina
4. chlamydial infection
5. *Trichomonas vaginalis*
6. candidal infection
7. other, non-sexually transmitted bacteria such as *Staphylococcus aureus*.

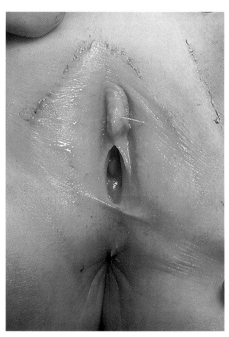

Figure 11.13 Gonococcal vulvovaginitis (reproduced from McMillan and Scott 2000[255])

Urethral gonorrhea

Urethral gonorrhea in the prepubescent boy is rare, but is usually the result of sexual abuse. The symptoms and signs are the same as those found in the adult male.

Oropharyngeal and rectal infection

Workers in the USA have described the occurrence of gonorrhea in these sites in a number of children[103].

Diagnosis

Microbiological tests are mandatory in making a diagnosis of gonorrhea. Because of the short incubation period and high infectivity, rapid diagnosis followed by immediate treatment and contact-tracing are important in the control of infection within the community.

Neisseria gonorrhoeae is a very fastidious organism and very careful techniques are necessary for the collection of specimens and their transport to the laboratory for culture and investigation. Ideally the patient is seen at a clinic with an adjacent or closely sited laboratory. Under these conditions the majority of infected patients (about 90% to 95% of males and 50% to 60% of females) can receive appropriate effective treatment on the first attendance after examination of Gram-stained smears. Cultural diagnosis of additional cases and confirmation of smear-positive cases can be made within 24 to 72 hours.

SPECIMENS REQUIRED FOR BACTERIOLOGICAL EXAMINATION
Specimens from males

In males, material for examination is obtained by inserting a sterile bacteriological loop into the everted urethral meatus and gently scraping the walls of the terminal part of the urethra. A loopful or less of the exudate obtained may be examined by microscopy of a Gram-stained smear and by culture. If recent anal intercourse is acknowledged or suspected a cotton wool-tipped applicator stick should be passed gently and blindly into the anal canal to a distance of 5 cm; a proctoscope should be passed and if mucopus is seen it may be examined microscopically and by culture. Direct microscopy of rectal material is often unhelpful as there are large numbers of other organisms in this site, and interpretation of a Gram-stained smear may be difficult. If there has been orogenital contact with a person who may possibly have been infected, material should be obtained for culture from the tonsillar crypts or bed and pharynx. Ideally, in every case of gonorrhea or in known contacts, it is wise to take this test without seeking details of sexual practice, which patients may be reluctant to discuss.

If the patient is known to have had sexual intercourse with an infected partner and he has no obvious signs of urethritis, it is often helpful to re-examine him when he has held his urine for several hours, preferably overnight. Any exudate which may have collected may then be massaged to the urethral orifice and examined by microscopy and culture. Even in the absence of an obvious discharge, specimens for culture should be obtained by gently scraping the urethral walls with a bacteriological loop. Occasionally examination of prostatic fluid may detect an asymptomatic infection.

Normally a single examination is sufficient to diagnose or exclude urethral gonorrhea in men. If rectal or pharyngeal infection are suspected, however, cultures should be repeated if the first tests are negative.

Specimens from females

In female patients specimens for cultural investigation should be taken from the urethra (traditionally specimens are taken from the urethra after massaging from above downwards to expel any discharge from the paraurethral glands), cervix (external cervical os and cervical canal), rectum, and throat. If pus is expressed from the orifice(s) of the ducts of the greater vestibular glands, this should be similarly examined. Smears should be taken from the urethra and endocervix for microscopic examination after Gram-staining. If the first set of culture tests is negative the tests should be repeated 1 week later before reassuring the patient that she does not have gonorrhea. A third set of tests is a justified additional precaution in the case of contacts of gonorrhea who have given two negative cultures. The use of non-selective medium should be considered for second and third tests in gonorrhea contacts.

TESTS IN DISSEMINATED GONOCOCCAL INFECTION

When disseminated gonococcal infection is suspected, the routine tests described and several blood cultures should be taken before commencing therapy. As procedures in routine blood culture may not be optimal for the gonococcus it is most important to inform the laboratory that disseminated gonococcal infection is a possible diagnosis. Although patients with suspected disseminated gonococcal infection may have no genital symptoms it is important to take anogenital (and pharyngeal) cultures as these are most likely to yield gonococci[96]. Skin lesions should be punctured with a sterile lancet and tissue fluid expressed[104] for culture and/or microscopy by specific immunofluoresence or Gram-staining; the latter will not distinguish between gonococci and meningococci. Fluid obtained by aspiration of a joint effusion should be examined by culture. For these investigations a non-selective medium should be employed in parallel with a selective medium containing lincomycin rather than vancomycin. The sensitivity of culture and microscopy is poor for detecting gonococci in skin lesions and joint fluids. Recently introduced molecular tests such as PCR or LCR are now the methods of choice for detecting gonococci in such specimens[105].

IMPORTANCE OF CULTURE SITE AND NUMBER OF DIAGNOSTIC TESTS

Repeated testing of multiple sites is necessary since not all infections in women will be detected on first attendance. The proportion of infected women detected at their first attendance has been variously reported as 66%[106], 90%[107] 91%[66] and 98%[108]. Provided that the microbiological service consistently reaches a high standard, only two sets of investigations need to be taken to diagnose or exclude gonorrhea in women[65, 108]. It is prudent, however, to carry out a third set of tests in the case of gonorrhea contacts.

The efficiency of detecting gonorrhea varies depending on factors such as the culture medium used. For example, a single endocervical culture detected 90% of infections when Modified New York City (MNYC) medium was used but only 78% when conventional Thayer–Martin (TM) medium was used[108]. A figure as low as 40% has been reported[109]. In terms of a screening schedule more infections are detected by testing additional sites at the first attendance than by re-screening by endocervical culture[108].

A 'high vaginal swab' is totally inadequate for diagnosing or excluding gonorrhea and if this is the only specimen taken, one in three infected women is likely to be missed[110]. The poor results with vaginal specimens are to be expected since this material detects only gonococci which may have contaminated the area, particularly from the cervix, a site of infection where gonococci are actively multiplying.

Rectal cultures are important in the female: approximately 25% to 50% of patients have anorectal involvement, and 5% to 10% may be positive only in this site[77]. Since rectal infection is usually asymptomatic, and may be an important cause of treatment failure, rectal cultures are essential in screening for infection and assessing effectiveness of treatment.

In males who may have acquired their infection through homosexual contact it is important to obtain screening cultures from all sites that might possibly be infected, regardless of the symptoms. For example, in a series of 278 homosexual men with gonorrhea[111] the urethra was infected in 61%, the anorectum in 41%, and the throat in 8%. This study also stressed the importance of repeat testing in diagnosing rectal and pharyngeal infection: by relying on only one set of tests 7% of patients with rectal gonorrhea and 26% of patients with pharyngeal gonorrhea would have been missed. Detection of rectal and pharyngeal gonorrhea in homosexual men is particularly important. Because the bio-

logical properties of gonococci associated with homosexually acquired infection tend to make them more resistant, treatment of rectal and pharyngeal gonorrhea in homosexual men requires higher penicillin dosage than does urethral infection or anogenital infection in women. Heterosexual men and women with pharyngeal gonorrhea also require higher penicillin dosage than those with uncomplicated infection. Pharyngeal infection may be much more common than previously considered: in 1991 the pharynx was infected in 56% of homosexual men, 17% of heterosexual men, and 31% of women with gonorrhea[112]. In all patients it is important to know which sites are infected in order to ensure appropriate therapy, to trace all contacts, and to ensure eradication of gonococci after treatment by sampling all infected sites.

MICROSCOPY

This is important as it enables a presumptive diagnosis to be made in the clinic so that appropriate treatment can be given immediately. Immediate treatment facilitates the prevention of spread of infection and progression of the disease to its more serious sequelae, particularly in those patients likely to default.

The Gram-stained smear

A smear of secretion or discharge is prepared and Gram-stained by standard bacteriological technique, but 0.1% neutral red is the preferred counterstain[113]. The stained and dried slide is examined under a 2 mm oil-immersion objective lens. A typical positive Gram-stained smear of urethral discharge from a male patient with gonorrhea usually shows a large number of characteristic kidney-shaped Gram-negative diplococci (GNDC) lying within the polymorphonuclear leukocytes with few extracellular organisms (Figure 11.14). If pleomorphic extracellular Gram-negative diplococci and bacilli with rare extracellular GNDC with morphology typical of *N. gonorrhoeae* are seen, the result of the smear examination is equivocal and not diagnostic. If no GNDC are seen the smear result is reported as negative.

Results in males

In patients whose Gram-stained smears of urethral discharge are unequivocally positive or negative this technique provides an immediate differential diagnosis between gonococcal and non-gonococcal urethritis in 85% of patients[114]. When the Gram-stained smear shows typical intracellular GNDC the culture is positive in over 95% of cases. Similarly, when the smear is unequivocally negative, the culture is also negative in over 95% of cases. In general, the sensitivity of Gram-staining urethral smears from symptomatic men ranges from 83% to 96% and the specificity from 95% to 99%[115]. The majority of false positive smears result from organisms, other than the pathogenic neisseriae, which fail to grow on selective medium. Very occasionally, however, usually in less than 0.1% of typical positive smears, the GNDC are shown to be meningococci on culture.

A diagnosis should not be made on the basis of equivocal results. As a general rule, Gram-staining is less reliable in the diagnosis of long-standing or asymptomatic infections or when the microscopist is inexperienced. Goodhart et al.[115] found that the probability of gonorrhea in men whose smears were reported as containing intracellular GNDC dropped from 94.8% to 53.9% when an inexperienced technician interpreted smears from patients with urethritis. The probability of gonorrhea in patients without symptoms whose smears were reported positive by an experienced observer was only 34.9%. This poor predictive value results from the low prevalence (2%) of gonorrhea in the population of men without symptoms. Because of the

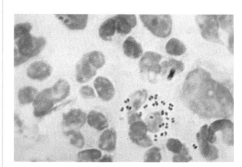

Figure 11.14 Gram-negative diplococci in polymorphonuclear leukocytes (reproduced from McMillan and Scott 2000[255])

complexity of the gut flora, rectal smears are only of value if pus or mucopus can be collected by proctoscopy. Gram-staining has no place in the diagnosis of pharyngeal infection.

Results in females

The sensitivity of Gram-staining of cervical smears ranges from 23% to 65% and the specificity from 88% to 100%[115]. According to Barlow and Phillips[116] and Thin and Shaw[117], Gram-staining of urethral smears made no significant difference to the diagnosis of gonorrhea in women. Rectal smears are not examined microscopically as a routine in the female patient.

In asymptomatic infection, which is common in women, the number of gonococci are less than in the male. The bacterial flora of the female genitourinary tract, also, is both qualitatively and quantitatively greater than in the male. Many of these organisms are small Gram-negative cocci and coccobacilli, sometimes appearing in pairs, and occasionally intracellularly, making interpretation of the smear difficult. When extracellular GNDC were considered as positive the sensitivity of Gram-staining increased from 31% to 51%, while the specificity decreased from 99% to 86%[115].

Comparing smear and culture results is an essential part of the quality control of gonorrhea diagnosis. In a small percentage of both male and female patients typical positive smear results will be obtained but gonococci will not be isolated on culture. This could arise when patients have taken an antibiotic before coming to the clinic, or it could be because the particular strain of gonococcus has a pronounced sensitivity to vancomycin, one of the antibiotics used in certain selective media: vancomycin sensitivity may vary from 2%[118] to as high as 30%[119]. If the proportion of patients giving positive smears but negative cultures is high, or increases, the culture procedures should be re-evaluated. For example when TM medium containing vancomycin was compared with MNYC medium containing lincomycin, 19% of infections in women gave positive smears but negative cultures using TM medium compared with 0%

when MNYC medium was used: the corresponding figures for men were 17% (TM medium) and 4% (MNYC medium)[108].

Lack of experience at interpreting smears may contribute to an unacceptably low proportion of women being detected and treated at their first visit to the clinic.

The decrease in prevalence of gonorrhea in the UK during the 1980s and early 90s has made it more difficult to ensure adequate experience for those involved in interpreting Gram-stained smears. A recent audit reported the sensitivity of Gram staining in women was 70% in 1971 when there were 441 cases of gonorrhea but had dropped to 29% in 1997 when there were only 70 cases[120]. Another study, however, reported no significant fall in sensitivity of Gram staining in women between 1993 when 66.7% (6/9) were positive compared with 1976 when 74.7% (65/77) were positive[121].

Simplified staining procedures

Attempts have been made to shorten the time taken for staining of genital smears by using single stains such as methylene blue or safranin, or a single reagent such as methyl green-pyronin. The time saved in staining with a single stain is lost by making the screening of smears much more difficult: the rapid exclusion of Gram-positive organisms saves more technician time than does shortening of the staining procedure[122].

Immunofluorescence staining

Monoclonal antibody reagents using antibodies against PI have replaced polyclonal antibody reagents for the direct fluorescent antibody staining of secretions direct from the patient. However, in view of the technical difficulties of immunofluorescence as a rapid on-the-spot test, costs, and lack of significantly increased diagnostic gain over the Gram film, the method is not widely used[104].

CULTURE

Immediate diagnosis must be supplemented as well as confirmed by culture if the maxi-

mum number of positive results is to be obtained. Cultures are obligatory in the diagnosis of rectal, oral, disseminated, and asymptomatic infections in both sexes, and are also essential in order to determine antibiotic sensitivities and to assess treatment efficiency. Cultures are also essential for medico-legal purposes.

Culture media

There are many variations of media in use but all contain a rich nutrient base supplemented with blood, either partially lysed by heat ('chocolate' agar) or completely lysed by the chemical saponin. Most laboratories now use one of the following selective media or their modifications.

Thayer–Martin (TM) selective medium

In comparison with a non-selective medium the selective medium of Thayer and Martin, formulated to allow growth only of gonococci and meningococci, increases the proportion of positive isolations from all sites. It is particularly valuable in isolating the gonococcus from heavily contaminated sites such as the rectum or pharynx. The antibiotics (vancomycin, colistin, and nystatin) present in the medium prevent other flora in the sample from overgrowing any gonococci present. *Proteus* species are resistant to these antibiotics, and occasionally their spreading growth completely covers a culture plate: trimethoprim added to the medium can inhibit the growth of *Proteus* species[123]. Although gonococci are sensitive to the sequential action of sulfamethoxazole and trimethoprim when combined in co-trimoxazole, they are much more resistant to trimethoprim alone than are most other bacteria.

Although widely used in many laboratories, TM medium has been criticized because a proportion of gonococcal strains are inhibited by vancomycin; growth is slow; and colonies are small on TM medium. Superior isolation of gonococci and complete inhibition of *Proteus* was achieved with a modified TM medium[124] which differs from TM medium in containing double the concentration of agar (2.0%), glucose (0.25%), and trimethoprim (5.0 mg/mL).

Modified TM medium does not overcome the problems of vancomycin sensitivity. Vancomycin sensitivity is not distributed evenly within the gonococcal population and certain strains, for example auxotype AHU, are much more sensitive than others[118]. The relative frequency of these auxotypes could account, in part, for the variations in the percentage of vancomycin sensitive strains which has been reported to be as high as 30%[119].

Martin–Lewis medium

This medium is similar to modified TM medium but contains anisomycin in place of nystatin to inhibit yeasts[125]. Anisomycin is more stable than nystatin, a property considered useful in providing commercially prepared selective media with a longer shelf life.

Modified New York City (MNYC) medium

This simply prepared modification of the original New York City (NYC) medium devised by Faur *et al.*[126], to provide a luxuriant growth of pathogenic neisseriae after incubation for 24 hours contains lincomycin, colistin, amphotericin and trimethoprim: lincomycin is less inhibitory to gonococci than vancomycin while amphotericin is more inhibitory to yeasts than nystatin. Modified New York City medium is also enriched with yeast dialysate and glucose so that growth is more rapid and the colonies are larger. In comparison with TM medium, MNYC medium improves the overall isolation rate and enables a larger percentage of isolates to be identified at 24 hours[127].

Others have also noted an improvement in culture results with MNYC medium and adopted it for routine use[128, 129]. As lincomycin is less inhibitory than vancomycin, it is important to examine cultures after 24 hours of incubation. If rectal cultures are not examined until 48 hours of incubation, contaminants could mask small numbers of gonococcal colonies. Lawton and Koch[130] compared commercially available NYC and Martin–Lewis media and found NYC medium to be much superior.

Although most laboratories now purchase commercially prepared media rather than prepare it themselves there is a lack of comparative performance data for commercial media. In a study comparing fourteen commercially prepared selective media none performed as well overall as the 'in-house' medium[131]. Only two of the commercial media supported the growth of all 105 gonococcal isolates but both these media were less effective than the 'in-house' medium in inhibiting non-pathogenic neisseriae and miscellaneous organisms. Failure to grow gonococci was significantly associated with

- serovar 1A isolates
- AHU auxotype
- the presence of vancomycin rather than lincomycin.

The use of 10% blood rather than 5% was also important in supporting the growth of all gonococci. Too many commercial media perform inadequately, probably because of a combination of factors including the level of nutrition, inappropriate choice of antibiotic supplements, and a shelf life that is too long.

Combination of a selective and non-selective medium

The combination of a selective and non-selective medium has been recommended to ensure the detection of gonococci with markedly increased susceptibility to antibiotics (*Env* mutants) as well as vancomycin-sensitive gonococci. Although this may be theoretically desirable it is too time consuming, technically demanding, and not cost-effective[132]. A more practical approach is to use lincomycin in place of vancomycin in selective media. In addition a non-selective medium can be included in the subsequent examination of contacts of infected patients if their initial tests were negative. A non-selective medium can always be used in sampling sites such as joint fluid or blood that are normally sterile. If non-selective media are used it is important that they are properly quality controlled to ensure their ability to culture clinical isolates of gonococci.

Transport and culture systems

As the gonococcus is very susceptible to drying, dry swabs should never be used. Best results are achieved by direct plating. Culture plates, preferably warmed beforehand to 37°C, are inoculated directly with patient's secretions and immediately incubated at 36° to 37°C in a moist atmosphere containing 5% to 10% carbon dioxide.

Culture plates should be date stamped and stored in the refrigerator at the clinic. Ratner *et al.*[133] showed that there was no significant difference in the isolation rate of *N. gonorrhoeae* on plates inoculated straight from the refrigerator and on those warmed to room temperature. After 24 hours incubation, however, gonococcal colonies tended to be larger and more numerous on the room temperature plates. As most identification methods for use with primary cultures work best with young, 18 to 24-hour cultures, rapid growth is an important advantage of pre-warming plates to 37°C.

The most suitable transport and culture system must be related to constraints imposed in individual localities. In general, direct plating is the system that most consistently produces the best results for specimens from all sites. One of the major problems in direct plating is ensuring the availability and appropriate storage (refrigeration) of medium with a short shelf life (normally a few weeks) at the point of use. Recently a new method of packaging medium has been developed which permits the storage of the medium for up to 1 year at room temperature and has a self-contained system for production of carbon dioxide. The plates consist of a rectangular tray with an inner well containing chocolate blood agar medium with antibiotics. A bonded seal over the well prevents evaporation and oxidation during storage[134]. Further evaluations are required with different media and selective antibiotics to determine the true utility of this development.

When direct plating and immediate incubation are impracticable conventional non-nutrient transport media or a nutrient transport and culture system should be used.

The simple non-nutrient transport media are cheap and easy to use. Amies medium is more effective than Stuart's at maintaining gonococcal viability[135]. Other advantages of Amies medium include the addition of charcoal to neutralize toxic ions produced by irradiation of commercial swab sticks, cotton wool, agar, and the by products of bacterial metabolism. Contamination is less of a problem with Amies medium, which includes an inorganic phosphate buffer rather than glycerol phosphate: the latter acts as an energy source and supports the growth of bacterial contaminants. Recently Amies medium has been included in the Copan transport swab system. An important feature of this system is a plastic-laminated film pouch that is flushed with nitrogen gas to expel atmospheric air. Swabs are placed into agar gel in a polypropylene tube that contains active scavenging agents that neutralize oxygen, superoxide, and free radicals[136]. The use of these agents may obviate the need for charcoal which may interfere with the interpretation of Gram-stained smears. The Copan system without charcoal performed as well as direct plating when transport time did not exceed 6 hours. Transport media are not recommended for overnight transit: transport for 24 and 48 hours can reduce the isolation rate by as much as 40% and 63% respectively[137].

Transport-cum-culture systems are also available but have not been widely used. These systems comprise a selective medium usually present in a small chamber containing carbon dioxide, for example Transgrow[138] or a carbon dioxide-generating system, for example JEMBEC[139]. These nutrient transport and culture systems are expensive and seem to offer little advantage when the transit time is less than 6 hours. When more prolonged transport is anticipated it may be best to use a transport growth system and to incubate it overnight in the clinic prior to sending to the laboratory.

Identification

After 24 hours of incubation, plates are examined and any colonies suspected as being gonococcal are tested by the cytochrome oxidase test and if positive by Gram staining. Negative cultures are incubated for a further 24 hours and the plate re-examined before the culture can be reported as negative.

Presumptive identification (oxidase positive Gram-negative diplococci)

The cytochrome oxidase test

This is a useful screening test since all neisseriae are oxidase positive, whereas many other organisms such as coliforms, staphylococci, and lactobacilli are negative. The test is conveniently carried out by touching the colony with a cotton swab soaked in a 1% (w/v) solution of tetramethyl-p-phenylenediamine dihydrochloride. A positive reaction is indicated by the colony turning purple within 5 to 15 seconds. This technique is so simple and quick that, when using a selective medium, virtually all colonies can be tested, thus minimizing the risk of missing gonococci because of an atypical colonial appearance. Colonies with the same morphology must be examined by Gram-staining since other organisms, for example *Kingella*, *Moraxella*, and *Haemophilus* spp. are also oxidase-positive.

Gram-stained smear from colony

The various members of the genus *Neisseria* are indistinguishable by microscopy: all appear as Gram-negative cocci, usually in pairs but sometimes in clumps or singly. A presumptive diagnosis of gonorrhea made on the basis of oxidase-positive GNDC growing on selective medium is approximately 99.5% accurate for urethral specimens from men and anogenital specimens from women. Smeltzer et al.[140] found presumptive diagnosis 98.5% accurate for endocervical specimens from a low prevalence population. Whilst this may be acceptable under certain circumstances, whenever resources allow further identification should be undertaken to provide a definitive diagnosis. Presumptive diagnosis is less reliable for rectal and urethral cultures from homosexual men as approximately 5% to 10% and 1% to 2% respectively of GNDC will be meningococci. As the vast majority of GNDC isolated from the throat are meningococci, presumptive diagnosis is inappropriate for this site.

Definitive diagnosis (a biochemical and an immunological test)

A definitive diagnosis has traditionally been made by carbohydrate utilization tests although one of a number of new biochemical tests for the identification of *Neisseria* species are often used nowadays. Immunological identification using reagents based on monoclonal antibodies should be performed in parallel with biochemical identification. Parallel testing will prevent misidentification because of an erroneous reaction in either type of test.

Carbohydrate utilization tests

These tests are based on the ability of *Neisseria* species to utilize various sugars. As neisseriae metabolize sugars oxidatively the term 'fermentation test', although widely used, is inaccurate. Gonococci produce acid from glucose only, whereas meningococci produce acid from glucose and maltose. *N. lactamica*, an organism found mainly in the throat, grows readily on selective media with a colonial morphology similar to the meningococcus. It utilizes lactose in addition to glucose and maltose. Commensal neisseriae do not normally grow on selective media but can usually be differentiated by their ability to utilize glucose and maltose, usually in combination with sucrose and/or fructose[141]. The exception is *N. cinerea* which is asaccharolytic in most sugar utilization tests. *Branhamella catarrhalis* (previously *N. catarrhalis*) is always asaccharolytic. Carbohydrate utilization tests are basically of two types, conventional and rapid.

Conventional tests for carbohydrate utilization

In conventional tests for carbohydrate utilization, a solid medium containing the appropriate carbohydrate and pH indicator is inoculated with the test organism. Although widely used, these tests are unsuitable since a positive reaction is dependent on adequate growth of the test organism which may take up to 72 hours. The main problem with these tests is finding a suitable medium to support the growth of all strains of gonococci while at the same time giving reproducible and clear-cut indicator changes.

Failure to support gonococcal growth is a significant problem with the commercially available cystine trypticase agar (CTA) system. Inconclusive results and other problems with CTA medium accounted for

44% of 141 gonococcal cultures sent to Centers for Disease Control and Prevention Atlanta for confirmation[142]. The poor performance of CTA medium has led to the acceptance of 'glucose-negative' gonococci, a concept which may cause diagnostic problems. Knapp *et al.*[143] described an asaccharolytic diplococcus which was isolated from the cervix of a patient with arthritis. The isolate was presumptively identified as a glucose negative gonococcus but was later identified as *Neisseria cinerea*.

Certain meningococci fail to give a positive reaction with maltose in the CTA system[144]. Colonization with 'maltose-negative' meningococci has been mis-diagnosed as pharyngeal gonorrhea[145].

Rapid carbohydrate utilization test (RCUT)

In the RCUT, pre-formed enzyme is measured by adding a suspension of the overnight growth of the suspect organism to a buffered, non-nutrient solution containing the sugar to be tested and a pH indicator[146]. Apart from rapidity, enabling identification of other neisseriae and confirmation of *N. gonorrhoeae* to be made within 24 to 72 hours of seeing the patient, the RCUT, in measuring pre-formed enzyme, has the advantage of being independent of growth. Results of the RCUT are usually available after 1 to 3 hours incubation at 37°C.

Provided that the test reagents are properly quality controlled and suspensions are prepared with young 18 to 24 hour cultures grown on media containing glucose, RCUT methods are more accurate than conventional tests[147].

RCUT methods have the additional advantage that isolates can be characterized, including detection of penicillinase, from the primary isolation plate[108]. Considerable saving in time and reagents can be made by performing the test in microtiter plates. Plates containing reagents can be prepared in batches and stored at −20°C for several months. Commercially available adaptations of the RCUT method include the Minitek system (BBL Microbiology Systems, Cockeys-yule, MD) and the Neisseria Kwik test (MicroBioLogics, St Cloud, MN).

Biochemical identification systems

Examples of these include the RapID NH System (Innovative Diagnostic Systems Inc., Atlanta, GA) and Gonocheck (E-Y Laboratories, San Mateo, CA), and the apiNH system (bioMerieux, Marcy-l'Etoile, France).

The RapID NH System is a 4-hour test designed to differentiate *Neisseria* spp., *Branhamella*, *Moraxella*, and *Haemophilus* spp. and is based on both sugar utilization tests and single-substrate chromogenic biochemical tests.

The Gonocheck test is designed to differentiate *N. gonorrhoeae*, *N. meningitidis*, *N. lactamica*, and *B. catarrhalis*. It is based upon the degradation of three substrates contained in one tube. The enzymes produced by *N. gonorrhoeae*, *N. meningitidis*, and *N. lactamica* are proline aminopeptidase, gamma-glutamylamino peptidase and beta-galactosidase respectively. *Branhamella catarrhalis* does not produce any of these enzymes.

The apiNH system employs a battery of thirteen tests including a range of chromogenic substrates and acidification resulting from utilization of a range of carbohydrates. *Neisseria gonorrhoeae* and a range of other bacteria can be identified by a numeric code computed from the results of the various groups of tests.

There is a lack of recent publications comparing the various identification systems although earlier studies suggest that certain of the tests may fail to differentiate between *N. gonorrhoeae* and *N. cinerea* and may occasionally mis-identify meningococci as gonococci[148].

IMMUNOLOGICAL IDENTIFICATION

Immunological confirmation of the identity of gonococci can be obtained rapidly and with very small amounts of bacterial growth. The development of reagents based on pools of monoclonal antibodies make these highly specific and sensitive tests. Two of the most widely used tests are the Phadebact® Monoclonal GC test (Boule Diagnostics AB, Huddinge, Sweden) and the MicroTrak test (originally marketed by Syva Co, Palo Alto, CA).

The Phadebact Monoclonal GC test is a very simple and rapid coagglutination (CoA) test. Coagglutination involves the attachment of anti-gonococcal IgG, by its Fc portion, to protein A on whole killed cells of *Staphylococcus aureus*. The test kit contains two separate reagents, WI and WII/WIII prepared with different pools of monoclonal antibodies reactive with epitopes on P1A and P1B respectively. When a boiled suspension made from a few suspect gonococcal colonies is mixed with each reagent, if epitopes of either P1A or P1B are present they will react with the antibody binding site on the specific IgG attached to the staphylococci and result in agglutination that is visible to the naked eye. A significantly stronger reaction in either the WI or WII/WIII reagents constitutes a positive result. The test is 100% specific and has a sensitivity in excess of 99.7%; false negative reactions are associated with gonococci belonging to the extremely rare serovar (1B17)[149, 150]. Further false negative reactions have not been reported.

The Syva MicroTrak test is a direct immunofluorescence test in which a pool of monoclonal antibodies conjugated to fluorescein isothiocyanate is used to stain a smear of suspect gonococci on a slide. It is technically more complex, time consuming, and subjective than CoA. Although initially considered to be of high sensitivity, false negative reactions have ranged from 4.6%[151] to 20%[152] and have involved several phenotypes of gonococci.

SUPPLEMENTARY IDENTIFICATION TESTS

The superoxol test

This is essentially a catalase test performed with 20% to 30% hydrogen peroxide in place of 3%, as used in the conventional method. A positive superoxol test is of limited diagnostic value as a considerable number of meningococci, other neisseriae and *B. catarrhalis* give a positive reaction[153]. On the other hand, a negative superoxol test result is a very simple and reliable method of excluding the gonococcus as 99.8% of gonococci are superoxol positive. Odugbemi and Arko[154, 142] found a negative superoxol test valuable in differentiating *Kingella denitrificans* from *N. gonorrhoeae*. *Kingella denitrificans* is oxidase positive and has a colonial morphology similar to that of the gonococcus. On Gram staining it may appear coccoid or short-rod shaped and be difficult to differentiate from neisseriae.

AccuProbe

The AccuProbe culture identification test for *N. gonorrhoeae* (Gen-Probe Inc, San Diego, CA) uses a chemiluminescent single-stranded DNA probe that is complementary to gonococcal rRNA. Test bacteria are lysed to release the rRNA which in the case of gonococci combines with the DNA to form a stable DNA-RNA hybrid. The labeled hybrids are detected using a luminometer. This test gave 100% sensitivity and specificity[155].

NON-CULTURAL DIAGNOSIS

The non-cultural diagnosis of gonorrhea is based upon the detection of gonococcal components in secretions. The need for non-cultural diagnosis is evident from the number of clinics that have to rely on culture results from specimens that have been transported, sometimes for prolonged periods. Non-cultural methods are particularly suited to large centralized laboratories serving peripheral populations, and have potential value in large-scale screening programs. Although several methods were investigated in the 1970s and 80s[148] none were sufficiently reliable to make an impact on diagnosis. Recently a variety of molecular detection methods have been developed; these are already widely used in the detection of chlamydia infection.

Ligase chain reaction (LCR)

The LCR for detection of gonococci is based on a target sequence of the *opa* gene. In an evaluation of 200 men the overall prevalence of gonococcal infection was 24.5%: 96% (47 of 49) were identified by culture, 100% by LCR of urethral specimens, and 98% (48 of 49) by LCR of first voided urine (FVU) – all LCR positive culture negative specimens were confirmed by a second LCR using target sequences based on the pilin gene[156]. The prevalence of infection in 125 women was 15.2%: 63.2% (12 of 19) were detected by urethral culture, 84.2% (16 of 19) by urethral LCR and 94.7% (18 of 19) by LCR of FVU, 84.2% (16 of 19) by endocervical culture and 89.5% (17 of 19) by endocervical LCR. All samples gave an LCR specificity of 100% apart from the endocervical LCR (99.1%)[156]. In a population with a prevalence of 16.8% (52 of 309). LCR testing of vaginal swabs (taken by patients themselves after demonstration) was 100% sensitive and 99.6% (256 of 257) specific compared with a sensitivity of 84.6% (44 of 52) for both cervical LCR and culture[156a]. In this study three vaginal swabs were taken before endocervical specimens were taken for endocervical LCR testing and cervical culture on modified TM medium. In a study by Buimer *et al.*[156b] the prevalence of gonorrhea was 5.9% (13 of 220) by culture for men and 2.9% (11 of 383) for women. The corresponding values were 8.2% (18 of 220) and 5.5% (21 of 383) respectively, by LCR testing of urethral and cervical swabs. Prevalence values by LCR testing of urine were 7.3% (16 of 220) for men and 2.9% (11 of 383) for women. The sensitivity of culture on modified TM medium was 72.2% (13 of 180) for men and 50% (11 of 220) for women. The sensitivities of LCR were 100% (18 of 18) with male urethral swabs, 95.4% (21 of 22) with cervical swabs, 88.9% (16 of 18) with male urine, and 50.0% (11 of 22) with female urine. The specificity of LCR was 100% for all specimen types. Others have confirmed the high specificity of LCR: 100% for endocervical and female urine specimens, 100% for male urethral swabs, and 99.6% for male urine specimens[157]. In this study LCR on urethral swabs from men gave higher sensitivity than LCR on urine (100% and 94.7% respectively) while the LCR on endocervical swabs and urine from women were the same (91.7%). A small proportion of urine specimens may give false negative results because of inhibition of amplification; inhibition may be overcome by freezing and thawing the urine before testing.

Ligase chain reaction and extragenital infection

A preliminary study demonstrated the potential value of LCR in detecting rectal and pharyngeal infection in gay men. Rectal and throat LCR both gave a sensitivity of 100% compared to direct plating on MNYC medium which gave a sensitivity of 52.9% and 46.9%[158]. Further studies on the detection of extragenital infection by molecular tests are required.

Polymerase chain reaction (PCR)

The Amplicor PCR assay (Roche Molecular Systems, Branchburg, NJ) uses primers based on the gonococcal cytosine methyltransferase gene. In a study involving STI clinic patients the sensitivities of urethral culture on modified TM medium, urethral PCR, and urine PCR were 76.6%, 97.3% and 94.4% respectively for male patients; corresponding specificities were 100%, 97%, and 98.5%[159]. In female patients, the sensitivities of endocervical culture, endocervical PCR, and urine PCR were 65.2%, 100% and 90%; corresponding specificities were 100%, 99.4%, and 95.9%. When sensitivities were calculated per patient rather than per specimen the sensitivity of urine PCR fell to 88.3% for men and 78.3% for women. The fully automated COBAS Amplicor (Roche Molecular Systems, Branchburg, NJ) was evaluated in a multi-center study involving both symptomatic and asymptomatic patients[160]. With the infected patient as the standard, endocervical PCR was 92.4% sensitive compared with 64.8% for urine PCR: there was no significant difference between symptomatic and asymptomatic women. In symptomatic men urine PCR was 94.1% sensitive and urethral swab PCR was 98.1% sensitive; for asymptomatic men the results were 42.3% and 73.1% respectively. The sensitivity of culture (details of culture procedures not stated) was 84.8% for endocervical specimens, 92.7% for symptomatic male urethral specimens, and 46.2% for urethral specimens from asymptomatic men. An internal control showed that 2% of specimens were inhibitory when tested initially. PCR specificity calculated on a patient basis was 99.5% for endocervical swabs, 99% for urethral swabs from asymptomatic men and 98.8% for symptomatic men; the corresponding specificities for urine PCR were 99.8% for women and 99.9% for men (both symptomatic and asymptomatic). A study among female sex workers in Benin found PCR had much lower sensitivity in testing urine (53.8%) than endocervical swabs (91.5%)[161]: corresponding specificities were 98.9% and 100%. A study from Perth, Western Australia, found the Amplicor PCR had a sensitivity and specificity of 100% when testing 73 men with a gonorrhea prevalence of 52.1%: the sensitivity of microscopy and/or culture using transport swabs was 86.8%[162]. Certain strains of *N. subflava* and *N. cinerea* may produce false positives with the Amplicor PCR test[163].

Digene Hybrid Capture II test and PACE 2 nucleic acid probe tests

The PACE 2 (Gen-Probe Inc, San Diego, CA) uses the same principle as the AccuProbe culture identification test for *N. gonorrhoeae* described above.

The Digene Hybrid Capture II (HC II) CT/GC Test (Digene Corp., Beltsville, MD) is a new nucleic acid signal amplification-based test for the detection of *C. trachomatis* and *N. gonorrhoeae* in specimens from the genital tract. The target DNA is hybridized with RNA probes. Hybrids are captured and detected using an antibody conjugate specific for RNA-DNA hybrids. Multiple enzymes are conjugated to each antibody molecule, and many antibodies bind to each RNA-DNA hybrid, resulting in a marked amplification of the signal. An initial positive result means that the specimen is positive for either *C. trachomatis* or *N. gonorrhoeae* or both. A second test is performed in parallel (HC II CT-ID and HC II GC-ID) to determine whether the initial signal was caused by the presence of chlamydial or gonococcal DNA.

Compared to culture of *N. gonorrhoeae* on TM medium the HC II CT/GC test had a sensitivity of 93% (87 of 94) and a specificity of 98.5% (1244 of 1263)[164]. Testing of some specimens with discrepant results by PCR suggested that test performance would be improved if it were compared to a nucleic acid amplification test. The proprietary cervical brush appeared to be better than dacron swabs for collecting specimens. In another study the relative sensitivity of the HC II test for the detection of 1750 swab specimens for *N. gonorrhoeae* was 100% with a specificity of 99.7%[165]. The relative sensitivity of the PACE 2 GC System was 86.5 % and the specificity 100%[165].

Comment

Molecular tests are already used in certain areas to diagnose gonococcal infection, and in future this usage will inevitably increase. Under these circumstances it is essential to develop a strategy to culture as many as possible of the patients who give positive molecular test results in order to ensure that antibiotic susceptibility surveillance is maintained.

DETECTION OF ANTIBODY

Although various attempts have been made to develop reliable antibody-based diagnostic tests none have gained acceptance. The advent of the molecular tests described above virtually obviated the need for such tests.

ANTIBIOTIC SUSCEPTIBILITY

Once the gonococcus has been fully identified, antibiotic sensitivity tests are carried out. Since the majority of patients with gonococcal infection will have been treated on the basis of a positive smear, antibiotic susceptibility tests are of little direct help in the initial management of the patient. However, they provide valuable epidemiological data and are extremely important in planning rational therapy for use in the geographical area concerned. Antibiotic susceptibility of an individual gonococcal isolate is important in the further treatment of patients whose infections have not been cured by initial therapy. Antibiotic

susceptibility testing, its interpretation, and subsequent action, must be considered in relation to the various types and degree of resistance found in individual gonococcal isolates and to the prevalence of resistance in the total gonococcal population circulating in a given area.

Definitions and mechanisms of antibiotic resistance in the gonococcus

Antibiotic susceptibility is usually defined quantitatively by determining the minimum inhibitory concentration (MIC) of an antibiotic to a particular strain: the MIC is the lowest concentration of drug that inhibits growth. The MIC value is used to define the categories sensitive, intermediate, and resistant depending on the probability of curing uncomplicated genital infection with the recommended dosage of antibiotic. The expected cure rate for the various categories is

- sensitive, greater than 95%
- intermediate, 90% to 95% (may be higher at increased dosage)
- resistant, less than 90% (even at increased dosage)[166].

Antibiotic resistance in the gonococcus results from mutations in chromosomal genes and/or from resistance mechanisms coded for by plasmids. The main types of clinically significant resistant gonococci are shown in Box 11.1.

Penicillin and the cephalosporins

Resistance to β-lactam antibiotics is caused by mutations at a series of loci on the chromosome resulting in small additive increases in penicillin resistance or to the inactivation of penicillin by a β-lactamase enzyme coded for by a plasmid.

Chromosomal resistance

The main genetic loci involved in chromosomal resistance are *penA*, *penB*, and *mtr*[167, 168]. *PenA* codes for PBP-2, a penicillin-binding protein which is a bifunctional enzyme with transpeptidase and transglycosylase activities; mutation, or genetic exchange with commensal neisseriae, results in low affinity forms of PBP-2 with decreased affinity for penicillin. The *PenB* locus is linked to the porin (*por*) gene; mutations affect the porin molecule and reduce the permeability to hydrophilic antibiotics including penicillin and tetracycline[169]. The *mtr* locus (multiple transferable resistance) is an operon that codes for an effective efflux system; mutations in the *mtrR* gene or the MtrR protein-binding region prevent binding of the repressor protein resulting in the Mtr phenotype with increased expression of the Mtr efflux system[170]. Antibiotics such as penicillin, fluoroquinolones, and tetracycline are pumped out as soon as they enter the bacterium and are unable to reach their intracellular target.

Mutation at the *penA* locus results in an eight-fold increase in resistance to penicillin alone. Mutation at the *mtr* locus results in a two- to four-fold increase in resistance to penicillin and to other antibiotics, dyes and detergents. Mutation in *penB* results in a four-fold increase in resistance to penicillin and tetracycline: *penB* is only expressed phenotypically when a mutation at *mtr* is present within the same cell. For the laboratory the accumulative effect of these three mutations is a 128-fold increase in penicillin resistance, a situation similar to that observed with clinical isolates over the last 50 years. As these mutations exert their effect by altering the permeability of the gonococcal cell envelope, isolates with clinically significant levels of resistance to penicillin are likely to be relatively resistant to a range of antibiotics such as erythromycin, tetracycline, and chloramphenicol. These isolates are termed chromosomally mediated resistant *Neisseria gonorrhoeae* (CMRNG). Reduced susceptibility to the cephalosporins such as cefuroxime, cefotaxime, and ceftriaxone appears to result from mutations in the same loci[171].

It is unlikely that the *mtr* system evolved to provide antibiotic resistance. The *mtr* system allows the gonococcus to regulate the permeability of its cell envelope in response to environmental signals, so that they can grow in the presence of toxic fecal lipids in the rectum as well as in the genital tract[172]. There is another set of gonococcal mutations termed *env*. Strains carrying these mutations are much more sensitive (hypersensitive) to antibiotics, dyes, and detergents[173, 174]. The *env* mutation suppresses the phenotypic expression of the *mtr* mutation if the two occur within the same strain[174]. The phenotypic expression of the *env* mutation is an alteration in the cell envelope so that it becomes more permeable to inhibitory substances. As *env* mutations are selected and maintained it has been speculated that the increased membrane permeability aids uptake of nutrients and gives a growth advantage *in vivo*: in contrast *mtr* mutations decrease permeability and may limit uptake of nutrients.

Plasmid mediated resistance

Gonococci may acquire one of several plasmids that code for the production of a TEM-1 type β-lactamase which will hydrolyse penicillins with a β-lactam ring structure to produce penicilloic acid which is inactive. Penicillinase plasmids probably originated in *Haemophilus* species[171]. Penicillinase-producing *Neisseria gonorrhoeae* (PPNG) were reported simultaneously in the UK and the USA in 1976; the respective isolates were linked epidemiologically with West Africa and South East Asia. The production of β-lactamase was shown to be due to the presence of a 3.2 Mdal plasmid in strains from Africa and Europe and a 4.4 Mdal plasmid in strains from Asia and the USA. Penicillinase-producing *N. gonorrhoeae* spread rapidly throughout the world and now the terms 'African' and 'Asian' can only be used to describe the plasmid type and not the geographical origin of the isolate. Additional plasmids have since been discovered: a 2.9 Mdal 'Rio' plasmid; a 3.05 Mdal 'Toronto' plasmid; a 4.0 Mdal 'Nimes' plasmid; a 6.0 Mdal 'New Zealand' plasmid; and a 2.2 Mdal 'Durban' plasmid[175]. These additional plasmids are related to the two original plasmids but are not so widespread.

Transfer of penicillinase plasmids can occur between strains of gonococci but requires the presence of a 24.5 Mdal conjugative plasmid. Originally this plasmid was found in association with the 4.4 Mdal plasmid but spread has now occurred and the conjugative plasmid can also be found in association with other resistance plasmids. In addition to the above plasmids most gonococcal strains carry a 2.6 Mdal plasmid. This was the first plasmid discovered in the gonococcus. No phenotypic character has been attributed to this plasmid and it is therefore termed 'cryptic'. A 7.8 Mdal plasmid is found in some strains and is thought to be a trimer of the 2.6 Mdal plasmid.

Tetracycline resistance

Chromosomal resistance to tetracycline is controlled by a specific locus (*tet*) as well as the non-specific loci *pen*B and *mtr* described above (see p. 334). High-level plasmid-mediated tetracycline resistant *N. gonorrhoeae* (TRNG) were reported in 1985. This is caused by the presence of a 25.2 Mdal plasmid resulting from the acquisition of the *tet*M resistant determinant by the 24.5 conjugative plasmid[176]. The *tet*M determinant encodes a 68 kDa cytoplasmic protein that protects the translational apparatus from tetracycline inactivation[177]. Restriction endonuclease analysis of the plasmid consistently produced one of two patterns termed the 'American' type and the 'Dutch' type, corresponding to where they originated. It is thought that two independent evolutionary events occurred at approximately the same time to produce the two plasmids.

Quinolone (ciprofloxacin) resistance

Resistance to the 4-quinolones is due to chromosomal mutations in the *gyrA* and *gyrB* genes of DNA gyrase, and in *parC* encoding topoisomerase IV[178]. DNA gyrase and topoisomerase IV are needed for maintaining and segregating the bacterial chromosome, they are essential for DNA replication and transcription. Increasing resistance to fluoroquinolones occurs by multi-step mutations. Low levels of resistance are due to single amino acid changes in *gyrA* while higher levels of resistance are found in isolates with double amino acid changes in *gyrA* and single amino acid changes in *parC*[179, 180]. Low-level resistance is also associated with amino acid changes in *gyrB*. Resistance mutations are readily transferred between gonococcal strains by transformation[181]. Furthermore, isolates containing the *gyrA* and *parC* mutations, if combined with mutations at the *penA*, *penB*, and *mtr* loci are likely to acquire resistance not only to fluoroquinolones but also to penicillins, cephalosporins, and tetracycline[182].

Spectinomycin resistance

Spectinomycin resistance results from chromosomal mutations in the 16S rRNA genes resulting in decreased binding of the drug to its ribosomal target[183]. High-level resistance occurs in a single step.

Erythromycin and azithromycin resistance

There is little information on the specific mechanisms of resistance of gonococci to macrolide antibiotics but it is generally considered to be caused by target site modification by methylation of adenine in 23S ribosomal RNA encoded by variants of the *erm* gene, which may reduce or prevent access of macrolide antibiotics to binding sites on the ribosome. Resistance is inducible by sub-inhibitory concentrations of macrolides. The long biological half-life of azithromycin results in long-term low levels of the drug which favors the selection of less susceptible strains[184].

Susceptibility testing

Susceptibility testing may be performed by disk diffusion, agar dilution (full MIC or breakpoint) or by the commercially available E-test. In disk diffusion, a small disk impregnated with a given concentration of antibiotic is placed on the surface of an agar plate inoculated with a bacterial suspension. After overnight incubation the size of the zone of inhibition indicates the susceptibility of the organism.

In the agar dilution method the antibiotic to be tested is serially diluted, and each dilution incorporated into one agar plate. A series of different antibiotics, each at several concentrations, can be used. Accurate amounts of antibiotic are available commercially in tablet form (Adatabs, Mast Laboratories, Bootle, Merseyside, UK) which, when added to an appropriate volume of medium, will give the required concentration. Normally twofold dilutions of antibiotic are used (for example penicillin from 4.0 to 0.015 mg/L); other antibiotics such as cefuroxime or ceftriaxone, ciprofloxacin, and spectinomycin can also be included. Approximately twenty isolates can be tested at the same time. A standardized suspension of each strain is inoculated onto the series of agar plates using a multi-point inoculator. Appropriate sensitive and resistant control organisms should be included with the series of test isolates. After overnight incubation the lowest concentration of antibiotic which inhibits growth is taken as the MIC. The breakpoint method is a form of agar dilution testing performed at a single antibiotic concentration chosen such that only resistant isolates will grow. The breakpoint method will give an accurate indication of clinical resistance but will not allow the detection of trends towards increasing resistance that can be detected by MIC testing.

The E-test is a novel method of determining the MIC. The E-test consists of a thin, plastic strip, the lower side of which contains a continuous concentration gradient of stabilized and dried antibiotic while the upper side is marked with a MIC scale. The strip is placed on an agar plate inoculated with a suspension of the test organism and after overnight incubation the intersection between the value printed on the edge of the strip and the inhibition zone is the MIC.

Methods for susceptibility testing of *N. gonorrhoeae* need strict standardization of medium and inoculum to produce reproducible results; more accurate results are obtained with the agar dilution method than with disk diffusion. Details of antibiotic susceptibility testing are reviewed elsewhere[185]. There are no universally accepted guidelines for susceptibility testing of gonococci although guidelines are provided by the WHO, the Australian Gonococcal Surveillance Programme, and the National Committee for Clinical Laboratory Standards (NCCLS) in the USA[171]. A recent survey of New York State laboratories found poor compliance with NCCLS guidelines[186].

The zone sizes and MIC values used to define the various categories of susceptibility are given in Table 11.3.

In the case of azithromycin, no category for resistance was proposed because none of 105 isolates tested had an MIC greater than 2 mg/L[187]. Subsequently, an isolate with an azithromycin MIC of 3 mg/L was isolated from a patient who had been treated with 1 g oral azithromycin[187a]; as the pre-treatment isolate had an MIC of 0.125 mg/L it was considered that resistance had developed during treatment. Other treatment failures have occurred in patients infected with isolates in the MIC range 0.125 to 0.25 mg/L, well within the current 'susceptible' category[188]. It was concluded that the antibiotic MIC/treatment outcome correlates that are usually found in gonorrhea do not apply for azithromycin.

In studies to establish the interpretive criteria for ceftriaxone, all strains, including those resistant to other antibiotics, gave an MIC of 0.125 mg/L or less[189]. It was

Table 11.3 Interpretative criteria for antibiotic susceptibility testing (the values are in accordance with NCCLS guidelines and were taken from: Jones *et al.* 1989[189]; Knapp *et al.* 1995[191]; Mehaffey *et al.* 1996[187]

Antibiotic (disk content)	Susceptible: MIC mg/L (zone diameter mm)	Intermediate: MIC mg/L (Zone diameter mm)	Resistant: MIC mg/L (Zone diameter mm)
Penicillin (6 μg)	≤ 0.06 (Ɛ 47)	0.12–1 (27–46)	≥ 2 (≤ 26)[a]
Ceftriaxone (30 μg)	≤ 0.25 (Ɛ 35)	Not categorized	Not categorized
Ciprofloxacin (5 μg)	≤ 0.06 (Ɛ 36)	0.125–0.5 (28–35)	≥ 1 (≤ 27)
Tetracycline (30 μg)	≤ 0.25 (Ɛ 38)	0.12–1 (31–37)	≥ 2 (≤ 30)[b]
Spectinomycin (100 μg)	≤ 32 (Ɛ 18)	64 (15–17)	≥ 128 (≤ 14)
Azithromycin (15 μg)	≤ 2 (Ɛ 25)	Not categorized	Not categorized

[a] PPNG usually give a zone size ≤ 19 mm.
[b] TRNG usually give a zone size ≤ 19 mm.

concluded that the definition of a resistant category must await the discovery of strains with MICs of 0.5 mg/L or more and treatment outcome results. Recently, 16.5% of 98 cases from Zhanjiang, China were reported to have an MIC of 2 mg/L or more[190].

Although an MIC of 1 mg/L or more is the proposed criteria for resistance to ciprofloxacin[191], monitoring in the UK includes strains with reduced susceptibility (MIC ≥ 0.05 mg/L) as treatment failure has occurred with infections from such strains[192, 193]. It is important to monitor treatment outcomes for isolates in this category to ensure that the criteria for clinical resistance (MIC ≥ 1 mg/L)[191] is not too stringent. An earlier study[194] noted that strains that fail to fall within the susceptible category (MIC ≤ 0.06 mg/L) were not necessarily resistant, but until data correlating clinical responses with higher MICs were obtained, such strains could not be considered susceptible.

Testing for plasmid resistance

Detection of penicillinase-producing Neisseria gonorrhoeae *(PPNG)*

In areas where penicillin is used for treatment, this is the most important aspect of sensitivity testing and it is best to screen all isolates as soon as possible. Even although

penicillin may not be used for treatment it is important to monitor the level of PPNG for epidemiological purposes.

Screening can be performed very simply by disk diffusion; using a 6 μg penicillin disk PPNG usually give a zone size up to 19 mm. Suspect PPNG can then be confirmed by one of the specific penicillinase detection methods[195]. One of the most sensitive and convenient methods uses commercially available paper strips impregnated with a chromogenic cephalosporin. When a few PPNG colonies are rubbed onto a test strip moistened with water the resulting hydrolysis of the β-lactamase ring causes a purple color to form around the area where the organisms were added; the test takes a few minutes. Other tests depend upon the bacterial breakdown of penicillin to penicilloic acid, which is detected by the ability of penicilloic acid to dissociate a starch–iodine complex, or by a pH indicator system. The latter method can be easily carried out alongside the rapid carbohydrate utilization test as part of the routine identification procedure, enabling all strains to be tested.

Detection of high-level plasmid-mediated tetracycline resistance (TRNG)

This is mainly of epidemiological interest and can easily be tested by disk diffusion; TRNG usually give a zone size up to 19 mm

to a 30 μg disk[189] or no zone around a 10 μg disk[171].

Epidemiology of resistance

There is considerable geographical variation in the proportion of strains showing some form of antibiotic resistance. Although regional or national programs for monitoring gonococcal susceptibility have been developed in some industrialized countries, in the developing world, where the burden of infection and resistance is the greatest, resistance data has mainly been derived from sentinel studies from individual laboratories with no continuous surveillance data[196]. With the extent of modern travel there is a continual influx of resistant strains with the potential for them to persist and become endemic amongst the indigenous gonococcal population. Recognizing that a program of continuous surveillance that crosses national boundaries would be of considerable benefit the WHO established a global surveillance network, the gonococcal antimicrobial-susceptibility program (GASP)[196]. The overall aim of GASP is to create a series of networks of laboratories based on WHO regions that will monitor gonococcal antimicrobial susceptibility and disseminate information on trends in susceptibility and emergence of resistance. These data can be used to direct the choice of appropriate treatment regimens. Although the development of GASP has been slow and constrained by lack of funds, significant progress has been made in the Americas and the Caribbean, the western Pacific region, and the southeast Asian region.

The establishment and outcomes of the WHO Western Pacific Region program, involving laboratories in 17 countries has been described[197]. About 20 000 gonococci were examined over the 3-year period 1992 to 1994. Resistance to the penicillins through β-lactamase production or chromosomal mechanisms was widespread. Spectinomycin resistance was infrequently encountered but high-level tetracycline resistance was present in most participating centers, with some having high proportions of tetracycline-resistant organisms. Quinolone resistance increased and became widespread throughout the region in the 3 years, ultimately involving all but one center. Both the number and MICs of quinolone-resistant isolates increased markedly. In Hong Kong, ciprofloxacin resistance has increased from 7.7% in 1995 to 24% in 1996, in Singapore from 0.3% in 1993 to 3.5% in 1996, and in Australia from 0.1% in 1992 to 2.6% in 1996[196].

The Gonococcal Isolate Surveillance Project (GISP) was established in 1986 to monitor trends in antimicrobial susceptibilities of strains of gonococci in the USA. This is a collaborative sentinel surveillance program: isolates are collected from the first twenty men with gonorrhea attending STI clinics each month in twenty-eight cities distributed across the USA[64]. Overall 29.4% (1384 of 4712) of isolates collected in 1998 were resistant to penicillin, tetracycline, or both; this proportion has been relatively constant since 1988. The percentage of PPNG declined from a peak of 11% in 1991 to 3% in 1998 while the prevalence of TRNG at 6.6% has varied little since 1990 (it increased from 4% in 1988 to almost 6% in 1990). The proportion of isolates with both resistance plasmids (PPNG-TRNG) was 0.7% in 1998 and has been decreasing from a peak of just over 2% in 1995. Therefore, in 1998, the total burden of plasmid-mediated resistance was 3.7% for penicillin and 7.3% for tetracycline. The percentage with chromosomal resistance to penicillin alone increased from 0.5% in 1988 to 5.1% in

1998. The prevalence of chromosomally mediated resistance to tetracycline alone was 6.8% and has been relatively stable since 1989. However, the presence of isolates with chromosomally mediated resistance to both penicillin and tetracycline increased from 3% in 1989 to 7.2% in 1998. The total level of chromosomal resistance to penicillin has therefore increased from 3.5% in 1998 to 12.3% in 1998. All isolates were susceptible to ceftriaxone although there was a drift to higher MICs (0.015 to 0.125 mg/L). The percentage of isolates with intermediate resistance (0.125 to 0.5 mg/L) or resistance (≥ 1 mg/L) to ciprofloxacin increased from 0.6% in 1997 to 1% in 1998 (only 0.1% had an MIC ≥ 1 mg/L). No isolates were resistant to spectinomycin.

Surveillance in the UK is performed by sentinel studies in London, the submission of resistant isolates to the Genitourinary Infections Reference Laboratory at Bristol from diagnostic laboratories throughout England and Wales, and the referral of all gonococci isolated in Scotland to the Scottish *Neisseria gonorrhoeae* Reference Laboratory (SNGRL). Within Scotland, the percentage of PPNG decreased slightly from 3.9% in 1991 to 2.4% in 1999; TRNG and PPNG-TRNG were absent in 1991 but accounted for 1.5% and 0.4% of isolates respectively in 1999. Therefore in 1999, the total burden of plasmid-mediated resistance was 2.8% for penicillin and 1.9% for tetracycline compared with levels of 3.7% and 7.3% respectively for the USA in 1998. Chromosomally mediated resistance to penicillin increased from 0% in 1991, peaked at 6% in 1995, and decreased to 0.4% in 1999 (compared with 12% for the USA in 1998). Chromosomally mediated tetracycline resistance increased from 6% in 1993, peaked at 20% in 1996 and decreased to 10% in 1999 (compared with 14% for the USA in 1998). The level of isolates with intermediate resistance (MIC 0.05 to 0.5 mg/L) or resistance (MIC ≥ 1 mg/L) to ciprofloxacin increased from 0.5% in 1991 to 4.8% in 1999 (2% had an MIC ≥ 1 mg/L compared with 0.1% in the USA in 1998). No isolates were resistant to spectinomycin. Epidemiological data on patients in Scotland infected with resistant isolates demonstrated that plasmid-mediated and ciprofloxacin resistant isolates usually

occurred in heterosexual men, belonged to unusual serovars, and were usually acquired outwith the UK, often in the Far East. In contrast chromosomally mediated penicillin and tetracycline-resistant isolates were usually associated with infection in homosexual men and were acquired in the UK.

Isolates collected from ten hospitals in the London area over a 3-month period in 1997 found a prevalence of 0.5% for PPNG, 2.4% for TRNG, and 1.3% for PPNG-TRNG[198]. Chromosomally mediated resistance to penicillin was found in 8% of isolates and resistance to ciprofloxacin (MIC ≥ 1 mg/L) in 0.4%.

Although the Genitourinary Infections Reference Laboratory at Bristol does not have denominator data, in 1998 it received 3% more isolates than in 1997 and the largest number of resistant isolates since 1988[199,199a]. Epidemiological data gathered on the resistant isolates showed that chromosomally mediated penicillin-resistant isolates were usually acquired in the UK while ciprofloxacin-resistant isolates were usually acquired in the Far East (39%); although the number of such infections acquired in the UK increased to 28% from 7% in 1997.

About half of the isolates with reduced susceptibility to ciprofloxacin were also PPNG. This is particularly important as ciprofloxacin has been widely used for treating infections considered to be acquired in areas where PPNG are common. A correlation between reduced susceptibility to ciprofloxacin and PPNG has also been reported from The Netherlands[199].

Sentinel surveillance in The Netherlands for isolates from 1997 to 1998 showed 11% of isolates were PPNG, 10% were chromosomally resistant to penicillin, 20% showed chromosomal resistance to tetracycline, 18% were consistent with TRNG, and 1.6% showed ciprofloxacin resistance[199a]. Different susceptibility patterns were found in isolates from consecutive male patients in Fukuoka, Japan[182]: in 1997 to 1998 2% of isolates were PPNG (decreased from 7.9% in 1993 to 1994), none were TRNG, 1.9% showed chromosomal resistance to penicillin (decreased from 12.6% in 1993 to 1994), 2% showed chromosomal resistance to tetracycline (decreased from 3.3% in 1993 to 1994), and 24.4% were ciprofloxacin resistant (increased from 6.6% in 1993 to 1994). Fluoroquinolones were the most frequently used first line treatment for gonorrhea during this period.

In developing countries antibiotic resistant isolates are much more common. With the caveat that resistant strains are likely to be over represented in culture studies in developing countries, the prevalence of PPNG has been reported as 28% in Thailand[200], 36% in Libya[201], 50% to 62% in Taiwan[202], 55% in the Philippines[203], 67% in Zimbabwe[204], 73% in Nigeria[205], 78% in Nicaragua[206], 77% in the Gambia[206a], 57%, 63%, and 67% in Rwanda, Zaire, and the Ivory Coast[207]. The frequency of TRNG was also extremely high at 64% in Rwanda, 41% in Zaire, and 65% in the Ivory Coast. Levels of TRNG of 84% were reported in the Gambia[206a]. Chromosomally mediated resistance to penicillin was also high in many of the above studies: 51% in Thailand[200], 50% in Nicaragua[206], and 55% in the Philippines[203].

EPIDEMIOLOGICAL MARKERS (TYPING OF GONOCOCCI)

Epidemiological typing is important in the control of infectious diseases. As 'contact tracing' is part of the overall control of gonorrhea, typing of isolates may be particularly valuable. Gonococcal typing allows the variety of organism types to be determined, as well as their distribution and prevalence in specific geographical areas, aiding

- recognition of new strains in a community
- detection of strains associated with antibiotic resistance
- differentiation between re-infection and treatment failure
- studies of sexual transmission networks
- comparisons between strains in medicolegal cases.

For many years only phenotypic typing methods that depend on a characteristic expressed by the bacteria on growth were available, more recently molecular methods that detect differences in the whole genome or particular genes have become available.

The main methods of typing are outlined before citing a few examples of their application in gonorrhea.

Phenotypic methods

A more detailed discussion of the various phenotypic methods and their application is given by Sarafian and Knapp[208].

Antibiograms

Antibiotic susceptibility patterns were used to distinguish between certain strains of gonococci before other typing methods were available. Although their value is very limited when used alone, in conjunction with other phenotypic methods they are essential for the description of the diversity of antimicrobial-resistant strains in a community and in allowing comparisons between geographical areas.

Auxotyping

Auxotyping was developed in 1973[209]. It is based upon the nutritional profile of gonococcal isolates growing on chemically defined media containing amino acids, nucleic acid bases, and certain vitamins. Auxotyping involves inoculating the gonococcus onto a series of plates containing 'complete' medium (on which all strains should grow) and media lacking single or multiple specific nutrients. Gonococci that grow on all media have no specific requirements and are termed non-requiring (NR), prototrophic (Proto), or wild type. Other strains are designated according to their specific growth requirements; those requiring proline are termed (P), arginine (A), hypoxanthine (H), and uracil (U). Strains with multiple requirements are designated according to the individual requirements, for example AHU strains. Although only a limited number of auxotypes are encountered, the gonococcus is heterogeneous with respect to distribution and prevalence of auxotypes and these are subject to temporal change.

Serotyping

The current typing system based on monoclonal antibodies was a natural development of the earlier classification systems based on polyclonal antibodies. The typing procedure is based on CoA that involves the attachment of anti-gonococcal IgG, by its Fc portion, to protein A on whole killed cells of *Staphylococcus aureus*. The addition

of gonococci which have determinants that react with the antibody-binding site on the specific IgG attached to the staphylococci results in agglutination which is visible to the naked eye. The method is used in the identification of cultured gonococci.

Two commercial groups produced monoclonal antibodies specific for epitopes on protein 1A and protein 1B. Separate panels of monoclonal antibodies were developed by the two groups and these are termed GS-antibodies (Genetic Systems Corporation, Seattle, WA) and Ph-antibodies (Pharmacia, Uppsala, Sweden)[210]. On the basis of the pattern of reaction of a gonococcal strain to the panel of reagents, particular serovars (serovariants) can be recognized. The GS system[143] uses six P1A specific (b,e,d,g,i,h) and six P1B (a,b,c,g,h,k) specific monoclonal antibody CoA reagents. The reaction pattern with the panel of reagents is then converted to a numerical code (prefixed by A or B) which was based on the frequency with which strains of a particular reaction pattern (serovar) were encountered in a worldwide survey of gonococci. For example, serovar 1A1 which reacts with monoclonal antibodies b,e,d, g,i,h was the most frequently occurring serovar, while serovar 1A24 which reacts with antibodies e,d,h was the rarest. Subsequently, serovar 1A2 which reacts with e,d,g,i,h but not b has been shown to be the most common 1A serovar in many geographical areas. The same system is used to designate 1B serovars with 1B1 which reacts with a,b,c,k being the most frequent and 1B32 which reacts only with k, being the rarest.

The system proposed by Bygdeman *et al.*[211] for the Ph panel names serovars by using the prefix A or B and listing the letters that denote the monoclonal antibodies with which the strain reacts. The Ph panel has five P1A reagents (r,o,s,t,v) and nine P1B reagents (r,o,p,y,u,v,s,t,x). The Ph panel gives greater discrimination and in one study[212] the Ph panel divided 1637 strains into 42 serovars compared with 28 by the GS panel. Using both serovar panels 81 serovar combinations could be obtained.

Following several years when both panels of antibodies were widely used, the GS system, as adopted by Centers for Disease Control and Prevention[143], became more widely used as workers wished to be able to compare data on serovars from different areas. Although typing with both panels does give greater discrimination it is very labor intensive. However, the Ph panel has a role in subtyping the common 1B serovars; for example 1B1 can be divided into the following main groupings: 1B1/Bropt, 1B1/Bropyt, 1B1/Bropst and 1B1/Brypust, while 1B2 can also be divided into 1B2/Brypust, 1B2/Bryput, 1B2/Bropyt and 1B2/Bypust[212].

Dual classification using auxotyping and serotyping

To overcome the individual limitations of auxotyping and serotyping an auxotype/ serovar (A/S) classification system was proposed[143]. This dual classification system based on two independent phenotypic characteristics that are stable *in vitro* provides greater resolution than does a system based on one phenotypic characteristic. An isolate that was non-requiring and belonged to serovar 1B1 would be designated NR/1B1.

Molecular methods

The first molecular typing methods involved characterization of the plasmids associated with penicillin resistance, and later tetracycline resistance. By extracting the DNA from the bacteria and separating it by gel electrophoresis under appropriate conditions it is possible to determine the size of the various β-lactamase plasmids discussed earlier (see p. 335), as well as determining whether the strain carries the 2.6 Mda cryptic plasmid and/or the 24.5 Mda conjugative plasmid or 25.2 Mda conjugative tetracycline resistance plasmid. More recently PCR has been used to amplify specific regions of the TetM plasmid and to differentiate them into the American and Dutch types[213].

PCR can also be used now to detect and differentiate between the Asian, African, and Toronto β-lactamase plasmids[214].

A variety of molecular methods have been used to analyze the entire gonococcal chromosome or specific genes. These include restriction endonuclease analysis[215], pulsed field gel electrophoresis[216], PCR and restriction fragment length poly-

morphism of outer membrane protein IB genes[217], arbitrarily primed PCR (AP-PCR), amplified ribosomal-DNA restriction analysis (ARDRA),[218], and ribotyping[219]. Because of the nature of these tests they have been restricted to a few highly specialized centers. Their more widespread use is also hampered by the lack of an agreed standard method and nomenclature that is needed to make epidemiological comparisons of the isolates from various geographical areas. In addition, methods such as restriction endonuclease analysis and pulsed-field gel electrophoresis that use the whole chromosome do not give a correlation between a particular restriction pattern and A/S class[220, 221].

More meaningful data are likely to be achieved by using the standard A/S phenotyping system first and then using a simple molecular method thereafter. A relatively simple subtyping scheme based on the *Lip* gene that is present in all gonococcal strains was described recently[222]. The *Lip* gene has a variable number of pentamer repeat sequences present. After PCR using specific primers, the product is run on a polyacrylamide gel and various sized bands are given depending on the number of repeat sequences in the gene from a particular strain. If required, isolates with the same number of repeats can be differentiated further by sequencing the PCR product. Among 46 strains examined 8 different Lip repeat numbers were identified; sequencing increased this to 17 subtype patterns.

For studying sexual networks and in medico-legal cases very high levels of discrimination are required. The extensive variation and rapid evolution of the *opa* gene repertoire (see p. 315) may provide a high-resolution typing method for studies of the short-term transmission of gonorrhea[223]. A single pair of primers from the *opa* genes are amplified by PCR, digested with frequently cutting restriction enzymes, and the fragments fractionated on polyacrylamide to provide an opa-type. The method appeared to be highly discriminatory as the opa-types of gonococci, isolated worldwide over the last 30 years, were all different. Opa-typing discriminated between isolates of the same A/S class. Similarly, there were 41 opa-types among 43 conse-

cutive isolates from an STI clinic. With one minor exception, identical opa-types were obtained from gonococci recovered from known sexual contacts, These results suggest that variation in the family of eleven *opa* genes evolves so rapidly that the opa-types of gonococci are distinguishable, unless the isolates are from sexual contacts or a short chain of disease transmission. The identification of gonococci with identical opa-types is therefore believed to be a good indicator that the individuals from which they were recovered were sexual partners, or part of a short chain of disease transmission.

Application of epidemiological markers

Auxotyping has demonstrated that AHU strains predominate in patients with disseminated gonoccocal infection. Strains with the AHU auxotype are usually hypersensitive to penicillin and resistant to the bactericidal action of normal human serum. The AHU strains predominate in men with asymptomatic gonococcal infection, thus allowing the strains a greater opportunity to disseminate.

The prevalence of AHU strains varies widely among different geographical areas. Although they are relatively common in the USA and parts of Europe they are rare in areas such as South East Asia and Africa where antibiotic resistance is common. As AHU strains are usually very sensitive to antibiotics, the use of gonococcal-selective media containing vancomycin may influence the prevalence of AHU strains in different areas as they would not be detected on such media. Isolates belonging to the PAU auxotype are of interest as they lack the 2.6 Mda cryptic plasmid found in most gonococcal isolates[224].

Serotyping has also shown some interesting correlations. Serovar 1A isolates tend to be particularly sensitive to antibiotics such as penicillin: excluding PPNG 74% of 1A isolates had a minimum inhibitory concentration (MIC) to penicillin of 0.015 mg/L or less compared with 4% of 1B isolates[225]. Serovars also correlate with sexual orientation, 1A serovars are almost exclusively associated with heterosexually acquired infection whereas 1B serovars are associated with both heterosexual and homosexually acquired infection. The following A/S classes were strongly associated with heterosexual transmission: PAU/1B2 (in 48% of female and 0% of male rectal isolates); A/1B3 (in 36% of female and 0% of male rectal isolates); H/1B3 (in 36% of female and 0% of male rectal isolates); H/1B6 (in 40% of female and 0% of male rectal isolates) and NR/1B31 (in 58% of female and 0% of male rectal isolates). Isolates associated with homosexual transmission include P/1B6 (in 98% of men with 16% involving rectal infection), NR/1B2 (in 91% of men with 23% involving rectal infection), and NR/1B6 (in 72% of men with 19% involving rectal infection).

Temporal changes also occur. 1B2 remains the most common isolate in Scotland accounting for 33% of isolates in 1998 compared with 44.8% in 1997. Serovar 1B3 accounted for 9% in 1998 but in 1995 it accounted for 22% of isolates. Serovar 1B6 increased to 28% in 1998 from 4% in 1995. Serovar 1B31 also increased markedly to 16% from 2% in 1997.

Serovar 1A2 has been shown to be more infectious but less symptomatic than other serovars[226]. Auxotype/serovar classes CU/1B1 and CU/1B3 (CU is similar to AU but the requirement for arginine is satisfied by citrulline but not ornithine) are extremely rare and have been associated with asymptomatic infection in men[227]. Gram-stained urethral smears of specimens from men infected with these isolates were more often negative than smears from men infected with other isolates and leading to a more frequent misdiagnosis of non-gonococcal urethritis.

Opa-typing was used to study an outbreak of ciprofloxacin-resistant gonococcal infection in England[228]. Of 73 NR auxotype ciprofloxacin-resistant isolates, 24 had unique opa-types (10 from infections acquired abroad) while 49 were indistinguishable (none were known to be acquired abroad). This cluster included 31 isolates from Oldham and Rochdale, 16 from elsewhere in the north of England, and 2 from southern England and south Wales with known epidemiological links to cases from Manchester and Rochdale respectively.

Opa-typing has also been used to study sexual networks and may be able to link

infections that would otherwise remain unlinked, thus aiding interventions to control endemic disease[229].

Pulsed field gel electrophoresis was used to demonstrate the emergence of a single clone of gonococcus with reduced susceptibility to ciprofloxacin (A/S class was not given) in Cleveland, OH. Between 1991 and 1994 the prevalence of this isolate increased from 2% to 16%. Patients infected with this strain were less likely to give positive Gram-stained urethral smears and were consequently less likely to be treated for gonorrhea at their initial visit. To date the increase in ciprofloxacin isolates with reduced susceptibility has not always been related to the spread of a single strain although there is clearly potential for this to happen. In Scotland, the prevalence of reduced susceptibility to ciprofloxacin increased from 0.5% in 1991 to 5% in 1999[193]: the 98 strains were represented by 25 different A/S classes, many of which were uncommon, supporting importation rather than endemic spread.

Epidemiology of plasmid mediated resistance

A combination of serovar analysis, auxotyping, and determination of plasmid profile has proved valuable in the epidemiology of PPNG. There has been a change from the early pattern observed among PPNG strains, where those originally described as African type were arginine requiring and contained a 3.2 Mdal plasmid, while those of the Asian type were non-requiring and contained a 4.4 Mdal plasmid, usually in conjunction with a 24.5 Mdal transfer plasmid. Strains of PPNG with a diversity of different auxotypes and serovars have since emerged, expressing the spread of the β-lactamase encoding plasmids between strains of different serovar/auxotype combinations. The evolution of certain of these changes has been reviewed for areas of the USA by Sarafian and Knapp[208]. During the years 1998 to 1996 the PPNG strain population in Miami, FL, consisted of a few dominant and many transient A/S classes; the predominant A/S classes also differed from one period to the next. It was speculated that the PPNG strain population in Miami underwent temporal changes influenced

by the introduction and eradication of different PPNG strains, rather than by transfer of the plasmids in the community. Similarly, TRNG strain populations have been characterized by the introduction and eradication of individual TRNG strains, although approximately 50% of isolates initially studied in the USA were NR/1B1 isolates. In 1998 plasmid analysis of isolates submitted to the Genitourinary Infections Reference Laboratory at Bristol demonstrated that 75% of PPNG-TRNG isolates contained the 3.2 MDa plasmid and 25% the 4.4 MDa plasmid[230]. Of the PPNG isolates, 37% had the 3.2 MDa plasmid, 13% the 4.4 Mda plasmid, and 50% the 3.05 MDa plasmid; this was the first year that the 3.05 MDa plasmid was more prevalent than the 3.2 MDa plasmid. The 3.05 MDa plasmid was also common in PPNG isolated in Scotland in 1998 but the distribution of other plasmids was different from that in England and Wales[225]: 33% of PPNG-TRNG strains contained the 3.2 MDa plasmid and 67% the 4.4 MDa plasmid, while among the PPNG-only isolates 25% had the 3.2 MDa plasmid, 17% the 4.4 MDa plasmid and 58% the 3.05 MDa plasmid.

The combination of serotype, auxotype, and plasmid profile (including subtyping of TRNG) showed a highly heterogeneous group with 14 different strains among 18 isolates; several of the infections were known to be acquired abroad, supporting the theory of importation to Scotland rather than endemic spread. In developing countries there tends to be much more restricted plasmid profile indicating endemicity. A study of isolates from Bangladesh in 1997 found that all PPNG had the 3.2 MDa plasmid[231] whilst, with one exception, all PPNG isolates from Sumatra, Indonesia in 1996 contained the 4.4 MDa plasmid[232].

Treatment

PRINCIPLES OF TREATMENT

The aim of treatment is to eradicate the organism from all infected anatomical sites as quickly as possible. A minimum criterion of efficacy of a drug is that it will cure more than 95% of uncomplicated gonococcal infections[233]. Ideally the treatment used should be based on the pattern of the sensitivity to antibiotic and chemotherapeutic agents observed amongst the strains of the organism in the population of the place of residence of the infecting partner. Regimens of treatment should be constantly reviewed, account being taken of the results of continuous monitoring of isolates for the emergence of drug resistance. For example, in a national sentinel surveillance system undertaken between September 1987 and December 1988, to estimate levels and monitor trends of antimicrobial resistance in gonococcal isolates, 16.8% of 6204 isolates evaluated from twenty-one clinics in the USA had chromosomally mediated resistance (minimum inhibitory concentration ≥ 2 μg/mL) to penicillin, tetracycline, or cefoxitin[234]. As treatment failure rates increase with increasing resistance to antimicrobial agents[235], the decision of the Centers for Disease Control and Prevention[236] to discontinue the recommendation of penicillins in the treatment of gonorrhea in the USA is vindicated.

A course of treatment with almost any antimicrobial drug to which the organism is sensitive will cure the majority of patients with gonorrhea. Patient adherence, however, is often unsatisfactory and tablets may be inadvisably shared with a partner. For example, within 1 or 2 days of commencing oral treatment with amoxicillin in doses, say, of 250 mg 8-hourly, symptoms of gonococcal urethritis may resolve and lead the patient to assume, wrongly, that he has been cured. Strains of organisms with increased resistance to antimicrobials may emerge when courses of treatment prescribed are not completed. For these reasons a single large dose of antibiotic, given under supervision either orally or parenterally, is the preferred treatment for uncomplicated infections. In most cases blood and tissue concentrations of the drug reach a high level and are maintained for sufficient time to eradicate the organism. Oral administration of antibiotic is preferred to intramuscular injections, which are not only painful but more liable to cause hypersensitivity reactions. Single-dose therapy with penicillins has not proved satisfactory, however, in the treatment of oropharyngeal gonorrhea or in complicated infections. In male anorectal gonorrhea infections single-dose treatment with ciprofloxacin and the newer cephalosporins is generally satisfactory.

ANTIMICROBIAL DRUGS USED IN THE TREATMENT OF GONORRHEA

Amoxicillin

Unwanted effects

Minor gastrointestinal symptoms, including nausea, vomiting, and diarrhea, are sometimes described by patients receiving amoxicillin. Skin rashes, pruritus, and urticaria may occur and, rarely, erythema multiforme may complicate the use of the drug. Severe hypersensitivity reactions including anaphylaxis, angio-neurotic edema, and vasculitis have been described, and amoxicillin should not be given to individuals with a history of penicillin hypersensitivity. Other side effects are rare.

Use in pregnancy and lactation

Animal studies have shown no teratogenic effects, and amoxicillin is suitable for use in pregnant women. As only trace amounts of the drug are found in breast milk there is no contraindication to its use in lactating women.

Preparations available

For the treatment of uncomplicated gonorrhea, amoxicillin is available in capsule form, each capsule containing 250 mg or 500 mg of amoxicillin trihydrate. A sucrose-free syrup containing 250 mg amoxicillin trihydrate per 5 mL is useful for those who have difficulty in swallowing capsules. A suspension containing 125 mg of amoxicillin trihydrate per 1.25 mL is available for pediatric use.

Note: probenecid

Probenecid inhibits the renal tubular secretion of many drugs, including the penicillins, resulting in a higher plasma concentration of that drug; the use of amoxicillin to treat gonorrhea takes advantage of this property. Probenecid is almost completely absorbed when given orally, the peak concentration being achieved within 2 to 4 hours. The plasma half-life is dose dependent, and varies between less than 5 hours to more than 8 hours.

Cephalosporins

As there may be cross hypersensitivity between the cephalosporins and penicillin or other non-cephalosporin β-lactam antibiotics, care should be exercised in treating individuals who have a history of reactions to these drugs, especially if this has been an anaphylactic reaction.

With the exception of cefixime, which can be given orally, the cephalosporins that are currently recommended for the treatment of gonorrhea must be given by the parenteral route.

Unwanted effects of the cephalosporins

Adverse events are generally mild and transient, the most common being gastrointestinal, including diarrhea or loose stools. Pancreatitis has occurred during treatment with ceftriaxone, but the evidence associating the drug with this complication is weak. Various skin rashes – maculopapular lesions, urticaria, and rarely, Stevens–Johnson syndrome – have been reported during treatment. Anaphylactic reactions are rare. Hematological abnormalities, including anemia, leukopenia, eosinophilia, and thrombocytopenia, have been reported, and transient elevations in plasma enzyme tests of liver function have been described. Increases in prothrombin times have been noted, and care should be taken in the co-administration of the cephalosporins with oral anticoagulants.

Very rarely, reversible urinary precipitates of calcium ceftriaxone have developed, particularly in dehydrated patients, and have been associated with anuria and renal impairment. If there is renal impairment, biliary excretion of ceftriaxone is increased, and in patients with hepatic dysfunction, renal excretion is increased (Roche Products Ltd Data Sheet 1999–2000). In severe renal impairment accompanied by hepatic insufficiency, the elimination half-life of ceftriaxone is increased, and, when multiple dosing schedules are required as in disseminated infection, plasma levels of the drug should be monitored during therapy, and the daily dose adjusted accordingly. In the case of cefixime, normal doses of drug can be given unless the creatinine clearance is less than 20 mL/min, in which case, no more than 200 mg per day should be administered (Rhone-Poulenc Rorer Ltd Data Sheet 1999–2000). As metabolism accounts for some 40% of elimination of cefotaxime, there is no need to reduce the dose of the drug used in the treatment of uncomplicated gonorrhea. When given for the treatment of complicated infection, however, an adjustment of dose is required if the patient has severe renal impairment (creatinine clearance < 5 mL/min). In patients with renal insufficiency, single-dose treatment with cefoxitin can be given in the usual dosage (Table 11.4). Similarly, the usual dose of ceftizoxime can be given.

Administration of high doses of cephalosporins may produce encephalopathy, particularly in those patients with renal insufficiency.

Rarely, arrythmias have developed following rapid intravenous infusion of cefotaxime.

Most adverse events have been reported amongst patients who have received courses of the drug, often given for serious infections. In the case of patients treated for gonorrhea by a single intramuscular injection, the risk of unwanted effects such as pseudomembranous colitis and super-infection with fungi is low. Pain or discomfort at the injection site, however, may occur.

Use in pregnancy and lactation

Although there are no adverse effects on fetal development in laboratory animals, the safety of cephalosporins in pregnancy has not been established, and they should only be used if there are no well-established safe alternatives. Animal studies suggest that placental transfer of cefixime is small, and teratogenic effects have not been shown. Cefotaxime crosses the placental barrier but animal model studies have not shown an adverse effect on the developing fetus. Similarly, fetal damage or impaired fertility have not been shown in rats or mice given cefoxitin. Although less than 2% of the administered dose of cefixime has been found in breast milk in lactating rats, it is not yet known if the drug is excreted in human breast milk. Only minimal concentrations of ceftriaxone are detected in breast milk. Cefotaxime and cefoxitin, however, are excreted in breast milk.

Preparations of cephalosporins available for use in the treatment of gonorrhea

Ceftriaxone

Vials containing 250 mg of ceftriaxone in the form of a crystalline powder consisting of 298.3 mg of the hydrated disodium salt. The powder is reconstituted with 1 mL of lidocaine (lignocaine) hydrochloride, 1% w/v, and the drug is administered by deep intramuscular injection. For use by the intravenous route, vials containing 1 g of ceftriaxone in the form of 1.19 g of the disodium salt are available. The powder is reconstituted with 10 mL of sterile Water for Injections.

Cefotaxime

Vials containing 500 mg cefotaxime sodium powder. The drug is reconstituted with 2 mL of Water for Injection. For intravenous use, 1 to 2 g of cefotaxime are dissolved in 40 to 100 mL of Water for Injection, or in infusion fluid. The prepared infusion may be administered over a 20 to 60 minute period.

Cefoxitin

Vials containing 2 g of cefoxitin as sodium salt. For intramuscular injection the drug may be reconstituted with 0.5% or 1.0% lidocaine (lignocaine) hydrochloride. In the treatment of uncomplicated gonorrhea, concomitant administration of probencid is recommended. Cefoxitin is excreted

Table 11.4 Treatment regimens for uncomplicated gonorrhea of the urethra, cervix, and rectum

Antimicrobial agent	Dosage
Amoxicillin[a]	3 g in a single oral dose, given with probenecid, 1 g by mouth
Ciprofloxacin[bc]	500 mg as a single oral dose
Ceftriaxone[bc]	125 mg as a single intramuscular injection
Cefixime[c]	400 mg as a single oral dose
Ofloxacin[bc]	400 mg as a single oral dose
Levofloxacin[bc]	250 mg as s single oral dose
Spectinomycin[d]	2 g as a single intramuscular injection
Cefotaxime[d]	500 mg as a single intramuscular injection
Ceftizoxime[d]	500 mg as a single intramuscular injection
Cefoxitin[d]	2 g as a single intramuscular injection together with probencid as a single oral dose of 1 g
Gatifloxacin[d]	400 mg as a single oral dose
Norfloxacin[d]	800 mg as a single oral dose
Lomefloxacin[d]	400 mg as a single oral dose

[a] Can be used where prevalence of penicillin resistant strains of *N. gonorrhoeae* is < 5%.
[b] Quinolones should not be used for infections acquired in Asia or the Pacific, including Hawaii.
[c] Regimens recommended by the Centers for Disease Control 2002[60].
[d] Alternative regimens recommended by the Centers for Disease Control and Prevention 2002[237].

virtually unchanged by the kidneys and probencid slows its tubular excretion, thereby increasing and prolonging blood levels of the drug.

Cefixime

Cefixime is available in tablet form, each tablet containing 200 mg of anhydrous cefixime. For pediatric use an oral suspension is available, each 5 mL of reconstituted suspension containing 100 mg cefixime.

Quinolones

Quinolones have been found useful in the treatment of gonorrhea, and although resistance has become problematic in some geographical areas, they are still widely used where the prevalence of resistant strains is low.

Unwanted effects of the quinolones

The most frequent unwanted effects include nausea, vomiting, abdominal pain, headache, restlessness, and dizziness (Bayer plc Data Sheet 1999–2000). The more serious adverse events are seen in patients who receive multiple dosing regimens. As convulsions have been reported following the use of ciprofloxacin, caution should be exercised in administering the drug to those with a history of epilepsy. In addition, plasma levels of phenytoin may be altered when the drugs are given concomitantly. Skin rash, including rarely, erythema multiforme, pruritus, urticaria, and anaphylaxis have also been reported. Photosensitivity is recognized as an unwanted effect of several quinolones. Transient increases in plasma bilirubin and plasma enzyme tests of liver function may occur, and in some patients, hepatitis and hepatic necrosis has developed. Arthralgia, joint swelling, and myalgia have all been recorded as adverse events, and rarely, tendinitis has led to tendon rupture. Patients must discontinue therapy if pain or inflammation of a tendon occurs. Ciprofloxacin and the other quinolones should not be used in patients who have a past history of tendinitis.

Transient hematological abnormalities may occur, and it should be appreciated that patients with a family history of glucose-6-phosphate dehyrogenase deficiency may develop hemolytic reactions with quinolones. The bleeding time may be prolonged when ciprofloxacin and oral anticoagulants are given concomitantly. The quinolones may also potentiate the action of glibenclamide, resulting in hypoglycemia.

Note: As arthropathy can be induced in immature animals, the use of the quinolones is contra-indicated in prepubertal children and adolescents.

Use in pregnancy and lactation

Although there is no evidence of teratogenicity, or of impairment of peri- and postnatal development in experimental animals, arthropathy may occur in young animals, and its use in human pregnancy should therefore be avoided. The drug is secreted in breast milk, and nursing mothers should not be treated with this agent.

Ciprofloxacin

The oral bioavailability of ciprofloxacin is between 50% and 80%; absorption is impaired by divalent cations, for example iron preparations and antacids.

Use in renal or hepatic impairment

In the case of multiple dose regimens, dosage adjustment is not usually necessary except when there is severe renal impairment (creatinine clearance < 20 mg/min). No dosage adjustment is needed when there is hepatic dysfunction.

Preparations available

Tablets, each containing 291 mg of ciprofloxacin hydrochloride monohydrate (equivalent to 250 mg ciprofloxacin) are available. A preparation containing ciprofloxacin (as lactate) 2 mg/mL, in sodium chloride 0.9% is available for intravenous infusion.

Ofloxacin

See Chapter 10.

Levofloxacin

As in the case of ciprofloxacin, absorption of levofloxacin is impaired by concomitant administration of iron preparations or antacids.

Use in hepatic or renal impairment

In the case of intravenous administration of levofloxacin, doage adjustment is necessary in the case of renal impairment (creatinine clearance < 50 mg/min). The excretion of the drug can also be impaired in hepatic dysfunction, necessitating a dosage adjustment.

Preparations available

Tablets, each containing levofloxacin hemihydrate 256.23 mg, equivalent to 250 mg of levofloxacin. A solution for intravenous infusion, containing levofloxacin 5 mg/mL. The infusion time should not be less than 30 minutes.

Norfloxacin

Iron preparations, antacids, and multivitamin tablets interfere with absorption and should not be given concomitantly or within 2 hours of administration of norfloxacin.

Preparations available

Tablets, each containing 400 mg of norfloxacin.

Use in renal or hepatic impairment

Such patients can be treated with the standard single-dose therapy (Table 11.4).

Gatifloxacin and lomefloxacin

These quinolones have been proposed by the Centers for Disease Control and Prevention[237] as being alternative treatments. Experience in their use is limited, and neither of these drugs appears to offer any significant advantage over the quinolones discussed above. They are not currently available in the UK.

Spectinomycin

Spectinomycin is given by intramuscular injection.

Unwanted effects

The most common unwanted effect is pain at the injection site. Nausea, chills, urticaria, dizziness, reduced urinary output, and, very rarely, anaphylaxis have been reported (Pharmacia and Upjohn Data Sheet 1999–2000).

Preparation available

Vials containing spectinomycin hydrochloride powder, equivalent to spectinomycin 2 g, are available. The drug is reconstituted with 3.2 mL Water for Injection.

TREATMENT SCHEDULES

Uncomplicated genital infections in men and women

Various regimens for single-dose treatment currently used in the treatment of uncomplicated anorectal gonorrhea are given in Table 11.4, and the results of treatment are shown in Table 11.5. The sensitivity of the infecting organisms may vary geographically and hence cure rates may not approach those cited. Although amoxicillin is used widely in the UK in the treatment of gonorrhea, penicillin therapy is no longer recommended by the Centers for Disease Control and Prevention[238].

Rectal and oropharyngeal gonorrhea

With the use of the cephalosporins or quinolones in the treatment of rectal gonorrhea in men and women, cure rates are identical to those obtained in the treatment of genital infection[239]. Oropharyngeal gonorrhea is generally considered to be more difficult to treat than infection at other anatomical sites. Moran[239] undertook a systematic review of

Table 11.5 Single-dose antimicrobial agents for the treatment of genital gonorrhea in men and women

Antimicrobial agent	Dosage	Number of patients		Reference
		Treated	**Cured**	
Penicillins				
Amoxicillin[a]	3 g orally	54	51 (94%)	Thin *et al.* 1977[256]
Cephalosporins				
Ceftriaxone	250 mg i.m.	94	92 (98%)	Handsfield *et al.* 1991[257]
Ceftriaxone	250 mg i.m	63	63 (100%)	Plourde *et al.* 1992[258]
Ceftriaxone	125 mg i.m.	110	109 (99%)	Handsfield and Hook 1987[259]
Cefixime	400 mg orally	93	89 (96%)	Handsfield *et al.* 1991[257]
Cefixime	400 mg orally	121	118 (98%)	Plourde *et al.* 1992[258]
Cefotaxime	500 mg i.m.	218	213 (98%)	McCormack *et al.* 1993[260]
Cefotaxime	1.0 g i.m.	102	102 (100%)	De Koning *et al.* 1983[261]
Cefoxitin[a]	2 g i.m.	140	136 (97%)	Veeravahu *et al.* 1983[262]
Ceftizoxime	500 mg i.m.	100	99 (99%)	Spencer *et al.* 1984[263]
Quinolones				
Ciprofloxacin	250 mg orally	83	83 (100%)	Bryan *et al.* 1990[264]
Ciprofloxacin	250 mg orally	284	268 (94%)	Thorpe *et al.* 1996[265]
Ofloxacin	400 mg orally	43	43 (100%)	Rajakumar *et al.* 1988[266]
Ofloxacin	400 mg orally	171	166 (97%)	Bogaerts *et al.* 1993[267]
Norfloxacin	800 mg orally	197	189 (96%)	Bogaerts *et al.* 1993[267]
Spectinomycin	2 g i.m.	52	52 (100%)	Tupasi *et al.* 1983[268]
Spectinomycin	2 g i.m.	51	47 (92%)	Crider *et al.* 1984[269]

[a] With 1 g probenecid by mouth

published therapeutic trials of various modern antimicrobial regimens in the treatment of uncomplicated gonorrhea (16 737 infections). He noted that although these schedules were highly successful in the eradication of *N. gonorrhoeae* from the genital tract and rectum of men and women – more than 95% of all infections were cured – only 79.9% and 83.7% of pharyngeal infections in men and women respectively were eradicated.

In the treatment of infection at this site, either ceftriaxone, given by intramuscular injection in a dose of 125 mg, of ciprofloxacin*, given in a single oral dose of 500 mg are currently recommended by the Centers for Disease Control and Prevention[237]. In his review, Moran[239] noted 61 (93.8%) of 65 pharyngeal infections were cured by ceftriaxone. A similar success rate (93%) was recorded in the treatment of 15 infections with ciprofloxacin.

Gonococcal conjunctivitis

Treatment is with ceftriaxone, given in a single intramuscular injection of 1 g[237]. It is also helpful to use saline lavage once.

Post-gonococcal urethritis in the male

The management of this complication is dealt with in Chapter 10. In an attempt to reduce the incidence of post-gonococcal urethritis, azithromycin (1 g as a single oral dose) or doxycycline (100 mg by mouth every 12 hours for 7 days) may be given†[237].

Complicated gonorrhea

Epididymo-orchitis

If inflammation is severe, the patient should be admitted to hospital and kept in bed. A scrotal support should be worn to relieve pain and adequate analgesia should be provided. Gonococcal epididymitis is treated with ceftriaxone 250 mg, given as a single intramuscular injection, and followed by doxycycline, given orally in a dose of 100 mg every 12 hours for 10 days[237]. Alternatively, ofloxacin 300 mg twice daily by mouth, or levofloxacin 500 mg once daily by mouth can be given for 10 days[238]. Scrotal support and analgesia are helpful adjuvants to antimicrobial therapy, and bed rest is recommended for patients with marked discomfort and fever.

Bartholinitis and abscess

The patient may need admission to hospital if the inflammation is severe. Although there have been no recent reports on the efficacy of newer treatment regimens in the management of gonococcal bartholinitis, the authors recommend that the woman should be treated with ceftriaxone and doxycycline in the dosages given for epididymo-orchitis. If an abscess persists, this is best treated by aspiration during antimicrobial therapy or by marsupialization if this fails.

Pelvic inflammmatory disease

See Chapter 12.

Disseminated gonococcal infection with or without arthritis and/or skin lesions

The patient should be admitted to hospital for initiation of treatment. Although recent studies on the treatment of disseminated gonococcal infection are lacking, the Centers for Disease Control[237] recommend the drugs shown in Box 11.2 for the initial treatment of this complication. Usually within 48 hours the condition of the patient improves and oral treatment may be substituted and continued for 10 to 14 days. The following oral antimicrobial agents have been recommended by the Centers for Disease Control[237]

1. ciprofloxacin 500 mg every 12 hours
2. ofloxacin 400 mg every 12 hours
3. cefixime 400 mg every 12 hours.
4. levofloxacin 500 mg once daily.

Note: fluoroquinolones should not be used for infections acquired in Asia or the Pacific, including Hawaii.

> **Box 11.2** Recommended regimens for initial treatment for disseminated gonococcal infection with arthritis (Centers for Disease Control 2002[238])
>
> ---
>
> ***Recommended initial treatment***
>
> Ceftriaxone 1 g by intravenous infusion or intramuscular injection every 24 hours
>
> ***Alternative initial regimens***
>
> Cefotaxime 1 g intravenously every 8 hours
>
> or
>
> Ceftizoxime 1 g intravenously every 8 hours
>
> or
>
> Ciprofloxacin[a] 500 mg intravenously every 12 hours
>
> or
>
> Ofloxacin[a] 400 mg intravenously every 12 hours
>
> or
>
> Levofloxacin 250 mg intravenously once daily
>
> Spectinomycin[a] 2 g by intramuscular injection every 12 hours
> [a] Suitable for use in patients with hypersensitivity to β-lactam antimicrobial agents)

Endocarditis and meningitis

In the preantibiotic era, 4% to 10% of all cases of endocarditis were due to *N. gonorrhoeae*[98] and in one series of 38 cases encountered over a 12-year period, 10 (26%) infections were caused by this organism[99]. Since deterioration may occur rapidly in endocarditis – despite apparently appropriate antibiotic treatment – and delay in valve replacement may prove fatal, it is strongly recommended that such patients should be referred early for expert management by a cardiologist and cardiac surgeon. Patients with fever and a heart murmur should have blood cultures – three specimens taken at intervals of a few hours – without delay before any antibiotic treatment is given, even if this means referral to hospital.

Ceftriaxone given by intravenous infusion in a dosage of 1 to 2 g every 12 hours is

---

* Unless the source of infection has been Asia or the Pacific, including Hawaii.

† If amoxicillin or other penicillin derivative has been used in the treatment of gonorrhea, doxycycline is given the day after, to avoid the mutually antagonistic effects of penicillins and tetracyclines.

recommended for the treatment of meningitis and endocarditis[237]. Treatment of meningitis should continue for 10 to 14 days, and of endocarditis for at least 4 weeks.

Treatment of pregnant women with gonorrhea

Care is needed in giving any drug in pregnancy. Treatment with quinolones or tetracyclines is contraindicated. The cephalosporins are generally considered safe and the standard dose can be given. Women who are intolerant of a cephalosporin should be given spectinomycin in a single intramuscular dose of 1 g[237]. Erythromycin, azithromycin, or amoxicillin should also be given for presumed or proven concurrent chlamydial infection (Chapter 10).

Treatment of gonorrhea in prepubertal children

Conjunctivitis of the newborn (ophthalmia neonatorum)

Infants with gonococcal ophthalmia should be admitted to hospital, and examined for signs of disseminated infection, such as meningitis or arthritis. Combined local and parenteral therapy is necessary.

1. *Local therapy*: frequent, repeated instillations of sterile isotonic saline into the affected eye. Topical antibiotic treatment may produce sensitization reactions and should, for this reason, be avoided.
2. *Parenteral therapy*: ceftriaxone 25 to 50 mg/kg given as a single intramuscular or intravenous injection, is the recommended treatment[237]. The dose should not exceed 125 mg. Some cephalosporins, including ceftriaxone, can displace bilirubin from serum albumin. Caution should therefore be exercised in administering the drug to an infant who is jaundiced, especially if he or she has been born prematurely. The efficacy of ceftriaxone was shown in a study from Kenya[240]; all 55 infants treated with the drug had clinical and microbiological cure.

In geographical areas where ceftriaxone is unavailable, kanamycin 25 mg/kg, given as a single intramuscular injection, to a maximum of 75 mg, is often effective[241].

Spectinomycin, 25 mg/kg by intramuscular injection as a single dose to a maximum of 75 mg, is an alternative treatment regimen[242].

Both parents must be examined and treated.

Disseminated gonococcal infection and scalp abscesses in the neonate

Neonates with disseminated infection or scalp abscesses should be treated with ceftriaxone 25 to 50 mg/kg once daily by intravenous or intramuscular injection for 7 days. If there are features of meningitis, the course should be continued for 10 to 14 days[237]. An alternative regimen is cefotaxime 25 mg/kg every 12 hours by intravenous or intramuscular injection for 7 days, or for 10 to 14 days, for those with and without meningitis respectively[237].

Gonococcal infection after the neonatal period

Vulvovaginal, cervical, urethral, rectal, or pharyngeal infection

Children who weigh more than 45 kg can be treated with one of the regimens recommended for adults. The possibility of joint damage caused by fluoroquinolones, however, should be borne in mind. Ceftriaxone 125 mg as a single intramuscular injection is recommended for the treatment of children who weigh less than 45 kg[237]. An alternative treatment is with spectinomycin given by intramuscular injection in a dose of 40 mg/kg to a maximum of 2 g. This regimen, however, is unsuitable for pharyngeal gonorrhea[238].

Disseminated gonococcal infection

Ceftriaxone is the treatment of choice, being given in a dose of 50 mg/kg as a single intramuscular or intravenous injection daily for 7 days; the maximum daily dose in children who weigh less than 45 kg should be 1 g, and in heavier children it should be 2 g[237].

Test of cure

After treatment every patient should be carefully examined to ensure that the infection has been cured. It is often difficult to distinguish between treatment failure and re-infection. By convention, the finding of positive tests within 2 weeks of treatment is regarded as treatment failure if the patient does not admit to further sexual contact.

Follow-up tests in the male

The majority of men with urethral gonorrhea are symptomatic, and with successful treatment symptoms resolve rapidly. Such resolution of symptoms, however, does not always equate with treatment success. In one study, it was found that 78 (1.9%) of 4080 symptomatic men who became asymptomatic 3 to 7 days after treatment had persistent infection[243]. Of 582 men who remained symptomatic after therapy, 103 (17.7%) had a positive culture for *N. gonorrhoeae*. It is therefore clear that if microbiological tests of cure had not been undertaken in all men after treatment, 43% of infections would not have been recognized as treatment failures. Although there are cost implications – in the early 1980s it has been estimated that at least $4,900 had to be spent to diagnose and cure each case of asymptomatic treatment failure[244], the authors consider it prudent to offer post-treatment testing of men with gonococcal urethritis even when they have become asymptomatic. In the case of men who were asymptomatic at the time of presentation, cure can only be established by undertaking a test after completion of therapy. The timing of the test of cure depends on the antibiotic used for treatment, but 72 hours is considered ideal[245].

Cure of rectal gonorrhea in men is not as certain as that of urethral gonorrhea, and test of cure is recommended. As 7% of infections at this site will not be identified if only one test is undertaken[111], it is the authors' practice to obtain two tests of cure at an interval of 7 days.

As treatment failure of pharyngeal gonorrhea is common – in a review of published therapeutic trials, only 79.2% of men with infection at this site were cured with standard antimicrobial treatment[239], tests of cure are mandatory. If only one test is taken for the diagnosis of pharyngeal gonorrhea, 25% of infections at this site will be missed[111]. Two tests of cure therefore should be performed at an interval of 7 days.

Follow-up tests in the female

As a single test may fail to identify up to 9% of infected women, two consecutive series of cultures from the urethra, cervix, and rectum should be taken at weekly intervals, the first test being performed 72 hours after completion of treatment. The case for routinely sampling the anorectum in assessing cure is strengthened by the study of Schroeter and Reynolds[246] who found that about a third of treatment failures in women would have been missed if only cervical material had been cultured. If positive on first attendance, the culture from the pharynx should be taken twice, at 1 week and at 2 weeks after treatment.

Treatment when diagnosis of gonorrhea is suspected on epidemiological grounds

Accurate diagnosis and treatment is the approach of choice when adequate facilites exist. Treatment before diagnosis is not desirable as a routine, even in contacts, except when there are special problems. For example, a contact of a known case of gonorrhea may be treated if unlikely to re-attend. In such a case a form of treatment known to produce high cure rates (say 95%) in the locality where the infection has been acquired may be justified. Follow-up with tests of cure should also be offered and, of course, partner notification should always be undertaken.

Prevention of gonorrhea

CONDOM USE

The use of condoms has been shown to reduce transmission of *N. gonorrhoeae* (see Chapter 2).

PREVENTION OF GONOCOCCAL OPHTHALMIA NEONATORUM

Towards the end of the nineteenth century, at a time when gonorrhea was the leading cause of blindness amongst European children, Crede introduced the practice of cleaning the neonate's eyes, followed by installation of a drop of silver nitrate solution into each conjunctival sac. As a result, the incidence of eye infection and blindness declined dramatically[247]. In countries such as the UK where the incidence of gonococcal ophthalmia is low, prophylaxis is not usually undertaken. Where the prevalence of gonorrhea is high, and in most states of the USA (where prophylaxis is required by law anyway), the installation of a prophylactic into the eyes of all newborn infants is recommended[237, 242]. When considered necessary, prophylaxis should be given as soon as possible after delivery, whether this was vaginal or by cesarean section. The infant's eyes should be carefully cleaned, and either silver nitrate solution (1% w/v), erythromycin ointment (0.5% w/w), or tetracycline ophthalmic ointment (1% w/w) should be applied once to each eye. The efficacy of silver nitrate and tetracycline prophyaxis was shown in a study from Nairobi, Kenya, involving more than 27 300 neonates[248]. Compared with historical controls, the incidence of gonococcal ophthalmia decreased 83% among infants treated with silver nitrate, and 93% among those treated with tetracycline. As silver nitrate can cause conjunctival irritation in a substantial number of children, many clinicians prefer to use tetracycline ointment for prophylaxis. Erythromycin also appears to be effective in prophylaxis against gonococcal ophthalmia, but efficacy in high-risk populations has not been fully assessed[249].

Although the installation of povidone iodine ophthalmic solution has been shown to be as effective in prophylaxis against gonococcal ophthalmia in a study from Kenya[250], there is insufficient experience to recommend it as a first-line prophylactic agent.

Infants born to mothers with untreated gonorrhea are at high risk of infection, and treatment with ceftriaxone is recommended (see page 347 for the dosage).

VACCINES

The various aspects of gonococcal vaccine development have been reviewed elsewhere[251, 252]. The following antigens have received the most attention as potential gonococcal vaccine candidates.

Pili

Anti-pilus antisera is known to reduce the adhesion of both piliated gonococci and purified pili to epithelial cells, opsonize gonococci for phagocytosis by polymorpho-nuclear leukocytes, and protect tissue-cultured cells form the cytotoxic effect of challenge with gonococci. Human volunteer studies demonstrated that immunization with pili protects against infection with the homologous but not heterologous strains of gonococci. These results, which are almost certainly due to the antigenic diversity of gonococcal pili, make the development of an effective pilus vaccine unlikely. Although pilin proteins have conserved regions as well as variable regions, the conserved regions (which would be the target of a vaccine) are buried deep in the interior of the pilus and are not accessible to antibodies[1].

Opa protein (PII)

The marked phase and antigenic variation of these proteins make them unattractive as vaccine candidates.

PI

Antibody to PI acquired during infection is bactericidal and prevents repeated attacks of salpingitis due to strains with the same type of PI[24]. Although evidence of serovar-specific immunity to uncomplicated mucosal infection has been suggested[42] this was not confirmed by others[43]. Any vaccine based on PI would have to contain a cocktail of PI molecules from gonococci of different serovars. Other limitations in the use of a PI vaccine include contamination of PI with small amounts of PIII; this may give rise to blocking antibodies that nullify the bactericidal effect of the anti-PIi antibodies. Sialylation of LOS abolishes the bactericidal effect of anti-PI antibodies by partially blocking surface exposure of PI epitopes and also by inhibiting complement activation. In spite of this Barbosa-Cesnik et al.[252] considered PI to be the most attractive candidate antigen owing to its relatively limited antigenic variation. The use of a recombinant vector such as *Salmonella typhimurium* expressing PI has potential as an oral vaccine that would stimulate both mucosal and humoral immunity.

PIII

Although PIII is highly immunogenic, its ability to produce blocking antibodies as described above may render an individual vaccinated with this antigen more vulnerable to the development of systemic infection.

References

1 Salyers AA, Whitt DD. *Neisseria gonorrhoeae*. In: *Bacterial Pathogenesis: A Molecular Approach*. Washington DC; American Society for Microbiology: 1994, pp. 244–259.

2 Harkness AH. The pathology of gonorrhoea. *Br J Vener Dis* 1948; **56**: 227–229.

3 Makino S, van Putten JP, Meyer TF. Phase variation of the opacity outer membrane protein controls invasion by *Neisseria gonorrhoeae* into human epithelial cells. *EMBO J* 1991; **10**: 1307–1315.

4 Meyer TF. Pathogenic neisseriae: Complexity of pathogen–host cell interplay. *Clin Infect Dis* 1999; **28**: 433–441.

5 Danielsson D. Biology of *Neisseria gonorrhoeae*. In: Oriel JD, Harris JRW (eds) *Recent Advances in Sexually Transmitted Diseases*. Edinburgh; Churchill Livingstone: 1986, pp. 1–21.

6 Mosleh IM, Boxberger HJ, Sessler MJ, Meyer TF. Experimental infection of native human ureteral tissue with *Neisseria gonorrhoeae*: Adhesion, invasion, intracellular fate, exocytosis, and passage through a stratified epithelium. *Infect Immun* 1997; **65**: 3391–3398.

7 Novotny P, Short JA, Hughes M, *et al.* Studies on the mechanism of pathogenicity of *Neisseria gonorrhoeae*. *J Med Microbiol* 1977; **10**: 347–363.

8 Jephcott AE. Gonorrhoea, chancroid and granuloma venereum. In: Collier L, Balows A, Sussman M (eds). *Topley and Wilson's Microbiology and Microbial Infections* vol. 3, 9th edition. London; Arnold Publishing: 1998, pp. 623–640.

9 Heckels JE, Blackett B, Everson JS, Ward ME. The influence of surface charge on the attachment of *Neisseria gonorrhoeae* to human cells. *J Gen Microbiol* 1976; **96**: 359–364.

10 Kallstrom H, Liszewski MK, Atkinson JP, Jonsson AB. Membrane cofactor protein (MCP or CD46) is a cellular pilus receptor for pathogenic Neisseria. *Mol Microbiol* 1997; **25**: 639–647.

11 Jawetz, Melnick and Adelberg. The Neisseriae. In: Brooks GF, Butel JS, Morse SA (eds) *Medical Microbiology* 4th edition. Connecticut; Appleton and Lange: 1998, pp. 258–266.

12 Seifert HS, Wright CJ, Jerse AE, Cohen MS, Cannon JG. Multiple gonococcal pili variants are produced during experimental infections. *J Clin Invest* 1994; **93**: 2744–2749.

13 Jonsson A-B, Liver D *et al.* Sequence changes in the pilus subunit lead to tropism variation of *Neisseria gonorrhoeae* to human tissue. *Mol Microbiol* 1994; **13**: 407–416.

14 Ilver D, Kallstrom H, Normark, S, Jonsson AB. Transcellular passage of *Neisseria gonorrhoeae* involves pilus phase variation. *Infect Immun* 1998; **66**: 469–473.

15 Kellogg DS, Cohen IR, Norins LC, Schroeter AL, Reisling G. *Neisseria gonorrhoeae* II. Colonial variation and pathogenicity during 35 months in vitro. *J Bacteriol* 1968; **96**: 596–605.

16 Swanson J. Outer membrane variants of *Neisseria gonorrhoeae*. In: Brooks GF, Gotschlich EC, Holmes KK, Sawyer WD, Young FE (eds) *Immunobiology of Neisseria gonorrhoeae*. Washington DC; American Society for Microbiology: 1978, pp. 130–137.

17 Stern A, Meyer TF. Common mechanism controlling phase and antigenic variation in pathogenic Neisseriae. *Mol Microbiol* 1987; **15**: 531–541.

18 Zak K, Diaz JL, Jackson D, Heckels JE. Antigenic variation during infection with *Neisseria gonorrhoeae*: detection of antibodies to surface proteins in sera of patients with gonorrhoea. *J Infect Dis* 1984; **149**: 166–174.

19 James JF, Swanson J. Studies on gonococcus infection XIII. Occurrence of colour/opacity colonial variants in clinical cultures. *Infect Immun* 1978; **19**: 332–340.

20 Sandstrom EG, Chen KCS, Buchanan TM. Serology of *Neisseria gonorrhoeae*. Coagglutination serogroups WI and WII/III correspond to different outer membrane protein I molecules. *Infect Immun* 1982; **38**: 462–470.

21 Gotschlich EC, Seiff ME, Blake MS, Koomey M. Porin protein of *Neisseria gonorrhoeae*; cloning and gene structure. *Proc Natl Acad Sci USA* 1987; **84**: 8135–8139.

22 Cooke SJ, Jolley K, Ison, CA, Young H, Heckels JE. Naturally occurring isolates of *Neisseria gonorrhoeae*, which display

anomalous serovar properties, express PIA/PIB hybrid porins, deletions in PIE or novel PIA molecules. *FEMS Microbiol Lett* 1998; **162**: 75–82.

23 Blake MS, Gotschlich EC. Functional and immunologic properties of pathogenic *Neisseria* surface proteins. In: Inouye M (ed.) *Bacterial Outer Membranes as Model Systems*. New York; Wiley: 1987, pp. 377–400.

24 Buchanan TM, Eschenbach DA, Knapp JS, Holmes KK. Gonococcal salpingitis is less likely to recur with *Neisseria gonorrhoeae* of the same principal outer membrane protein antigenic type. *Am J Obstet Gynecol* 1980; **138**: 978–980.

25 Wolff K, Stern A. Identification and characterisation of specific sequences encoding pathogenicity associated proteins in the genome of commensal *Neisseria* species. *FEMS Microbiology Letters* 1995; **125**: 255–264.

26 Klugman KP, Gotschlich EC, Blake MS. Sequence of the structural gene (rmpM) for the class 4 outer membrane protein of *Neisseria meningitidis*, homology of the protein to gonococcal protein III and *Escherichia coli* OmpA, and construction of meningococcal strains that lack class 4 proteins. *Infect Immun* 1989; **57**: 2066–2071.

27 Blake MS, Wetzler LM *et al.* Protein III: structure, function and genetics. *Clin Microbiol Rev* 1989; **2** (Suppl): S60–S63.

28 Rice PA, McQuillen DP, Mcquillen DP, *et al.* Serum resistance of *Neisseria gonorrhoeae*. Does it thwart the inflammatory response and facilitate the transmission of infection? *Ann NY Acad Sci* 1994; **730**: 7–14.

29 Mintz CS, Apicella MA, Morse SA. Electrophoretic and serological characteristics of the lipooligosaccharide produced by *Neisseria gonorrhoeae*. *J Infect Dis* 1984; **149**: 544–552.

30 Rice PA, Kasper DL. Characterisation of gonococcal antigens responsible for induction of bactericidal antibody in disseminated infection. *J Clin Invest* 1977; **60**: 1149–1158.

31 Parsons NJ, Boons GJ, Ashton PR. Lactic acid is the factor in blood cell extracts which enhances the ability of CMP-NANA to sialylate gonococcal lipooligosaccharide

and induce serum resistance. *Microbiol Pathogenesis* 1996; **20**: 87–100.

32 Apicella MA, Shero M, Jarvis GA, Griffiss JM, Mandrell RE, Schneider H. Phenotypic variation in epitope expression of the *Neisseria gonorrhoeae* lipooligosaccharide. *Infect Immun* 1987; **55**: 1755–1761.

33 Gotschlich EC. Genetic locus for the biosynthesis of the variable portion of *Neisseria gonorrhoeae* lipooligosaccharide. *J Exp Med* 1994; **180**: 2181–2190.

33a Apicella MA, Mandrell RE, Shero M, *et al*. Modification by sialic acid of *Neisseria gonorrhoeae* lipooligosaccharide epitope expression in human urethral exudates: an immunoelectron microscopic analysis. *J Infect Dis* 1990; **162**: 506–512.

34 Johannsen DB, Johnston DM, Koymen HO, Cohen MS, Cannon JGA. *Neisseria gonorrhoeae* immunoglobulin A1 protease mutant is infectious in the human challenge model of urethral infection. *Infect Immun* 1999; **67**: 3009–3013.

35 Morse SA, Genco CA. Neisseria. In: *Topley & Wilson's Neisseria Microbiology and Microbial Infections* vol. 2, 9th edition. London; Arnold Publishing: 1998, pp. 877–899.

36 Watt PJ, Medlen AR. Generation of chemotaxins by gonococci. In: Brooks GF, Gotschlich EC, Holmes KK, Sawyer WD, Young FE (eds) *Immunobiology of Neisseria gonorrhoeae*. Washington DC; American Society for Microbiology: 1978, pp. 239–241.

37 Casey SG, Shafer WM, Spitznagel JK. *Neisseria gonorrhoeae* survive intraleukocytic oxygen-independent antimicrobial capacities of anaerobic and aerobic granulocytes in the presence of pyocin lethal for extracellular gonococci. *Infect Immun* 1986; **52**: 384–389.

38 Cohen IR. Natural and immune human antibodies reactive with antigens of virulent *Neisseria gonorrhoeae*: immunoglobulins G, M and A. *J Bacteriol* 1967; **94**: 141–148.

39 Schoolnik GK, Ochs HD, Buchanan TM. Immunoglobulin class responsible for gonococcal bactericidal activity of normal human sera. *J Immunol* 1979; **122**: 1771–1779.

40 Lammel CJ, Sweet RL, Rice PA, *et al*. Antibody-antigen specificity in the immune response to infection with *Neisseria gonorrhoeae*. *J Infect Dis* 1985; **152**: 990–1001.

41 Brooks GF, Lammel CJ. Humoral immune response to gonococcal infections. *Clin Microbiol Rev* 1989; **2** (Suppl) S5–S10.

42 Plummer FA, Simonsen JN, Chubb H, *et al*. Epidemiologic evidence for the development of serovar-specific immunity after gonococcal infection. *J Clin Invest* 1989; **83**: 1472–1476.

43 Ross JDC, Moyes A, Young H. Serovar specific immunity to *Neisseria gonorrhoeae*: Does it exist? *Genitourin Med* 1995; **71**: 367–369.

44 Buchanan TM, Eschenbach DA, Knapp JS, Holmes KK. Gonococcal salpingitis is less likely to recur with *Neisseria gonorrhoeae* of the same principal outer membrane protein antigenic type. *Am J Obstet Gynecol* 1980; **138**: 978–980.

45 Hedges SR, Mayo MS, Mestecky J, Hook EW, Russell MW. Limited local and systemic antibody responses to *Neisseria gonorrhoeae* during uncomplicated genital infections. *Infect Immun* 1999; **67**: 3937–3946.

46 Simpson SD, Ho Y, Rice PA, Wetzler LM. T lymphocyte response to *Neisseria gonorrhoeae* porin in individuals with mucosal gonococcal infections. *J Infect Dis* 1999; **180**: 762–773.

47 Crawford G, Knapp JS, Hale J, Holmes KK. Asymptomatic gonorrhea in men: caused by gonococci with unique nutritional requirements. *Science* 1977; **196**: 1352–1353.

48 Knapp JS, Holmes KK. Disseminated gonococcal infections caused by *Neisseria gonorrhoeae* with unique nutritional requirements. *J Infect Dis* 1975; **132**: 204–208.

49 O'Brien JP, Goldenberg DL, Rice PA. Disseminated gonococcal infection: a prospective analysis of 49 patients and a review of pathophysiology and immune mechanisms. *Medicine* 1987; **62**: 395–406.

50 Rompalo AM, Hook EW, Roberts PL, Ramsey PG, Handsfield HH, Holmes KK. The acute arthritis-dermatitis syndrome. The changing importance of *Neisseria gonorrhoeae* and *Neisseria meningitidis*. *Arch Intern Med* 1987; **147**; 281–283.

51 Rice PA, Goldenberg DL. Clinical manifestations of disseminated infection caused by *Neisseria gonorrhoeae* are linked to differences in bactericidal reactivity of infecting strains. *Ann Intern Med* 1980; **95**: 175–178.

52 Schoolnik GK, Buchanan TM, Holmes KK. Gonococci causing disseminated infection are resistant to the bactericidal action of normal human serum. *J Clin Invest* 1976; **58**: 1163–1173.

53 Wiesner PJ, Tronca E, Bonin P, Pedresen AHB, Holmes KK. Clinical spectrum of pharyngeal gonococcal infection. *N Engl J Med* 1973; **288**: 181–185.

54 Wise CM, Morris CR, Wasilauskas BL, Salzer WL. Gonococcal arthritis in an era of increasing penicillin resistance. Presentations and outcomes in 41 recent cases. *Arch Intern Med* 1994; **154**: 2690–2695.

55 Harriman GR, Podak ER, Braude AI, Corbeil LC, Essex AF, Curd JG. Activation of complement by serum-resistant *Neisseria gonorrhoeae*. *J Exp Med* 1982; **156**: 1235–1249.

56 Petersen BH, Lee TJ, Snyderman R, Brooks GF. *Neisseria meningitidis* and *Neisseria gonorrhoeae* bacteremia associated with C6, C7, or C8 deficiency. *Ann Intern Med* 1979; **90**: 917–920.

57 Gerbase AC, Rowley JT, Heymann DHL, Berkley SFB, Piot P. Global prevalence and incidence estimates of selected curable STDs. *Sex Transm Inf* 1998; **74** (Suppl. 1): S12–S16.

58 Van der Heyden JH, Catchpole MA, Paget WJ, Stroobant A. Trends in gonorrhoea in nine western European countries, 1991–1996. European Study Group. *Sex Transm Inf* 2000; **76**: 110–116.

59 PHLS, DHSS&PS and the Scottish ISD(D)5 Collaborative Group. *Trends in Sexually Transmitted Infections in the United Kingdom, 1990–1999*. London: Public Health Laboratory Service: 2000.

60 Centers for Disease Control and Prevention. Gonorrhea – United States, 1998. *MMWR* 2000; **49**: 538–542.

61 Paris M, Gotuzzo E, Goyzueta G, *et al*. Prevalence of gonococcal and chlamydial infections in commercial sex workers in a Peruvian Amazon city. *Sex Transm Dis* 1999; **26**: 103–107.

62 Ndoye I, Mboup S, De Schryver A, *et al*. Diagnosis of sexually transmitted infections in female prostitutes in Dakar, Senegal. *Sex Transm Inf* 1998; **74** (Suppl. 1): S112–S117.

63 Fennema JS, Cairo I, Coutinho RA. Substantial increase in gonorrhoea and syphilis among clients of Amsterdam sexually transmitted diseases clinic. *Ned Tijd Geneeskunde* 2000; **144**: 602–603.

64 Centers for Disease Control and Prevention. Sexually Transmitted Disease Surveillance 1998 Supplement: *Gonococcal Isolate Surveillance Project (GISP) Annual Report – 1998*. Division of STD Prevention, Department of Health and Human Services, Public Health Service, Atlanta: 1999.

65 Barlow D, Nayyar K, Phillips I, Barrow J. Diagnosis of gonorrhoea in women. *Br J Vener Dis* 1976; **52**: 326–328.

66 Chipperfield EJ, Catterall RD. Reappraisal of Gram-staining and cultural techniques for the diagnosis of gonorrhoea in women. *Br J Vener Dis* 1976; **52**; 36–39.

67 Evans BA. Detection of gonorrhoea in women. *Br J Vener Dis* 1976; **52**: 40–42.

68 Holmes KK, Johnson DW, Trostle HJ. An estimate of the risk of men acquiring gonorrhea by sexual contact with infected females. *Am J Epidemiol* 1970; **91**: 170–174.

69 Hooper RR, Reynolds GH, Jones OG, *et al*. Cohort study of venereal disease. I. The risk of gonorrhea transmission from

infected women to men. *Am J Epidemiol* 1978; **108**: 136–144.

70 Blackwell CC, Winstanley FP, Weir DM, Kinane DF. Host–parasite interactions influencing susceptibility to diseases caused by the pathogenic *Neisseria* species. In: Schoolnik GK, Brooks GF, Falkow S, Frasch E, Knapp JS, McCutchan JA, Morse SA (eds) *The Pathogenic Neisseriae*. Washington DC; American Society for Microbiology: 1985, pp. 452–455.

71 Tramont EC, Boslego JW, Chung R, *et al*. In: Schoolnik GK, Brooks GF, Falkow S, Frasch E, Knapp JS, McCutchan JA, Morse SA (eds) *The Pathogenic Neisseriae*. Washington DC; American Society for Microbiology: 1985, pp. 316–322.

72 Young H, Sarafian SK, Harris AB, McMillan A. Non-cultural detection of *Neisseria gonorrhoeae* in cervical and vaginal washings. *J Med Microbiol* 1983; **16**: 183–191.

73 Sherrard J, Barlow D. Gonorrhoea in men: clinical and diagnositc aspects. *Genitourin Med* 1996; **72**: 422–426.

74 Wallin J. Gonorrhoea in 1972. A 1-year study of patients attending the VD Unit in Uppsala. *Br J Vener Dis* 1975; **51**: 41–47.

75 Soendjojo A. Gonococcal urethritis due to fellatio. *Sex Transm Dis* 1983; **10**: 41–42.

76 McMillan A, Young H, Moyes A. Rectal gonorrhoea in homosexual men: source of infection. *Int J STD AIDS* 2000; **11**: 284–287.

77 Bhattacharyya MN, Jephcott AE. Detection of gonorrhoea in women. Role of the rectal sample. *Br J Vener Dis* 1974; **50**: 109–112.

77a Laga M, Plummer FA, Nzanze H, *et al*. Epidemiology of ophthalmia neonatorum in Kenya. *Lancet* 1986; **ii**: 1145–1149.

78 Wasserheit JN. Epidemiological synergy: interrelationships between human immunodeficiency virus and other sexually transmitted diseases. *Sex Transm Dis* 1992; **19**: 61–77.

79 Laga M, Manoka A, Kivuvu M, *et al*. Non-ulcerative sexually transmitted diseases as risk factors for HIV-1 transmission in women: results from a cohort study. *AIDS* 1993; **7**: 95–102.

80 Beck EJ, Mandalia S, Leonard K, Griffith RJ, Harris JRW, Miller DL. Case–control study of sexually transmitted diseases as cofactors for HIV-1 transmission. *Int J STD AIDS* 1996; **7**: 34–38.

81 Craib KJP, Meddings DR, Strathdee SA, *et al*. Rectal gonorrhoea as an independent risk factor for HIV infection in a cohort of homosexual men. *Genitourin Med* 1995; **71**: 150–154.

82 Grosskurth H, Mosha F, Todd J, *et al*. Impact of improved treatment of sexually transmitted diseases on HIV infection in rural Tanzania: randomised controlled trial. *Lancet* 1995; **346**: 530–536.

83 Mostad SB, Overbaugh J, DeVange D, *et al*. Hormonal contraception, vitamin A deficiency, and other risk factors for shedding of HIV-1 infected cells from the cervix and vagina. *Lancet* 1997; **350**: 922–927.

84 Garnett GP, Anderson RM. Strategies for limiting the spread of HIV in developing countries: conclusions based on studies of the transmission dynamics of the virus. *JAIDS* 1995; **9**: 500–513.

85 Moss GB, Overbaugh J, Welch M, *et al*. Human immunodeficiency virus DNA in urethral secretions in men: association with gonococcal urethritis and CD4 cell depletion. *J Infect Dis* 1995; **172**: 1469–1474.

86 Atkins MC, Carlin EM, Emery VC, Griffiths PD, Boag F. Fluctuations of HIV load in semen of HIV positive patients with newly acquired sexually transmitted diseases. *Br Med J* 1996; **313**: 341–342.

87 Cohen MS, Hoffman IF, Royce RA, *et al*. Reduction of concentration of HIV-1 in semen after treatment of urethritis: implications for prevention of sexual transmission of HIV-1. *Lancet* 1997; **349**: 1868–1873.

88 Stolz E, Schuller J. Gonococcal oro- and nasopharyngeal infection. *Br J Vener Dis* 1974; **50**: 104–108.

89 McMillan A, McNeillage G, Gilmour HM, Lee FD. Histology of rectal gonorrhoea in men, with a note on anorectal infection with *Neisseria meningitidis*. *J Clin Pathol* 1983; **36**: 511–514.

90 Osoba AO, Alausa O. Gonococcal urethral stricture and watering-can perineum. *Br J Vener Dis* 1976; **52**: 387–393.

91 Holmes KK, Counts GW, Beaty HN. Disseminated gonococcal infection. Clinical review. *Ann Intern Med* 1971; **74**: 979–993.

92 Bayer AS. Gonococcal arthritis syndromes: an update on diagnosis and management. *Postgrad Med* 1980; **67**: 200–204 and 207–208.

93 Muralidhar B, Rumore PM, Steinman CR. Use of the polymerase chain reaction to study arthritis due to *Neisseria gonorrhoeae*. *Arthritis Rheum* 1994; **37**: 710–717.

94 Ackerman AB, Miller RC, Shapiro L. Gonococcemia and its cutaneous manifestations. *Arch Dermatol* 1965; **91**: 227–232.

95 Seifert MH, Warin AP, Miller A. Articular and cutaneous manifestations of gonorrhoea. *Ann Rheum Dis* 1974; **33**: 140–146.

96 Barr J, Danielsson D. Septic gonococcal dermatitis. *Br Med J* 1971; **i**: 482–485.

97 Sayeed ZA, Bhaduri U, Howell E, Meyers HL. Gonococcal meningitis. A review. *JAMA* 1972; **219**: 1730–1731.

98 John JF, Nichols JT, Eisenhower EA, Farrar WE. Gonococcal endocarditis. *Sex Transm Dis* 1977; **4**: 84–88.

99 Williams RH. Gonococcal endocarditis. A study of twelve cases with ten postmortem examinations. *Arch Int Med* 1938; **61**: 26–38.

100 Holmes KK, Counts GW, Beaty HN. Disseminated gonococcal infection. Clinical review. *Ann Intern Med* 1971; **74**: 979–993.

101 Kohen DP. Neonatal gonococcal arthritis: three cases and review of the literature. *Pediatrics* 1974; **53**: 436–440.

102 Brook I, Rodriguez WJ, Controni G, Gold B. Gonococcal scalp abscess in a newborn. *South Med J* 1980; **73**: 396–397.

103 Nelson JD, Mohs E, Dajani AS, Plotkin SA. Gonorrhea in preschool- and school-aged children. Report of the Prepubertal Gonorrhea Cooperative Study Group. *JAMA* 1976; **236**: 1359–1364.

104 Jephcott AE. Microbiological diagnosis of gonorrhoea. *Genitourin Med* 1997; **73**: 245–252.

105 Liebling MR, Arkfeld DG, Michelini GA, *et al*. Identification of *Neisseria gonorrhoeae* in synovial fluid using the polymerase chain reaction. *Arthritis Rheum* 1994; **37**: 702–709.

106 Catterall RD. Diagnosis of vaginal discharge. *Br J Vener Dis* 1970; **46**: 122–124.

107 Thin RN, Williams IA, Nicol CS. Direct and delayed methods of immunofluorescent diagnosis of gonorrhoea in women. *Br J Vener Dis* 1971; **47**: 27–30.

108 Young H. Cultural diagnosis of gonorrhoea with modified New York City (MNYC) medium. *Br J Vener Dis* 1978; **54**: 36–40.

109 Norins LC. The case for gonococcal serology. *J Infect Dis* 1974; **230**: 677–679.

110 Bhattacharyya MN, Jephcott AE, Morton RS. Diagnosis of gonorrhoea in women: comparison of sampling sites. *Br Med J* 1973; **ii**: 748–750.

111 McMillan A, Young H. Gonorrhea in homosexual men: frequency of infection by culture site. *Sex Transm Dis* 1978; **5**: 146–150.

112 Young H, Moyes A, Ross JDC. Pharyngeal gonorrhoea: an increase in clinical and microbiological significance? In: Conde-Glez CJ, Morse S, Rice P, Sparling F, Calderon E (eds) *Pathobiology and Immunobiology of Neisseriaceae*. Mexico; Instituto Nacional de Salud Publica: 1994, pp. 140–141.

113 Duguid JP. Neisseria: Staining methods. In: Collee JG, Fraser AG, Marmion BP, Simmons A (eds) *Mackie and McCartney Practical Medical Microbiology*. New York; Churchill Livingstone: 1996, pp. 793–812.

114 Jacobs NF, Kraus SJ. Gonococcal and non-gonococcal urethritis in men. Clinical and laboratory differentiation. *Ann Intern Med* 1975; **82**: 7–12.

115 Goodhart ME, Ogden J, Zaidi AA, Kraus SJ. Factors affecting the performance of smear

and culture tests for the detection of *Neisseria gonorrhoeae*. *Sex Transm Dis* 1982; **9**: 63–69.

116 Barlow D, Phillips I. Gonorrhoea in women. Diagnostic, clinical and laboratory aspects. *Lancet* 1978; **I**: 761–764.

117 Thin RN, Shaw EJ. Diagnosis of gonorrhoea in women. *Br J Vener Dis* 1979; **55**: 10–13.

118 Mirret S, Keller LB, Knapp JS. *Neisseria gonorrhoeae* strains inhibited by vancomycin in selective media and correlation with auxotype. *J Clin Microbiol* 1981; **14**: 94–99.

119 Windall JJ, Hall MM, Washington JA, Douglass TJ, Weed LA. Inhibitory effect of vancomycin on *Neisseria gonorrhoeae* in Thayer-Martin medium. *J Infect Dis* 1980; **142**: 775.

120 Evans JK, Mercey DE, French PD, Prince, MV. Audit of diagnosis of gonorrhoea at first visit to a London genitourinary medicine clinic. *Genitourin Med* 1994; **70**: 291–292.

121 Edwards S, Dockerty G. Diagnosis of gonorrhoea by microscopy. *Genitourin Med* 1995; **71**: 200–201.

122 Oxtoby MJ, Arnold AJ, Zaidi AA, Kleris GS, Kraus SJ. Potential shortcuts in the laboratory diagnosis of gonorrhea: a single stain for smears and nonremoval of cervical secretions before obtaining test specimens. *Sex Transm Dis* 1982; **9**: 59–62.

123 Seth A. Use of trimethoprim to prevent overgrowth by *Proteus* in the cultivation of *N. gonorrhoeae*. *Br J Vener Dis* 1970; **46**: 201–202.

124 Martin JE, Armstrong JH, Smith PB. New system for cultivation of *Neisseria gonorrhoeae*. *Appl Microbiol* 1974; **27**: 802–808.

125 Martin JE, Lewis JS. Anisomycin: improved antimycotic activity in modified Thayer-Martin medium. *Pub Health Lab* 1977; **35**: 53–60.

126 Faur YC, Weisburd MH, Wilson ME, May PS. A new medium for the isolation of pathogenic *Neisseria* (NYC medium). I. Formulation and comparisons with standard media. *Health Lab Sci* 1973; **10**: 44–54.

127 Young H. Advances in routine laboratory procedures for diagnosis of gonorrhoea. In: Harris JRW (ed) *Recent Advances in Sexually Transmitted Diseases 2*. Edinburgh; Churchill Livingstone: 1981, pp. 59–71.

128 Svarva PL, Maeland JA. Comparison of two selective media in the cultural diagnosis of gonorrhoea. *Acta Pathol Microbiol Scand* 1979; **87B**: 391–392.

129 Holmes KK, Counts GW, Beaty HN. Disseminated gonococcal infection. Clinical review. *Ann Intern Med* 1971; **74**: 979–993.

130 Lawton WD, Koch LW. Comparison of commercially available New York City and Thayer-Martin medium for recovery of *Neisseria gonorrhoeae* from clinical specimens. *J Clin Microbiol* 1982; **18**: 1264–1265.

131 Young H, Moyes A. An evaluation of pre-poured selective media for the isolation of *Neisseria gonorrhoeae*. *J Med Microbiol* 1996; **44**: 253–260.

132 Bonin P, Tanino TT, Handsfield HH. Isolation of *Neisseria gonorrhoeae* on selective and non-selective media in a sexually transmitted diseases clinic. *J Clin Microbiol* 1984; **19**: 218–220.

133 Ratner HB, Tinsley H, Keller RE, Stratton CW. Comparison of the effect of refrigerated versus room temperature media on the isolation of *Neisseria gonorrhoea* from genital specimens. *J Clin Microbiol* 1985; **21**: 127–128.

134 Beverly A, Bailey-Griffin JR, Schwebke JR. In tray GC medium versus modified Thayer-Martin agar plates for diagnosis of gonorrhoea from endocervical specimens. *J Clin Microbiol* 2000; **38**: 3825–3826.

135 Human RP, Jones GA. Survival of bacteria in swab transport packs. *Med Lab Sci* 1986; **43**: 14–18.

136 Olsen CC, Schwebke JR, Benjamin WH, Beverly A, Waites KB. Comparison of direct inoculation and Copan transport systems for isolation of *Neisseria gonorrhoeae* from endocervical specimens. *J Clin Microbiol* 1999; **37**: 3583–3585.

137 Ebright JR, Smith KE, Drexler L, Ivsin R, Krogstad S, Farmer SG. Evaluation of modified Stuart's medium in culturettes for transport of *Neisseria gonorrhoeae*. *Sex Transm Dis* 1982; **9**: 44–47.

138 Martin JE, Lester A. Transgrow: a medium for transport and growth of *Neisseria gonorrhoeae* and *Neisseria meningitidis*. *Health Services and Mental Health Administration Report* 1971; **86**: 30–33.

139 Martin JE, Jackson RL. Biological environmental chamber for the culture of *Neisseria gonorrhoeae*. *J Am Vener Dis Assoc* 1975; **2**: 28–30.

140 Smeltzer MP, Curran JW, Brown ST, Pass J. Accuracy of presumptive criteria for culture diagnosis of *Neisseria gonorrhoeae* in low prevalence populations of women. *J Clin Microbiol* 1980; **11**: 485–487.

141 Fallon RJ, Young H. Neisseria: Acinetobacter: Moraxella (Branhamella) catarrhalis. In: Collee JG, Fraser AG, Marmion BP, Simmons A (eds) *Mackie and McCartney Practical Medical Microbiology*. New York; Churchill Livingstone: 1996, pp. 283–297.

142 Arko RJ, Odugbemi T. Superoxol and amylase inhibition tests for distinguishing gonococcal and nongonococcal cultures growing on selective media. *J Clin Microbiol* 1984; **20**: 1–4.

143 Knapp JS, Tam MR, Nowinski RC, Holmes KK, Sandstrom EG. Serological classification of *Neisseria gonorrhoeae* with use of monoclonal antibodies to gonococcal outer membrane protein I. *J Infect Dis* 1984; **150**: 44–48.

144 Saez-Nieto JA, Fenoll A, Vazquez J, Casal J. Prevalence of maltose-negative *Neisseria meningitidis* variants during an epidemic period in Spain. *J Clin Microbiol* 1982; **15**: 78–81.

145 Noble RC, Cooper RM. Meningococcal colonisation misdiagnosed as gonococcal pharyngeal infection. *Br J Vener Dis* 1979; **55**: 336–339.

146 Young H, Paterson IC, McDonald DR. Rapid carbohydrate utilisation test for the identification of *Neisseria gonorrhoeae*. *Br J Vener Dis* 1976; **52**: 172–175.

147 Tapsall JW, Cheng J. Rapid identification of pathogenic species of *Neisseria* by carbohydrate degradation tests: importance of glucose in media for preparation of inocula. *Br J Vener Dis* 1981; **57**: 249–252.

148 Robertson DHH, McMillan A, Young H. Diagnosis of gonorrhoea: laboratory and clinical procedures. In: *Clinical Practice in Sexually Transmissible Diseases*. Edinburgh; Churchill Livingstone: 1989.

149 Moyes A, Young H. Fluorescent monoclonal antibody test for the confirmation of *Neisseria gonorrhoeae*. *Med Lab Sci* 1989; **46**: 6–10.

150 Young H, Moyes A. Utility of monoclonal antibody coagglutination to identify *Neisseria gonorrhoeae*. *Genitourin Med* 1989; **65**: 8–13.

151 Beebe, JL, Rau MP, Flageolle S, Calhoon B, Knapp JS. Incidence of *Neisseria gonorrhoeae* isolates negative by Syva direct fluorescent-antibody test but positive by Gen-Probe accuprobe test in a sexually transmitted disease clinic population. *J Clin Microbiol* 1993; **31**: 2535–2537.

152 Turner A, Gough KR, Jephcott AE. Comparison of three methods for culture confirmation of *Neisseria gonorrhoeae* strains currently circulating in the UK. *J Clin Pathol* 1995; **48**: 919–923.

153 Young H, Harris AB, Tapsall JW. Differentiation of gonococcal and non-gonococcal neisseriae by the superoxol test. *Br J Vener Dis* 1984; **60**: 87–89.

154 Odugbemi T, Arko RJ. Differentiation of *Kingella denitrificans* from *Neisseria gonorrhoeae* by growth on semisolid medium and sensitivity to amylase. *J Clin Microbiol* 1983; **17**: 389–391.

155 Young H, Moyes A. Comparative evaluation of AccuProbe culture identification test for *Neisseria gonorrhoeae* and other rapid methods. *J Clin Microbiol* 1993; **31**: 1996–1999.

156 Stary A, Ching SF, Teodorowicz L., Lee H. Comparison of ligase chain reaction and culture for detection of *Neisseria gonorrhoeae* in genital and extragenital

specimens. *J Clin Microbiol* 1997; **35**: 239–242.

156a Hook EW, Ching SF, Stephens J, Hardy KF, Smith KR, Lee HH. Diagnosis of *Neisseria gonorrhoeae* infections in women by using the ligase chain reaction on patient-obtained vaginal swabs. *J Clin Microbiol* 1997; **35**: 2129–2132.

156b Buimer M, Vandoornum GJJ, Ching S, *et al*. Detection of *Chlamydia trachomatis* and *Neisseria gonorrhoeae* by ligase chain reaction-based assays with clinical specimens from various sites: implications for diagnostic testing and screening. *J Clin Microbiol* 1996; **34**: 2395–2400.

157 Carroll KC, Aldeen WE, Morrison M, Anderson R, Lee D, Mottice S. Evaluation of the Abbott LCx ligase chain reaction assay for detection of *Chlamydia trachomatis* and *Neisseria gonorrhoeae* in urine and genital swab specimens from a sexually transmitted disease clinic population. *J Clin Microbiol* 1998; **36**: 1630–1633.

158 Young H, Moyes A, McMillan A. Detection of Male Rectal and Pharyngeal Gonorrhoea by the Ligase Chain Reaction (LCR). International Congress of Sexually Transmitted Diseases, Seville; Spain: 1997.

158a Young H, Moyes A, McMillan A. Azithromycin and erythromycin resistant *Neisseria gonorrhoeae* following treatment with azithromycin. *Int J STD AIDS* 1997; **8**: 299–302.

159 Crotchfelt KA, Welsh LE, De Bonville D. Rosenstraus M, Quinn TC. Detection of *Neisseria gonorrhoeae* and *Chlamydia trachomatis* in genitourinary specimens from men and women by a coamplification PCR assay. *J Clin Microbiol* 1997; **35**: 1536–1540.

160 Martin DH, Cammarata C, van der Pol B, *et al*. Multicenter evaluation of Amplicor and automated Cobas Amplicor CT/NG tests for *Neisseria gonorrhoeae*. *J Clin Microbiol* 2000; **38**: 3544–3549.

161 Mukenge-Tshibaka L, Alary M, Bernier F, *et al*. Diagnostic performance of the Roche Amplicor PCR in detecting *Neisseria gonorrhoeae* in genitourinary specimens from female sex workers in Cotonou, Benin. *J Clin Microbiol* 2000; **38**: 4076–4079.

162 Palladino S, Pearman JW, Kay ID, *et al*. Diagnosis of *Chlamydia trachomatis* and *Neisseria gonorrhoeae* genitourinary infections in males by the Amplicor PCR assay of urine. *Diagn Microbiol Infect Dis* 1999; **33**: 141–146.

163 Farrell DJ. Evaluation of AMPLICOR *Neisseria gonorrhoeae* PCR using cppB nested PCR and 16S rRNA PCR. *J Clin Microbiol* 1999; **37**: 386–390.

164 Schachter J, Hook III EW, McCormack WM, *et al*. Ability of the Digene Hybrid Capture II test to identify *Chlamydia trachomatis* and

Neisseria gonorrhoeae in cervical specimens. *J Clin Microbiol* 1999; **37**: 3668–3671.

165 Modaress KJ, Cullen AP, Jaffurs WJ, *et al*. Detection of *Chlamydia trachomatis* and *Neisseria gonorrhoeae* in swab specimens by the hybrid capture II and PACE 2 nucleic acid probe test. *Sex Transm Dis* 1999; **26**: 303–308.

166 Lind I, Riou JY, Sng EH, Bentzon MW. *Antimicrobial Susceptibility Testing of* Neisseria gonorrhoeae: *Guidelines for Use of the WHO Reference Strains*. WHO Collaborating Centre for Reference and Research in Gonococci, Statens Seruminstitut; Copenhagen: 1984.

167 Sarubbi FA, Blackman E, Sparling PF. Genetic mapping of linked antibiotic resistance loci in *Neisseria gonorrhoeae*. *J Bacteriol* 1974; **120**: 1284–1292.

168 Sparling PF, Sarubbi FA, Blackman E. Inheritance of low-level resistance to penicillin, tetracycline and chloramphenicol in *Neisseria gonorrhoeae*. *J Bacteriol* 1975; **124**: 740–749.

169 Gill MJ, Simjee S, AlHattawi K, Robertson BD, Easmon CSF, Ison CA. Gonococcal resistance to beta-lactams and tetracycline involves mutation in loop 3 of the porin encoded at the penB locus. *Antimicrob Agents Chemother* 1998; **42**: 2799–2803.

170 Hagman KE, Lucas CE, Balthazar JT, *et al*. The MtrD protein of *Neisseria gonorrhoeae* is a member of the resistance/nodulation/division protein family constituting part of an efflux system. *Microbiology UK* 1997; **143**: 2117–2125.

171 Ison CA. Antimicrobial agents and gonorrhoea: Therapeutic choice, resistance and susceptibility testing. *Genitourin Med* 1996; **72**: 253–257.

172 Pan WB, Spratt BG. Regulation of the permeability of the gonococcal cell envelope by the Mtr system. *Mol. Microbiol* 1994; **11**: 769–775.

173 Maness MJ, Sparling PF. Multiple antibiotic resistance due to a single mutation in *Neisseria gonorrhoeae*. *J Infect Dis* 1973; **128**: 321–330.

174 Sarubbi FA, Sparling PF, Blackman E, Lewis E. Loss of low-level antibiotic resistance in *Neisseria gonorrhoeae* due to *env* mutations. *J Bacteriol* 1975; **124**: 750–756.

175 Pillay M, Chenia HY, Hoosen AA, Pillay B, Pillay D. A novel beta-lactamase plasmid in *Neisseria gonorrhoeae*. *Med Sci Res* 1997; **25**: 435–436.

176 Morse SA, Johnson SR, Biddle JW, Roberts MC. High-level tetracycline resistance in *Neisseria gonorrhoeae* is result of acquisition of streptococcal tetM determinant. *Antimicrob Agents Chemother* 1986; **30**: 664–670.

177 Chopra I, Hawley PM, Hinton M. Molecular mechanisms of tetracycline resistance in *Neisseria gonorrhoeae*. *Antimicrob Agents Chemother* 1992; **29**: 245–277.

178 Deguchi T, Yasuda M, Nakano M, *et al*. Quinolone-resistant *Neisseria gonorrhoeae*: correlation of alterations in the GyrA subunit of DNA gyrase and the ParC subunit of topoisomerase IV with antimicrobial susceptibility profiles. *Antimicrob Agents Chemother* 1996; **40**: 1020–1023.

179 Deguchi T, Yasuda M, Nakano M, *et al*. Rapid detection of point mutations of the *Neisseria gonorrhoeae* gyrA gene associated with decreased susceptibilities to quinolones. *J Clin Microbiol* 1996; **34**: 2255–2258.

180 Deguchi T, Yasuda M, Nakano M. Rapid screening of point mutations of the *Neisseria gonorrhoeae* parC gene associated with resistance to quinolones. *J Clin Microbiol* 1997; **35**: 948–950.

181 Belland RJ, Morrison SG, Ison C, Huang WM. *Neisseria gonorrhoeae* acquires mutations in analogous regions of gyrA and parC in fluoroquinolone-resistant isolates. *Mol Microbiol* 1994; **14**: 371–380.

182 Tanaka M, Nakayama H, Haraoka M, Saika T, Kobayashi I, Naito S. Antimicrobial resistance of *Neisseria gonorrhoeae* and high prevalence of ciprofloxacin-resistant isolates in Japan, 1993 to 1998. *J Clin Microbiol* 2000; **38**: 521–525.

183 Galimand M, Gerbaud G, Courvalin P. Spectinomycin resistance in *Neisseria* spp. due to mutations in 16S rRNA. *Antimicrob Agents Chemother* 2000; **44**: 1365–1366.

184 Ehret JM, Nims LJ, Judson FN. A clinical isolate of *Neisseria gonorrhoeae* with in vitro resistance to erythromycin and decreased susceptibility to azithromycin. *Sex Transm Dis* 1996; **23**: 270–272.

185 Fekete T. Antimicrobial susceptibility testing of *Neisseria gonorrhoeae* and implications for epidemiology and therapy. *Clin Microbiol Rev* 1993; **6**: 22–33.

186 Kiehlbauch JA, Hannett GE, Salfinger M, Archinal W, Monserrat C, Carlyn C. Use of the National Committee for Clinical Laboratory Standards Guidelines for disk diffusion susceptibility testing in New York State laboratories. *J Clin Microbiol* 2000; **38**: 3341–3348.

187 Mehaffey PC, Putnam SD, Barrett MS, Jones RN. Evaluation of in vitro spectra of activity of azithromycin, clarithromycin, and erythromycin tested against strains of *Neisseria gonorrhoeae* by reference agar dilution, disk diffusion, and E test methods. *J Clin Microbiol* 1996; **34**: 479–481.

188 Tapsall JW, Shultz TR, Limnios EA, Donovan B, Lum G, Mulhall BP. Failure of azithromycin therapy in gonorrhea and discorrelation with laboratory test parameters. *Sex Transm Dis* 1998; **25**: 505–508.

189 Jones RN, Gavan TL, Thornsberry C, *et al*. Standardization of disk diffusion and agar dilution susceptibility tests for *Neisseria*

gonorrhoeae: interpretive criteria and quality control guidelines for ceftriaxone, penicillin, spectinomycin, and tetracycline. *J Clin Microbiol* 1989; **27**: 2758–2766.

190 Guoming L, Qun C, Shengchun W. Resistance of *Neisseria gonorrhoeae* epidemic strains to antibiotics: report of resistant isolates and surveillance in Zhanjiang, China: 1998 to 1999. *Sex Transm Dis* 2000; **27**: 115–118.

191 Knapp JS, Hale JA, Neal SW, Wintersheid K, Rice RJ, Whittington WL. Proposed criteria for interpretation of susceptibilities of strains of *Neisseria gonorrhoeae* to ciprofloxacin, ofloxacin, enoxacin, lomefloxacin, and norfloxacin. *Antimicrob Agents Chemother* 1995; **39**: 2442–2445.

192 Turner A, Jephcott AE, Gough KR. Laboratory detection of ciprofloxacin resistant *Neisseria gonorrhoeae*. *J Clin Pathol* 1991; **44**: 169–170.

193 Forsyth A, Moyes A, Young H. Increased ciprofloxacin resistance in gonococci isolated in Scotland. *Lancet* 2000; **356**: 1984–1985.

194 Fuchs PC, Barry AL, Baker C, Murray PR, Washington JA. Proposed interpretive criteria and quality control parameters for testing in vitro susceptibility of *Neisseria gonorrhoeae* to ciprofloxacin. *J Clin Microbiol* 1991; **29**: 2111–2114.

195 World Health Organization Scientific Group. Neisseria gonorrhoeae *and Gonococcal Infections.* Technical Report. Series 616, Geneva; World Health Organization: 1978.

196 Ison CA, Dillon JR, Tapsall JW. The epidemiology of global antibiotic resistance among *Neisseria gonorrhoeae* and *Haemophilus ducreyi. Lancet* 1998; **351**: 8–11.

197 Tapsall JW, Rahim N, Ye SZ, *et al.* Surveillance of antibiotic susceptibility of *Neisseria gonorrhoeae* in the WHO Western Pacific Region 1992–4. *Genitourin Med* 1997; **73**: 355–361.

198 Ison CA, Martin IMC. Susceptibility of gonococci isolated in London to therapeutic antibiotics: establishment of a London surveillance programme. *Sex Transm Inf* 1999; **75**: 107–111.

199 Van de Laar MJW, van Duynhoven YTHP, Dessens M, van Santen M, van Klingeren B. Surveillance of antibiotic resistance in *Neisseria gonorrhoeae* in the Netherlands, 1977–95. *Genitourin Med* 1997; **73**: 510–517.

199a de Neeling AJ, van Santen-Verheuvel M, Spaargaren J, Willems RJL. Antimicrobial resistance of *Neisseria gonorrhoeae* and emerging ciprofloxacin resistance in the Netherlands, 1991 to 1998. *Antimicrob Agents Chemother* 2000; **44**: 3184–3185.

200 Clendennen TE, Echeverria P, Saengeur S, Kees S, Boslego JW, Wignall FS. Antibiotic

susceptibility survey of *Neisseria gonorrhoeae* in Thailand. *Antimicrob Agents Chemother* 1992; **36**: 1682–1687.

201 Elghoul MT, Joshi RM. Antimicrobial susceptibility of non-penicillinase and penicillinase-producing *Neisseria gonorrhoeae* strains isolated in Tripoli, Libya. *Int J STD AIDS* 1990; **1**: 343–345.

202 Chu ML, Ho LJ, Lin HC, Wu YC. Epidemiology of penicillin-resistant *Neisseria gonorrhoeae* isolated in Taiwan, 1960–1990. *Clin Infect Dis* 1992; **14**: 450–457.

203 Clendennen TE, Hames CS, Kees ES, *et al.* In vitro antibiotic susceptibilities of *Neisseria gonorrhoeae* isolates in the Philippines. *Antimicrob Agents Chemother* 1992; **36**: 277–282.

204 Mason PR, Gwanzura L, Latif AS, Marowa E. Antimicrobial susceptibility of *Neisseria gonorrhoeae* in Harare, Zimbabwe. Relationship to serogroup. *Sex Transm Dis* 1990; **17**: 63–66.

205 Otubu JA, Imade GE, Sagay AS, Towobola OA. Resistance of recent *Neisseria gonorrhoeae* isolates in Nigeria and outcome of single-dose treatment with ciprofloxacin. *Infection* 1992; **20**: 339–341.

206 Castro I, Bergeron MG, Chamberland S. Characterization of multiresistant strains of *Neisseria gonorrhoeae* isolated in Nicaragua. *Sex Transm Dis* 1993; **20**: 314–320.

206a Adegbola RA, Sabally S, Corrah T, West B, Mabey D. Increasing prevalence of penicillinase-producing *Neisseria gonorrhoeae* and the emergence of high level, plasmid-mediated tetracycline resistance among gonococcal isolates in the Gambia. *Trop Med Int Health* 1997; **2**: 428–432.

207 Van Dyck E, Crabbe F, Nzila N, *et al.* Increasing resistance of *Neisseria gonorrhoeae* in West and Central Africa. *Sex Transm Dis* 1997; **24**: 32–37.

208 Sarafian SK, Knapp JS. Molecular epidemiology of gonorrhea. *Clin Microbiol Rev* 1989; **2** (Suppl.): S49–S55.

209 Catlin BW. Nutritional requirements and auxotyping. In: Roberts (ed.) *The Gonococcus.* New York; John Wiley: 1977, pp. 91–109.

210 Bygdeman SM. Polyclonal and monoclonal antibodies applied to the epidemiology of gonococcal infection. In: Young H, McMillan A (eds) *Immunological Diagnosis of Sexually Transmitted Diseases.* New York; Marcel Dekker: 1988, pp. 77–116.

211 Bygdeman SM. A comparison between two different sets of monoclonal antibodies for the serological classification of *Neisseria gonorrhoeae.* In: Schoolnik GK, Brooks GF, Falkow S, Frasch CE, Knapp JS, McCutchan JA, Morse SA (eds) *The Pathogenic Neisseriae.* Washington, DC; American Society for Microbiology: 1985, pp. 31–36.

212 Moyes A, Young H. Epidemiological typing of *Neisseria gonorrhoeae*: a comparative analysis of three monoclonal, antibody serotyping panels. *Eur J Epidemiol* 1991; **7**: 311–319.

213 Turner A, Gough KR, Leeming JP. Molecular epidemiology of tetM genes in *Neisseria gonorrhoeae. Sex Transm Inf* 1999; **75**: 60–66.

214 Dillon JR, Li H, Yeung KH, Aman TA. A PCR assay for discriminating *Neisseria gonorrhoeae* beta-lactamase-producing plasmids. *Mol Cell Probe* 1999; **13**: 89–92.

215 Falk, ES, Bjorvatn B, Danielsson D, Kristiansen BE, Melby K, Srensen B. Restriction endonuclease fingerprinting of chromosomal DNA of *Neisseria gonorrhoeae. Acta Pathol Microbiol Immunol Scand [B]* 1984; **92**: 271–278.

216 Poh CL, Lau QC. Subtyping of *Neisseria gonorrhoeae* auxotype-serovar groups by pulsed-field gel electrophoresis. *J Med Microbiol* 1993; **38**: 366–370.

217 Lau QC, Chow VTK, Poh CL. Differentiation of *Neisseria gonorrhoeae* strains by polymerase chain reaction and restriction fragment length polymorphism of outer membrane protein IB genes. *Genitourin Med* 1995; **71**: 363–366.

218 Van Looveren M, Ison CA, Ieven M, *et al.* Evaluation of the discriminatory power of typing methods for *Neisseria gonorrhoeae. J Clin Microbiol* 1999; **37**: 2183–2188.

219 Li H, Dillon JAR. Utility of ribotyping, restriction endonuclease analysis and pulsed-field gel electrophoresis to discriminate between isolates of *Neisseria gonorrhoeae* of serovar IA-2 which require arginine, hypoxanthine or uracil for growth. *J Med Microbiol* 1995; **43**: 208–215.

220 Poh CL, Ocampo JC, Sng EH, Bygdeman SM. Rapid in situ generation of DNA restriction endonuclease patterns for *Neisseria gonorrhoeae. J Clin Microbiol* 1989; **27**: 2784–2788.

221 Marquez C, Xia MS, Borthagaray G, Roberts MC. Conjugal transfer of the 3.05 beta-lactamase plasmid by the 25.2 Mda plasmid in *Neisseria gonorrhoeae. Sex Transm Dis* 1999; **26**: 157–159.

222 Trees DL, Schultz AJ, Knapp JS. Use of the neisserial lipoprotein (Lip) for subtyping *Neisseria gonorrhoeae. J Clin Microbiol* 2000; **38**: 2914–2916.

223 Orourke M, Ison CA, Renton AM, Spratt BG. Opa-typing: A high-resolution tool for studying the epidemiology of gonorrhea. *Mol Microbiol* 1995; **17**: 865–875.

224 Dillon JR, Pauze M. Relationship between plasmid content and auxotype in *Neisseria gonorrhoeae* isolates. *Infect Immun* 1981; **33**: 625–628.

225 Young H, Moyes A, Noone A. *Gonococcal Infections in Scotland, 1998.* Scottish Centre for Infection and Environmental Health Weekly Report 1999; **33**: 298–304.

226 Ross JDC, Young H . Infectivity and clinical features of gonorrhoea: a serovar analysis. In: Conde-Glez CJ, Morse S, Rice P, Sparling F, Calderon E, (eds) *Pathobiology and Immunobiology of Neisseriaceae*. Mexico; Instituto Nacional de Salud Publica: 1994, pp. 111–115.

227 Whittington WLH, Holmes KK. Unique gonococcal phenotype associated with asymptomatic infection in men and with erroneous diagnosis of nongonococcal urethritis. *J Infect Dis* 2000; **181**: 1044–1048.

228 Palmer HM, Leeming JP, Turner A. Investigation of an outbreak of ciprofloxacin resistant *Neisseria gonorrhoeae* using a simplified opa-typing method. *Epidemiol Infect* 2001; **126**: 219–224.

229 Ward H, Ison CA, Day SE, *et al*. A prospective social and molecular investigation of gonococcal transmission. *Lancet* 2000; **356**: 1812–1817.

230 Communicable Disease Surveillance Centre. Laboratory reports of antimicrobial resistant isolates of *Neisseria gonorrhoeae*. Communicable Disease Report 1999; 271–272.

231 Bhuiyan BU, Rahman M, Miah MRA, *et al*. Susceptibilities and plasmid contents of *Neisseria gonorrhoeae* isolates from commercial sex workers in Dhaka, Bangladesh: Emergence of high-level resistance to ciprofloxacin. *J Clin Microbiol* 1999; **37**: 1130–1136.

232 Su X, Hutapea N, Tapsall JW, Lind I. *Plasmid mediated resistance in* Neisseria gonorrhoeae *strains isolated from female sex workers in North Sumatra, Indonesia 1996*. Abstract 216, Twelfth International Pathogenic Neisseria Conference, Galveston, Texas: 2000

233 Moran JS, Levine WC. Drugs of choice for the treatment of uncomplicated gonococcal infections. *Clin Infect Dis* 1995; **20** (Suppl. 1): S47–S65.

234 Schwarcz SK, Zenilman JM, Schnell D, *et al*. National surveillance of antimicrobial resistance in *Neisseria gonorrhoeae*. The Gonococcal Isolate Surveillance Project. *JAMA* 1990; **264**: 1413–1417.

235 Guinan ME, Biddle J, Thornsberry C, Reynolds G, Zaidi A, Wiesner P. The national gonorrhea therapy monitoring study: I. Review of treatment results and of in vitro antibiotic susceptibility, 1972–1978. *Sex Transm Dis* 1979; **6** (Suppl. 2): 93–102.

236 Centers for Disease Control. Sexually transmitted diseases treatment guidelines. *MMWR* 1989; **38**; 1–38.

237 Centers for Disease Control and Prevention. Increases in unsafe sex and rectal gonorrhea among men who have sex with men – San Francisco, California, 1994–1997. *MMWR* 2001; **48**: 45–48.

238 Centers for Disease Control and Prevention. 2002 Guidelines for treatment of sexually transmitted diseases. *MMW* 2002; **51**: RR–6.

239 Moran JS. Treating uncomplicated *Neisseria gonorrhoeae* infections: is the anatomic site important? *Sex Transm Dis* 1995; **22**: 39–47.

240 Laga M, Naamara W, Brunham RC, *et al*. Single-dose therapy of gonococcal ophthalmia neonatorum with ceftriaxone. *N. Engl J Med* 1986; **315**: 1382–1385.

241 Fransen L, Nsanze H, D'Costa L, Brunham RC, Ronald AR, Piot P. Single-dose kanamycin therapy of gonococcal ophthalmia neonatorum. *Lancet* 1984; **ii**: 1234–1236.

242 WHO 1999. Unpublished draft recommendations of a Steering Group.

243 Schmid GP, Johnson RE, Brenner ER, and the Cooperative Study Group. Symptomatic response of men with gonococcal urethritis: do all need post-treatment cultures? *Sex Transm Dis* 1987; **14**: 37–40.

244 Braun P, Sherman H, Komaroff AL. Urethritis in men: benefits, risks, and costs of alternative strategies of management. *Sex Transm Dis* 1982; **9**: 188–199.

245 Fitzgerald M, Bedford C. National standards for the management of gonorrhea. *Int J STD AIDS* 1996; **7**: 298–300.

246 Schroeter AL, Reynolds G. The rectal culture as a test of cure of gonorrhea in the female. *J Infect Dis* 1972; **125**: 499–503.

247 Foster A, Klauss V. Ophthalmia neonatorum in developing countries. *N Engl J Med* 1995; **332**: 600–601.

248 Laga M, Plummer FA, Piot P, *et al*. Prophylaxis of gonococcal and chlamydial ophthalmia neonatorum. A comparison of silver nitrate and tetracycline. *N. Engl J Med* 1988; **318**: 653–657.

249 Rothenberg R. Ophthalmia neonatorum due to *Neisseria gonorrhoeae*. Prevention and treatment. *Sex Transm Dis* 1979; **6** (Suppl.): 187–191.

250 Isenberg SJ, Apt L, Wood M. A controlled trial of povidone-iodine as prophylaxis against ophthalmia neonatorum. *N. Engl J Med* 1995; **332**: 562–566.

251 Cohen MS, Cannon JG, Jerse AE, Charniga LM, Isbey SF, Whicker LG. Human experimentation with *Neisseria gonorrhoeae*: rationale, methods, and implications for the biology of infection and vaccine development. *J Infect Dis* 1994; **169**: 532–537.

252 Barbosa-Cesnik CT, Gerbase A, Heymann D. STD Vaccines – an overview. *Genitourin Med* 1997; **73**: 336–342.

253 Hanenberg RS, Rojanapithayakorn W, Kunasol P, Sokal DC. Impact of Thailand's HIV-control programme as indicated by the decline of sexually transmitted diseases. *Lancet* 1994; **344**: 243–245.

254 Rein MF (ed) *Atlas of Infectious Diseases, Volume V, Sexually Transmitted Diseases*. Churchill Livingstone; Philadelphia: 1996.

255 McMillan A, Scott GR. *Sexually Transmitted Infections, Colour Guide*. Churchill Livingstone; Edinburgh: 2000.

256 Thin RN, Symonds MAE, Shaw EJ, Wong J, Hopper PK, Slocombe B. A double-blind trial of amoxycillin in the treatment of gonorrhoea. *Br J Vener Dis* 1977; **53**: 118–120.

257 Handsfield HH, McCormack WM, Hook EW, *et al*. A comparison of single-dose cefixime with ceftriaxone as treatment for uncomplicated gonorrhea. The Gonorrhea Treatment Study Group. *N Engl J Med* 1991; **325**: 1337–1341.

258 Plourde PJ, Tyndall M, Agoki E, *et al*. Single-dose cefixime versus single-dose ceftriaxone in the treatment of antimicrobial-resistant *Neisseria gonorrhoeae* infection. *J Infect Dis* 1992; **166**: 919–922.

259 Handsfield HH, Hook EW. Ceftriaxone for treatment of uncomplicated gonorrhea: routine use of a single 125-mg dose in a sexually transmitted disease clinic. *Sex Transm Dis* 1987; **14**: 227–229.

260 McCormack WM, Mogabgab WJ, Jones EW, Hook EW, Wendel GD, Handsfield HH. Multicenter, comparative study of cefotaxime and ceftriaxone for treatment of uncomplicated gonorrhea. *Sex Transm Dis* 1993; **20**: 269–273.

261 De Koning AJ, Tio D, van den Hoek JAR, van Klingeren B. Single 1 g dose of cefotaxime in the treatment of infections due to penicillinase-producing *Neisseria gonorrhoeae*. *Br J Vener Dis* 1983; **59**: 100–102.

262 Veeravahu M, Sumathipala AHT, Clay JC. Cefoxitin v. procaine penicillin in the treatment of uncomplicated gonorrhoea. *Br J Vener Dis* 1983; **59**: 406.

263 Spencer RC, Smith T, Talbot MD. Ceftizoxime in the treatment of uncomplicated gonorrhoea. *Br J Vener Dis* 1984; **60**: 90–91.

264 Bryan JP, Hira SK, Brady W, *et al*. Oral ciprofloxacin versus ceftriaxone for the treatment of urethritis from resistant *Neisseria gonorrhoeae* in Zambia. *Antimicrob Agents Chemother* 1990; **34**: 819–822.

265 Thorpe EM, Schwebke JR, Hook EW, *et al*. Comparison of single-dose cefuroxime axetil with ciprofloxacin in treatment of uncomplicated gonorrhea caused by penicillinase-producing and non-penicillinase-producing *Neisseria gonorrhoeae* strains. *Antimicrob Agents Chemother* 1996; **40**: 2775–2780.

266 Rajakumar MK, Ngeow YF, Khor BS, Lim KF. Ofloxacin, a new quinolone for the treatment of gonorrhea. *Sex Transm Dis* 1988; **15**: 25–26.

267 Bogaerts J, Tello WM, Akingeney J, Mukantabana V, Van Dyck, E, Piot P.

Effectiveness of norfloxacin and ofloxacin for treatment of gonorrhoea and decrease of in vitro susceptibility to quinolones over time in Rwanda. *Genitourin Med* 1993; **69**: 196–200.

268 Tupasi TE, Crisologo LB, Torres CA, Calubrian OV, De Jesus I. Cefuroxime, thiamphenicol, spectinomycin and penicillin G in uncomplicated infections due to penicillinase-producing strains of *Neisseria gonorrhoeae*. *Br J Vener Dis* 1983; **59**: 172–175.

269 Crider SR, Kilpatrick ME, Harrison WO, Kerbs SBJ, Berg SW. A comparison of penicillin G plus a beta-lactamase inhibitor (Sulbactam) with spectinomycin for treatment of urethritis caused by penicillinase-producing *Neissseria gonorrhoeae*. *Sex Transm Dis* 1984; **11**: 314–317.

Chapter 12

Pelvic inflammatory disease
A McMillan

Salpingitis or, more strictly, pelvic inflammatory disease (PID), resulting from ascending infection of the cervix and uterus is a well-recognized complication of infections due to *Neisseria gonorrhoeae* and *Chlamydia trachomatis*, the most common causes of PID.

Pelvic inflammatory disease

Pelvic inflammatory disease, in its acute form, is mainly a disease of sexually active young women and usually results from an ascending infection of the cervix and uterus. In developed countries the annual incidence, which has been rising over the past 35 years in women aged 15 to 39 years, varies from 10 to 13 per 1000, with a peak incidence of 20 per 1000 women in the 20 to 24-year age group.

In pathogenesis and prognosis with regard to fertility, it differs from pelvic inflammatory disease arising as a sequel to previous surgical manipulation. Although inflammation of the uterine tubes (salpingitis) is clinically the most prominent feature, the supporting structures of the uterus share in the inflammation to a greater or lesser extent, so PID is strictly the more accurate term and may be used synonymously.

ETIOLOGY

Gonococcal pelvic inflammatory disease

Pelvic inflammatory disease is a complication in about 10% of women with untreated gonorrhea[1], the exact figure for its incidence depends on the criteria used for diagnosis, the population group studied, and accessibility to medical care. In the UK where, in a recent study[2] *N. gonorrhoeae* was found to be the causative organism in 14% of 104 women with acute PID, gonococcal PID is less prevalent than in many areas of the USA. For example, in Richmond, VA, *N. gonorrhoeae* was associated with acute PID in 62 (74%) of 84 women with laparoscopically proven PID[3]. Although recovery of *N. gonorrhoeae* from the endocervix correlates with recovery from the uterine tubes, the correlation is not good since the gonococcus is isolated from the tubes in only 10% of women with untreated gonorrhea and PID. This low recovery rate might be explained by a bactericidal action in the inflammatory exudate, or by the possibility that another organism is responsible. *Chlamydia trachomatis* may be isolated from the endocervix of about 40% of women with untreated gonorrhea[4], and dual infection has recently been recorded in 7% of women with acute PID[2].

While recovery of *N. gonorrhoeae* from an endocervical culture of a patient with PID does not prove conclusively that the gonococcus caused the disease in the uterine tubes, there is little doubt that, at least in some cases, the gonococcus is the primary pathogen. *In vitro* studies have shown that *N. gonorrhoeae* can infect tubal mucosa and invade and destroy epithelial cells[5].

Chlamydial pelvic inflammatory disease

There is little doubt that *C. trachomatis* is an important cause of pelvic inflammatory disease. The organism can be recovered from the cervix, endometrium and uterine tubes of patients with PID[3], and salpingitis can be established in primates[6]. It is estimated that about 20% of women with untreated chlamydial infection develop PID. *Chlamydia trachomatis* is the most common causative organism in women from populations with a low prevalence of gonorrhea. In a recent British study, *C. trachomatis* was the etiological agent in 45% of 104 women with acute PID[2]. Where gonorrhea is highly prevalent, however, the proportion of cases of acute PID associated with *C. trachomatis* is significantly smaller, for example 13 (15%) of 84 women in Soper's series[3].

Other possible bacterial causes of pelvic inflammatory disease

Mycoplasma hominis has been isolated from the uterine tubes of just under 10% of women with acute PID[7] and, although its growth in human fallopian tube organ cultures is associated with swelling of the cilia (but no loss of ciliary activity)[8], its role in the causation of PID is uncertain. Similarly, the role of *M. genitalium* in the etiology of some cases of PID remains uncertain. The organism can cause salpingitis in primates[9], but to date *M. genitalium* has not been detected in the upper genital tract of women.

Ureaplasma urealyticum has been cultured from the uterine tubes of about 4% of women with PID[7], but its etiological role is unclear.

Facultative and anaerobic bacteria, including those associated with bacterial vaginosis (Chapter 17) may be cultured from the uterine tubes of women with acute PID[10]. The proportion of women with these bacteria varies from 13% to 78%[11], this wide variation being accounted for by differences in patient populations, severity of the disease, and microbiological methods. It has been postulated that bacterial vaginosis (BV) may alter the cervicovaginal environment, thereby increasing the risk of ascending infection by the organisms of BV and/or *C. trachomatis* or *N. gonorrhoeae*[3]. Several observations support this hypothesis[11].

1. BV is more common in women with PID than in matched controls: Paavonen et al.[12] found BV in 9 of 31 women with endometritis and/or laparoscopic evidence of salpingitis compared with none of 14 controls. There is also a good relationship between the presence of BV and endometritis, even in the absence of gonococcal or chlamydial infection. In one series[13], 10 of 22 women with BV had plasma cell endometritis compared with only 1 of 19 who were not affected. There was also a significant difference in the isolation rates of BV-associated organisms between women with and women without plasma cell endometritis: these organisms were cultured from the endometrium of 9 of 11 women with, but from only 8 of 30 women without endometritis.

2. BV-associated organisms are frequently isolated from the upper genital tract of women with PID (14% of 84 women with acute salpingitis studied by Soper et al.[3]).

3. Mucinase and sialidase activity in vaginal fluid samples is detected significantly more frequently in women with BV than in those without[14]. Briselde et al.[15] showed that *Prevotella* spp. and *Bacteroides* spp. accounted for the sialidase activity in most of the vaginal washings examined. Sialidase activity could alter the mucous barrier at the cervical os, and predispose to ascending infection. In other anatomical sites, mucolytic enzymes have been implicated in the pathogenesis of infection. With respect to genital tract infection, it is interesting to note that sialidase digestion of *N. gonorrhoeae* exposes an epitope, which is similar to the precursor of human erythrocyte *i* antigen, that may facilitate adherence to epithelial cells[16].

Bacteroides spp. can damage the cilia in human fallopian tube organ cultures, but the mechanism of tissue damage is unknown.

PATHOGENESIS

In gonococcal and chlamydial salpingitis, the inflammatory process chiefly affects the endosalpinx, the organisms having ascended by way of the endometrium, where a marked inflammation may be induced[17]. Ascent of organisms from the endocervix may be facilitated by uterine contractions that, during the follicular phase of the menstrual cycle, move from the cervix to the fundus, and increase in amplitude and frequency until ovulation; thereafter, the contractions are less well coordinated until menstruation, when they move from the fundus to the cervix[18]. There is destruction of tubal epithelium and a purulent exudate fills the lumen. Pus may escape from the fimbriated end of the tube and track down to the rectovaginal pouch, where a pelvic abscess may form. With continued inflammation the ostia become occluded by edema and pus collects in the cavity of the tube forming a pyosalpinx. If untreated, fibrous adhesions form within the tube with relatively few external adhesions. Occasionally a hydrosalpinx (an accumulation of serous fluid in the tube) is found; its pathogenesis is uncertain, but it may result from recurrent episodes of subacute salpingitis.

Mechanisms of disease in gonococcal pelvic inflammatory disease

There is some evidence that certain strains of *N. gonorrhoeae* are more likely to be associated with PID than others. The MICs of various antibiotics were noted to be significantly higher amongst isolates from women with upper genital tract infection than from those who had uncomplicated disease[19]. In addition, the same workers found that there were significant differences in auxotype patterns between isolates from salpingitis cases and uncomplicated cases. In fallopian tube organ culture, gonococci attach to the microvilli of non-ciliated cells which they rapidly enter[20]. Multiplication occurs within these cells which the organisms exit by exocytosis from the basal surfaces. In addition, there is loss of ciliary activity, and ciliated cells adjacent to non-ciliated cells undergo necrosis. *In vitro* studies have shown that lipopolysaccharide and peptidoglycan fragments from *N. gonorrhoeae* can interfere with ciliary function. An acute inflammatory reaction follows binding of antibody to gonococcal lipopolysaccharide and peptidoglycan in the fallopian tubes, with activation of complement and initiation of the prostaglandin cascade[21].

Mechanisms of disease in chlamydial pelvic inflammatory disease

T_{H2}-type CD4+ T cells appear to be associated with scarring trachoma and cytokines appear to be implicated in the disease process. Microscopical examination of conjunctival biopsies from patients with trachoma show that B cells predominate in tissue from those with fibrosis confined to the deep substantia propria. More extensive fibrosis, however, is associated with a predominantly CD4+ T cell infiltrate. It has been proposed that up-regulated local production of cytokines contributes to the scarring of severe trachoma. This is probably also true of uterine tube fibrosis in humans. Endometrial biopsies from women with upper genital tract infection show a significantly higher frequency of lymphoid follicle formation than those with uncomplicated cervical infection. As these follicles are formed by B cell expansion, this would suggest that T_{H2}-type cytokines (IL-4, IL-5, IL-6, and IL-10) are important driving forces in this regard.

Repeated or chronic infection with *C. trachomatis* increases the likelihood of long-term sequelae. In women with repeated episodes of PID, the risk of permanent tubal damage doubles with each recurrent episode[22]. It was shown in the macaque monkey model that repeated genital tract infection is necessary to produce uterine tube damage[23]. In guinea pigs, primary vaginal infection with the guinea pig inclusion conjunctivitis agent results in an acute inflammatory response, but repeated infection produces chronic inflammation and oviduct scarring[24]. High levels of tumor necrosis factor-α (TNF-α) which is important in cell-mediated immune responses and is known to be chlamydiastatic, were found in the genital secretions within the first 2 weeks of infection, correlating with the acute inflammatory reaction, but not thereafter, and not in chronically infected animals. The mechanism for the production of fibrosis is unclear, but transforming growth factor-β (TGF-β), produced by activated macrophages, T and B cells might be important. TGF-β is produced in a latent form, formation of which can be induced by heat shock proteins (Hsps) or by lipopolysaccharide. After formation and activation by proteolytic enzymes of macrophages or by the plasminogen activator-plasmin system[25], TGF-β induces synthesis of extracellular matrix proteins and hence fibrosis. In experimental animals, neutralizing antibody against TGF-β can prevent scarring.

Heat shock proteins* may play a role in chronic chlamydial infection, as suggested by the more severe inflammation found in mice who had been immunized with Hsp60 and subsequently challenged by the intravaginal inoculation of live chlamydiae[26]. Domeika et al.[27] examined the association between humoral immunity to unique and conserved epitopes of C. trachomatis Hsp60 and immunity to human Hsp60 in 129 with laparoscopically proven PID. They found that about 50% of the women had antibodies to human Hsp60 and these cross reacted with the chlamydial Hsp60 peptide 260–271;

---

* Heat shock proteins (Hsps) are a family of closely related proteins that are found in all eukaryotic and prokaryotic cells where they have a role in assembly, folding, and transport of other molecules. Higher levels of these proteins are expressed in cells that are subjected to stress, for example high temperatures, thereby stabilizing protein structure. Remarkably, Hsps from different taxa show amino acid sequence homology. There are four main groups based on their molecular weights: Hsp90, Hsp70, Hsp 60, and the small Hsps.

antibodies to peptide 260–271 were associated with IgG and IgA antibodies against chlamydiae. Although by no means conclusive evidence, it was postulated that an autoimmune response to human Hsp60 was the consequence of an immune response to an epitope of chlamydial Hsp60 cross-reactive with the human Hsp60. A further study of the role of Hsps in chronic chlamydial disease showed that the prevalence of antibody against Hsp60 in the sera of patients with scarring endemic trachoma was twice as high as in individuals without signs of the disease, even after correcting for raised antibody to whole C. trachomatis[28]. The problem as to whether serum antibodies to Hsps reflect a pathogenic role for Hsps or result from hyperimmunization by chronic infection remains unresolved[29].

Genetic factors appear to play some part in determining the severity of clinical disease in humans, but their overall importance in immunity to chlamydial infection, or in its pathogenesis, is unknown. In a study of sex-industry workers in Kenya, Kimani et al.[30], however, observed that MHC class I HLA-A31 was independently associated with PID in women infected with C. trachomatis.

EPIDEMIOLOGY

Incidence and prevalence

Available data on incidence and prevalence of PID in different communities are difficult to interpret. There are no universally accepted criteria for diagnosis, and many cases are asymptomatic. Most reports concern hospital in-patient data. In England and Wales the incidence of PID appears to have been increasing over the past 35 years, the increase being greatest in the 16 to 24-year age group[31]. In contrast, the number of episodes of hospital admission for PID in Sweden has fallen steadily in the 15 to 29-year age group since the late 1970s, during which time a concerted effort was made to control chlamydial infection in the community[32].

Risk factors

The peak age incidence of PID is in the 20 to 24-year old group, which corresponds to the age group with the highest incidence of

chlamydial infection and gonorrhea. After adjusting for these infections, age is no longer associated with PID. Oral contraception has been recognized as providing some degree of protection against PID in women with chlamydial infection: a 70% reduction was noted in Wolner-Hanssen's study[33]. A possible explanation for the protective effect of these agents is that they reduce the inflammatory response in the uterine tubes. Women who use intrauterine contraceptive devices (IUD) may be at increased risk of PID – due to both C. trachomatis and N. gonorrhoeae, and to non-sexually transmitted organisms – compared with women using other means of contraception[10]. The risk of symptomatic PID following insertion of an IUD in a woman with untreated chlamydial or gonococcal infection has been reported as ranging from 3.1% to 5.3%[34, 35], most of the increased risk occurring during the first few months after insertion. A recent analysis, however, has shown that the estimated risk of PID following insertion of an IUD, even when the prevalence of STIs is high, is low (0.15%)[36]. A clearly defined risk factor for the development of PID is instrumentation of the uterus: up to 25% of women with untreated chlamydial infection of the cervix develop PID after termination of pregnancy[37].

The clinical presentation of PID in HIV-1-infected women is generally similar to that in HIV-non-infected individuals[37a]. However, tubo-ovarian abscess formation is more likely amongst the former group of women, particularly if they are severely immunocompromised[38]. An interesting observation is that, following stimulation with C. trachomatis elementary bodies, peripheral blood mononuclear cells from HIV-1-infected women secrete significantly less interferon-γ than those from HIV-non-infected women[38a]. As interferon-γ plays a role in protection against chlamydial infection (Chapter 10), decreased production of this cytokine may enhance susceptibility of HIV-infected women to PID.

In the USA an association between vaginal douching and PID has been shown, and Wolner-Hanssen et al.[39] found that when cases were compared with controls, those who douched at least three times per month were 3.6 times more likely to have PID than those who douched less than once per month. The reasons for the increased risk associated with douching are uncertain, but changes in the microflora balance and pH, and removal of protective immune components have all been cited[11]. As vaginal douching appears to be less common in the UK, this factor is likely to be less important there.

Cigarette smoking is stated as a risk factor for PID[40], possibly by suppressing the local immune system. The relationship, however, is not entirely clear, and smoking may only be an indication of risk-taking behavior.

CLINICAL FEATURES

Mild to moderate pelvic inflammatory disease

Most women with mild to moderately severe PID are young and have either gonococcal or chlamydial infection. The onset of pain, which is usually felt in the lower abdomen, is usually subacute. Additional features include increased vaginal discharge, dysuria, and, less commonly, nausea and vomiting. Irregular menstruation occurs in about 40% of women with PID, particularly if this is associated with *C. trachomatis* (this may be because of the endometritis associated with chlamydial infection). Deep dyspareunia is common.

Pyrexia is found in about 50% of cases, particularly when the PID is associated with *N. gonorrhoeae*. There is adnexal tenderness and a mass may be found in about 50% of women with gonococcal PID[41].

Although the results of laboratory tests may show non-specific changes, they can give some useful information to support a provisional diagnosis of acute PID. In about two-thirds of patients the white cell count in the peripheral blood is elevated, particularly in the PID associated with *N. gonorrhoeae*. The erythrocyte sedimentation rate is raised, most frequently in women with chlamydial PID in about 75% of patients. The C-reactive protein (CRP) concentration is elevated in PID, the level reflecting the severity of the PID[42].

Severe pelvic inflammatory disease

The symptoms of severe PID usually occur during or shortly after menstruation or in the puerperium. The patient complains usually of lower abdominal pain, often exacerbated by movement of the psoas muscle, fever, malaise, anorexia, and vomiting. With the increased use of laparoscopy, it has become apparent that whilst abdominal pain is the most reliable symptom, it may be minimal in at least 5% of cases[43]. Pyrexia (temperature of 38°C or greater) may be found in only about two-thirds of women with acute PID, and more commonly in cases caused by *N. gonorrhoeae*[44].

There is usually tenderness and a variable degree of muscular guarding over the lower abdomen. Pain is elicited by moving the cervix during bimanual examination. Palpation of the uterus and tubes is usually impossible on account of tenderness and guarding.

In about half the cases of acute PID, the white cell count in the peripheral blood is elevated. The erythrocyte sedimentation rate is raised in about 75% of cases, especially when the salpingitis is associated with *C. trachomatis*[41].

Paralytic ileus, presenting with abdominal distention and vomiting, may occur in 1% of cases. In such cases fluid levels are noted on the plain film of the abdomen, taken with the patient in an upright position.

Chronic pelvic inflammatory disease

Chronic PID may be asymptomatic and undiscovered until the patient is investigated for infertility. Symptoms, when they occur, consist of intermittent lower abdominal pain or discomfort, discomfort in the groin, backache, malaise, and frequent heavy menstrual periods. The tubes may not be palpable or they may be irregularly thickened, and the uterus may be retroverted and fixed.

COMPLICATIONS

Tubo-ovarian and pelvic abscess

This is usually a late complication of untreated PID, and is associated with infection with facultative anaerobes and anaerobes. In HIV-1-infected women, however, tubo-ovarian abscess formation is more common than in those who are uninfected. In a study from Nairobi, Kenya[38], tubo-ovarian abscesses were found in 33% of 52 HIV-seropositive women, compared with 15% of 81 HIV-uninfected women, a significant difference. It was also shown in that study that abscess formation was more likely amongst those who were severely immunocompromised than amongst those who were less immunosuppressed.

Infertility

Infertility is a risk after PID, and to examine the magnitude of this risk, a large prospective study was undertaken in Sweden[45]. Women who presented with pelvic pain suggestive of PID between 1960 and 1984 and who underwent laparoscopy were followed-up. The patient group consisted of 1732 women who had had a laparoscopically confirmed diagnosis of PID, and the control group of 601 women had had no evidence of PID. The patients were followed for a mean of 94.3 months after the index episode, and the control group for a mean of 80.1 months. Of the women attempting pregnancy, 16% of 1309 women who had had PID failed to conceive, compared with 2.7% of 451 control women. Tubal factor infertility was confirmed in 141 (67.6%) of 209 infertile patients, but in none of the control women. For patients with only one episode of PID, the incidence of tubal infertility was higher amongst those who had severe infection at laparoscopy, and this finding was confirmed in a recent study.

Fifty-eight women were contacted by telephone 2 to 9 years after their index episode of PID; 19 (40%) of 48 women not using contraception were involuntarily infertile after the episode[46]. These investigators found that at the time of the index episode these women were more likely to have had occluded or partially occluded tubes and peri-tubal adhesions compared with women who had a pregnancy in the intervening period. Westrom *et al.*[45] also found that the rate of tubal infertility doubled with each repeated episode of PID. On average, after one episode of PID, 8% of 991 women had tubal infertility; compared with 19.5% of 185, and 40% of 65 women who had two and three or more episodes respectively.

Ectopic pregnancy

Westrom and colleagues[45] found that the first pregnancy after the index episode of PID was ectopic in 100 (9.1%) of the 1309 patients attempting pregnancy, compared with 6 (1.4%) of the control women. In this study it was also noted that the risk of ectopic pregnancy increased directly with the severity of the index episode and with the number of episodes of PID[47]. Previous PID also increases the risk of subsequent ectopic pregnancy even if the first one is intrauterine, the risk increasing with the severity of the initial episode[48]. It does not, however, appear to add any incremental risk in the case of a woman whose first pregnancy after an episode of PID was ectopic.

Chronic pain

Pelvic or abdominal pain persisting for more than 6 months is reported in about 12% of patients who have had one episode of PID, but in about one-third and two-thirds of women who have had two and three episodes respectively[49].

DIFFERENTIAL DIAGNOSIS
Ectopic pregnancy

In the case of a ruptured ectopic pregnancy, there is usually sudden onset of pain in an iliac fossa or hypogastrium, often with syncope. Tracking of blood to the upper abdominal cavity may induce pain referred to the shoulder. Symptoms usually develop after a short period of amenorrhea during which there may have been cramping discomfort in one iliac fossa; vaginal spotting of blood may also be a feature in early ectopic pregnancy. If intra-abdominal hemorrhage is severe, the patient presents a state of shock, with pallor, tachycardia, and hypotension. There is tenderness over the lower abdomen, and on vaginal examination (which must not be performed in patients with signs of severe hemorrhage) there is irregular, tender enlargement of the tube on the affected side. Pelvic hematoma may be detected in the rectovaginal pouch. Urine tests for pregnancy may be either positive or negative depending upon the secretory activity of the trophoblast.

Measurement of the serum concentration of β human chorionic gonadotropin (βHCG) together with transvaginal ultrasonography has improved diagnosis. In the presence of an ectopic mass or fluid in the pouch of Douglas, a serum concentration of βHCG of 1500 IU/L strongly suggests an ectopic pregnancy. In the absence of ultrasound signs, the higher concentration of 2000 IU/L should be the cut-off point before a diagnosis is made[50]. The serum concentration of βHCG is generally lower in ectopic than in intrauterine pregnancy, and the normal doubling of the concentration every 48 hours during the eighth to twelfth week does not occur. The examination of paired sera taken at an interval of 48 hours can be helpful in diagnosis. Ultrasonic examination of the pelvis, particularly transvaginal ultrasonography, can give useful information. Using the latter method there is direct visualization of the ectopic embryo in 16% to 32% of cases. In many cases, a ring-like structure has been found in the adnexae and free fluid may be seen in the pelvis. Although a definitive diagnosis of ectopic pregnancy is more commonly made using intravaginal transducers, the majority of ectopic pregnancies cannot be diagnosed by ultrasonic examination alone[51].

Specialist gynecological advice is indicated in this surgical emergency.

Acute appendicitis

Abdominal pain commences usually in the umbilical area and after some hours localizes to the right iliac fossa. Menstrual irregularities are unusual but nausea and anorexia are more pronounced than in acute PID.

Ruptured ovarian or endometriotic cyst

There is usually sudden onset of lower abdominal pain, most commonly occurring about the time of menstruation. The patient is usually afebrile.

Acute pyelonephritis

There is generally a sudden rise in temperature, often with rigors, and pain in the loins and iliac fossae. Commonly there are urinary symptoms such as frequency of micturition, urgency, strangury, dysuria, nocturia, and hematuria. The urine contains pus and there is a polymorphonuclear leukocytosis in most cases.

Intestinal obstruction

Pain is colicky in nature and is felt in the umbilical or hypogastric areas. It is associated with vomiting and the absence of passage of flatus. Bowel sounds are hyperactive. There may be a history of previous abdominal surgery.

Septic abortion

A history of amenorrhea is followed by symptoms and signs of abortion – either complete or incomplete. There is uterine bleeding, painful uterine contractions, pyrexia, tachycardia, offensive vaginal discharge, uterine tenderness, and general systemic upset. The white cell count and erythrocyte sedimentation rate are raised. Vaginal examination may show a dilated cervix.

Diagnosis of pelvic inflammatory disease

A presumptive diagnosis of acute PID may be made from the patient's history and the clinical and laboratory findings. However, a diagnosis made on clinical features is imprecise. Confirmation of the diagnosis requires the use of laparoscopy, except when a presumptive diagnosis of gonorrhea has been made by smear examination or confirmed by culture. Jacobson and Westrom[43] demonstrated that only 60% of clinically diagnosed cases of acute PID were confirmed by laparoscopy. In their series, acute appendicitis, pelvic endometriosis, and intrapelvic hemorrhage were the conditions most commonly mimicking acute salpingitis. The laparoscopic findings in acute PID include tubal erythema, swelling and exudate (Figure 12.1); the tubes, however, may look normal in women with chronic or plasma cell salpingitis.

Laparoscopy, however, requires the administration of a general anesthetic and

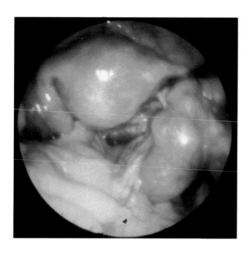

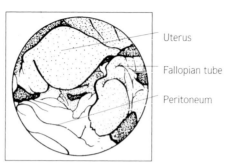

Figure 12.1 Laparoscopic view of uterus and swollen uterine tubes in acute pelvic inflammatory disease (reproduced from Rein 1996[79])

is not without hazard. Rawlings and Balgobin[52] reported a complication rate of 6%. Complications included perforation of the bowel, mesenteric hemorrhage, hematoma of the abdominal wall, and pelvic abscess formation. Laparoscopy should only be undertaken by gynecologists experienced in its use.

Some time ago, Paavonen et al.[53] showed that there was a good relationship between the laparoscopic diagnosis of acute PID and a histological diagnosis of plasma cell endometritis. In their study of 27 women, they found that endometrial biopsy had a sensitivity of 89%, a specificity of 67%, a positive predictive value of 84%, and a negative predictive value of 22%. As the procedure is easily undertaken in a clinic setting, it was proposed that it could form a good alternative to laparoscopy. Histological changes, however, may be focal and therefore missed, thereby reducing the sensitivity of the test, and, other than in research settings, endometrial biopsy is not widely used in the diagnosis of PID.

In more than 90% of women with severe PID, pelvic ultrasound examination shows dilated uterine tubes, tubo-ovarian abscess formation, fluid in the rectovaginal pouch, and enlarged polycystic ovaries[54]. The ultrasonic findings, however, are less obvious in mild PID, and the principal application of ultrasonography in such cases is to assist in the exclusion of other pathology. Transvaginal ultrasonography has been evaluated as a possible method for the diagnosis of PID. Cacciatore et al.[55] examined 51 women with suspected PID by transvaginal ultrasonography and endometrial biopsy. They found that of the 13

women who had plasma cell endometritis, 11 had thickened fluid-filled tubes, while none of the women with a histologically normal endometrium had such findings. Other findings associated with plasma cell endometritis were polycystic-like ovaries and free fluid in the pelvis. None of the patients with a normal scan had endometritis. Khalife and colleagues[56] showed that transvaginal ultrasonography is a sensitive method of detecting the presence of more than 8 mL of free pelvic fluid, and should be useful in the diagnosis of pelvic pathology associated with increased peritoneal fluid.

Magnetic resonance imaging (MRI) has recently been evaluated in the diagnosis of PID. Tukeva et al.[57] working in Helsinki, Finland, undertook MRI, transvaginal ultrasonography, and laparoscopy in 30 women suspected of having PID. Twenty-one women had laparoscopically confirmed PID, and the imaging findings agreed with the laparoscopic diagnosis in 20 (95%) of these women. By contrast, the findings on transvaginal ultrasonography agreed with those of laparoscopy in 17 (81%) patients. Although MRI appears to be more accurate than ultrasound in the diagnosis of PID, it is a costly procedure that is not widely available.

When a young woman attends an STI clinic complaining of lower abdominal pain that started within 10 days of the onset of menstruation, and when examination reveals tenderness in both fornices, the most likely diagnosis is PID. Every effort must be made to identify chlamydial and gonococcal infection (see Chapters 10 and 11). Although the presence of mucopus at

the cervical os is common in women attending STI clinics, its absence, or the absence of polymorphonuclear leukocytes in a Gram-stained smear of endocervical material, should alert the clinician to the possibility of an alternative diagnosis. Treatment should be started on the result of examination of Gram-stained smears and altered, if necessary, when culture reports become available.

TREATMENT

Cases of acute PID with systemic disturbance should be admitted to hospital. The decision is not so straightforward in patients with less severe symptoms and signs. If there is any doubt as to the diagnosis, or about the patient's reliability in taking the antibiotic or chemotherapy prescribed, admission to hospital is indicated. Pregnant women are best treated in hospital. As complications of PID are more common in women who are immunocompromised, such patients should also be admitted to hospital.

Supportive measures such as rest and the provision of adequate analgesia are important. In an individual case, there is often some uncertainty about the precise cause of lower abdominal or pelvic pain. When suggestive clinical features are present in a sexually active young woman, it is better not to delay treatment until the results of laboratory tests are available. Prompt treatment with the appropriate antimicrobial agents reduces the risk of long-term sequelae[58].

Most studies on the treatment of PID have concerned parenteral therapy, and have had, as outcome measures, clinical and microbiological cure. Clinical trials have provided limited information of the effect of treatment on long-term complications of PID such as infertility. The choice of an appropriate regimen of therapy should take into consideration the following[59]

- severity of the illness
- prevalence in the community of the most likely pathogens, viz. C. trachomatis and N. gonorrhoeae
- antimicrobial susceptibility patterns of the prevalent strains of N. gonorrhoeae
- patient preference and likelihood of adherence
- cost.

PARENTERAL TREATMENT

In severe disease in the immunocompromised patient, and in the pregnant woman, initial treatment by the parenteral route is preferred to oral therapy. Twenty-four hours after clinical improvement, oral treatment can be substituted[60]. Irrespective of the results of Gram-smear microscopy of endocervical material, the following regimens are recommended [59, 60]:

Cefoxitin, given in an intravenous dose of 2 g every 6 hours, or *cefotetan* given intravenously in a dosage of 2 g every 12 hours, plus *doxycycline*, preferably given orally, in a dosage of 100 mg every 12 hours. If the woman cannot tolerate oral doxycycline, the drug can be given in a similar dose by the intravenous route. Subsequent treatment is with *doxycycline* (100 mg every 12 hours) and *metronidazole* (400 mg twice daily), both given orally and continued for 14 days. If there is pelvic or tubo-ovarian abscess formation, anaerobic bacteria are likely to be present, and metronidazole, given in an intravenous dose of 500 mg every 8 hours, should be added to the initial parenteral regimen.

An alternative regimen[60] is *clindamycin*, given in a dosage of 900 mg by intravenous infusion every 8 hours, with *gentamicin**, as an intravenous or intramuscular loading dose of 2 mg/kg of body weight, followed by a maintenance dose of 1.5 mg/kg every 8 hours. Oral treatment can be substituted 24 hours after the patient improves clinically. This consists of either *clindamycin* 450 mg every 6 hours for 14 days, or *doxycycline* 100 mg every 12 hours, plus *metronidazole* 400 mg every 12 hours, for 14 days.

In a multicenter, open-label clinical trial that compared the efficacy of the three parenteral regimens recommended by the Centers for Disease Control and Prevention, almost identical cure rates were produced by each regimen; 275 (94.2%) of women did not require alteration of their initial therapeutic regimen[61].

Other parenteral regimens that have broad spectrum antimicrobial activity, and have been shown to have at least short-term efficacy in the treatment of acute PID include the following.

- *Ofloxacin*, given by intravenous infusion every 12 hours, plus *metronidazole* 500 mg intravenously every 8 hours. In a series of 36 women, *N. gonorrhoeae* or *C. trachomatis* were isolated from at least one anatomical site from 25 and 6 of these women respectively, parenteral ofloxacin was shown to be effective, and all patients responded to therapy[62]. The quinolones, however, have minimal activity against anaerobes[63] and therefore it seem prudent to include metronidazole in ofloxacin-containing regimens.
- *Ampicillin/sulbactam* given by intravenous infusion in a dosage of 3 g every 6 hours, plus *doxycycline* given orally or intravenously in a dosage of 100 mg every 12 hours. The clinical response rate (cure or improvement) has been shown to be similar to that of cefoxitin with doxycycline[64].
- *Ciprofloxacin*, by intravenous infusion in a dosage of 200 mg every 12 hours, plus *doxycycline*, 100 mg every 12 hours by mouth or by intravenous infusion, plus *metronidazole* 500 mg intravenously every 8 hours. Limited data exist on the efficacy of this regimen, but in a small series of women, Heinonen *et al.*[65] reported success in 9 women with chlamydial or gonococcal PID and in 6 of 7 women with non-gonococcal, non-chlamydial PID.

Oral or intramuscular treatment regimens

Evidence for the efficacy of oral regimens in the treatment of acute PID is limited. *Ofloxacin*, in a dosage of 400 mg every 12 hours, plus *metronidazole* 400 mg, both drugs being given orally for 14 days, is effective against *C. trachomatis* and many strains of *N. gonorrhoeae*, and anaerobe infection is covered by the metronidazole. In a well-designed study from Texas, USA, short-term follow-up of treatment with ofloxacin alone showed that the drug produced clinical improvement or cure in 95% of 128 women[66].

In the out-patient treatment of mild to moderate PID, a single intramuscular 250 mg dose of *ceftriaxone* plus *doxycycline*, given orally in a dose of 100 mg every 12 hours for 14 days has given a cure rate of about 95%[66]. Alternative cephalosporins effective against strains of *N. gonorrhoeae* that have chromosomally or plasmid-mediated resistance to penicillin and other antimicrobial agents, include 1) *cefoxitin* given as a single intramuscular dose of 2 g with probenecid (1 g orally), and 2) *cefotaxime* given as a single intramuscular infection of 1 g. As there is some uncertainty about the effect of these antimicrobial agents on anaerobe infection, *metronidazole*, given by mouth in a dosage of 400 mg every 12 hours should be added to this regimen.

Doxycycline given with metronidazole for 14 days is a common regimen in the management of PID in the UK[67]. Despite the drugs being given parenterally, however, studies have shown that clinical and microbiological cure with this regimen is achieved in only 75% of cases[11]. It is thus difficult to justify their continuing use in clinical practice[67].

Treatment of pregnant women with pelvic inflammatory disease

Treatment with fluoroquinolones, gentamicin, and tetracyclines are contraindicated in pregnant and lactating women. A parenteral cephalosporin such as cefoxitin, given intravenously in a dose of 2 g every 8 hours, with erythromycin lactobionate* given as an intravenous infusion of 50 mg/kg, with the possible addition of metronidazole, 500 mg every 8 hours by intravenous infusion is recommended[59].

---

* Gentamicin is available as 1 or 2 mL vials, each containing gentamicin 40 mg (as sulfate)/mL. It is given by *slow* intravenous injection; alternatively, it can be diluted in up to 100 mL of 5% glucose or 0.9% sodium chloride and given by infusion over about 30 minutes. Ototoxicity and nephrotoxicity are the most common side effects, and in renal impairment the dose should be modified.

---

* Erythromycin lactobionate is dispensed as a vial containing 1.0 g of erythromycin as erythromycin lactobionate; when reconstituted with sterile water, each 20 mL contains 1.0 g of erythromycin. The preparation is further diluted in 5% glucose or 0.9% sodium chloride to a concentration of 1 mg per mL.

Follow-up of treated patients

It is recommended that women are reviewed within 72 hours of initiation of treatment. Failure to produce improvement in clinical features at that time should prompt the clinician to reconsider the diagnosis, to institute parenteral therapy, or to consider surgical intervention. A further review is often undertaken 4 weeks later to ensure

1. complete resolution of symptoms and signs
2. that there had been adherence to the prescribed medication
3. that there had been no further risk of infection.

Management of sexual partners

In most instances, acute PID in young women has resulted from an STI, and it is important that the possible primary and any secondary sexual contacts are offered screening for chlamydial and gonococcal infection. As these infections may not be identified in either partner, the authors believe that the male should be treated on epidemiological grounds with the appropriate antibiotic.

Perihepatitis

The increasing incidence of chlamydial infection in men and women has focused attention on another manifestation of *C. trachomatis* infections, namely perihepatitis, with its main presentation of pain in the upper right quadrant of the abdomen and it is particularly associated with PID in women. The relationship between upper abdominal peritonitis, perihepatitis, and salpingitis was first described in 1919 in Uruguay by Carlos Stanajo. The recognition by Curtis[68] of perihepatic adhesions resulting from perihepatitis, and their association with gonococcal salpingitis, was followed by a further description of the acute clinical features by Fitz-Hugh, of the University of Pennsylvania[69].

Subsequently the condition of acute right upper quadrant pain in association with perihepatitis became known as the Curtis–Fitz-Hugh syndrome. In more recent years renewed interest followed its increasing incidence and the recognition that *C. trachomatis* as well as *N. gonorrhoeae* may be causative organisms.

Curtis, a Chicago gynecologist, noticed that 'violin string' adhesions were frequently found between the anterior surface of the liver and the adjacent anterior abdominal wall.

The use of the laparoscope has enabled confirmation of the findings of Curtis and Fitz-Hugh. In the acute stage of perihepatitis 'violin string' adhesions form (Figure 12.2) that are fragile and friable and may be easily broken at laparoscopy, either by insufflation of carbon dioxide or by instrumentation, leaving the appearance of white fibrous plaques and tiny hemorrhages[70]. In Curtis' description he emphasized that the adhesions were numerous, often of sufficient length to allow considerable movement between the liver and parietal peritoneum, and that they occupied an area of several inches in diameter. Characteristically, the condition occurred in female patients with symptoms suggestive of gall bladder disease or pleurisy.

ETIOLOGY

The evidence assembled by Bolton and Darougar[70] for the association between genital tract infection and perihepatitis is very strong. Stanley[71] described the successful treatment of three female patients with perihepatitis in whom acute pain developed in the upper part of the

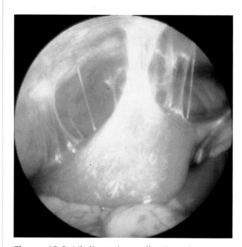

Figure 12.2 Violin-string adhesions in chlamydial pelvic inflammatory disease and perihepatitis (reproduced from Rein 1996[79])

abdomen, especially on the right side, in whom gonococci were cultured from the cervix or urethra or both. In the context of a surgical ward in Helsinki, von Knorring and Nieminen[72] describe 6 female patients with symptoms indistinguishable from acute cholecystitis, and in all 6 the diagnosis was established by obtaining *N. gonorrhoeae* on culture from the cervix.

In more recent years cases have been reported in which the clinical picture of the Curtis–Fitz-Hugh syndrome was present, the diagnosis of perihepatitis was supported by laparoscopy, but in whom the gonococcus could not be found. In these cases *C. trachomatis* is probably the cause. Of 11 cases in Zurich, reported by Muller-Schoop et al.[73], in women aged 17 to 38 years with acute peritonitis proven by laparoscopy, 7 also had perihepatitis, and only 2 had signs of salpingitis on gynecological examination. Micro-immunofluorescence tests showed extremely high titers (≥ 2048) of IgG antibody in 6 patients, and in 4 there was strong evidence of recent chlamydial infection; the gonococcus was detected on cervical culture in 3 women.

In 1982, Wolner-Hanssen et al.[74] succeeded in isolating *C. trachomatis* by swabbing the surface of the liver capsule in a patient whose laparoscopic findings indicated acute salpingitis and perihepatitis, i.e. the Curtis–Fitz-Hugh syndrome, and who had presented because of a 10-day history of abdominal pain in the right upper quadrant. In this case *C. trachomatis* was also isolated from the cervix but not from the uterine tube; *N. gonorrhoeae* was not isolated from any site.

The route by which organisms affecting the genital tract may reach the liver surface has been the subject of much speculation. Transcoelomic, bloodstream, and lymphatic spread have all been considered. *C. trachomatis* may ascend through the genital tract without causing salpingitis in some cases. A peritoneal reaction with exudate may facilitate spread of the organism.

The Curtis–Fitz-Hugh syndrome was first reported in a male in whom the gonococcus was cultured by Kimball and Knee[75]. In a case in Ibadan, Nigeria, the syndrome was accompanied by proven gonococcal urethritis, fever, and arthritis of the left knee, both ankles, and right wrist[76]. In the case of a male bisexual described by Davidson and Hawkins[77], *N. gonorrhoeae* was cultured from the throat, and the presence of a widespread pustular rash thought to be typical of a disseminated gonococcal infection suggested that spread had occurred by the bloodstream.

CLINICAL FEATURES

Characteristically the Curtis–Fitz-Hugh syndrome almost always occurs in young women. Pain, often severe and acute, is the main symptom and it is felt in the right upper quadrant of the abdomen. Similar severe pain may have been present in the preceding 1 to 2 weeks and occasionally there is a longer history of chronic pain. Patients with the acute and severe pain may be admitted as acute surgical emergencies and the condition confused with cholecystitis, biliary colic, pleurisy, pneumonia, or pulmonary embolism.

The pain is typical of peritoneal inflammation – being made worse by movement, deep breathing, and abdominal palpation – and patients prefer to lie still. The pain often radiates to the back and right shoulder. Nausea and vomiting sometimes accompany the pain, but vomiting is unusual. Tenderness in the right upper abdominal quadrant is always present and patients exhibit guarding and a positive Murphy's sign*. A hepatic friction rub may be heard over the right anterior costal margin. Signs of generalized peritonitis are usually absent but evidence of pelvic peritonitis should be sought. About half the patients have a low-grade pyrexia and the erythrocyte sedimentation rate may be raised.

Careful questioning will elicit a history of previous genital tract infection or PID in at least two-thirds of patients, and the majority will have symptoms and signs of pelvic infection[70].

DIAGNOSIS

In patients with Curtis–Fitz-Hugh syndrome a sexual history should be obtained,

---

* Murphy's sign: the examining hand is placed just below the right costal margin midway between the xiphisternum and anterior axillary line. In patients with acute cholecystitis deep inspiration is associated with a sudden accentuation of pain.

and the examination necessary to exclude gonococcal and chlamydial disease, and other STIs should be carried out. Hematological, biochemical, and radiological investigations (white cell count in the peripheral blood, erythrocyte sedimentation rate, radiological and ultrasonic investigations of the biliary tract, radiological examination of the chest, and liver-related enzymes and bilirubin) will enable the exclusion of alternative explanations of the patient's symptoms and signs.

Antichlamydial antibody levels in the blood may be useful retrospectively. Antibodies to *C. trachomatis* may also be sought in discharges from the cervix and urethra, using the micro-IF test[70].

TREATMENT

The management of perihepatitis is as described above for PID (see pp. 362–363). Immediate relief of pain may be obtained when pain persists, in spite of antimicrobial treatment, by the division surgically by cauterization and division of perihepatic adhesions under direct laparoscopic visualization[78].

References

1 Eschenbach DA, Holmes KK. Acute pelvic inflammatory disease: current concepts of pathogenesis, etiology and management. *Clin Obstet Gynecol* 1975; **18**: 35–36.

2 Bevan CD, Johal BJ, Mumtaz G, Ridgway GL, Siddle NC. Clinical, laparoscopic and microbiological findings in acute salpingitis: report of a United Kingdom cohort. *Br J Obstet Gynaecol* 1995; **102**: 407–414.

3 Soper DE, Brockwell NJ, Dalton HP, Johnson D. Observations concerning the microbial etiology of acute salpingitis. *Am J Obstet Gynecol* 1994; **170**: 1008–1017.

4 Woolfit JMG, Watt L. Chlamydial infection of the urogenital tract in promiscuous and non-promiscuous women. *Br J Vener Dis* 1977; **53**: 93–95.

5 Ward ME, Watt PJ, Robertson JN. The human fallopian tube; a laboratory model for gonococcal infection. *J Infect Dis* 1974; **129**: 650–659.

6 Patton DL. Immunopathology and histopathology of experimental chlamydial salpingitis. *Rev Infect Dis* 1982; **7**: 746–750.

7 Mardh P-A, Westrom L. Tubal and cervical cultures in acute salpingitis with special reference to mycoplasma and T-strain mycoplasmas. *Br J Vener Dis* 1970; **46**: 179–186.

8 Mardh P-A, Westrom L, von Mecklenburg C, Hammar E. Studies on ciliated epithelia of the human genital tract. I. Swelling of the cilia of Fallopian tube epithelium in organ cultures infected with *Mycoplasma hominis. Br J Vener Dis* 1976; **52**: 52–57.

9 Tully JG, Taylor-Robinson D, Rose DL, Furr PM, Graham CE, Barile MF. Urogenital challenge of primate species with *Mycoplasma genitalium* and characteristics of infection induced in chimpanzees. *J Infect Dis* 1986; **153**: 1046–1054.

10 Eschenbach DA, Harnisch JP, Holmes KK. Pathogenesis of acute pelvic inflammatory disease: role of contraception and other risk factors. *Am J Obstet Gynecol* 1977; **128**: 838–850.

11 Walker CK, Workowski KA, Washington AE, Soper D, Sweet RL. Anaerobes in pelvic inflammatory disease: implications for the Centers for Disease Control and Prevention's guidelines for treatment of sexually transmitted diseases. *Clin Infect Dis* 1999; **28** (Suppl. 1): S29–S36.

12 Paavonen J, Teisala K, Heinonen PK, *et al.* Microbiological and histopathological findings in acute pelvic inflammatory disease. *Br J Obstet Gynaecol* 1987; **94**: 454–460.

13 Korn AP, Bolan G, Padian N, Ohm-Smith M, Schachttere J, Landers DV. Plasma cell endometritis in women with symptomatic bacterial vaginosis. *Obstet Gynecol* 1995; **85**: 387–390.

14 McGregor JA, French JI, Jones W, *et al.* Bacterial vaginosis is associated with prematurity and vaginal fluid mucinase and sialidase: results of a controlled trial of topical clindamycin cream. *Am J Obstet Gynecol* 1994; **170**: 1048–1060.

15 Briselden AM, Moncla BJ, Stevens CE, Hillier SL. Sialidases (neuraminidases) in bacterial vaginosis and bacterial vaginosis-associated microflora. *J Clin Microbiol* 1992; **30**: 663–666.

16 Apicella MA, Mandrell RE, Shero M, *et al.* Modification by sialic acid of *Neisseria gonorrhoeae* lipoligosaccharide epitope expression in human urethral exudates: an immunoelectron microscopic analysis. *J Infect Dis* 1990; **162**: 506–512.

17 Mardh P-A, Moller BR, Engerselv HJ, Nussler E, Westrom L, Wolner-Haussen P. Endometritis caused by *Chlamydia trachomatis. Br J Vener Dis* 1981; **57**: 191–195.

18 Brosens JJ, de Souza NM, Barker FG. Uterine junctional zone: function and disease. *Lancet* 1995; **346**: 558–560.

19 Draper DL, James JF, Hadley WK, Sweet RL. Auxotypes and antibiotic susceptibilities of *Neisseria gonorrhoeae* from women with acute salpingitis: comparison with gonococci causing uncomplicated genital tract infections in women. *Sex Transm Dis* 1981; **8**: 43–50.

20 Taylor-Robinson D, Whytock S, Green CJ, Carney FE. Effect of *Neisseria gonorrhoeae* on human and rabbit oviducts. *Br J Vener Dis* 1974; **50**: 279–288.

21 Rice PA, Schachter J. Pathogenesis of pelvic inflammatory disease. What are the questions? *JAMA* 1991; **266**: 2587–2593.

22 Lehtinen M, Paavonen J. Heat shock proteins in the immunopathogenesis of chlamydial pelvic inflammatory disease. In: Orfila J (ed.) *Chlamydial Infections.* Proceedings of the 7th international symposium on human chlamydial infections. Bologna; Esculapio: 1994.

23 Patton DL, Wolner-Hanssen P, Cosgrove SJ, Holmes KK. The effects of *Chlamydia trachomatis* on the female reproductive tract of the *Macaca nemestrina* after a single tubal challenge following repeated cervical inoculations. *Obstet Gynecol* 1990; **76**: 643–650.

24 Rank RG, Sanders MM, Patton DL. Increased incidence of oviduct pathology in the guinea pig after repeat vaginal inoculation with the chlamydial agent of guinea pig inclusion conjunctivitis. *Sex Transm Dis* 1995; **22**: 48–54.

25 Darville T, Andrews CW, Kishen LR, Rank RG, Williams DM. Transforming growth factor-beta is associated with increased pathology in gamma-interferon gene knockout mice infected with chlamydiae. In: Stephens RS, Byrne GI, Christiansen G, *et al.* (ed.) *Chlamydial Infections.* Proceedings of the 9th international symposium on human chlamydial infection. San Francisco; International Chlamydia Symposium: 1998.

26 Blander SJ, Amortegui A, Wagar E. Mice sensitised to the 60 kDa heat shock protein have increased inflammation after genital chlamydial infection. *Clin Res* 1994; **42**: 150–157.

27 Domeika M, Domeika K, Paavonen J, Mardh PA, Witkin SS. Humoral immune response to conserved epitopes of *Chlamydia trachomatis* and human 60-kDa heat-shock protein in women with pelvic inflammatory disease. *J Infect Dis* 1998; **177**: 714–719.

28 Peeling RW, Bailey RL, Conway DJ, *et al.* Antibody response to the 60 kDa heat shock protein is associated with scarring trachoma. *J Infect Dis* 1998; **177**: 256–259.

29 Ward ME. Mechanisms of chlamydia-induced disease. In: Stephens RS (ed.) *Chlamydia. Intracellular Biology, Pathogenesis, and Immunity.* Washington DC; ASM Press: 1999.

30 Kimani J, Maclean IW, Bwayo JJ, *et al.* Risk factors for *Chlamydia trachomatis* pelvic inflammatory disease among sex workers in Nairobi, Kenya. *J Infect Dis* 1996; **173**: 1437–1444.

31 Simms I, Stephenson JM. Pelvic inflammatory disease epidemiology: what do we know and what do we need to know. *Sex Transm Infect* 2000; **76**: 80–87.

32 Kamwendo F, Forslin L, Bodin L, Danielsson D. Decreasing incidences of gonorrhea and chlamydia-associated acute pelvic inflammatory disease. A 25-year study from an urban area of central Sweden. *Sex Transm Dis* 1995; **23**: 384–391.

33 Wolner-Hanssen P, Eschenbach DA, Paavonen J, *et al.* Decreased risk of symptomatic chlamydial pelvic inflammatory disease associated with oral contraceptive use. *JAMA* 1990; **263**: 54–59.

34 Sinei SK, Morrison CS, Sekkade-Kigondu C, Allen M, Kokonya D. Complications of use of intrauterine devices among HIV-1 infected women. *Lancet* 1998; **351**: 1238–1241.

35 Faundes A, Telles E, Cristofoletti M, Faundes D, Castro S, Hardy E. The risk of inadvertent intrauterine device insertion in women carriers of endocervical *Chlamydia trachomaits. Contraception* 1999; **58**: 105–109.

36 Shelton JD. Risk of pelvic inflammatory disease attributable to an intrauterine device. *Lancet* 2001; **357**: 443.

37 Qvigstad E, Skaug K, Jerve F, Vik ISS, Ulstrup JC. Therapeutic abortion and *Chlamydia trachomatis* infection. *Br J Vener Dis* 1982; **58**: 182–183.

37a Irwin KL, Moorman AC, O'Sullivan MJ, *et al.* Influence of human immunodeficiency virus infection on pelvic inflammatory disease. *Obstet Gynecol* 2000; **95**: 525–534.

38 Cohen CR, Sinei S, Reilly M, *et al.* Effect of human immunodeficiencey virus type 1 infection upon acute salpingitis: a laparoscopic study. *J Infect Dis* 1998; **178**: 1352–1358.

38a Cohen CR, Nguti R, Bukusi EA, *et al.* Human immunodeficiency virus type 1-infected women exhibit reduced interferon-gamma secretion after *Chlamydia trachomatis* stimulation of peripheral blood lymphocytes. *J Infect Dis* 2000; **182**: 1672–1677.

39 Wolner-Hanssen P, Eschenbach DA, Paavonen J, *et al.* Association between vaginal douching and acute pelvic inflammatory disease. *JAMA* 1990; **263**: 1936–1941.

40 Scholes D, Daling J, Stergachis A. Current cigarette smoking and risk of acute pelvic inflammatory disease. *Am J Public Health* 1992; **82**: 1352–1355.

41 Svensson L, Westrom L, Ripa KT, Mardh PA. Differences in some clinical and laboratory parameters in acute salpingitis related to culture and serologic findings. *Am J Obstet Gynecol* 1980; **138**: 1017–1021.

42 Lehtinen M, Laine S, Heinonen PK, *et al.* Serum C-reactive protein determination in acute pelvic inflammatory disease. *Am J Obstet Gynecol* 1986; **154**: 158–159.

43 Jacobson L, Westrom L. Objectivized diagnosis of acute pelvic inflammatory disease. *Am J Obstet Gynecol* 1969; **105**: 1088–1098.

44 McCormack WM, Nowroozi K, Alpert S, *et al.* Acute pelvic inflammatory disease: characteristics of patients with gonococcal infection and evaluation of their response to treatment with aqueous procaine penicillin G and spectinomycin hydrochloride. *Sex Transm Dis* 1977; **4**: 125–131.

45 Westrom L, Joesoef R, Reynolds G, Hagdu A, Thompson SE. Pelvic inflammatory disease and fertility. A cohort study of 1,844 women with laparoscopically verified disease and 657 control women with normal laparoscopic results. *Sex Transm Dis* 1992; **19**: 185–192.

46 Pavletic AJ, Wolner-Hanssen P, Paavonen J, Hawes SE, Eschenbach DA. Infertility following pelvic inflammatory disease. *Infect Dis Obstet Gynecol* 1999; **7**: 145–152.

47 Westrom L. Influence of sexually transmitted diseases on sterility and ectopic pregnancy. *Acta Eur Fertil* 1985; **16**: 21–24.

48 Joesoef MR, Westrom L, Reynolds G, Marchbanks P, Cates W. Recurrence of ectopic pregnancy: the role of salpingitis. *Am J Obstet Gynecol* 1991; **165**: 46–50.

49 Westrom L, Svensson L. Chronic pain after acute pelvic inflammatory disease. In: Belfort *et al.* (eds) *Advances in Gynecology and Obstetrics.* Proceedings of the XIIth world congress in gynecology and obstetrics. Lancashire UK; Casterton Hall: 1988.

50 Mol BWJ, Hajenuis PJ, Engelsbel S, *et al.* Serum human chorionic gonadotrophin measurement in the diagnosis of ectopic pregnancy when transvaginal sonography is inconclusive. *Fertil Steril* 1998; **70**: 972–981.

51 Filly RA. Ectopic pregnancy. In: Callen PW (ed.) *Ultrasonography in Obstetrics and Gynecology.* Philadelphia; WB Saunders; 1994.

52 Rawlings EE, Balgobin B. Complications of laparoscopy. *Br Med J* 1975; **i**: 727–728.

53 Paavonen J, Aine R, Teisala K, Heinonen PK, Punnonen R. Comparison of endometrial biopsy and peritoneal fluid cytologic testing with laparoscopy in the diagnosis of acute pelvic inflammatory disease. *Am J Obstet Gynecol* 1985; **151**: 645–650.

54 Swayne LC, Love MB, Karasick SR. Pelvic inflammatory disease: sonographic-pathologic correlation. *Radiology* 1984; **151**: 751–755.

55 Cacciatore B, Leminen A, Ingman-Friberg S, Ylostalo P, Paavonen J. Transvaginal sonographic findings in ambulatory patients with suspected pelvic inflammatory disease. *Obstet Gynecol* 1992; **80**: 912–916.

56 Khalife S, Falcone T, Hemmings R, Cohen D. Diagnostic accuracy of transvaginal ultrasound in detecting free pelvic fluid. *J Reprod Med* 1998; **43**: 795–798.

57 Tukeva TA, Aronen HJ, Karjalainen PT, Molander P, Paavonen T, Paavonen J. MR imaging in pelvic inflammatory disease: comparison with laparoscopy and US. *Radiology* 1999; **210**: 209–216.

58 Hillis SD, Joesoef R, Marchbanks PA, Wasserheit JN, Cates W, Westrom L. Delayed care of PID as a risk factor for impaired fertility. *Am J Obstet Gynecol* 1993; **168**: 1503–1509.

59 Clinical Effectiveness Group (Association of Genitourinary Medicine and the Medical Society for the Study of Venereal Diseases. 2001 Guidelines for the management of pelvic infection and perihepatitis. www.mssvd.org.uk/ceg.html.

60 Centers for Disease Control and Prevention. 2002 Guidelines for treatment of sexually transmitted diseases. *MMWR* 2002; **51**; RR-6.

61 Hemsell DL, Little BB, Faro S, *et al.* Comparison of three regimens recommended by the Centers for Disease Control and Prevention for the treatment of women hospitalized with acute pelvic inflammatory disease. *Clin Infect Dis* 1994; **19**: 720–727.

62 Soper DE, Brockwell NJ, Dalton HP. Microbial etiology of urban emergency department acute salpingitis: treatment with ofloxacin. *Am J Obstet Gynecol* 1992; **167**: 653–660.

63 Wolfson JS, Hooper DC. Fluoroquinolone antimicrobial agents. *Clin Microbiol Rev* 1989; **2**: 378–424.

64 McGregor JA, Crombleholme WR, Newton E, Sweet RL, Tuomala R, Gibbs RS. Randomized comparison of ampicillin-sulbactam to cefoxitin and doxycycline or clindamycin and gentamicin in the treatment of pelvic inflammatory disease or endometritis. *Obstet Gynecol* 1994; **83**: 998–1004.

65 Heinonen PK, Teisala K, Miettinen A, Aine R, Punnonen R, Gonroos P. A comparison of ciprofloxacin with doxycycline plus metronidazole in the treatment of acute pelvic inflammatory disease. *Scand I Infect Dis* 1989; **60** (Suppl.): 66–73.

66 Arrendondo JL, Diaz V, Gaitan H, *et al.* Oral clindamycin and ciprofloxacin versus intramuscular ceftriaxone and oral doxycycline in the treatment of mild-to-moderate pelvic inflammatory disease in outpatients. *Clin Infect Dis* 1997; **24**: 170–178.

66 Martens MG, Gordon S, Yarborough DR, Faro S, Binder D, Berkeley A. Multicenter randomized trial of ofloxacin versus cefoxitin and doxycycline in outpatient treatment of pelvic inflammatory disease. Ambulatory PID Research Group. *South Med J* 1993; **86**: 604–610.

67 Ross JDC. Outpatient antibiotics for pelvic inflammatory disease. *Br Med J* 2001; **322**: 251–252.

68 Curtis AH. A cause of adhesions in the right upper quadrant. *JAMA* 1930; **94**: 1221–1222.

69 Fitz-Hugh T. Acute gonococcal peritonitis of the right upper quadrant in women. *JAMA* 1934; **102**; 2094–2096.

70 Bolton JP, Darougar S. Perihepatitis. *Br Med J* 1983; **39**: 159–162.

71 Stanley MM. Gonococcic peritonitis of the upper part of the abdomen in young women. *Arch Int Med* 1946; **78**: 1–13.

72 von Knorring J, Nieminen J. Gonococcal perihepatitis in a surgical ward. *Ann Clin Res* 1979; **11**: 66–70.

73 Muller-Schoop JW, Wang SP. Munzinger J. Schlapfer HU, Knoblauch M, Wammann RW. *Chlamydia trachomatis* as a possible cause of peritonitis and perihepatitis in young women. *Br Med J* 1978; **I**: 1022–1024.

74 Wolner-Hanssen P, Svensson L, Westrom L, Mardh P-A. Isolation of *Chlamydia trachomatis* from the liver capsule in Fitz-Hugh–Curtis syndrome. *N Engl J Med* 1982; **306**: 113.

75 Kimball MW, Knee S. Gonococcal perihepatitis in the male. *N Engl J Med* 1970; **282**: 1082–1084.

76 Francis TI, Osoba O. Gonococcal hepatitis Fitz-Hugh–Curtis syndrome in a male patient. *Br J Vener Dis* 1972; **48**: 187–188.

77 Davidson AC, Hawkins DA. Pleuritic paIn: Fitz-Hugh–Curtis syndrome in a man. *Br Med J* 1982; **284**: 808.

78 Reichart JA, Valle RF. Fitz-Hugh–Curtis syndrome. *JAMA* 1976; **236**: 266–268.

79 Rein MF (ed.). *Atlas of Infectious Diseases, Volume V, Sexually Transmitted Diseases.* Churchill Livingstone; Philadelphia: 1996.

Chapter 13

Prostatitis, orchitis, and epididymitis
A McMillan

Prostatitis and chronic pelvic pain syndrome in men

In those with clinical features, particularly episodes of pain characteristic of inflammation of the prostate, it may not be possible to confirm a diagnosis of prostatitis because histological findings and the results of examination of the prostatic fluid, including attempts to isolate organisms, are often inconclusive. 'Acute prostatitis' caused by organisms isolated by conventional bacteriological techniques and referred to here as 'eubacteria', is, however, more clearly defined as an entity than 'chronic prostatitis', where no organisms can be isolated either by conventional bacteriological methods, or even by the special methods required for other organisms that may have an etiological role. As the diagnosis of 'prostatitis' tends therefore to be made on symptoms, it is necessary to consider first the symptom of 'prostatic pain'.

PROSTATIC PAIN

Prostatic pain may be felt in the suprapubic region, the back, the groins, and the spermatic cord and testis of one or both sides. It may also radiate to the inner thighs. It may radiate to the perineum and to the penis, where it may be felt in the urethra and in the penile meatus, usually at the beginning and on completion of micturition. There may also be urgency, frequency, dysuria, painful ejaculation, abnormal urine flow, alteration in color of the semen, and, occasionally, hematospermia.

In view of the common segmental autonomic innervation of the kidneys, urethra, bladder, and prostate, the distribution of pain may be the same in pathology of any part of the upper and lower urinary tract; for these reasons imaging of the urinary tract and cystourethroscopy may be necessary to exclude such pathology when the prostate itself, so far as can be ascertained, is not the cause of the pain[1].

The variability of symptoms in the prostatitis syndromes has led the National Institute of Diabetes and Digestive and Kidney Diseases, USA[2] to reclassify the prostatitis syndromes (Table 13.1) and to develop a practical instrument (chronic prostatitis symptom index) that measures the symptoms of 'chronic prostatitis' and can be used in a clinical or research setting[3]. The universal adoption of this index should allow comparison of studies from different centers, for example, on the effects of treatments.

PROSTATITIS WITH DEMONSTRABLE INFECTION

Acute prostatitis

Histologically, there is diffuse edema and hyperemia, and a marked polymorpho-

Table 13.1 Classification system for prostatitis (National Institute of Diabetes and Digestive and Kidney Diseases 1995[3])

Type	Classification	Definition
I	Acute bacterial prostatitis	Evidence of acute bacterial infection
II	Chronic bacterial prostatitis	Evidence of recurrent bacterial infection
III	Chronic pelvic pain syndrome	No demonstrable infection
III A	Inflammatory (formerly chronic abacterial prostatitis)	White blood cells in semen, expressed prostatic secretions or voided bladder urine 3 (sediment from initial 10 mL urine after prostatic massage during Meares-Stamey 4 glass test)
III B	Non-inflammatory (formerly prostatodynia)	No white blood cells in semen, expressed prostatic secretions or voided bladder urine 3 (sediment from initial 10 mL urine after prostatic massage during Meares–Stamey 4 glass test)
IV	Asymptomatic inflammatory prostatitis	No symptoms, incidental diagnosis during prostatic biopsy or presence of white blood cells in prostatic secretions during evaluation for other disorders

nuclear leukocyte infiltration of either part of or the entire gland[4]. The inflammatory cell infiltrate is seen within and around the acini, and lymphocytes, plasma cells, and macrophages also invade the stroma. Micro-abscesses are common, and larger abscesses may develop.

Acute prostatitis is characterized by pyrexia, rigors, frequency and urgency of micturition, and dysuria. There is pain in the distribution described, although perineal pain itself is uncommon in the acute phase, since the accompanying malaise encourages bed rest and relaxation of pelvic floor musculature[1]. Gentle palpation of the gland per rectum may show that it is tender, swollen, irregular, and indurated. On transrectal ultrasonography, the gland is slightly and symmetrically enlarged and there is a heterogeneous echo pattern with multiple echo-poor areas. There is a prominent peri-urethral halo and prominent peri-prostatic veins may be seen[5]. Bacteriological examination of the urine by conventional techniques generally demonstrates the causative organisms, which may be *Escherichia coli*, *Klebsiella* spp., *Pseudomonas aeruginosa*, or *Proteus* spp. Gonococcal prostatitis is rare.

If acute prostatitis is untreated a prostatic abscess may develop and cause perineal pain of great intensity. A more common symptom, however, is acute retention of urine[4]. Additional features of prostatic abscess formation may be apparent and include fever, frequency, dysuria, and hematuria. Prostatic abscesses may be associated with a variety of organisms, including *Escherichia coli*, staphylococci, *Pseudomonas* spp., *Brucella* spp., and *Staphylococcus aureus*, and are most commonly found in diabetic men, immunocompromised individuals, and those with in-dwelling catheters. Transrectal ultrasonography or CT imaging are the investigations of choice. A hypoechoic mass, often with contained echoes, crossing septa and a thick wall are seen by the former method, and CT scanning reveals a low-density collection with septa, and an enclosing rim[6].

Chronic prostatitis

This is one of the most common causes of relapsing urinary tract infection due to eubacteria in any age group but, more commonly, in middle age. Accounting for less than 5% of cases, however, chronic bacterial prostatitis is not the most common cause of chronic pelvic pain syndrome (CPPS) in men[7]. The histology of the gland is non-specific and the inflammatory changes are less marked than in acute prostatitis and are often focal. There is a variable infiltrate of plasma cells and macrophages within and around acini, and focal invasion by lymphocytes[4]. It may be associated with a variety of organisms, most commonly Gram-negative bacilli, but occasionally Gram-positive organisms. Obligate anaerobes are only rarely associated with chronic prostatitis. Chronic bacterial (eubacterial) prostatitis is characterized by a relapsing urinary tract infection caused by the same pathogen[8] and although some patients present with an asymptomatic bacteriuria, symptoms of 'prostatic' pain and dysuria also occur.

Viral prostatitis

In the immunocompromised patient, viral prostatitis is rare, but herpes simplex virus has been detected in prostatic fluid from patients with symptoms of chronic prostatitis[9], and cytomegalovirus infection of the prostate has been reported in immunocompromised patients.

Granulomatous prostatitis

Granulomatous prostatitis, that can only be diagnosed by histology, may be idiopathic or be caused by *Mycobacterium tuberculosis*, Bacillus Calmette-Guerin (BCG), following intravesical installation of BCG as adjuvant therapy for bladder cancer, or fungal infections, including *Cryptococcus* spp. and histoplasmosis.

Trichomonas vaginalis and prostatitis

Using an immunoperoxidase method, Gardner and colleagues[10] demonstrated *T. vaginalis* in the human prostate gland.

They described a variety of inflammatory changes within the prostatic urethra and parenchyma, ranging from focal aggregates of polymorphonuclear leukocytes to micro-abscesses, and there is focal denudation of the glandular epithelium. A chronic inflammatory response, including lymphocytes and macrophages, may also be seen in the stroma of the gland. As concurrent infection was not excluded in the study, however, it cannot be assumed that the protozoan caused these inflammatory changes.

CHRONIC PELVIC PAIN SYNDROME

In its clinical presentation this chronic condition is associated with recurrent episodes of pain, and it has been referred to in terms such as chronic idiopathic prostatitis, prostatodynia, or chronic non-bacterial prostatitis. The patient is usually young to middle-aged, most affected individuals being between 35 and 45 years. Symptoms are those described in 'prostatic pain' (page 369) but malaise and pyrexia are absent, and the perineal pain, particularly, is not as severe as in acute bacterial prostatitis. Bacterial culture of the urine yields negative results, and in contrast to chronic bacterial prostatitis, recurrent episodes of cystitis and epididymitis do not tend to occur. Increased numbers of polymorphonuclear leukocytes may or may not be found in expressed prostatic secretions. In a recent study[11], inflammation was found in 29% of biopsies from 97 men with CPPS. The inflammatory infiltrate was composed predominantly of mononuclear cells distributed in a diffuse stromal pattern; neutrophils were rare and only found in the lumina of the glands. Moderate to severe inflammation was only found in 5% of these men. However, histological evidence of prostatic inflammation is extremely common in men without pelvic pain[12].

Etiology

The detection of bacterial gene sequences in prostatic tissue from some patients with

CPPS using a broad spectrum PCR, suggested a bacterial etiology for this condition[13]. However, bacterial DNA sequences have also been identified in transperineal prostatic biopsies from men without CPPS. Using nested primers for a highly conserved region of the bacterial 16s rRNA gene, bacterial sequences were found in 11 of 18 biopsies of 8 of 9 patients with adenocarcinoma of the prostate[14]. The genera and species of the bacteria from which the DNA has been derived remain to be identified.

The following organisms have been proposed as playing an etiological role in CPPS.

1. Chlamydia trachomatis

Chlamydia trachomatis is unlikely to play a causative role in CPPS. In an investigation of 53 cases of non-acute prostatitis in Sweden, Mardh[15] isolated *C. trachomatis* from the urethra in only one case and failed to find this organism in any of the 28 specimens of prostatic fluid examined. From this result, and from those of micro-immunofluorescent tests, they considered that in their study *C. trachomatis* appeared to play only a minor role, if any, in 'non-acute' prostatitis. Isolation difficulties might, however, be analogous to the situation of ocular hyperendemic trachoma, where it is possible to isolate *C. trachomatis* from 70% of acute cases but from only 5% of chronic cases[16]. *Chlamydia trachomatis* has rarely been cultured from prostatic aspirates or antigen detected in such material from patients who did not have urethral chlamydial infection[17], further casting doubts about a chlamydial etiology for chronic idiopathic prostatitis. The report of the detection of chlamydial DNA in prostatic tissue by *in situ* hybridization in 3 of 11 biopsy specimens[18] needs confirmation before conclusions can be drawn on the significance of the finding.

2. Ureaplasma urealyticum

The role of *Ureaplasma urealyticum* in CPPS is controversial. Although Brunner *et al.*[7] found possible prostatic infection with ureaplasmas in about 14% of over 500 patients, these findings have not been confirmed in more recent studies in which expressed prostatic secretions and biopsy tissue were examined[19].

3. Staphylococcus species

Coagulase-negative *Staphylococcus* spp., including *S. epidermidis* and *S. haemolyticus*, have recently been implicated in the etiology of the chronic idiopathic prostatitis. Lowentritt *et al.*[20] cultured these organisms from the expressed prostatic secretions more frequently from men with CPPS than from control subjects. As coagulase-negative *Staphylococcus* spp. are known to adhere to urothelial cells and to cellular proteins, it is postulated that after adherence they ascend and colonize the prostate gland. In addition, an extracellular slime substance that has anti-phagocytic properties and impairs proliferative responses by T lymphocytes is secreted by these organisms and may protect against host defenses. This slime substance may also protect the bacteria from exposure to antibiotics, resulting in treatment failure.

4. Gram-variable, pleomorphic bacteria

Gram-variable, pleomorphic bacteria are sometimes noted in stained smears of expressed prostatic secretions, and there has been a recent report on the culture of two species of *Corynebacterium*, *C. minutissimum* and *Corynebacterium* group ANF, from this fluid[21]. Culture of these bacteria requires particular growth factors and extended cultivation, and, as laboratories generally do not use the media described, it is likely that the presence of these organisms has previously been overlooked. The significance of these bacteria, and of a recently described species of *Corynebacterium* [22] in the etiology of CPPS remains unknown.

Higher mean levels of the pro-inflammatory cytokines tumor necrosis factor-α (TNF-α) and interleukin-1β (IL-1β) have been found in the semen of some patients with chronic prostatitis or CPPS than in semen from normal men[23]. There was no correlation between the concentrations of these cytokines and the number of leukocytes in expressed prostatic secre-tions. These findings suggest that inflammation of the genital tract is a feature of the condition, irrespective of the presence or absence of leukocytes in expressed prostatic fluid.

Reflux of sterile urine into the prostatic parenchyma as a result of incomplete relaxation of the bladder neck and proximal urethra with resulting inflammation has been postulated as a mechanism for the production of symptoms[24].

DIAGNOSIS OF ACUTE AND CHRONIC PROSTATITIS AND CHRONIC PELVIC PAIN SYNDROME

Acute prostatitis

As the causative organism of acute prostatitis is almost always detected in the urine and prostatic massage may lead to bacteremia, this procedure should be avoided.

Chronic bacterial prostatitis

Traditionally, the diagnosis of chronic prostatitis due to eubacteria has been made by quantitative bacteriological techniques[8, 25]. The following procedures are necessary.

1. Intercourse should be proscribed for at least 24 hours[26], and preferably for 48 hours, before testing.
2. The patient should have a full bladder and a desire to micturate (e.g. after retaining urine overnight or for about 8 hours).
3. Skin preparation is usually unnecessary in the circumcised male. The uncircumcised male is instructed to retract his foreskin and maintain retraction throughout collection of the specimens. The glans is cleansed with detergent; all soap is washed away with a swab soaked in sterile saline.
4. The first 5 to 10 mL of urine passed is collected in a sterile tube (specimen 1: voided bladder urine 1).
5. A midstream specimen of urine (MSU) is obtained after the patient has urinated about 200 mL (specimen 2: voided bladder urine 2).
6. The patient stops voiding and, by gentle prostatic massage, a few drops

of prostatic fluid* are collected in a wide-mouthed container (specimen 3: prostatic fluid).

7. The patient then voids, and 5 to 10 mL urine is collected (specimen 4: voided bladder urine 3 after prostatic massage).

As cultures for eubacteria must be quantitative, it is essential that there is good liaison between the clinician and the microbiologist.

The diagnosis of bacterial prostatitis (or, *sensu stricto*, eubacterial) is made when the bacterial counts in specimen 3 (prostatic fluid) or specimen 4 (urine after prostatic massage) are more than tenfold those in specimens 1 and 2. Recent studies, however, have cast doubts on the validity of these localization studies. For example, Lee et al.[28] found no correlation between bacteria found in specimen 4 (voided bladder urine), and those cultured from prostatic tissue biopsies.

Chronic pelvic pain syndrome

The diagnosis of CPPS is made when the characteristic symptoms have been present for at least 3 months, and other conditions that may mimic prostatitis have been excluded. Pain is central to the diagnosis. Urethral smears, including early morning urethral smears and cultures, should be taken to exclude gonococcal infection; tests should also be taken, when possible, to exclude *Chlamydia trachomatis*, *Ureaplasma urealyticum*, *Trichomonas vaginalis* and herpes simplex virus.

Theoretically, enumeration of the polymorphonuclear leukocytes in the expressed prostatic secretions and in urine specimens 1, 2, and 4 (see above) should differentiate between *CPPS, inflammatory*, and *CPPS, non-inflammatory*. These tests, however, are unreliable. An assessment of prostatic inflammation based on the number of leukocytes per high-power microscope field (× 40 objective) and on the cell count in expressed prostatic secretions was reported by Simmons and Thin[29]. They estimated that the upper limit of normal for the number of leukocytes was 5 per oil immersion field, or $0.5 \times 10^9/L$. These values are lower than those reported by others, but dilution of secretion with residual urine in the method may explain this discrepancy. To base a diagnosis on microscopy findings alone, however, is not reliable[8]; counts of more than 10 leukocytes per high-power field have been found in 6% of healthy volunteers in the Royal Navy[26]. Cellular content varies from day to day and on occasions not enough may be found in a sample. A recent study has shown clearly that the leukocyte counts in expressed prostatic secretions from men with CPPS do not differ significantly from comparison subjects[28].

In any case, there is really no evidence that the management of men with CPPS, inflammatory, and CPPS, non-inflammatory should be different, and the authors consider that the performance of prostatic massage or localization studies referred to above, with enumeration of leukocytes, is unnecessary.

Other tests for prostatic inflammation have been proposed are as follows.

Enumeration of leukocytes in semen

The results of semen analysis for inflammation are difficult to interpret. In a study of 100 men who attended a special prostatitis clinic in Seattle, USA,[30] 6 (26%) of 23 men with more than 10 leukocytes/mL in seminal fluid had what would now be classed as CPPS, inflammatory, and 17 (74%) had a diagnosis of CPPS, non-inflammatory (based on the finding of less than 5 leukocytes/mL in expressed prostatic secretions). Of 77 men who did not have an excess of leukocytes in the seminal fluid, 15 (19%) had CPPS, inflammatory. These findings, and the difficulty in differentiating leukocytes from other cells, make examination of seminal fluid unreliable for the diagnosis of prostatitis.

pH of expressed prostatic fluid

A change in the pH of the prostatic fluid is related to the inflammatory response and not to the organisms isolated[31, 32] and thus may be of value as a clinical test. Although a prostatic fluid pH of 8 or higher is likely to be associated with prostatitis, other tests are required to confirm this diagnosis.

Imaging studies

Transrectal ultrasonography may show diffuse symmetrical enlargement of the gland with a heterogeneous echo pattern. There are focal areas of increased or reduced echogenicity, especially in the peripheral gland, and prostatic calcification is common[33]. None of these changes is specific, and focal lesions in the peripheral region of the prostate that have an identical appearance may be seen in adenocarcinoma. The two conditions can only be differentiated by histology. In men over the age of 50 years, the ultrasonic appearance of benign prostatic hyperplasia makes it difficult to detect inflammatory foci in the central gland.

Magnetic resonance imaging (MRI) provides precise delineation of the prostate, applied in the sagittal plane it demonstrates very clearly the relation of the gland to the base of the bladder, and in the coronal plane the gland's lateral margins. Confident differentiation, however, between prostatitis and neoplasia is not possible, and the application of MRI appears to be in the staging of prostatic carcinoma.

---

* *Technique in obtaining specimens of prostatic secretion.*

As a general rule it is best for the patient to be placed in the left lateral position, with the buttocks at the edge of the bed and the knees well drawn up, although some doctors prefer to have the patient in the dorsal or knee–elbow position. The patient should be asked to breathe freely through the mouth, as this will relax the abdominal muscles and avoid the Valsalva maneuver, i.e. causing increased intrathoracic pressure by forcible exhalation effort against a closed glottis. The well-lubricated forefinger should be introduced slowly. Each lateral lobe of the prostate receives two or three gentle strokes with the palmar surface of the finger, commencing at the periphery of the gland and ending at the midline. This is followed by two downward strokes in the midline over the prostatic urethra. Finally the finger is withdrawn slowly through the anal canal. Slow insertion and withdrawal of the finger lessens discomfort considerably. If no secretion appears at the external urethral meatus, even after gentle milking of the penile urethra, a further attempt may be made at a later date.

A number of adverse reactions to prostatic palpation have been described. Bilbro[27] recorded eight episodes of syncope or faintness, occurring within 30 seconds to 2 minutes, in 2500 prostatic examinations on US Army personnel in Korea during a 13-month period. The patients turned pale and had a bradycardia of 36 to 48 beats per minute. As the patients showed a sudden loss of consciousness if they were not placed supine, it must be assumed they were not lying down when rectal examination was carried out.

Video urodynamic findings

In men with CPPS, peak and average urinary flow rates may be reduced, and there is incomplete relaxation of the bladder neck and proximal urethra to a point just proximal to the external urinary sphincter[4]. Abnormally high maximal urethral closure pressures at rest are also found.

Imaging of the urinary tract and cystourethroscopy

Although imaging of the urinary tract by ultrasonography or excretion urography, or cystourethroscopy are useful in the exclusion of other urological conditions, neither chronic bacterial prostatitis nor CPPS can be confirmed by such methods.

Prostatic biopsy

This procedure is rarely indicated in the investigation of the prostatitis syndromes.

Differential diagnosis of persistent prostatic pain

Causes of persistent prostatic pain include neoplasm, urethral stricture, benign prostatic hyperplasia, radiolucent or opaque bladder calculi, and other causes of functional obstruction to urinary flow.

The pain of prostatitis differs from that of proctalgia fugax, which may be defined as pain, seemingly arising in the rectum, recurring at irregular intervals and being unrelated to organic pain[34]. Among the diagnostic features of this condition are

1. unaccountable occurrence of pain at very irregular intervals in the day or night in a patient in perfect health
2. spontaneous disappearance of the pain
3. localization of pain in the rectal region above the anus, always in the same place in the same patient, but varying somewhat in different patients
4. the severity is variable but the pain may be intense
5. the pain is described as gnawing, aching, cramp-like, or stabbing.

Asymptomatic inflammatory prostatitis

The discovery of excess leukocytes in the expressed prostatic secretion has been taken as the sole criterion in making a diagnosis of prostatitis in patients without prostatic pain. Using this finding, prostatitis has been diagnosed after treatment of urethritis, both gonococcal and non-gonococcal, and treatment of other conditions of uncertain etiology such as

- most (83%) cases of ankylosing spondylitis
- most (95%) cases of sexually acquired reactive arthritis.

For reasons given above, there is doubt over the significance of both the diagnosis and of the findings of 'excess' pus cells in the expressed prostatic secretion.

TREATMENT OF PROSTATITIS

Acute prostatitis

After obtaining a mid-stream specimen of urine for culture, treatment should be initiated before the results become available. In the presence of acute inflammation, penetration of antibiotics into the prostate gland is good. If the symptoms are mild to moderate, oral therapy may be satisfactory. Ciprofloxacin[35], given in an oral dose of 500 mg at 12-hour intervals, or trimethoprim given orally in a dosage of 400 mg every 12 hours, are often satisfactory. In serious infections, gentamicin given by the intravenous route in a dosage of 1.0 to 1.7 mg/kg every 8 hours *and* cefotaxime given by intravenous infusion of 1 g every 12 hours may be used. If there is a good clinical response to the latter regimen and the patient has been afebrile for 48 hours, the antibiotics can be changed to an oral agent to which the infecting pathogen is sensitive. In all cases, treatment should be continued for up to 30 days.

In the treatment of prostatic abscess, drainage is indicated in addition to the use of the above antimicrobial agents. Acute retention of urine should be managed by the insertion of a suprapubic catheter, avoiding urethral instrumentation.

Chronic bacterial prostatitis

The choice of antimicrobial drug should be based on the sensitivities of the infecting organism. Many antimicrobial agents that are active against Gram-negative bacteria, penetrate the prostate poorly. Although most drugs achieve significant levels in the prostatic stroma, in cases of bacterial prostatitis the level achieved in the prostatic secretions correlates best with cure[4]. Tissue levels of the fluoroquinolones are generally higher than those in plasma[36], and for trimethoprim the ratio of the concentration in prostatic tissue to that in serum ranges from 2:1 to 3:1[37]. Ciprofloxacin (500 mg), or ofloxacin (200 mg), or norfloxacin (400 mg), each given by mouth every 12 hours for 28 days, are suitable first-line treatments[38–40].

TREATMENT OF CHRONIC PELVIC PAIN SYNDROME

The treatment of CPPS can be difficult, and the several therapeutic approaches that are described attest to the lack of consensus on optimal therapy. In all cases, however, the patient must be strongly reassured about the benign nature of the condition, and a full explanation about the possible causes should be given. The following strategies may be helpful.

1. As there is some evidence that at least some cases of CPPS are associated with bacterial infection (see pp. 370–371), perhaps as an initiating event, a trial of antimicrobial treatment as described for chronic bacterial prostatitis and given for 28 days is probably justified. There is also some evidence that the tetracyclines, for example, doxycycline, given in an oral dose of 100 mg every 12 hours, are helpful[41].
2. Non-steroidal anti-inflammatory drugs such as ibuprofen may be required for pain relief.
3. The bladder neck and prostate are rich in α-adrenergic nerves, and α-blocking agents that relax the bladder neck and prostate, and improve voiding dysfunction, elevated intra-prostatic pressure, and ejaculatory duct reflux, have been used successfully in the treatment of CPPS[4]. Alfuzosin given in an oral dosage of 2.5 mg every 8 hours, or terazosin given in an initial dose of 1 mg at bedtime, and increased at weekly intervals to a maximum of 10 mg daily, are examples of α-adrenergic drugs that have been used[4]. Postural hypotension, particularly after the first dose is

common, and the patient should be forewarned of this effect. Sedation, weakness, dry mouth, tachycardia and palpitations, and retrograde ejaculation are other side effects. The aim of treatment with α-adrenergic blocking agents is to minimize symptoms without causing troublesome side effects. Treatment should be given for at least 6 months, but, as recurrence of symptoms often develops on discontinuation of the drug, long-term treatment is usually necessary.

4. As there are some anecdotal reports stating that such agents may be useful in the management of troublesome CPPS, and as depression is common amongst affected men[42], a trial of amitriptyline, given as a single dose of 25 to 50 mg before retiring may be justified.

Inflammation of the testis and epididymis

Acute epididymitis in older men (over 35 years of age) usually occurs as a result of a complicated urinary tract infection, commonly caused by coliform organisms. In the case of younger men, in whom such infection is rare, epididymitis is usually caused by the sexually transmitted organisms, *C. trachomatis* or *N. gonorrhoeae*. The prevalence of coliform infection in epididymo-orchitis in young homosexual men who have had unprotected insertive anal intercourse, however, is higher than in heterosexual men[43]. In countries where medical attention and antibiotic or chemotherapy are readily available, gonococcal epididymitis is rare. Coliforms may reach the epididymis as a result of urethral instrumentation[44]. As anatomical abnormalities of the urinary tract are common in men with Gram-negative bacterial infections, especially in those aged 50 years and over[45], urological investigations are indicated in this group of patients. Acute epididymitis due to coliform organisms tends to extend into the testis only in advanced disease, when there may be abscess formation.

In epididymitis complicating a general infection, as in leprosy and mumps, and in the now rare late-stage syphilis, there is almost invariably substantial testicular involvement[46]. It is therefore important to try to distinguish between acute epididymitis and orchitis by careful examination and to detect STIs.

Patients who have a frank urethral discharge may tend to reach departments of genitourinary medicine, whereas those who do not have such a discharge or who may have only a slight discharge may be referred to surgical units. The approach to the diagnosis may therefore differ and there is a need for each discipline to collaborate in the diagnosis and management of epididymitis, as special microbiological facilities required for isolation of the organisms responsible are not always widely available.

ACUTE EPIDIDYMITIS, A COMPLICATION ARISING FROM INFECTION OF THE URINARY TRACT

In countries where antibiotics are freely available acute epididymitis is an uncommon complication of gonorrhea[46]. In young men, however, acute epididymitis is clearly associated with sexually transmitted organisms. In the investigation of a group of 18 men under 32 years of age with epididymitis, culture from the urethra yielded *N. gonorrhoeae* in 6 and *C. trachomatis* in 6 men: both organisms were isolated in an additional patient[47]. Isolations of herpes virus, cytomegalovirus and *U. urealyticum* were also made from urethral specimens in this group[47].

In a study of acute epididymitis (conducted in hospital clinics of the University of Washington, Seattle, USA) involving 13 men under the age of 35 years and 10 men over that age, it was found that in the case of the younger men *C. trachomatis* was the likely cause, as this organism was found in the aspirated material from the affected epididymis in 5 of the 6 tested. In 4 of the 5 patients with chlamydia isolated from the urethra the organism was also obtained from the epididymis. In 5 of the 10 older men examined, only coliform organisms were found in material aspirated from the epididymis[48]. In addition, in 9 of 15 men with epididymitis not due to coliform organisms, *U. urealyticum* was found

in the first-voided urine but aspirated material from the epididymis provided no evidence that *U. urealyticum* reached the epididymis[48].

In men 30 years or older with no obvious risk of an STI, epididymitis is usually associated with bacteriuria due to *Escherichia coli*, *Klebsiella* spp., *Pseudomonas aeruginosa* or *Proteus* spp. In such cases urological investigation is indicated and this should include an excretion urogram and urethrocystoscopy. When epididymitis is associated with a chronic cystitis there is always some predisposing cause of the infection, such as obstruction, stone, or neurological disorder and it is important to exclude pyelonephritis, renal tuberculosis, or analgesic nephropathy. Chronic eubacterial prostatitis may also be a cause.

PATHOLOGY OF EPIDIDYMITIS

At surgical exploration of the scrotum, acute epididymitis shows as an enlarged and tense organ with prominent blood vessels and a fibrinous exudate. Histologically, there is a polymorphonuclear infiltration of the organ with vascular congestion and occasionally abscess formation[49]. Chronic inflammation of the epididymis is characterized by interstitial fibrosis with a chronic inflammatory cell infiltrate, and sometimes lymphoid follicle formation. Although the epididymis is the predominant site of the acute inflammatory process, many patients have concomitant involvement of the testis.

Complications of untreated gonococcal or chlamydial infections include testicular infarction, abscess formation (especially with gonococcal infection), and infertility from fibrosis of the epidididymes or vasa deferentia[50], or from destruction of the testicular parenchyma[51].

ORCHITIS OR EPIDIDYMO-ORCHITIS IN GENERALIZED INFECTIONS

Orchitis and epididymo-orchitis secondary to generalized infections may seldom be seen in STD clinics, but knowledge of their pathology[46] as well as that of other inflammatory lesions of the epididymis and testis is necessary for differential diagnosis.

In syphilis the testicular lesion may be a diffuse chronic interstitial inflammation proceeding to atrophy or a gumma. Clinically, this now rare late-stage effect presents as a painless smooth enlargement of the testis, which is characteristically not tender. Eventually the testis becomes hard because of fibrosis.

In leprosy, particularly lepromatous leprosy, involvement of the testis and, to a lesser extent, the epididymis is very common. *Mycobacterium leprae* proliferates freely in the testes and testicular atrophy is associated with sterility, impotence, and gynecomastia.

Tuberculous epididymitis may begin quickly and be indistinguishable from the infections described, but it is usually insidious. The epididymis enlarges and becomes hard and craggy but is only slightly tender. The vas deferens may be elongated and beaded. Later the epididymis becomes fixed to the skin.

A tuberculous orchitis, generally accompanied by an epididymitis, is always secondary to lesions elsewhere, especially in the lungs, bones, joints, or lymph nodes. It is often preceded by tuberculosis of the prostate and seminal vesicles.

In mumps, epididymo-orchitis complicates 20% of cases in adults, with 1 in 6 showing bilateral involvement. Scrotal swelling is usually noted within a week of parotid enlargement, but sometimes only when the clinical signs of mumps have disappeared. Focal inflammatory changes in the testis become diffuse and there is suppuration in severe cases. The epididymis is involved in 85% of cases and on rare occasions epididymitis occurs by itself. Bilateral orchitis followed by atrophy results in sterility or serious impairment of fertility. If there is no atrophy, even in bilateral cases, fertility does not appear to be impaired. The onset of orchitis is associated with fever and headache. The testis is extremely painful and tender.

Appearing at any stage of brucellosis, an orchitis is clinically more evident than an epididymitis. Morgan[46] reports on an incidence of 5% to 18% and records that it may be five times more common in *Brucella melitensis* infections than in those due to *Br. abortus*. In coxsackie virus B infections orchitis is common, sometimes involving one-third of those infected.

Orchitis may be a complication of systemic fungal infections such as histoplasmosis, blastomycosis, and coccidiodomycosis[49].

A sperm granuloma is caused by extravasation of spermatozoa into surrounding tissue causing a characteristic cellular reaction followed by fibrosis. Sometimes such a granuloma may be seen in the spermatic cord, especially since vasectomy has become more common.

A granulomatous orchitis is a chronic inflammatory lesion of uncertain etiology leading to a hard swelling of the testis in men 50 to 60 years old[46].

In an inflamed hydrocele, proliferation of mesothelial cells in the inflammatory exudate is frequently seen, and is an observation of importance to the pathologist, who wishes to differentiate this change from a true mesothelioma.

Hard non-tender masses of nodular periorchitis may be palpable through the scrotal wall. These may be 0.2 to 2.0 cm in diameter, projecting from either or both layers of the tunica. Sometimes they form loose bodies and histologically they consist of concentrically laminated hyaline collagen[46].

In infestations with *Wuchereria bancrofti, W. pacifica, Brugia malayi,* and related filariae, the clinical manifestations are slow to develop and change in each successive age group. As the infection develops, the adult worms in the lymph nodes may be associated with an adenopathy and sometimes fever and an allergic inflammatory reaction in the catchment areas of the nodes. A lymphangitis spreads centrifugally, for example, from the affected lymph glands in the abdomen, down the spermatic cord and testis, producing a funiculitis and orchitis. An effusion may develop within the tunica vaginalis and eventually elephantiasis of the scrotum may develop. Filariasis due to *W. bancrofti* will be seen in those from Africa and throughout the tropics. In filariasis due to *W. pacifica* (from the islands of the Southern Pacific, particularly Samoa) clinical manifestations are more severe. In filariasis due to *B. malayi* (from coastal regions of India, from Malaya, Indo-China, Indonesia, and New Guinea) genital involvement is rare[52].

CLINICAL FEATURES OF ACUTE EPIDIDYMITIS

The onset of acute epididymitis due to pyogenic organisms, including *N. gonorrhoeae* or associated with *C. trachomatis,* is usually acute, and the pain on the affected side is severe. An associated purulent or mucopurulent urethral discharge is usual in this condition in young men, and there may be malaise and fever. It tends to occur during the second to third week of urethritis, affecting the tail first then the whole of the epididymis, which becomes painful, swollen, and tender, while the overlying skin appears red and shiny. There may be an inflammatory hydrocele. After a few days the inflammation subsides but the epididymis may be left swollen and indurated.

After excluding the gonococcus as a cause, clinical findings may help to distinguish epididymitis due to coliform organisms from that due to chlamydia. Although a urethral discharge may be present in those with chlamydial infection, the patient may not be aware of it; the first urine specimen voided will contain more pus cells than the second, and threads may be present. In coliform urinary infection pyuria will be present in all urine specimens and there will often be visible turbidity in the first voided specimen as well as in the second. Inguinal pain may be more pronounced in the chlamydia-positive cases than in the coliform cases. Scrotal edema and erythema may be more pronounced in patients with coliform infection.[48]

DIAGNOSIS IN EPIDIDYMITIS

Gonococcal infections are recognized by the methods already outlined (Chapter 11). Non-gonococcal epididymitis may be associated with chlamydial infections and the diagnosis is usually reached by

1. detection or exclusion of the gonococcus as a cause
2. examination of urethral or urine specimens for *C. trachomatis,* epididymal aspirations are not advised as a routine procedure
3. detection or exclusion of *E. coli, Klebsiella* spp., *Pseudomonas* or *Proteus* spp. by bacterial examination of a midstream specimen of urine.

There are many potential causes of acute scrotal pain, but differentiation of acute epididymitis from testicular torsion is a common dilemma. Although Blandy *et al.*[53] advise that surgical exploration should be carried out in every apparent 'epididymitis' if there is no infection of the urinary tract, particularly when the swelling is not obviously confined to the epididymis, the use of ultrasonography has obviated this necessity in the majority of patients. The incidence of intravaginal testicular torsion is about 1 in 4000 males under the age of 25 years; about 85% of cases occur in the 12 to 18-year age group. In the typical patient with torsion, there is a sudden onset of pain in the affected side of the scrotum, sometimes with nausea and vomiting. The cremasteric reflex is absent, the testis lies more horizontal than usual and is high in the scrotum. The lower pole of the affected testis is exquisitely tender. When these features are present, surgical exploration is mandatory. The viability of the testis that has undergone torsion depends on the degree of torsion and the duration of symptoms, and surgical intervention should be undertaken as soon as possible after onset of symptoms. It has been estimated[54] that if symptoms have been present for less than 4 hours, the testis remains viable in 95% of cases, if present for less than 8 hours in 90%, if present for less than 12 hours 80%, and if present for more than 24 hours, less than 10% of cases. Clinical signs are not always trustworthy, but imaging studies may give valuable assistance (see below).

It must be emphasized that in any undiagnosed thickening, irregularity, nodule, or enlargement of the testis or epididymis, surgical exposure of the testis is necessary for the exclusion or detection of a malignant neoplasm, although the surgeon will have ultrasonography as an important aid to diagnosis.

Tuberculous epididymitis is rare, but the examination of three consecutive early morning specimens of urine by microscopy of the centrifuged deposit and by culture should detect mycobacterium tuberculosis.

The diagnosis of infection with *Wuchereria bancrofti*, *W. pacifica* or *B. malayi* can be established with certainty only by identifying the microfilariae in the peripheral blood or by recovering an adult worm from an infected lymph node.

Scrotal ultrasonography

The advent of high-frequency real-time ultrasound is now recognized as providing a highly accurate investigation of scrotal pathology[55] and is advocated in all patients referred with scrotal symptoms and signs. In the diagnosis of malignant disease its accuracy, sensitivity, and specificity are clearly superior to clinical methods. Hypoechoic malignant lesions can be discovered within the testicular substance and small central and impalpable tumors can be revealed.

In orchitis the testis is diffusely hypo-echoic. In acute epididymitis the epididymis is swollen and hypoechoic. The differentiation between solid and cystic lesions enables the easy diagnosis of epididymal cysts. Ultrasound is of great value in the examination of a testis rendered impalpable by a surrounding hydrocele. In varicoceles blood flow can be 'visualized'.

Torsion of the testis, however, is not easy to diagnose by real-time scrotal ultrasonography. Color Doppler ultrasound, however, is useful in differentiating acute torsion from epididymo-orchitis, particularly when sophisticated equipment and 'power' Doppler are used. In torsion, blood flow is either absent or reduced whereas in epididymo-orchitis it is increased. However, the detection of color flow in all testes is not always possible, and, especially in small-volume testes, the absence of color may not reflect the presence of impaired perfusion[56]. Conversely, false negative results may occur in the diagnosis of torsion for a variety of reasons, including inexperience of the operator, the often intermittent nature of torsion, and difficulty in obtaining blood flow in small testes. When there is diminished or absent flow to a testis, immediate surgery is required. If the scrotal contents are normal with intratesticular flow demonstrated, the possibility of intermittent torsion cannot be excluded, and the whole clinical picture should be considered together with the ultrasound findings. Thus, the main purpose of color Doppler ultrasonography is the exclusion of causes of testicular pain other than torsion.

TREATMENT OF ACUTE EPIDIDYMITIS

Treatment will depend upon the cause. In the case of acute epididymitis the patient should rest in bed. A bandage or jock strap with a cotton-wool pad supporting the testis will limit movement and prevent pain, and it is helpful to prescribe a non-steroidal anti-inflammatory drug such as ibuprofen.

Treatment for epididymitis is indicated before the results of microbiological tests, with the exception of Gram-smear microscopy, are available. When gonorrhea is suspected, the patient may be given either a single intramuscular injection of ceftriaxone in a dose of 250 mg, or ciprofloxacin in a single oral dose of 500 mg*. As a chlamydial infection may co-exist with gonorrhea, this is followed by doxycycline given as an oral dose of 100 mg every 12 hours for 10–14 days[57,58]. If the patient is hypersensitive to cephalosporins or to tetracyclines, ofloxacin can be given orally in a dose of 200–300 mg every 12 hours for 10–14 days. If the etiology is thought to be *C. trachomatis*; doxycycline is the treatment of choice. Ofloxacin in the above dosage, or levofloxacin, 500 mg given as a single oral dose, each drug being given for 10–14 days should be used for epididymitis associated with enteric bacteria. Improvement is rapid, and failure to improve within 72 hours should prompt reconsideration of the diagnosis of epididymitis. Cragginess or induration of the epididymis, however, may persist for weeks or months. Box 13.1 indicates the conditions that may be associated with failure to respond to antimicrobial therapy. Imaging studies may be helpful in the differential diagnosis, but it is recommended that a surgical opinion should be sought early. The tracing and treatment of contacts is essential in both gonococcal and chlamydial infections as well as in those in which the organismal diagnosis is uncertain.

---

* The quinolones should not be used to treat gonococcal infections that have been acquired in Asia or the Pacific (Chapter 11).

MALIGNANT TUMORS OF THE TESTICLE

Surgical exploration is very important when there is doubt about the diagnosis of any swelling of the testis; some 4% to 16% or more of seminomas or teratomas may present as inflammatory painful lesions[53], and 74% of testicular tumors occur in the age group 20 to 49 years[59]. Scrotal ultrasonography has been shown to be highly accurate in comparison to clinical examination (see page 376).

The usual symptoms of testicular cancer include a lump in the testicle, painless swelling, or altered consistency of the testis. In many cases the tumor is discovered incidentally during medical examination and the mildness of early symptoms together with fear of cancer may lead patients to delay seeking advice. Typically testicular cancer is stony hard with 'a suggestion of weightiness' on palpation. It is of prime importance when the diagnosis is suspected, to refer patients promptly for surgical advice. In addition to assessment by inspection at operation the surgeon will have available the results of serum assays of various tumor markers of malignant germ-cell tumors, namely alpha fetoprotein, beta subunit of human chorionic gonadotropin (HCG) and placental alkaline phosphatase[60]. About 90% of patients with non-seminomatous testicular tumors have elevated serum concentrations of serum alpha fetoprotein and/or HCG; serum levels are elevated in only 5% to 10% of individuals with pure seminomas. The measurement of these markers is useful in the staging of disease and the monitoring of treatment response in those with germ-cell tumors.

The incidence and mortality rates for testicular cancer tend to be bimodal, with prominent peaks in the age group 25 to 34 years and a lesser peak beginning after the age of 75 years. The incidence of testicular cancer is four times greater in whites than in Afro-Caribbean people in the USA[61]. Worldwide, over the past three decades, there has been a rise in the incidence of testicular cancer in young men of about 50%, and in the age group 20 to 34 years testicular cancer is now the most common malignancy although mortality has been reduced by improvement in treatment.

The majority of testicular tumors are germ-cell tumors, broadly classified further into seminoma and malignant teratoma. At present cure rates for seminomas, when patients are seen early, approximate to 80% and early-stage teratoma can be cured by orchidectomy. For metastatic disease effective cytotoxic chemotherapy is available.

Testicular maldescent is recognized as being associated with an increased risk of tumor formation. Another recognized factor that predisposes to testicular cancer is a history of malignancy in the contralateral testis. Random biopsy with special histological techniques may show premalignant cells –carcinoma *in situ* – believed to be precursors of most germ-cell tumors. This technique applied more widely has revealed carcinoma *in situ* in about 5% of patients with unilateral testicular germ-cell cancer[62], 2% of adult men with a history of maldescent of the testis, up to 1% of infertile men, and in up to 80% of men with the rare condition of gonadal dysgenesis[63].

References

1 Blacklock NJ. Prostatic pain. *Br J Hospital Med* 1978; **20**: 80–81.
2 Executive summary. *NIH Workshop on Chronic Prostatitis*. Bethesda, Maryland. 1995. Appendix 1: 1–5.
3 Litwin MS, McNaughton-Collins M, Fowler FJ, *et al*. The National Institutes of Health chronic prostatitis symptom index: development and validation of a new outcome measure. *J Urol* 1999; **162**: 369–375.
4 Meares EM. Prostatitis and related disorders. In: Walsh PC, Retik AB, Darracott Vaughan E, Wein AJ (eds) *Campbell's Urology* 7th edition. Philadelphia: WB Saunders: 1998.
5 Griffiths GJ, Crooks AJR, Roberts EE, *et al*. Ultrasonic appearances associated with prostatic inflammation: a preliminary study. *Clin Radiol* 1984; **35**: 343–345.
6 Thornhill BA, Morehouse HT, Coleman P, Hoffman-Tretin JC. Prostatic abscess: CT and sonographic findings. *Am J Roentgenol* 1987; **148**: 899–900.
7 Brunner H, Weidner W, Schiefer HG. Studies on the role of *Ureaplasma urealyticum* and *Mycoplasma hominis* in prostatitis. *J Infect Dis* 1983; **147**: 807–813.
8 Meares EM. Prostatitis: diagnosis and treatment. *Drugs* 1978; **15**: 472–479.
9 Doble A, Harris JRW, Taylor-Robinson D. Prostatodynia and *Herpes simplex* virus infection. *Urology* 1991; **38**: 247–248.
10 Gardner WA, Culberson DE, Bennett BD. *Trichomonas vaginalis* in the prostate gland. *Arch Pathol Lab Med* 1986; **110**: 430–432.
11 True LD, Berger RE, Rothman I, Ross SO, Krieger JN. Prostate histopathology and the chronic prostatitis/chronic pelvic pain syndrome: a prospective biopsy study. *J Urol* 1999; **162**: 2014–2018.
12 Nickel JC, Young ID, Boag AH. Asymptomatic inflammation and/or infection in benign prostatic hyperplasia. *Br J Urol Int* 1999; **84**: 976–981.
13 Krieger JN, Riley DE, Roberts MC, Berger RE. Prokaryotic DNA sequences in patients with chronic idiopathic prostatitis. *J Clin Microbiol* 1996; **34**: 3120–3128.
14 Keay S, Zhang CO, Baldwin BR, Alexander RB. Polymerase chain reaction amplification of bacterial 16s rRNA genes in prostate biopsies from men without chronic prostatitis. *Urology* 1999; **53**: 487–491.
15 Mardh P-A, Ripa KT, Colleen S, Treharne JD, Darougar S. Role of *Chlamydia trachomatis* in non-acute prostatitis. *Br J Vener Dis* 1978; **54**: 330–334.
16 Darougar S, Woodland RM, Forsey T, Cubitt S, Allami J, Jones BR. Isolation of *Chlamydia* from ocular infections. In: Hobson D, Holmes KK (eds) *Nongonococcal Urethritis and Related Infections*. Washington DC:

American Society for Microbiology: 1977, pp. 295–298.

17 Doble A, Thomas BJ, Walker MM, *et al.* The role of *Chlamydia trachomatis* in chronic abacterial prostatitis: a study using ultrasound guided biopsy. *J Urol* 1989; **141**: 332–333.

18 Kadar A, Bucsek M, Kardos M, Corradi G. Detection of *Chlamydia trachomatis* in chronic prostatitis by in situ hybridization (preliminary methodical report). *Orv Hetil* 1995; **136**: 659–662.

19 Doble A, Thomas BJ, Furr PM, *et al.* A search for infectious agents in chronic abacterial prostatitis utilising ultrasound guided biopsy. *Br J Urol* 1989; **64**: 297–301.

20 Lowentritt JE, Kawahara K, Human LG, Hellstrom WJG, Domingue GJ. Bacterial infection in prostatodynia. *J Urol* 1995; **154**: 1378–1381.

21 Domingue GJ, Human LG, Hellstrom WJG. Hidden microorganisms in 'abacterial' prostatitis/prostatodynia. *J Urol* 1997; **157**: 243.

22 Riegel P, Ruimy R, De Brief D, *et al.* *Corynebacterium seminale* sp. nov., a new species associated with genital infections in male patients. *J Clin Microbiol* 1995; **33**: 2244–2249.

23 Alexander RB, Ponniah S, Hasday J, Hebel JR. Elevated levels of proinflammatory cytokines in the semen of patients with chronic prostatitis/chronic pelvic pain syndrome. *Urology* 1998; **52**: 744–749.

24 Kirby RS, Lowe D, Bultitude MI, Shuttleworth KED. Intra-prostatic urinary reflux: an aetiological factor in abacterial prostatitis. *Br J Urol* 1982; **54**: 729–731.

25 Meares EM, Stamey TA. Bacteriologic localization patterns in bacterial prostatitis and urethritis. *Invest Urol* 1968; **5**: 492–518.

26 Blacklock NJ. Some observations on prostatitis. In: Williams DC, Briggs MH, Standford M (eds) *Advances in the Study of the Prostate.* London; Heinemann: 1969, pp. 37–61.

27 Bilbro RH. Syncope after prostatic examination. *N Engl J Med* 1970; **282**: 167–168.

28 Lee JC, Muller CH, Rothman I, *et al.* Prostatic bacteria and inflammation in male chronic pelvic pain syndrome: a case-control study. *J Urol* 2000; **163**: S23, Abstract 101.

29 Simmons PD, Thin RN. A method for recognising non-bacterial prostatitis: preliminary observations. *Br J Vener Dis* 1983; **59**: 306–310.

30 Krieger JN, Berger RE, Ross SO, Rothman J, Muller CH. Seminal fluid findings in men with nonbacterial prostatitis and prostatodynia. *J Androl* 1996; **17**: 310–318.

31 Blacklock NJ, Beavis JP. The response of the prostatic fluid in inflammation. *Br J Urol* 1974; **46**: 537–542.

32 White MA. Change in pH of expressed prostatic secretion during the course of prostatitis. *Proc Roy Soc Med* 1975; **68**: 511–513.

33 Doble A. Prostatitis. In: Harris JRW, Forster SM (eds) *Sexually Transmitted Diseases.* London; Churchill Livingstone: 1991.

34 Douthwaite AH. Proctalgia fugax. *Br Med J* 1962; **ii**: 164–165.

35 Naber KG. The role of quinolones in the treatment of chronic bacterial prostatitis. *Infection* 1991; **19** (Suppl. 3): S170–S177.

36 Larsen EH, Grasser TC, Dorflinger T, *et al.* The concentration of various quinolones in the human prostate. In: Weidner W, Brunner H, Krause W, Rothauge CF (eds) *Therapy of Prostatitis.* Munich; Verlag: 1986.

37 Meares EM. Prostatitis: review of pharmacokinetics and therapy. *Rev Infect Dis* 1982; **4**: 475.

38 Weidner W, Schiefer HG, Brahler E. Refractory chronic bacterial prostatitis: a re-evaluation of ciprofloxacin treatment after a median follow up of 30 months. *J Urol* 1991; **146**: 350–352.

39 Remy G, Roouger C, Chavanet P, *et al.* Use of ofloxacin for prostatitis. *Rev Infect Dis* 1988; **10** (Suppl. 1): 173–174.

40 Schaeffer AJ, Darras FS. The efficacy of norfloxacin in the treatment of chronic bacterial prostatitis refractory to trimethoprim-sulfamethoxazole and/or carbenicillin. *J Urol* 1990; **144**: 690–693.

41 Nickel JC, Corcos J, Afridi S, *et al.* Antibiotic therapy for chronic inflammatory (NIH category II/IIIA) prostatitis. *J Urol* 1998; **159**: S272.

42 Berghuis JP, Heiman JR, Rothman I, Berger RE. Psychologoical and physical factors involved in chronic idiopathic prostatitis. *J Psychosomatic Res* 1996; **41**: 313–325.

43 Berger R, Kessler D, Holmes KK. Etiology and manifestations of epididymitis in young men: correlations with sexual orientation. *J Infect Dis* 1987; **155**: 1341–1343.

44 Berger RE, Holmes KK, Mayo ME, *et al.* The clinical use of epididymal aspiration cultures in the management of selected patients with acute epididymitis. *J Urol* 1980; **124**: 60–61.

45 Bullock KN, Hunt JM. The intravenous urogram in acute epididymo-orchitits. *Br J Urol* 1981; **53**: 47–49.

46 Morgan AD. Inflammation and infestation of the testis and paratesticular structures. In: Pugh RCE (ed.) *Pathology of the Testis.* Oxford; Blackwell Scientific Publications: 1976, pp. 79–138.

47 Harnisch JP, Bergen RE, Alexander ER, Monda G, Holmes KK. Aetiology of acute epididymitis. *Lancet* 1977; **i**: 819–821.

48 Berger RE, Alexander ER, Monda GD, Ansell J, McCormick G, Holmes KK. *Chlamydia trachomatis* as a cause of acute 'idiopathic' epididymitis. *N Eng J Med* 1978; **298**: 301–304.

49 Krieger JN. Epididymitis, orchitis, and related conditions. *Sex Transm Dis* 1984; **11**: 173–181.

50 Sufrin G. Acute epididymitis. *Sex Transm Dis* 1981; **8**: 132–139.

51 Nilsson S, Obrant KO, Persson PS. Changes in the testes parenchyma caused by acute nonspecific epididymitis. *Fertil Steril* 1968; **19**: 748–757.

52 Kershaw WE. Filariasis due to infection with *Wuchereria bancrofti, W. pacifica, Brugia malayi* and related filaria. In: Jelliffe DB, Stansfield JP (eds) *Diseases of Children in the Subtropics and Tropics* 3rd edition. London; Edward Arnold: 1978, pp. 915–919.

53 Blandy JP, Hope-Stone HF, Dayan AD. *Tumours of the Testicle.* London; William Heinemann Medical Books: 1970.

54 Sheldon CA. Symposium on pediatric surgery. 1. Undescended testes and testicular torsion. *Surg Clin N Am* 1985; **65**: 1303–1329.

55 Fowler RC, Chennells PM, Ewing R. Scrotal ultrasonography: a clinical evaluation. *Br J Radiol* 1987; **60**: 649–654.

56 Sidhu PS. Clinical and imaging features of testicular torsion: role of ultrasound. *Clin Radiol* 1999; **54**: 343–352.

57 Centers for Disease Control and Prevention. 2002 Guidelines for treatment of sexually transmitted diseases. *MMWR* 2002; **51**; RR-6.

58 Clinical Effectiveness Group. National guideline for the management of epididymo-orchitis. ww.mssvd.org.uk/ceg.htm.

59 Pugh RCB (ed.) *Pathology of the Testis. Testicular Tumours — Introduction.* Oxford; Blackwell Scientific Publications: 1976, pp. 139–159.

60 Kohn J, Raghavan D. Tumour markers in malignant germ-cell tumours. In: Peckham MJ (ed.) *The Management of Testicular Tumours.* London; Arnold: 1981, pp. 50–69.

61 Mettlin C. Cancer of the prostate and testis. In: Bourke GJ (ed.) *The Epidemiology of Cancer.* Kent; Croom Helm: 1983, pp. 245–259.

62 Von Der Maase H, Rørth M, Walbom-Jørgensen S, *et al.* Carcinoma in situ of contralateral testis in patients with testicular germ cell cancer: study of 27 cases in 500 patients. *Br Med J* 1986; **293**: 1398–1401.

63 Hargreaves TB. Carcinoma in situ of the testis. *Br Med J* 1987; **293**: 1389.

Chapter 14

Sexually acquired reactive arthritis
A McMillan

Introduction

Although Hans Reiter described the disease, which now bears his name, in 1916, this disorder had been reported more than a century earlier by Stoll in 1776 and later by Sir Benjamin Brodie in 1818. Reiter described the occurrence of urethritis, conjunctivitis, and arthritis in a young man. Since then, many cases have been recorded and it has become apparent that there is a spectrum of clinical features, but not all three signs are necessarily present. It is for this reason that many physicians prefer the term sexually acquired reactive arthritis (SARA) to describe the illness.

Following the first acute attack, the patient may appear to recover completely, and may have no further episodes. Other individuals, however, may have multiple recurrences, with remissions varying from months to years. Generally, with each recurrence fewer features accompany the arthritis, which may be the sole indication of the disease in the later stages. Patients with SARA who develop persistent arthropathy are those most likely to be human leukocyte antigen B27 (HLA-B27) positive.

Etiology

In the UK, and in the USA, urethritis (usually non-specific) is the condition that most often shows itself before the manifestations of reactive arthritis. Sexually acquired reactive arthritis is associated with genitourinary infection with sexually transmissible organisms, particularly Chlamydia trachomatis, and, much less frequently, Ureaplasma urealyticum, Mycoplasma genitalium, and, possibly, Neisseria gonorrhoeae. As reactive arthritis is defined as a sterile inflammation of the synovial membrane, tendons, and fascia, triggered by an infection at a distant site, and, as metabolically active organisms may be detected in synovial membrane of the former two infections, SARA may be a misnomer. Reactive arthritis is an uncommon complication of non-specific urethritis (less than 1% of cases). Although C. trachomatis has been isolated from the urethra in about 30% of cases in men with SARA, it has been cultured from the synovial fluid during the acute episode only on rare instances. Chlamydial antigens and nucleic acids, however, have been found in the synovial membrane and fluid of patients with SARA (see page 380). Ureaplasma urealyticum infection has been associated with persistent infectious arthritis in patients with hypogammaglobulinemia[1], but there is some evidence that at least some cases of SARA are associated with this infection. Although rarely isolated from synovial fluid, U. urealyticum has been detected much more frequently in the urethra or cervix of some individuals with SARA who have no microbiological evidence of chlamydial or enteric infection[2]. In addition, U. urealyticum DNA has been detected by PCR in synovial fluid from a few patients with SARA or persistent reactive polyarthritis[3, 4]. Further evidence that at least some cases of reactive arthritis are caused by U. urealyticum comes from the observations that some individuals have high serum antibody levels against U. urealyticum, and that peripheral blood and synovial fluid lymphocytes from some patients show a specific proliferative response to ureaplasma antigens[2]. Mycoplasma genitalium DNA has been detected by PCR and in the synovial fluid of a patient with SARA[5]. There is much uncertainty about the role of N. gonorrhoeae in the etiology of reactive arthritis. Csonka[6], however, reported that the onset of Reiter's disease was preceded by gonococcal urethritis that had responded to penicillin therapy without the development of post-gonococcal urethritis.

On the continent of Europe, shigella dysentery has more commonly preceded the appearance of the disease, and in the famous study by Paronen[7] of 344 cases of reactive arthritis (Reiter's disease) following dysentery due to Shigella flexneri, the incidence was low (0.2%). In most countries, however, it is likely that both sexually transmitted and post-dysenteric forms co-exist. Reactive arthritis may also complicate salmonella infection, and in a recent outbreak of salmonellosis associated with Salmonella enterica subsp. enterica 6.9% of 224 patients developed arthritis[8]. Infection with Yersinia enterocolitica usually produces a mild gastrointestinal illness, complicated uncommonly by arthritis, including sacro-iliitis. About 90% of patients infected with the organism who had arthritis were found to have HLA-B27 antigen, compared with only 15% of patients developing diarrhea but no arthritis[9]. It may be that individuals who have this antigen are more likely to develop arthritis on challenge with a particular organism. Recently, reactive arthritis has been reported as a complication of Clostridium difficile infection following antibiotic treatment to eradicate Helicobacter pylori[10].

Pathogenesis

Reactive arthritis is triggered either by Chlamydia trachomatis (the most common cause of SARA), or by intestinal infection by *Salmonella* spp., *Shigella* spp., *Campylobacter* spp., *Yersinia enterocolitica*, or *Clostridium difficile*.

CHLAMYDIA TRACHOMATIS-ASSOCIATED ARTHRITIS

Circulating immune complexes can be detected in the sera of about two-thirds of patients with SARA[11], but in the absence of other features of immune complex disease, they are unlikely to be important in the pathogenesis of the condition.

Although *C. trachomatis* cannot be cultured from the synovial fluid or membrane of individuals with SARA, chlamydial antigen and nucleic acids can be detected[12, 13]. Using PCR, intact specific DNA has been found in synovial tissue, and mRNA has been detected by Northern analysis[14]. By electron microscopy, chlamydia-like structures have been identified in synovial membrane from patients with SARA, but the morphology has not been typical of chlamydial cells[15, 16]. These findings, however, cannot tell whether the chlamydia are alive and metabolically active in the synovium. An elegant study to help resolve this uncertainty was undertaken by Gerard *et al*[17]. They argued that since primary rRNA transcripts are produced only in actively growing bacterial cells, and are short lived, the detection in synovial tissue would be strong evidence for the presence of metabolically active chlamydiae. Using reverse transcription PCR and primers targeting primary transcripts from the rRNA operons, they obtained positive results from 14 of 16 samples that contained chlamydial DNA, indicating that viable chlamydiae were present. It was further shown that in each of the 14 samples, messengers from other genes required for assembly and function of the chlamydial protein synthesis system were also present. On the other hand, transcripts for *omp1*, encoding the immunodominant surface antigen MOMP of *C. trachomatis*, and normally expressed at high rate during bacterial growth, were not detected. It has been postulated that repression of synthesis of this protein results in the aberrant morphology of the chlamydia-like struc-

tures seen in the synovial membrane by electron microscopy.

As chlamydiae can be detected in peripheral blood mononuclear cells[17a], it is postulated that the organisms are phagocytosed by macrophages or dendritic cells in the genital tract, that then enter the circulation, and are recruited subsequently to the synovial membrane[18]. There is a high rate of recruitment of macrophages to inflamed joints, and chlamydiae have been detected, for example, in the synovium of patients with rheumatoid disease in a population with a high prevalence of chlamydial infection[19].

The reasons for persistence of chlamydiae within synovial tissue are unknown, but, as IL-4 expression is increased in the synovial fluid of patients with reactive arthritis[20], T_{H2}-type responses may contribute. T_{H1}-type immune responses with the production of cytokines such as interferon-γ and interleukin-2 (IL-2) are thought to be important in the elimination of bacteria, while T_{H2}-type responses, with the production of IL-4 and other cytokines, including, possibly IL-10, that inhibit clearance and produce a delayed hypersensitivity reaction. This has been shown clearly in mice that lack the interferon-γ gene. Another T lymphocyte-derived cytokine, interleukin-17, which can damage cartilage and stimulate osteoclastogenesis, has been found in the joints of patients with reactive arthritis[21], and may play a role in its pathogenesis.

Transcripts for the heat shock protein, Hsp60, that may play an important part in the host inflammatory response to chlamydial infection, were also found in the RNA preparations from the 14 samples. A recent study showed that, although CD4+ T cells from synovial fluid from 4 of 15 patients with SARA proliferated in response to a 57 kDa heat shock protein, none responded to MOMP[22]. An attractive hypothesis, therefore, that remains to be proven, is that the chlamydial Hsp60 product is largely responsible for the joint inflammation of SARA. Studies of T cell recognition of Hsp60 have shown that the epitope identified in *C. trachomatis* Hsp60 is identical to that in *C. pneumoniae*[23]. It has been postulated that infection with *C. pneumoniae* in earlier life primes the

immune system so that on infection with *C. trachomatis*, an immune response to Hsp60 is elicited[18]. This situation may be analogous to scarring trachoma in which recurrent infection is necessary for disease; certainly, disease can be produced by challenging primed animals with Hsp60 (Chapter 12).

The mechanisms that lead to persistent reactive arthritis in some patients are unknown.

The pathogenesis of the reactive arthritis associated with *U. urealyticum*, *M genitalium*, or *N. gonorrhoeae* is unknown.

Although there is an association between reactive arthritis and HLA-B27, this appears to be weaker than previously supposed. In addition, no more than a quarter of HLA-B27-positive patients develop reactive arthritis following exposure to potential triggering agents. A possible explanation for this may be that in earlier studies, more severely affected individuals were investigated[24]. It has been proposed that HLA-B27 might be a marker for disease severity rather than susceptibility, and might be more closely associated with classic spondyloarthropathic features such as sacro-iliitis than with synovitis[24]. Although several hypotheses have been proposed[25], the underlying mechanism for the association of HLA-B27 with disease is unknown.

Clinical features

Sexually acquired reactive arthritis is a disorder of young adults, the age of onset usually being between 18 and 50 years. Very rarely children under the age of 12 years are involved. Males are affected some fifty times more frequently than females.

The pre-patent period is variable, but the disease usually manifests itself 10 to 30 days after sexual intercourse or after an attack of dysentery. The mode of onset is variable, but commonly urethritis precedes the appearance of conjunctivitis, which is followed by arthritis. Any of the three principal features, however, may appear initially.

The duration of the first episode of SARA varies from between 2 weeks and several years. In general (more than 70% of cases) first episodes resolve within 12 weeks.

At least half of the patients develop recurrences, the interval between the initial episode and the recurrence varying between 3 months and up to 36 years. Although recurrence may be precipitated by urethritis or dysentery, other factors have been identified and include surgical operations on the urinary tract. The clinical manifestations may be classified as follows.

INFLAMMATION OF THE GENITOURINARY TRACT IN THE MALE

Non-specific urethritis

Non-specific urethritis is the most common form of urinary tract inflammation in this disease, and in about 70% of cases is also associated with the post-dysenteric form of the disease[7, 26]. In a series of 144 cases of Reiter's disease associated with urethritis, the urethritis in the initial episode was gonococcal in 17%, non-gonococcal in 43%, both gonococcal and non-gonococcal in 36%, and undiagnosed in 4% of cases.

In patients who have a mixed gonococcal and non-gonococcal urethritis a urethral discharge usually persists following treatment of the gonorrhea with penicillin. Occasionally a patient who has had gonorrhea and has been adequately treated develops SARA but shows no evidence of post-gonococcal urethritis even on careful examination.

The clinical features of the associated non-specific urethritis are identical to those of uncomplicated urethritis; in both conditions the severity varies considerably. If untreated, the urethritis usually subsides after some 2 to 4 weeks, but occasionally may persist for several months.

During the recurrent episodes of SARA, there may be no clinical evidence of urinary tract inflammation. Csonka[26], who studied 156 recurrences of the disease, recorded urethritis in about 58% of these cases. When urethritis is associated with a recurrence, it is most often non-gonococcal in nature, and an integral feature of the recurrence, rather than the apparently initiating factor of the first attack. It is clear, however, that in some patients re-infection with gonorrhea or with non-gonococcal urethritis following sexual intercourse may precipitate a recurrence of signs and symptoms of SARA. Urethritis resulting from re-infection may not always be followed by a recurrence of the arthritis.

Cystitis

Cystitis, often mild and causing little inconvenience, may be associated with SARA, Csonka[27] reported an incidence rate of 20%.

A much more severe, but fortunately rare, form of cystitis is that of acute hemorrhagic cystitis. This is characterized by the rapid onset of frequency of micturition, nocturia, strangury, urgency, hematuria, and suprapubic or perineal pain, which may radiate to the penis or testes. Occasionally the patient may be ill with pyrexia, malaise, and a polymorphonuclear leukocytosis. In some patients there may be a preceding urethritis[28]. The urine contains many leukocytes and red cells, but is sterile by conventional bacteriological examination.

Cystoscopy ought to be avoided during the acute stage, but it has revealed edema of the bladder mucosa (including the trigone), superficial membranous sloughs, diffuse petechial hemorrhages, and multiple discrete ulcers.

Intravenous urography in most cases of acute hemorrhagic cystitis shows unilateral or bilateral dilatation of the ureters and renal pelves and calyces. This is probably because of obstruction of the ureteric orifices by mucosal edema, although in a few cases the inflammatory process may extend proximally from the bladder. Following resolution of the cystitis, the hydronephrosis usually, but not always subsides, generally within 2 months.

Without treatment, hemorrhagic cystitis may persist for long periods, often with exacerbations and remissions. Hemorrhagic cystitis may occasionally precede, by weeks or months, the appearance of other features of the syndrome or may be the sole feature of a recurrence.

Acute prostatitis

Acute prostatitis, which may be followed by the formation of prostatic abscesses, has been described in SARS, but is excessively rare.

The incidence of 'chronic prostatitis' is difficult to determine as there is controversy as to how such a diagnosis is made. Chronic prostatitis has been defined as being present when there are ten or more pus cells per high-power field in samples of the expressed prostatic fluid examined as a wet film. Using this criterion, chronic prostatitis has been diagnosed in 95% of cases of SARA[29].

Epididymo-orchitis

Epididymo-orchitis, probably secondary to concomitant chlamydial infection occurs uncommonly.

Renal parenchymal involvement

Renal parenchymal involvement is a rarity[7].

INFLAMMATION OF THE GENITOURINARY TRACT IN THE FEMALE

In the female, evidence of inflammation of the urinary tract and/or reproductive system is less obvious and less easily defined. Urethritis rarely shows a definite discharge because the female urethra is shorter than the male one. Non-specific inflammation as a sign may show by cystitis, on occasions hemorrhagic and of intense severity, vaginitis, or cervicitis[30].

OCULAR INFLAMMATION

The most common ocular manifestation of SARA is conjunctivitis (occurring in about 30% of cases), which may be unilateral or, more frequently, bilateral (Figure 14.1). The severity of the conjunctivitis varies widely, ranging from a mild irritation with few objective signs to a severe inflammation with subconjunctival hemorrhage (Figure 14.2). Resolution occurs spontaneously within 1 to 4 weeks, although occasionally conjunctivitis may persist for several months. Mild episcleritis may be associated with conjunctivitis.

During a recurrent episode of the disease, and occasionally late on in the course of an initial severe acute episode, anterior uveitis may develop in about 8% of

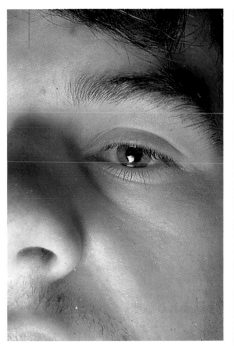

Figure 14.1 Bilateral conjunctivitis in a man with sexually acquired reactive arthritis (reproduced from McMillan and Scott 2000[54])

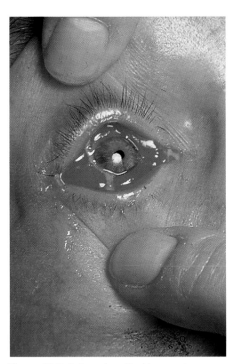

Figure 14.2 Subconjunctival hemorrhage associated with sexually acquired reactive arthritis (reproduced from McMillan and Scott 2000[54])

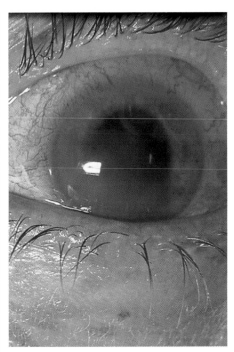

Figure 14.3 Acute anterior uveitis in sexually acquired reactive arthritis (reproduced from McMillan and Scott 2000[54])

patients. This complication is usually confined to one eye, when the patient complains of gradual onset of pain and blurring of vision in that eye. On inspection the affected eye is red, particularly at the margin of the cornea, because there is congestion of anterior ciliary blood vessels (Figure 14.3). As a result of edema, the normal pattern of the iris is obscured, the pupil is small, reacting poorly to light, and is irregular because of adhesions forming between the iris and the anterior surface of the lens.

It has been demonstrated that anterior uveitis occurs more commonly when a patient has radiological evidence of sacro-iliitis than when they do not. In one study[31] of 15 patients with SARA who had anterior uveitis, 12 had sacro-iliitis.

In a patient with SARA, uveitis is frequently recurrent, and is often the sole manifestation of a recurrence, during which objective evidence of arthritis is found infrequently. Indeed, uveitis may be the presenting feature of the disease, and hence all young people with uveitis should have a full physical examination to determine the etiology of the ocular inflammation.

ARTHRITIS AND OTHER CONNECTIVE TISSUE DISORDERS ASSOCIATED WITH SARA

Arthritis

During the acute initial episode of SARA, some 95% of patients develop symptoms of joint involvement. Although a number of patients (about 15%) may complain of arthralgia without objective evidence of inflammation such as joint swelling, the majority develop acute arthritis. The histological appearance of the synovial membrane is not characteristic, being indistinguishable from that of rheumatoid arthritis.

There is rapid onset of pain in, and swelling of, the affected joint, with limitation of movement. The skin overlying the joint may be reddened (Figure 14.4). There is thickening of the joint capsule and evidence of effusion into the joint. Atrophy of the muscles adjacent to the joint develops rapidly.

Although occasionally only one joint, usually the knee, may be affected, SARA is most commonly associated with polyarthritis (more than 95% of cases), with asymmetrical involvement of the peripheral large joints. The incidence of joint involvement during the initial episode of SARA in 50 cases is illustrated in Figure 14.5. The joints of the lower limbs are predominantly affected. Usually the arthritis does not

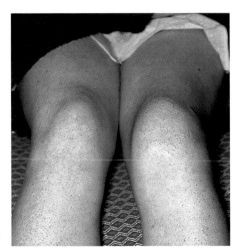

Figure 14.4 Arthritis of the knee joint in sexually acquired reactive arthritis (reproduced from McMillan and Scott 2000[54])

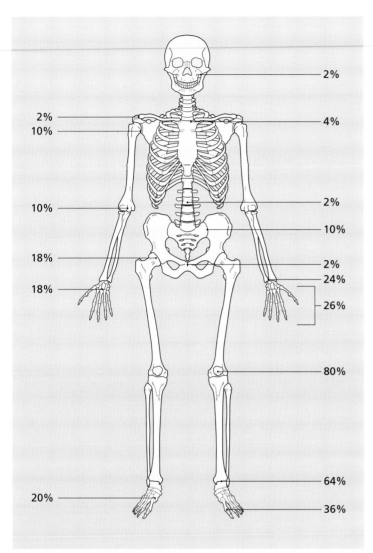

Figures annotated on the skeleton: 2%, 2%, 10%, 4%, 10%, 2%, 10%, 18%, 2%, 24%, 26%, 18%, 80%, 20%, 64%, 36%

Figure 14.5 Distribution of affected joints in a series of fifty men with sexually acquired reactive arthritis

involve the joints simultaneously, as there is generally an interval of some days between one joint and another becoming inflamed. After reaching maximum severity, 10 to 14 days after its onset, the arthritis gradually resolves, but recovery may be punctuated by acute exacerbations, perhaps associated with recrudescence of other manifestations of the disease.

Following the acute arthritis of the initial episode, there may be no clinical evidence of joint damage. In some cases, with each recurrent episode of arthritis, permanent damage is done to the joint that may ultimately show the features of chronic arthritis. Uncommonly, in less than 5% of cases, following the initial episode of arthritis, resolution of the inflammatory process is incomplete and chronic arthritis rapidly develops in the affected joints. The patient complains of pain, stiffness, and swelling of the joint, the severity of symptoms being subject to exacerbations and remissions; deformity is the ultimate fate of joints affected in this way. Most frequently it is the joints of the lower limbs and the sacroiliac joints which bear the brunt of chronic arthritis in this disease. Generally, as chronic arthritis develops, other manifestations of the disease become less obvious, with the possible exception of anterior uveitis.

In a disease in which there may be periods of activity separated by long periods of apparent quiescence, it is not possible to give an accurate prognosis after a single episode of SARA. In one study of 100 patients who had suffered from Reiter's disease some 20 years previously, 18% had chronic arthritis[32].

As a rare complication, spontaneous rupture of a joint, usually the knee joint, may occur; joint rupture is thought to occur from a cystic formation in the popliteal fossa. There is sudden onset of pain in the calf, and examination reveals a swollen leg which feels warm; the signs resemble thrombophlebitis which may itself also occur during the course of SARA (see page 386). Ultrasound examination is of great value in differentiating between the two conditions.

Radiology of joints in SARA

In the early stage of an acute episode of SARA, no radiological abnormalities may be observed; alternatively there may be non-specific, reversible changes such as thickening of the peri-articular tissues[33]. If the inflammatory process is mild, no further changes may occur, but as the disease progresses, radiological abnormalities develop in at least one joint in more than 40% of cases. These changes are most noticeable in the joints and bones of the lower limbs, especially the feet and in the sacroiliac joints.

Destructive lesions ('erosions') are found at the periphery of the articular surface of the affected joint, they appear as small well-demarcated areas of bone destruction. As the condition progresses, the area of destruction increases and the articular surface of the joint is eventually destroyed, with radiological narrowing of the joint space. Erosions are most commonly found in the metatarsal, tarsal, and interphalangeal joints of the feet, and on the posterior aspect of the calcaneum.

In cases where radiological abnormalities are found, periostitis is frequent. Most commonly the periostitis affects the neck of the metatarsals and metacarpals, the distal parts of the tibia and fibula, and the shafts of the proximal phalanges. It appears on X-ray as a thin linear opacity running parallel to the cortex of the bone. In the bones of the tarsus and carpus, the sharp outline of the bone may be replaced by an irregular contour.

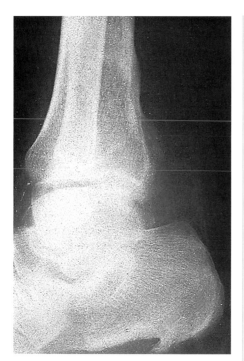

Figure 14.6 Plantar spur in sexually acquired reactive arthritis (reproduced from McMillan and Scott 2000[54])

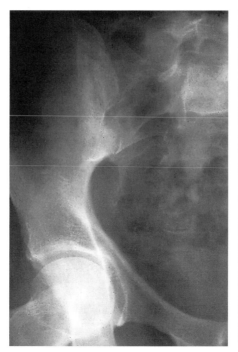

Figure 14.7 Sacroiliitis in sexually acquired reactive arthritis (reproduced from McMillan and Scott 2000[54])

Periostitis affecting the calcaneum is a common radiological finding, occurring in more than 50% of cases[33]. The changes involve the posterolateral and plantar aspects of the bone. In chronic cases, as periosteal new bone is formed on the plantar surface of the calcaneum at the insertion of the plantar fascia, a 'spur' develops with a characteristic 'fluffy' appearance because of the diffuse nature of the periostitis (Figure 14.6).

Plantar spurs of a different character may be found in normal individuals, in those suffering from osteoarthrosis, in rheumatoid arthritis, and in ankylosing spondylitis. These spurs, representing ossification at the site of attachment of plantar ligaments, are clearly defined and not associated with changes beyond the base of the spur.

Interpretation of radiographs of the sacroiliac joints is often difficult, as some asymmetry of the joints is common, and leads to differences in appearance of the joints. Sacro-iliitis is found in about 50% of cases, most frequently in recurrent cases, the incidence rising with the duration of the disease. It manifests radiologically as loss of the normal outline of the joint, irregularity of the joint margins because of erosions, and sclerosis beyond the area of the erosion. Although sometimes unilateral (less than 20%), these changes are usually seen in both joints (Figure 14.7). Complete obliteration of the joint, as is seen in ankylosing spondylitis, is uncommon, but when it occurs it is indistinguishable from that condition. Occasionally, radiological changes, in the form of narrowing of joint space, irregularity of the joint margin and ossification of joint ligaments may be noted in the symphysis pubis.

Spinal changes may be noted uncommonly in SARA. Syndesmophytosis (i.e. the appearance of strips of bone joining adjacent vertebrae) occurs in cases of long-standing disease, and, rarely, radiological changes indistinguishable from those found in ankylosing spondylitis.

In the chronic arthritis of SARA, joint deformities such as lateral dislocation of the proximal phalanges on the metatarsals may be noted on X-ray.

Enthesitis, tendonitis, and bursitis

Enthesitis, that is, inflammation at the point of ligament, tendon, or capsule insertion into the bone, is found most commonly at the insertion of the Achilles tendon or plantar fascia. Clinical evidence of plantar fasciitis is found in about 20% of patients suffering an acute episode of the disease. The patient complains of pain in the sole of the foot. In the most severely affected cases, the skin overlying the fascia is reddened and swollen. More commonly, there is only tenderness of the fascia, particularly close to the heel. Although usually involving both feet, one may be more severely affected than the other. Plantar fasciitis generally resolves within several weeks of its onset, but occasionally may be very persistent.

Although any tendon and its synovial sheath may become inflamed during the course of SARA, the Achilles tendon most often produces clinical signs (about 10% of cases in the acute stage). Tendonitis is most often accompanied by adjacent bone or joint disease.

Rarely, inflammation of bursae, especially the prepatellar bursa, may occur during the acute stages of the disease. On a radiograph tendonitis and tenovaginitis may appear as a broad soft-tissue shadow.

SKIN LESIONS

Pustular psoriasis (keratoderma blenorrhagica) is the typical skin lesion found in SARA, occurring in up to 30% of cases. Although the soles of the feet are most commonly affected (Figure 14.8), keratoderma may also occur anywhere on the body (dorsa of the feet, palms, extensor surfaces of the legs and forearms, trunk, scalp, scrotum, shaft of penis, umbilicus (Figure 14.9)) and occasionally presents as a generalized skin rash.

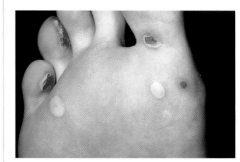

Figure 14.8 Pustular psoriasis of the soles of the feet in a man with sexually acquired reactive arthritis

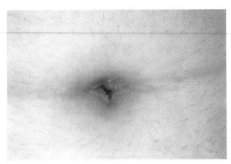

Figure 14.9 Psoriatic papules around the umbilicus in a man with sexually acquired reactive arthritis

The initial lesion is a brown macule 2 to 4 mm in diameter, which rapidly becomes papular. The center of the papule becomes pustular and the roof becomes thickened. Increase in size occurs from the accumulation of parakeratotic scales on the surface of the lesion and from lateral growth of the base; this is the typical limpet-like lesion of keratoderma. Most commonly the skin manifestations of SARA are less florid, and few typical keratoderma lesions are to be seen. In such cases, pustular lesions on the soles of the feet may be the only skin lesions to be found, and these subside generally within 3 to 4 weeks of their appearance. On the weight-bearing areas of the soles, lateral spread of the pustule produces a thick-walled bulla. Generally lesions on the trunk, arms, legs, and shaft of penis are less typical, and consist of firm, dull-red papules (the hard parakeratotic nodule).

Keratoderma usually heals within 6 to 10 weeks from its onset, but may occasionally take much longer. 'Cropping' is characteristic during the course of an acute episode, various stages of development of the lesions of keratoderma being present at the same time.

Although the physical appearance of keratoderma may cause the patient distress, the lesions themselves do not usually produce discomfort unless there is secondary bacterial infection.

The finger and toe nails may be involved in about 10% of cases of SARA. In mild cases, the nail plate becomes opaque, thickened, ridged, and brittle. When the nails are more severely affected, in addition to the latter changes, sterile, subungual abscesses develop and, as these dry out,

yellow debris accumulates under the distal half of the nail. As this process continues, the nail becomes elevated from its bed, turns brown, and is often shed. The skin adjacent to the nail base and the nail fold takes part in the reaction. These changes may be mistaken for fungal infection of the nails.

The Köbner phenomenon has been described as occurring in SARA (non-specific trauma induces skin changes in the affected site of a type present at the same time elsewhere on the body). The Köbner phenomenon is found in many skin diseases for example, lichen planus, molluscum contagiosum, and warts.

ORAL LESIONS

Lesions of the mucous membranes of the buccal cavity occur in about 10% of cases of SARA. The site most commonly affected is the palate, followed by the buccal mucosa, gingiva, and tongue. Such lesions are asymptomatic, have to be looked for carefully, and generally heal within a few weeks of their appearance.

On the palate the lesions usually appear as whitish, slightly elevated macules, not

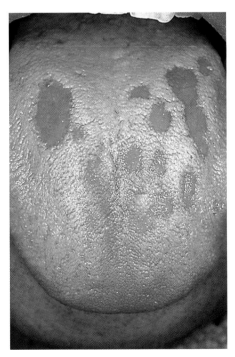

Figure 14.10 Lesions of the tongue in sexually acquired reactive arthritis (reproduced from McMillan and Scott 2000[54])

covered by inflammatory exudate, and surrounded by a narrow erythematous zone. Occasionally, multiple purpuric spots may appear.

Similar lesions may be noted on the buccal mucosa. On the tongue, round or oval reddened areas appear, sharply demarcated from the surrounding normal epithelium 'bald patches' (Figure 14.10).

PENILE LESIONS

Reference has already been made to keratoderma of the shaft of the penis and the outer aspect of the prepuce. Psoriatic lesions may also be found in about 25% of cases on the glans penis and on the mucous surface of the prepuce, which usually precede other mucocutaneous manifestations.

On the glans, the appearance of the lesion depends on whether or not the individual has been circumcised. If he is circumcised, the lesions are dry and appear as slightly elevated, scaling macules sharply demarcated from the surrounding skin (Figure 14.11). When a prepuce is present, scale formation is inhibited, and the lesions appear as moist, glistening, red, sharply defined macules, which become confluent producing a polycyclic margin known as circinate balanitis (Figure 14.12). Unless there is secondary bacterial infection, which is a common complication, pain is absent, and healing tends to occur within 4 weeks of the appearance of the lesions. Circinate lesions of the labia minora have also been described[34].

VISCERAL LESIONS OF SARA

Clinical evidence of involvement of organs of the body, other than those previously

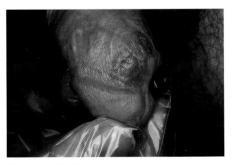

Figure 14.11 Psoriatic lesions of the glans penis in a circumcised male with sexually acquired reactive arthritis

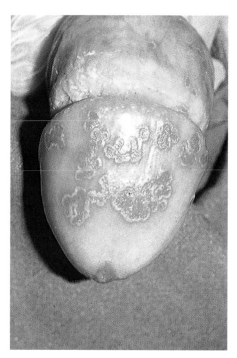

Figure 14.12 Circinate balanitis in sexually acquired reactive arthritis (reproduced from McMillan and Scott 2000[54])

mentioned, is uncommon. It is quite possible that, in a disease with such a broad spectrum of symptoms and signs, many organs are involved in the inflammatory process without producing obvious abnormalities.

Cardiovascular system

Pericarditis

This occurs uncommonly (in less than 5% of cases) during an acute episode of SARA. The patient may or may not have chest pain when there is pericarditis[35].

Myocarditis

The incidence of myocarditis is difficult to determine, but is less than 5%. The most common finding is first degree heart block, i.e. a P–R interval greater than 0.20 seconds. Rarely other conduction defects such as second degree heart block, left bundle-branch block, and complete heart block occur.

Although usually transient, these ECG abnormalities may persist unchanged for years, or one abnormality may supervene on another[36].

Aortitis

This is a rare complication, having been adequately described in the literature in fewer than 30 patients. It is usually associated with recurrent episodes of the disease, which has been present for at least 8 years, with sacro-iliitis and conduction defects[37]. Aortic incompetence is the usual presenting feature.

Thrombophlebitis of the deep veins of the leg

This may be found during an acute episode of SARA in about 3% of cases[38]. Patients complain of pain in the affected calf and there is tenderness, induration of the calf muscles, and edema of the leg. Thrombophlebitis occurs within a few days of the onset of the arthritis and the knee joint on the affected side is always involved.

The most important condition to be distinguished from thrombophlebitis is spontaneous rupture of the knee joint. Ultrasonic examination of the veins of the calf, and venography are useful aids to diagnosis.

Respiratory system

Pleurisy has been described as occurring in the acute stages of SARA, having been found in about 8% of cases described by Paronen[7]. Transient opacities may be observed on chest radiographs of patients, but their significance is uncertain[39].

Reticuloendothelial system

Generalized enlargement of lymph nodes has been observed uncommonly in SARA (less than 1% of cases). Histological examination reveals non-specific reactive hyperplasia. Rarely there is moderate enlargement of the spleen.

Nervous system

Various neurological abnormalities have been described in association with SARA, but these are seen in less than 2% of cases. Meningoencephalitis, multiple peripheral neuropathy, and amyotrophic lateral sclerosis have been well documented as occurring during an acute episode of the

disease, occasionally reappearing during recurrences[40].

In long-standing cases, the occurrence of Parkinsonism and other neuro-psychiatric abnormalities is difficult to evaluate, as these disorders also affect the general population[41].

Amyloidosis

This is a very rare complication of severe SARA[42].

Laboratory tests in SARA

There is no diagnostic test for SARA, but the investigations given here aid the differential diagnosis.

BLOOD TESTS
Red cells

Hemoglobin concentration, packed cell volume, mean corpuscular hemoglobin concentration, and mean corpuscular volume are tested.

In severe cases, the results of these tests indicate mild normocytic, normochromic anemia, i.e. the hemoglobin concentration is less than 135 g/l but the mean corpuscular volume is normal (76–96 fl) as is the mean corpuscular hemoglobin concentration (30–35 g/dL).

White cell count

In the acute episode, there is a polymorphonuclear leukocytosis (i.e. a white cell count of greater than 11.0×10^9/L) in 25% to 30% of cases.

Erythrocyte sedimentation rate and C-reactive protein

This is elevated in more than 90% of cases of acute SARA, being in the early stages greater than 50 mm per hour (Westergren) in about 40% of cases. The erythrocyte sedimentation rate falls slowly during the first month of the acute episode, and, although becoming normal by about the sixth to tenth week after the onset, may remain elevated in about 15% of patients for much longer. During the acute inflammatory phase, C-reactive protein is elevated.

Plasma-protein changes

During the acute episode, in about 30% of cases, the plasma albumin is lower than normal, and the alpha globulin fraction is elevated. There is only slight elevation in the gamma globulin fraction. In the acute stage, serum concentrations of IgM and IgA may be raised, but fall to normal as the inflammatory process resolves.

Antibody against *Chlamydia trachomatis*

Titers of anti-chlamydial IgG in the serum are higher in patients with SARA than in men with uncomplicated non-specific urethritis[43, 44]. The specificity of these antibodies, however, has been questioned, and tests based on IgG antibody detection have not proved useful in clinical practice[45]. A substantial proportion of patients with chlamydia-associated SARA do not have detectable antibodies[46], further calling into question the value of serological tests.

Human leukocyte antigen B27

About 30% of patients with SARA are HLA-B27 positive.

Rheumatoid factor

The incidence of rheumatoid factor in the normal population is about 4%, and in SARA the incidence is similar. The rheumatoid arthritis latex particle agglutination test and the sheep red cell agglutination tests are usually negative (96%) in SARA. Although these tests for IgM rheumatoid factor are usually negative, IgG antiglobulin may be demonstrated in the serum of some patients.

Anti-streptolysin O titer

The results of this test are within normal limits.

Antinuclear antibodies

These tests usually give negative results.

Uric acid

The differential diagnosis from gout may be difficult in 2% of cases of SARA when the serum uric acid is elevated.

Smooth-muscle antibody

This may be detected in about 50% of cases, and it should be noted that this test is not specific for active chronic hepatitis.

URINALYSIS

The detection of proteinuria, microscopic hematuria, and sterile pyuria are found in up to 50% of acute episodes of SARA.

SYNOVIAL FLUID

Joint aspiration is needed only if the diagnosis is in doubt, or if there is considerable discomfort from a large effusion. Fluid aspirated from an affected joint is yellow and turbid, clotting spontaneously. The white cell count varies considerably from 1000 to 5000×10^6/L. The normal white cell count in joint fluid is less than 200×10^6/L. Although the inflammatory exudate is initially composed mainly of polymorphonuclear leukocytes, as the duration of the arthritis increases, lymphocytes predominate.

The protein content of the fluid is high, about 40 to 50 g/L (reference value for synovial fluid 10 to 20 g/L). Synovial fluid glucose concentration is low (about 4.2 mmol/L) in about a third of patients. The total hemolytic complement activity in synovial fluid in SARA is normal or high (c.f. rheumatoid arthritis where it is low).

Differential diagnosis of the acute episode of sexually acquired reactive arthritis (SARA)

The differential diagnosis of oligoarthritis is broad and a simple diagnostic test for the reactive arthritis associated with STIs, such as *Chlamydia trachomatis*, is not currently available. In many cases, a careful sexual history may indicate that there has been

risk of exposure to an STI, but the history may be unreliable and, in patients with SARA, symptoms or signs of genital tract inflammation are often lacking. Serological tests for IgA or IgG antibodies against chlamydiae are unreliable for the diagnosis of SARA[46]. Erlacher *et al*[45], however, found that microbiological examination of material from the genital tract for chlamydial infection was a useful diagnostic test in those men and women who had oligoarthritis, even when genitourinary symptoms were absent.

The following diseases must be considered in the differential diagnosis.

GONOCOCCAL ARTHRITIS

This is the disease with which SARA is most often confused. Both conditions have urethritis and arthritis in common. In any urethritis it is important to exclude the gonococcus, but it should be remembered that there may be dissemination of this organism from the pharynx or rectum in the absence of urethral infection.

In gonococcal arthritis, isolation of *Neisseria gonorrhoeae* from the synovial fluid is often unsuccessful.

The skin lesions of the bacteremic stage of a disseminated gonococcal infection should not be confused with keratoderma.

Urethral gonorrhea may be a precipitating factor in SARA and immediate differentiation may be difficult. Within 2 to 3 days of commencing antibiotic treatment, however, gonococcal arthritis will have improved considerably, whereas improvement does not necessarily occur in SARA.

RHEUMATOID ARTHRITIS

This disease is more commonly found in females and usually presents in middle age. In contrast to SARA, the onset tends to be insidious and joints are affected in a symmetrical fashion. Any synovial joint may be involved, but particularly the metacarpophalangeal (80%), wrist (85%), elbow (70%), metatarsophalangeal (70%), and knee joints (80%). Although sacroiliitis may be demonstrated radiologically, the appearances are rarely as striking as those found in SARA. Chronic prostatitis may be diagnosed in about 20% of males with rheumatoid disease. Anterior uveitis may occur in about 20% of patients. Rheumatoid factor is present in the serum in at least 80% of patients. Subcutaneous nodules, which occur in 30% of cases of rheumatoid arthritis, are never found in SARA.

The systemic form of juvenile rheumatoid arthritis (Still's disease) may appear in adults either as a recrudescence of a childhood disease, or *de novo*. The onset is acute, often with a sore throat, and sometimes with spiking fever and chills. Migratory synovitis during the early stages of the illness is followed later by chronic arthritis. A transient macular rash is often a feature, and hepatic and splenic enlargement, and generalized lymphadenopathy may be found. There is a polymorphonuclear leukocytosis but tests for rheumatoid factor and antinuclear antibodies are negative.

RHEUMATIC FEVER

Although usually preceded by pharyngitis, a proportion (up to 30%) of patients with rheumatic fever do not give this history. The onset of arthritis, which is usually polyarticular, is acute, when large joints are chiefly affected. Classically the arthritis is migratory, affected joints returning to normal within a few days of the onset. Joints, however, may remain inflamed for weeks.

Erythema marginatum is found in about 10% of children affected, and in severe cases, subcutaneous nodules of various sizes may be found. Erythema nodosum may also be associated with rheumatic fever.

Ocular and urinary tract inflammation does not occur. Serum antistreptolysin O titers rise above normal limits in 80% of patients with rheumatic fever.

LYME DISEASE

Early in infection, when dissemination of *Borrelia burgdorferi* occurs, there may be fever, a migratory arthralgia without obvious joint swelling, and the characteristic erythema migrans. Arthritis, which is usually episodic, develops weeks to months later, and principally affects the large joints. During the acute stage, the diagnosis is made by the detection of specific IgM in the serum, and in those with the later onset arthritis, serum IgG is usually detectable.

ACUTE SEPTIC ARTHRITIS (EXCEPTING GONOCOCCAL ARTHRITIS)

Acute septic arthritis may be caused by numerous organisms, for example *Staphylococcus aureus*, *Streptococcus pyogenes*, *Neisseria meningitidis*, *Salmonella* spp., and *Streptococcus pneumoniae*.

Any joint may become inflamed, but most often the knee, wrist, and elbow are affected. Aspiration of the effusion, with appropriate bacteriological examination of the aspirated fluid, is usually diagnostic.

OTHER REACTIVE ARTHRITIDES

Reactive arthritis may follow intestinal infection with *Yersinia enterocolitica*, *Shigella* spp., *Salmonella* spp., *Campylobacter* spp., and *Clostridium difficile*. The diagnosis is made by culture of the bacteria from the feces or, in the case of yersinia, by the detection of IgM antibodies in acute-phase sera. In relation to intestinal infection, it is worth remembering that patients may not have diarrhea when they present with arthritis. By finding a specific proliferative lymphocyte response of synovial lymphocytes to shigella antigen, Sieper *et al.*[46a] made a presumptive diagnosis of shigella-related reactive arthritis in a group of patients who gave a recent history of diarrhea but who had negative stool cultures for bacterial pathogens.

BACTERIAL ENDOCARDITIS

Arthritis, affecting only a few joints, may be a feature of bacterial endocarditis. The joints may be swollen and painful, or there may be symptomless effusions. Organisms are seldom isolated from synovial fluid.

TUBERCULOUS ARTHRITIS

In the UK this is a rare disease, encountered most commonly in the elderly. The onset is insidious and most often the arthritis is monoarticular. Synovial biopsy, with bacteriological and histological examination is necessary for diagnosis.

BRUCELLOSIS

Bone and joints are frequently affected in this disease. Peripheral arthritis, sacro-iliitis, and spondylitis occur. The arthritis may affect any joint, but most commonly the shoulders, knees, and elbows. Sacroiliitis occurs in about 30% of patients, and may affect one or both sides.

In a patient with arthritis, particularly if there has been contact with farm animals, the following serological tests for brucellosis should be done to exclude this infection: a standard agglutination test, the anti-human globulin (Coombs) test for non-agglutinating antibodies, and the complement fixation test.

VIRAL ARTHRITIS

Arthritis is a feature of systemic viral infections, including rubella, EB virus, HIV, hepatitis B virus, and human parvovirus. The arthritis of parvovirus resembles that of rubella, with sudden onset of a symmetrical polyarthritis, particularly affecting the hands. In both infections, the arthritis is self limiting and the diagnosis is made by the detection of specific IgM in the serum. The arthritis of HIV infection is discussed in Chapter 7, and the diagnosis of hepatitis B and Epstein–Barr virus infections is considered in Chapters 8 and 9 respectively.

TRAUMA

Non-specific urethritis is common in young men, and it is not uncommon to find urethritis in association with a traumatized joint.

ERYTHEMA MULTIFORME AND STEVENS–JOHNSON SYNDROME

Erythema multiforme is a self-limiting skin disease associated in many cases with some underlying condition, such as herpes simplex infection or drug idiosyncrasy. When severe the condition is termed Stevens–Johnson syndrome and is associated with mucous membrane ulceration (oral and genital) bullous lesions of the skin, conjunctivitis, and arthritis.

SYSTEMIC LUPUS ERYTHEMATOSUS

Usually it is females that are affected by this condition. Symmetrical peripheral joint involvement is usual although there is much variation in the pattern of affected joints. There are additional features such as fever and rash. Antinuclear factor is found in the blood, and DNA antibodies are present in the active stage of this disease; antibody to double-stranded DNA is characteristic.

GOUT AND PSEUDOGOUT

Acute episodes of gout usually affect a single peripheral joint, especially the first metatarsophalangeal joint. In the rarer polyarticular gout, fever is common, and many patients give a history of typical gouty attacks. Pseudogout, acute synovitis associated with the deposition of calcium pyrophosphate crystals in articular cartilage, may resemble septic arthritis with fever. It is a condition found in the elderly, and the diagnosis is often made by the radiological appearance of chondrocalcinosis; alternatively, microscopical examination of the fluid shows a leukocytosis and typical crystals.

SYSTEMIC VASCULITIS

Fever and polyarthritis are common features of systemic vasculitis but there are usually other clues as to the diagnosis such as skin lesions and microscopic hematuria.

SARCOIDOSIS

Acute arthritis often associated with erythema nodosum may be a feature of sarcoidosis. Hilar lymphadenopathy is usually found in such cases and indicates the diagnosis. Angiotensin-converting enzyme levels in the blood are significantly elevated in about two-thirds of patients with active sarcoidosis.

OTHER SERONEGATIVE SPONDARTHRITIDES

Acute arthritis may be associated with ankylosing spondylitis, psoriatic arthritis, ulcerative colitis, Crohn's disease, Behçet's syndrome, and Whipple's disease. The relationships of these conditions require separate consideration and may be important in the differential diagnosis, particularly of the chronic episode of arthritis.

Differential diagnosis of chronic spondyloarthropathy

The differentiation of the chronic arthropathy that may develop in some patients with SARA from other spondyloarthropathies is often difficult.

IDIOPATHIC ANKYLOSING SPONDYLITIS

Peripheral arthritis occurs in about 60% of patients, and sacro-iliitis is found in all patients with ankylosing spondylitis.

Evidence of inflammation of the urinary or reproductive system is found in at least 80% of cases of ankylosing spondylitis. Anterior uveitis, too, is a complication of about 20% of cases of ankylosing spondylitis, and aortitis is a rare complication.

Idiopathic ankylosing spondylitis is not usually associated with psoriasis or other mucocutaneous lesions.

PSORIATIC ARTHRITIS

Psoriasis may uncommonly be associated with a seronegative, radiologically erosive polyarthritis (about 5% of cases). Except in those patients with distal interphalangeal joint involvement, the anatomical distribution of joints affected by arthritis is not a helpful factor in reaching a diagnosis. Radiological evidence of sacro-iliitis is found also in at least 20% of patients with psoriatic arthritis.

ULCERATIVE COLITIS, CROHN'S DISEASE, AND WHIPPLE'S DISEASE

Peripheral arthritis, sacro-iliitis, anterior uveitis, and diarrhea are features of this group of conditions.

Management

The natural history of reactive arthritis should be explained to the patient who should be reassured that, in the majority of cases, the condition is self limiting.

The individual should be screened for potential sexually transmissible causes of reactive arthritis, including microbiological tests for *Chlamydia trachomatis*, *Neisseria gonorrhoeae* and, perhaps, *Ureaplasma urealyticum*. When there is a history of diarrhea, a stool sample should be examined for bacterial pathogens, and serological tests for *Yersinia enterocolitica* should also be undertaken. Radiographs of the joints, including the sacroiliac joints and lateral views of the heels may yield useful information. An electrocardiograph and echocardiography are useful ancillary tests, particularly when cardiac involvement is suspected. It is the authors' practice to refer every patient to an ophthalmologist for slit-lamp examination to detect anterior uveitis. When the diagnosis is uncertain, additional tests for other causes of arthritis may be required (Table 14.1).

Treatment

At present, treatment for SARA is not curative but is aimed at relieving symptoms. When the patient first attends, other STIs should be excluded and the course of the disease fully explained. They should be told particularly that the acute episode may last for at least 6 weeks, but that sometimes it may last for twice as long.

As viable, metabolically active chlamydiae are found in the synovial membrane of patients with chlamydia-associated SARA, antimicrobial therapy might be expected to influence the course of the arthritis. The benefits of therapy with respect to alteration of the natural history of the arthritis, however, are uncertain. Certainly, SARA can develop in patients treated for chlamydial urethritis[47]. The results of trials of antimicrobial agents have been contradictory. In a small study on the use of lymecycline for 3 months in chlamydia-associated SARA, significantly more patients who had been treated with lymecycline had recovered by 15 weeks compared with placebo recipients[48]. Sieper et al[49], however, found no difference in the rate of resolution of arthritis between patients treated with ciprofloxacin

Table 14.1 Investigations that may be helpful in the diagnosis of sexually acquired reactive arthritis (SRA) and the exclusion of other conditions

Investigation	Conditions in which the investigation may be helpful in the diagnosis or exclusion of SRA
Culture for *Neisseria gonorrhoeae*	Gonococcal arthritis
Genital tests for *Chlamydia trachomatis*	*Chlamydia trachomatis*-associated reactive arthritis
Tests on blood:	
full blood count	
erythrocyte sedimentation rate	
C-reactive protein	
plasma enzyme tests of liver function	
blood culture	Septic arthritis and endocarditis
serological tests for:	
Yersinia enterocolitica	Reactive arthritis of yersinia infection
Borrelia burgdorferi	Arthritis of Lyme disease
Brucella spp.	Brucellosis
viral infections, including rubella, parvovirus, EB virus, hepatitis B virus, HIV	Arthritis of viral infections
fasting serum uric acid	Gout
rheumatoid factor	Rheumatoid arthritis
anti-streptolysin O titer	Rheumatic fever
angiotensin-converting enzyme	Sarcoidosis
antinuclear antibody and anti-double stranded DNA	Systemic lupus erythematosus
anti-neutrophil cytoplasmic antibody	Wegener's granulomatosis
HLA-B27	See text
Urinalysis	Microscopic hematuria and protein may indicate systemic vasculitis
Stool culture	Reactive arthritis associated with enteric bacterial pathogens
Synovial fluid	Crystal-related arthropathies (microscopy using polarized light)
	Septic arthritis (Gram-stained smear and culture)
Chest X-ray	Tuberculosis (culture)
	Sarcoidosis
Radiology of joints	

for 3 months and those given placebo. The latter finding may be explained by persistence of *C. trachomatis* in the synovial membrane, despite antimicrobial therapy[15].

URETHRITIS

The management of non-gonococcal urethritis has already been discussed (Chapter 10). The presence of the complication of SARA does not alter the general approach. Although of value in aiding resolution of urethritis, treatment with a tetracycline does not alter the course of the disease.

CONJUNCTIVITIS

This is a self-limiting condition, generally resolving within a few weeks of its onset. Although the use of topical steroid preparations may produce symptomatic relief, it is generally agreed that they should be withheld to prevent a possible viral keratitis.

ANTERIOR UVEITIS

Advice should be obtained from an ophthalmologist for the management of this complication. Mydriasis is maintained by the use of atropine sulfate eye drops,

1% w/v twice daily, with phenylephrine eye drops, three times daily. Dilatation of the pupil produces relief of pain and reduces the risk of the development of iris adhesions.

Steroids should be applied topically, for example in the form of betamethasone sodium phosphate eye drops, three or four times daily.

ARTHRITIS

During the acute stage of the illness, when the joints are markedly inflamed, bed rest is advisable. It is of great importance to ensure that the correct posture is assumed during this period of rest. The patient should be nursed on a firm mattress, with adequate support given for their back. A bed cage to keep the weight of the bed clothes off the lower limbs is useful. Pillows must not be placed behind the knees as this favors the development of flexion deformities.

Local immobilization of an affected joint by means of a plaster of Paris splint, held in place by a bandage, may be a useful aid in relieving the patient's discomfort. Gentle active movement of the joint twice daily reduces the risk of stiffness developing in the splinted joint. By supervising these exercises, a physiotherapist can help with the patient's management.

Various non-steroidal anti-inflammatory drugs (NSAIDs) drugs have been used in the management of the arthritis of SARA. The authors have experience of the drugs mentioned below.

Aspirin and salicylates

The dosage of aspirin must be determined by trial and error, the minimum dose effective in relieving the pain being used. To maintain adequate blood levels of the drug, 4-hourly oral administration is necessary. The total daily dose varies between 3 and 6 g.

Side effects of aspirin are common, and dyspepsia is the most common complaint (in at least 30% of patients).

Aspirin administration may result in chronic gastrointestinal bleeding and, rarely, acute massive hemorrhage. The use of salicylates should be avoided in all patients with a history of peptic ulceration. Hypersensitivity reactions to aspirin are very rare.

Indomethacin

This is a powerful analgesic and anti-inflammatory agent. The dosage is 25 mg three times daily by mouth. To relieve morning stiffness, a single tablet containing 75 mg indomethacin given before retiring may be useful.

The side effects of this drug are dose related and include headache, especially in the morning, dizziness, tinnitus, drug rashes, nausea, and anorexia. Occasionally gastrointestinal hemorrhage from a peptic ulcer has occurred and sometimes even perforation.

It is recommended that, when a patient is seen with mild arthritis, aspirin should be used initially, and if there is a poor response to this drug, one of the other agents employed. In more severe cases, indomethacin may be required from the start, and continued until the inflammatory process begins to abate. Aspirin may then be substituted for this agent.

Corticosteroids

The use of corticosteroid preparations, such as prednisolone, is rarely necessary, most cases responding to the measures already outlined. A short course of prednisolone, given orally in a dose of 10 to 25 mg daily may be useful when severe symptoms arise from several joints[50]. When posterior uveitis or symptomatic pericarditis occur, specialist advice should be sought, as systemic steroids are indicated.

The aspiration of a tense effusion in the knee joint followed immediately by the instillation of 40 mg of methylprednisolone acetate has proved useful in alleviating joint symptoms, but prospective and controlled trials are difficult and have not yet been done.

When disabling arthritic symptoms persist for more than 3 months or there is erosive joint damage, the opinion of a rheumatologist on further management should be sought. The following additional therapies may be indicated[50].

Sulfsalazine

This drug is generally used as second-line therapy when either the above measures have failed and the arthritis persists, or there is evidence of erosive joint damage. The drug is given in an oral dose of 500 mg daily, increased at weekly intervals to a maximum of 2 g per day in divided doses. A large number of adverse effects have been described in patients treated with sulfasalazine, particularly amongst patients who are slow acetylators. Anorexia, nausea, and fever are common side effects, and hematological abnormalities, including Heinz body (particularly in patients with glucose-6-phosphate dehydrogenase deficiency) and megaloblastic anemia, leukopenia, and thrombocytopenia may develop. Hyersensitivity reactions are possible complications. There is no contraindication to the use of the drug in pregnancy.

Methotrexate

Although its use in SARA is not well established, case reports suggest that it may occasionally be helpful. The drug is given orally in an initial dose of 2.5 mg once weekly, increasing slowly to 7.5 to 15 mg once weekly. An oral dose of folic acid, 5 mg, given once weekly with the methotrexate is recommended. Myelosuppression and hepatitic cirrhosis are important adverse effects, and careful monitoring is mandatory. A full blood count, and renal and liver function tests should be undertaken before initiation of therapy, and repeated weekly until therapy has been stabilized. If there are pre-existing abnormalities of liver function tests, methotrexate should not be used, and if these tests become abnormal during therapy, the drug must be discontinued. The drug is contraindicated in pregnancy.

Azathioprine

Azathioprine has been used successfully in the management of persistent arthritis[51]. It is generally given in an oral dose of 1 to 4 mg/kg of body weight. Myelosuppression is the principal adverse effect, and regular blood counts are required weekly for the first 4 weeks of therapy and 3 monthly thereafter. Hypersensitivity reactions, including fever, cholestatic jaundice, interstitial nephritis, and rash, are well-recognized complications of therapy. Use of the drug in pregnancy should be avoided.

The use of gold salts or D-penicillamine in the treatment of the chronic arthritis of associated with SARA is not established. Synovectomy and arthroplasty may be required in exceptional cases.

ENTHESITIS

Rest, physiotherapy, and ultrasound therapy are often helpful, but NSAIDs are also required. Local injection of a steroid, such as methylprednisolone 40 mg/mL, combined with lidocaine (lignocaine) hydrochloride 10 mg/mL, can give rapid relief of symptoms, but repeated injections may be necessary.

PSORIASIS OF THE PENIS (CIRCINATE BALANITIS)

This condition usually resolves spontaneously within a few weeks of its onset, but healing may be facilitated by the use of a topical steroid preparation, combined with an antimicrobial agent, for example betamethasone ointment with clioquinol applied twice daily for 1 to 2 weeks.

When there is secondary bacterial infection, the use of local saline lavages, and dressings soaked in normal saline applied to the glans are of value.

KERATODERMA BLENORRHAGICA

Although there is no specific treatment for this self-limiting manifestation, calcipotriol, a vitamin D derivative that is used in the management of plaque psoriasis may be helpful[52]. The cream or ointment (50 μg/g) is applied once or twice daily. The skin should be kept dry. Oral retinoids have been used in the management of severe psoriatic lesions in HIV-infected individuals[53], but they should only be used in consultation with a dermatologist.

THROMBOPHLEBITIS AND RUPTURE OF THE KNEE JOINT

The use of a supporting stocking and anti-inflammatory drugs (e.g. indomethacin) is sufficient to produce relief of symptoms. To reduce the possibility of phlebothrombosis developing in the deep veins of the calf, patients with this complication should not be immobilized longer than necessary. When synovial membrane rupture occurs, bed rest with immobilization of the joint for 2 to 3 days is all that is required.

References

1 Lehmer RR, Andrews BS, Robertson JA, Stanbridge EJ, de la Maza L, Friou GJ. Clinical and biological characteristics of *Ureaplasma urealyticum* induced polyarthritis in a patient with common variable hypogammaglobulinaemia. *Ann Rheum Dis* 1991; **50**: 574–576.

2 Horowitz S, Horowitz J, Taylor-Robinson D, *et al. Ureaplasma urealyticum* in Reiter's syndrome. *J Rheumatol* 1994; **21**: 877–872.

3 Li F, Bulbul R, Schumacher HR, *et al.* Molecular detection of bacterial DNA in venereal-associated arthritis. *Arthritis Rheum* 1996; **39**: 950–958.

4 Vittecoq O, Schaeverbeke T, Favre S, *et al.* Molecular diagnosis of *Ureaplasma urealyticum* in an immunocompetent patient with destructive reactive polyarthritis. *Arthritis Rheum* 1997; **40**: 2084–2089.

5 Taylor-Robinson D, Gilroy CB, Horowitz S, *et al. Mycoplasma genitalium* in the joints of two patients with arthritis. *Eur J Clin Microbiol Infect Dis* 1994; **13**: 1066–1069.

6 Csonka GW. The course of Reiter's syndrome. *Br Med J* 1958; **i**: 1088–1090.

7 Paronen I. Reiter's disease. *Acta Medica Scandinavica* 1948; **131**: Suppl. 212.

8 Matilla L, Leirisalo-Relo M, Koskimies S, Granfers K, Siitonen A. Reactive arthritis following an outbreak of Salmonella infection in Finland. *Br J Rheumatol* 1994; **33**: 1136–1141.

9 Aho K, Ahvonen P, Lassus A, Sievers K, Tiilkainen A. HLA-A27 in reactive arthritis. A study of Yersinia arthritis and Reiter's disease. *Arthritis Rheum* 1974; **17**: 521–526.

10 Soderlin MK, Alasaarela E, Hakala M. Reactive arthritis as a complication of *Clostridium difficile* after eradication of *Helicobacter pylori. Clin Rheumatol* 1999; **18**: 337–338.

11 Rosenbaum JT, Theofilopoulos AN, McDevitt HO, Cereira AB, Carson D, Calin A. Presence of circulating immune complexes in Reiter's syndrome and ankylosing spondylitis. *Clin Exp Immunol* 1981; **18**: 291–297.

12 Keat A, Thomas B, Dixey J, Osborn M, Sonnex C, Taylor-Robinson D. *Chlamydia trachomatis* and reactive arthritis: the missing link. *Lancet* 1987; **i**: 72–74.

13 Taylor-Robinson D, Gilroy CB, Thomas BJ, Keat ACS. Detection of *Chlamydia trachomatis* DNA in joints of reactive arthritis patients by polymerase chain reaction. *Lancet* 1992; **340**: 81–82.

14 Rahman MU, Cheema MA, Schumacher HR, Hudson AP. Molecular evidence for the presence of chlamydia in the synovium of patients with Reiter's syndrome. *Arthritis Rheum* 1992; **35**: 521–529.

15 Beutler AM, Hudson AP, Whittum-Hudson JA. *Chlamydia trachomatis* can persist in joint tissue after antibiotic treatment in chronic Reiter's syndrome/reactive arthritis. *J Clin Rheum* 1997; **3**: 125–130.

16 Nanagara R, Li F, Beutler AM, Hudson AP, Schumacher HR. Alteration of *Chlamydia trachomatis* biological behavior in synovial membranes: suppression of surface antigen production in reactive arthritis and Reiter's syndrome. *Arthritis Rheum* 1995; **38**: 1410–1417.

17 Gerard HC, Branigan PJ, Schumacher R, Hudson AP. Synovial *Chlamydia trachomatis* in patients with reactive arthritis/Reiter's syndrome are viable but show aberrant gene expression. *J Rheumatol* 1998; **25**: 734–742.

17a Kuipers JG, Jurgenssaathoff B, Bialowons A, *et al.* Detection of *Chlamydia trachomatis* in peripheral blood leukocytes of reactive arthritis patients by polymerase chain reaction. *Arthritis Rheum* 1998; **41**: 1894–1895.

18 Gaston JSH. Immunological basis of chlamydia induced reactive arthritis. *Sex Transm Inf* 2000; **76**: 156–161.

19 Schumacher H, Arayssi T, Branigan P, *et al.* Surveying for evidence of synovial *Chlamydia trachomatis* by polymerase chain reaction (PCR). A study of 411 synovial biopsies and synovial fluids. *Arthritis Rheum* 1997; **40**: S270.

20 Simon AK, Seipelt E, Sieper J. Divergent T-cell cytokine patterns in inflammatory arthritis. *Proc Natl Acad Sci USA* 1994; **91**: 8562–8566.

21 Yao ZB, Painter SL, Fanslow WC, *et al.* Human IL-17: a novel cytokine derived from T cells. *J Immunol* 1995; **155**: 5483–5486.

22 Campbell F, Birkelund S, Ward ME, Panayi GS, Kingsley GH. Sexually acquired reactive arthritis synovial T cells respond to *Chlamydia trachomatis* 57 kD heat shock protein but not the major outer membrane protein (abstract). *Arthritis Rheum* 1996; **39** (Suppl 9.): S184.

23 Deane K, Jecock R, Pearce J, *et al.* Identification and characterization of a DR4-restricted T cell epitope within chlamydia hsp60. *Clin Exp Immunol* 1997; **109**: 439–445.

24 Sieper J, Kingsley G. Recent advances in the pathogenesis of reactive arthritis. *Immunol Today* 1996; **17**: 160–163.

25 Nuki G. Ankylosing spondylitis, HLA-B27, and beyond. *Lancet* 1998; **351**: 767–769.

26 Csonka GW. Recurrent attacks in Reiter's disease. *Arthritis Rheum* 1960; **3**: 164–169

27 Csonka GW. Reiter's syndrome. *Ergebnisse der Inneren Medizin und Kinderheilkunde* 1965; **23**: 139–189.

28 Berg RL, Weinberger H, Dienes L. Acute hemorrhagic cystitis. *Am J Med* 1957; **22**: 818–858.

29 Mason RW, Murray RS, Oates JK, Young AC. Prostatitis and ankylosing spondylitis. *Br Med J* 1958; **i**: 748–752.

30 Oates JK, Csonka GW. Reiter's disease in the female. *Ann Rheum Dis* 1959; **18**: 37–44.

31 Oates JK, Young AC. Sacro-iliitis in Reiter's disease. Br Med J 1959; **i**: 1013–1015.

32 Sairanen E, Paronen I, Mahonen H. Reiter's syndrome: a follow-up study. *Acta Med Scand* 1969; **185**: 57–63.

33 Murray RS, Oates JK, Young AC. Radiological changes in Reiter's syndrome and arthritis associated with urethritis. *J Faculty Radiologists* 1958; **9**: 37–43.

34 Thamber N, Dunlop R, Thin RN, Huskisson EC. Circinate vulvitis in Reiter's syndrome. *Br J Vener Dis* 1977; **53**: 260–262.

35 Csonka GW, Oates JK. Pericarditis and electrocardiographic changes in Reiter's syndrome. *Br Med J* 1957; **i**: 867–869.

36 Rossen RM, Goodman DJ, Harrison DC. A.V. conduction disturbances in Reiter's syndrome. *Am J Med* 1975; **58**: 280–284.

37 Block SR. Reiter's syndrome and acute aortic insufficiency. *Arthritis Rheum* 1972; **15**: 218–220.

38 Csonka GW. Thrombophlebitis in Reiter's syndrome. *Br J Vener Dis* 1966; **42**: 93–95.

39 Gatler RA, Moskowitz RW. Pneumonitis associated with Reiter's disease. *Dis Chest* 1962; **42**: 433–436.

40 Oates JK, Hancock JAH. Neurological symptoms and lesions occurring in the course of Reiter's disease. *Am J Med Sci* 1959; **238**: 79–83.

41 Good AE. Reiter's disease: a review with special attention to cardiovascular and neurologic sequelae. *Sem Arthritis Rheum* 1974; **3**: 253–286.

42 Caughey DE, Wakem CJ. A fatal case of Reiter's disease complicated by amyloidosis. *Arthritis Rheum* 1973; **16**: 695–700.

43 Kousa M, Saikku P, Richmond S, Lassus A. Frequent association of chlamydial infection with Reiter's syndrome. *Sex Transm Dis* 1978; **5**: 57–61.

44 Keat AC, Thomas BJ, Taylor-Robinson D, Pegrum GD, Maini RH, Scott JT. Evidence of *Chlamydia trachomatis* infection in sexually acquired reactive arthritis. *Ann Rheum Dis* 1980; **39**: 431–437.

45 Erlacher L, Wintersberger W, Menschik M, *et al.* Reactive arthritis: urogenital swab culture is the only useful diagnostic method for the detection of the arthritogenic infection in extra-articularly asymptomatic patients with undifferentiated oligoarthritis. *Br J Rheumatol* 1995; **34**: 838–842.

46 Bas S, Vischer TL. *Chlamydia trachomatis* antibody detection and diagnosis of reactive arthritis. *Br J Rheumatol* 1998; 37: 1054–1059.

46a Sieper J, Braun J, Wu P, Hauer R, Laitko S. The possible role of shigella in sporadic enteric reactive arthritis. *Br J Rheumatol* 1993; **32**: 582–585.

47 Keat A, Thomas BJ, Taylor Robinson D. Chlamydial infection in the aetiology of arthritis. *Br Med Bull* 1983; **39**: 168–174.

48 Lauhio A, Leirisalo Repo M, Lahdevirta J, Saikku P, Repo H. Double-blind, placebo-controlled study of three-month treatment with lymecycline in reactive arthritis with special reference to Chlamydia arthritis. *Arthritis Rheum* 1991; **34**: 6–14.

49 Sieper J, Fendler C, Eggens U, *et al.* Long term antibiotic treatment in reactive arthritis and undifferentiated oligoarthritis: results of a double-blind placebo-controlled randomized study. *Arthritis Rheum* 1997; **40**: S227.

50 Clinical Effectiveness Group. National guideline for the management of sexually acquired reactive arthritis. www.mssvd.org.uk/ceg.htm.

51 Calin A. A placebo-controlled, cross-over study of azathioprine in Reiter's disease. *Ann Rheum Dis* 1986; **45**: 653–655.

52 Thiers BH. The use of topical calcipotriene/calcipotriol on conditions other than plaque-type psoriasis. *J Am Acad Dermatol* 1997; **37**: S69–S71.

53 Louthrenoo W. Successful treatment of severe Reiter's syndrome associated with human immunodeficiency virus infection with etretinate. Report of two cases. *J Rheumatol* 1993; **20**: 1243–1246.

54 McMillan A, Scott GR. *Sexually Transmitted Infections, Colour Guide.* Churchill Livingstone; Edinburgh: 2000.

Chapter 15

Syphilis and the endemic treponematoses
H Young, A McMillan

Introduction

Syphilis is an infectious disease caused by the bacterium *Treponema pallidum*. It is spread principally by sexual intercourse but may also be acquired congenitally, that is to say, the fetus becomes infected by its mother while *in utero*. The disease is systemic from the onset and fluctuates between short symptomatic and prolonged asymptomatic stages. The natural course of infection may span several decades.

Syphilis is conveniently divided into two stages, the early infectious and the late non-infectious stages. In the early infectious stage of the disease lesions occur on the moist mucocutaneous parts of the body, particularly the genitalia. These lesions contain many treponemes and enable transmission to occur by sexual intercourse. Even if untreated, these lesions tend to heal but may recur during the first 2 to 4 years, after which they heal and the disease becomes latent or hidden. The latent form or the non-infectious late stage of the disease may persist for decades without producing obvious clinical changes, but a proportion of patients will unpredictably develop active involvement of the cardiovascular system (about 10%), the central nervous system (about 10%), or localized gummatous destructive lesions which can affect the musculoskeletal system (about 10%), the viscera, and the mucous membranes (about 15%).

In both early and late stages of syphilis an infected mother can communicate the disease to her unborn fetus. Although the disease can be transmitted to the fetus transplacentally long after a mother has ceased to be sexually infectious, the longer she has had the disease the less likely is this to occur.

If treated in the early stage clinical cure can be achieved with penicillin treatment and with certain other antibiotics. In the late stages curative effects are often spectacular in some forms of neurosyphilis and in gummatous syphilis. In cardiovascular forms of the disease the effects of antibiotic therapy are not easy to define. Mucocutaneous lesions of syphilis may facilitate transmission of HIV infection, and HIV may affect the natural history of syphilis.

Etiology

The causative organism of syphilis, *Treponema pallidum*, is a delicate spiralled filament 6 to 20 μm in length. Members of the genus *Treponema* (treponemes) are found in the oral cavity, intestinal tract, and genital areas of humans and other animals. Whereas commensal species of treponeme can be cultured by employing appropriate cell-free culture media, the treponemes that are pathogenic to man cannot. Inability to cultivate these pathogenic treponemes has hindered our understanding of their biology but applications of modern methods, such as electron microscopy and DNA reassociation assays have enabled progress to be made. Miao and Fieldsteel[1] demonstrated 100% homology between the DNA of *T. pallidum* and *T. pertenue* and as a result of this finding and other similarities both are now considered to be the same species; because of the different degrees of virulence and clinical symptoms in man and their different ability to infect various laboratory animals, *T. pertenue* is considered to be a subspecies of *T. pallidum*.

The entire genome of *T. pallidum* subsp. *pallidum* has now been determined and shown to be 1 138 006 base pairs containing 1041 predicted coding sequencies[2]. Systems for DNA replication, transcription, translation, and repair are intact, but catabolic and biosynthetic activities are minimized. These findings are in keeping with an obligate human parasite that cannot be cultured continuously *in vitro*.

Polymerase chain reaction (PCR) analysis can now show a degree of difference between *T. pallidum* subsp. *pallidum* and *T. pallidum* subsp. *pertenue*. Identification and sequence analysis of *tprJ*, a member of a polymorphic multigene family showed only 87.3% identity between the two subspecies indicating significant sequence differences[3]. Differences in the 5′ flanking region of TpN15 lipoprotein gene can distinguish between the subspecies *pallidum*, *pertenue*, and *endemicum*[4]. Polymerase chain reaction of the acidic repeat protein (arp) gene has allowed the development of the first epidemiological typing system for *T. pallidum* subsp. *pallidum*.

The main differential characteristics of the non-cultivable treponemes are given in Table 15.1.

Diseases caused by the three subspecies of *T. pallidum* and *T. carateum* are referred to collectively as the treponematoses.

1. *T. pallidum* subsp. *pallidum* is the only pathogenic treponeme indigenous to Britain. It is the cause of venereal and congenital syphilis in man. It is the most virulent with the capacity to

Table 15.1 Characteristic features of infection by non-cultivable 'subspecies' of the genus *Treponema* (in 1984)

Feature	*Treponema pallidum*				
	subsp. pallidum	subsp. pertenue	subsp. endemicum	*T. carateum*	*T. poralu- iscuniculi*
Natural host					
Homo sapiens	+	+	+	+	–
Oryctolagus cuniculus (rabbit)	–	–	–	–	+
Nature of infection, potential to affect:					
skin, bone, viscera, and CNS	+	–	–	–	–
skin and bone only	–	+	+	–	–
skin only	–	–	–	+	+
Transmission					
sexual intercourse	+	–	–	–	+
close contact, mainly in childhood	–	+	+	+	–
Geographical distribution					
worldwide	+	–	–	–	
restricted (Middle East, SE Asia, previously in Yugoslavia)	–	–	+	–	
tropical, W and E hemispheres	–	+	–	–	
tropical, W hemisphere	–	–	–	+	
Cutaneous lesions produced experimentally in					
Oryctolagus cuniculus	+	+	+	–	
Mesocricetus auratus (hamster)	–	+	+	–	
Mus musculus (mouse)	–	–	–	–	
Cavia porcellus (guinea pig)	–	–	+	–	

cause pathological effects in the skin, bone, viscera, and central nervous system.

2. *T. pallidum* subsp. *pertenue* is the cause of yaws, a non-venereal but communicable disease, found in tropical countries. It is regarded as intermediate in virulence of the three subspecies with the capacity to involve the skin and bone.

3. *T. pallidum* subsp. *endemicum* is the cause of non-venereal endemic syphilis known as 'bejel' in the Middle East.

4. *T. carateum* is the cause of pinta, a mild contagious disease similar to yaws but confined to Central and South America. It is regarded as the least virulent of the three species with the capacity to involve only the skin.

5. *T. paraluiscuniculi* produces benign venereal spirochetosis (rabbit spirochetosis or rabbit syphilis) in rabbits.

Many commensal species of *Treponema* occur in the mouth (for example *T. denticola, T. vincentii,* and *T. scolodontum*) and on the mucous surfaces of the genitalia (for example *T. refringens, T. minutum,* and *T. phagedenis*) where their differentiation is important in the diagnosis of primary syphilis.

TREPONEMA PALLIDUM
Morphology and staining

Treponema pallidum is a delicate tightly coiled spiralled filament 6 to 10 μm (average 10 to 13 μm) by 0.1 to 0.18 μm in diameter (average 0.13 to 0.15 μm) with 6 to 12 regular coils: the wavelength of the coils is 1.1 μm and the amplitude 0.2 to 0.3 μm. The ends of the cells are pointed and covered with a sheath.

Treponema pallidum is feebly refractile and too narrow to be seen well by ordinary light microscopy. Dark ground illumination is normally used to examine the organism and this was the technique described by Fritz Schaudinn and Erich Hoffmann in 1905 to demonstrate that *T. pallidum* was the cause of syphilis. Special techniques such as silver impregnation may be used to demonstrate the organism, particularly in tissue, but this tends to alter the morphology. Immunofluorescent techniques can now be used to demonstrate the organism in tissues and body fluids. The presence of a capsular or slime layer has been observed occasionally on the surface of *T. pallidum* and this may explain the lack of serological reactivity of organisms freshly isolated from animal tissues. Treponema-associated mucopolysaccharides may be part of the capsular layer or may be derived from tissue constituents of the host.

Treponema pallidum, like other spirochetes, comprises a central protoplasmic cylinder consisting of cytoplasmic and nuclear regions enclosed by a cytoplasmic membrane and a cell wall containing peptidoglycan. When isolated, the peptidoglycan retains a helical configuration indicating that it determines the shape of the cell.

Between the cell wall and the outer envelope lie the axial filaments or internal flagella which are presumed to be responsible for motility although there is no direct evidence for this. There are three movements that propel spirochetes: slow undulation, corkscrew-like rotation and a sluggish backwards and forwards motion. *Treponema pallidum* often displays a characteristic tendency to bend at right angles near its midpoint. Spirochetal motion persists at high viscosity which blocks the flagellar motion of ordinary bacteria, suggesting a possible basis for the evolution of the complex structure of spirochetes.

A multilayered membrane encloses the cell. Compared with the outer membranes of enteric Gram-negative bacteria, the *T. pallidum* outer membrane lacks lipopolysaccharide, is far more labile, and appears to have a substantially lower protein:lipid ratio. The highly immunogenic *T. pallidum* lipoproteins are not surface exposed. The poor antigenicity of virulent *T. pallidum* is a function of both the lipid composition and the low protein content of its outer membrane[5]. A physical feature of *T. pallidum* is its striking low density of membrane-spanning outer membrane proteins (*T. pallidum* rare outer membrane proteins (TROMPs)) which are believed to contribute to the pathogenic properties of this organism including its ability to cause chronic infection and elicit a relatively slow-developing protective immune response. Cardiolipin, present in the lipid fraction of treponemes, brings about the production of an antibody which cross reacts with host tissue antigens. This is important in the diagnosis of treponemal infection.

Norris and colleagues[6] described a standard nomenclature for *T. pallidum* polypeptides to aid the correlation of experimental results from various laboratories that may use different terminology to refer to the same protein. The nomenclature consists of the prefix TpN (for *T. pallidum* Nichols strain, the reference strain) followed by a consensus M_r (relative molecular mass) and, if necessary, a letter to distinguish between polypeptides with a similar M_r. The main polypeptides of importance in diagnosis are given in Table 15.2.

Propagation and *in vitro* cultivation

Pathogenic treponemes can grow in the testicular tissue of rabbits, and this is the normal way of maintaining them in the

Table 15.2 Major *Treponema pallidum* subsp. *pallidum* polypeptides (modified from Norris 1993[6])

Standard designation	*Mr*	Other designations/ molecular weights	Properties
TpN15	15 000	15.5 kDa; 12 kDa	Lipoprotein; induces antibody response during infection; recombinant antigen used in diagnosis (EIA)
TpN17	17 000	14 kDa;Tpp17	Major membrane lipoprotein; induces antibody response; recombinant antigen used in diagnosis (EIA)
TpN37	37 000	38 kDa; 37 kDa	Flagellin; recombinant antigen available; homolog in commensal treponemes; several other flagellar associated proteins; e.g. Tpn27.5; TpN29; TpN30; TpN33; TpN34.5
TpN44.5a	42 000	42 000; 44 000; TmpA	Membrane lipoprotein; recombinant antigen available; homolog in commensal treponemes
TpN47	45 000	47 000; 46 000; 45 000; TpS	Major membrane protein; highly immunogenic; early antibody response; recombinant antigen used in diagnosis (EIA)

laboratory. Apart from ethical considerations intratesticular inoculation and weekly passage is a difficult, expensive, and time-consuming process. These factors, while limiting basic studies on the biology of *T. pallidum*, have produced strong incentives to elucidate the appropriate requirements for *in vitro* cultivation. The production of several recombinant *T. pallidum* polypeptides has, to some extent at least, overcome the limitations that inability to culture imposed on the production of antigens for diagnosis.

Most experiments with pathogenic treponemes employ Nichols strain of *T. pallidum* subsp. *pallidum*: this strain was isolated in 1913 from the cerebrospinal fluid of a patient with neurosyphilis and is still virulent for humans.

The discovery that *T. pallidum* is microaerophilic, rather than a strict anaerobe like the cultivable treponemes, greatly aided culture studies. Successful replication of

Nichols strain of *T. pallidum* was reported by Fieldsteel *et al.*[7]. Treponemes were shown to attach and replicate on the surface of tissue culture cells of cottontail rabbit epithelium (Sf1Ep) growing as conventional monolayers. Extract of rabbit testis and selection of appropriate batches of fetal bovine serum were key factors in successful multiplication. The number of treponemes increased reaching a plateau between days 9 and 12 of incubation, with increases ranging up to 100-fold and averaging 49-fold. Organisms harvested after 7-days incubation remained virulent for rabbits with the inoculation of an average of six to seven organisms producing erythematous, indurated treponeme-containing lesions.

Cultivation of *T. pallidum* under the conditions described above was independently corroborated by Norris[8]: although total increase in treponemes was lower (8.9 to 26.2-fold) and treponemes retained motility and virulence over a 12-day incubation period. The doubling time (30 to 33 hours) approached that observed *in vivo* in rabbits. Further work by Fieldsteel et al.[9] suggests that *T. pallidum* is not as fastidious as was formerly believed, treponemal replication occurring over a fairly wide range of temperatures and oxygen concentrations. The extent of treponemal multiplication was dependent on the initial inoculum: it was greatest when the inoculum was 10^6 and least at 10^8. For all inocula the maximum ceiling of multiplication was 2×10^8. It seems likely that the ceiling of multiplication is because of a combination of factors including exhaustion in the medium of some essential components, the accumulation of toxic products and exhaustion of oxygen, which both cells and treponemes need for survival and replication.

It may be necessary for *T. pallidum* to attach to a cell surface before the treponemes can divide. If this is the case, one of the newly divided treponemes will remain attached to one end, while the other end will be set free or will be attached to another site on the host cell after division. This process may be the method by which *T. pallidum* multiplies *in vivo* and *in vitro*, making tissue culture essential for successful *in vitro* propagation.

Epidemiology

OCCURRENCE OF DISEASE
Acquired syphilis

Syphilis is worldwide in its distribution but it is difficult to compare the incidence from one country to another. The extent to which available statistics reflect the incidence of the disease depends upon the efforts made in case finding, the variations in notification practices, and social factors that may increase or reduce the interaction between infected individuals and health services.

United Kingdom

Trends for early syphilis in the UK for the period 1975–1998 (Figure 15.1) reached a peak of 4886 in 1978 but this was less

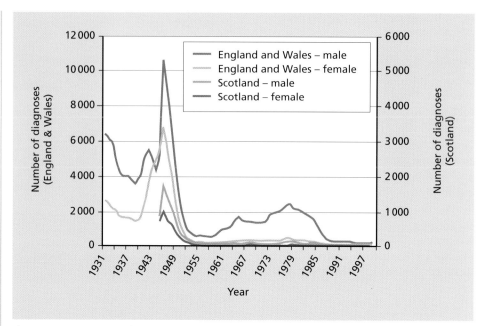

Figure 15.1 Diagnosis of syphilis (primary, secondary, and latent in the first 2 years of infection) seen in GUM clinics England, Scotland[a], and Wales, 1931 to 1999[b]

than one-fifth of the post-war peak of 27 761 in 1946. The increase in the detection of early syphilis in the late 1970s may have been partly because of the increased use of serological tests that were more sensitive and specific than the older methods such as the Wassermann Reaction and partly because of the number of tests carried out, particularly in homosexual men. The rise in numbers of infections in men who had had sex with men was probably another factor because of the tendencies of 'open-coupled' or functional members of the group to casual and often numerous sexual contacts. In a large-scale survey in 1977, 54% of syphilis infections were reported as homosexually acquired compared with 42% in 1971[10]. With changing sexual behavior amongst men who have sex with men, the number of homosexually acquired cases of early syphilis has fallen. Between 1998 and 1999, however, the number of cases of homosexually acquired infectious syphilis almost doubled (from 43 to 80 cases)[11], with sporadic outbreaks of early syphilis being described in several English cities[11a].

In the UK mortality from neurosyphilis declined progressively from the beginning of the twentieth century, the decline being accelerated in the early 1950s with the introduction of penicillin into clinical practice. Death rates from cardiovascular syphilis, less easy to detect or reverse with treatment, declined more slowly. Late-stage syphilis is now rare in the industrialized world.

United States of America

In the USA since a nadir in 1956, syphilis epidemics have peaked and troughed in approximately 10-year cycles[12]. The increase in the number of cases of infectious syphilis that was observed between 1969 and 1976 was almost exclusively amongst men; at the same time the proportion of men with early syphilis who named other men as sexual partners increased by about 200%[13]. As in the UK, the incidence of infection amongst homosexual men declined markedly with the advent of AIDS. The recent resurgence of primary and secondary syphilis in Washington State amongst men who have sex with men[14], however, reinforces the need for vigilance and continued education programs for this population.

In the USA, in the late 1980s, there was an increase in the number of cases of heterosexually acquired primary and secondary syphilis, that peaked in 1990 with an incidence rate of 20.3 per 100 000 population before declining steadily to 3.2 cases per 100 000 population in 1997. The infection rate in 1990 was particularly high amongst African-Americans (142.6 cases per 100 000 population) who accounted for about 80% of infected individuals; 10% to 12% of these people were adolescents[12]. This epidemic was attributed to the use of crack cocaine, the exchange of sex for drugs[15], and, possibly, the use of spectinomycin (an antibiotic that is not treponemicidal) to treat gonococcal infection. Even after the height of the epidemic, infection rates amongst African-Americans (30.2 persons per 100 000 population in 1996) remain some fifty times higher than amongst non-Hispanic whites, possibly reflecting poorer access to health care and a greater degree of poverty[12].

There are regional differences in the incidence of early syphilis in the USA, with higher rates being found in the larger cities than in rural areas[12]. Interestingly, rates of syphilis for African-Americans in various regions peak at similar levels but in different years. It has been proposed that syphilis epidemics may begin by the introduction of infection into a core group of susceptible individuals with multiple sexual partners. This core group would then transmit infection to a larger number of partners. As the disease progresses, the affected individuals become less infectious, or are treated, thereby limiting the spread of infection. The temporal differences in the peaking of the epidemics may be explained by the differential development of susceptible populations[16].

Eastern Europe

An epidemic of syphilis was reported from the Russian Federation in the mid-1990s[17]. In the last quarter of the twentieth century, the infection rate rose from a nadir of 4.2 cases per 100 000 population in 1988 to 263 cases per 100 000 in 1996. The male to female ratio was approximately 1. Amongst both men and women, proportionately larger increases in rates of new cases were noted in those aged 15 to 19 years than in the older age groups. The reasons for the epidemic are uncertain, but changes in both sexual behavior and sexual health services may have contributed. The propensity for spread of infection from epidemic areas is clearly shown by the finding that 25% of cases of early syphilis in the UK between 1994 and 1996 were associated with the Russian epidemic[18].

Developing world

It has been estimated that at any one time there are 27 million people with syphilis in the world, and that the majority of these infected individuals are in developing countries. Reflecting the global population distribution, southeast Asia, which accounts for 57.2% of the world's population in the 15 to 49-year age group (1995 figures), accounts for 48.7% of new infections. Sub-Saharan Africa accounts for another 21.1%, and Latin America and the Caribbean 9.7%[19]. The prevalence of syphilis is high amongst workers in occupations such as long-distance lorry driving and prostitution, and those who have had little education also appear to be at increased risk[20]. As a result of health education programs and the promotion of condom use, the incidence of infection in some countries such as Thailand has fallen[21].

Congenital syphilis

In the UK congenital syphilis has virtually disappeared as a cause of death in children under the age of 1 year. The death rate started to decline when arsenical treatment became widely available and accelerated with the advent of penicillin. It is an uncommon disease in the UK. In England during the 12 months ending in December 1996 there were two reported cases[11]. Antenatal examination routinely includes serological tests for syphilis and this screening, together with adequate treatment of infected mothers, accounts for the low incidence of the disease in this country.

In the late 1980s in the USA there was a marked increase in the incidence of congenital syphilis that paralleled the increasing infection rate amongst women. In New York City, the incidence rate was 357 per 100 000 live births. African-American infants have accounted for over 70% of cases of congenital syphilis[22].

In Africa and South America congenital syphilis is still common, although in regions where yaws is endemic an immune effect may modify the consequences of syphilis in the adult female and its transmissibility to the fetus. Syphilis, however, remains a risk factor for fetal death in developing countries[23]. It can be prevented *in utero* by treatment of the infected woman with penicillin during early pregnancy or cured later in pregnancy; its occurrence in a community is an indicator of defective antenatal care and the result of insufficient primary medical care.

TRANSMISSION OF INFECTION

Sexual

Treponema pallidum is so feebly viable outside its host that syphilis is ordinarily acquired by sexual intercourse. The organism has little intrinsic invasiveness and usually gains entry to its new host through minute abrasions in the epithelial surfaces that come into contact with the moist mucocutaneous lesions of an infected partner. An infected person usually ceases to be sexually infectious 2 to 4 years after acquiring the disease. Some individuals appear resistant to infection since not everyone exposed to early syphilis acquires the disease: Schober *et al.*[24] reported that just over 50% of at risk sexual contacts developed syphilis.

Accidental

Acquisition by means other than sexual intercourse usually involves direct contact. In such cases the organisms may gain entry through a small skin abrasion. Accidental inoculation has occurred under the following circumstances

- in doctors and nurses who have examined a syphilitic lesion without wearing gloves
- in laboratory workers by needle prick when inoculating pathogenic *T. pallidum* into rabbits or when handling large numbers of treponemes during isolation and purification procedures
- in patients being transfused with blood from a donor suffering from early syphilis[25].

Many cases of transfusion-acquired syphilis were reported prior to the 1950s. During the last few decades the number of cases reported has been very low. The decline is partly because of the lower incidence of syphilis and more thorough screening of blood donors. More important, however, is the fact that nowadays fresh blood is rarely used. In usual practice, when infected blood is stored at 4°C in citrate anticoagulant, infectivity is lost after 96 to 120 hours. The actual survival time may depend on the number of treponemes initially present in the donor blood[26]. Treponemes are not viable after storage for a few days to a few weeks at –10°C to –20°C. Treponemes are, however, viable when stored for extended periods at –45°C and infectious for an indefinite period when stored at –78°C. Freezing followed by desiccation kills the organism[25].

The risk of accidental infection by infected blood is highest when fresh heparinized blood is used. Such blood is favored for exchange transfusion in neonates because it practically guarantees normal pH, electrolyte composition, and concentration of glucose and ionized calcium. An infant girl acquired syphilis in this way in Rotterdam in 1977[27]. She showed typical features of early infectious syphilis 3.5 months after the transfusion. Although the blood donor had negative serological tests for syphilis 5 days before giving the blood, later tests were positive indicating that he must have become infected shortly before donating the blood.

Congenital

Although it has previously been considered that *T. pallidum* was not transmitted to the fetus before the fourth month of gestation, possibly through the protective effect of the cytotrophoblastic (Langhan's) layer, studies have clearly demonstrated that infection of the fetus can occur before the tenth week. *In utero* infection is supported by the detection of anti-treponemal IgM in cord blood obtained at birth from affected infants[28]. Transplacental transmission of *T. pallidum* is suggested by the finding of treponemes, in association with the typical histological changes of syphilis, in the placentas and umbilical cords of affected infants[29, 30], and in the umbilical cord blood[31]. As treponemes can also be found in the amniotic fluid of about 75% of

women with early syphilis, even as early as 14 weeks[32, 33], it may be that congenital infection can also result from nasopharyngeal and gastrointestinal colonization with *T. pallidum*.

Infection of the fetus is more likely to occur when the mother's infection is in the early stage, as at this time considerable numbers of organisms are present in the circulation. During the first year of infection in an untreated woman there is an 80% to 90% chance that the infection will be transmitted to the fetus. The probability of fetal infection declines rapidly after the second year of infection in the mother and becomes rare after the fourth year. In general, the greater the duration of syphilis in the mother, the less chance there is of the fetus being affected. If a mother with early-stage syphilis is not treated, 25% to 30% of fetuses die *in utero*, 25% to 30% die after birth, and of the infected survivors 40% develop late symptomatic syphilis. Up to 14% of pregnant women who have been treated for syphilis during their pregnancy deliver a stillbirth or an infant with signs of disease. Most of these women have been treated for secondary syphilis late in their pregnancy[34].

Non-venereal

Endemic treponematosis is transmitted by direct or indirect non-venereal contact in early childhood, for example by playing, by sharing eating or drinking utensils, and by close skin contact. It usually occurs in communities living in overcrowded and unhygienic conditions. Once common in parts of Europe, for example Yugoslavia, it is seen mainly in Africa as yaws, and in the Middle East as bejel, and in certain parts of Central and South America as pinta. There is no certain evidence of transmission from an infected mother to the fetus *in utero*.

COURSE OF UNTREATED SYPHILIS IN NON-HIV-INFECTED INDIVIDUALS

The natural course of infection in the non-HIV-infected individual may span many decades and present a variety of clinical forms. The classification of the stages of syphilis is shown in Box 15.1. The possible

impact of HIV infection on the course of syphilis is discussed on page 444.

Acquired infection

Clinical features are dealt with in detail later (see pp. 416–427) but the infection, if untreated, may run a course outlined diagrammatically in Figure 15.2.

The clinical horizon in this figure separates the stages when clinical features are absent from those when these are present. The period before the disease shows itself (pre-patent or incubation period) is usually about 25 days (range 9 to 90 days).

If the disease is not detected and treated in the primary stage, it progresses to the secondary stage, usually 6 to 12 weeks after contact, but occasionally this process may take up to 12 months. Secondary syphilis, characterized by a variety of macular, papular, papulo-squamous, and other skin lesions, results from the generalized spread and multiplication of *T. pallidum* throughout the body; the treponemes may be carried to virtually every organ and tissue.

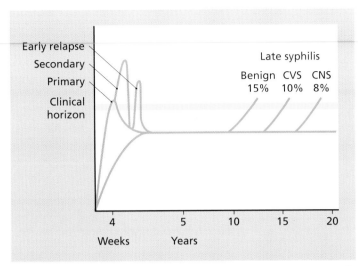

Figure 15.2 Simplified diagrammatic representation of the course of untreated syphilis from the time of infection. The early stages, whether primary, secondary, or early relapse of latent syphilis, are indicated together with the subsequent development of late-stage effects, whether late benign or gummatous, cardiovascular, central nervous system, or late-stage latent syphilis. The percentage of effects may vary in different populations (modified from Kampmeier 1964[250])

After the primary or secondary stage and probably also *ab initio* the infection becomes latent but mucocutaneous relapses may recur over a two-year period and render the infected person infectious again. Once the early infectious stage of the disease has run its course it enters the late non-infectious stage about 2 years after the initial contact. There may be no clinical evidence of this disease and latency, when disease is hidden, may persist for several decades, even for life, but a proportion of patients (30% to 40%) will unpredictably develop either gummatous lesions or, more seriously, cardiovascular or neurological disorders, bringing very serious disability and sometimes death.

The data in Figure 15.2 pertaining to late-stage syphilis are based on the famous Oslo study of untreated syphilis[35]. During the period 1891 to 1910 approximately 2000 patients with primary and secondary syphilis were isolated in hospital when infectious, but otherwise they were not treated. The patients were those of Professor Boeck, who, convinced about the inadequacies of current therapy, withheld treatment. Later a study group analyzed case histories of 1404 of Professor Boeck's original admissions to hospital.

As shown in Figure 15.2, infection may not run the 'typical' course, it may remain below the clinical horizon. Patients who are completely unaware of having experienced primary or secondary symptoms are diagnosed with latent infection. Symptoms are often suppressed during pregnancy. Antibiotics prescribed for other conditions may abort or delay early-stage infection, minimizing or abolishing early symptoms.

Congenital infection

In congenital syphilis resulting from blood-borne infection of the fetus via the placenta there is no stage analogous to primary acquired syphilis. Clinically congenital infection is divided into the early stage, the late stage, and the late latent stage with or without stigmata: the division between early and late stages is an arbitrary one.

Early stage pertains to the first 2 years of life and produces infectious lesions similar to those in the secondary stage of acquired syphilis. Lesions of late-stage congenital infection generally occur from 2 to 3 years of age and include gummata identical with those of benign tertiary acquired syphilis. The stigmata are scars and deformities of early or late lesions that

are no longer active; these include the saddle-shaped nose, interstitial keratitis, Hutchinson's teeth, and eighth nerve deafness. These differences in early and late-stage congenital syphilis may reflect the stage of infection of the mother and child during the pregnancy.

Pathology

PRIMARY SYPHILIS

The initial lesion noted in primary syphilis is a dull red papule, resulting from infiltration of the dermis with lymphocytes and plasma cells (Figure 15.3). As the disease progresses, thrombotic obstruction of blood vessels, whose walls show marked inflammatory changes (endarteritis obliterans), leads to necrosis of the overlying epidermis, and hence ulceration.

SECONDARY SYPHILIS

The classical description of the histopathology of secondary syphilis is that of swelling and proliferation of the endothelium of the superficial and deep dermal blood vessels, and of intense perivascular infiltration with plasma cells and lymphocytes. Recent studies suggest, however, that the histological appearances are more variable[36]. The dermis shows some abnormality in all cases. Infiltration with lymphocytes and plasma cells in both the superficial and deep dermis is usual, particularly near dermal blood vessels (Figure 15.4). Immunochemical staining

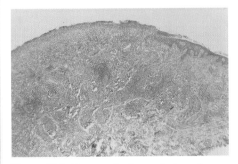

Figure 15.3 Biopsy of primary lesion of syphilis showing disruption of epithelium and dense infiltration of the submucosa with plasma cells and, to a lesser extent, lymphocytes (hematoxylin and eosin, × 40

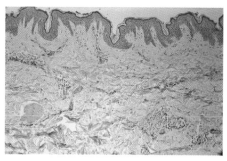

Figure 15.4 Biopsy of maculopapular lesion of secondary syphilis, showing infiltration of superficial and deep dermis with lymphocytes and plasma cells, particularly in relation to dermal blood vessels (hematoxylin and eosin, × 40)

has shown that histiocytes and cytotoxic CD8+ lymphocytes predominate in this infiltrate[37]. Vasodilatation is common, and activation of endothelial cells is shown by the expression of HLA-DR and swelling of these cells. Endothelial proliferation is rare.

Considerable emphasis has been placed, when making a histological diagnosis of syphilis, on the presence of plasma cells in the dermal infiltrate. In at least 25% of biopsies, however, these cells are either inconspicuous or absent. Edema of the epidermis can be observed in about 75% of biopsies, and acanthosis, an increase in the number of cells in the Malpighian layer, is found in about 30% of cases. Hyperkeratosis that is seen in some biopsies may be induced by cytokines such as interferon-γ, tumor necrosis factor-α, interleukin-6, and interleukin-8[37]. Exocytosis, that is, the presence of inflammatory cells within the epidermis, is seen in at least 80% of biopsies; there are polymorphonuclear leukocytes but lymphocytes usually predominate. In skin biopsies from individuals with secondary syphilis, there is no apparent correlation between the degree of cellularity and either the patient's HIV status or, in people with HIV infection, the CD4+ cell count in the peripheral blood[37].

In the lymphadenopathy of secondary syphilis, the glands show follicular hyperplasia with prominent germinal centers and epithelial cell clusters. Fibrosing endarteritis and periarteritis are marked, and fibrosis of the trabeculae and capsule is common. Treponemes are rarely found within the affected lymph nodes.

GUMMATA

In the localized lesion there is a central area of necrosis that is surrounded by a zone of granulation tissue that, in turn, is surrounded by a narrow zone of fibrous tissue. The granulation tissue contains lymphocytes and plasma cells, particularly around small blood vessels. There is intimal thickening and occlusion of some vessels, resulting in necrosis of tissue. Diffuse interstitial fibrosis results from gummatous involvement of organs such as the tongue and testis.

NEUROSYPHILIS

In all forms of meningovascular syphilis there is a widespread, often diffuse, thickening of the pia-arachnoid and infiltration with lymphocytes and plasma cells. The basal meningitis of the secondary stage may be carried into the late stage with increased fibrosis and the formation of small miliary gummata. This can lead to hydrocephalus and papilledema. The basal meningitis may be continued over the upper cervical segments of the spinal cord, or a diffuse spinal arachnoiditis may reveal its presence by root signs and symptoms. Meningeal gummata are very rare.

Lesions of the cerebral vessels may accompany any form of neurosyphilis but syphilitic vascular disease is not a common cause of cerebral vascular accidents. The classical lesion is endarteritis obliterans with fibroblasts and eventually collagenous thickening of the intima.

In tabes dorsalis the lesions are concentrated on the dorsal roots and columns, most often at the lumbosacral and lower thoracic levels. In classical paretic dementia (general paralysis of the insane), in a patient who dies demented after several years of illness, the brain is shrunken and covered with an opaque thickened arachnoid membrane. Microscopical examination at any stage shows the lesions to be concentrated in the cerebral cortex, corpus striatum, and hypothalamus. In the cerebral cortex, particularly in the prefrontal cortex, all cellular elements are involved with a striking loss of cortical architecture. The meningeal and perivascular infiltrations, microglial and astrocytic hyperplasia, and the degeneration and disappearance of nerve cells are similar to those found in other forms of subacute or chronic encephalitis such as African trypanosomiasis (due to *Trypanosoma brucei rhodesiense* or, more particularly, in that due to *T. b. gambiense*) and subacute sclerosing panencephalitis.

CARDIOVASCULAR SYPHILIS

Involvement of the aorta is the commonest manifestation of late-stage syphilis. There is an endarteritis obliterans with a cellular reaction that radiates at some distance round the lesion in the form of a cuff within the periarterial tissues. The most severe lesions are usually in the aortic ring and the ascending part of the aorta, possibly because the vasa vasorum with their circumvascular lymphatics are most numerous in these portions of the vessel. The elastic tissue and muscle of the tunica media are destroyed and hence there is weakening of the aortic wall and loss of its elastic recoil. As the vessel becomes unable to withstand the force of the blood pressure it dilates. The dilatation often affects the root of the aorta and hence widens the ring of the aortic valve. This is not the only cause of incompetence, for the cusps suffer damaging changes of a distinctive kind. There is an ingrowth of fibroblasts from the intima of the aorta along the free margin of the valve, which is given a cord-like or 'rolled-edge' deformity, and the coronary ostia are often involved[38].

Granulomatous lesions often involve the openings of the coronary arteries particularly in those patients in whom, as a developmental anomaly, the vessels arise above the level of the aortic sinus and are consequently nearer to the region of the greatest damage to the aorta.

Weakening of the media in syphilis often leads to general dilatation of the aorta and, in addition, localized dilatation may occur almost always in the ascending thoracic aorta. Such an aneurysm may press on neighboring structures, including the vertebrae, sternum, and ribs, that can be eroded by continuing pressure. The recurrent laryngeal nerve may be stretched and the esophagus compressed. Rupture of the aueurysm is a common cause of death.

INVOLVEMENT OF THE EAR IN CONGENITAL SYPHILIS

In sections of the temporal bone of individuals with long-standing sensori-neural deafness which has resulted from congenital syphilis, there is patchy osteitis with inflammation of all three layers of the otic capsule. Hydrops of the cochlear duct, saccule, and utricle occurs and there is degeneration of the organ of Corti with loss of cochlear neurons. Similar changes may affect the sensory epithelium or neurons of the vestibular system[39].

PLACENTAL AND UMBILICAL CORD IN UNTREATED EARLY SYPHILIS

The placenta from women with untreated early syphilis is often enlarged and pale. Histologically, there is a variety of changes, including proliferative vascular changes, chronic villitis, relative immaturity of the villis, and, less commonly, acute villitis[39a]. However, none of these changes is specific. Necrotising funiculitis, characterised by perivascular concentric rings of inflammatory cells, necrotic debris or calcium deposits whilst associated in some cases with syphilis, is not pathognomic of this infection[39b].

Pathogenesis and immunology

ENTRY, ATTACHMENT, AND DISSEMINATION

Treponema pallidum subsp. *pallidum* enters the tissues most commonly through abrasions or minor breaks in the skin, often not at mucosal sites. There is no evidence for the colonization of mucosal surfaces before penetration. After entering the body, the organisms multiply slowly at the site of penetration, initially causing no overt pathogenic effect. However, animal studies have shown that treponemes appear in the blood and lymphatics within minutes and disseminate widely within hours. The chancre eventually appears at the site of the inoculum; the larger the inoculum the shorter the pre-patent period before the chancre develops. Syphilis can be described as a generalized infection of vascular tissues. Within lesions in each stage of syphilis treponemes localize primarily in vascular areas.

Attachment to host tissues is an important initial step in many infections at mucosal surfaces and is also generally considered to be important in syphilis. *In vitro* studies have shown that that *T. pallidum* subsp. *pallidum* and *T. pallidum* subsp. *pertenue* attach to numerous and different types of tissues. Non-pathogenic treponemes do not attach and this factor substantiates attachment as a prerequisite for pathogenesis. Attachment may be by specific attachment ligands such as fibronectin although attachment also occurs to other structural components of basement membranes and extracellular matrices such as laminin, collagen IV, collagen I, and hyaluronic acid[40].

To move away from the initial site of entry, and gain access to the blood and lymphatic channels, treponemes must traverse the viscous ground substance or gel-like matrix between tissue cells. *Treponema pallidum* subsp. *pallidum* has a hyalouronidase that degrades the hyaluronic acid within the ground substance to facilitate the spread of the organisms. To gain access to the blood and lymphatics, treponemes must degrade the intact basement membrane surrounding these vessels and then pass between endothelial cells to enter the lumen. At distant sites, the process is reversed and organisms eventually localize perivascularly.

Experimental models involving isolated rabbit capillary tissues support the importance of treponemal hyaluronidase in disseminating the organism by degrading the hyaluronic acid enzymatically thereby splitting the endothelial cell junctions[41]. Treponemal hyaluronidase may also play a role in capillary destruction. Ground substance provides structural support for capillaries. With extensive perivascular multiplication of organisms degradation of the hyaluronic acid would damage capillary structural support. In turn collapsed vessels would result in the inhibited blood supply, necrosis, and ulceration that are characteristic of syphilitic histopathology.

Treponema pallidum subsp. *pallidum* has strategies to aid survival and spread within the host. Glycosaminoglycans similar to hyaluronic acid coat the outer surface of the organism and inhibit complement of the classic (antibody dependent) pathway. Treponemal surface-associated sialic acid inhibits complement activation by the alternative (antibody independent) pathway. *Treponema pallidum* subsp. *pallidum* can synthesize its own prostaglandin E2 which down regulates early immune processing by stimulating macrophage suppressor activity.

With the exception of the gummata, clinical manifestations of syphilis result from multiplication of treponemes within tissues. Fitzgerald[42] proposed a model for pathogenesis of syphilis in which treponemal multiplication is dependent on ground substance polysaccharide. This model helps explain the following

- the primary stage involving dermal tissue which contains relatively high concentrations of mucopolysaccharides
- the secondary stage involving most tissues, all of which contain varying amounts of ground substance
- the late stage involving the aorta which also contains relatively high levels of mucopolysaccharides and nerve tissue which is composed of nerve fibers separated by ground substance.

At least some of the birth defects of congenital syphilis may result from treponemal interference with ground substance mucopolysaccharide production during the very active fetal growth period.

HOST RESPONSE

It has been known for some time that humans exert some degree of natural resistance to *T. pallidum*; only 50% of at-risk sexual contacts of primary and secondary syphilis develop infection[24]. The proportion reported is similar to that in the pre-antibiotic era.

Normal human serum contains a heat-stable cross-reactive treponemicidal antibody elicited by the non-pathogenic, host-indigenous *T. phagedenis*. This antibody and the extent of the treponemal challenge dose may account in part for the relatively low infection rate[43]. Acquired immunity is slow to evolve and requires relatively prolonged periods of antigenic stimulation. In the Sing Sing study[44] 62 patients with syphilis were experimentally challenged with Nichols strain of *T. pallidum* subsp. *pallidum*. The immunity of these patients was related to the duration of the initial infection; as the duration of untreated syphilis increased, lesions following challenge occurred less frequently. Also, as shown in the Oslo study[35] 65% of untreated patients did not progress beyond the primary stage, implying a certain degree of immunity. Clinical observation and experimental studies suggest that a vigorous, but imperfect, immune response develops during syphilis infection that is successful in clearing most but not all of the treponemes infecting the host, thus allowing the disease to progress through the various stages.

Cellular and humoral factors

Histologic studies of human and rabbit syphilis lesions have shown that the inflammation resembles a delayed-type hypersensitivity response[45]. The predominant cell types infiltrating syphilis lesions are T lymphocytes (CD4+ and CD8+). Activated macrophages play a major role in the clearance of *T. pallidum* from early syphilis. Sensitized T lymphocytes which arise early in infection produce migration inhibition factor as well as macrophage activation factor[46]. Living *T. pallidum* can be phagocytosed by macrophages *in vitro* in the presence of specific antibody. Opsonic antibodies are directed against pathogen-specific antigens. Peak production of macrophage activation factor by lymphocytes correlates with bacterial clearance in primary lesions of experimentally infected rabbits. In both primary and secondary lesions the infiltrating cells predominantly express the T_{h1} cytokines interleukin-2, interferon-γ and interleukin-12. Arroll and colleagues[45] considered that the role of the T cell response during early syphilis infection is to develop a T_{h1} cytokine

environment that promotes macrophage activation and bacterial clearance. T cell responses later in syphilis are believed to play a role in the development of immunity to infection but the late development of immunity (in the rabbit at least) is a separate process from the bacterial clearance described above. Studies with recombinant antigens in experimental syphilis showed that the membrane proteins TpN17 and TpN47, as well as the endoflagellar sheath protein TpN37, induced strong proliferation responses through most of the syphilis infection. An unexpected drop in proliferative response to these antigens at day 90 of infection (after clearing of treponemes from the initial lesions), followed by a dramatic increase in response at day 180, suggests that there may be a secondary dissemination of *T. pallidum* which induces a recall response. The intensity of the proliferation and T_{h1} cytokine response to TpN37 (which recognized new epitopes during infection) correlates with both the lesion-clearing response (days 10 to 30) and resistance to re-infection (day 180). These findings with recombinant antigens differ from the proliferative response to a sonicate of *T. pallidum* which was maintained at high levels for 2 years. It was suggested that a late T cell response to a different subset of antigens masks the down regulation observed with the TpN17, TpN37, and TpN47 antigens.

It has also been shown that a close quantitative relationship exists between the development of acquired resistance and the level of treponemicidal antibody, suggesting that killing antibody plays a key role in the acquisition of protective immunity[47]. The low density of membrane-spanning outer membrane proteins (*T. pallidum* rare outer membrane proteins (TROMPs)) are believed to contribute to the pathogenic properties of this organism including its ability to cause chronic infection and elicit a relatively slow-developing protective immune response. *Treponema pallidum* rare outer membrane proteins are major targets of protective immunity that develops during the course of experimental syphilis: complete immunity correlated with antibody that killed *T. pallidum* and aggregated TROMPs. Although antibody against TROMPS with complement effectively kills

T. pallidum it is conceivable that other antibody-mediated mechanisms, such as opsonization, or antibody dependent cellular cytoxicity may play key roles in an antibody protective response[47].

Humoral immune response

Specific anti-*T. pallidum* IgM is detectable during the second week of infection while production of specific anti-treponemal IgG begins around the fourth week after infection and usually reaches much higher titers than those for IgM[48]. Recently many investigators have applied immunoblotting to analyze the immune response in experimental and human infection[49–52]. The IgG and IgM reactivity in patients with primary syphilis is variable but generally the number of molecules recognized by antibodies and the intensity of reactivity, reflect the duration of clinical symptoms. Sera from patients with secondary and early latent syphilis uniformly demonstrated reactivity to twenty-two separate polypeptide antigens[49]; decreased reactivity was seen in late latent syphilis. In a recent study[52] nine pathogen-specific polypeptides (15, 17, 33, 37, 39, 43, 45, 47, 49 kDa) were commonly recognized by the time chancre immunity developed – minor differences in the molecular masses of some of these antigens have been described by different investigators[53]; some of the antigens above will equate to TpN15, TpN17, TpN33, TpN37, TpN39, TpN44.5, and TpN47 using the newer standard nomenclature.

In primary infection a strong antibody response to TpN47 was reported by Baker-Zander and colleagues[49] as well as reactivity against six other bands including TpN15. In secondary and early latent syphilis the main serological response is associated with TpN15, TpN17, TpN33, TpN37, TpN44.5, and TpN47. In late latent syphilis reactivity against the TpN47, TpN17, and TpN15 predominates, but there is a decreased spectrum and intensity of IgG reactivity[49, 51].

Although early replication is primarily extracellular at least some treponemes become intracellular following attachment and penetration[43]. The inflammatory response to primary infection in both the human and experimental rabbit disease consists essentially of infiltration by lymphocytes, plasma cells, and macrophages with a distribution depending upon the stage of lesion development versus healing. Healing may occur as a result of inactivation of *T. pallidum* by specific antibodies, with resultant enhanced phagocytosis and destruction by macrophages.

Phagocytosis

In infections such as listeriosis, toxoplasmosis, and tuberculosis destruction of the infecting organism is mediated by macrophages which have been activated by soluble products of specifically sensitized T lymphocytes. Sensitized T lymphocytes which arise early in infection produce migration inhibition factor as well as macrophage activation factor[46]. Living *T. pallidum* can be phagocytosed by macrophages *in vitro* in the presence of specific antibody. Macrophages play a major role in the clear-ance of organisms from the local site of infection.

Although degradation of ingested organisms within phagocytic vacuoles has been described, the direct killing of *T. pallidum* by macrophages has not yet been demonstrated.

Electron microscopic studies have documented the rapid uptake of *T. pallidum* into membrane-bound vacuoles in human polymorphonuclear leukocytes (PMNLs) *in vitro* after incubation for as little as 5 minutes. Leukocyte degranulation and loss of treponemal integrity was observed within a few hours. Intradermal injection of *T. pallidum* into rabbits caused a rapid accumulation of PMNLs. Thus, although PMNLs are attracted to, and appear to ingest *T. pallidum* they fail to eradicate the organisms following inoculation[54].

Diagnosis

Microbiological tests are essential in making, or excluding, a diagnosis of syphilis but they must be interpreted in relation to the patient's history and physical examination. Serology is the main method of diagnosis at all stages of infection although the direct detection of *T. pallidum* is also used in early infection, particularly in the diagnosis of primary syphilis. *Treponema pallidum* may be demonstrated in the lesions of primary syphilis before an antibody response is detectable. Diagnosis of syphilis is covered in several recent reviews[55–58]. All current tests for syphilis are in fact tests for infection with a pathogenic treponeme and do not differentiate between syphilis (*T. pallidum* subsp. *pallidum*), yaws (T. *pallidum* subsp. *pertenue*), endemic syphilis (*T. pallidum* subsp. *endemicum*), and pinta (*T. carateum*).

DEMONSTRATION OF *TREPONEMA PALLIDUM* IN LESION EXUDATES

Several methods are available for detecting *T. pallidum* in lesions and tissues although few are used routinely in current practice. The relative performance characteristics of several methods are summarized in Table 15.3.

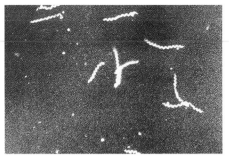

Figure 15.5 Dark ground appearance of *Treponema pallidum* (× 1000) (reproduced from McMillan and Scott 2000[251])

Dark ground/darkfield microscopy

Dark ground/darkfield microscopy (DGM) of exudate from genital ulcers has long been regarded as standard practice in the diagnosis of primary syphilis (Figure 15.5). It has the advantage over other methods in that it can be performed in less than 30 minutes in any clinic equipped with a microscope with a dark ground condenser, and with experienced personnel good results are obtained (see Table 15.3). Because of interference from commensal spirochetes that are found in the normal flora of the genital and rectal mucosae, DGM is considered to be less reliable in examining rectal and non-penile genital lesions. Dark ground/darkfield microscopy is not suitable for examining oral lesions because of the many commensal treponemes that occur in the mouth. It can, however, be applied to the moist mucous lesions (condylomata lata or mucous

Table 15.3 Sensitivity and specificity of methods to detect *Treponema pallidum*

Study	Detection method			
	DGM	DFA-TP	Visuwell EIA	M-PCR
Hook *et al.* 1985[249]	Sensitivity 97% Specificity 77%	Specificity 100% Sensitivity 100%		
Romanowski *et al.* 1987[253]	Sensitivity 79% Specificity 100%	Sensitivity 73% Specificity 100%		
Cummings *et al.* 1996[257]	Sensitivity 86% Specificity 100%	Sensitivity 92% Specificity 100%	Sensitivity 82% Specificity 90%	
Orle *et al.* 1996[64]	Sensitivity 81% Specificity 100%			Sensitivity 91% Specificity 99%

patches) of secondary syphilis but as sero-logical tests are virtually 100% sensitive at this stage there is little need for it.

After cleansing the surfaces of the primary or secondary lesions with a swab soaked in physiological saline, serum obtained from the depth of the lesion is examined by DGM using the oil-immersion objective. *Treponema pallidum* is distin-guished from other spirochetes by its slender structure, the tightness of its spirals, and characteristic motion: slow deliberate forward and backward move-ment with rotation about the longtitudinal axis and occasional angulation or bending to about 90⁰. It must be carefully distin-guished from the many other treponemes that are part of the normal genital flora (for example *T. refringens* and *T. phagedenis*)[56] although these tend to be surface organisms and are not found in the depth of lesions. If the initial test is negative the procedure should be repeated daily for at least 3 days: antibiotics should be withheld during this period, although local saline lavage may be used to reduce local sepsis.

Adequate training and experience in taking specimens, setting up the dark-ground microscope and interpretation of findings is essential for good performance of this method as there are many technical reasons for false negative results

- too little material on the slide may cause quick drying
- too much fluid may cause difficulty in observing the movement of the treponemes
- improper thickness of slide or coverslip may cause difficulty in focusing[58]
- too many blood cells, air bubbles, or tissue fragments make the specimen unsatisfactory.

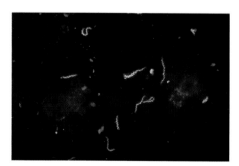

Figure 15.6 Direct immunofluorescence for *Treponema pallidum* (× 1000) (reproduced from McMillan and Scott 2000[251])

A downside of the decrease in primary syphilis in many areas has been a con-comitant decrease in DGM experience. Great care is required in performing DGM as the need to maintain viability of *T. pallidum* means that the material being processed may contain potentially infec-tious agents such as HIV.

Direct fluorescent antibody test for *Treponema pallidum*

The direct fluorescent-antibody staining for *T. pallidum* (DFA-TP) test (Figure 15.6) whereby a smear of exudate is made on a slide, fixed in acetone, and sent to the laboratory alleviates the problem of examining potentially infectious material. Originally, smears were stained with a conjugated syphilitic serum made specifically for *T. pallidum* but in spite of absorption with cultivable treponemes the DFA-TP test gave non-specific results and was less reliable than DGM[59]. A newer version of the DFA-TP test employing a fluorescein-labeled pathogen-specific monoclonal antibody to TpN47 or TpN37, is at least as sensitive and more specific than DGM (see Table 15.3). Like DGM the test is also subject to sampling variation and obstruction of treponemes by debris and erythrocytes. Lesions should be examined on 3 consecutive days before being considered negative. Evaluation of the diagnostic potential of DFA-TP in routine practice awaits the availability of commercial kits. Theoretically this test could be applied to chancres from any site, but as pathogen-related oral spirochetes have antigenic determinants thought to be unique to pathogenic treponemes[60] findings from oral lesions should be interpreted with caution.

Although DFA-TP can also be used to detect *T. pallidum* in tissues this remains a highly specialized procedure[61] and is best restricted to specialized laboratories or research centers.

Other staining methods

Methods such as indian ink staining and silver staining are essentially obsolete. Silver staining does not give a clear differentiation between *T. pallidum* and tissue fibers shaped like treponemes.

Polymerase chain reaction

Polymerase chain reaction for *T. pallidum* requires standardization and further evaluation to determine if it provides a significant advantage over DFA-TP. Using experimentally infected rabbits it was shown that whole blood in heparin or EDTA (but not serum as treponemes may be trapped during clotting), lesion exudate, punch biopsy, and swabs of lesions were useful specimens[62]. There are few studies on the use of PCR to detect early syphilis in humans. Jethwa and colleagues[63] used a PCR (primers based on the gene for TpN47) to detect *T. pallidum* DNA extracted from slides containing touch preparations of lesion exudate for examination by DFA-TP (using fluorescein-conjugated monoclonal antibody against TpN37) and found similar reactivity with a concordance between DFA-TP and PCR of 96%. An interesting development is a multiplex PCR (M-PCR) assay that uses three different sets of primers for the simultaneous detection of *T. pallidum*, *Haemophilus ducreyi*, and herpes simplex virus (HSV)[64]. In a study of geni-tal ulcer disease in New Orleans, M-PCR gave a sensitivity of 91% for *T. pallidum* (target based on gene for TpN47) compared with 81% for DGM. Although not yet available commercially the M-PCR has been used to study the etiology of genital ulcers in India[65] and Madagascar[66].

Polymerase chain reaction has also been used to detect *T. pallidum* in non-primary lesions. A PCR based on the gene for the TpN47 detected treponemal DNA in skin lesions from the scalp of a patient with secondary syphilis and diffuse alopecia: treponemes were not detected by silver staining or DFA[67]. Conventional tech-niques also failed to detect spirochetes in the skin lesions of late secondary and gummatous syphilis although the presence of *T. pallidum* DNA could be demonstrated by PCR[68]. Polymerase chain reaction also detected *T. pallidum* DNA (target based on gene for the TpN 44.5a antigen) in pseudo-lymphomatous gastric lesions from two patients[69]: silver staining was negative in both patients while one patient gave a positive indirect fluoresent antibody test result. The use of PCR in neurosyphilis and congenital syphilis is discussed on p. 415.

Reverse transcriptase polymerase chain reaction

Whereas the above PCR assays are thought to target single-copy genes, the advantage of reverse transcriptase PCR (RT-PCR) is the high number of copies of 16S rRNA per cell. *In vitro* experiments showed that the RT-PCR reproducibly detected one organism and was more sensitive than a TpN47 DNA PCR[70]. Because of the sensitivity of the assay higher dilutions of lysed organisms can be used thus minimizing the effect of PCR inhibitors that may be present in some patient samples. It is also possible that RT-PCR may be able to distinguish between live and dead organisms because RNA is usually rapidly degraded once the cells die. This technique remains to be evaluated in the clinical setting.

Rabbit infectivity test)

This research tool is the most sensitive method for detecting infectious treponemes. Fresh clinical specimens such as cerebrospinal fluid (CSF) are inoculated into the testes of rabbits that are then monitored for the development of orchitis or a serological response[56]. The technical complexity of the procedure and the long incubation period makes the rabbit infectivity test impractical other than in a research setting.

DEMONSTRATION OF ANTIBODIES IN THE SERUM

Infection with *T. pallidum* produces antibodies to over twenty different polypeptide antigens. The number of antigens recognized by antibodies and the intensity of reactivity increases initially and reflects the duration of clinical symptoms. By the time clinical signs develop most patients have both IgG and IgM antibodies[49]. Specific anti-*T. pallidum* IgM is detectable during the second week of infection while production of IgG begins around the fourth week after infection and usually reaches much higher titers than those for IgM. The spectrum and intensity of reactivity decreases with the duration of infection, even in the absence of treatment. Although IgM is undetectable in many cases of late syphilis, IgG

Table 15.4 Use of main serological tests in syphilis serology

Antigen	Test	Screening	Confirmation	Activity of infection/ Response to treatment
Cardiolipin	VDRL//RPR	✓	–	✓
Cardiolipin	SpiroTek Reagin II EIA	✓	–	–
Treponema pallidum native	TPHA/TPPA	✓	✓	–
Treponema pallidum native and recombinant	EIA	✓	✓	–
Treponema pallidum native	FTA-abs	–	✓	–
Treponema pallidum native and recombinant	Immunoblotting	–	✓	–[a]
Treponema pallidum native	IgM EIA	–	–	✓
Treponema pallidum native	IgM SPHA	–	–	✓
Treponema pallidum native	19S IgM FTA-abs	–	–	✓

[a] Recombinant antigen immunoblotting may prove to have some value in the future.

reactivity usually persists. Therapeutic intervention causes a generalized loss of antibodies against individual antigens but again low levels of specific IgG usually remain detectable.

Serological tests for syphilis are of two main types (cardiolipin antigen or treponemal antigen) and can be used in one or more ways, for example as screening and/or confirmatory tests or to help assess the activity of infection and the response to treatment (see Table 15.4). The following section outlines the antigens involved and the principles of the main tests before discussing their performance criteria and application in clinical practice. Several reviews discuss the various serological tests in greater detail[48, 56, 58, 71].

Cardiolipin antigen tests

These tests are sometimes referred to as nontreponemal antigen tests, but as cardiolipin is present in treponemes the authors prefer the term cardiolipin antigen tests.

All cardiolipin antigen tests are cheap, simple, and quick to perform and can be used for screening. The antigen used in the modern cardiolipin antigen tests, which have evolved from the original Wassermann complement fixation test, is an alcoholic solution containing cardiolipin, lecithin, and cholesterol. The antigen in the original Wassermann test consisted of a saline extract of syphilitic tissues obtained from stillborn fetuses with congenital infection. It was assumed that *T. pallidum* present in the infected tissue was responsible for the positive reactions obtained in patients with syphilis. Later it was shown that the same results were obtained with an alcoholic extract of heart muscle. In 1941 the diphospholipid cardiolipin was identified as the active component in beef heart extract, and for over 50 years cardiolipin and lecithin have been isolated and purified from beef hearts although synthetic antigens are now being evaluated[72]. The discovery of cardiolipin as the active antigenic component allowed more standardized and reproducible antigen preparations and gave rise to the Venereal Disease Research Laboratory (VDRL) slide test[73]. Cardiolipin is widespread in nature and can be isolated from many mammalian tissues: it is a component of the inner membrane of the mammalian mitochondrion which accounts for the success of beef heart, which is rich in mitochondria, as a source of antigen. Historically the type of antibody reacting in the Wassermann reaction was termed reagin at a time when little was known of the nature of the reactions involved. The antibody produced during treponemal infection is directed against cardiolipin present in treponemes as well as against host tissue cardiolipin released during treponemal infection.

'Biological false positive' reactions

Because of the widespread nature of cardiolipin, antibodies reacting with it are occasionally found in the sera of healthy individuals (less than 1% of the population) or patients without any clinical evidence of syphilis. Traditionally these reactions have been termed biological false positive reactions (BFP). A high frequency of BFP reactions occurs in drug addicts, although the exact significance of this is not clear. Biological false positive reactions are classified as acute if they disappear spontaneously within 6 months and chronic if they persist for longer.

The acute or transient BFP may occur shortly after an acute febrile infectious disease (for example infectious mononucleosis, infective hepatitis, measles, or upper respiratory tract infection) or be provoked by strong immunological stimuli such as vaccination and pregnancy. The acute BFP disappears within a few weeks or months after the acute illness has subsided. Approximately 60% of acute BFP reactors are under 30 years of age.

In contrast, the chronic BFP reaction persists longer than 6 months, and approximately 60% of reactors are over 30 years of age. Chronic BFP reactions are also more common in women than men. They may be associated with autoimmune and related diseases, for example rheumatoid arthritis, systemic lupus erythematosus (SLE), Sjögren's disease, autoimmune thyroiditis, and autoimmune hemolytic anemia. The anticardiolipin antibodies present in patients with SLE and/or phospholipid antibody syndrome differ in specificity from the anticardiolipin antibodies produced in syphilis[74, 75]. However, as these antibodies are not 'biologically false' it has been suggested that they should be referred to as nontreponemal-infection associated phospholipid antibodies (NTPA)[58]. Immunoglobulin G antiphospholipid antibodies may cross the placenta and be detected in the neonate by cardiolipin antigen tests: on serial testing the antibody should disappear and the tests become negative in 2 to 3 months.

Venereal Disease Research Laboratory slide test

In this test the patient's serum, previously heated to inactivate complement, is mixed with a freshly prepared suspension of cardiolipin-lecithin-cholesterol antigen on a glass slide. The mixture is rotated, usually mechanically, and after a few minutes flocculation (aggregation of antigen–antibody complexes in suspension) is detected microscopically using a low-power objective. The VDRL slide test is rarely used for screening nowadays but is retained for examining the CSF[56].

The addition of choline chloride and EDTA to the VDRL antigen enhanced the reactivity of the test, stabilized the antigen so that it did not need to be made up fresh each day, and allowed unheated serum or plasma to be tested (the USR or unheated serum regain test). By incorporating charcoal particles in the antigen the results of the reaction, which took place in a teardrop-shaped area on a plastic-coated card, could be read microscopically (the original RPR or rapid plasma regain test). The RPR teardrop card is still used to test plasma in field studies but testing serum by the RPR 18 mm circle card test is more sensitive.

Rapid plasma regain 18 mm circle card test or Venereal Disease Research Laboratory carbon antigen test

This is the most widely used form of cardiolipin antigen test. In the USA the test is referred to as the RPR while in Europe the test is usually referred to as the VDRL carbon antigen test or RPR carbon antigen test. To take account of these differences the term VDRL/RPR is used throughout. Serum is spread over a defined circle on a card, antigen added and the card placed on a mechanical rotator for about 8 minutes before examining the area for agglutination. Screening is normally performed using undiluted serum and the test is interpreted subjectively as reactive or nonreactive. Quantitative tests can be performed using doubling dilutions of serum: the titer is the reciprocal of the final serum dilution that is reactive.

SpiroTek Reagin II enzyme immunoassay

None of the standard cardiolipin tests is suitable for current methods of automation. Enzyme immunoassay (EIA) is widely used in diagnostic laboratories and is readily automated (see EIA under treponemal antigen tests below). The SpiroTek Reagin II EIA is more sensitive than the RPR and could substitute for the RPR test as a screening test[76].

Treponemal antigen tests

The antigen used in these tests is derived from Nichols strain of *T. pallidum* subsp. *pallidum* or recombinant antigens in the case of certain of the newer tests. Nichol's strain, isolated in 1913 from the cerebrospinal fluid of a patient with neurosyphilis, is still virulent for humans and is maintained in rabbits by intratesticular inoculation and weekly passage. The early treponemal antigen tests were used as verification tests to confirm the treponemal nature of a positive cardiolipin antigen test but many of the newer treponemal antigen tests are used for screening. The *Treponema pallidum* immobilization (TPI) test, once the only reliable test for distinguishing between treponemal and nontreponemal cardiolipin-antibody responses, has now been superseded by the widespread use of the fluorescent treponemal antibody absorbed (FTA-abs) test.

The fluorescent treponemal antibody absorbed test

Historically, this is the standard confirmatory test. In the fluorescent treponemal antibody absorbed (FTA-Abs) test[77], the patient's serum is absorbed with a sonicate of *T. phagedenis* (Reiter's treponeme) in order to remove group-specific antibody. Binding to *T. pallidum* of antibody specific for pathogenic treponemes is then demonstrated by the indirect immunofluorescence technique. The indirect immunofluorescence technique is carried out in two stages.

1. a smear of *T. pallidum* is incubated with patient's serum: any anti-treponemal antibody in the patient's serum reacts with the treponemes on the slide
2. fluorescein-labeled anti-human immunoglobulin (either polyvalent anti-human IgG/IgM/IgA or anti-human IgG) is added to reveal any antibody which was bound in the first stage.

Treponemes are located by dark ground microscopy and then examined by ultraviolet illumination. If the serum is positive the treponemes give bright apple-green fluorescence. Scoring of the test is based on the degree of fluorescence and is highly subjective.

A modification of the FTA-abs, the fluorescent treponemal antibody absorbed double staining procedure (FTA-abs DS), was introduced to update the FTA-abs test for new microscopes equipped with incident illumination. The procedure incorporates a rhodamine-labeled class-specific anti-human immunoglobulin G primary stain and fluorescein-labeled anti-treponemal globulin as counterstain[78]. The double staining method should overcome the difficulty of demonstrating the presence of antigen on non-reactive slides. Although considered to be less time consuming and easier on the eyes than the conventional FTA-abs, and to result in fewer borderline reactions, the double-staining method has not been widely adopted.

The Treponema pallidum hemagglutination assay

In the USA the *Treponema pallidum* hemagglutination assay (TPHA) is often referred to as the MHA-TP (microhemagglutination assay for *T. pallidum*). The TPHA is simple to perform and the availability of commercial kits based on sheep and fowl erythrocytes made this the first of the treponemal antigen tests to be used for routine screening. Basically erythrocytes coated with an extract of *T. pallidum* are agglutinated by antibody from the serum of patients with syphilis: pre-absorption of sera with components of Reiter treponemes, rabbit testis, and erythrocyte membranes is used to eliminate hemagglutination due to antibody against any of these agents. Any serum giving a positive reaction is tested against control erythrocytes (i.e. not coated with *T. pallidum* antigen) to check the specificity of the agglutination. In spite of the absorption procedure about 0.1% of specimens agglutinate erythrocytes in the absence of antigen: this non-specific agglutination makes the individual test result invalid. The use of fowl erythrocytes in the TPHA test may decrease the number of non-specific agglutination reactions. Sera are normally screened at a dilution of 1 in 80 and the degree of hemagglutination interpreted subjectively. Quantitative tests using serial doubling dilutions can also be performed if desired. Recently, a *T. pallidum* particle agglutination assay (TPPA) that uses gelatin particles as a carrier rather than erythrocytes became available commercially and has already replaced the TPHA in some laboratories.

Enzyme immunoassay

Enzyme immunoassay (EIA) is a relatively simple method that is widely used in the diagnosis of many infections. Patients' serum is allowed to react with antigen coated on the surface of wells in a microtiter plate. Specific antibodies binding to the antigen are then quantitated by means of anti-immunoglobulin conjugated to an enzyme such as alkaline phosphatase or horseradish peroxidase. By use of appropriate enzyme substrates color changes can be measured spectrophotometrically allowing objective interpretation of the results. Another advantage of EIA is the potential for automation and electronic report generation. Several EIAs are available commercially[79] including some that use recombinant *T. pallidum* antigens[80–82] to coat the wells rather than a sonicate of *T. pallidum* cultured in rabbits. Enzyme immunoassays are read objectively by a spectrophotometer and scored as positive or negative on the basis of the optical density (OD) of the test serum relative to a 'cut-off OD' that is either based on a positive control serum or determined from the kit negative control. The result is often expressed as an antibody index (OD of test serum/cut-off OD).

Immunoblotting

This method is based on electrophoretic separation of *T. pallidum* proteins according to their size. The separated proteins are transferred onto a nitrocellulose membrane and incubated with patients' serum. Resulting antibody–antigen complexes are detected by adding an anti-human globulin enzyme substrate. Although potentially this is a valuable confirmatory test the reaction patterns may include non-relevant proteins and the criteria for determining a positive result need to be established; reactivity with three of four major antigens as suggested in some studies gives poor sensitivity[83].

Test for specific anti-treponemal immunoglobulin M

19S immunoglobulin M fluorescent treponemal antibody absorbed test

This test employs the same indirect fluorescence principle as the FTA-abs but the test is performed not with whole serum but with the 19S IgM fraction (after separation by gel filtration or ultracentrifugation) which is detected by a mono-specific anti-human IgM conjugate. The test is highly demanding technically and is restricted to a few research or reference centers. An earlier version of this test, the IgM-FTA-abs test which used a mono-specific anti-human IgM conjugate to detect the IgM component in whole serum, is unreliable. It should not be used because false positive and false negative results severely limit its clinical value. False positive reactions may result because of rheumatoid factor (IgM antibody) in the serum reacting with treponemes already coated with anti-treponemal IgG[84]. False negative reactions are prone to arise when there are very high levels of IgG as at the beginning of the secondary stage and after re-infection: the smaller IgG molecules react with the receptors on the surface of *T. pallidum* before the larger IgM molecules can attach. The following tests depends upon IgM capture and are not subject to interference by rheumatoid factor or by competition from anti-treponemal IgG thus obviating the need to fractionate the serum.

Solid-phase hemadsorption test

In the IgM solid-phase hemadsorption (SPHA) test microtiter plate wells act as the solid phase for μ-chain capture; the anti-treponemal component of the captured IgM is detected by TPHA reagents[85]. Although this was one of the first specific anti-treponemal IgM tests which was simple and cheap enough to be applied on a large scale it has not been used widely.

Captia Syphilis M® enzyme immunoassay

This commercially available test (Trinity Biotech) is the most widely used method to detect anti-treponemal IgM. Rabbit antibodies against human IgM (μ-chain-specific) are coated on the inner surface of microtiter wells. When diluted sera are incubated in the wells a portion of the total IgM is captured. After washing to remove unbound antibodies and other serum proteins specific anti-treponemal IgM within the total bound IgM is detected by adding a tracer system comprising *T. pallidum* antigen, biotinylated monoclonal antibody reactive with an epitope on the TpN37 antigen, and streptavidin-horse radish peroxidase conjugate. After further washing, bound horse radish peroxidase is detected by adding tetramethylbenzidine substrate. The intensity of the colored reaction product is directly proportional to the amount of anti-*T. pallidum* IgM in the original serum.

The rationale of screening and confirmatory tests

Syphilis serodiagnosis depends on the principle of dual-level testing. Traditionally treponemal antigen tests were considered necessary to confirm that the reactivity given by cardiolipin antigen tests was due to anti-treponemal antibodies. However, confirmatory tests remain necessary even when screening with highly specific treponemal antigen tests. This is because the prevalence of syphilis is very low in most developed countries which means that a poor positive predictive value results even when tests of high specificity (greater than 99%) are used for screening. For example, a test with 99% specificity has a positive predictive value (PPV) of only 50% (i.e. only half of all positive screening tests will be true positives) when the prevalence of syphilis is 1%. With antenatal patients, where the prevalence of syphilis may be 0.1% or lower, a test with 99% specificity has a positive predictive value of around 10% (i.e. only 1 in 10 screening tests will be true positives). Because confirmatory tests are only performed on sera reactive on screening the prevalence of syphilis is higher in this population. In the first example given above, screening has increased the prevalence of disease from 1% in the initial population to 50% in the confirmatory population, and the use of a second (confirmatory) test of the same specificity (99%) increases the PPV to 99% (i.e. 99 of 100 confirmatory tests are true positives). Approximately 10 000 sera will have been screened to give rise to the one specimen giving a reactive confirmatory test that is not due to treponemal antibodies. Because the negative predictive value is dependent on the sensitivity of the test as well as prevalence of the disease, if the confirmatory test has a lower sensitivity than the screening method then some sera may be classified falsely as non-treponemal.

Performance criteria of screening tests and strategies

There are three main choices
1. a cardiolipin antigen test
2. a *T. pallidum* antigen test
3. a combination of both.
Table 15.5 summarizes the sensitivity of serological tests at various stages of infection. The advantages and disadvantages of these approaches are discussed below.

Cardiolipin antigen tests

Antibodies to cardiolipin become detectable early in the infection around 7 to 10 days after the appearance of the primary chancre or 3 to 5 weeks after infection. Overall sensitivity for the VDRL/RPR is approximately 70% to 80% and may reach 100% in the secondary stage. Titers gradually increase to 8 to 16 during the primary stage while titers of 16 to 128 are commonly found in secondary syphilis and in active cardiovascular or neurosyphilis. After the secondary stage titers decline and eventually become negative in around 30% of patients with late syphilis, although high titers are found in some patients with late active disease. Cardiolipin antigen tests also tend to become negative after treatment. Cardiolipin tests when used alone provide an effective screen for early infection only and are often used in areas of high prevalence and limited resources. The VDRL/RPR is particularly suitable as an immediate test and has been advocated for

Table 15.5 A guide to the sensitivity of serological tests at various stages of infection (based on the authors' experience using treponemal antigen tests for screening)

Test	Primary	Secondary[a]	Late latent	Late active	Treated
VDRL/RPR	70–80%	95–100%[b]	50–60%	60–70%	10–50%[c]
TPHA/TPPA	70–80%	100%	100%	100%	98–99%[d]
EIA (treponemal)	85–90%	100%	100%	100%	98–99%[d]
FTA-abs	85–90%	100%	100%	100%	95–98%[d]

[a] Sensitivities in early latent similar to secondary.
[b] Allowance for false negative reactions due to the prozone phenomenon.
[c] Varies depending on time since treatment and stage at which treated.
[d] 20–30% if coexisting HIV.

testing pregnant patients who have had no prenatal care, when they present at an emergency department with any complaint, in the hope of reducing the incidence of congenital syphilis[86].

Disadvantages of cardiolipin antigen tests include the occurrence of BFP reactions in around 0.3% to 0.9% of all sera examined. The most serious, and often underestimated disadvantage, is the occurrence of the prozone phenomenon: i.e. false negative reactions resulting from inhibition of agglutination because of excess antibody in the serum. The prozone phenomenon is generally considered to occur in 1% to 2% of patients with secondary syphilis[48, 87]. This may be an underestimate: a policy of performing a quantitative VDRL/RPR test on any serum with a TPHA titer of 5120 or over that gave a negative VDRL/RPR on screening, gave a prozone rate of 8% in patients with secondary and 10% in patients with early latent infection[112].

The tendency of the prozone phenomenon to occur in sera with high VDRL/RPR titers could be particularly important in patients with concomitant HIV infection as sera from many such patients have unusually high antibody levels[88, 89]. Unusually high titers are also found in patients undergoing re-infection, even in cases of primary syphilis[112]; the increased risk of the prozone phenomenon occurring in sera from these patients makes detection of re-infection by cardiolipin antigen tests less reliable.

False negative results are also important in antenatal screening. Four cases with false negative serological tests because of the prozone phenomenon were encountered in women who gave birth to infants with a congenital infection[90]. Although serum dilution prior to testing was recommended as a routine procedure for all seronegative women in an area of high syphilis prevalence[90] this is not a practical solution. These findings suggest that, because of the prozone phenomenon, cardiolipin tests based on agglutination should not be used alone to screen for untreated early infection. Enzyme immunoassay using cardiolipin (for example the SpiroTek Reagin II EIA) should overcome the problem of the prozone reaction but it

would still be a poorer screen for late infection than treponemal antigen tests.

As the VDRL/RPR test is very rapid it is ideal for use in emergency departments.

In these circumstances diluted as well as undiluted serum should be tested as part of the standard procedure.

Screening with a combination of cardiolipin and Treponema pallidum antigen tests

The activities of the TPHA and VDRL tests are complimentary and the combined use of the two tests provides an excellent screen for the detection or exclusion of syphilis at all stages[91, 92]. Treponema pallidum hemagglutination assay reactivity may be detectable around the fourth week of infection. The overall sensitivity in untreated primary infection is in the 70% to 80% range. The TPHA titer tends to be low in primary syphilis (80 to 320) but rises sharply in the secondary stage reaching 5120 or greater. The titer declines during the latent stage but invariably remains positive, often at low titer (80 to 1280). Titers may decline after therapy but, with the exception of patients co-infected with HIV[93], the test almost always remains positive.

According to Luger[48] the TPHA, with an overall margin of error in the range of 0.07% false positive reactions and 0.008% false negative reactions, is the most sensitive and specific method for detecting antibodies to T. pallidum. When false negative reactions occur they are usually associated with early primary infection and this is the main reason why the TPHA has not been widely used as a single screening test in laboratories serving STI clinics. Serological detection of primary syphilis is increased by the combination of tests as they are complimentary in their activity with regard to primary syphilis[112]: for example the VDRL/RPR test gave a sensitivity of 72.7% compared with 70.5% for the TPHA, whereas the two tests gave a combined sensitivity of 84.1%. Although several studies have suggested that antibody detected by the TPHA appears later, or is of relatively lower titer, than that detected by cardiolipin antigen tests[94] in one large retrospective analysis of routine

practice the TPHA gave a sensitivity of 73.9% (487/659) in primary infection compared with 70.4% for the VDRL/RPR[95]. In using the combination of tests, apart from increasing the detection of primary infection, the TPHA will detect high titer sera that may give a false negative reaction because of the prozone phenomenon.

Although the test combination cannot be faulted with regard to performance, it requires more labor than a single test, interpretation is subjective, and the combination does not lend itself readily to automation.

Screening with a single Treponema pallidum antigen test

Treponema pallidum hemagglutination assay

The TPHA on its own is a good screen for syphilis at all stages beyond the early primary stage. Because of the importance attached to detecting early primary infection the TPHA has not been advocated as a single screening test for diagnostic laboratories. Non-reactivity of the TPHA in primary syphilis may be attributable to poor binding of IgM antibodies to the antigen coating the erythrocytes. Certain TPHA tests may be more sensitive than others in detecting primary infection.

Treponema pallidum particle agglutination assay

An early developmental report[96] found that the microcapsule agglutination method was superior to the TPHA in detecting cases of primary syphilis. This improvement may be partially attributable to improved binding of insoluble antigens to microcapsules as opposed to erythrocytes. More recently, Pope and colleagues in the USA[76] reported that the TPPA was an appropriate substitute for the TPHA.

Enzyme immunoassay

Enzyme immunoassay as a single screening test was shown to give similar results to the RPR and TPHA combination some years ago[81] and is already used by many laboratories, particularly those with large workloads. Even when tests that detect only

IgG are used the sensitivity in untreated primary syphilis can be good. The original Captia Syphilis G® test gave a sensitivity of 82%, or 88% if equivocal results are scored positive as would happen on screening[97]. Schmidt and colleagues[79] evaluated eight commercially available EIAs, that detect IgG or total antibody, on 52 highly selected sera (all TPHA negative) from patients with primary syphilis. Seven of these tests showed greater sensitivity (range 49% to 77%) than the VDRL (44%). The only test to give poorer sensitivity than the VDRL was the Captia Syphilis G® test (23%). The highest sensitivities were given by Trepanostika (77%), a competitive EIA that uses a lysate of *T. pallidum* as antigen, and immune capture enzyme immunoassay (ICE) syphilis (75%) that uses three recombinant antigens (TpN15, TpN17, and TpN47) in a capture EIA that detects both IgG and IgM. Very few of the EIAs described in this study have been subjected to peer-reviewed evaluation of general performance criteria. A new EIA that uses two unstated recombinant antigens and detects IgG and IgM gave a sensitivity of 100% and a specificity of 99.6% compared with a sensitivity and specificity of 99.4% and 99.8% respectively: the sensitivity of the TPPA was 99.4% and the FTA-abs 94.5%[82]

Recommended screening procedures

Modern guidelines for the serological diagnosis for syphilis are long overdue. The last guidelines that were produced by WHO in 1982[91] recommended the use of a cardiolipin antigen test such as the VDRL or RPR test and the TPHA for screening for syphilis. The new Public Health Laboratory Service recommendations[98] extend the WHO guidelines by suggesting that treponemal antigen-based EIAs are an appropriate alternative to the combined VDRL/RPR and TPHA screen. Screening with a cardiolipin antigen test alone is not recommended because of the potential for false negative results caused be the prozone phenomenon[99].

Whilst the detection of early infectious syphilis is the priority of any syphilis-testing program it must also be recognized that in the UK most newly diagnosed cases are late-stage infections[100]. The screening schedules proposed in the guidelines take account of this and achieve high sensitivity in all stages of infection. However, depending on the particular tests used and the quality of the clinical/laboratory liaison there may be a failure to detect a small proportion of untreated early primary infections at one end of the spectrum and markers of long-standing treated treponemal infection at the other. The risk of missing early primary infection is minimized by encouraging clinicians to maintain a high index of suspicion and to request a specific anti-treponemal EIA test whenever lesions that could represent early primary syphilis are present. The use of any of the treponemal antigen tests will detect virtually 100% of untreated infections beyond the primary stage including late latent infection.

The above guidelines differ from those in the USA where screening in hospital laboratories is based on cardiolipin antigen tests (usually the RPR) to identify active cases of syphilis. Treponemal antigen tests are used to confirm the treponemal nature of the RPR reactivity. Interestingly treponemal antigen tests are used for screening in bloodbanks[56].

Clearly the two approaches place a different emphasis on the group of patients that are cardiolipin antigen test negative but treponemal antigen test positive. Studies have shown that these patients can have clinically significant infections[48]. Although the majority of patients in this group will have treated rather than late infections, nevertheless in Europe it is generally accepted that the additional cases of late syphilis, including late latent, detected by screening with *T. pallidum* antigen tests, outweighs the difficulties that may arise in differentiating between untreated or inadequately treated patients and those who have a well-documented history of appropriate therapy. In the USA the definition of latent syphilis states 'No past diagnosis of syphilis, a reactive nontreponemal test (i.e. VDRL or RPR), and a reactive treponemal test (i.e. FTA-ABS or MHA-TP)'[101].

However, treponemal antigen tests have already been advocated for the screening of certain groups of patients such as psychiatric patients[102] and are recognized as important in determining whether HIV-infected patients have ever been exposed to syphilis[103]. These differences outlined in the screening approach have an important bearing when new treponemal antigen tests are being evaluated and on the performance of confirmatory tests in routine practice.

Confirmatory tests and strategies

Fluorescent treponemal antibody absorbed test

The FTA-Abs test is currently the standard confirmatory test. It becomes reactive around the third week of infection and in primary infection has an overall sensitivity of around 85% to 90% but may give higher or lower values depending on how long the primary lesion has been present. It is positive in almost 100% of untreated infections in the secondary and later stages. Reactivity persists after adequate therapy although the test may occasionally become non-reactive if treatment is given early in the disease.

The FTA-abs is considered to be a very specific test. However, the test is not endowed with the high level of specificity usually accorded to it. The reputation for high specificity stems from the principle of dual testing described earlier, i.e. the FTA-abs is used to test sera that have been pre-selected thus considerably increasing the probability that they contain anti-treponemal antibodies. The overall specificity of the FTA-abs test is around 97% and ranges from 94% to 100%[56]. The total prevalence of false reactivity is around 1% in normal persons, but higher rates have been reported in hospital patients[48]. Diseases and clinical entities associated with false reactivity include lupus erythematosus, rheumatoid arthritis, HSV infection, hepatic cirrhosis, diabetes, tuberculosis, abnormal globulins, intravenous drug abuse, thyroiditis, and cancer. The FTA-abs gave a specificity of only 68% in a group of patients with rheumatic diseases[104]. Reactivity only in the FTA-abs test must be treated with caution. An evaluation of 43 such patients found that only 3 had primary or treated syphilis, 21 (49%) had clinical and/or serological signs of Lyme disease, 7 (16%) had genital HSV infection, and the remaining 12 (28%) had miscellaneous disorders[105]. In the same study an isolated positive FTA-abs reaction was found in 43% (13 of 30) of control patients with Lyme disease. Conversely false negative FTA-abs reactions have been reported in HIV-seropositive individuals with positive VDRL/RPR tests[106] who were initially classified as BFP reactors but later confirmed as having treponemal infection by imunoblotting. Further problems with the FTA-abs test include kit variation and subjectivity of reading. Most laboratories use commercial kits for performing the FTA-abs test and this is an area where much greater standardization is required. The ability of four different kits to detect reactive samples varied from 83% to 95%, and the agreement with non-reactive and borderline samples ranged from 81% to 96.4%[107]. In another study, agreement between four kits was 63% for treponemal and 50% for non-treponemal sera[108]. Discrepancies with treponemal sera were associated with low levels of antibody characterized by TPHA titers of 160 or less and a negative VDRL test. Discrepancies with non-treponemal sera were significantly associated with false reactivity on screening with EIA.

The degree of reactivity in a subjective test such as the FTA-abs is also important and can have a very significant effect on the utility of the test. Borderline reactions are common and in the USA it has been recommended that the borderline report should be eliminated[109]. This change increased the specificity of the test from 83% to 89% but only decreased the sensitivity from 100% to 99.5% in the case of VDRL-positive sera. However, discounting borderline reactions in the case of treponemal sera that were mainly VDRL negative had a different effect. Depending on the kit used specificity varied from 52% to 83% when borderline reactions were scored positive and from 71% to 96% when they were scored negative: the corresponding sensitivity ranges were 91% to 95%, and 74% to 90%.

These findings suggest that if the Centers for Disease Control recommendations are applied to sera selected on the basis of screening by a treponemal antigen test then a significant number of treponemal sera will fail to be confirmed. However, it should be stressed that these are unlikely to be active cases of syphilis.

Treponema pallidum *hemagglutination assay/Treponema pallidum particle assay*

The possibility of using the TPHA as a confirmatory test in Europe has only arisen because laboratories are changing from screening with the TPHA to screening with EIA. Recent evaluations of the newer EIAs with other treponemal antigen tests show that the TPHA is more sensitive than the FTA-abs: 97% versus 92%[109a] as is the TPPA: 99% versus 95%[82]. Specificity of the TPHA is superior to that of the FTA-abs[48].

Enzyme immunoassay

Based on practical issues such as personnel costs and the number of tests to be run, Pope and colleagues considered the Syphilis-G and TPPA tests to be appropriate alternatives to the MHA-TP for use as confirmatory tests. In a study comparing the Captia Syphilis G® test and the FTA-abs the highly subjective nature of the FA-abs test was noted[110]. When the technologist knew the VDRL/RPR result there was a 15% (76/89) discrepancy between Captia G® EIA and the FTA-abs giving Captia a sensitivity of 70.7% and a specificity of 97.9%. Re-testing when the technologist was unaware of the RPR result and chart review, reduced discrepancies to 2% (87/89) giving Captia a sensitivity of 96.7% and a specificity of 98.3%. It was concluded that the Captia G® EIA is a reliable method for syphilis testing and that personnel performing the FTA-abs test which depends on subjective interpretation may be biased by the RPR results and over interpret the degree of FTA-abs reactivity. The potential problem of subjective interpretation of test results is obviated by the EIA procedure.

Immunoblotting

Test kits based on native *T. pallidum* antigen are available commercially but these have not yet been subjected to peer-reviewed evaluation[58]. It is likely that they will be superseded by tests based on recombinant antigens before imunoblotting is more widely used as a confirmatory test. A newly developed kit (INNO-LIA Syphilis Kit®, Innogenetics NV) which determines an antibody response to three recombinant antigens (TpN15, TpN17, and TpN47) as well as a synthetic peptide based on TpN44.5a (TmpA) deposited as distinct lines on a strip should make interpretation easier and may also help in disease staging[111].

Guidelines for confirmatory testing

The recent UK guidelines[98] suggest that a reactive screening result should be confirmed with a treponemal antigen test of a different type from that used in screening (for example TPHA if EIA is used for screening). Indeed the FTA-abs is not recommended as the first line confirmatory test. The specificity of the FTA-abs is poorer than that of the other treponemal antigen screening tests[48, 55] while certain newer EIAs are significantly more sensitive than the FTA-abs[113] in detecting markers of past infection, which means that the FTA-abs will fail to confirm a small number of genuinely reactive EIAs. The sensitivity of the TPHA/TPPA is very similar to that of the newer EIAs, which means that the most accurate confirmation of treponemal antibodies will result from using either the TPHA/TPPA to confirm a reactive EIA or an EIA to confirm a reactive TPHA/TPPA (the practicalities of laboratory testing mean that the former scenario is more likely). Although the FTA-abs may have slightly greater sensitivity in early primary infection a positive FTA-abs result alone has poor specificity. The use of an anti-treponemal IgM to supplement standard screening and confirmatory procedures is a better approach to maximizing the detection of early primary infection than relying on the FTA-abs. Quantitative non-treponemal tests (VDRL/RPR) are recommended to help stage the disease and are of course necessary to monitor the efficacy of treatment. On the rare occasion when the first-line confirmatory test does not support the result of the treponemal antigen screening test then an additional confirmatory test is recommended. In future, imunoblotting with recombinant antigens is likely to fulfill this role. In all categories of treponemal infection a repeat specimen is advised to confirm the findings; this will normally be a week or so after the initial specimen.

The guidelines make recommendations on test type only. Which particular test a laboratory uses will be based on many factors including cost, ease of use, suitability for automation, compatibility with the format of other tests already in use in the laboratory, as well as performance characteristics. There is an enormous choice of test reagents, manufactured and/or supplied by different companies. Published performance criteria following stringent evaluation in independent centers is available for very few of the numerous tests (and their modifications) produced by different manufacturers. It is important that laboratories do not change reagents frequently in order that they and their users such as genitourinary medicine physicians become fully conversant with the performance characteristics of the particular tests used.

NEUROSYPHILIS

Invasion of the CNS appears to be fairly common in early syphilis and occurred in 30% of patients with untreated primary or secondary infection as demonstrated by the rabbit infectivity test[114]. Although this may not always equate or lead to pathological changes in the CSF there is obviously potential for it to do so.

It is unnecessary to perform serological tests for syphilis on the CSF of patients with symptoms referable to the central nervous system (CNS) in whom there is no suspicion of syphilis. A negative treponemal antigen test on serum will virtually exclude neurosyphilis and is a better screen for all forms of late syphilis than examination of the CSF. In cases selected on clinical grounds and backed by a positive treponemal antigen test on blood, however, investigations should be carried out on the CSF to detect early invasion of the CNS. Because invasion of the CNS can be detected before symptoms develop, and also because the (early) effects of syphilis on the CNS can often be reversed by penicillin

treatment, CSF examinations are important in the assessment of patients with the disease. It has also been suggested that the serum TPHA titer is a useful criterion when selecting non-HIV-infected patients for lumbar puncture[115]. In this study, taking a TPHA titer of 1280 as a cut-off would have reduced the number of lumbar punctures by 68% and given considerable savings in cost. A more cautious approach would be to perform lumbar puncture on patients with a TPHA titer of 640 or more, as in one series of 45 patients with neurosyphilis (including asymptomatic neurosyphilis) TPHA titers were 640 (1), 1280 (1), 2560 (4) and more than 5120 (39)[116]. Because the TPPA test is usually more sensitive than the TPHA by one doubling dilution a TPPA cut-off of 1280 may be appropriate.

Cerebrospinal fluid examination

A total volume of 8 to 10 mL of CSF is usually sufficient for the tests required, which should be carried out as soon as possible after collection; note that contamination of the CSF specimen with even a small amount of blood can give misleading results. Investigation of the CSF should include

- serological tests
- a cell count
- an estimation of total protein, IgG, IgM, and albumin.

Serological tests and estimation of IgG and albumin should be performed in parallel on serum. Although RPR, TPHA, EIA, and FTA-abs are regularly performed on CSF in many laboratories, the VDRL slide test is the only test to have Centers for Disease Control approval for testing CSF.

Exclusion of neurosyphilis

A negative treponemal antigen test on CSF virtually excludes neurosyphilis, and neurosyphilis is most improbable at CSF TPHA titers below 320[116].

A non-reactive CSF VDRL slide test, however, does not exclude neurosyphilis as the overall sensitivity is only around 50% with a range of 10% for asymptomatic cases to 90% for symptomatic cases[91, 116, 117]. Apart from non reactivity because of

insufficient antibody being present false negative CSF VDRL reactions because of the prozone may occur in HIV-positive patients with neurosyphilis[89].

Confirmation of neurosyphilis

Whilst parameters such as a raised cell count ($> 5 \times 10^6$/L) and raised total protein (> 0.4 g/L) are often found in neurosyphilis patients they are non-specific tests and indicate inflammation without disclosing its cause. These parameters are even less specific indicators of neurosyphilis in HIV-infected patients as 40% to 60% of such patients without syphilis have abnormalities of CSF protein or cell counts[118].

A positive treponemal antigen test result in the CSF is of limited value without knowledge of the levels of serum antibody and the degree of impairment of the serum–CSF barrier since reactivity may be caused by normal transudation of immunoglobulins from the serum into the CSF or by leakage through a damaged blood–brain barrier resulting from conditions other than syphilis. Parameters such as the TPHA index (see below) allow for impaired barrier function and lead to more accurate diagnosis. In the large study of neurosyphilis undertaken by Luger[116] all 67 patients with adequately treated syphilis without involvement of the CSF gave a reactive TPHA and 49% were reactive in the FTA-abs. A positive CSF VDRL slide test, although lacking sensitivity, is a good predictor of neurosyphilis as it was reactive in only 6% of the adequately treated patients. More recently it was noted that a TPHA index over 70 (see below) and a CSF TPHA titer over 320 gave the most reliable results for supporting the diagnosis of neurosyphilis[116a]. The following parameters are helpful in establishing a definitive diagnosis of neurosyphilis.

Albumin quotient

Albumin quotient = CSF albumin (mg/dL) $\times 10^3 \div$ serum albumin (mg/dL)
This quotient provides a means of defining the normality or degree of impairment of the blood–CSF barrier. Normal values range from 3.0 to 8.0 depending on the age of the patient.

Treponema pallidum hemagglutination assay index

TPHA index = CSF TPHA titer ÷ albumin quotient

The TPHA index compares the actual amount of treponemal antibody in the CSF with the amount that would be expected from normal transudation. A value below 70 is considered normal, values from 70 to 500 are strongly suggestive of neurosyphilis, and above 500 are proof of active neurosyphilis. Extreme disorders of the blood–CSF barrier at albumin quotient levels above 20 may cause false non-reactive results in the TPHA index. The use of the TPHA index in HIV-infected patients doubled the number of patients diagnosed with neurosyphilis[119]: 2 patients were CSF-VDRL positive but TPHA index negative; 3 were CSF-VDRL and TPHA index positive; 5 were TPHA index positive and CSF-VDRL negative.

Immunoglobulin G index

IgG index = IgG quotient ÷ albumin quotient

The IgG quotient is analogous to the albumin quotient described above, i.e.

CSF IgG (mg/dL) × 10^3/ serum IgG (mg/dL).

The IgG index estimates whether the IgG antibody concentration in the CSF is greater than the concentration that could be accounted for by mere transudation from the serum to the CSF. Because of their different molecular weights, two molecules of albumin will cross the barrier for every one molecule of globulin, giving a normal IgG index of 0.5. An IgG index above 0.85 is usually taken to indicate intrathecal production of IgG because its concentration in the CSF is greater than can be accounted for by transudation from the serum.

Detection of anti-treponemal IgM

The detection of anti-treponemal IgM in CSF in patients with normal blood–brain barrier function is indicative of neurosyphilis. Unfortunately, the commercially available Captia Syphilis M® EIA has very poor sensitivity in neurosyphilis while the small volumes of CSF make immunoglobulin fractionation for testing by the 19S IgM FTA-abs impractical. The IgM SPHA performs well on CSF giving a sensitivity of 95% in patients with neurosyphilis while not reacting with adequately treated patients without CSF involvement.

Detection of Treponema pallidum in cerebrospinal fluid by polymerase chain reaction

Variable results have been reported for PCR detection of *T. pallidum* in the CSF of patients suspected as having CNS invasion by *T. pallidum*[120]. Polymerase chain reaction had a sensitivity of 47% and a specificity of 93% for detecting a known history of syphilis[121]: in 19 patients with treponemal disease undergoing lumbar puncture to look for evidence of neurosyphilis, the PCR was positive in 75% of patients with neurosyphilis or possible asymptomatic neurosyphilis, but it was also positive in 50% of patients with latent infection. Another study also found the PCR undersensitive: treponemal DNA was detected in 71% (5 of 7) patients with acute neurosyphilis, in none of 4 patients with chronic symptomatic neurosyphilis, and in 13% (2 of 16) of patients with asymptomatic neurosyphilis[122]: DNA was also often detected in CSF long after intravenous treatment with penicillin, in one case after 3 years. In a later study *T. pallidum* DNA was not consistently detected in any sample, even when the CSF-VDRL was reactive[123]. Further studies using more highly standardized methods are required to determine the utility of PCR in the diagnosis of neurosyphilis.

Resolution of tests following treatment

After treatment for neurosyphilis the CSF cell count should return to normal first, followed by the CSF protein concentration, followed by serological tests. The CSF should be entirely normal by 2 years. A study of 22 patients with neurosyphilis (13 infected with HIV) suggested slower resolution of CSF abnormalities in the HIV-infected group[124].

CONGENITAL SYPHILIS

The diagnosis of congenital syphilis can present a considerable problem since it depends mainly on the results of serological tests and also because most neonates so affected are asymptomatic at birth. As the standard serological tests for syphilis depend on responses involving IgG and IgM antibodies their interpretation is extremely difficult; the IgG found in the serum of neonates is largely passively acquired through the placenta and does not represent the infant's own response. The demonstration of anti-treponemal IgM in neonatal serum correlates well with congenital infection. The simple and widely available Captia Syphilis M® EIA gave better results than the technically complex 19S IgM-FTA-abs test[125], and was also superior to IgM immunoblotting[126]. Although PCR may be a useful adjunct its sensitivity was slightly lower than that of immunoblotting[127].

Because of the possibility of a delayed IgM response or suppression of IgM synthesis in the neonate because of high levels of circulating maternal anti-treponemal IgG[128], IgM testing should be repeated after 4, 8, and 12 weeks.

Whereas a rising or higher titer in the neonate than in the mother is suggestive of infection, lower titers in neonates when compared to their mothers are suggestive of passively transferred antibody. In the absence of infection passively transferred antibody detected by the VDRL/RPR will decrease and the tests will become negative in approximately 3 months. In the case of the treponemal antigen tests it may take up to 6 or 9 months for the test to become negative.

Congenital syphilis is preventable through antenatal screening and appropriate action in the case of positive results. Unfortunately, this does not always happen[129, 130]. These failures to act on positive serological results highlight the importance of close collaboration between medical microbiologists, obstetricians, genitourinary medicine physicians, and pediatricians to ensure that the pregnancy is managed optimally and that appropriate follow-up of infants occurs.

In late-stage infection, either treated or untreated, test results tend to fluctuate over a period of months or years. The VDRL/RPR test often remains positive at low titer in association with a low TPHA titer and positive FTA-abs test. Data on specific anti-treponemal IgM in late-stage congenital infection are inadequate.

GUIDE TO THE INTERPRETATION OF SEROLOGICAL TEST RESULTS IN VARIOUS STAGES OF INFECTION

The main patterns of serological results that may result from screening and confirmatory testing are shown in Table 15.6.

Primary syphilis

Usually one or more of the screening tests may be positive and should be supported by a positive FTA-abs and a positive anti-treponemal IgM EIA. During the primary stage the VDRL titer may rise to 8 or 16 while TPHA/TPPA titers of 80 to 320 can be expected: in re-infection much higher titers may be observed. Around 10% to 15% of patients with primary syphilis, particularly very early infection, may be seronegative with routine screening tests at first presentation and the diagnosis will depend on a positive dark ground investigation. In

the absence of a positive dark ground, reactivity only in the FTA-abs or IgM should be interpreted with caution; early testing of a further specimen is advised. When cardiolipin antigen tests are used for screening, sera positive only in the VDRL/RPR are most likely to be BFPs. A further specimen of blood should be taken and the test repeated to exclude technical error or an atypical primary pattern. In screening for early syphilis, tests should be repeated over a period of at least 3 months.

Secondary and early latent syphilis

Secondary syphilis will commonly give VDRL/RPR titers of 16 to 128. During the secondary stage TPHA/TPPA titers also rise sharply and usually reach 5120 or greater. Titers tend to decline after the secondary stage. Therefore when quantitative VDRL/RPR and TPHA/TPPA tests are positive to high titer and the FTA-abs and IgM EIA tests are also positive the most likely diagnosis is secondary syphilis or early latent syphilis. The same pattern of results can be obtained in recently treated second-

ary or early latent syphilis before the VDRL/RPR titer and IgM response declines so it is clear that interpretation of syphilis serology is dependent on the history and clinical findings of the patient. Although the anti-treponemal IgM EIA test is usually positive in patients with untreated secondary and early latent infection, a negative result does not exclude the need for specific treatment. Antibiotics taken for conditions other than syphilis may result in negative-specific IgM tests.

Late-stage syphilis

The VDRL/RPR titer declines after the secondary stage and eventually becomes negative in approximately 30% of untreated latent and late infections; specific IgM tests are also usually negative but the treponemal antigen screening tests (EIA and TPHA/TPPA) and the FTA-abs should all be positive. The VDRL/RPR titers may be high (16 to 128) in active cardiovascular and neuro-syphilis and in those with gummatous lesions. The TPHA titer declines during the latent stage but unlike the VDRL/RPR test it invariably remains positive at low titer (80 to 640). High titers (5120 or greater) can be expected in active late syphilis. Therefore, when quantitative VDRL/RPR and TPHA tests are positive regularly over a period of time at low titer in patients without signs then the infection is likely to be beyond the early latent stage and may have been modified by coincidental curative or subcurative antibiotic treatment. Adequately treated infections may give a similar pattern of results so again patient history is important.

Occasionally, many years after adequate treatment, one or more of the treponemal antigen tests, EIA, TPHA/TPPA, or FTA-abs (more often the FTA-abs) may be negative but in the absence of HIV infection this is probably of little clinical significance.

Table 15.6 Pattern of results of serological tests in different stages of acquired syphilis

VDRL/RPR	EIA	TPHA/TPPA	FTA-abs	IgM	Most likely interpretation
+	–	–	–	–	False positive reaction, repeat to exclude primary infection
+/–	+/–	+/–	+/–	+	Primary infection; darkground investigation of lesion may be positive
+	+	+	+	+	Untreated (or recently treated) secondary or early latent
+/–	+	+	+	–/+	Untreated late or latent, treated or partially treated at any stage
-	+/–	+/–	+/–	–	History of treated syphilis (probably many years previously)

+ Positive.
– Negative.
+/– Usually positive at low titer but may be negative.
–/+ Usually negative but may be positive at low titer.

Clinical features of acquired syphilis

The clinical features of early and late syphilis may be altered by concurrent infection with HIV and this issue is considered on pp. 443–445.

EARLY STAGE
Primary syphilis

Following a pre-patent period of about 3 weeks (range 10 to 90 days), the primary lesion or chancre develops at the site of inoculation of *T. pallidum*.

The chancre is typically a single ulcer (Figures 15.7, 15.8), well demarcated from the surrounding tissue, with a smooth, flat, dull-red surface which may be covered by a thin yellow or brown crust. Characteristically the ulcer is painless, not tender and on pressure serous fluid, but no blood, exudes from the lesion. Induration of the ulcer is often marked giving it a cartilaginous consistency. Occasionally there may be considerable edema of the adjacent tissues.

Many lesions of primary syphilis are atypical[131]. The patient may complain of painful tender ulceration which is a result of secondary bacterial infection. Multiple chancres may occur. In the anal region primary lesions may resemble slightly indurated anal fissures (Figure 15.9) (see Chapter 18 for a fuller discussion of anorectal syphilis). In any patient with an ulcer, particularly in an oral or anogenital site, it is essential to exclude syphilis by dark ground examination when appro-

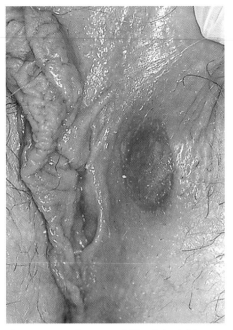

Figure 15.8 Primary syphilis of the labium majus (reproduced from McMillan and Scott 2000[251])

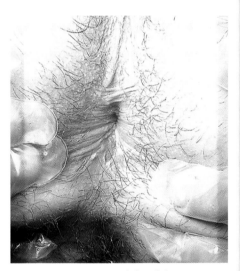

Figure 15.9 Primary syphilis of the anus (reproduced from McMillan and Scott 2000[251])

priate and by serological tests repeated over a 3-month period.

Within a few days of the appearance of the chancre there is usually regional lymph node enlargement. When the chancre is on the genitalia, bilateral inguinal lymphadenitis is usual, but when the lesion is extragenital it is more common to find unilateral enlargement. The enlarged lymph nodes are discrete, rubbery, and

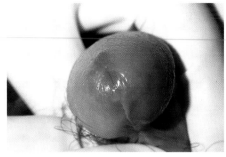

Figure 15.10 Primary syphilis of the urethral meatus, note erythematous swelling that was markedly indurated on palpation

unless the chancre is secondarily infected, painless. Without treatment the primary lesion heals within 3 to 8 weeks leaving a thin atrophic scar.

Sites of primary lesions in males

The chancre may be found on any part of the external genitalia, but especially in the coronal sulcus, on the inner surface of the prepuce, on the glans, or on the shaft of the penis. Rarely an intra-urethral chancre may occur (Figure 15.10) producing symptoms of urethritis. In men who have had receptive anal intercourse the chancre may be found at the anal margin or, less frequently, in the rectum where it may be mistaken for carcinoma. Primary lesions in the latter sites may produce no symptoms and as a result the patient may first present with manifestations of secondary syphilis.

Chancres may also occur in the lips, buccal cavity, tongue, tonsil, and pharynx. Lesions of the tonsil and pharynx may be painful. In these sites the diagnosis by dark ground microscopy may be difficult because there are often saprophytic treponemes. Lesions elsewhere, such as on a finger, are rare.

Sites of primary lesions in females

Chancres may occur on the labium majus, labium minus, fourchette, clitoris, or cervix. Lesions of the cervix usually produce no symptoms and since the lymph drains to the iliac nodes, these nodes may be found to be enlarged on abdominal examination. Extragenital chancres are uncommon.

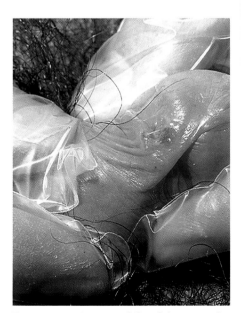

Figure 15.7 Primary syphilis of the coronal sulcus and frenum (reproduced from McMillan and Scott 2000[251])

Secondary syphilis

Signs of secondary syphilis usually appear 7 to 10 weeks after infection or 6 to 8 weeks after the appearance of the primary lesion, which may not have been noticed by the patient (see above). In about a third of patients with early secondary syphilis a primary lesion will still be present.

Lesions of secondary syphilis result from the spread of *T. pallidum* throughout the tissues of the body and the immunological reactions of the host. Without treatment the features of secondary syphilis may appear and regress spontaneously at intervals over a period of about 2 years. During such relapses mucocutaneous lesions in the anogenital area contain *T. pallidum*, enabling further transmission during sexual intercourse. After the secondary stage or after the chancre or even in the absence of these stages, the infection persists as a hidden disease, that is, as latent syphilis.

Many atypical cases of early syphilis have been described, and although this may be caused by a change in the disease itself, it is as likely that clinicians have become more aware of the possibility of syphilis and have access to more sensitive and more specific diagnostic tests. Widespread use of antibiotics may have a modifying effect and produce more atypical cases.

Symptoms

The patient often feels generally unwell, with mild fever, malaise, headache, and anorexia. He/she may complain of a non-itchy skin rash, patchy loss of hair, hoarseness, swollen lymph nodes, bone pain, and, rarely, deafness or other evidence of neural damage.

Signs

Skin lesions (syphilides)

Skin lesions are seen in over 80% of patients with secondary syphilis. Mucocutaneous lesions particularly, contain many treponemes and are infectious.

Skin eruptions are often polymorphic – several types of eruption appear simultaneously – during the course of secondary syphilis and, although early skin lesions are usually symmetrically distributed, later lesions are not always in this pattern. Just

over 40% of patients with secondary syphilis complain of pruritus[132].

The diagnosis of secondary syphilis usually depends upon clinical and serological findings but, when biopsies have been taken in a histological approach to the diagnosis of skin disease, the pattern of changes seen on microscopy may suggest such a diagnosis. Except in condylomata lata, *T. pallidum* is only occasionally found in histological sections[133].

Macular syphilide (roseola)

These lesions are usually the earliest to appear but, being faintly colored, are often overlooked. The individual macules are rose-pink in color, about 1 cm in diameter, discrete, and with indistinct margins (Figure 15.11). Pressure obliterates the lesion. The rash progresses daily, becoming more widely distributed, but occasionally it may last only a few days. It is common to find macules or papules in the generalized eruption.

Papular and papulosquamous syphilide

These are the commonest lesions to be detected in secondary syphilis. Papules are dull red lesions, variable in size, distributed

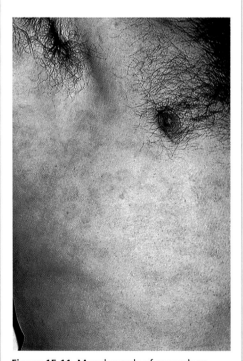

Figure 15.11 Macular rash of secondary syphilis (reproduced from McMillan and Scott 2000[251])

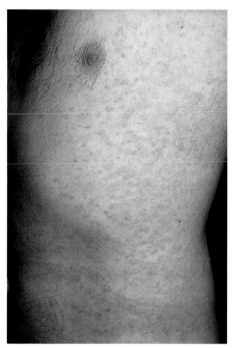

Figure 15.12 Maculopapular lesions of secondary syphilis

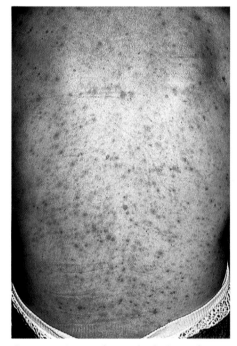

Figure 15.13 Maculopapular lesions of secondary syphilis (reproduced from McMillan and Scott 2000[251])

symmetrically (during the early stages of secondary syphilis) over the body (Figures 15.12, 15.13), and are especially prominent on flexor aspects. They are firm to touch and initially have a shiny surface.

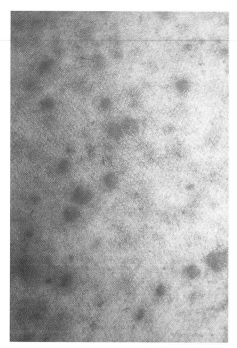

Figure 15.14 Papules of secondary syphilis showing minor scaling on the surface (reproduced from McMillan and Scott 2000[251])

Later, as the papule ages, scaling is noted on the surface (Figure 15.14). When scaling papules predominate in the eruption, the term papulosquamous syphilide (Figure 15.15) is applied.

Although papules may be found anywhere on the body the following sites require special mention.

1. *Face* This is often affected, papules being especially prominent in the nasolabial folds and on the chin. Occasionally a group of papules may be noted on the forehead just below, and parallel to, the hairline, sometimes described as corona veneris.

2. *Scalp* When a hair follicle is involved in the inflammatory changes in the skin, hair growth is arrested and shedding of the contained hair occurs. Hair loss in secondary syphilis is characteristically irregular, the scalp having a 'moth-eaten' appearance – syphilitic alopecia (Figure 15.16). Occasionally, as a non-specific reaction to a systemic disease, there may be a more diffuse hair loss (telogen effluvium) after recovery from the secondary stage (Figure 15.17). This results from interference with hair growth at the time

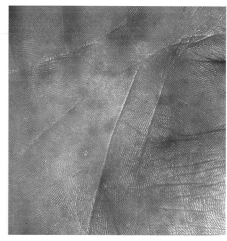

Figure 15.18 Palmar lesion of secondary syphilis (reproduced from McMillan and Scott 2000[251])

of the illness with the abnormal hair being shed 3 to 5 months afterwards as the new hair starts to grow.

3. *Palms and soles* Palmar (Figure 15.18) and plantar syphilide. Papular lesions on these sites do not project much above the surface of the skin, but appear as firm lesions, dull red in color, associated with thickening and peeling of the overlying epidermis.

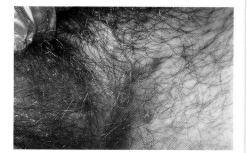

Figure 15.15 Papulosquamous lesions of secondary syphilis

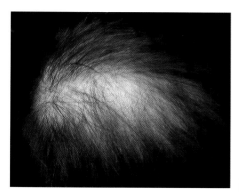

Figure 15.16 Syphilitic alopecia

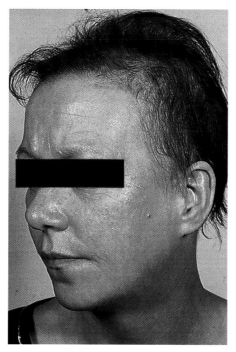

Figure 15.17 Telogen effluvium in a woman with secondary syphilis (reproduced from McMillan and Scott 2000[251])

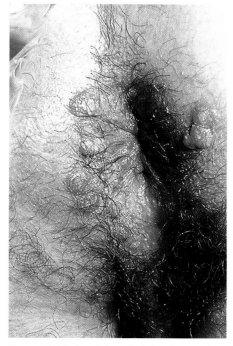

Figure 15.19 Condylomata lata of secondary syphilis (reproduced from McMillan and Scott 2000[251])

Frequently a collar of scales surrounds individual lesions.

4. *External genitalia* On moist areas such as the vulva and perianal region, papules may become hypertrophied, flat-topped, moist, wart-like lesions called condylomata lata (Figure 15.19). The surface is often eroded and the exudate from the erosion contains large numbers of *T. pallidum*. In such lesions the infection is highly contagious. Commonly papules encircle the free margin of the foreskin, and, as a result of moisture, trauma, and secondary infection, deep painful fissures develop. Papulosquamous lesions are often found on the shaft of the penis and on the scrotum.

In the later stages of secondary syphilis, papules become fewer in number and asymmetrical in distribution. Nummular lesions, 1 to 3 cm in diameter, are commonly found at this time and are frequently surmounted by a thick layer of scales resembling the plaques of psoriasis (Figure 15.20). Coalescence of papules in the later secondary stage may produce annular lesions, especially in dark-skinned people. Occasionally a large papule may be found, surrounded by smaller satellite lesions –

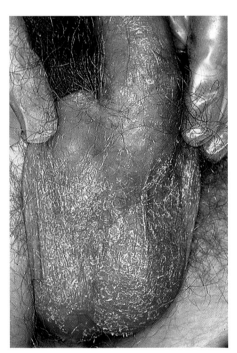

Figure 15.20 Psoriasiform lesions of secondary syphilis (reproduced from McMillan and Scott 2000[251])

corymbose syphilide. Such lesions may be the only ones noted in late secondary syphilis.

Nail growth may be affected, particularly in the late secondary stage. The nail loses its lustre, becomes brittle, and may be shed.

Pustular syphilide

Rarely papules become pustular because of necrosis of the upper dermis and epidermis, which is caused by occlusion of the lumen of blood vessels. Multiple pustular lesions are very seldom found in western countries[134], but may be seen in patients suffering from some concomitant debilitating disease such as tuberculosis.

With the exception of pustular syphilide, the skin lesions of secondary syphilis heal without leaving scars. Areas of faint pigmentation may persist for months. Occasionally, depigmentation of the skin of the neck may be noted, particularly in dark-haired women – leukoderma colli. This residual depigmentation lasts for life.

Lesions of the mucous membranes

Such lesions are found in about 30% of patients with secondary syphilis. The characteristic lesion is the so-called 'mucous patch' which appears at the same time as the skin rash. Both skin and mucosal lesions have similar histological appearances.

The mucosal lesions appear as round or oval gray areas surrounded by a narrow zone of erythema. Shedding of the gray necrotic membrane reveals superficial ulceration, and if several patches coalesce a 'snail-track ulcer' may result (Figure 15.21).

Mucosal lesions are generally painless and resolve within a few weeks or, less commonly, within a few days.

The following sites may be involved in secondary syphilis.

- *Tonsils* Usually the mucous patches are symmetrically arranged.
- *Cheeks palate and lips* Lesions appear as gray-white patches.
- *Tongue* Mucous patches on the tongue appear as round or oval, smooth areas, sharply demarcated from the surrounding epithelium, the smoothness of the lesions results from the loss of filiform papillae.
- *Larynx* Lesions are most often found on the epiglottis and aryepiglottic folds, surrounding tissue edema produces

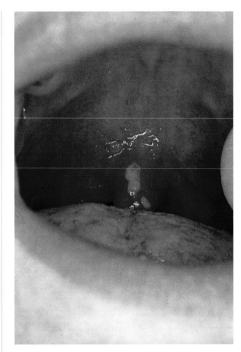

Figure 15.21 Mucosal lesions of secondary syphilis (mucous patch) (reproduced from McMillan and Scott 2000[251])

hoarseness, a common symptom of secondary syphilis.

- *Nasal mucosa* Mucous patches of the nasal mucosa may produce serous nasal discharge.
- *Mucous membranes of the genitalia* Patches may be found on the glans penis, sub-preputial surface of the prepuce (Figure 15.22), vulva, fourchette, and cervix.

Lymph node enlargement

Generalized lymph node enlargement is found in at least 60% of cases of secondary syphilis. Cervical, suboccipital, axillary,

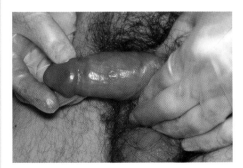

Figure 15.22 Mucosal lesions of secondary syphilis on the penis

epitrochlear, and inguinal nodes are often palpably enlarged. The glands are discrete with a rubbery consistency and are not tender. Not uncommonly the spleen is enlarged in secondary syphilis.

Periostitis

This is said to be an uncommon manifestation of secondary syphilis, although bone pain may occasionally be the presenting feature of the disease[135]. Periostitis is usually a localized process most commonly affecting the anterior tibia. Localized bone pain, especially at night, relieved by movement and exacerbated by immobilization, is the chief symptom and localized tenderness may be noted on examination. Radiological examination usually reveals no abnormalities although osteolytic foci and periostitis may be seen. Bone scanning, using ^{99}Tc, may show areas of increased bone uptake; the superficial bones, including the skull, are chiefly affected. These changes resolve within about 9 months of completion of therapy.

Arthritis and bursitis

Painless effusion into joints and bursae occurs rarely during the course of secondary syphilis. Arthralgia, however, either localized or generalized is more common affecting at least 6% of patients.

Hepatitis

Rarely, jaundice may be associated with secondary syphilis. With respect to the plasma enzyme tests for hepatocellular damage in the form of hepatitis, the level of serum alkaline phosphatase – of hepatic origin – is often disproportionately elevated, in comparison with only a moderate elevation in the case of alanine aminotransferase. These serum enzyme abnormalities may also be noted in patients with secondary syphilis who are not jaundiced. In about half of those with early syphilis there are minor abnormalities of the hepatic histology, the most common findings being mild to moderate Kupffer cell hyperplasia and focal liver cell necrosis, sometimes with portal lymphoid hyperplasia[136]. It should be noted, however, that most studies on hepatitis in syphilis were undertaken at a time when serological tests for hepatitis C virus (HCV) infection were not available, and it is possible that several patients with so-called syphilitic hepatitis may have been infected with HCV. The histology of the liver does not correlate with serum biochemical findings. Usually within 6 weeks of treatment the plasma enzyme activities revert to normal.

Glomerulonephritis and the nephrotic syndrome

Patients with secondary syphilis frequently have mild albuminuria, possibly as the result of immune complexes trapped by the glomeruli setting up an inflammatory reaction there. Such changes are usually mild and transient, but rarely a membranous glomerulonephritis results, being manifest as the nephrotic syndrome. Nodular lumps on the epithelial side of the basement membrane are found on electron microscopy of glomeruli in renal biopsy specimens; immunofluorescence studies show deposition of IgG and complement component (C3) in these lumps. Anti-treponemal antibody can be demonstrated in affected glomeruli by using elution techniques. These findings suggest that the glomerulonephritis of secondary syphilis is due to the presence of treponemal antigen – anti-treponemal antibody complexes from the circulation being deposited within the glomeruli[137].

If untreated the nephrotic syndrome appears to resolve spontaneously.

Iridocyclitis and choroidoretinitis

Iritis, usually discovered late in secondary syphilis, is now a rare complication in western countries (less than 1% of cases)[138]. Uveitis and choroidoretinitis may be precipitated by the use of corticosteroid preparations for some other complication (for example glomerulonephritis) or for some intercurrent illness.

Treponeme-like forms have been identified in the aqueous humour of patients suffering from iridocyclitis[139].

Neurological abnormalities in secondary syphilis

Headache that is especially noticeable in the morning, is a common complaint and probably reflects meningeal inflammation. Although transitory abnormalities of the white cell count and protein content in the CSF occur in only about 5% of patients with secondary syphilis, frank meningoencephalitis may rarely be encountered[140]. A CT scan or MRI shows meningeal enhancement.

Peripheral neuritis may be a rare complication. Perceptive nerve deafness with or without vestibular dysfunction, is another uncommon complication. It is usually associated with tinnitus, and the CSF tends to show some abnormality. Improvement, both subjective and objective, occurs following antibiotic treatment[141]. Although pure-tone, speech and impedance audiometry is usually normal in patients with early syphilis, brain-stem electrical response audiometry often indicates subclinical brain-stem disease[142].

Parotitis

Unilateral parotitis has been described as a complication of secondary syphilis[143].

Differential diagnosis of secondary syphilis

The appearance of the rash of secondary syphilis is variable and as a result many dermatological conditions have to be considered in the differential diagnosis. Table 15.7 indicates the more common conditions to be considered; the problem is generally resolved by the serological tests for syphilis and by the generally rapid response to antibiotic treatment.

EARLY LATENT SYPHILIS

The lesions of early syphilis may heal and the disease may become latent. During this stage, known as early-stage latent syphilis, recurrence of infectious mucocutaneous lesions may be seen. Latency may, however, persist, and early-stage latent syphilis is arbitrarily taken to last for 2 years.

LATE STAGE

In the early years of a syphilis infection the lesions already described (chancre, mucous patch, condyloma latum) are infectious and there is evidence of a recurrent spirochetemia and recurring mucocutaneous

Table 15.7 Differential diagnosis of secondary syphilis

Lesions	Diseases to be differentiated	
Macular syphilide	Drug eruptions	History of intake, pruritus present in drug eruptions.
	Measles Rubella	May be difficult to differentiate from secondary syphilis.
	Pityriasis rosea	'Herald patch', lesions of generalized eruption, discrete, oval, dull red, with collarette of scales. Usually on trunk or proximal areas of limbs. Palmar/plantar lesions exceptional.
Papular syphilide	Psoriasis Lichen planus Pityriasis lichenoides	Lesions are small firm lichenoid papules, reddish brown in color. On detaching overlying scale, shiny brown surface revealed.
	Condylomata acuminata Ulcerated hemorrhoids Herpes simplex infection	May resemble mucous patches, but herpes lesions are usually painful.
	Impetigo contagiosa	Facial papules of syphilis may resemble impetigo.
	Tinea pedis	Plantar syphilide and hypertrophic papules between toes require differentiation from tinea.
	Trichophytides	Micropapular syphilides may resemble these.
	Keratotic eczema	Resembles plantar or palmar syphilide.
Mucosal lesions of syphilis	Aphthous ulcers Herpetic gingivostomatitis	Generally painful and tender.
	Infectious mononucleosis	May be difficult to differentiate clinically from secondary syphilis – macular rash, tonsillar/palatal lesions, lymph node and splenic enlargement; occasionally jaundice. Cardiolipin tests (VDRL) may be positive.

lesions. In pregnant women, also, infection of the fetus *in utero* is inevitable in untreated early-stage syphilis. Syphilis then enters a subclinical stage of latency in which the only readily detectable evidence of infection is serological, and this latency may persist for years or even for life. Transmission of the disease by sexual intercourse does not occur although in the case of pregnancy the woman can infect her fetus long after she has ceased to be infectious sexually. Further activity of the disease may, at any time during latency, cause profound effects and lead to death as long as three decades or more after infection. The main forms of late-stage syphilis are described below, although the protean manifestations call for the consideration of syphilis in the differential diagnoses of many diseases, particularly those involving the cardiovascular or central nervous system.

Late-stage latent syphilis

The diagnosis rests on the finding of positive specific serological tests for syphilis, and the absence of other evidence of disease. In western industrialized countries, the discovery of positive serological tests in an otherwise healthy person often raises the question as to whether syphilis has been acquired before birth or later. This problem is difficult as stigmata appear to be rare now. A family history may be misleading. Patients should, however, be carefully examined for the presence of obvious stigmata, and slit-lamp microscopy of the cornea should be included in the investigation to search for ghost vessels, as a trace of previous interstitial keratitis[144]. Nerve deafness may be obvious or, if mild, demonstrable by audiography. In doubtful cases, serological examination of parents or brothers and sisters may be helpful, and to avoid serious social upset consultation, collaboration with the general practitioner is advised.

Before reaching a diagnosis of late latent syphilis, the CSF should be examined and the aorta screened by CT scanning to exclude changes due to involvement of the aortic valve and the first part of the aorta particularly. Latent syphilis is the commonest manifestation of late syphilis, probably made more common because the patient will have had courses of antibiotics for other conditions which will have prevented the emergence of the late effects such as neurosyphilis. In people from geographical areas where the endemic treponematoses are common, it may be impossible to differentiate past infection with these infections from venereal syphilis.

Late-stage gummatous syphilis

This is now very rare. It is characterized by gumma formation (syphilitic granulation tissue) which may develop because there is reactivation of residual treponemes in sensitized persons who have been untreated or inadequately treated.

Serological tests for syphilis give positive results. Gummatous lesions tend to be solitary or few in number. They are asymmetrical, indurated and indolent. On the skin late-stage lesions tend to be arcuate in

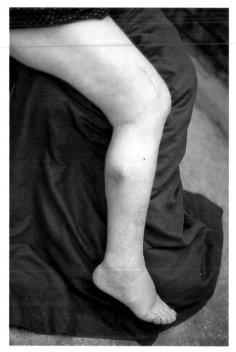

Figure 15.23 Gummatous nodule on the leg

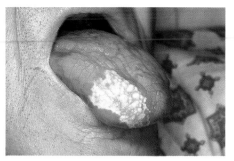

Figure 15.25 Chronic superficial glossitis with leukoplakia (reproduced from McMillan and Scott 2000[251])

outline because without treatment they tend to heal partially in the center and extend peripherally. Atrophic or hyper-pigmented scars form. Gummatous lesions respond rapidly to treatment. A gumma may form a nodule in the subcutaneous tissue (Figure 15.23) that increases in size, breaks down and may produce a gummatous ulcer (Figure 15.24), often described as 'punched out' as it tends to have vertical walls. The granular floor of such an ulcer may have a 'wash leather'

appearance because of slough. The sites commonly involved are the upper part of the leg below the knee, the scalp, face, sternoclavicular region, or the buttocks.

The mouth and throat are much less frequently involved by a gummatous lesion than the skin and bones. The submucosa is involved first but either the soft or hard palate may be affected, leading to perforation. A gumma of the tongue can develop but a diffuse lesion with infiltration and a chronic superficial glossitis is more common. In such a case the patchy epithelial necrosis and the leukoplakia which develops, produce white areas of adherent epithelium on the tongue (Figure 15.25). Mouth lesions should always be biopsied as malignant change is not uncommon and a careful life-long follow-up is necessary. Infiltration of the laryngeal mucosa may occur with or without ulceration.

Two main types of late syphilis of bone are recognized. Gummatous periostitis without destruction but with bony proliferation may lead to the development of 'saber tibia'. Gummatous osteitis may cause a destructive lesion. Clinically, in late syphilis of the bone, the patient may have boring pain and localized redness or swelling.

Gummata of the liver may occur in late syphilis. A gumma of the testis produces a smooth painless swelling; the testis must be removed surgically to exclude malignant neoplasm. Lesions of the esophagus, stomach, and intestine have been reported. Opacity, however, detected in a chest X-ray of a patient with syphilis is nearly always caused by a carcinoma as a gumma is very rare in this site. Gummatous lesions generally respond rapidly to treatment although when fibrosis is marked resolution will be slow. Reference has already been made to the importance of biopsy and a careful follow-up in cases of mouth lesions where malignant change is a recognized hazard.

Neurosyphilis

Although *T. pallidum* may invade the central nervous system and involve particularly the meninges during early syphilis, causing minor changes in the CSF, overt manifestations may occur only in about 5% of cases. In those cases, meningeal symptoms or signs may appear abruptly (headache or drowsiness, amaurosis with papilledema, cranial nerve palsies or hemiplegia). Neurological abnormalities in early syphilis have been referred to on page 421.

Neurosyphilis of the late stage is uncommon, but its sporadic appearance and often very good response to antibiotic therapy make it vitally important to make a diagnosis as early as possible. It may appear in a form with more localized and less striking clinical effects than were seen in the classical forms of parenchymatous neurosyphilis that were so much more common in times before antibiotic and chemotherapy, when the wards of every mental hospital were crowded with cases in various stages of mental and physical deterioration. Although late-stage neurosyphilis can be classified into various forms there may be considerable overlap.

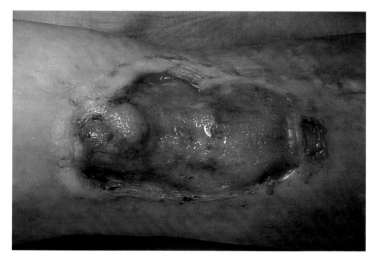

Figure 15.24 Gummatous ulcer of the leg (reproduced from McMillan and Scott 2000[251])

It is clearly important in all hospital departments to consider syphilis in diagnosis and to use treponemal serological tests (for example EIA) as non-treponemal serological tests (for example VDRL) are sometimes negative in late syphilis.

Although neurosyphilis is classified as parenchymatous or meningovascular, overlapping processes are found. The classification of tabes dorsalis among the parenchymatous forms of neurosyphilis is justified by the concentration of the lesions in the dorsal roots and columns. In most cases of tabes dorsalis in which cerebral symptoms appear and which are diagnosed clinically as taboparesis, the cerebral lesions are those of meningovascular syphilis. Again, primary optic atrophy is commonly associated with tabes dorsalis and sometimes with meningovascular syphilis, but rarely with general paralysis of the insane.

Clinical forms of acquired late-stage neurosyphilis

Asymptomatic neurosyphilis

The diagnosis rests on CSF findings, indicative of syphilis of the CNS in the absence of clinical symptoms or signs. It is reasonable to conclude that the inflammatory process is more restricted than in those forms of the disease with overt signs and symptoms. The investigation in such a case should not be restricted to serological tests for syphilis and CSF examination but should include a full clinical examination and chest X-ray to exclude signs of syphilis in other systems.

Meningovascular syphilis

Symptoms and signs of meningovascular involvement may develop even during the secondary stage when the effect is predominantly meningeal with signs discussed already.

Meningovascular syphilis of the late stage may produce headache associated with cranial nerve palsies, particularly of the third and sixth; the auditory or vestibular nerves may also be affected. The optic nerves or chiasma may be involved in a basal meningitis. If cerebral vessels are affected, mental deterioration and focal signs such as aphasia or hemiplegia will occur. If the gummatous infiltration involves the spinal cord progressive paraplegia can develop and occasionally there is a transverse myelitis due to occlusion of the anterior spinal artery. In meningovascular and, indeed, all forms of late-stage neurosyphilis pupillary abnormalities are common and the fully developed sign is the Argyll Robertson pupil.

Argyll Robertson pupil In December 1868, at a meeting of the Edinburgh Medico-Chirurgical Society[145], Douglas Argyll Robertson described reflex pupillary paralysis to light in a case of spinal disease and later he defined the sign now known by his name: although the retina is quite sensitive, and the pupil contracts during the act of accommodation for near objects, yet an alteration of the amount of light admitted into the eye does not influence the size of the pupil.

In all forms of late neurosyphilis, overt or latent, pupillary abnormalities in the presence of good vision are common. In more than 80% of cases and in tabes in particular, pupil abnormalities develop in the course of time. The fully developed condition already described and known as the Argyll Robertson pupil is a valuable sign, although not pathognomonic of neurosyphilis as it has been described as a curiosity in conditions such as diabetes, alcoholic neuropathy, hypertrophic polyneuropathy, and tumors of the pineal region when there is also, as a rule, a defect of upward conjugate gaze.

Earlier manifestations of reflex iridoplegia (failure to react to light) may be found in neurosyphilis, and during neurological examination the eye should be examined carefully to discover whether

1. reaction to light is reduced in amplitude
2. reaction to light is not sustained
3. the latent period is longer than usual
4. reaction may be brisker in one eye
5. the consensual reflex is brisker than the direct reflex
6. rarely a dilatation may occur in response to light.

In addition, oculosympathetic paralysis may be seen with no dilatation of the pupil in response to a scratch on the neck. Ptosis with compensatory wrinkling of the brow may also occur. Patchy depigmentation of the iris may give it a watery blue color. Both pupils are usually affected but unequally.

The fully developed Argyll Robertson pupil may best be described as 'small, constant in size and unaltered by light or shade; it contracts promptly and fully on convergence and dilates again promptly when the effort to converge is relaxed; it dilates slowly and imperfectly to mydriatics.'

The method of testing is important. To test the light reflex

1. ask the patient to look at a distant object
2. cover the other eye to eliminate the consensual reaction
3. test by shining light into the eye and look for contraction of the pupil.

To test the accommodation reflex

1. ask the patient to look at distant object, then
2. ask him to look at examiner's finger that is brought gradually to within 2 inches of the eyes, the reaction consists of contraction of the medial recti muscles and contraction of the pupil.

The site of the lesion continues to excite controversy and is not entirely settled. The reflex paths in the midbrain are the most popular site for the causal injury, although a peripheral lesion in the iris has been suggested. The location of a lesion in the periaqueductal region of the midbrain by MRI in a patient with Argyll Robertson pupils due to neuro-ophthalmic complications of acute sarcoidosis[146] was in keeping with the midbrain theory. The suggestion is that the Argyll Robertson syndrome is caused by interruption of the light reflex pathway and inhibitory supranuclear pathways to the Edinger-Westphal nucleus at a point dorsorostral to the oculomotor complex, while fibers controlling accommodation, being placed more ventrally, are left unaffected.

Subcortical or cortical infarction may be found on neuroimaging.

Gummata of the brain

This form of neurosyphilis is exceedingly rare. The presentation is that of a space-occupying lesion. Multiple ring-enhancing lesions may be found on CT or MRI examination[147].

General paresis (dementia paralytica, general paralysis of the insane, or GPI)

This can develop 7 to 15 years after a primary infection. The clinical syndrome now encountered is often one of simple mental deterioration, sometimes with depression, not distinguishable from the more common and less specific pre-senile dementia. In the classical form of GPI the disease is insidious in its development and is characterized by episodes of strange behavior at variance with the previous good character of the individual. Comprehension and esthetic feelings are dulled and the alterations in the patient's personality distress their friends and relatives. Grandiose delusions and euphoria used to be commonly seen but are rare now. Writing may be tremulous and tremors of the tongue, hands, and facial muscles may develop. Pronunciation difficulties may distort words beyond recognition. Epileptic fits and transient attacks of hemiplegia and aphasia are frequent. Tremor of the hands and a slow slurred speech are characteristic as the disease progresses. Spastic weakness of the legs develops and the final stage is that of paralysis and dementia.

Neurosyphilitic psychosis most commonly presents now as a depressive illness or a simple dementia, and patients presenting with grandiose delusions are very rare.

Tendon reflex abnormalities are common and degrees of iridoplegia, irregularity, and inequality of the pupils are valuable signs. The fully developed Argyll Robertson pupil may be found in 25% of cases.

A CT scan or MRI shows atrophy with no specific features.

Tabes dorsalis

The lesions in tabes dorsalis are concentrated on the dorsal spinal roots and dorsal columns of the spinal cord, most often at the lumbosacral and lower thoracic levels. The dorsal roots are thin and gray and contrast with the thick white ventral roots. The dorsal columns show shrinkage although the dorsal root ganglia show less definite atrophy. The reasons for this selective degeneration are not understood.

Among the subjective manifestations are lightning pains, so called from their sudden brief stabbing quality. A brief jab of severe pain striking a localized point of one leg may make the patient wince. Such pains can be felt as girdle pains around the trunk or in the area supplied by the trigeminal nerve. The patient may complain of paresthesiae, saying that he feels as if he is walking on cotton wool. He may have

defects in his sensation of the need to defecate or to empty his bladder.

Various paroxysmal painful disorders of the viscera known as tabetic crises, probably reflecting irritation of the dorsal roots, may occur as a result of spasm of smooth muscle. In gastric crises attacks of epigastric pain and ceaseless vomiting may mimic the 'acute abdomen' and last for several days. Laryngeal crises present with dyspnea, cough, and stridor. Tenesmus, and bladder and penis pain occur in rectal and vesical crises respectively.

Other symptoms and signs are explained in terms of loss of sensory function. The patient is ataxic as there is loss of position sense, he tends to walk on a broad base, staggering and lifting his feet with a stamping gait. In Romberg's sign the patient demonstrates his inability to keep his balance with his eyes closed and his feet together. Muscles are hypotonic, the tendon reflexes are diminished or absent. Vibration sense, deep pain sense, and position sense are all diminished or absent.

Trophic changes may be seen. In the neuropathic joint (Charcot's joint) affecting a hip (Figure 15.26), knee, wrist, or other joints, there is bone destruction with

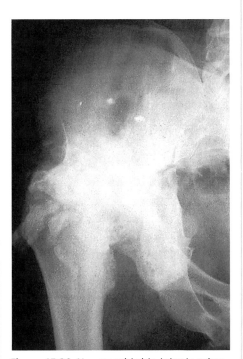

Figure 15.26 Neuropathic hip joint in tabes dorsalis, showing destruction of the joint (reproduced from McMillan and Scott 2000[251])

osteophyte formation. The joint is swollen and deformed with marked crepitus but quite painless. Collapse of the lumbar spine can cause nerve root compression. Perforating trophic ulcers may develop on the soles of the feet (Figure 15.27).

Charcot's joints are not pathognomonic of syphilis, being found in other neurological conditions such as syringomyelia, subacute combined degeneration of the spinal cord, diabetic neuropathy, or following intra-articular injections of corticosteroids.

Optic atrophy and a bilateral ptosis with compensatory wrinkling of the brow are common in tabes. Optic atrophy as an isolated condition occurs as blindness in a third form of late-stage neurosyphilis. The discs are small and pale. The atrophy may progress to cause complete blindness in about one-third of patients, even with penicillin treatment. Atrophic fibers cannot regenerate whatever treatment is given. Recognition of syphilis at an early stage and penicillin therapy are vital in the prevention of these serious late-stage effects.

Modified late-stage forms of neurosyphilis

In western countries, since the introduction and widespread use of antibiotics, the classical clinical picture of late-stage neurosyphilis is seldom seen, but the disease may appear as modified neurosyphilis[148] with more isolated, localized and less striking signs. The diagnosis is backed by the sensitive and highly specific serological tests such as the FTA-ABS and/or TPHA tests. In such modified forms the differential diagnosis needs careful thought.

Ophthalmological signs indicative of neurosyphilis An Argyll Robertson pupil or an irregular, unequal fixed pupil sometimes with synechiae of the iris and with positive serological tests for syphilis are indicative of neurosyphilis.

Ophthalmological signs in which positive serum treponemal antibody tests may be coincidental. Such findings should not be attributed automatically to syphilis, although full treatment for late-stage syphilis is nevertheless mandatory.

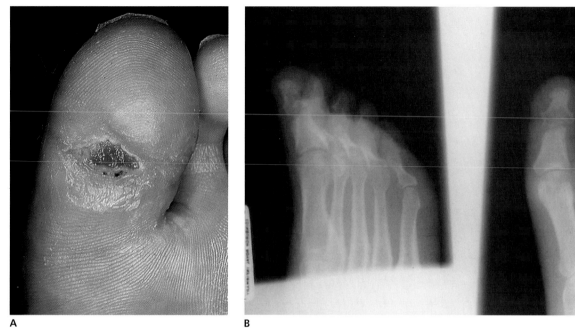

Figure 15.27 (a) Perforating ulcer of the sole of the foot in tabes dorsalis, (b) radiograph of (a) showing bony involvement (Fig. 15.27a reproduced from McMillan and Scott 2000[251])

1. *Choroidoretinitis* This is a manifestation of posterior uveitis and is now more commonly due to *Toxocara* spp. or *Toxoplasma* spp. infestation than to syphilis.

2. *Secondary pigmentary degeneration of the retina* This may be a sequel to syphilitic neuroretinitis and resemble retinitis pigmentosa, an entity where there is a family history of the condition, and the patient will complain of night blindness. There is concentric constriction of the visual fields and pigmentation obscures the choroidal blood vessels, which are narrowed.

3. *Ptosis* In bilateral ptosis consider also myasthenia gravis or a rare localized ocular myopathy. If the ptosis is unilateral, a neoplasm or aneurysm in the chest or neck, or diabetes are possibilities as well as syphilis.

4. *Optic atrophy* This may be associated with an insidious glaucoma, multiple sclerosis, or the result of injury or retro-orbital neoplasm or inflammation. In cases of optic atrophy associated with temporal arteritis the patient is ill, has a continuous headache and a high erythrocyte sedimentation rate.

Neurological features attributable to localized inflammatory lesions of syphilis In this group patients may present with epileptiform fits or as incomplete tabes with tendon reflex changes such as absent ankle jerks or a Babinski sign. Some may have a sensory abnormality and in some the signs of cervical spondylosis are caused by syphilitic pachymeningitis rather than arthropathy.

Psychiatric disorders Here it may be difficult to attribute depression, mania, personality disorder, or dementia, to syphilis unless there are definite CSF changes.

Cardiovascular syphilis

Reference has already been made to the decline in the numbers of deaths from cardiovascular syphilis in England and Wales, a decline common in all forms of late-stage syphilis, although the improvement in incidence has been much more apparent in its neurological than in its cardiovascular forms.

Gummata tend to occur in the interatrial septum or in the upper portion of the interventricular septum. Because of

their proximity to the atrioventricular node, they may disturb the conducting system of the heart and provide one of the rare causes of the Stokes–Adams syndrome (complete heart block).

The second category of cardiac lesions in acquired syphilis are those which lead to aortic-valve insufficiency. In all stages of syphilis arteritis is a constant feature. The coronary ostial stenosis, coupled with the low diastolic pressure accompanying the valvular insufficiency, gravely lessens the blood supply to the myocardium. The ischemia may cause angina and sudden death because of infarction.

Aortic lesions in syphilis are maximal in the first part of the aorta and the arch, they are absent below the diaphragm. In contrast, in atheroma the lesions increase progressively from the arch to the bifurcation. In syphilis an aneurysm is usually thoracic and the aortic valve incompetent; in atheroma the aneurysm is usually abdominal and if the aortic valve is involved it is stenosed.

Clinical features

Compensation for aortic regurgitation is so efficient that patients may live for many years with minimal symptoms. They may be aware of the heaving cardiac impulse in bed and may notice transient dizziness following changes in posture. The compensation is achieved because the refluxing blood augments that which enters the left ventricle through the mitral valve to produce increased stretching and hence more powerful contraction of the ventricle. Gross hypertrophy and dilatation of the left ventricle has produced some of the largest hearts to be found at autopsy.

The symptoms and signs depend upon the site and the anatomical nature of the lesion. Coronary ostial stenosis will cause angina. Dilatation of the aorta may cause an aortic systolic murmur and a characteristic loud aortic component of the second sound. Aortic regurgitation is responsible for an early diastolic murmur, often best heard in the second right intercostal space with the patient leaning forward and holding his breath.

An aortic aneurysm may cause pulsation of the anterior chest wall or occasionally obstruction of the superior vena cava, causing facial edema. Pressure of the aneurysm on the bronchi can cause a tracheal tug felt by the examiner as a downward pull on the thyroid cartilage. Hoarseness, dysphagia, and bone pain are other symptoms.

Electrocardiogram changes may show evidence of myocardial ischemia or signs of left ventricular hypertrophy. The radiograph of the chest shows dilatation of the aorta (Figure 15.28), and linear calcification of the surrounding portion is a useful early sign. The most useful diagnostic measure is CT angiography that demonstrates the degree of reflux into the ventricle in diastole. As long as compensation is maintained cardiac catheterization will show that the end diastolic pressure in the left ventricle and the left atrial pressures are normal.

Diagnosis

In any case of aortic regurgitation or aneurysmal dilatation of the ascending aorta syphilis should be suspected. Syphilis seldom causes ischemic heart disease alone without producing aortic regurgitation. Serological tests for syphilis will indicate the etiology.

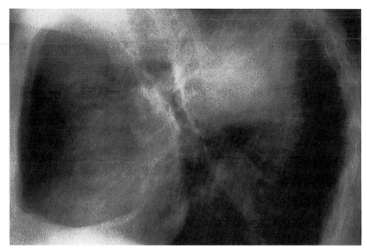

Figure 15.28 Syphilitic aneurysm of the ascending aorta (reproduced from McMillan and Scott 2000[251])

Clinical features of congenital syphilis

Fetal syphilis can be detected *in utero* in a mother who has positive serological tests for syphilis. Ultrasonography shows hydrops fetalis with hydramnios, placental thickening, skin thickening, serous cavity effusions, hepatomegaly, and splenomegaly[149–151].

After birth, the manifestations of congenital syphilis may conveniently be divided into two stages, early and late; the end of the second year of life is the arbitrary point of division between the two stages. Fuller details of the clinical features of congenital syphilis may be found in Nabarro's book[152] and in a review by Robinson[153] as well as by reference to the individual papers cited.

EARLY-STAGE CONGENITAL SYPHILIS

When congenital syphilis was common it was rare to find acute signs of syphilis in the newborn and in cases that occurred, death usually followed within a few days. Infants were often born prematurely or, if full-term, were often of low birth weight. The skin was wrinkled and there was a bullous skin rash (syphilitic pemphigus) particularly on the soles and palms. The clear or purulent fluid from the bullae contained large numbers of *T. pallidum* and

was highly infectious. Other skin lesions, most often maculopapules, were usually present and were found around the body orifices. Rhinitis produced a mucoid or mucopurulent nasal discharge, and a hoarse cry resulted from laryngitis. Abdominal distention was common and hepatic and splenic enlargement almost invariably found. Hemorrhagic manifestations occasionally occurred caused by thrombocytopenia and macroglobulinemia[154].

The majority of infants infected with syphilis appear healthy at birth, as the characteristic clinical features do not develop until between 2 and 12 weeks. After a period of normal development, the child fails to thrive and the clinical picture of congenital syphilis becomes apparent.

It is convenient to describe the manifestations according to the particular part of the body affected.

Cutaneous manifestations

Skin rashes of varied character are found in 70% to 90% of infants with congenital syphilis. The rash is symmetrical in distribution and erythematous macular, papular, and papulosquamous lesions may exist together in different parts of the body. On the face the eruption is particularly prominent around the mouth. Where the skin is moist, for example on the buttocks and external genitalia, the rash appears eczematous (Figure 15.29). In these sites

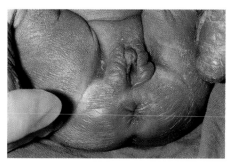

Figure 15.29 Perianal lesions of congenital syphilis (reproduced from Rein 1996[252])

hypertrophic lesions resembling condylomata lata may appear, usually as a manifestation of a recurrence following resolution of the initial rash. Deep fissures develop round the body orifices, and healing of these lesions leaves characteristic scars (rhagades).

The skin of the palms and soles may show peeling. In severe cases the hair becomes scanty and brittle and involvement of the nails leads to shedding and replacement by narrow, atrophic nails.

In addition to the eruptions described, the skin may show wrinkling from weight loss and there is 'café-au-lait' pigmentation.

If an infant is not treated, or is inadequately treated, the skin lesions usually heal within a year, but there may be recurrences during the second year. Recurrent lesions usually differ from those seen in the original rash and include condylomata lata.

Mucosal lesions

Clinical evidence of rhinitis is found in 70% to 80% of infected infants. There is nasal obstruction and a mucoid nasal discharge which becomes mucopurulent and occasionally blood stained (syphilitic snuffles) (Figure 15.30). Numerous treponemes may be demonstrated in the discharge which is highly infectious. Arrested development of nasal structures, and continued pressure changes within the nose as a result of obstruction lead to deformities of the nose (saddle nose).

Mucous patches resembling those seen in secondary acquired syphilis may occur in the mouth and pharynx. Laryngitis produces a hoarse or aphonic cry.

Lymphadenitis and splenic enlargement

Although not a constant accompaniment of early congenital syphilis, moderate generalized enlargement of the lymph nodes is common. The spleen is enlarged in at least 60% of infected infants.

Bone and joint manifestations

Bone disease, diagnosed by clinical or radiological examination, or both, occurs in at least 85% of infected infants under the age of 1 year[152]. In only about 40% of cases is there clinical evidence of bone involvement. Bones are usually affected symmetrically, but one side may be more involved than the other. The child cries when adjacent joints are passively moved and he/she rarely moves affected limbs (Parrot's pseudoparalysis).

Radiological examination of infected infants under the age of 12 months, who have no clinical evidence of bone involvement, demonstrates abnormalities in at least 75% of cases. Multiple long-bone involvement is most commonly found, the metaphyses being particularly affected. Variable degrees of calcification at the growing ends of the bone result in a variety of radiological changes[155]. Most commonly there is an irregular (saw tooth) dense zone of calcification overlying an osteoporotic area at the metaphysis. Peripheral osteoporosis of the metaphysis is less often observed, as is the appearance of dense bands sandwiching such zones.

Irregular patchy areas of loss of bone density are commonly found in both metaphyses and diaphyses. A characteristic sign is the loss of density of the upper medial aspect of the tibiae (Wimberger's sign). In severe cases there may be a fracture at the site of bone destruction in the metaphysis, with impaction or displacement of the epiphysis.

Periostitis appears radiologically either as a single layer or as multiple layers of new-bone formation along the cortex of the shaft of the bone (Figure 15.31); it is common in early congenital syphilis, particularly amongst children aged 4 weeks and over[155]. Although any long bone may be affected, the distal femur and radius, and the proximal tibia and humerus are the most often involved. The changes described are not specific for syphilis, similar radiological findings being encountered in rubella, cytomegalovirus infection, rickets, and hemolytic disease of the newborn. Occasionally in early congenital syphilis lens-shaped areas known as Parrot's nodes appear around the anterior fontanelle on the frontal and parietal bones. These nodes are probably caused by periostitis. Usually the changes described resolve within the second 6 months of life, but periostitis persists and may become more pronounced.

During the later stages of early congenital syphilis, dactylitis, manifesting clinically as painless, spindle-shaped swellings of the fingers, may occur in a small number of cases (less than 5%). Radiographic examination shows that up to 25% of all infected children under the age of 2 years have dactylitis.

Hepatic and pancreatic involvement

The liver is almost invariably enlarged, usually in association with the spleen, in

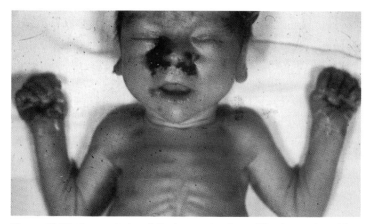

Figure 15.30 Congenital syphilis: hemorrhagic snuffles (reproduced from Rein 1996[252])

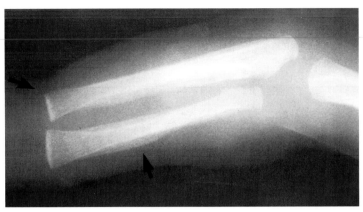

Figure 15.31 Bony lesions in early congenital syphilis, note periosteal new bone formation (reproduced from Rein 1996[252])

congenital syphilis appearing in the neonatal period, and in at least 60% of older infants. Jaundice is an uncommon feature, but its presence in the neonate should alert the physician practising in areas where syphilis is common, to the possibility that syphilis may be the cause of the jaundice.

Although not clinically apparent, pancreatitis is a common finding at autopsy of infants dying of congenital syphilis in the neonatal period[156].

Renal involvement

The nephrotic syndrome may rarely be associated with early congenital syphilis, and is thought to be the result of deposition of soluble complexes of treponemal antigen and anti-treponemal antibody in the glomeruli[157]. Acute nephritis is a rarity[158].

Bronchopulmonary involvement

In the aborted fetus and stillborn infant, the lungs are always affected, as bronchi and lung parenchyma have developed abnormally.

Neurological involvement

Although meningitis is common in early congenital syphilis, particularly during the exanthem stage, clinical signs relating to the nervous system are uncommon. Epileptiform seizures, irritability, and bulging of the anterior fontanelle may occur. There may be focal changes in the cerebral tissue because of thrombotic occlusion of blood vessels affected by a panarteritis. These cerebral lesions may produce hemiplegia, monoplegia, and cranial nerve palsies.

In about a third of infants under the age of 12 months, the cerebrospinal fluid is abnormal with respect to cell content and protein levels, and gives positive results when examined by the serological tests for syphilis.

Ocular manifestations

Iritis is rare in early congenital syphilis. Choroidoretinitis is considerably more common during the first year of life. Examination with an ophthalmoscope shows small spots of pigment surrounded by yellow areas (salt and pepper fundus). If untreated the inflammatory process progresses, and if the macular or optic disc regions are involved, blindness may result.

Hematological abnormalities

Anemia of varying severity occurs in at least 20% of infants with congenital syphilis. Normocytic, normochromic anemia reflects depression of hematopoiesis in the bone marrow as a result of the chronic infection. Increased hemolysis probably plays a small part in the development of the anemia. Secondary iron deficiency produces a microcytic, hypochromic anemia. Occasionally a leuko-erythroblastic anemia occurs.

Thrombocytopenia, associated with a bleeding disorder during the first few weeks of life, has been described[159]. Macroglobulinemia may be associated with the bleeding diathesis[154].

In early congenital syphilis, the white cell count is usually elevated, with lymphocytosis.

Assessment of the infant in the first month of life who has been born to a mother with positive serological tests for syphilis

Infants born to mothers with positive serological tests for syphilis should be carefully examined for clinical evidence of congenital infection. Serological tests should be undertaken on the infant's serum (not cord blood) (see above), and if there are bullous lesions or serous discharges from body orifices, dark-field microscopy or direct immunofluorescent antibody tests should be performed to identify *T. pallidum*, although the sensitivity of these tests is low because of the sparcity of organisms. In addition, it has been found helpful to examine the placenta and umbilical cord for histological evidence of syphilis (see above), and to detect *T. pallidum*-specific DNA by PCR[159a]. When infection is confirmed or strongly suspected, examination of the CSF for cell count and protein concentration, and by VDRL is recommended[172]. A full blood count should also be performed, and, when clinically indicated, additional tests such as radiological examination of the long bones.

Assessment of the older (age > 4 weeks) child with positive serological tests for syphilis

It is helpful to examine the mother's obstetrical records to note if she had had positive serological tests for syphilis during the pregnancy. The child should be examined carefully for evidence of congenital syphilis, and it may be helpful to undertake other investigations such as radiography of the long bones and chest, abdominal ultrasound and auditory brain stem response[172]. Haemotological examination and estimation of plasma bilirubin, alanine aminotransferase should be performed. The CSF should be examined for abnormalities in cell count and protein concentration, and by the VDRL.

LATE-STAGE CONGENITAL SYPHILIS

In at least 60% of affected children there are no clinical signs of the disease, the only abnormal finding being positive serological tests, that is latent congenital syphilis.

Interstitial keratitis

This is the most common clinical manifestation of late congenital syphilis, occurring in about 40% of affected children. Interstitial keratitis appears to be the result of immunological reaction in the cornea to the treponeme, penicillin treatment having no influence on the course of this manifestation. In most cases this develops between the ages of 6 and 14 years, but it may occur earlier or very much later (even over the age of 30 years). Although commencing in one eye, both become involved in more than 90% of cases; the second eye shows features of the condition a few days to several months after the first. The patient complains of pain in the affected eye, photophobia with excessive lacrimation and dimness of vision. A diffuse haziness near the center of the cornea of one eye is the earliest clinical sign, but within a few weeks the whole cornea becomes opaque. This is usually associated with circumcorneal sclerotic congestion.

Examination by slit-lamp microscopy shows that these corneal changes are attributable to blood vessels extending into the cornea from the sclera, and to exudation of cells from these vessels.

The condition gradually improves over a period of 12 to 18 months, leaving a variable degree of corneal damage that may lead to blindness or that may only be detectable by slit-lamp examination. This latter investigation may show empty blood vessels (ghost vessels) within the cornea of patients who have had interstitial keratitis earlier in life, but have no apparent residual scarring[144].

After resolution of the initial episode of interstitial keratitis, 20% to 30% of patients suffer a relapse of this condition.

Bone lesions

The essential bone lesion in late congenital syphilis is hyperplastic osteoperiostitis, a process which may be diffuse (resulting in sclerosis of bone) or localized (periosteal node or gumma). Gumma formation may lead to necrosis of the underlying cortex with softening of the bone. The tibiae are most commonly affected by these changes.

Usually bone lesions develop between the fifth and twentieth year of life, when the patient complains of pain in the affected bone. Palpation may reveal nodules on the anterior surface of the bone, and rarely ulceration may be observed where a gumma has involved skin and bone. In older children, thickening of the anterior surface of the tibia may result in forward bowing of that bone (saber tibia).

Painless gummatous lesions may be found on the hard and soft palates or in the pharynx. These are often extensive, with considerable necrosis of tissue. Perforation of the palate, absence of the uvula, and scarring about the oropharynx may be the result.

Destructive gummatous lesions of the nasal septum may cause perforation of the septum with or without deformity of the lower part of the nose.

Joint lesions

The commonest type of joint lesion (Clutton's joints), seen in about 20% of untreated children, is bilateral effusion into the knee joints. This condition, like interstitial keratitis, is unaffected by antibiotic treatment and appears to be an immunological reaction to *T. pallidum*. Less commonly, other joints are similarly affected. Although most frequently occurring in children between the ages of 5 and 10 years, joint involvement may be seen at any age from 3 years to the mid-20s.

The onset of the arthritis is acute, often with a history of antecedent trauma. Although most commonly painless, the affected joints may be acutely painful, particularly at the onset. Radiological examination reveals no specific changes in the joint.

There is gradual resolution of the arthritis over many months, with recovery of full function.

Neurosyphilis

In about 20% of infected children over the age of 1 year neurosyphilis is latent or hidden and diagnosis depends upon the detection of abnormalities in the cerebrospinal fluid.

As a late result of the meningitis of early-stage congenital syphilis, epileptiform seizures, mental deficiency, and cranial nerve palsies may be found in children over

the age of 2 years. Parenchymatous involvement produces two main clinical conditions: juvenile general paralysis of the insane and tabes dorsalis.

Juvenile general paralysis (juvenile GPI)

This occurs in about 1% of affected children, appearing about the age of 10 years, but occasionally much earlier or much later, as in middle age. The sexes are affected equally (in contrast to the GPI of acquired syphilis in which males are more often affected than females). There is usually a gradual onset of symptoms, the child becoming dull, irritable, apathetic and forgetful. Later, delusions, usually paranoid in type, occur and speech becomes disturbed. The voice is monotonous, articulation becomes stumbling and tremulous, and speech is eventually lost. There is generally tremor of the lips, hands, and legs. Handwriting becomes indistinct. Epileptiform seizures are common at a late stage of the disease.

Pupillary abnormalities are seen in over 90% of cases; the pupils are of the Argyll Robertson type or immobile and dilated. Optic atrophy occurs in between 10% and 35% of cases.

Other physical findings resemble those found in general paralysis of acquired syphilis.

Juvenile tabes

This is much rarer than general paralysis. The onset of the condition is generally between the ages of 10 and 17 years. Failing vision and paraesthesiae are the most common symptoms; lightning pains and ataxia are rare. Later in the course of the disease headaches, photophobia, and diplopia occur frequently. Sphincter disturbances are uncommon although enuresis may be found. Clinical examination may detect nystagmus, pupillary abnormalities, optic atrophy, and absent or diminished tendon reflexes. Trophic disturbances are rare and it is unusual to find evidence of loss of cutaneous sensation.

Ear disease

The middle ear may be affected by a painless otolabyrinthitis, showing as a slight purulent aural discharge. Conduction deafness may result without treatment. The deafness of congenital syphilis, however, is predominantly sensory.

Even after what has been considered adequate penicillin treatment, treponemes have been demonstrated in endochondral bone, a dense structure into which antibiotics do not readily diffuse.

Subjective hearing impairment is commonly a late manifestation, often not occurring until adult life, although it can occur in childhood. In addition the patient may not be seen first until middle age, when the diagnosis of congenital syphilis may not come readily to mind unless there are other stigmata of the disease.

Vestibular disease is frequent in patients with congenital syphilis. The symptoms, which include dizziness, unsteadiness of gait, and paroxysmal vertigo, usually begin with the onset of deafness[160].

Audiograms show a variety of patterns. The most common (35%) is high-tone loss, followed by a flat audiogram (25% of cases) and low-tone loss (15% of cases)[160]. There is progressive deterioration of deafness although spontaneous fluctuation may occur. The most severe difficulty is in discrimination of speech. It is usually an isolated finding, bilateral, although one side is often more severely affected than the other. There are usually no abnormalities in the CSF.

Skin lesions

Gummata similar to those occurring in late acquired syphilis may be found.

Cardiovascular lesions

Myocarditis may be found in children dying of congenital syphilis, but aortitis is exceedingly rare.

Liver disease

Gummata of the liver are rarely found.

Paroxysmal cold hemoglobinuria

This rare condition, occurring in less than 1% of patients with late congenital syphilis, may be seen also in acquired syphilis. Large quantities of hemoglobin are excreted in the urine after exposure to cold.

Shivering or a rigor heralds the attack and this is rapidly followed by fever, head-ache and pains in the back or limbs. A generalized urticarial rash may also develop. Within the next few hours the urine becomes dark brown in color and contains hemoglobin, methemoglobin, but few red blood cells. In most cases, the clinical features described resolve within several hours, but occasionally mild jaundice may develop and persist for some days. This condition is liable to recur periodically when the patient is exposed to cold of varying severity.

Cold hemolysins are found in the blood, and demonstrated by the Donath Landsteiner test. The basis of this test is the ability of the hemolysin to unite with red cells when the blood is chilled. When the blood is then warmed to 37°C, these sensitized cells are lysed in the presence of complement.

STIGMATA OF CONGENITAL SYPHILIS

Lesions of early and late congenital syphilis may heal leaving scars and deformities characteristic of the disease. Such scarring and deformities constitute the stigmata of congenital syphilis, but they only occur in some 40% of patients.

Stigmata of early lesions

Facial appearance

The 'saddle-nose' deformity (Figure 15.32) may result from rhinitis. The palate may appear high arched as a result of under-development of the maxilla.

Teeth

The tooth germs of deciduous teeth are fully differentiated by the tenth week of gestation before tissue reaction to treponemes appears to occur; hence these teeth are usually unaffected. Teeth that develop later may, however, be affected. Two groups of teeth bear the brunt, the upper central incisors and the first molars.

Typically the affected upper incisor is smaller than normal, darker in color, and peg-like, instead of being flat, with the sides converging to the cutting edge which classically has a notched center (Figure 15.33), the so-called Hutchinson's incisor[161]. Affected incisors do not always show this typical appearance but may often be

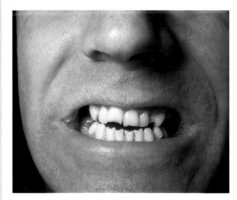

Figure 15.33 Hutchinson's incisors

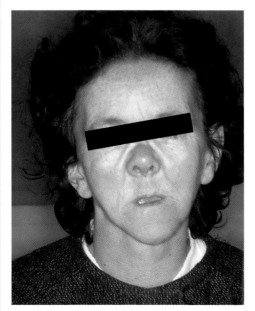
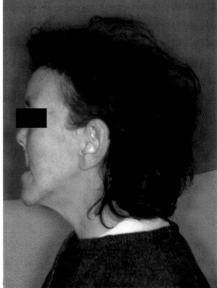

Figure 15.32 Saddle-nose deformity, a stigma of congenital syphilis

thickened anteroposteriorly, with rounding of the incisal angles, they may have a shallow depression on the incisal edge rather than a notch.

The typically affected molar, Moon's molar, shows a constricted occlusal surface and rounded angles. The cuspules of the molar are poorly developed and appear crowded together. Such teeth are prone to dental caries and as a result are lost early.

In one series[162], in 45% of patients with congenital syphilis the upper central incisors were affected, and in about 20% of patients the first molars were involved. The incidence of dental changes is high in patients who also develop interstitial keratitis.

Rhagades

The deep cutaneous lesions around the orifices of the body heal, producing scars radiating from the orifice known as rhagades.

Nails

Atrophy and deformity of the nails may be seen in adult life as a result of nail-bed inflammation in infancy.

Choroidal scarring

Healing of choroidoretinitis produces white scarred areas surrounded by pigmentation on the retina.

Stigmata of late lesions

Corneal lesions

Opacities of the cornea and ghost vessels observed on slit-lamp examination are the result of interstitial keratitis[144].

Bone lesions

Saber tibia resulting from osteoperiostitis may be observed, as may the scars of destructive lesions of the oropharyngeal and nasal regions. Broadening of the skull may result from osteoperiostitis of the frontal and parietal bones.

Optic atrophy

This may occur as a single entity without iridoplegia (for example Argyll Robertson pupils)[153].

Nerve deafness

Treatment of syphilis

Among the kaleidoscopic changes in medical practice since 1946 when penicillin first became easy to obtain, the effect of this antibiotic has been more spectacular in the treatment of syphilis than in anything else. It continues to be the antibiotic of first choice for the treatment of all stages of syphilis, effectively having replaced arsenicals and bismuth.

PRINCIPLES OF PENICILLIN THERAPY IN SYPHILIS

One layer of the cell wall of prokaryotes, including the treponeme, consists of a complex macromolecule, peptidoglycan, the component of bacterial cell walls responsible for their mechanical strength[163]. It is a fortunate fact for the development of chemotherapy that peptidoglycan is unique to the prokaryotic cell wall, as are its characteristic monomer components, N-acetyl muramic acid, diaminopimelic acid and some D-amino acids.

The final cross-linking stage in peptidoglycan synthesis involves a transpeptidation reaction between adjacent peptide chains with the elimination of a molecule of D-alanine per linkage. The cross-linking results in the production of a vast sponge-like macromolecule of considerable strength, but penicillin inhibits this final stage. If synthesis of the peptidoglycan is inhibited by penicillin whilst synthesis of other cell components and the action of autolysins – enzymes which bring about minor removal of wall substances necessary for remodelling of the cell wall in the course of growth – continue, then gradually increasing numbers of weaknesses appear in the cell wall until the hydrostatic pressure within cause the organism to rupture.

Penicillin is thought to be a structural analogue of D-alanyl-D-alanine and this may explain its effect on the final transpeptidation reaction involving the two terminal D-alanines on the pentapeptide. It is important to appreciate that penicillin is only effective against actively growing

bacteria, the optimum effect being achieved when there is unhindered and rapid multiplication. It follows that penicillin will be most effective against the treponeme during early syphilis where there is rapid multiplication of the organism. Treponemes, like other bacteria, can exist in a resting phase when there is minimal cell wall synthesis and when penicillin effects are minimal[164].

In the case of rapidly growing bacteria, such as gonococci, the organism will be particularly sensitive to the action of penicillin many times over a 24-hour period. In organisms with a longer generation time these phases of optimal sensitivity are correspondingly less frequent, for example in *T. pallidum* in the experimentally infected rabbit testicle where the generation time is given as 33 hours[165]. During a treatment period of, say, 10 to 14 days, these phases might well occur 7 to 10 times; as the treponemes do not reproduce synchronously in the infected host these phases of maximum sensitivity to penicillin are conceivably spread diffusely over the period of treatment[164]. It is, therefore, an important determinant for therapeutic success to ensure that effective plasma concentrations are maintained over an adequate time.

Treponema pallidum is one of the most penicillin-sensitive micro-organisms known. For penicillin to be effective in the therapy of syphilis, however, two requirements are essential

1. a minimal benzylpenicillin concentration of 0.018 mg/L of serum, which gives several times the serum and tissue levels needed to kill *T. pallidum*, should be maintained for at least 7 to 10 days in early syphilis
2. penicillin-free or sub-treponemicidal intervals during treatment should not exceed 24 to 30 hours in order that treponemes still surviving can be prevented from re-multiplying[166].

Although *T. pallidum* is extremely sensitive to penicillin (healing of lesions occurs rapidly and treponemes disappear from early-stage lesions), biological cure, that is total eradication of treponemes, is difficult to prove, however, as *T. pallidum* cannot be cultured *in vitro*.

Although lesions of early-stage syphilis heal spontaneously, the disease can remain as a latent (concealed) infection for many years, even for a lifetime, while a proportion, unpredictable in the individual, develop overt forms of late syphilis. The passage of time has, however, given confidence that individuals treated for early syphilis will not suffer ill effects from late syphilis provided that they have had a course of penicillin that gives adequate blood levels over a sufficient length of time.

Clinical and serological follow-up after treatment has always been maintained as important in clinical practice and there are occasional reports of failure after a generally acceptable course of penicillin.

After treatment of some early, but especially of latent or late-stage syphilis with penicillin, or indeed after treatment with any anti-treponemal agent, the T. pallidum immobilization test, positive before treatment, remains positive afterwards and often remains thus for life[167], although cardiolipin antigen tests, such as the VDRL, become negative. The explanation of this persistence of immobilizing antibody in these circumstances was sought by the French team, Collart, Borel, and Durel[168, 169]. This team came to the conclusion that the persistence of immobilizing antibody was due to the persistence of treponemes in the tissues after treatment.

Their conclusions were based on careful experimental work in which testes of rabbits were inoculated with T. pallidum. In most of these rabbits a syphiloma developed and in the others a persistently positive TPI result indicated latent syphilis. A popliteal lymph node was removed from some of the rabbits 18 to 24 months after inoculation and implanted subscrotally into other uninfected rabbits. After 40 days approximately 75% (29 of 38) of these rabbits developed a syphiloma. The experiment and its continuation showed that in experimental syphilis there is a progressive lessening of virulence of the treponeme with the duration of the infection. It was clear, however, that lymph node transplants alone could not be relied upon to confirm sterilization of a treponemal infection.

In rabbits infected with T. pallidum 2 years previously and then treated with penicillin, the titer of the TPI dropped faster than that in the untreated controls but in no animal, however, did the TPI

become negative. Collart et al.[168–170], found that in both untreated controls and in those treated with penicillin 2 years after infection, occasional treponemes could be found in histological sections. In the treated group, however, lymph node transplants were seldom successful in producing a syphiloma. The authors concluded from their experiments that viable treponemes, particularly if long resident in the host, persist after treatment, although these organisms appear to have lost their virulence.

Continuing their study in humans, they examined 10 patients (3 with latent syphilis, 6 with tabes dorsalis and 1 with taboparesis). All but 1 patient had had different treatments, including penicillin, over periods varying from 1 to 16 years. All showed a positive TPI test. Treponemes were seen in the lymph nodes from all cases, in 6 cases the treponemes were typical and in 4 they were considered atypical. Lymph nodes transplanted to healthy rabbits produced syphilomas with spiral organisms considered to be T. pallidum.

With careful search, too time-consuming to apply in clinical practice, tests of aqueous humor, cerebrospinal fluid and other sites for treponeme-like forms have given a small yield in undoubted cases of late syphilis. In a few cases these organisms have been shown to be T. pallidum but in many their nature is uncertain[171]. The finding of treponemes, apparently avirulent and incapable of causing further clinical disease, persisting after treatment of late syphilis, does not alter the fact that the treatment of early syphilis produces a clinical cure and prevents the emergence of late effects and that it is only in early syphilis with moist lesions that transmission can occur by sexual contact.

Worldwide experience in the use of penicillin in the treatment of syphilis over three decades has been fully and valuably considered by Idsoe et al.[166] in a World Health Organization publication. There are a multiplicity of empirically developed treatment plans but, in spite of the variations in the case of long-acting penicillins, results have been good[164]. Imperfections in the understanding of penicillin effects in late and latent syphilis, and more particularly in the long-term value of alternative antibiotics, leave some questions unanswered.

After intramuscular injection of the salts of benzylpenicillin absorption occurs within a few minutes to produce a high concentration in the blood. Excretion is rapid, and in order to maintain a blood level at over 0.1 mg/L for 2, 4, and 8 hours, dosages have been shown to be 30, 141, and 840 mg respectively. Thus, if a continuous effect is required, large and frequent dosages are necessary. Probenecid prolongs the action of each dose by interfering with tubular excretion of penicillin.

Long-acting forms of benzylpenicillin and expressions of dosage

Long-acting forms of penicillin diminish the need for repeated injections and consist of procaine penicillin, an equimolecular compound of penicillin and procaine; benethamine penicillin; and benzathine penicillin; with these forms relatively low concentrations are produced for periods respectively of 24 hours, 5 days, or some weeks.

In this chapter the terms benzylpenicillin, procaine penicillin and benzathine penicillin are respectively synonymous with crystalline penicillin G (either as the sodium or potassium salt), procaine penicillin G, and benzathine penicillin G. The approximate weight equivalents in milligrams of the long-acting forms of penicillin to 600 mg of benzylpenicillin, calculated on the basis of molecular weights, are given in Table 15.8. Where reference is made in this chapter to the dosage of long-acting penicillins, the dose is given in milligrams or grams, together with the approximate weight equivalents in milligrams or grams and in units of benzylpenicillin. This will help to reconcile the current USA practice of referring to penicillin dosage in units and the advised practice in the UK of expressing dosages in milligrams.

GUIDELINES IN TREATMENT

The UK National Guidelines produced by the Clinical Effectiveness Group of the Association of Genitourinary Medicine and the Medical Society for the Study of Venereal Diseases, and the guidelines established by a group of experts and the staff of the Centers for Disease Control, US

Table 15.8 Long-acting penicillins and their equivalents to benzylpenicillin megaunit or 600 mg, calculated on the basis of molecular weights (Prasad 1986, personal communication)*

	Benzyl penicillin sodium	Benethamine penicillin	Benzathine penicillin	Procaine penicillin	Phenoxymethyl penicillin
Molecular weight	356.4	545.7	$909.1 \times \frac{1}{2}$[a]	588.7	350.4
Weight equivalent to 1 000 000 units	600 mg	919 mg	765 mg	991 mg	590 mgL

[a] This salt is 'bivalent' in terms of penicillin; the effective molecular weight is therefore half of the actual molecular weight.
* Various approximate equivalents to units or mg of benzylpenicillin are given for various long-acting forms of penicillin in manufacturers' data on commercial products, but a more 'scientific' approach to the determination of equivalents (on the basis of weight) is to use calculations based on molecular weights (mol. wt.). In order to determine the weight of, say, procaine benzylpenicillin (procaine penicillin) equivalent to 600 mg of benzylpenicillin sodium the following relationship may be used:

$$\text{weight of procaine benzylpenicillin (procaine penicillin)} = \frac{\text{mol. wt of procaine benzylpenicillin (procaine penicillin)} \times 600 \text{ mg}}{\text{mol. wt of benzylpenicillin sodium}}$$

NB the unit is defined in terms of benzylpenicillin sodium (mol. wt. = 356.4) not benzylpenicillin (mol. wt. = 334.4). The above approach bypasses the intermediate stage of having to convert weight to units and then back to the weight of a different salt.

Public Health Service[172] form a valuable source of guidance when considering therapy. As already discussed, other empirically developed regimens are numerous in the treatment of syphilis. In keeping with practice in the UK, the authors tend to place less reliance on single-dose schemes than that given in current recommendations in the USA. In all cases regular clinical and serological follow-up is advised after treatment.

Treatment of early syphilis (primary, secondary, latent syphilis of less than 1 year's duration) in non HIV-infected individuals

In Europe, procaine penicillin is available as Jenacillin A®, containing both procaine penicillin G and benzylpenicillin. The drug is dispensed in vials containing 1.5 g procaine penicillin and 300 mg benzylpenicillin sodium, and is reconstituted with 4.6 ml water for injections, the final volume being 6 ml. An intramuscular infection of 3 ml of Jenacillin is given daily for 10 days. If interruption of therapy for two to three days is necessary, for example, over a weekend, the long-acting penicillin Biclinocillin® (containing benethamine penicillin 1 MIU) may be given as a single intramuscular injection of 1.67 MIU[173] to maintain plasma and tissue penicillin

concentrations until the next dose of procaine penicillin*.

In the USA, benzathine penicillin 1.836 g (approximately equivalent to 1.44 g or 2.4 MIU of benzylpenicillin) given intramuscularly once is the treatment of choice for early syphilis[172]. When there are doubts about adherence to the treatment regimen, benzathine penicillin is also recommended in the UK but a second injection 7 days after the first is advised[173].

In the treatment of children with acquired syphilis, the adult dose of procaine penicillin can be given to those whose weight exceeds 25 kg. Proportionately lower doses should be given to children who weigh less than 25 kg. The dose of benzathine penicillin G is 50 000 units/kg by intramuscular injection, up to the adult dose of 2.4 MIU in a single dose[172].

A patient who has clinical evidence of neurological involvement or has uveitis or other ocular manifestations should be treated as for neurosyphilis (see pp. 436–437).

In early latent syphilis it is difficult to obtain direct information regarding the duration of the disease and it is advisable in cases of doubt to examine the CSF, because

---

* Neither benethamine penicillin nor benzathine penicillin are manufactured in the UK. Supplies may be obtained, however, from Laboratoires Clin Midi, 32–34 Rue Masbeuf, 75008, Paris, France.

when it is abnormal a diagnosis of asymptomatic neurosyphilis can be made, and treatment given as indicated below. Kern[164] in Berlin set the desirable duration of the long-acting penicillin course at 15 days in the case of all forms of early-stage syphilis and at 30 days for later stages.

Treatment of patients who refuse parenteral treatment

Amoxicillin in an oral dosage of 500 mg every 6 hours, given with probenecid 500 mg every 6 hours, is said to be effective in the treatment of early syphilis[174], and has been recommended for individuals who refuse parenteral therapy[173]. Oral antimicrobial agents that are useful in those who are hypersensitive to penicillin are possible alternatives (see below).

Treatment in patients who are hypersensitive to penicillin

In the treatment of men and non-pregnant women, doxycycline 100 mg or 200 mg, given as a single oral dose every 12 hours for 14 days has given promising results[175]. The higher dose is recommended so that plasma concentrations should not reach suboptimal concentrations should the patient miss a dose[173]. Although tetracycline hydrochloride, 500 mg four times a day by mouth for 14 days is recommended[172], patient adherence may be less than optimal, and the authors have discontinued the use of this agent in the treatment of syphilis. Children under the age of 8 years should not be given tetracyclines.

Ceftriaxone has been proposed as a useful alternative for the treatment of syphilis in those patients who are hypersensitive to penicillin. In the rabbit model of infectious syphilis, ceftriaxone has activity against *T. pallidum*[174a], and several trials involving small numbers of patients have shown that the drug is effective in the treatment of early syphilis[174b, 174c]. The optimal dose of ceftriaxone, however, has not been established. In treatment of primary syphilis, the dose reportedly used by American physicians varies between 2 g given by intramuscular or intravenous injection once daily for 2 to 10 days[174d]. These physicians use somewhat higher doses and longer duration of therapy in the treatment of secondary syphilis: 1–2 g once or twice daily for 3 to 21 days. It should be borne in mind that there is some cross-reactivity between the cephalosporins and the penicillins. About 8% of individuals with a history of hypersensitivity to penicillins have reactions to cephalosporins[174e].

Azithromycin has also been evaluated in the treatment of syphilis in those hypersensitive to penicillin. Successful treatment has been reported amongst patients given azithromycin in an oral dose of 500 mg, either daily or every other day, for 10 days[174f, 174g].

Satisfactory results have been obtained with erythromycin treatment of early syphilis[176]. The usual dose is 500 mg by mouth every 6 hours for 14 days[173].

These antibiotics appear to be effective, but results have been evaluated less fully than in the case of penicillin therapy. Clinical and serological follow-up are therefore very important.

Treatment of syphilis of more than 1 year's duration (latent syphilis of indeterminate duration or more than 1 year's duration, cardiovascular or late benign syphilis) except neurosyphilis

In patients who do not have neurosyphilis, Jenacillin (see above) is given daily as a 3 mL intramuscular injection for 17 to 21 days. Good results have been reported with this regimen[177].

In the USA, benzathine penicillin 1.836 g (approximately equivalent to 1.44 g or 2.4 MIU of benzylpenicillin) given intramuscularly weekly for 3 successive weeks is recommended by the Centers for Disease Control[172].

Optimal treatment schedules for syphilis of more than 1 year's duration are less well established than those for early syphilis. Cerebrospinal fluid examinations are mandatory in suspected symptomatic neurosyphilis and desirable in other patients with syphilis of more than 1 year's duration.

Treatment of cardiovascular syphilis with penicillin should take the form advised for late-stage syphilis (other than neurosyphilis) although objective evidence of cardiovascular improvement can seldom be obtained. None the less, such a course of treatment should be given and it should be remembered that neurosyphilis may co-exist with cardiovascular syphilis, when a longer course is advised. In surgery of aneurysm of the ascending aorta, a mortality rate as high as 40% may be expected. Resection of an aneurysm of the aortic arch is the most demanding operation in surgery and carries a very high mortality rate.

In coronary ostial stenosis surgical intervention can produce dramatic relief and although antibiotic treatment is given, as in other forms of cardiovascular syphilis, a decision about the advisability of surgery will require a cardiological assessment including a coronary angiogram.

Treatment of patients who are hypersensitive to penicillin or who refuse parenteral therapy

Alternative antibiotics recommended by the Centers for Disease Control, USA[172] are as follows.

- Doxycycline given in an oral dose of 100 mg every 12 hours for 28 days is satisfactory, but a twice daily dose of 200 mg is recommended in the UK National Guidelines[173]. The lower dosage regimen is probably adequate, but it is argued that the higher dose is just as well tolerated and allows better therapeutic safety if doses are missed.

- Tetracycline hydrochloride 500 mg four times daily by mouth for 30 days (oxytetracycline in the same dose may be used as an alternative to tetracycline.) Compliance may be difficult to ensure with this regimen – reattendance and successive issues of 1 week's treatment may assist in this regard. Examination of CSF and follow-up are important in patients being treated with these regimens as their efficacy in the long term is not yet clear.

- In those who refuse parenteral treatment, but who are not hypersensitive to penicillin, amoxicillin, given in an oral dose of 2 g every 8 hours plus probenecid 500 mg, also given orally, every 6 hours, both drugs being administered for 28 days. This recommendation by the Clinical Effectiveness Group[173] is supported by the experimental work reported by Morrison *et al.*[190]. Cure was effected in each of 7 infected rabbits given amoxicillin in an intravenous dosage of ≥ 0.1 mg/kg; this dose achieving a serum concentration of ≥ 0.11 mg/L. In the same study, 17 patients with latent syphilis were treated with amoxicillin 2 g three times per day, with probencid. Treponemicidal concentrations in the CSF were achieved after the third or fourth dose.

Treatment of neurosyphilis

Early diagnosis and the rapid institution of treatment are of prime importance in neurosyphilis. Results of treatment depend to a very great extent upon how much irreversible damage to the CNS has occurred before treatment has begun, and it is clear that any patient should be seen as a matter of urgency. For a long time it seemed that in neurosyphilis there was little evidence that more clinical benefit could be obtained by using doses higher than those recommended[178] or by giving benzylpenicillin rather than long-acting forms such as benzathine penicillin or procaine penicillin. Furthermore, Wilner and Brodie[179] found that in 40% of cases of general paresis treated with penicillin new neurological signs would develop subsequently after months or years. Such progression of disease occurred in the absence of deterioration in the CSF findings and was thought to be due to irreversible cerebrovascular damage before treatment, with further loss of neurons as a result of aging. Currently this explanation is under challenge, as is the practice of using long-acting or repository forms of penicillin in the treatment of neurosyphilis.

Some clinicians have never wholly relied upon long-acting forms of penicillin for treating neurosyphilis and now there is a strong movement in clinical practice in the USA, and elsewhere, to use specifically benzylpenicillin and, furthermore, to give it intravenously rather than intramuscularly. It is known that, although blood levels may be adequate and treponemicidal, penetration of penicillin into the CSF is poor. In normal circumstances about 0.2% to 2.0% of the blood concentration of penicillin is achieved, whereas in the presence of inflammation, as in the case of purulent meningitis, the ratio is higher namely 2.0% to 6.0%[180]. Mohr *et al.*[181] treated 13 patients with neurosyphilis with 2.754 g of benzathine penicillin (equivalent to 2.160 g or 3.6 MIU of benzylpenicillin) once-weekly for four weeks. In 12 patients there was no detectable penicillin in the CSF, while in 1 there was 0.1 mg/L CSF. Encouraging CSF values in 2 patients were obtained after giving 5 and 10 MIU (respectively 3.0 g and 6.0 g) benzylpenicillin daily intravenously. Ethical and practical difficulties surround the problem of conducting trials of treatment, and arguments for using intravenous penicillin tend to be based on pharmacological and bacteriological rather than clinical criteria for determining its effectiveness. Benzylpenicillin given intramuscularly fails to achieve a steady penicillin level, but when given in large doses by continuous intravenous (vena cava) infusion maintained by an automatic injection unit it was possible to do so[182]. By this means a serum level of 30 to 42 mg/L (50 000 to 70 000 units/L) was sufficient to maintain CSF levels of 1.8 to 3.0 mg/L (3000 to 5000 units/L). Ritter *et al.* thought that giving benzylpenicillin in doses of 12 g/4 h (20 MIU/4 h) – with an infusion time of 30 min each and a total dosage of 72 g/day (120 MIU/day) – over a period of several treponemal generation cycles (say 3 to 5 days) might prevent the high failure rates seen with 'insufficient' dosage of depot or long-acting forms of penicillin.

Tramont[183] reported the isolation of *T. pallidum* in rabbits inoculated with CSF from a patient who had been treated intramuscularly with 918 mg benzathine penicillin (approximately equivalent to 720 mg or 1.2 MIU benzylpenicillin) three times weekly for 3 weeks. After intravenous penicillin, however, subsequent attempts at isolation by the inoculation of CSF into rabbits were unsuccessful. Again, in a case of neurosyphilis[184], progressive deterioration occurred despite treatment with benzathine penicillin, but subsequently after intravenous therapy with high doses of benzylpenicillin both subjective and objective improvement occurred. In their study in Montreal, Ducas and Robson[185] found that in patients with latent syphilis – none of whom had evidence of neurosyphilis – none of the 18 cases treated weekly for 3 weeks with 1.836 g benzathine penicillin (approximately equivalent to 1.44 g or 2.4 MIU of benzylpenicillin) intramuscularly and only 2 of 15 given 3.672 g (approximately equivalent to 2.88 g or 4.8 MIU of benzylpenicillin) had adequate penicillin levels in the CSF. Probenecid 500 mg by mouth four times daily gave rise to problems in patient compliance and did not regularly produce CSF levels greater than 0.018 mg/L (30 units/L) CSF. As a result it was considered that benzathine penicillin should not be employed as a first-line agent in the treatment of neurosyphilis.

Unwanted effects of a high dosage of penicillin

A cautionary note is needed. A number of individuals have received benzylpenicillin intravenously in doses of 24 to 48 g (40 to 80 MIU) daily for as long as 4 weeks without untoward effects, but parenteral administration of benzylpenicillin in daily doses of more than 12 g (20 MIU), or less in the case of those patients with renal insufficiency, may produce confusion, twitching, multifocal myoclonus, or generalized epileptiform seizures. These are most apt to occur in the presence of localized central nervous system lesions, hypo-natremia, or renal insufficiency. When concentration of benzylpenicillin in the CSF exceeds 10 mg/L significant dysfunction of the central nervous system is frequent. The injection of 12 g (20 MIU) of benzyl-penicillin potassium which contains 34 mmol of potassium may lead to severe or even fatal hyperkalemia in persons with renal dysfunction[163]. Risks, also, of hemolytic anemia developing in those given benzylpenicillin intravenously in doses of about 6 g or more should be considered[186].

Probenecid

The proposition that probenecid may be used in neurosyphilis requires consideration. Fishman's data from experiments in dogs[187] supported the theory of the existence of a transport system close to the CSF, presumably in the choroid plexus, that actively transports organic acids, such as penicillin, from the CSF. Probenecid achieves higher CSF levels of penicillin by

1. raising the blood level
2. inhibiting the active transport of penicillin from CSF
3. increasing the diffusible penicillin in plasma by competition for binding to serum protein.

Probenecid may actually interfere with the accumulation of penicillin in the brain tissue; in Fishman's experiments in rats there was evidence of competition between penicillin and probenecid for entry into the brain. The suggestion is that probenecid may achieve higher CSF and blood levels but may not necessarily be a useful adjunct in the treatment of bacterial infection of the nervous system. The special permeability characteristics of the brain depend upon the net transfer characteristics of multiple complex membranes, that constitute the cerebral capillaries, glia, and neurons, and on brain metabolism which serves also to stabilize neuronal environments[187].

Penicillin therapy in neurosyphilis: recommendations in current practice

In the UK procaine penicillin given in a daily dosage of 1.8 to 2.4 g (1.8 to 2.4 MIU) by intramuscular injection, plus probenecid 500 mg by mouth every

6 hours, for 17 to 21 days is the preferred treatment[173]. This regimen has been shown to produce treponemicidal concentrations of penicillin in the CSF[188]. An alternative regimen is intravenous benzyl-penicillin*, 1.8 to 2.4 g (3 to 4 MIU) every 4 hours for 17 to 21 days.

The United States Centers for Disease Control[172] guidelines give two potentially effective regimens, none of which has been adequately studied, these are

1. benzylpenicillin 1.8 to 2.4 g (3 to 4 MIU) intravenously every 4 hours for 10 to 14 days
2. procaine penicillin 2.378 g (approximately equivalent to 1.44 g or 2.4 MIU benzylpenicillin) intramuscularly once daily plus probenecid 500 mg by mouth 4 times daily, both for 10 to 14 days.

After completion of these drug regimens, many physicians administer a single intramuscular injection of benzathine penicillin 1.836 g (approximately equivalent to 1.44 g or 2.4 MIU benzylpenicillin).

As treponemicidal concentrations are consistently obtained by the oral administration of doxycyline and amoxicillin[189, 190], the following regimens are considered as second-line therapies for neurosyphilis[173]

1. doxycycline 200 mg by mouth every 12 hours for 28 days
2. amoxicillin 2 g by mouth every 8 hours plus probenecid 500 mg every 6 hours, both given for 28 days.

Ceftriaxone, given in a daily intramuscular or intravenous dose of 2 g for 10 to 14 days, has been recommended as an alternative treatment for neurosyphilis[172]. However, when ceftriaxone was administered intramuscularly to 8 rabbits infected with *T. pallidum*, viable organisms were recovered from the brain of one animal[190a].

---

* Benzylpenicillin for Injection BP (either as benzylpenicillin sodium or benzylpenicillin potassium) is prepared by dissolving the sterile contents of the sealed container in the required amount of water for injections. Intravenous doses above 1.2 g (2 MIU) should be administered slowly at a rate of not more than 300 mg/min to avoid irritation of the CNS. A slow intravenous infusion technique with very high doses over the 3 to 5-day period described by Ritter *et al.*[182] is an approach which requires further study.

The significance for human infection of this finding is uncertain.

A Jarisch–Herxheimer reaction with pyrexia occurs in over 90% of patients with general paresis with grossly abnormal CSFs but in other forms of neurosyphilis it is much less frequent (less than 40%). Clinical reactions are of special importance in general paresis when 10% of patients may be expected to develop a sudden intensification of somatic or psychotic symptoms (convulsions, coma, focal vascular accidents, excitement, confusion, mania, hallucinations or paranoid delusions)[191].

The complications of neurosyphilis may be managed as follows.

Meningitis

Where there is a labyrinthitis, prednisolone in a high initial dosage together with penicillin is justified as an attempt to reduce the chance of an irreversible deafness[141].

Tabes dorsalis

This condition is rare and may present in an incomplete form. In some patients the disease is recognized as a result of a chance medical examination or because the patient has sought advice for ataxia or lightning pains. Treatment with penicillin sometimes appears to halt the progress but deterioration often occurs in spite of treatment. Lightning pains, tabetic crises, bladder dysfunction, Charcot's arthropathy, and optic atrophy, may progress after treatment. In the follow-up of a case of tabes dorsalis there are particular points to consider. The paroxysmal painful disorders of visceral function known as crises can be cut short by an injection of pethidine hydrochloride 100 mg, but this and other potentially addictive drugs should be avoided unless absolutely essential. In the case of a gastric crisis the patient should be endoscoped since the failure to diagnose a gastric ulcer in a tabetic may be more disastrous for the patient than to mistake an organic lesion of the stomach for a gastric crisis. In severe recurrent cases benefit has followed section of lower thoracic spinal dorsal roots[192]. The loss of circulatory reflexes and orthostatic hypotension may result from interruption on the afferent side of the

reflex arc from baroreceptors as part of the deep sensory loss characteristic of tabes. Such patients learn that they can rise to their feet only slowly if they are to avoid fainting but few have more than an occasional loss of consciousness. Tabetic pains can be controlled sometimes by analgesics although the assessment of the value of individual drugs in the relief of the characteristic lightning pains is notoriously difficult in this now rare condition. In some cases analgesics are effective and their use should follow the principles of analgesic medication. If the antipyretic analgesic, acetyl salicylic acid (as aspirin soluble tablets) in a dose of 0.6 g (up to 0.9 g) every 4 to 6 hours is ineffective or unsuitable because of gastrointestinal side effects, paracetamol 0.5 g repeated every 4 to 6 hours may be tried. Mefenamic acid in a total daily dose of 1.0 g (each capsule contains 250 mg) may be used as an alternative; repeated changes within this group will delay tolerance and minimize side effects. If the pains are very intense, one of the weak narcotics, dihydrocodeine tablets BP in an oral dose of 30 mg can be tried, or alternatively the narcotic antagonist with analgesic activity, pentazocine (as tablets BP) in the oral dose of 25 to 50 mg may be given after food.

The pains of tabes are paroxysmal, brief, and often very intense and this similarity to the pains of trigeminal neuralgia suggested the use of carbamazepine. It appeared to be effective when given as an initial dose of 200 mg twice daily, increasing to a maximum maintenance dose of 400 to 800 mg daily[193].

In tabes the bladder becomes atonic and distended because there is damage to the posterior roots and ganglia which gives loss of both deep pain and deep postural sensation including that of the bladder. If there is no evidence of hydronephrosis the patient should be instructed to empty the bladder every 3 hours during the day by the clock, before retiring and again early in the morning. Precipitancy of micturition may be relieved by propantheline 15 mg three times daily[192]. Attempts may be made to empty an atonic bladder by giving an anticholine-sterase (for example distigmine bromide 5 mg by mouth half an hour before breakfast or by an intramuscular injection of 0.5 mg for the first few days), or by reducing the resistance at the bladder neck with a transurethral resection. Manual compression can be dangerous as more urine may pass up the ureter than is expelled. When renal function is impaired, or there is urinary infection which has failed to respond to chemotherapy, surgery may be necessary[192]. Permanent drainage with a urethral or suprapubic catheter may be advised or the urine can be diverted to the skin. Urine must not be diverted into the colon in tabes as it will leak from the anus that is supplied by the same nerve roots as the bladder.

In Charcot's arthropathy attempts are made to reduce the weight carried by the joint and improve its stability. Various calipers are available for the patient to use while walking. Perforating ulcers should be prevented by wearing well-fitting socks and shoes and by careful treatment of corns on the feet. When ulcers do develop, rest, clean dressings, and antibiotic treatment may aid healing .

Ataxia may be improved by careful exercises to give confidence, supervised by a physiotherapist.

Optic atrophy

Acute optic neuritis in secondary syphilis will respond well to penicillin and the visual prognosis is good when there is acute visual loss. In optic atrophy the prognosis is poor although prednisone 30 to 60 mg daily with penicillin therapy may be given in an attempt to halt its progress. The help of an ophthalmologist should be sought in all such cases.

TREATMENT OF SYPHILIS DURING PREGNANCY

In localities where the number of reported cases of transplacental (congenital) syphilis are more than very rare the antenatal care, with regular serological testing, of pregnant women is a matter of major importance and will enable the eradication of congenital syphilis.

Procaine penicillin or benzathine penicillin are recommended for pregnant women in dosages appropriate for the stage of syphilis.

Pregnant women should be followed up carefully clinically and have monthly quantitative cardiolipin antigen serological tests, preferably the VDRL, for the remainder of the current pregnancy. A fourfold rise in titer is an indication for retreatment.

It is the authors' practice to give a single 10-day course of procaine penicillin during early pregnancy in any patient who has had syphilis, even if adequately treated in the past. This 'insurance course' is justified on the grounds that treponemes appear to persist in the host in spite of treatment and might be transmitted transplacentally. It is difficult, however, to test the validity of this argument and doubtful whether it is ethical to do so if it brings a risk of transmission to the fetus.

Alternative antibiotic therapy in pregnant women with a history of hypersensitivity to penicillin

As a general rule patients giving a history of allergy to penicillin should be treated with an antibiotic of a different type. In those gravid women allergic to penicillin, tetracyclines should not be used.

Erythromycin has been offered as a suitable alternative to penicillin and may be given in an oral dose of 500 mg four times daily for 20 days[194]. It is recommended that all babies born to women so treated should be treated at birth[173]. With oral erythromycin serum levels may be unsatisfactory and even after multiple maternal doses the average fetal blood level may only be 0.06 µg/mL. As placental transfer is unpredictable and the problem of patient compliance very serious, the evidence suggests that oral erythromycin is not a good agent in the treatment of *in utero* syphilis[195]. South *et al.*[196] first recorded this problem in a pregnant woman who was treated for secondary syphilis with erythromycin estolate in an oral dose of 500 mg three times daily for 10 days; her syphilis was apparently controlled but the infant had severe congenital syphilis. In view of the unpredictable placental transfer of erythromycin during treatment of the pregnant woman for syphilis with this antibiotic, full treatment of the infant with penicillin, beginning at birth, is an essential

precaution[195, 172] and it is clear that admission to hospital is desirable to ensure that the prescribed dosage is in fact taken at the required intervals.

Erthromycin treatment is no longer recommended by the Centers for Disease Control and Prevention[172]. Another option, however, that has been recommended by the Clinical Effectiveness Group[173] is the use of azithromycin, in a daily dosage of 500 mg for 10 days, *and* treatment of the neonate at birth.

As there are insufficient data on efficacy of treatment of pregnant women with azithromycin or ceftriaxone, the Centers for Disease Control and Prevention[172] do not currently recommend these agents for use in this setting. Their recommendation is that women who have a history of penicillin allergy should be desensitised and treated with penicillin (see below).

Desensitization

In the case of syphilis in the pregnant woman who gives a history of hypersensitivity to penicillin, treatment is problematic. Treatment with erythromycin may control the infection in the gravid patient but it may fail to prevent or cure the infection in her fetus.

Type 1 hypersensitivity reactions (anaphylactic sensitivity) to penicillin are very rare indeed and occur in about 3 in every 100 000 cases, with fatalities in less than 2 in every 100 000. The rare and fatal reactions occur mainly in those known to have had a prior reaction to penicillin or an allergic diathesis[197]. In unusual instances where treatment with penicillin is essential, skin tests may be of some help[198]. The question of management of the patient who gives a history of penicillin hypersensitivity has been addressed by the staff and experts of the United States Centers for Disease Control[172]. The following discussion is based on their deliberations.

With the passage of time after a hypersensitivity reaction to penicillin, most individuals cease to produce specific IgE and can safely be given the drug. About 10% of people, however, remain hypersensitive. Skin testing with the major and minor antigenic determinants (Appendix 15.1) can reliably identify individuals who are at high risk, and if testing has yielded negative results, penicillin therapy can be given. Skin test-positive patients should be desensitized (Appendix 15.2).

If negative results are obtained in testing with only the major determinant, benzylpenicilloyl poly-L-lysine (Pre-Pen, Taylor Pharmacal Company, Decatur, IL) and penicillin G (the only reagents available commercially), reactions may still occur (up to 10% of hypersensitive patients fail to be identified unless the minor determinants are included in the test system). Caution must therefore be exercised in giving penicillin to patients who have negative reactions with limited testing, and it has been suggested that these individuals should be considered as hypersensitive and desensitized before receiving full-dose treatment (Appendix 15.2). Others propose that those with a negative skin test can be test dosed gradually with oral penicillin in hospital.

The problem is not, however, wholly solved.

TREATMENT OF CONGENITAL SYPHILIS

In addition to the treatment of infants with clinical features of syphilis at birth, the Centers for Disease Control[172] recommend treatment if the child is born to a mother who meets certain criteria (Box 15.2). If there is clinical or serological evidence of syphilis the Centers for Disease Control advise that the CSF should be examined before treatment, and a full blood count should be obtained to provide a baseline for follow-up. Regardless of the CSF results, children should be treated with a regimen effective for neurosyphilis. The regimens recommended are as follows

1. Benzylpenicillin 60–90 mg (100 000–150 000 units) per kg body weight intravenously daily in two divided doses of 30 mg for the first 7 days of life, and 30 mg (50 000 units) per kg every 8 hours thereafter for a total of 10 days, or

2. Procaine penicillin G 49.55 mg (approximately equivalent to 30 mg or 50 000 units benzylpenicillin) per kg body weight intramuscularly daily in single dose for 10 to 14 days.

Box 15.2 Maternal characteristics that suggest the necessity to treat the infant (Centers for Disease Control 2002[172])

The mother:

had untreated syphilis at delivery

had serological evidence of a relapse or re-infection after treatment

was treated with a non-penicillin-containing regimen during pregnancy

was treated for syphilis within 1 month of delivery

did not have a well-documented history of treatment for syphilis

was treated for syphilis during pregnancy with the appropriate penicillin regimen, but cardiolipin antibody titers did not decrease fourfold

was treated appropriately before pregnancy but had insufficient serological follow-up to ensure an adequate treatment response and lack of current infection.

After the neonatal period (i.e. at more than one month of age) benzylpenicillin should be used in a dosage of 120–180 mg (200 000–300 000 units) per kg per day given by intravenous infusion 50 000 units/kg every 4 to 6 hours[172]. Alternatively, procaine penicillin can be given in the same dosage as that used in infection in the first month of life[173]. If hypersensitive to penicillin, the child should be desensitised. Tetracyclines should not be used in children under 8 years of age.

Treatment, however, does not prevent the development or course of interstitial keratitis, hydrarthrosis, and neural deafness.

Management of interstitial keratitis

Patients with interstitial keratitis should be managed in hospital, in consultation with an ophthalmologist.

Topically applied corticosteroids rapidly suppress the inflammatory reaction in the cornea and anterior uveal tract, and their use, until spontaneous cure occurs, has

revolutionized the management of this condition. Although the infiltration of the cornea by inflammatory cells resolves, scarring from previous episodes of keratitis is not affected.

Betamethasone eye drops, 0.1%, instilled into the affected eye(s) every 1 to 2 hours, is a useful preparation. Treatment should be continued until the corneal inflammatory infiltrate has cleared, and visual acuity restored to the patient's normal level. Slit-lamp examination is essential before steroid treatment is discontinued, as mild degrees of keratitis may not otherwise be apparent. Regular examination is required after cessation of treatment, as corneal scarring may result from continuing mild inflammation.

During steroid treatment, mydriatics such as atropine eye drops 1%, may be useful adjuvants by reducing ciliary muscle tension.

Corneal grafting may be required in patients with corneal scarring acquired during attacks of interstitial keratitis.

Management of hydrarthrosis (Clutton's joints)

This is a self-limiting disorder and does not require any specific therapy.

Management of nerve deafness

Despite previous treatment of congenital syphilis with what have been regarded as adequate doses of penicillin, progressive neural deafness may develop at any age, but most commonly in the adult of middle age. This may be the result of failure of the drug to reach adequate concentrations in the perilymph or endolymph.

Morrison[160] advocated the use of benzylpenicillin in a dosage of 300 mg (500 000 units) given by intramuscular injection every 6 hours for 17 days, together with probenecid in a dose of 1 g every 6 hours by mouth. During the first week of treatment, 30 mg of prednisone is given orally, the dose thereafter being reduced to 25 mg daily for 3 weeks. As a response to treatment is seen within the first month, treatment may be discontinued if there has been no improvement at that time. When the response has been satisfactory, steroids may be continued for 3 to 6 months in gradually diminishing doses. A further course of penicillin is then given. Occasionally patients have required maintenance treatment with low doses of steroids to abolish vertigo and maintain hearing.

Ampicillin in a dosage of 1.5 g every 6 hours for 4 weeks, together with prednisolone 30 mg daily for 10 days, tailing off over the succeeding 10 days has been used in the management of this condition[199].

Audiometry may give useful information regarding response to treatment. The value of treatment has not been fully assessed. In some cases the disease process may be arrested, but in others improvement in hearing may only be temporary.

In advanced cases where there has been considerable tissue damage, however, no response to medical treatment occurs.

TREATMENT ON EPIDEMIOLOGICAL GROUNDS

Patients who have clearly been exposed to infectious syphilis and who are not likely to cease sexual intercourse for 3 months, or to attend for surveillance, should be considered on epidemiological grounds for treatment and followed up; the regimen advised is that for early syphilis. It is the authors' practice to treat couples such as husband and wife simultaneously if possible, if one partner develops early syphilis. Every effort is made, however, in such cases to establish a diagnosis beforehand.

In the case of early-stage syphilis immediate treatment for the infected person or 'epidemiologic' treatment for potentially infected contacts will interrupt a possible chain of infection. Although about one-third of recently exposed persons will develop syphilis and two-thirds will not, the United States Public Health Service has advocated 'epidemiologic' treatment (preventive) of all contacts because of the inability to identify quickly those who will develop the disease[200]. The Centers for Disease Control[172] guidelines recommend that those exposed to infectious syphilis within the preceding 3 months and those who, on epidemiological grounds are at high risk for early syphilis should be treated as for early.

Response to treatment and assessment of cure

RESPONSE TO TREATMENT

Penicillin in a sufficient dosage causes disappearance of *T. pallidum* from early surface lesions within 6 to 26 hours[166]. Infectivity appears to be lost very soon and lesions heal often within a few days. Obvious induration, depth, size, and number of lesions will vary in relation to the duration of the disease and healing may be correspondingly longer. The infection can no longer be transmitted by sexual contact and relapse after adequate treatment is exceedingly rare, recurrences usually being caused by re-infection.

Cardiolipin antigen tests

Because there is no microbiological 'test for cure' patients treated for syphilis are assessed by serial quantitative cardiolipin antigen tests such as the VDRL/RPR[93]. All cardiolipin antigen tests tend to become negative after treatment, particularly in early syphilis while the rate of decline in titer depends on the stage of infection, the initial titer, and the history of previous syphilis[93]. In interpreting a fall or rise in titer a fourfold change is considered significant but a twofold change is not. It has been suggested that in primary and secondary syphilis the titer should decline approximately fourfold in 3 months and eightfold in 6 months[201]. Others considered these criteria too stringent and suggested that a fourfold decline by 6 months and an eightfold decline by 12 months was acceptable[202]. In early latent syphilis the decrease was only fourfold at 12 months[202]. The mean period of reactivity after treatment is 4 months for primary syphilis, 17 months for secondary, 13 months for early latent disease and 60 months for latent infection of indeterminate duration[48]. After adequate treatment of late infection the VDRL test will show a slow decline in titer, some cases eventually becoming negative while others may remain reactive (titer < 16) for many years. Ideally, all follow-up tests should be performed in the same laboratory, by the same method, and using reagents from the

same manufacturer. There is no satisfactory method of assessing efficacy of treatment in the infections with a negative VDRL/RPR test.

Anti-treponemal IgM

An appreciable decrease in specific IgM may be interpreted as evidence of therapeutic success[48]: of the various methods of detecting anti-treponemal IgM described earlier, reactivity in the 19S (IgM)-FTA-abs provides the most reliable correlation with treatment status in all stages of infection[203]. Effective treatment is indicated by a negative 19S (IgM)-FTA-abs test: within 3 months of the beginning of treatment in cases of early syphilis, and within 12 to 18 months of the beginning of treatment in cases of late disease. Unfortunately experience with the 19S (IgM)-FTA-abs test is restricted to a very few laboratories. Although IgM detected by the Captia M® declined after treatment, EIA was not recommended as a replacement for the VDRL test to monitor patients treated for syphilis[204].

Activity of infection

Only the rabbit infectivity test described earlier gives categorical proof of active infection. Normally the clinician must rely on guidance from quantitative VDRL/RPR and specific IgM tests although in future molecular approaches may be helpful.

The Centers for Disease Control[172] guidelines advise that quantitative non-treponemal tests should be taken 6 and 12 months after treatment. If the disease is of more than 1 year's duration, serological tests for syphilis should be repeated 24 months afterwards. Follow-up, possibly for life, is especially important in patients treated with antibiotics other than penicillin, and the CSF should be examined about 1 year after completion of treatment with alternative antibiotics.

Re-infection with syphilis is a possibility, particularly in those who have multiple casual sexual relationships. Neither the humoral or cell-mediated immune responses that occur during an initial infection with *T. pallidum* give rise to protective immunity and when syphilis was prevalent re-infection was common. During re-infection VDRL/RPR titers are consistently higher than during the corresponding stage of the first infection, and the serological responses to treatment are always slower. Demonstration of a reproducible fourfold increase in VDRL/RPR titer is the normal laboratory method of diagnosing re-infection or clinical relapse. Because antibody levels may be particularly high in re-infection the possibility of false negative reactions due to the prozone phenomenon should be kept in mind. A positive anti-treponemal IgM result in the serum of a patient previously IgM negative also supports re-infection. Although the 19S (IgM)-FTA-abs has reasonable sensitivity in re-infection (87%) that of the Captia Syphilis M® is poor (57%)[97].

Patients should be retreated if

- cardiolipin antibody titers increase fourfold
- an initially high titer (≥ 32) fails to decline at least fourfold within 12 to 24 months
- symptoms or signs of syphilis develop in the patient.

In cases where retreatment is thought to be necessary, a CSF examination should be carried out before retreatment unless re-infection and a diagnosis of early syphilis is clearly established.

Abstinence from sexual intercourse is advised in a patient being treated for early syphilis until the disease cannot be transmitted. This is usually achieved within a few days, but it is wise for the patient to abstain until after the course of antibiotic when all lesions will be healed, and possibly for 1 month after treatment if resumption of intercourse with an uninfected partner is to take place. If one partner is infected and has put the other at risk simultaneous treatment of both is advisable as re-infection of the treated by the untreated can occur. Such treatment on epidemiological grounds in a person at very high risk will call for the same follow-up and assessment of cure as in the patient in whom a diagnosis is established.

Follow-up and prognosis of neurosyphilis

The Centers for Disease Control[172] recommend follow-up after treatment with periodic quantitative cardiolipin tests (e.g.

VDRL), clinical evaluation and a repeat CSF examination every 6 months until the cell count is normal. If the cell count has not decreased after 6 months, or if the CSF is not entirely normal after 2 years, retreatment is advised. Changes in the cardiolipin antibody titers in the CSF are slower to resolve and are of less use in assessing the need for retreatment.

The prognosis and follow up after treatment depend upon the type of neurosyphilis[178] and the amount of permanent damage caused before treatment is started.

Syphilitic meningitis

With the predominantly meningeal involvement which occurs in early-stage syphilis beyond the primary stage, treatment is very effective. When there is an acute labyrinthitis with eighth cranial nerve dysfunction recovery may be slow and deafness can persist. Recovery from other meningitic effects is usual.

Meningovascular neurosyphilis

In late-stage meningovascular neurosyphilis the effects are caused by foci of ischemia due to the syphilitic arteritis, and although there is often considerable recovery after penicillin and an arrest of the disease process, ischemic effects will persist and together with gliosis will cause persistent focal neurological effects such as aphasia, hemiplegia, and cranial nerve involvement. In patients with predominantly psychiatric disorders differentiation from other psychosis is most important. Early treatment produces often remarkable improvement, but complete recovery is not to be expected.

General paresis (dementia paralytica, general paralysis of the insane)

Early diagnosis and the rapid institution of treatment are vital. In patients who have an acute onset of symptoms and are seen within weeks, treatment can be spectacular in its effect. Patients have been able to resume the practice of a profession within weeks of treatment and have remained efficient subsequently.

In those with a greater degree of damage recovery is often remarkable and

the patients will feel much better, wishing to return to work as soon as possible. Sometimes their enthusiasm is not matched by the return of their intellectual ability, and psychological assessment is a necessary prelude to retraining for an occupation requiring less intellectual effort and less responsibility.

In patients who have become demented over a few years, and in whom the disease has presented with a more insidious course, there is often a serious loss of cortical neurons. Although treatment will arrest part of the disease process new signs of neurological disease may develop in a third of patients[179] and these signs of progression do not seem to be limited by further courses of penicillin or by larger amounts of this antibiotic. The new signs described include grand-mal epilepsy, hand paraplegia, hemiparesis, amyotrophy, tabes dorsalis, optic atrophy, or oculomotor palsy

Follow-up of cardiovascular syphilis

In uncomplicated syphilitic aortitis, diagnosed on the detection of dilatation of the aorta in the absence of aortic incompetence, there is no appreciable threat to life during the first 7 years after the discovery. Progression to aortic incompetence occurs in about a third of patients within 4 years, and the quantity of penicillin treatment given does not appear to influence these changes.

The progression of uncomplicated aortitis to aortic incompetence is not certainly halted by antibiotic treatment. Compensation for aortic regurgitation is so efficient that patients may live for many years with minimal symptoms such as an awareness of the heaving cardiac impulse in bed or transient dizziness following sudden changes in posture. Failure of compensation is indicated by angina and shortness of breath. As life expectancy is so good and the long-term effects of valve replacement are still unpredictable, physicians may be reluctant to refer patients for surgery until they develop symptoms. This excessive conservatism has its disadvantages as the results of surgery will be adversely affected if the operation is deferred until the ventricle has become irreparably damaged.

Treatment on epidemiological grounds

Patients who have clearly been exposed to infectious syphilis and who are not likely to cease sexual intercourse for three months, or to attend for surveillance, should be considered on epidemiological grounds for treatment and followed up; the regimen advised is that for early syphilis. It is our practice to treat couples such as husband and wife simultaneously, if possible, if one partner develops early syphilis. Every effort is made, however, to establish a diagnosis beforehand in such cases.

In the case of early-stage syphilis immediate treatment for the infected person or 'epidemiologic' treatment for potentially infected contacts will interrupt a possible chain of infection. Although about one-third of recently exposed persons will develop syphilis and two-thirds will not, the United States Public Health Service has advocated 'epidemiologic' treatment (preventive) of all contacts because of the inability to identify quickly those who will develop the disease[200]. The Centers for Disease Control[172] guidelines recommend that those exposed to infectious syphilis within the preceding three months and those who, on epidemiological grounds, are at high risk for early syphilis should be treated as for early infection.

JARISCH–HERXHEIMER REACTION

The Jarisch–Herxheimer reaction (JHR) is a complication that usually follows within a day of the initial treatment of a number of organismal diseases, including syphilis, it is characterized by fever and an aggravation of existing lesions together with their attendant symptoms and signs.

In 1895 Jarisch recorded the fact that the spots of roseolar syphilis became clearer and more numerous after treatment with mercury. Later, in 1902, Herxheimer and Krause pointed out that the reaction followed soon after an adequate dose of mercury and was accompanied by a rise in temperature. The reaction is generally confined to the first day of treatment and it occurs also after treatment with antibiotics such as penicillin; it can be evoked twice in the same patient if the first injection of penicillin is only 1 020 units per kg body weight[208]. The JHR develops in about 55% of cases of VDRL-negative primary syphilis, also in 95% of patients with general paralysis of the insane – in those with high CSF cell counts, the JHR may be expected to occur after treatment when there may be exacerbation of mental signs or symptoms. Generally no reaction is noted following treatment of very early and late-stage latent syphilis. The JHR may occur in early-stage congenital syphilis, most frequently in children under the age of 6 months, but is rare after treatment of late-stage congenital syphilis.

The salient features of the JHR are as follows[209].

1. A rise and then a fall in body temperature, the rise is accompanied by a chill and the fall by sweating.
2. Aggravation of pre-existing lesions and their attendant symptoms and signs, for example flaring of the rash in syphilis, and acute myocarditis in louse-borne relapsing fever.
3. Characteristic physiological changes which include early vasoconstriction, hyperventilation, and a rise in blood pressure and cardiac output, and later a fall in blood pressure associated with a low peripheral resistance.

The cause of the JHR is not completely understood. In 1895 Jarisch postulated that the cause of the reaction was a toxin liberated from degenerating treponemes, but it was not until 1961 that endotoxin-like activity was detected in a spirochete, *Borrelia vincentii*, and only in 1973 was a lipopolysaccharide, resembling that of Gram-negative organisms, identified in *T. pallidum*[210]. In louse-borne relapsing fever, due to *Borrelia recurrentis*, the JHR is much more severe than in syphilis and Bryceson et al.[209] found that in 1 case out of the 4 examined, the plasma taken from a patient during the JHR induced fever 60 minutes after transfusion into that patient on the following day. In addition endotoxin has been detected by the limulus amoebo-cyte lysate assay in the plasma of patients at the time they were undergoing the JHR and this was accompanied by depression of the third component of complement[211]. It has been shown that *T. pallidum* bears proteolipids that can induce the synthesis of tumor necrosis factor-α (TNF-α)[212]. These proteolipids use a signaling pathway that is somewhat distinct from that used by lipopolysaccharides and that may not be susceptible to glucocorticoid suppression. Recent studies[213] have shown that after initiation of therapy for louse-borne relapsing fever, the plasma concentrations of the cytokines, TNF-α, interleukin-6 (IL-6), and interleukin-8 (IL-8) rise transiently, coinciding with the pathophysiological changes.

In neurosyphilis exacerbation of signs may occur in patients treated with penicillin and this may resemble, but be less severe than, the reactive encephalopathy seen in patients with *Trypanosoma brucei rhodesiense* or *T. b. gambiense* meningoencephalitis treated with melarsoprol. In neither general paralysis of the insane nor in secondary syphilis, however, are these JHRs as severe as in louse-borne relapsing fever. In a number of instances a possible flare up of local lesions is feared, as for example in acute labyrinthitis of early syphilis when irreversible deafness is a threat[141]. In the now rare gummata of the brain and larynx, which contain numerous treponemes, treatment has proved on occasions fatal. In local lesions of the aorta involving the coronary ostia a JHR may have serious consequences.

The late lesions of syphilis described are now rare in western countries. The use of prednisolone in high initial dosage is advised on rather limited evidence in acute labyrinthitis and may be considered, again on limited evidence of its efficacy, in late forms of disease where exacerbation of local inflammation is feared. In the louse-borne relapsing fever model of the JHR, high-dose hydrocortisone infused before and during the JHR reduced the patient's baseline temperature but did not mitigate the febrile, physiological, or local inflammatory features of the JHR in any way[214]. The clinical value of steroids remains unproven. The use of polyclonal antibody against TNF-α to ameliorate the JHR has been assessed in a randomized, double-blind placebo-controlled clinical trial in patients with louse-borne relapsing fever treated with penicillin. Compared with control subjects, the peak plasma concentrations of IL-6 and IL-8, and the incidence of the reaction was reduced[215]. Adverse effects of TNF blocking, however, outweigh its usefulness[216]. Interleukin-10 inhibits the production of interferon-γ, inhibits antigen presentation and macrophage production of IL-1, IL-6, and TNF-α, and might be expected to have a role in the treatment of cytokine-associated inflammatory conditions, including the JHR. A recent study in patients treated for louse-borne relapsing fever, however, failed to show any effect on cytokine concentrations or on the physiological changes associated with the reaction[217].

Clinical phases of the Jarisch–Herxheimer reaction

There are four clinical phases, and the effects are greatest in secondary syphilis and in general paralysis of the insane. In primary syphilis the effects are usually mild. The reaction develops within 4 hours of starting treatment, becomes most intense at 6 to 8 hours and resolves within 24 hours.

The clinical phases are

1. a prodromal phase with aches and pains
2. rigor or chill, when the patient's temperature rises by an average of 1°C (range 0.2 to 2.7°C) 4 to 8 hours after treatment
3. flush, the temperature reaches a peak, usually at about 8 hours after the first injection, and is associated with hypotension
4. defervescence, which lasts up to 12 hours.

Other clinical and physiological observations

The patient may feel discomfort in the local lesions, which become more pronounced and show an acute transient inflammatory reaction. Histologically it is found that neutrophil and mononuclear cells appear and migrate through the swollen vascular endothelium into the surrounding edematous tissue.

There is a leukocytosis and a fall in the lymphocyte count. The metabolic rate is increased and peaks with the rigor. Pulmonary ventilation and cardiac output exceed metabolic requirements and pulmonary oxygen uptake is impaired.

During the rigor phase there is early hyperventilation; the systemic arterial blood pressure rises due to vasoconstriction, but falls in the flush phase due to a decrease in vascular resistance as a result of vasodilatation.

The reaction to specific treatment, whether antibiotic or not, is seen in diseases other than syphilis, namely in louse-borne relapsing fever, rat-bite fever, leptospirosis, yaws, brucellosis, tularemia, glanders, anthrax, and in African trypanosomiasis, particularly in that due to *Trypanosoma brucei rhodesiense*. In relapsing fever and leptospirosis the reaction is much more severe than in syphilis, and it can be fatal.

Between 40% and 67% of pregnant women who have a JHR after initiation of penicillin treatment for syphilis, develop uterine contractions and decreased fetal movement. These events coincide with the onset of fever and usually abate within 16 to 24 hours[218, 219]. In about 40% of these women, recurrent, variable decelerations of the fetal heart rate are observed. In the reported series, however, none of the women required delivery at the time of treatment, but if the fetus is severely affected, preterm labor or fetal death may occur[218]. Fewer than 1% of infants treated for presumed congenital syphilis develop a JHR[34].

ADVERSE EFFECTS OF PENICILLIN

Penicillins are virtually non-toxic in the doses discussed, but by far the most serious reactions are due to hypersensitivity – Type 1 anaphylactic sensitivity – and penicillin is one of the most common causes of this and other forms of hypersensitivity.

Anaphylactic reactions may occur at any age. Their incidence is thought to be 0.04% to 0.2% of patients treated with penicillins, and about 0.001% of patients treated may die from anaphylaxis, most often following *injection* of penicillin. Anaphylaxis has also been observed after oral ingestion of the drug and has even resulted from the intradermal instillation of a very small quantity for the purpose of testing for the presence of hypersensitivity. There appears to be no completely safe and reliable practical method of detecting sensitivity to penicillin, but inquiry concerning reactions to previous treatment should always be made. Patients who suffer from sensitivities to other agents are more liable to react adversely to penicillin, and sensitivity induced by one penicillin may lead to similar reactions to others. Reactions include skin rashes of all types, fever, arthralgia, lymphadenopathy, stomatitis, and glossitis, but Type 1 hypersensitivity (anaphylactic reaction) with severe hypotension and rapid death is the most dramatic and sudden. Bronchospasm with severe asthma, or abdominal pain, nausea, and vomiting, or extreme weakness and fall in blood pressure, or diarrhea and purpuric skin eruptions have characterized anaphylactic episodes in other instances[163].

Occasionally very serious reactions and even death, occurring during or shortly after an injection of penicillin, may result from accidental intravenous injection with subsequent pulmonary embolism. Some of these reactions may simulate anaphylaxis. Injection of procaine penicillin may result in an immediate reaction, characterized by dizziness, tinnitus, headache, hallucinations, and sometimes seizures. This is caused by the rapid liberation of toxic concentrations of procaine[197]. It has been reported to occur in 1 of 200 patients receiving 4.757 g procaine penicillin (approximately equivalent to 2.88 mg or 4.8 MIU benzylpenicillin) for an STI[163].

Syphilis and HIV infection

Syphilis and HIV infection may interact in several ways: mucocutaneous lesions of syphilis may facilitate transmission of the virus, the natural history of syphilis may be altered by HIV infection, and standard treatment may be inadequate.

SYPHILIS AND SEROCONVERSION FOR HIV

Amongst women in Abidjan, Cote d'Ivoire, Ghys et al.[220] showed that there was a significant association between the presence of genital ulceration, including that caused by *T. pallidum*, and shedding of HIV-1 from the genital tract. This finding may help to explain the finding by Otten et al.[221] that syphilis was a marker for HIV seroconversion. These workers examined the records of 5164 men and women who attended STI clinics in Miami, and who had at least two HIV antibody tests between late

1987 and 1990. The HIV seroconversion rate was 12.8 per 100 person years for patients with primary or secondary syphilis, compared with 2.3 for patients who never had syphilis, and 3.1 for those who had had syphilis before their first HIV test. Several other studies have examined the role of syphilis in the acquisition of HIV, and these have been reviewed critically by Fleming and Wasserheit[222].

NATURAL HISTORY AND CLINICAL FEATURES OF SYPHILIS IN HIV-INFECTED INDIVIDUALS

The clinical presentation of early syphilis in the majority of patients who have concurrent infection with HIV is similar to that in non-HIV-infected individuals. Although not observed in every study, however, HIV-seropositive men, but not women, are more likely to present with secondary syphilis than primary stage disease, and primary lesions persisting into the secondary stage are more likely in those with dual infection[223]. There have been many reports on unusual skin features of syphilis in HIV-infected individuals. Hyperkeratotic lesions on the soles have been described, as have ulcerative, non-granulomatous lesions, and gummata[224–226]. As syphilis was highly variable in its clinical presentation in the pre-HIV era, it is difficult to draw conclusions from these case reports.

Similarly, because denominator data are unavailable, it is difficult to draw firm conclusions on the role of HIV in altering the natural history of neurosyphilis. Numerous reports have suggested that neurosyphilis in the HIV-infected individual is more likely to develop earlier, and to have a more atypical presentation than that in non-HIV infected people[227, 147]. Compared with the pre-antibiotic era, neurosyphilis in HIV-infected individuals is more likely to present as meningeal and meningovascular disease than general paralysis of the insane or tabes dorsalis[228]. Musher and colleagues[228] noted that 16 of the 42 patients reviewed had been treated for syphilis prior to the development of neurosyphilis; in 5 cases the neurological features were apparent within 6 months of therapy. In San Francisco between 1985 and 1992, 90% of 83 patients with

neurosyphilis were seropositive for HIV[229] and, as noted by others, meningitis and meningovascular syphilis were the most common presentations. Uveitis often accompanies these forms of syphilis, and in HIV-positive individuals this is the most common ocular manifestation of ocular syphilis[230].

INFLUENCE OF HIV ON SYPHILIS SEROLOGY

Serodiagnosis

The initial report that an HIV-infected patient who acquired syphilis failed to produce anti-treponemal antibodies[231] had extremely serious implications for the diagnosis and control of syphilis. A few other early reports described a similar phenomenon but when the patients were followed for longer they did develop an antibody response, albeit slower than normal, and are more accurately classified as 'delayed seropositivity' rather than seronegative[232]. In one patient, although treponemal and cardiolipin antigen tests were reactive imunoblotting revealed antibodies to far fewer treponemal antigens than are usually present in secondary syphilis sera[224]. Fortunately, the vast majority of HIV-infected patients who acquire syphilis appear to have a normal serological response to *T. pallidum*[233]. Indeed many HIV-infected patients who acquire syphilis produce very high levels of anti-treponemal antibodies[88]; this may be a result of polyclonal B-cell activation but the fact that many such patients are likely to be experiencing re-infection with syphilis might also contribute to high antibody levels. However, higher VDRL/RPR titers have been reported in patients with HIV infection with no previous syphilis[234] as well as in patients with previous syphilis[235]. On balance, there would seem more risk of false negative VDRL/RPR results due to the prozone phenomenon[99, 236] than to the failure to produce an antibody response.

Serological tests for monitoring therapy

There is the possibility that the polyclonal B-cell activation that occurs in HIV infection might interfere with the reliability

of treatment monitoring by quantitative VDRL/RPR tests. In one of the early studies to address this issue it was found that co-existing HIV infection had no influence in on post-treatment titers, at least when patients were in the early stages of HIV infection[235a]. Another retrospective study in a cohort of intravenous drug abusers found no difference by HIV status in the rate of decrease of RPR titers after treatment across all stages of syphilis[235]. A similar study, but including non-intravenous drug abusers, also found that HIV had no effect on the rate of decline of RPR titers following treatment[223]. A prospective study of HIV-positive and HIV-negative women in Zaire found no difference in serological response to therapy[237]. Recently, a further small prospective study reported a normal response to treatment in HIV-infected patients[238].

A few studies have reported that HIV does have an effect on serological response following treatment. An early retrospective analysis[239] found that HIV-infected patients with primary syphilis, when compared with HIV-negative controls, were less likely to have a fourfold or greater decrease in cardiolipin antibody titer, or seroreversion, within 6 months of treatment. Cases and controls with secondary syphilis had similar serological responses after treatment. Another retrospective study reported the decrease in RPR titer was slower in HIV-positive compared to HIV-negative patients[240]. A multicenter, randomized double-blind trial to assess two treatments for early syphilis found that serologically defined treatment failure was more common in HIV-infected than in non-HIV-infected patients but the reverse occurred in early latent stage disease although clinical failure was uncommon in both groups[241]. The RPR titers decreased more slowly among HIV-infected than non-infected patients with primary syphilis.

Further studies are required to determine definitively whether HIV alters the serological response to therapy in patients with early syphilis. However, as no consensus has been reached to date it suggests that coexisting HIV does not seriously limit the value of post-treatment monitoring by quantitative VDRL/RPR tests.

Serological markers for past syphilis

There are several reports to suggest that serological evidence of treated syphilis may disappear after patients become infected with HIV. Johnson and colleagues[242] found that 10% of AIDS patients lost reactivity to the TPHA and FTA-abs tests over a 3-year period. In another study it was found that none of a group of HIV-negative individuals lost reactivity to a treponemal test whereas 7% of HIV-positive asymptomatic individuals, and 38% of those with symptomatic HIV infection, had lost reactivity to either the TPHA or FTA-abs test: the mean duration since the last documented episode of syphilis was 52 months for the seronegative patients and 62.9 for the seropositive patients. Comparing HIV-infected and non-infected patients by the TPHA, Captia G® EIA and FTA-abs tests it was found that 11% of the HIV-positive patients were negative by all three tests and 25% were negative in at least one test: the period since treatment for syphilis ranged from 2 months to approximately 22 years (average approximately 8 years)[243]. None of the HIV-negative patients were negative in all three tests while 6% were negative in at least one test. Although each of the treponemal tests gave lower sensitivity in the HIV-positive than in the HIV-negative group the difference was only significant with regard to the FTA-abs, 79% versus 97%. Clearly there is a reduction in levels of specific anti-treponemal antibody to *T. pallidum* in some HIV-infected individuals as they progress through their illness. This means that a negative treponemal antigen test does not necessarily exclude a past syphilis infection in patients with AIDS. Exclusion of a past history of syphilis in HIV-infected patients may be more reliable if more than one test is used. The ICE recombinant EIA was positive in all 15 patients with co-existing HIV (antibody index above 5 in 12 patients) whereas three were negative by the Captia Select Syph-G® EIA and the FTA-abs, and one by the TPHA[113].

Whilst the above studies mainly involve patients treated several years earlier, loss of a treponemal antibody response has been noted within 2 years of treatment for secondary syphilis and before the onset of AIDS[244]. In this case the loss of antibody response was not linked to serious humoral immune deficit since IgG responses to other infections such as rubella, cytomegalovirus, hemolytic streptococci, and staphylococci remained detectable. Interactions between syphilis serology and HIV may be different depending on whether the two infections are acquired simultaneously, HIV is acquired after an individual has been treated for syphilis, or syphilis is acquired by an individual with HIV.

False positive reactions

Attention was drawn to high RPR titer (≥ 16) false positive reactions in eight HIV-infected intravenous drug abusers as such patients could be initially misdiagnosed as syphilis[245]; biological false positive reactors usually give a titer of less than 8. More recently, a number of patients with positive RPR over 8 who were initially classified as BFP reactors were later confirmed as having treponemal infection by imunoblotting[106]. Although one report involving a group of STI clinic attenders that included intravenous drug abusers, found that BFP RPR results were more common in HIV-seropositive patients (4%) compared with HIV-seronegative patients (0.8%)[246], this was not supported in another population. A review of 1077 HIV-seropositive patients in the United States Air Force, a population with a low risk of intravenous drug abuse, found a BFP rate of only 1%.

TREATMENT OF SYPHILIS IN HIV-INFECTED INDIVIDUALS

Early syphilis

As there have been few prospective studies, there is still some doubt as to the most effective treatment for syphilis in HIV-infected patients[12]. Rolfs and colleagues[241] compared standard benzathine penicillin treatment for early syphilis with standard therapy enhanced with oral amoxicillin and probenecid given three times per day to 541 patients, 101 of whom were HIV infected. There was one clinically defined treatment failure in an HIV-seropositive patient. The authors concluded that benzathine penicillin was adequate for treating patients with early syphilis whether or not they have concurrent HIV infection. The Centers for Disease Control[172] recommend the same dosage of penicillin for early syphilis in HIV-infected individuals as that given for early syphilis in non-HIV infected people.

Late syphilis

Although there are few studies on which to advise on the management of late syphilis, including neurosyphilis, in HIV-infected patients, the Centers for Disease Control[172] advise CSF examination in those with late latent syphilis or in people who have syphilis of unknown duration. This advice has been challenged, however, as it has been shown that HIV-infected individuals with neurosyphilis are more likely to have high cardiolipin antibody (RPR) titers in the serum than those without neurological involvement[119]. It has been proposed that CSF examination is only necessary when the RPR titer is above 32[12].

When the CSF is examined and there are no changes suggestive of neurosyphilis, benzathine penicillin in three weekly doses of 2.4 MIU each is advised. Patients who have neurosyphilis, either asymptomatic or associated with neurological abnormalities, should be treated as for neurosyphilis in the non-HIV-infected individual. Notwithstanding the use of high-dose intravenous penicillin, treatment failures have been reported[247].

Although the use of ceftriaxone by intravenous infusion has shown promise in the treatment of neurosyphilis in HIV-infected patients[248], data are only available on small numbers of patients and, currently, penicillin should be the drug of choice. In the case of those who have apparent hypersensitivity to penicillin, skin testing and, if indicated, desensitization, may be helpful.

Patients should be evaluated at 6, 12, 18, and 24 months after completion of therapy. If there is a fourfold rise in titer in the cardiolipin antibody tests, or if clinical features suggestive of neurosyphilis develop, the CSF should be examined and the patient treated again. Similarly, if the cardiolipin antibody titer does not decline fourfold between months 12 and 24 post-treatment, the CSF should be examined.

In the case of the treatment of congenital syphilis, there are no data on which to offer advice. The authors recommend the treatment regimens used for non-HIV-infected infants (see page 439).

Endemic treponematoses

The geographical distribution of the endemic treponematoses in the early 1950s (Figure 15.34) is contrasted with that in the early 1980s (Figure 15.35).

PINTA

(synonyms: ***pinta***; ***mal de pinto*** (in Mexico); ***carate*** (in Colombia and Venezuela); ***azul*** (in Chile and Peru))

This is a disease of remote rural communities affecting the skin (blue-stain disease) and it is the least damaging of the human treponematoses. The causative organism is *Treponema pallidum* subsp. *carateum*, the most attenuated of the pathogenic treponemes. Pinta used to be prevalent in semi-arid regions of Brazil, Colombia, Cuba, southern Mexico, and Venezuela, with scattered foci in Central and South American countries and the Caribbean islands; today only scattered foci remain in northern South America and Mexico[258]. It differs from yaws and endemic syphilis in that it affects children and adults of all ages. Throughout its course the disease is confined to the skin where pigmented and achromic lesions may remain infective for years, permitting spread by direct skin-to-skin contact.

Clinical features

The primary or initial lesion develops usually after 2 to 3 weeks, often on an uncovered part of the body, as a lenticular and slightly scaly papule which enlarges to form a plaque; mostly the initial lesion is to be found on the legs, the dorsum of the foot, the forearm, or the back of the hands. At first pink in color in fair skins, the lesion becomes pigmented or hypochromic to a variable degree as it enlarges; lymph nodes draining the area also enlarge. After 2 months or up to a year later, secondary lesions develop, some on occasions appearing on the same site as the initial lesion. At

first erythematous and afterwards copper colored, these 'pintids' become pigmented to a varying degree, changing slowly from a copper color to lead-gray and slate-blue as a result of photosensitization, and areas of erythema, hypopigmentation, and leuko-

derma develop. The polychromic lesions become keratotic.

In late-stage pinta, residual areas of hyperchromia and achromia develop in isolated patches to form multicolored lesions; the depigmentation process occurs

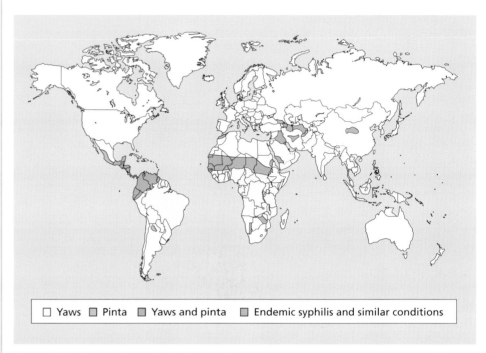

Figure 15.34 Geographical distribution of the endemic treponematoses in the early 1950s. World map, Peters projection (data from WHO Scientific Group 1982[261])

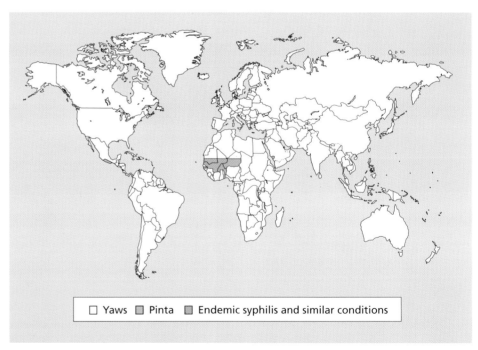

Figure 15.35 Geographical distribution of the endemic treponematoses in the early 1980s. World map, Peters projection (data from WHO Scientific Group 1982[261])

at different rates even within the same lesion. No disability or complication other than leukoderma occurs[258].

The causative organism, *T. pallidum* subsp. *carateum*, is detected by dark ground illumination microscopy in serum obtained from the base of a lesion after abrading the surface; although numerous in early-stage lesions, treponemes persist through to the late dyschromic stage[259].

YAWS

(synonyms: ***pian*** (French); ***framboesia*** (German, Dutch); ***bouba*** (Portuguese); ***buba*** (Kiswahili))

Yaws has shown the greatest changes in regional prevalence since the mass treatment campaigns of the 1950s. In South America only scattered foci of active yaws persist; Brazil and Surinam are almost yaws free, and in Colombia, Ecuador, French Guiana, and Guyana only a few dozen or a hundred cases are reported annually. In southeast Asia yaws still exists in Indonesia and Papua New Guinea, and sporadic outbreaks have been reported from Thailand[260]. Africa remains the part of the world most affected, although where there is improved rural medical care and improved standards of living, as in the Ivory Coast and Nigeria, the numbers of clinical cases are declining[261]. In Ghana, however, resurgence of yaws occurred following cessation of active yaws surveillance; the numbers of reported cases of infectious yaws increased 21-fold between 1969 and 1976[262].

In a WHO survey in the Central African Republic, Congo, and Gabon, clinical yaws was detected in over 20% of the pygmy population and positive serological tests in 80%[261]. Out of a total pygmy population of 100 000 to 200 000, two major groups have undergone less assimilation than the others – the Binga of the tropical rain forests to the west of the Ubangi River, and the Mbuti, several hundred miles to the east in the Ituri Forest[263]. In a survey (486 examined) of the former group in 1978 to 1979, in the dry season, a time when these nomadic forest people were accessible, it was found that there were clinical signs of yaws in 50% of individuals, and serological tests (VDRL and TPHA) were positive in 86% of the children and 95% of the adults. In the

Table 15.10 Classification of yaws lesions (Hackett 1951, 1957, Perine 1984).

Yaws lesions	Examples	'Infectiousness' + to +++
Early-stage cutaneous (often pruritic; tendency to cropping; often polymorphous; modified by climate; if lesions moist then infectious)		
Initial lesion	Papule, papilloma	+++
Papillomata	papilloma; some serpiginous; some ulcerated	+++
Macules		++
Micropapules, papules		+++
Squamous macules		+
Squamous micropapules, papules		++
Polymorphous or mixed		++
Plaques		+
Nodules	e.g. front of knees	+
Hyperkeratosis	palmar, plantar (as in crab yaws – painful)	–
Early-stage bone Osteoperiostitis	polydactylitis tibia goundou (osteitis of nasal processes of maxilla)	– –
Early-stage joint	ganglion, hydrarthrosis	–
Late-stage cutaneous Hyperkeratosis Ulcer with characteristic tissue destruction (gummatous)	palmar, plantar	–
Late-stage bone Gummatous osteoperiostitis	sabre tibia; monodactylitis gangosa	– –
Late-stage joint	ganglion hydrarthrosis bursitis juxta-articular nodes	– – – –

case of neighboring non-pygmy peasant cultivators clinical evidence of yaws was also common (30%) and 78% of the children and 98% of the adults had positive serological tests[264]. Eradication campaigns had clearly not reached such isolated populations, and total mass treatment (see antibiotics in treatment and control in endemic treponematoses) would be the appropriate medical strategy. To achieve success, however, anthropological understanding would be an essential, as the forest pygmies have no formal social structure and organization and small bands constantly change in size and composition throughout the year[265, 263].

Yaws predominantly affects children, particularly those aged between 6 and 10 years.

Clinical features

Yaws is a contact disease of childhood, caused by *Treponema pallidum* subsp. *pertenue*[266], and is characterized by crops of highly infectious and relapsing skin lesions in the first 5 or 6 years of the natural course of the infection. The classification and nomenclature for the lesions of yaws were established in an illustrated monograph of the World Health Organization[267] and the bone lesions were discussed more fully by Hackett[268]. A classification of lesions and the degrees of infectiousness of such lesions, based on Perine *et al.*[258], are summarized in Table 15.10.

The most characteristic lesion in early yaws is the papilloma, and in the exudate of all early lesions, which may be macular, maculopapular, or papular (Figure 15.36), treponemes are numerous. The early papule enlarges to form a papillomatous lesion bearing some resemblance to a raspberry (a synonym is *framboesia*). There may also be adenitis. After 2 to 6 months the initial lesion heals, often without scarring. Further papillomata, often in crops, develop most often around the body orifices, near the nose, mouth, anus, and vulva. A change in climate may influence the number and morphology of yaws lesions: in the dry season lesions tend to be fewer in number and macular in form, and papillomata tend to be more concentrated in moist areas of the skin such as the axilla and anal cleft. Hyperkeratotic

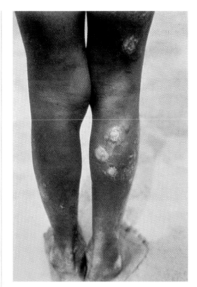

Figure 15.36 Papular lesions of yaws on posterior legs and thigh (courtesy of Dr O Arya, reproduced from McMillan and Scott 1991[277])

lesions occur on the soles of the feet and palms of the hands. On the feet plaques develop, which are painful, and walking becomes difficult (crab yaws) (Figure 15.37).

A periostitis may affect long bones or cause a polydactylitis affecting the phalanges and metacarpals. An osteitis of the nasal processes of the maxilla produces paranasal swellings (goundou) and is common in Africa. The tibia may become

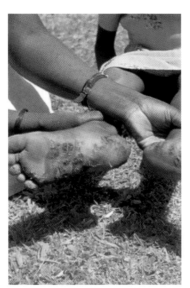

Figure 15.37 Keratotic lesions of yaws on soles of feet (crab yaws) (reproduced from McMillan and Scott 1991[277])

saber-shaped. Nocturnal bone pain and tenderness of the tibial shaft are common in early yaws.

Ganglions, particularly at the wrist, and hydrarthrosis can also occur in early yaws. There is also an early latent stage which may be interrupted by relapses of active early lesions.

Late-stage lesions (Table 15.10) develop 5 or more years after the infection, and the characteristic late lesion is a destructive ulcer, which may involve skin, subcutaneous tissue, the mucosae and the bones and joints. Deep destructive lesions are typified by the hideous mutilation of the central part of the face (rhinopharyngitis mutilans) called gangosa (Figure 15.38), in which there is destruction of cartilage and bone structures of the septum, palate, and posterior part of the pharynx[269]. It is probable, however, that there is no bone lesion that occurs in yaws that does not also occur in syphilis[268].

There is no certain evidence of transplacental or congenital infection in yaws. Serologically it cannot be distinguished from syphilis.

ENDEMIC SYPHILIS

(synonyms: **bejel** (Arabic); **njovera**, **dichuclzwa** (in Zimbabwe); **endemic syphilis** (in Bosnia)) (extinct forms of the

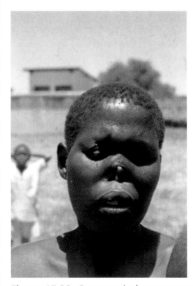

Figure 15.38 Gangosa in late-stage yaws (effect due to gummatous lesions of late yaws) (courtesy of Dr O Arya, reproduced from McMillan and Scott 1991[277])

disease: **sibbens** (in Scotland); **radesyge** (in Norway); **skerljevo** (of the Croatian coast, Yugoslavia))

Endemic syphilis is prevalent today primarily among the semi-nomads in the Arabian peninsula and along the southern border of the Sahara desert. A survey found thousands of cases of early endemic syphilis in Mali, Mauretania, Niger, and Upper Volta; in sub-Saharan Africa the disease may be a greater problem today than it was formerly[261]. It used to be found also in scattered foci in Central Asia, Australia, and India but these have been eliminated by the mass penicillin treatment campaigns of the 1950s[258].

The infection may be spread in the early stage through the use of recently contaminated drinking vessels[270]; by direct skin-to-skin contact; or by the fingers contaminated with saliva and mucus from infective lesions containing treponemes[258].

In Arabia endemic syphilis, known as bejel, presents in its early stage and generally in children aged 2 to 15 years, with a mucocutaneous eruption and exuberant papules, predominantly around the genitalia and anus. Mucous papules or shallow ulcerations (mucous patches) appear on the lips, in the mouth and in the fauces. Symptoms such as hoarseness, dysphagia, or dyspnea have been attributed to extension of the mucous patches to the larynx. Condylomata may be seen in the moist areas of the skin. Periostitis also occurs[271].

Late lesions are granulomatous and destructive, and the nose and its bony structure, the oral cavity and the hard palate and larynx are favorite sites. Hudson[271] remarks that in his time 'cleft-palate voices were common in the market place'. Destructive skin ulcers, plantar keratosis, juxta-articular nodes, and depigmented lesions are common late manifestations.

CONTROL OF ENDEMIC TREPONEMATOSES

Although the treatment of whole communities with long-acting penicillin preparations for the control of endemic treponematosis of childhood was followed initially by a remarkable regression of the community disease, early clinical yaws has not been eliminated in large endemic areas where transmission continues and periodic focal outbreaks tend to occur[272, 261]. Without renewed control programs gains made by mass treatment campaigns of the 1950s and afterwards may be lost, particularly for yaws in some African countries[258].

In the 1950s, on the basis of pilot studies on yaws in Haiti, endemic syphilis in Yugoslavia, and pinta in Mexico, mass treatment campaigns with penicillin were undertaken in forty-six countries in the context of the World Health Organization Treponematoses Campaign. Until 1970 some 160 million people had been examined and in 50 million clinical cases, latent cases, and contacts, treatment had been given. In Western Samoa, for example, the prevalence of clinically active yaws was about 11% in 1955, with about 3% with infectious lesions. On re-survey of the population a year after mass treatment, clinically active yaws was found in only 0.06% and infectious cases in 0.02% of individuals. In Bosnia, the prevalence of endemic syphilis varied from district to district and was highest in northeastern Bosnia, where about 14% of the population were infected. Of all those found during the campaign to have the treponemal disease, about 10% had early infectious lesions, 0.2% congenital, 85% latent, and 5% late lesions[270]. During the follow-up period after mass treatment it soon became evident that the chief risk of perpetuating the disease lay, not in treatment failures, but rather in infected persons escaping examination, in migrants from other districts with early lesions, in those with latent infections or those incubating the disease at the time of examination. In Yugoslavia the careful campaign, follow-up, and progressive environmental changes reduced the rate of endemic syphilis to nil. In Haiti more than 1.3 million clinical cases, latent cases, and contacts were treated, and surveys showed steady progress to low infectious levels of 0.01% in 1961.

Clinical surveys for active yaws may be conducted without any sophisticated laboratory test, but surveys for latent disease require serological tests[273]. The original indices were clinical, and the detection of cases of active yaws is likely to continue to be the mainstay of surveillance and most appropriate for economic and logistic reasons. Age-specific seroreactor rates are, however, useful to define areas as hyperendemic, mesoendemic, and hypoendemic, and in surveys after mass treatment such profiles demonstrate the age at which infections are occurring. In areas where very well-conducted campaigns have been carried out, an occasional seroreactive child is discovered with no evidence of past or present clinical disease, so there is a possibility of persisting subclinical infection. If the proportion of the population examined and treated is too low then seroreactors will be common in early age groups of a sample and a further mass campaign will be necessary.

False seroreactions in cardiolipin tests (biological false-positives) become relatively important when the seroreactor rates are declining, and particularly so in childhood. Special techniques of storing serum in liquid nitrogen[274] and other facilities have been developed to ensure that reliable specific antibody tests (TPHA or FTA tests) can be carried out for those working in the field.

The socioeconomic status of a large segment of the populations in the rural areas of West Africa has either not improved or has actually regressed in the last two decades. In these areas, patients with reported yaws infection now number tens of thousands, but epidemiological estimates place the true incidence as four times higher. In areas of increasing prevalence, atypical early yaws lesions may be under-diagnosed owing to the inexperience of clinicians unfamiliar with the manifestations of the disease[261].

Antibiotics in treatment and control in endemic treponematoses

Benzathine benzylpenicillin has been recommended by a WHO Expert Committee on Venereal Diseases and is preferred to other forms of penicillin for the treatment of treponemal diseases. Since a single deep intramuscular injection of benzathine benzylpenicillin 1.836 g (approximately equivalent to 1.44 g or 2.4×10^6 IU benzylpenicillin) in a healthy ambulant adult produces a penicillinemia above the treponemicidal level for more than 3 weeks, this dose is effective not only for curing treponemal diseases but also for providing protection against re-infection during this period. Currently schedules for the endemic treponematoses (not including venereal syphilis) are: a single intramuscular injection of 459 mg benzathine benzylpenicillin (approximately equivalent to 360 mg or 600 000 IU of benzylpenicillin) for patients and contacts aged under 10 years; and 918 mg benzathine benzylpenicillin (approximately equivalent to 720 mg or 1.2×10^6 IU benzylpenicillin) for those over 10 years[258].

The extent of treatment given to a community, village, or other group living close to one another, is based on the prevalence of clinically active yaws in the community. For hyperendemic areas (approximate prevalence of clinically active yaws in the community of over 10%) World Health Organization treatment policies recommend benzathine benzylpenicillin treatment to the entire population, namely total mass treatment (TMT);

for mesoendemic areas (approximate prevalence of clinically active yaws in the community of 5% to 10%) treatment with benzathine benzylpenicillin in all active cases, all children under 15 years of age, and obvious contacts of infectious patients, namely juvenile mass treatment (JMT); and for hypoendemic areas (approximate prevalence of clinically active yaws in the community under 5%) treatment with benzathine benzylpenicillin in all active cases and all household or other obvious contacts. In isolated and remote villages TMT may be appropriate even if the prevalence of active yaws is less than 10 per cent[258].

Penicillin treatment always carries the risk of serious side effects including fatal anaphylaxis. During the initial mass treatment campaigns, when almost all those treated were receiving penicillin for the first time, risks were very low. Those undertaking such campaigns should be prepared to treat such drug reactions. Alternatives have been suggested (for

example, tetracycline or erythromycin 500 mg orally four times daily for 15 days is probably effective). Children between 8 and 15 years of age may be given half doses of either drug, and those under 8 years of age only erythromycin in doses appropriate to their body weight. Tetracycline is not recommended in pregnancy[258].

Three cases of yaws that did not respond to penicillin therapy were reported from Ecuador by Anselmi et al.[275]; treatment with doxycycline was effective. Despite receiving recommended therapy, 11 of 39 children who had been treated for yaws in Papua New Guinea developed clinical and/or serological evidence of relapse within 22 months of treatment[276]. In this case, re-infection cannot be entirely excluded.

Adults who may have acquired yaws in childhood may be seen in the clinics of western countries, when the results of serological tests will not differentiate it from syphilis; in such cases, treatment appropriate for syphilis is advised.

References

1 Miao R, Fieldsteel AH. Genetic relationship between *Treponema pallidum* and *Treponema pertenue*, two noncultivable human pathogens. *J Bacteriol* 1980; **141**: 427–429.

2 Fraser CM, Norris SJ, Weinstock CM, *et al.* Complete genome sequence of *Treponema pallidum*, the syphilis spirochete. *Science* 1998; **281**:375–388.

3 Stamm LV, Greene SR, Bergen HL, Hardham JM, Barnes NY. Identification and sequence analysis of *Treponema pallidum* tprJ, a member of a polymorphic multigene family. *FEMS Microbiol Lett* 1998; **169**: 155–163.

4 CenturionLara A, Castro C, Castillo R, Shaffer JM, VanVoorhis WC, Lukehart SA. The flanking region sequences of the 15-kDa lipoprotein gene differentiate pathogenic treponemes. *J Infect Dis* 1998; **177**: 1036–1040.

5 Radolf JD, Robinson EJ, Bourell KW, *et al.* Characterization of outer membranes isolated from *Treponema pallidum*, the syphilis spirochete. *Infect Immun* 1995; **63**: 4244.

6 Norris SJ. Polypeptides of *Treponema pallidum*: Progress toward understanding their structural, functional, and immunologic roles. *Microbiol Rev* 1993; **57**: 750–779.

7 Fieldsteel AH, Cox DL, Moeckli RA. Cultivation of virulent *Treponema pallidum* in tissue culture. *Infect Immun* 1981; **32**: 908–915.

8 Norris SJ. *In vitro* cultivation of *Treponema pallidum*: independent confirmation. *Infect Immun* 1982; **36**: 437–439.

9 Fieldsteel AH, Cox DL, Moeckli RA. Further studies on replication of virulent *Treponema pallidum* in tissue cultures of Sf1Ep cells. *Infect Immun* 1982; **32**: 449–455.

10 British Co-operative Clinical Group. Homosexuality and venereal disease in the United Kingdom, a second study. *Br J Vener Dis* 1980; **56**: 6–11.

11 PHLS, DHSS&PS and the Scottish ISD(D)5 Collaborative Group. Trends in sexually transmitted infections in the United Kingdom 1990–1999. London; Public Health Laboratory Service: 2000.

11a Anonymous. Increased transmission of syphilis in Brighton and Greater Manchester among men who have sex with men. *Comm Dis Rep CDR Weekly* 2000; **10**: 383, 386.

12 Singh AE, Romanowski B. Syphilis: review with emphasis on clinical, epidemiologic, and biological features. *Clin Microbiol Rev* 1999; **12**: 187–209.

13 Henderson RH. Improving sexually transmitted diseases health service to gays:

a national perspective. *Sex Transm Dis* 1977; **4**: 58–62.

14 Williams LA, Klausner JD, Whittington WLH, Hunter Handsfield, Celum C, Holmes KK. Elimination and reintroduction of primary and secondary syphilis. *Am J Public Health* 1999; **89**: 1093–1097.

15 Rolfs RT, Goldberg M, Sharrar RG. Risk factors for syphilis: cocaine use and prostitution. *Am J Public Health* 1990; **80**: 853–857.

16 Nakashima AK, Rolfs RT, Flock ML, Kilmarx P, Greenspan JR. Epidemiology of syphilis in the United States, 1941–1993. *Sex Transm Dis* 1996; **23**: 16–23.

17 Tichinova L, Borisenko K, Ward H, Meheus A, Gromyko A, Renton A. Epidemics of syphilis in the Russian Federation: trends, origins, and priorities for control. *Lancet* 1997; **350**: 210–213.

18 Ratcliffe L, Nicoll A, Carrington D, *et al.* Reference laboratory surveillance of syphilis in England and Wales, 1994 to 1996. *Comm Dis Public Health* 1998; **1**: 14–21.

19 Gerbase AC, Rowley JT, Heymann DHL, Berkley SFB, Piot P. Global prevalence and incidence estimates of selected curable STDs. *Sex Transm Inf* 1998; **74** (Suppl. 1): S12–S16.

20 Newell J, Senkoro K, Mosha F, Grosskurth H, Nicol A, Barongo L. A population-based study of syphilis and sexually transmitted disease syndromes in north-western Tanzania. 2. Risk factors and heatlh seeking behaviour. *Genitourin Med* 1993; **69**: 421–426.

21 Hanenberg RS, Rojanapithayakorn W, Kunasol P, Sokal DC. Impact of Thailand's HIV control programme as indicated by the decline of sexually transmitted diseases. *Lancet* 1994; **344**: 243–245.

22 Centers for Disease Control and Prevention. Surveillance for gonorrhea and primary and secondary syphilis among adolescents, United States 1988–1992. *Morbid Mortal Weekly Rep* 1993; **42**: 1–11.

23 Folgosa E, Osman NB, Gonzalez C, Hagerstrand I, Bergstrom S, Ljungh A. Syphilis seroprevalence among pregnant women and its role as a risk factor for stillbirth in Maputo, Mozambique. *Genitourin Med* 1996; **72**: 339–342.

24 Schober PC, Gabriel G, White P, Felton WF. How infectious is syphilis? *Br J Vener Dis* 1983; **59**: 217–219.

25 Chambers RW, Foley HT, Schmidt PJ. Transmission of syphilis by fresh blood products. *Transfusion* 1969; **9**: 32–34.

26 van der Sluis JJ, Menke HE, Kothe FC. Transfusion syphilis: survival of *Treponema pallidum* in donor blood. *Antonie van Leeuwenhoek* 1982; **48**: 487–488.

27 Risseeuw-Appel IM, Kothe FC. Transfusion syphilis: a case report. *Sex Transm Dis* 1983; **10**: 200–201.

28 Sanchez PJ, McCracken GH, Wendel GD, Olsen K, Threlkeld N, Norgard V. Molecular analysis of the fetal IgM response to *Treponema pallidum* antigens: implications for improved serodiagnosis of congenital syphilis. *J Infect Dis* 1989; **159**: 508–517.

29 Jacques SM, Qureshi F. Necrotising funisitis: a study of 45 cases. *Hum Pathol* 1992; **23**: 1278–1283.

30 Qureshi F, Jacques SM, Reyes MP. Placental histopathology in syphilis. *Hum Pathol* 1993; **23**: 779–784.

31 Sanchez PJ, Wendel GD, Grimprel E, *et al.* Evaluation of molecular methodologies and rabbit infectivity testing for the diagnosis of congenital syphilis and neonatal central nervous system invasion by *Treponema pallidum*. *J Infect Dis* 1993; **167**: 148–157.

32 Lucas MJ, Theriot SK, Wendel GD. Doppler systolic–diastolic ratios in pregnancies complicated by syphilis. *Obstet Gynecol* 1991; **77**: 217–222.

33 Nathan L, Bohman VR, Sanchez PJ, Leos NK, Twickler DM, Wendel GD. In utero infection with *Treponema pallidum* in early pregnancy. *Prenat Diag* 1997; **17**: 119–123.

34 Sanchez PJ. Syphilis in pregnancy. In: Hitchcock PJ, Trent MacKay H, Wasserheit JN. (eds) *Sexually Transmitted Diseases and Adverse Outcomes of Pregnancy.* Washington DC; ASM Press: 1999, pp. 125–150.

35 Gjestland T. The Oslo study of untreated syphilis – an epidemiologic investigation of the natural course of untreated syphilis based on a study of the Boeck-Bruusgard material. *Acta Dermatol Venereol* 1955; **35**: Suppl. 34.

36 Abell E, Marks R, Wilson Jones E. Secondary syphilis: a clinico-pathological review. *Br J Dermatol* 1975; **93**: 53–61.

37 McBroom RL, Styles AR, Chiu MJ, Clegg C, Cockerell CJ, Radolf JD. Secondary syphilis in persons infected with and not infected with HIV-1. *Am J Dermatopathol* 1999; **21**: 432–441.

38 Heggtveit HA. Syphilitic aortitis. *Circulation* 1964; **29**: 346–355.

39 Karmody CS, Schuknecht HF. Deafness in congenital syphilis. *Arch Otolaryngol* 1966; **83**: 18–27.

39a Qureshi F, Jacques SM, Reyes MP. Placenta histopathology in syphillis. *Hum Pathol* 1993; **23**: 779–784.

39b Jacques SM, Qureshi F. Necrotizing funiculitis: a study of 45 cases. *Hum Pathol* 1992; **23**: 1278–1283.

40 Fitzgerald TJ, Repesh LA, Blanco DR, Miller JN. Attachment of *Treponema pallidum* to fibronectin, laminin, collagen IV, and collagen I, and blockage of attachment by immune rabbit IgG. *Br J Vener Dis* 1984; **60**: 357–363.

41 Quist EE, Repesh LA, Zeleznikar R, Fitzgerald TJ. Interaction of *Treponema pallidum* with isolated rabbit capillary tissues. *Br J Vener Dis* 1983; **59**: 11–20.

42 Fitzgerald TJ. Pathogenesis and immunology of *Treponema pallidum*. *Ann Rev Microbiol* 1981; **35**: 29–54.

43 Bishop NH, Miller JN. Humoral and immune mechanisms in acquired syphilis. In: Schell RF, Musher DF (eds) *Pathogenesis and Immunology of Treponemal Infection.* New York: Marcel Dekker: 1983, p. 241.

44 Magnusson HJ, Thomas EW, Olansky S, Kaplan BI, De Mello L, Cutler JC. Inoculation of syphilis in human volunteers. *Medicine* 1956; **35**: 33–82.

45 Arroll TW, CenturionLara A, Lukehart SA, VanVoorhis WC. T-cell responses to *Treponema pallidum* subsp *pallidum* antigens during the course of experimental syphilis infection. *Infect Immun* 1999; **67**: 4757–4763.

46 Lukehart SA. Macrophages and host resistance. In: Schell RF, Musher DF (eds) *Pathogenesis and Immunology of Treponemal Infection.* New York: Marcel Dekker: 1983.

47 Lewinski MA, Miller JN, Lovett MA, Blanco DR. Correlation of immunity in experimental syphilis with serum-mediated aggregation of *Treponema pallidum* rare outer membrane proteins. *Infect Immun* 1999; **67**: 3631–3636.

48 Luger AFH. Serological diagnosis of syphilis: current methods. In: Young H, McMillan A (eds) *Immunological Diagnosis of Sexually Transmitted Diseases.* New York and Basel: Marcel Dekker: 1988.

49 Baker-Zander SA, Hook EW, Bonin P, Handsfield HH, Lukehart SA. Antigens of *Treponema pallidum* recognized by IgG and IgM antibodies during syphilis in humans. *J Infect Dis* 1985; **151**: 264–272.

50 Baker-Zander SA, Roddy RE, Handsfield HH, Lukehart SA. IgG and IgM antibody reactivity to antigens of *Treponema pallidum* after treatment of syphilis. *Sex Transm Dis* 1986; **13**: 214–220.

51 Isaacs RD and Radolf JD. Molecular approaches to improved syphilis serodiagnosis. *Serodiag Immunotherapy Infect Dis* 1989; **3**: 299–306.

52 Wicher V, Zabek J, Wicher K. Pathogen-specific humoral response in *Treponema pallidum*-infected humans, rabbits, and guinea pigs. *J Infect Dis* 1991; **163**: 830–836.

53 Norris SJ, Aldereete JF, Axelsen NH, *et al.* Identity of *Treponema pallidum* subsp. *pallidum* polypeptides: correlation of sodium dodecylsulfate-polyacrylamide gel electrophoresis results from different laboratories. *Electrophoresis* 1987; **8**: 77–92.

54 Musher DM, Hague-Park M, Gyorkey F, Anderson DC, Baughn RE. The interaction between *Treponema pallidum* and human polymorphonuclear leucocytes. *J Infect Dis* 1983; **147**: 77–86.

55 Young H, Moyes A, McMillan A, Paterson J. Enzyme immunoassay for anti-treponemal IgG: screening or confirmatory test? *J Clin Pathol* 1992; **45**: 37–41.

56 Larsen SA, Steiner BM, Rudolph AH. Laboratory diagnosis and interpretation of tests for syphilis. *Clin Microbiol Rev* 1995; **8**: 1–21.

57 Young H. Syphilis serology. *Dermatologic Clinics* 1998; **16**: 691–698.

58 Wicher K, Horowitz HW, Wicher V. Laboratory methods of diagnosis of syphilis for the beginning of the third millennium. *Microbes Infect* 1999; **1**: 1035–1049.

59 Luger A. Diagnosis of syphilis. *Bulletin of the World Health Organisation* 1981; **59**: 647–655.

60 Tzagaroulaki E, Riviere G. Antibodies to *Treponema pallidum* in serum from subjects with periodontitis: relationship to pathogen-related oral spirochetes. *Oral Microbiol Immunol* 1999; **14**: 375–378.

61 Ito F, Hunter EF, George RW, Swisher BL, Larsen SA. Specific immunofluorescence staining of *Treponema pallidum* in smears and tissues. *J Clin Microbiol* 1991; **29**: 444–448.

62 Wicher K, Noordhoek GT, Abbruscato F, Wicher V. Detection of *Treponema pallidum* in early syphilis by DNA amplification. *J Clin Microbiol* 1992; **30**: 497–500.

63 Jethwa HS, Schmitz JL, Dallabetta G, *et al.* Comparison of molecular and microscopic techniques for detection of *Treponema pallidum* in genital ulcers. *J Clin Microbiol* 1995; **33**: 180–183.

64 Orle KA, Gates CA, Martin DH, Body BA, Weiss JB. Simultaneous PCR detection of *Haemophilus ducreyi*, *Treponema pallidum*, and Herpes Simplex virus types 1 and 2 from genital ulcers. *J Clin Microbiol* 1996; **34**: 49–54.

65 Risbud A, ChanTack K, Gadkari D, *et al.* The etiology of genital ulcer disease by multiplex polymerase chain reaction and relationship to HIV infection among patients attending sexually transmitted disease clinics in Pune, India. *Sex Transm Dis* 1999; **26**: 55–62.

66 Behets FMT, Andriamiadana J, Randrianasolo D, *et al.* Chancroid, primary syphilis, genital herpes, and lymphogranuloma venereum in Antananarivo, Madagascar. *J Infect Dis* 1999; **180**: 1382–1385.

67 Schlupen EM, Meurer M, Schirren CG, Baumann L, Volkenandt M. Alopecia specifica in secondary syphilis. Molecular detection of *Treponema pallidum* in lesional skin. *Eur J Dermatol* 1996; **6**: 19–22.

68 Zoechling N, Schluepen EM, Soyer HP, Kerl H, Volkenandt, M. Molecular detection of *Treponema pallidum* in secondary and tertiary syphilis. *Br J Dermatol* 1997; **136**: 683–686.

69 Inagaki H, Kawai T, Miyata M, Nagaya S, Tateyama H, Eimoto T. Gastric syphilis: Polymerase chain reaction detection of treponemal DNA in pseudolymphomatous lesions. *Hum Pathol* 1996; **27**: 761–765.

70 CenturionLara A, Castro C, Shaffer JM, VanVoorhis WC, Marra CM., Lukehart SA. Detection of *Treponema pallidum* by a sensitive reverse transcriptase PCR. *J Clin Microbiol* 1997; **35**: 1348–1352.

71 Young H, Penn CW. Syphilis, yaws and pinta. In: Smith GR, Easmon CSF (eds) *Topley and Wilson's Principles of Bacteriology, Virology and Immunology* vol. 8. Kent; Edward Arnold: 1990.

72 Castro, AR, Morrill WE, Shaw WA, *et al.* Use of synthetic cardiolipin and lecithin in the antigen used by the Venereal Disease Research Laboratory for serodiagnosis of syphilis. *Clin Diagnostic Lab Immunol* 2000; **7**: 658–661.

73 Harris A, Rosenberg AA, Riedel MM. A microflocculation test for syphilis using cardiolipin antigen. *J Vener Dis Information* 1946; **27**: 169–175.

74 Bernard C, de Moerloose P, Tremblet C, Reber G, Didierjean L. Biological true and false serological tests for syphilis: their relationship with anticardiolipin antibodies. *Dermatologica* 1990; **180**: 151–153.

75 Merkel PA, Chang YC, Pierangeli SS, Harris EN, Polisson RP. Comparison between the standard anticardiolipin antibody test and a new phospholipid test in patients with connective tissue diseases. *J Rheumatol* 1999; **26**: 591–596.

76 Pope V, Fears MB, Lukehart SA, Morrill WE, Castro AR, Kikkert SE. Comparison of the Serodia *Treponema pallidum* particle agglutination, Captia Syphilis G, and SpiroTek Reagin II tests with standard test techniques for diagnosis of syphilis. *J Clin Microbiol* 2000; **38**: 2543–2545.

77 Hunter EF, Deacon WE, Meyer PE. An improved FTA test for syphilis, the absorption procedure (FTA-ABS). *Public Health Report* 1964; **79**: 410–412.

78 Farshy CE, Kennedy EJ, Hunter EF, Larsen SA. Fluorescent treponemal antibody absorption double-staining test evaluation. *J Clin Microbiol* 1983; **17**: 245–248.

79 Schmidt BL, Edjlalipour M, Luger A. Comparative evaluation of nine different enzyme-linked immunosorbent assays for determination of antibodies against *Treponema pallidum* in patients with primary syphilis. *J Clin Microbiol* 2000; **38**: 1279–1282.

80 Zrein M, Maure I, Boursier F, Soufflet L. Recombinant antigen-based enzyme immunoassay for screening of *Treponema pallidum* antibodies in blood bank routine. *J Clin Microbiol* 1995; **33**: 525–527.

81 Young H, Moyes A, McMillan A, Robertson DHH. Screening for treponemal infection by a new enzyme immunoassay. *Genitourin Med* 1989; **65**: 72–78.

82 Young H, Aktas G, Moyes A. Enzywell recombinant enzyme immunoassay for the serological diagnosis of syphilis. *Int J STD AIDS* 2000; **11**: 288–291.

83 Young H, Walker PJ, Merry D, Mifsud A. A preliminary evaluation of a prototype Western blot confirmatory test kit for syphilis. *Int J STD AIDS* 1994; **5**: 409–414.

84 Wilkinson AE. Some aspects of research on syphilis: serological evidence of activity of the disease. In: Catterall RD, Nicol CE (eds) *Sexually Transmitted Diseases*. London; Academic Press: 1976.

85 Schmidt BL. Solid phase hemadsorption: a method for rapid detection of *Treponema pallidum*-specific IgM. *Sex Transm Dis* 1980; **7**: 53–58.

86 Samuels J, Ernst A. Stat RPRs. *Ann Emerg Med* 1991; **20**: 108–109.

87 Spangler AS, Jackson J, Fiumara NJ, Warthin TA. Syphilis with a negative blood test reaction. *JAMA* 1964; **189**: 113–116.

88 Rufli T. Syphilis and HIV infection. *Dermatologica* 1989; **179**: 113–117.

89 Feraru ER, Aronow HA, Lipton RB. Neurosyphilis in AIDS patients: initial CSF VDRL may be negative. *Neurology* 1990; **40**: 541–543.

90 Berkowitz K, Baxi L, Fox HE. False-negative syphilis screening: the prozone phenomenon, nonimmune hydrops, and diagnosis of syphilis during pregnancy. *Am J Obstet Gynecol* 1990; **63**: 975–977.

91 World Health Organization. *Treponemal Infections*. Technical report series 674. World Health Organization; Geneva: 1982.

92 Robertson DHH, McMillan A, Young H. Diagnosis of syphilis. In: *Clinical Practice in Sexually Transmissible Diseases* 2nd edition. Edinburgh; Churchill Livingstone: 1989, p. 118.

93 Lukehart SA. Serologic testing after therapy for syphilis: is there a test for cure? *Ann Intern Med* 1991; **114**: 1057–1058.

94 Young H, Penn CW. Syphilis, yaws and pinta. In: Smith GR, Easmon CSF (eds) *Topley and Wilson's Principles of Bacteriology, Virology and Immunology* vol. 8. Kent; Edward Arnold: 1990.

95 Anderson J, Mindel A, Tovey SJ and Williams P. Primary and secondary syphilis, 20 years' experience. 3: Diagnosis, treatment, and follow up. *Genitourin Med* 1989; **65**: 239.

96 Kobayashi S, Yamaya S-I, Sugahara T, Matuhasi T. Microcapsule agglutination test for *Treponema pallidum* antibodies: a new serodiagnostic test for syphilis. *Br J Vener Dis* 1983; **59**: 1–7.

97 Lefevre JC, Bertrand MA, Bauriaud R. Evaluation of the Captia enzyme immunoassays for detection of immunoglobulins G and M to *Treponema pallidum* in syphilis. *J Clin Microbiol* 1990; **28**: 1704–1707.

98 Egglestone SI, Turner AJL, and for the PHLS Syphilis Serology Working Group. Serological diagnosis of syphilis. *Communicable Disease and Public Health* 2000; **3**: 158–162.

99 Jurado RL, Campbell J, Martin PD. Prozone phenomenon in secondary syphilis. Has its time arrived? *Arch Intern Med* 1993; **153**: 2496–2498.

100 Lamagni TL, Hughes G, Rogers PA, Paine T, Catchpole M. New cases seen at genitourinary medicine clinics: England 1998. *Communicable Disease Report* 2000; **9** (Suppl. 6), S1–S12.

101 Centers for Disease Control and Prevention. Case definitions for public health surveillance. *MMWR* 1990; **39**: 34–38.

102 Reeves RR, Pinkofsky HB, Kennedy KK. Unreliability of current screening tests for syphilis in chronic psychiatric patients. *Am J Psychiatry* 1996; **153**: 1487–1488.

103 Haas JS, Bolan G, Larsen SA, Clement MJ, Bacchetti P, Moss AR. Sensitivity of treponemal tests for detecting prior treated syphilis during human immunodeficiency virus infection. *J Infect Dis* 1990; **162**: 862–866.

104 Murphy FT, George R, Kubota K, Fears M, Pope V, Howard RS, Dennis GJ. The use of Western blotting as the confirmatory test for syphilis in patients with rheumatic disease. *J Rheumatol* 1999; **26**: 2448–2453.

105 Carlsson B, Hanson HS, Wasserman J, Brauner A. Evaluation of the fluorescent treponemal antibody-absorption (FTA-Abs)

test specificity. *Acta Derm Venereol* 1991; **71**: 306–311.

106 Erbelding EJ, Vlahov D, Nelson KE, *et al.* Syphilis serology in human immuno-deficiency virus infection: Evidence for false-negative fluorescent treponemal testing. *J Infect Dis* 1997; **176**: 1397–1400.

107 Beebe JL, Nouri NJ. Comparative evaluation of commercial fluorescent treponemal antibody-absorbed test kits. *J Clin Microbiol* 1984; **19**: 789–793.

108 Chronas G, Moyes A, Young H. Syphilis diagnosis: screening by enzyme immunoassay and variation in fluorescent antibody absorbed (FTA-ABS) confirmatory test performance. *Med Lab Sci* 1992; **49**: 50–55.

109 Larsen SA, Farshy CE, Pender BJ, Adams MR, Pettit DE, Hambie EA. Staining intensities in the fluorescent treponemal antibody-absorption (FTA-Abs) test: association with the diagnosis of syphilis. *Sex Transm Dis* 1986; **13**: 221–227.

109a Young H, Moyes A, Seagar L, McMillan A. Novel recombinant-antigen enzyme immunoassay for serological diagnosis of syphilis. *J Clin Microbiol* 1998; **36**: 913–917.

110 Halling VW, Jones MF, Bestrom JE, *et al.* Clinical comparison of the *Treponema pallidum* CAPTIA syphilis-G enzyme immunoassay with the fluorescent treponemal antibody absorption immunoglobulin G assay for syphilis testing. *J Clin Microbiol* 1999; **37**: 3233–3234.

111 Ebel A, Vanneste L, Cardinaels M, *et al.* Validation of the INNO-LIA syphilis kit as a confirmatory assay for *Treponema pallidum* antibodies. *J Clin Microbiol* 2000; **38**: 2215–2219.

112 Young H. Syphilis: new diagnostic directions (editorial). *Int J STD AIDS* 1992; 3: 391–413.

113 Young H, Moyes A, Seagar L, McMillan A. Novel recombinant-antigen enzyme immunoassay for serological diagnosis of syphilis. *J Clin Microbiol* 1998; **36**: 913–917.

114 Lukehart SA, Hook EW, Baker-Zander SA, Collier AC, Critchlow CW, Handsfield HH. Invasion of the central nervous system by *Treponema pallidum*: implications for diagnosis and treatment. *Ann Intern Med* 1988; 109: 855–862.

115 De Silva Y, Walzman M, Shahmanesh M. The value of serum TPHA titres in selecting patients for lumbar puncture. *Genitourin Med* 1991; **67**: 37–40.

116 Luger A, Marhold I, Schmidt BL. Laboratory support in the diagnosis of neurosyphilis. World Health Organization WHO/VDT/RES/88. 1988: 379.

116a Luger AF, Schmidt BL, Kaulich M. Significance of laboratory findings for the diagnosis of neurosyphilis. *Int J STD AIDS* 2000; **11**: 224–234.

117 Larsen SA, Hambie EA, Wobig GH, Kennedy EJ. Cerebrospinal fluid serologic test for syphilis: treponemal and non-treponemal tests. In: Morisset R, Kurstak E, (eds) *Advances in Sexually Transmitted Diseases*. Utrecht, The Netherlands; VNU Science Press; 1985, pp. 157–162.

118 Hollander H. Cerebrospinal fluid normalities and abnormalities in individuals infected with human immunodeficiency virus. *J Infect Dis* 1988; **158**: 855–858.

119 Tomberlin MG, Holtom PD, Owens JL, Larsen RA. Evaluation of neurosyphilis in human immunodeficiency virus-infected individuals. *Clin Infect Dis* 1994; 18: 288–294.

120 Villanueva AV, Podzorski RP, Reyes MP. Effects of various handling and storage conditions on stability of *Treponema pallidum* DNA in cerebrospinal fluid. *J Clin Microbiol* 1998; **36**: 2117–2119.

121 Hay PE, Clarke JR, Taylor Robinson D, Goldmeier D. Detection of treponemal DNA in the CSF of patients with syphilis and HIV infection using the polymerase chain reaction. *Genitourin Med* 1990; **66**: 428–432.

122 Noordhoek GT, Wolters EC, de Jonge ME, van Embden JD. Detection by polymerase chain reaction of *Treponema pallidum* DNA in cerebrospinal fluid from neurosyphilis patients before and after antibiotic treatment. *J Clin Microbiol* 1991; **29**: 1976–1984.

123 Marra CM, Gary DW, Kuypers J, Jacobson MA. Diagnosis of neurosyphilis in patients infected with human immunodeficiency virus type 1. *J Infect Dis* 1996; **174**: 219–221.

124 Marra CM, Longstreth WT, Maxwell CL, Lukehart SA. Resolution of serum and cerebrospinal fluid abnormalities after treatment of neurosyphilis – influence of concomitant human immunodeficiency virus infection. *Sex Transm Dis* 1996; **23**: 184–189.

125 Stoll BJ, Lee FK, Larsen S, Hale E, *et al.* Clinical and serologic evaluation of neonates for congenital syphilis: a continuing diagnostic dilemma. *J Infect Dis* 1993; **167**: 1093–1099.

126 Schmitz JL, Gertis KS, Mauney C, Stamm LV, Folds JD. Laboratory diagnosis of congenital syphilis by immunoglobulin M (IgM) and IgA immunoblotting. *Clin Diag Lab Immunol* 1994; **1**: 32–37.

127 Sanchez PJ, Wendel GD, Grimprel E, *et al.* Evaluation of molecular methodologies and rabbit infectivity testing for the diagnosis of congenital syphilis and neonatal central nervous system invasion by *Treponema pallidum*. *J Infect Dis* 1993; **167**: 148–157.

128 Johnston NA. Neonatal congenital syphilis. Diagnosis by the absorbed fluorescent treponemal antibody (IgM) test. *Br J Vener Dis* 1972; **48**: 465–469.

129 Lackmann GM, Willnow U, Wahn V, Schroten H. The importance of reading test results. *Lancet* 1999; **353**: 290.

130 Lyon DJ. Congenital syphilis – when the medium fails to transmit the message. *Med J Aust* 1994; **160**: 94–95.

131 Chapel TA. The variability of syphilitic chancres. *Sex Transm Dis* 1978; **5**: 68–70.

132 Chapel TA. The signs and symptoms of secondary syphilis. *Sex Transm Dis* 1980; **7**: 161–164.

133 Lomholt G. Syphilis, yaws and pinta. In: Rook A, Wilkinson DS, Ebling FJG (eds) *Textbook of Dermatology* 3rd edition. Blackwell Scientific Publications; Oxford; 1979, pp. 701–747.

134 Miller RL. Pustular secondary syphilis. *Br J Vener Dis* 1974; **50**: 459–462.

135 Waugh MA. Bony symptoms in secondary syphilis. *Br J Vener Dis* 1976; **52**: 204–205.

136 Terry SI, Hanchard B, Brooks SEH, McDonald H, Siva S. Prevalence of liver abnormality in early syphilis. *Br J Vener Dis* 1984; **60**: 83–86.

137 Gamble CN, Reardan JB. Immunopathogenesis of syphilitic glomerulonephritis. Elution of antitreponemal antibody from glomerular immune-complex deposits. *N Engl J Med* 1975; **292**: 449–454.

138 Tait IA. Uveitis due to secondary syphilis. *Br J Vener Dis* 1983; **59**: 397–401.

139 MacFaul PA, Catterall RD. Acute choroidoretinitis in secondary syphilis. Presence of spiral organisms in the aqueous humour. *Br J Vener Dis* 1971; **47**: 159–161.

140 Parker JDJ. Uncommon complications of early syphilis. *Br J Vener Dis* 1972; **48**: 32–36.

141 Vercoe GS. The effect of early syphilis on the inner ear and auditory nerves. *J Laryngol Otol* 1976; **90**: 853–861.

142 Rosenhall U, Roupe G. Auditory brain-stem responses in syphilis. *Br J Vener Dis* 1981; **57**: 241–245.

143 Hira SK, Hira RS. Parotitis with secondary syphilis. A case report. *Br J Vener Dis* 1984; **60**: 121–122.

144 Dunlop EMC, Zwink FB. Incidence of corneal changes in congenital syphilis. *Br J Vener Dis* 1954; **30**: 201–209.

145 Robertson DMCL Argyll. (a) On an interesting series of eye-symptoms in a case of spinal disease, etc. *Edinburgh Med J* **14**: 696–708. (b) Four cases of spinal myosis, etc. *Edinburgh Med J* 1869; **15**: 487–493.

146 Poole CJM. Argyll Robertson pupils due to neurosarcoidosis: evidence for site of lesion. *Br Med J* 1984; **289**: 356.

147 Horowitz HW, Valsmis MP, Wicher V, *et al.* Cerebral syphilitic gumma confirmed by the polymerase chain reaction in a man with human immunodeficiency virus *N Engl J Med* 1994; **331**: 1488–1491.

148 Hooshmand H, Escobar MR, Koff SW. Neurosyphilis: a study of 241 patients. *JAMA* 1972; **219**: 729.

149 Wendel DG, Sanchez PJ, Peters MT et al. Identification of *Treponema pallidum* in amniotic fluid and fetal blood from pregnancies complicated by congenital syphilis. *Obstet Gynecol* 1991; **78**: 890–895.

150 Hallak M, Peipert JF, Ludomirsky A, Byers J. Nonimmune hydrops fetalis and fetal congenital syphilis: a case report. *J Reprod Med* 1992; **37**: 173–176.

151 Nathan L, Twickler DM, Peters MT, Sanchez PJ, Wendel GD. Fetal syphilis: correlation of sonographic findings and rabbit infectivity testing of amniotic fluid. *J Ultrsound Med* 1993; **2**: 97–101.

152 Nabarro D. *Congenital Syphilis*. Edward Arnold, London 1954.

153 Robinson RCV Congenital syphilis. Review article. *Arch Dermatol* 1969; **99**: 599–610.

154 Marchi AG, Tambussi AM, Famularo L. Un insolito guadro della disprotidemia luetica connatale: la crioglobulinemia. Present azrione di un caso. *Minerva Pediatrica* 1966; **18**: 1155–1157.

155 Hira SK, Bhat GJ, Patel JB, et al. Early congenital syphilis: clinico-radiologic features in 202 patients. *Sex Transm Dis* 1985; **12**: 177–183.

156 Oppenheimer EH, Hardy JB. Congenital syphilis in the newborn infant: Clinical and pathological observations in recent cases. *Johns Hopkins Med J* 1971; **129**: 63–82.

157 Yuceoglu AM, Sagel I, Tresser G, Wasserman E, Lange K. The glomerulopathy of congenital syphilis. *JAMA* 1974; **229**: 1085–1089.

158 Taitz LS, Isaacson C, Stein H. Acute nephritis associated with congenital syphilis. *Br Med J* 1961; **2**: 152–153.

159 Freiman I, Super M. Thrombocytopenia and congenital syphilis in South African Bantu infants. *Arch Dis Child* 1966; **41**: 87–90.

159a Genest DR, Choi-Hong SR, Tate JE, Qureshi F, Jacques SM, Crum C. Diagnosis of congenital syphilis from placental examination: comparison of histopathology, Steiner stain, and polymerase chain reaction for *Treponema pallidum* DNA. *Hum Pathol* 1996; **27**: 366–372.

160 Morrison AW. *Management of Sensorineural Deafness*. Butterworths, London. 1975, pp. 109–144.

161 Hutchinson J. On the influence of hereditary syphilis on the teeth. *Trans Odontol Soc* 1858; **2**: 95.

162 Putkonen T. Dental changes in congenital syphilis. Relationship to other stigmata. *Acta Dermato-venereol* 1962; **42**: 44–62.

163 Gilman AC, Goodman LS, Rall TW, Murad F (eds) *Goodman and Gilman's, the Pharmacological Basis of Therapeutics.* McMillan, New York, 1985, pp. 1115–1137.

164 Kern A. Grundlagen und gestaltung der penicillin-therapie der syphilis. *Medicamentum Berlin.* 1971; **12**: 194.

165 Turner TB, Holland DH. *Biology of the Treponematoses.* World Health Organisation, Monograph Series 1957; **35**: 43.

166 Idsoe O, Guthe E, Willcox RR. Penicillin in the treatment of syphilis: the experience of three decades. *Bulletin of the World Health Organisation* 1972; **47** (Suppl.).

167 Moore JE, Mohr CF. Biologically false positive serologic tests for syphilis. Type, incidence and cause. *JAMA* 1952; **150**: 467–473.

168 Collart P, Borel L-J, Durel P. Etude de l'action de la penicilline dans la syphilis tardive: persistence du treponeme pale. Premiere partie. La syphilis tardive experimentale apres traitement. *Annales de l'Institut Pasteur de Lille* 1962; **102**: 596–615.

169 Collart P, Borel L-J, Durel P. Etude de l'action de la penicilline dans la syphilis tardive: persistence du treponeme pale. Seconde partie. La syphilis tardive humaine apres traitement. *Annales de l'Institut Pasteur de Lille* 1962; **102**: 693–704.

170 Collart P, Borel L-J, Direl P. Significance of spiral organisms found after treatment in late human and experimental syphilis. *Br J Vener Dis* 1964; **40**: 81–89.

171 Dunlop EMC. Persistence of treponemes after treatment. *Br Med J* 1972; **2**: 577–580.

172 Centers for Disease Control and Prevention. 2002 Guidelines for treatment of sexually transmitted diseases. *MMWR* 2002; **51**: RR-6.

173 Clinical Effectiveness Group. UK national guidelines on sexually transmitted infections and closely related conditions. *www.mssvd.org.uk/ceg.htm*.

174 Onoda Y. Therapeutic effect of oral doxycycline on syphilis. *Br J Vener Dis* 1979; **55**: 110–115.

174a Johnson RC, Bey RF, Wolgamot SJ. Comparison of the activities of ceftriaxone and penicillin G against experimentally induced syphilis in rabbits. *Antimicrob Agents Chemother* 1982; **21**: 984–989.

174b Moorthy TT, Lee C-T, Lim K-B, Tan T. Ceftriaxone for treatment of primary syphilis in men: a preliminary study. *Sex Transm Dis* 1987; **14**: 116–118.

174c Hook EW, Roddy RE, Handsfield HH. Ceftriaxone therapy for incubating and early syphilis. *J Infect Dis* 1988; **158**: 881–884.

174d Augenbraun M, Workowski K. Ceftriaxone therapy for syphilis: report from the emerging infections network. *Clin Infect Dis* 1999; **29**: 1337–1338.

174e Kelkar PS, Li JT-C. Cephalosporin allergy. *N Engl J Med* 2001; **345**: 804–809.

174f Verdon MS, Handsfield HH, Johnson RB. Pilot study of azithromycin for treatment of primary and secondary syphilis. *Clin Infect Dis* 1994; **19**: 486–488.

174g Mashkilleyson AL, Gomberg MA, Mashkilleyson N, Kutin SA. Treatment of syphilis with azithromycin. *Int J STD AIDS* 1996; **7** (Suppl 1): 13–15.

175 Harshan V, Jayakumar W. Doxycycline in early syphilis: a long term follow-up. *Ind J Dermatol* 1982; **27**: 119–124.

176 Fernando WL. Erythromycin in early syphilis. *Br J Vener Dis* 1969; **45**: 200–201.

177 Hellerstrom S, Skog E. Outcome of penicillin therapy for syphilis. *Acta Dermatol Venereol* 1962; **42**: 179–193.

178 Kelly R. The treatment of neurosyphilis. *Practitioner* 1964; **192**: 90–95.

179 Wilner E, Brodie JA. Prognosis of general paresis after treatment. Lancet 1968; **ii**: 1370–1371.

180 Barling RWA, Skelton JB. The penetration of antibiotics into cerebrospinal fluid and brain tissue. *J Antimicrob Chemother* 1978; **4**: 203–227.

181 Mohr JA, Griffiths W, Jackson R, Saaddah H, Bird P, Riddle J. Neurosyphilis and penicillin levels in cerebrospinal fluid. *JAMA* 1976; **236**: 2208–2209.

182 Ritter G, Volles E, Muller F, Nabert-Bock G. Blut-liquor-kinetik von penicillin-G bei neurosyphilis. *Munchenen Medizinische Wochenschrift* 1975; **117**: 1383–1386.

183 Tramont EC. Persistence of *Treponema pallidum* following penicillin G therapy: Report of two cases. *JAMA* 1976; **236**: 2206–2207.

184 Greene BM, Miller NR, Bynum TE. Failure of penicillin G benzathine in the treatment of neurosyphilis. *Arch Int Med* 1980; **140**: 1117–1118.

185 Ducas J, Robson HG. Cerebrospinal fluid penicillin levels during therapy for latent syphilis. *JAMA* 1981; **246**: 2583–2584.

186 Ries CA, Rosenbaum JJ, Garatty G, Petz LD, Fudenberg H. Penicillin-induced hemolytic anaemia. *JAMA* 175; **233**: 432–435.

187 Fishman RA. Blood–brain and CSF barriers to penicillin and related organic acids. *Arch Neurol* 1966; **15**: 113–124.

188 Dunlop EM, Al-Egaily SS, Houang ET. Penicillin levels in blood and CSF achieved by treatment of syphilis. *JAMA* 1979; **241**: 2538–2540.

189 Yim CW, Flynn NM, Fitzgerald FT. Penetration of oral doxycycline into the cerebrospinal fluid for patients with latent or neurosyphilis. *Antimicrob Agents Chemother* 1985; **28**: 347–348.

190 Morrison RE, Harrison SM, Tramont EC. Oral amoxycillin, an alternative treatment for neurosyphilis. *Genitourin Med* 1985; **61**: 359–362.

190a Marra CM, Slatter V, Tartaglione TA, Baker–Zander SA, Lukehart SA. Evaluation of aqueous penicillin G and ceftriaxone for experimental neurosyphilis. *J Infect Dis* 1992; **165**: 396–397.

191 Moore JE, Farmer TW, Hockenga MT. Penicillin and the Jarisch-Herxheimer reaction in early, cardiovascular, and neurosyphilis. *Transactions of the Association of American Physicians* 1948; **61**: 176–183.

192 Walton Sir John. *Brain's Diseases of the Nervous System* 9th edition. Oxford University Press; Oxford: 1985, pp. 104, 271–272.

193 Ekbom K. Carbamazepine in the treatment of tabetic lightning pains. *Arch Neurol* 1972; **26**: 374–378.

194 Spence MR. Genital infections in pregnancy. *Med Clin North Am* 1977; **61**: 139–151.

195 Fenton LJ, Light IJ. Syphilis after maternal treatment with erythromycin. *Obstet Gynecol* 1976; **47**: 492–494.

196 South MA, Short DH, Knox JM. Failure of erythromycin estolate therapy in *in utero* syphilis. *JAMA* 1964; **190**: 70–72.

197 Green GR. In: Stewart GT, McGovern JP (eds) *Penicillin Allergy: Clinical and Immunological Aspects*. CC Thomas; Springfield IL: 1974, p. 162.

198 Solley GO, Gleich GJ, van Dellen RG. Penicillin allergy: clinical experience with a battery of skin-test reagents. *J Allergy Clin Immunol* 1982; **69**: 238–244.

199 Kerr AG, Smyth GDL, Cinnamond MJ. Congenital syphilitic deafness. *J Laryngol Otol* 1973; **87**: 1–12.

200 Kaufman RE, Blount JH, Jones OG. Epidemiologic treatment in early syphilis. *Public Health Reviews* 1974; **3**: 175–198.

201 Brown ST, Zaidi A, Larsen SA, Reynolds GH. Serological response to syphilis treatment. A new analysis of old data. *JAMA* 1985; **253**: 1296–1299.

202 Romanowski B, Sutherland R, Fick GH, Mooney D, Love EJ. Serologic response to treatment of infectious syphilis. *Ann Intern Med* 1991; **114**: 1005–1009.

203 Muller F, Lindenschmidt E-G. Demonstration of specific 19S (IgM) antibodies in untreated and treated syphilis: comparative studies of the 19S (IgM)-TPHA test and the solid-phase haemadsorption assay. *Br J Vener Dis* 1982; **58**: 12–17.

204 Ijsselmuiden OE, van der Sluis JJ, Mulder A, Stolz E, Bolton KP, van Eijk RV. An IgM capture enzyme linked immunosorbent assay to detect IgM antibodies to treponemes in patients with syphilis. *Genitourin Med* 1989; **65**: 79–83.

205 Muller F, Wollemann G. Analysis of specific immunoglobulin M immune response to *Treponema pallidum* before and after penicillin treatment of human syphilis. *Eur J Sex Transm Dis* 1985; **2**: 67–72.

206 Shannon R, Copley CG, Morrison GD. Immunological responses in late syphilis. *Br J Vener Dis* 1980; **56**: 372–376.

207 Schmidt BL, Gschnait F, Luger A. Comparison of three different *Treponema pallidum* specific IgM-tests. *Biology and pathogenicity of treponemes* conference sponsored by the World Health Organization 1989 (abstract).

208 Gudjonsson H, Skog E. The effect of prednisolone on the Jarisch-Herxheimer reaction. *Acta Dermatol Venereol* 1968; **48**: 15–18.

209 Bryceson ADM, Cooper KE, Warrell DA, Perine PL, Parry EHO. Studies on the mechanism of the Jarisch-Herxheimer reaction in louse-borne relapsing fever: evidence for the presence of circulating *Borrelia* endotoxin. *Clin Sci* 1972; **43**: 343–354.

210 Jackson SW, Zey PN. Ultrastructure of lipopolysaccharide isolated from *Treponema pallidum. J Bacteriol* 1973; **114**: 838–844.

211 Gelfland JA, Elin RJ, Berry FW, Frank MM. Endotoxaemia associated with the Jarisch-Herxheimer reaction. *N Engl J Med* 1976; **295**: 211–213.

212 Radolf JD, Norgard MV, Brandt ME, Isaacs RD, Thompson PA, Beutler B. Lipoproteins of *Borrelia burgdorferi* and *Treponema pallidum* activate cachectin/tumor necrosis factor synthesis: analysis using a CAT reporter construct. *J Immunol* 1991; **147**: 1968–1974.

213 Negussie Y, Remick DG, DeForge LE, Kunkel SL, Eynon A, Griffin GE. Detection of plasma tumor necrosis factor, interleukin 6, and 8, during the Jarisch-Herxheimer reaction of relapsing fever. *J Exp Med* 1992; **175**: 1207–1212.

214 Warrel DA, Pope HM, Parry EHO, Perine PL, Bryceson ADM. Cardiorespiratory disturbances associated with infective fever in man: studies of Ethiopian louse-borne relapsing fever. *Clin Sci* 1970; **39**: 123–145.

215 Coxon RE, Fekade D, Knox D, et al. The effect of antibody against TNF alpha on cytokine response in Jarisch-Herxheimer reactions of louse-borne relapsing fever. *QJM* 1997; **90**: 213–221.

216 Griffin GE. Cytokines involved in human septic shock – the model of the Jarisch-Herxheimer reaction. *J Antimicrob Chemother* 1998; **41** (Suppl. A): 25–29.

217 Cooper PJ, Fekade D, Remick DG, Wherry J, Griffin GE. Recombinant human interleukin-10 fails to alter proinflammatory cytokine production or physiologic changes associated with the Jarisch-Herxheimer reaction. *J Infect Dis* 2000; **181**: 203–209.

218 Klein VR, Cox SM, Mitchell MD, Wendel GD. The Jarisch-Herxheimer reaction complicating syphilotherapy in pregnancy. *Obstet Gynecol* 1990; **75**: 375–380.

219 Myles TD, Elam G, Park-Hwang E, Nguyen T. The Jarisch-Herxheimer reaction and fetal monitoring changes in pregnant women treated for syphilis. *Obstet Gynecol* 1998; **92**: 859–864.

220 Ghys PD, Fransen K, Diallo MO, et al. The associations between cervicovaginal HIV shedding, sexually transmitted diseases and immunosuppression in female sex workers in Abidjan, Cote d'Ivoire. *AIDS* 1997; **11**: F85–F93.

221 Otten MW, Zaidi AA, Peterman TA, Rolfs RT, Witte JJ. High rate of HIV seroconversion among patients attending urban sexually transmitted disease clinics. *AIDS* 1994; **8**: 549–553.

222 Fleming DT, Wasserheit JN. From epidemiological synergy to public health policy and practice: the contribution of other sexually transmitted diseases to sexual transmission of HIV infection. *Sex Transm Inf* 1999; **75**: 3–17.

223 Hutchinson CM, Hook EW, Shepherd M, Verley J, Rompalo AM. Altered clinical presentation of early syphilis in patients with human immunodeficiency virus infection. *Ann Intern Med* 1994; **121**: 94–100.

224 Radolf JD, Kaplan RP. Unusual manifestations of secondary syphilis and abnormal humoral immune response to *Treponema pallidum* antigens in a homosexual man with asymptomatic human immunodeficiency virus infection. *J Am Acad Dermatol* 1988; **18**: 423–428.

225 Bari MM, Shulkin DJ, Abell E. Ulcerative syphilis in acquired immunodeficiency syndrome: a case of precocious tertiary syphilis in a patient with human immunodeficiency virus. *J Am Acad Dermatol* 1989; **21**: 1310–1312.

226 Tucker SC, Yates VM, Thambar IV. Unusual skin ulceration in an HIV-positive patient who had cutaneous syphilis and neurosyphilis. *Br J Dermatol* 1997; **136**: 946–948.

227 Katz DA, Berger JR, Duncan RC. Neurosyphilis. A comparative study of the effects of infection with human immunodeficiency virus. *Arch Neurol* 1993; **50**: 243–249.

228 Musher DM, Hamill RJ, Baughn RE. Effect of human immunodeficiency virus (HIV) infection on the course of syphilis and on the response to treatment. *Ann Intern Med* 1990; **113**: 872–881.

229 Flood JM, Weinstock HS, Guroy ME, Bayne L, Simon RP, Bolan G. Neurosyphilis during the AIDS epidemic, San Francisco. *J Infect Dis* 1998; **177**: 931–940.

230 McLeish WM, Pulido JS, Holland S, Culbertson WW. Winward K. The ocular manifestations of syphilis in the human immunodeficiency virus type 1 infected host. *Ophthalmology* 1990; **97**: 196–203.

231 Hicks CB, Benson PM, Lupton GP, Tramont EC. Seronegative secondary syphilis in a

patient infected with the human immunodeficiency virus (HIV) with Kaposi sarcoma. A diagnostic dilemma published erratum appears in *Ann Intern Med* 1987; **107**: 492–495 and 946 (erratum).

232 Zalka A. Grossman ME, Silvers DN. 'Seronegative' syphilis in AIDS. *Ann Intern Med* 1991; **114**: 521–522.

233 Anonymous. Recommendations for diagnosing and treating syphilis in HIV-infected patients. *MMWR* 1988; **37**: 600–602, 607–608.

234 Hutchinson CM, Rompalo AM, Reichart CA, Hook EW. Characteristics of patients with syphilis attending Baltimore STD clinics. Multiple high-risk subgroups and interactions with human immunodeficiency virus infection. *Arch Intern Med* 1991; **151**: 511–516.

235 Gourevitch MN, Selwyn PA, Davenny K, *et al.* Effects of HIV infection on the serologic manifestations and response to treatment of syphilis in intravenous drug users. *Ann Intern Med* 1993; **118**: 350–355.

235a Terry PM, Page ML, Goldmeier D. Are serological tests of value in diagnosing and monitoring response to treatment of syphilis in patients infected with human immunodeficiency virus? *Genitourin Med* 1988; **64**: 219–222.

236 Jurado RL. Use of nontreponemal tests in the diagnosis of syphilis – reply. *Arch Intern Med* 1994; **154**: 2616.

237 Goeman J, Kivuvu M, Nzila N, *et al.* Similar serological response to conventional therapy for syphilis among HIV-positive and HIV-negative women. *Genitourin Med* 1995; **71**: 275–279.

238 Bordon J, Martinez-Vazquez C, Alvarez M, Miralles C, Ocampo A, de la Fuente-Aguado J, Sopena-Perez Arguelles, B. Neurosyphilis in HIV-infected patients. *Eur J Clin Microbiol Infect Dis* 1995; **14**: 864–869.

239 Telzak EE, Greenberg MS, Harrison J, Stoneburner RL, Schultz S. Syphilis treatment response in HIV-infected individuals. *AIDS* 1991; **5**: 591–595.

240 Yinnon AM, Coury-Doniger P, Polito R, Reichman RC. Serologic response to treatment of syphilis in patients with HIV. *Arch Intern Med* 1996; **156**: 321–325.

241 Rolfs RT, Joesoef R, Hendershot EF, *et al.* A randomized trial of enhanced therapy for early syphilis in patients with and without human immunodeficiency virus infection. *N Engl J Med* 1997; **337**: 307–314.

242 Johnson PD, Graves SR, Stewart L, Warren R, Dwyer B, Lucas CR. Specific syphilis serological tests may become negative in HIV infection. *AIDS* 1991; **5**: 419–423.

243 Young H, Moyes A, Ross JDC. Markers of past syphilis in HIV infection comparing Captia syphilis G anti-treponemal IgG enzyme immunoassay with other treponemal antigen tests. *Int J STD AIDS* 1995; **6**: 101–104.

244 Sjovall P, Flamholc L, Kroon BM, Bredberg A. HIV infection and loss of treponemal test reactivity. *Acta Derm Venereol* 1991; **71**: 458.

245 Glatt AE. Stoffer HR, Forlenza S, Altieri RH. High-titer positive nontreponemal tests with negative specific treponemal serology in patients with HIV infection and/or intravenous substance use. *J Acquir Immune Defic Syndr* 1991; **4**: 861–864.

246 Rompalo AM, Cannon RO, Quinn TC, Hook EW. Association of biologic false-positive reactions for syphilis with human immunodeficiency virus infection. *J Infect Dis* 1992; **165**: 1124–1126.

247 Gordon SM, Eaton ME, George R, *et al.* The response of symptomatic neurosyphilis to high-dose penicillin G in patients with human immunodeficiency virus infection. *N Engl J Med* 1994; **331**: 1469–1473.

248 Marra CM, Boutin P, McArthur JC, *et al.* A pilot study evaluating ceftriaxone and penicillin G as treatment agents for neurosyphilis in human immunodeficiency virus-infected individuals. *Clin Infect Dis* 2000; **30**: 540–544.

249 Hook EW, Roddy RE, Lukehart SA, Hom J, Holmes KK, Tam MR. Detection of *Treponema pallidum* in lesion exudate with a pathogen-specific monoclonal antibody. *J Clin Microbiol* 1985; **22**: 241–244.

250 Kampmeier RJ. Late manifestations of syphilis: skeletal, visceral and cardiovascular. *Med Clin N Am* 1964; **48**: 667–697.

251 McMillan A. Scott GR. *Sexually Transmitted Infections, Colour Guide.* Churchill Livingstone; Edinburgh: 2000.

252 Rein MF (ed.). *Atlas of Infectious Diseases, Volume V, Sexually Transmitted Diseases.* Churchill Livingstone; Philadelphia: 1996.

253 Romanowski B, Forsey E, Prasad E, Lukehart S, Tam M, Hook EW. Detection of *Treponema pallidum* by a fluorescent monoclonal antibody test. *Sex Transm Dis.* 1987; **14**: 156–159.

254 Saxon A, Beall GN, Rohr AS, Adelman DC. Immediate hypersensitivity reactions to beta-lactam antibiotics (clinical conference). *Ann Intern Med* 1987; **107**: 204–215.

255 Smibert RM. Genus III Treponema. In: Kreig NR, Holt JG, eds. *Bergey's Manual of Systematic Bacteriology.* Baltimore & London. Williams and Wilkins. 1984, pp. 290–296.

256 Wendel GD, Stark BJ, Jamison RB, Molina RD, Sullivan TJ. Penicillin allergy and desensitization in serious infections during pregnancy. *N Engl J Med* 1985; **312**: 1229–1232.

257 Cummings MC, Lukehart SA, Marra C, *et al.* Comparison of methods for the detection of *Treponema pallidum* in lesions of early syphilis. *Sex Transm Dis* 1996; **23**: 366–369.

258 Perine PL, Hopkins DR, Niemel PLA. St John RK, Causse G, Antal GM. *Handbook of Endemic Treponematoses.* Geneva; World Health Organization: 1984.

259 Marquez F. Pinta. In: Canizares O (ed.) *Clinical Tropical Dermatology.* London; Blackwell: 1975, pp. 86.

260 Tharmaphornpilas P, Srivanichakorn S, Phraesrisakul N. Recurrence of yaws outbreak in Thailand, 1990. *S E Asia T Trop Med Public Health* 1994; **25**: 152–156.

261 WHO Scientific Group Endemic treponematoses making a comeback. *WHO Chronicle* 1982; **36**: 77–78.

262 Agadzi VK, Aboagye-Atta Y, Nelson JW. Perine PL, Hopkins DR. Resurgence of yaws in Ghana. *Lancet* 1983; **ii**: 389–390.

263 Anonymous. *Peoples of Africa. Pygmies.* London; Marshall Cavendish: 1978, pp. 154–157.

264 Widy-Wirski R, D'Costa J, Meheus J. Prevalence du pian chez les pygmees en Centrafique. *Annales de la societe Belge de medecine tropicale (Bruxelles)* 1980; **60**: 61–67.

265 Turnbull CM. *The Forest People.* London; Reprint Society: 1963.

266 Chambers HD. *Yaws (framboesia tropica).* London; Churchill: 1938.

267 Hackett CJ. *An International Nomenclature of Yaws Lesions.* Geneva; World Health Organization: 1957.

268 Hackett CJ. *Bone Lesions of Yaws in Uganda.* Oxford; Blackwell Scientific Publications: 1951.

269 Kerdel-Vegas F. Yaws. In: Rook A, Wilkinson DS, Ebling FIG, Champion RH, Burton IL (eds) *Textbook of Dermatology* 4th edition, vol. 1. London; Blackwell: 1986, pp. 871–878.

270 Grin EI. *Epidemiology and Control of Endemic Syphilis.* WHO, Monograph Series No. 11; Geneva: 1953.

271 Hudson FH. *Non-venereal Syphilis.* Edinburgh; Livingstone: 1958.

272 Guthe I, Ridet J, Vorst F, D'Costa J, Grab B. Methods for surveillance of endemic treponematoses and sero-immunological investigations of 'disappearing' disease. *Bull WHO* 1972; **46**: 1–14.

273 WHO Scientific Group. Multipurpose serological surveys and WHO Serum Reference Banks. *WHO Technical Report Series*; No 454: 1970.

274 WHO Scientific Group. *Treponematoses Research.* WHO Technical Report Series. No 455, 1970. p. 61.

275 Anselmi M, Araujo E, Narvaez A, Cooper PJ, Guderian RH. Yaws in Ecuador: impact of control measures on the disease in the Province of Esmeraldas. *Genitourin Med* 1995; **71**: 343–346.

276 Backhouse JL, Hudson BJ, Hamilton PA, Nesteroff SI. Failure of penicillin treatment of yaws on Karkar Island, Papua New Guinea. *Am J Trop Med Hyg* 1998; **59**: 388–392.

277 McMillan A. Scott GR. *Colour Aids in Sexually Transmitted Diseases.* Churchill Livingstone; Edinburgh: 1991.

APPENDICES

APPENDIX 15.1

PENICILLIN ALLERGY SKIN TESTING (SAXON *et al.* 1987[254] WITH KIND PERMISSION OF THE PUBLISHERS OF THE *ANNALS OF INTERNAL MEDICINE*).

Reagents

Major determinant

- Benzylpenicilloyl poly-L-lysine (Pre-Pen, Taylor Pharmaceutical Company, Decatur, Illinois) (6×10^{-5} M).

Minor determinants

- Benzylpenicillin G (10^{-2} M, 3.3 mg/mL, 6000 units/mL).
- Benzylpenicilloate (10^{-2} M, 3.3 mg/mL).
- Benzylpenicilloate (or penicilloyl propylamine) (10^{-2} M, 3.3 mg/mL).

Positive control

- Commercial histamine for epicutaneous skin testing.

Negative control

- Diluent used to dissolve other reagents, usually phenol saline.

Procedures

The use of antihistamines before testing should be avoided (for example, chlorpheniramine, discontinuation for at least 24 hours should precede testing).

Patients with a history of penicillin anaphylaxis or those receiving β-adrenergic blocking agents should be tested with 100-fold dilutions of the full-strength skin-test reagents before being tested with full-strength reagents. Otherwise if the patient has had another type of immediate reaction to penicillin within the preceding year, the antigens should be diluted tenfold.

Epicutaneous (prick) tests

Duplicate drops of skin-test reagents are placed on the ventral aspects of the forearm. The underlying epidermis is pricked with a fine needle (26-gauge) without drawing blood. The test is positive if the average wheal diameter after 15 minutes is 4 mm larger than that of negative controls. The histamine controls should be positive.

Intradermal tests

If the epicutaneous tests are negative, duplicate 0.02 mL intradermal injections of negative control and antigen solutions are made into the ventral aspects of the forearm, using a 26-gauge needle on a syringe. A test is positive if the average wheal diameter 15 minutes after injection is more than 2 mm larger than the negative controls.

APPENDIX 15.2

DESENSITIZATION

Desensitization and a state of unresponsiveness by host cells to specific antigen may be induced with increasing doses of antigen. Using phenoxymethylpenicillin (penicillin V) by the oral route, a safer desensitization procedure than with parenteral benzylpenicillin. Wendel *et al.*[256] have followed a protocol (Table 15.9) which was effective therapeutically in pregnant women with syphilis. In this procedure an elixir of phenoxymethylpenicillin was given orally in doses of initially 0.059 mg (approximately equivalent to 0.06 mg or 100 IU of benzylpenicillin) and increasing by approximately doubling the oral dose every 15 minutes for 14 doses. During the desensitization procedure in hospital, intravenous lines were established and close personal medical supervision was maintained for 24 hours. Mild cutaneous reactions were allowed to resolve spontaneously or were treated with diphen-

Table 15.9 Oral desensitization protocol for patients with a positive skin test (from Wendel *et al.* 1985[256] copyright with 1985 Massachusetts Medical Society. All rights reserved)

Phenoxymethyl penicillin dose[a]	Amount (units/mL)	Volume (mL)	Units	Cumulative dose (units)
1	1000	0.1	100	100
2	1000	0.2	200	300
3	1000	0.4	400	700
4	1000	0.8	800	1 500
5	1000	1.6	1600	3 100
6	1000	3.2	3200	6 300
7	1000	6.4	6400	12 700
8	10 000	1.2	12 000	24 700
9	10 000	2.4	24 000	48 700
10	10 000	4.8	48 000	96 700
11	80 000	1.0	80 000	176 700
12	80 000	2.0	160 000	336 700
13	80 000	4.0	320 000	656 700
14	80 000	8.0	640 000	1 296 700

[a] Interval between doses, 15 minutes, elapsed time 3 hours and 45 minutes, cumulative dose 1.3 MIU.

hydramine 25 mg intravenously. After the desensitization process patients were able to tolerate intramuscular benzathine penicillin treatment in doses appropriate to their infec- tion, although close observation was given on re-admission for an oral test dose of 236 mg phenoxymethylpenicillin (equivalent to 240 mg or 400 000 IU of benzyl peni- cillin) followed by observation for 1 hour. The injection of benzathine penicillin was then given and the patients were monitored overnight.

Chapter 16

Tropical bacterial sexually transmissible infections
A McMillan, R C Ballard

Chancroid

Chancroid is an STI caused by the bacterium *Haemophilus ducreyi*. There is a high incidence in tropical countries, particularly in areas where living standards are low. Prostitutes constitute an important reservoir of infection. Although chancroid may occur in temperate climates, most infections have been imported from the tropics.

After a pre-patent period, usually less than 1 week, one or more ulcers develop on the genitalia, and are associated, in about half of the cases, with inguinal and/or femoral lymphadenitis. Untreated, an abscess develops in the affected lymph nodes and this may rupture through the skin, producing a sinus. Extensive tissue destruction is a distressing complication of the disease. Chancroid is a risk factor for the heterosexual spread of HIV.

In the past a diagnosis of chancroid was generally based on clinical findings and the exclusion of other conditions. This is no longer acceptable, and a definitive diagnosis of chancroid should be made only where *H. ducreyi* is recovered from genital ulcers, or specific nucleic acid sequences are detected in material obtained from lesions.

ETIOLOGY

Haemophilus ducreyi

Morphological and cultural characteristics

The causative organism, *Haemophilus ducreyi*, was first described in 1889 by Ducrey[1]. It is a small Gram-negative coccobacillus which tends to occur in clumps or chains. In smears made from lesions, or material aspirated from swollen regional lymph glands, intracellular as well as extracellular bacteria may be noted. Typically *H. ducreyi* is seen as short rods in a mucous matrix forming a 'rail-road track' or 'shoal of fish' pattern. A similar characteristic pattern is obtained when growth is taken from solid media, crushed on a slide and Gram-stained[2].

Haemophilus ducreyi is a fastidious organism: a humid atmosphere enriched with 5% to 10% carbon dioxide, incubation at 33°C to 35°C, and a pH of 6.5 to 7.0 are required for optimum growth. For primary isolation culture, methods with liquid or clotted-blood media have been superseded by solid selective media containing vancomycin. Rabbit, horse, sheep, or human blood may be used for enrichment.

Taxonomy and biochemical characterization

Our knowledge of the taxonomy of *H. ducreyi* is meager. Kilian[3] examined nine strains of *H. ducreyi* in the course of his impressive study of 426 strains of the genus *Haemophilus*. There were differences between the strains of *H. ducreyi*, all of which were originally isolated from cases of chancroid. Kilian divided them into two strains which he felt were acceptable as members of the *Haemophilus* genus, and seven that were unacceptable. However, as he was unable to judge which of the two groups agreed with Ducrey's original description, he recorded all nine strains as *H. ducreyi*.

Although new isolation and identification procedures have been developed, some properties of the species are still not clearly defined and its nutritional requirements, biochemical reactions, and colony characteristics are still debated[4]. For example, *H. ducreyi* has been considered to be both oxidase negative[3] and oxidase positive[5]. However, Nobre[4] noted that the oxidase test was positive when using the tetramethyl-p-phenylenediamine dihydrochloride but negative with the dimethyl compound.

By definition, the genus *Haemophilus* requires X factor (hemin or certain other porphyrins), or V factor (nicotinamide adenine dinucleotide), or both for growth. Although there have been reports that *H. ducreyi* does not require X factor, this is most likely a reflection of the culture medium and the strength of the disks used in the test. Hammond *et al.*[6] found that *H. ducreyi* requires a greater hemin concentration for growth than that required by other *Haemophilus* spp.

The need for exogenous hemin was confirmed by a negative porphyrin test thus demonstrating the lack of enzymic capability of *H. ducreyi* to synthesize hemin from aminolevulinic acid.

Haemophilus ducreyi tends to be inert in biochemical tests. Most investigators have reported little active carbohydrate fermentation. Nitrate reduction is a useful positive character. However, depending on the test conditions, isolates may be nitrate negative[2]. Alkaline phosphatase activity is another useful positive identification feature. Nitrate reduction and phosphatase activity form the basis of the rapid identification of *H. ducreyi* in a commercially available system[7]; lack of biochemical activity apart from nitrate reduction and phosphatase activity allowed differentiation between *H. ducreyi*, *H. influenzae*, *H. parainfluenzae*, and *H. aphrophilus*.

A major outer membrane protein with a molecular weight of 40 kDa is present in all strains of *H. ducreyi* and belongs to the OmpA family of proteins[8]. Very fine pili, consisting of a protein of molecular weight about 24 kDa are also found[9].

Hemolysin that is related to the calcium independent hemolysin produced by *Proteus mirabilis* is produced by *H. ducreyi*[10].

Plasmid-mediated β-lactamase production

The first reports of β-lactamase activity in *H. ducreyi* were published in 1978 soon after the discovery of β-lactamase production in *Neisseria gonorrhoeae*. Hammond et al.[6] examined the antibiotic susceptibility of nineteen strains of *H. ducreyi* isolated during an outbreak of chancroid in Winnipeg, Manitoba, Canada. They found that three strains were resistant to ampicillin (MIC >128 μg/mL) and produced β-lactamase. Later the β-lactamase activity of these strains was shown to be mediated by a 6.0×10^6 Da (6 MDa) non-conjugative plasmid[11]. Further characterization[12] suggested that the β-lactamase produced by *H. ducreyi* was a TEM-1 β-lactamase coded for by a plasmid containing a Tn2 type transposon. Although the Tn2 type transposon is possibly of enteric origin, it has been transposed into a small non-self-transmissible plasmid shared by members of the genera *Haemophilus* and *Neisseria*. Ampicillin resistance plasmids in *H. ducreyi* can be transferred by conjugation to *Haemophilus* recipients, provided that the donor cell also harbors a 23.5 MDa plasmid with the ability to mobilize the smaller resistance plasmid[13].

Handsfield et al.[14] studied plasmids from *H. ducreyi* isolated in Seattle, USA. All strains had an ampicillin resistance plasmid with a molecular weight of either 7.3, 5.7, or 3.6 MDa. Plasmid molecular weights were identical for isolates from epidemiologically linked cases and differed according to the geographical origins of the strains.

Although there are varying size estimates of plasmids reported by different authors, there are clear similarities between the plasmids of *H. ducreyi* and those of *N. gonorrhoeae*. The 5.7 (or 6.0) MDa *H. ducreyi* plasmid carries the entire sequence of pFA7, the 3.2 MDa β-lactamase-specifying plasmid found in isolates of *N. gonorrhoeae* linked originally to West Africa. Plasmids of 7.0 (or 7.3)

MDa carry the entire sequence of pFA3, the 4.4 MDa β-lactamase-specifying plasmid found in strains of *N. gonorrhoeae* originally isolated in the Far East[15]. The 3.2 (or 3.6) MDa *H. ducreyi* plasmid has also been shown to be the same as that found in gonococci[16]. Production of β-lactamase is common among *H. ducreyi* isolates from diverse geographical areas, for example Orange County, California,[16], Singapore[17], Johannesburg, South Africa[18], and Nairobi, Kenya[19].

Virulence and pathogenicity

Although there are several possible virulence factors, including lipo-oligosaccharide, pili, hemolysin, cytotoxin, and a hemoglobin-binding outer membrane protein, the mechanisms are little understood. In cultured human epithelial cell lines, *H. ducreyi* adheres to cells, adherence reaching a peak after 2 to 3 hours incubation[20]. These eukaryotic cells must be viable with native surface structures for adherence to occur. Some adherent bacteria can be seen invading epithelial cells, and later cell death and damage to the monolayer results. The cytotoxin produced by *H. ducreyi* that causes destruction of eukaryotic cells[21] can be neutralized by immune serum[21a], and may play an important part in pathogenesis. Isogenic mutants of *H. ducreyi* 35 000, a wild-type clinical strain, have now been constructed, and animal model systems, reviewed by Lewis[22], should provide invaluable insight into the virulence of the organism.

An experimental model of infection with *H. ducreyi*, that has proved useful in some studies, has been described by Spinola and colleagues[23]. Bacterial suspensions are loaded onto a Multi-Test applicator (this contains nine individual tines that penetrate the skin to about 2 mm) and pressed into the upper arm. The probabilities of pustule formation are dose dependent, and increasing the estimated delivered dose results in a higher probability of papule and pustule formation[24].

When bacterial suspensions are inoculated into the skin of human volunteers, papular lesions, that sometimes become pustular, develop. There is an infiltrate of polymorphonuclear leukocytes, macro-

phages, and CD4+ T cells. Human leukocyte antigen DR is expressed on the keratinocytes, probably as the result of expression of interferon-γ[25]. Messenger RNA for interleukin-8, a powerful inducer of neutrophil chemotaxis, and for tumor necrosis factor-α are also found in papules and pustules[26]. These immune responses resemble delayed-type hypersensitivity reactions.

PATHOLOGY

There is a superficial necrotic layer of polymorphonuclear leukocytes with fibrin and red cells that forms the base of the ulcer[27]. Beneath this there are one or two deeper layers recognizable histologically. The deep zone shows a dense infiltration of plasma cells and lymphocytes, above which there is a marked endothelial proliferation, palisading of blood vessels, degeneration of their walls, and occasional thrombosis[28]. The lymphocytic infiltrate contains macrophages, CD4+ and CD8+ T cells[29].

EPIDEMIOLOGY

On a global scale chancroid is a more frequent cause of genital ulceration than syphilis. The incidence of chancroid is highest in tropical and subtropical countries, particularly in southern, central, and eastern Africa. *Haemophilus ducreyi* has been isolated from up to 68% of cases of genital ulcer disease in South Africa[30]. Cases reported in temperate climates are usually in patients who have acquired their infection in the tropics (and their subsequent contacts). Chancroid is a rare disease in the UK but within the past 25 years there have been outbreaks in Canada[31], The Netherlands[32], Greenland[33], and in the USA[34]. In a recent outbreak of genital ulcer disease in Jackson, Mississippi[35], *H. ducreyi* was identified as the cause of the ulceration in 56 (39%) of 143 men. *Haemophilus ducreyi* has also been shown to be an important cause of genital ulceration in patients attending STI clinics in other US cities[36]: in Memphis, Tennessee, and in Chicago, Illinois, *Haemophilus ducreyi* was identified as the causative organism in 20% and 12% respectively of patients with genital ulcer disease. As these clinics tend to serve selected populations, however, care should be exercised in extrapolating these results to the general population.

It has long been considered that there is an association between chancroid, poverty and poor standards of hygiene. Its incidence decreases as the standard of living improves. Chancroid is more prevalent in war-time, and prostitutes are thought to constitute an important reservoir of infection. Among American troops in the Korean War it was fourteen to twenty-one times more common than gonorrhea[37], while in the Vietnam conflict the incidence of chancroid was second to that of gonorrhea among venereal diseases[38]. Over a 12-month period Hart[39] reported 269 cases of gonorrhea, 253 of non-gonococcal urethritis, 163 of chancroid, 5 of syphilis, and 62 of genital herpes among Australian troops in Vietnam. Unfortunately the diagnosis of chancroid was not made by isolation of *H. ducreyi* but by the appearance of the penile lesion, the presence of Gram-negative coccobacilli on Gram-stained smears, a negative dark ground examination, negative serological tests for syphilis, and the lack of other demonstrable pathogens.

To this day, prostitutes are considered an important reservoir of infection[40]. In a study of 300 men in Nairobi with culture-proven chancroid, 57% had acquired their infection from prostitutes. There was geographical clustering of areas where infection was acquired in the city center and in several poorer residential areas, suggesting geographical and social integrity of high-frequency transmission groups. Thirty-nine contact pairs, in whom the male partner had positive cultures, were examined. In 10 pairs the woman was designated the source contact; 8 of the 10 women had symptomatic chancroid and 6 were culture positive. These findings suggest that most female transmitters of *H. ducreyi* have genital ulcers. Of 29 women who were considered to be secondary contacts, 16 had symptomatic ulcers, 1 an asymptomatic ulcer and 12 had no ulcers. Of the 17 women with ulcers, 10 had positive cultures. Three of the 12 women with no evidence of genital ulceration on clinical examination had positive cervical cultures. In nearly half of the women in whom chancroid developed after exposure to the index man, sexual exposure occurred only while the man was incubating chancroid. As shown by the presence of *H. ducreyi* or genital ulceration, the infectivity of *H. ducreyi* for women from a single sexual contact with an infected man was estimated to be 63%. *Haemophilus ducreyi* infection in women was highly pathogenic, 10 of 13 infected women had genital ulcers.

Among prostitute populations implicated in the transmission of chancroid, genital ulcers were detected in 10% and asymptomatic genital carriage of *H. ducreyi* in 4% of the women. These women could either be transient or persistent carriers of *H. ducreyi* or could be incubating chancroid. Genital ulcers were less common in prostitutes not implicated in chancroid transmission and *H. ducreyi* carriage was not found in such women. Although the study was not designed to measure asymptomatic carriage of *H. ducreyi*, Hawkes et al.[41], using PCR to detect *H. ducreyi*-specific nucleic acids, found that 2% of 213 sex-industry workers in The Gambia, carried the organism without symptoms or signs.

DiCarlo and colleagues[34] examined the epidemiology of chancroid amongst 118 men with culture-proven *H. ducreyi* infection in New Orleans. They noted that by comparison with men with genital herpes, patients with chancroid were much more likely to have used cocaine, to have had sex with a prostitute, and to have traded drugs for sex. By the use of ribotyping, plasmid content and the antimicrobial sensitivity of the isolates, it was shown that these cases were caused by a limited number of strains[42]. This finding suggested that there was a limited introduction of *H. ducreyi* into the New Orleans community. The same workers[42] showed that isolates from patients with chancroid in Jackson, Mississippi, had ribotype patterns that differed from those of the New Orleans patients, suggesting that the two outbreaks were probably unrelated.

Association of chancroid with HIV infection

Several studies from Africa that have been reviewed by Wasserheit[43] have shown that genital ulcer disease, the majority of cases being associated with *H. ducreyi*, is a risk factor for the heterosexual transmission of HIV. After controlling for sexual behavior, two prospective studies showed that there is a significantly increased risk of HIV sero-conversion among patients with ulcerative genital disease (odds ratio 4.7 for men and 3.7 for women)[44, 45]. Using culture or PCR, HIV-1 can be detected in chancroid lesions[46, 35], and the recruitment of CD4+ T cells and macrophages into the lesions may partly explain the facilitation of HIV transmission in patients with chancroid.

CLINICAL FEATURES

The pre-patent period of chancroid is short, usually 2 to 3 days, although it may vary from as little as 24 hours to longer than 5 days[47].

The earliest lesion is a papule that soon becomes a pustule and ulcerates as a result of thrombotic occlusion of underlying dermal blood vessels. Characteristically, the superficial ulcer so formed is painful and tender. A gray membrane covers its floor and removal of this membrane reveals glistening granulation tissue that bleeds easily. The edges are ragged and undermined, and a narrow zone of erythema surrounds the ulcer. Unlike the primary lesion of syphilis, the lesions of chancroid are not indurated. The size of the individual ulcers varies from 3 to about 20 mm in diameter.

As a result of autoinoculation of surrounding tissues, multiple ulcers are often produced (Figure 16.1), and lesions at various stages of development are commonly seen in the same patient. Although single ulcers may occur, multiple ulcers are more common.

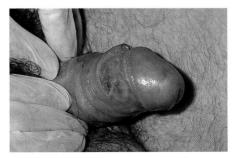

Figure 16.1 Sub-preputial chancroid (reproduced from McMillan and Scott 2000[119])

In the male, the lesions of chancroid most commonly occur at the preputial orifice, the resulting inflammation producing phimosis and, less frequently, a paraphimosis. Less frequently ulceration may occur on the glans penis, the shaft of the penis, or the distal urethra. Chancroid of the anal region may occur in male homosexuals, and autoinoculation from penile lesions may produce lesions of the scrotum and thighs.

The labia majora, introitus, vagina, and perianal regions are most commonly affected in the female. Rarely, cervical lesions have been described.

Extragenital lesions of chancroid are rare, and disseminated *H. ducreyi* infection is unknown.

In at least 60% of patients with chancroid, inguinal lymph nodes become enlarged on one or both sides within days to weeks of the appearance of the genital lesions. Initially the nodes are discrete and not tender. In about half of those who develop lymphadenopathy, suppuration occurs in the nodes, which become tender, matted together and show evidence of unilocular abscess formation (bubo) (Figure 16.2). The overlying skin, to which the inflamed glands adhere, becomes erythematous and if the inflammatory process continues, the bubo ruptures through the skin, forming a sinus. Bubo and sinus formation are usually unilateral[38].

Occasionally, ulceration becomes extensive, with considerable tissue destruction. In such cases secondary bacterial infection, particularly with *Treponema vincentii*, *Fusobacterium nucleatum*, and *Leptotrichia buccalis*, probably plays an important role in the destructive process.

In some cases ulceration may be more superficial, but covers a considerable area. Tissue destruction is minimal but healing is slow, with months or years elapsing before resolution is complete. Recurrent chancroid, although described, is a rarity.

DIAGNOSIS

The clinical diagnosis of chancroid is unreliable, particularly in geographical areas where the prevalence of infection is low. In Detroit, Michigan, the accuracy of clinical diagnosis was only 33%[48]; this compares with 80% in South Africa[49] where the index of suspicion was much higher. In the past, diagnosis has often been made by exclusion of other causes of genital ulceration. A definitive diagnosis of chancroid, however, should only be made when *H. ducreyi* is detected in genital ulcers.

Microscopy

A presumptive diagnosis may be made by finding organisms morphologically resembling *H. ducreyi* in stained smears prepared from material aspirated from a bubo or taken from the undermined edge of the ulcer: the lesions should be cleansed first with normal saline. Several staining methods can be used, for example Gram's or Giemsa's stain. In preparing a smear, the swab should be rolled through 180° in one direction only, never back and forth, to maintain the arrangement of the organisms. Typically *H. ducreyi* is seen as short rods in a mucous matrix forming a 'railroad track' or 'shoal-of-fish' pattern. The bacteria may exhibit bipolar staining. Unfortunately, many cases of genital herpes or syphilis may become colonized with Gram-negative rods, thus microscopy lacks diagnostic specificity.

Giemsa's stain may be helpful in identifying the giant balloon cells, frequently multinucleate, and the eosinophilic intracellular inclusion bodies characteristic of HSV infections in secondarily infected cases of genital herpes. Improvements in cultural and molecular methods for diagnosis have shown that direct microscopy may also lack sensitivity: in patients in whom no characteristic Gram-negative rods were seen, over 50% (22 of 41) of cultures grew *H. ducreyi*[50].

Culture

Material from the base of the ulcer is best inoculated directly on to suitable media. Culture plates should be transported to the laboratory as soon as possible and incubated at 33 to 35°C in a moist carbon dioxide-enriched (5%) microaerophilic atmosphere. Plates should be incubated for at least 72 hours. *Haemophilus ducreyi* colonies have a characteristic coherence and can be moved as an entire colony across the plate with an inoculating loop. The identity of the organisms may be confirmed by a negative porphyrin test[51] and positive tests for alkaline phosphatase and nitrate reduction.

Media

For primary isolation, culture methods with liquid or clotted-blood media have been superseded by solid selective media containing vancomycin (3 μg/mL). Hammond et al.[52], using a gonococcal agar base supplemented with 1% bovine hemoglobin, 1% IsoVitaleX™ enrichment and vancomycin (3 μg/mL), isolated *H. ducreyi* from

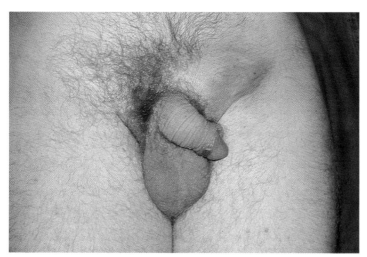

Figure 16.2 Penile chancroid with bubo (reproduced from McMillan and Scott 2000[119])

8 of 16 genital ulcers in Winnipeg, Canada. Addition of fetal calf serum to agar media improves the rates of isolation[53]. However, fetal calf serum is expensive and 5% sheep serum may be an acceptable alternative[50].

As yet no single medium provides an optimal rate of isolation of *H. ducreyi* from genital ulcers. Nsanze *et al.*[50] compared Mueller–Hinton agar base containing 5% chocolated horse blood (MH-HB) with a gonococcal agar base supplemented with 2% bovine hemoglobin and 5% fetal calf serum (GC-HgS): vancomycin (3 μg/mL) and 1% CVA™ enrichment (Gibco) were added to both media.

GC-HgS medium yielded positive cultures for *H. ducreyi* from 143 (71%) of 201 patients with clinical chancroid, in comparison with 122 (61%) positive cultures with MH-HB medium. 41 patients gave positive cultures only on GC-HgS medium, while 20 were positive only on MH-HB medium. The combination of both media increased the yield of positive cultures to 81%. It was concluded that the use of both media on a single split plate would optimize the detection of *H. ducreyi*. It should be noted, however, that inhibition of some strains of *H. ducreyi* by vancomycin has been described[54].

Antigen detection

A few investigators have studied the use of monoclonal antibodies in the detection of *H. ducreyi* antigen. Karim *et al.*[55] raised a monoclonal antibody to *H. ducreyi* that reacted with a single polypeptide band of 29 kDa molecular weight in the outer membrane protein of the bacterium, and used it in a direct immunofluorescent test. Compared with culture of clinical material, the test had a sensitivity of up to 93%, but a specificity of only 56% to 63%. As PCR for the detection of nucleic acids was not available at that time for confirmatory testing, it is probable that the specificity was significantly higher. Ahmed *et al.*[56] raised a monoclonal antibody (MAHD7) against *H. ducreyi* lipo-oligosaccharide that reacted with each of sixty strains of the organism, and used it in an indirect immunofluorescent test. They found that, compared with a PCR assay, the sensitivity

and specificity of the test on clinical material from Zambian patients were 89% and 81% respectively. It was also shown that the sensitivity of the test was 100% when compared with culture. Cross-reactivity with *H. influenzae* strain 2019 and strains of *Aeromonas hydrophila* may limit the use of the test in areas of low prevalence of *H. ducreyi*[57].

DNA amplification methods

Polymerase chain reaction methods have been developed to improve the sensitivity of the diagnosis of chancroid. Primers have been designed to amplify sequences from the *H. ducreyi* 16S ribosomal RNA gene, the *rrs* (16S)-*rrl* (23S) ribosomal intergenic spacer region, an anonymous fragment of cloned *H. ducreyi* DNA, or the *groEL* gene that encodes the GroEL heat shock protein of *H. ducreyi*[57]. A multiplex PCR (M-PCR) has been developed for the simultaneous amplification of DNA sequences from *Treponema pallidum*, *H. ducreyi*, and HSV[58]. Using this test in the diagnosis of genital ulcer disease in 105 patients from Lesotho, Africa, Morse *et al.*[59] found that the sensitivity in the detection of *H. ducreyi* was 95%, compared with 75% for culture. The presence of *Taq* polymerase inhibitors, however, may lower the sensitivity of the PCR methods[60]. When PCR assays have been compared with culture, some studies have shown an apparent lack of specificity[58]. This observation, however, is probably the result of the low sensitivity of culture.

Nucleic acid probes

Using labeled *H. ducreyi* probes, bacterial DNA can be detected by DNA-DNA hybridization. There are no data, however, on their use in clinical practice[57].

Serological tests

The presence of serum antibodies that cross-react with other species of *Haemophilus* has made interpretation of serological tests difficult. Using an enzyme immunoassay (EIA) with ultrasonicated whole-cell antigen of *H. ducreyi*, antibodies could be detected in the sera of Canadians

who had not been exposed to this organism[61]. As adsorption with *H. influenzae* and *H. parainfluenzae* effectively removed these antibodies, the anti-*H. ducreyi* response was shown to have been caused by cross-reacting antibodies. This is the rationale behind the adsorption EIA tests studied[61, 62]. Using an EIA after adsorption of serum with *Haemophilus* spp., Alfa and colleagues[61] showed that residual antibody was found in the sera from African people, suggesting that they had been exposed at some time to *H. ducreyi*. In the rabbit model system and in humans, infection with *H. ducreyi* results in a rapid antibody response that is predominantly of the IgG class, with a relative lack of specific IgM[61, 63]. This is explained by previous exposure to other *Haemophilus* spp. that have cross-reactive antigens, exposure to *H. ducreyi* resulting in an anamnestic response. IgG levels remain elevated for several months after therapy.

Although serological tests are of limited diagnostic value, recently described tests may be of some value in studying the epidemiology of chancroid. Elkins *et al.*[64] have recently described the development of a test, using as antigens recombinant outer membrane proteins of *H. ducreyi* strain 35 000, namely hemoglobin receptor (HgbA), heme receptor (TdhA), and *H. ducreyi* D15 homolog (D15). They found that antibodies to HgbA and to D15 correlated well with the clinical diagnosis of chancroid, and that cross-reactivity with *H. influenzae* was insignificant.

The value of serological tests in the diagnosis of genital ulcer disease is limited. Using two EIAs (adsorption EIA and lipo-oligosaccharide (LOS) EIA, Chen *et al.*[65] found that the sensitivity and specificity of the former test performed on an acute serum specimen were 53% and 71% respectively, and of the latter test they were 48% and 89% respectively. When convalescent sera were examined, the sensitivity and specificity of the adsorption EIA increased to 78% and 84% respectively. The proportion of patients testing positive for *H. ducreyi* increased with the duration of the infection. This observation is in keeping with human volunteer experiments: when the disease is terminated at the pustular stage of infection by antimicrobial therapy, there is no significant systemic antibody response[23].

Other immunological techniques are no longer used in the diagnosis of chancroid. The Ito-Reenstierna skin test involved the intradermal inoculation of a suspension of killed *H. ducreyi* into one site and a control suspension alone at another site. The value of the test was limited because of cross-reaction with other bacteria.

Biopsy

Routine biopsy is not justifiable as a diagnostic method.

Differential diagnosis

Other conditions that produce ulceration of the genitalia (Chapter 20) must be considered in the differential diagnosis of chancroid, and syphilis must be excluded in all cases as these diseases may co-exist in the individual patient. Details regarding the tests required to exclude syphilis are to be found in Chapter 15, but it is important to stress the need for searching for *Treponema pallidum* by dark ground microscopic examination of serum squeezed gently from the depth of the lesions. *Treponema pallidum* may be identified in such exudates after drying, fixation in acetone, and the application of tests based on monoclonal antibody (Chapter 15).

Infection with HSV produces superficial multiple tender ulcers, which are not indurated, and this condition must be carefully excluded. In the absence of suitable laboratory facilities it may be impossible to differentiate between the two diseases, especially in HIV-infected patients.

It is possible that some chancroid-like ulcers may be a non-specific host reaction to a variety of organisms rather than a single entity. Lymphogranuloma venereum may co-exist with chancroid, as may other STIs.

TREATMENT

Chemotherapy

Resistance to sulfonamides and tetracyclines, the traditional treatments for chancroid, is now common in Africa and the Far East. Susceptibility testing is usually undertaken by the plate dilution method described by Bilgeri *et al.*[66]. In addition to chromosomally mediated resistance to sulfonamides, some strains of *H. ducreyi* contain a 4.9 MDa sulfonamide resistance plasmid[67]. Most clinical isolates also produce a β-lactamase of the TEM type mediated by small non-conjugative plasmids. Co-trimoxazole was used previously for the treatment of chancroid, but the development of resistance to both sulfonamides and to trimethoprim[27a] have rendered this drug unsuitable for routine use.

The currently recommended drug treatments include azithromycin, ceftriaxone, ciprofloxacin, and erythromycin (Table 16.1).

Azithromycin is currently the treatment of choice. The drug has high *in vitro* activity against *H. ducreyi*, the MIC being 0.004 mg/L[68], and, of course, its pharmacokinetic properties permit single-dose therapy. Tyndall *et al.*[69] reported the results of a randomized, comparative study of azithromycin in men with culture-proven *H. ducreyi* genital ulceration. The

study was undertaken in Nairobi, Kenya, and the treatment response to azithromycin was compared with that to erythromycin, given orally in a dose of 500 mg every 6 hours for 7 days. The overall cure rates were 73 (89%) of 82 men treated with azithromycin and 41 (91%) of 45 men given erythromycin. Treatment failure was associated with HIV seropositivity and lack of circumcision. Equally good results were reported in a non-comparative study of single-dose azithromycin in the treatment of chancroid in migrant mine workers in South Africa[70]: 34 (89%) of 38 men were cured. An interesting observation on the prevention of chancroid in human volunteers was made by Thornton *et al.*[71]. These workers found that azithromycin, given in a single oral dose of 1 g, prevented re-infection for nearly 2 months, compared with ciprofloxacin (500 mg as a single oral dose) which gave protection for only 1 week.

The majority of isolates of *H. ducreyi* are susceptible to ceftriaxone, with a MIC of 0.25 mg/L or less[72], and clinical trials have shown that this drug is effective in the treatment of chancroid. In a randomized study, Martin and colleagues[73] found that each of 33 patients with culture-proven disease who were treated with ceftriaxone in a dose of 250 mg given by intramuscular injection were cured or had clinical improvement at follow-up.

The MICs of ciprofloxacin for most isolates of *H. ducreyi* are less than 0.125 mg/L[72], and excellent results have been obtained in clinical trials of this agent. In an oral dosage of 500 mg twice daily for 3 days, ulcers and buboes healed rapidly in all of 40 patients treated by Naamara and colleagues[74], and there were no treatment failures in the 16 patients treated by D'Souza *et al.*[75] in India. Single-dose therapy with ciprofloxacin (500 mg) has also been studied. In one study clinical cure or improvement was observed in only 32 (76%) of 42 patients[76], while more recently[77] a cure rate of 92% was achieved.

Erythromycin is active *in vitro* against the majority of isolates of *H. ducreyi*, the MIC of the drug being 0.25 mg/L or less[72]. The drug is usually given in an oral dosage of 500 mg every 6 hours for 7 days.

Table 16.1 Recommended treatment regimens for chancroid (Centers for Disease Control and Prevention 2002[114])

Antimicrobial agent	Dosage
Azithromycin *or*	1 g as a single oral dose
Ceftriaxone *or*	250 mg as a single intramuscular injection
Ciprofloxacin *or*	500 mg by mouth every 12 h for 3 days
Erythromycin base	500 mg by mouth every 6 h for 7 days

Treatment efficacy has generally been in excess of 90%[70, 75, 78]. A lower dose of erythromycin (250 mg every 6 hours for 7 days) has been shown to be equally effective in a study of 219 patients, 26.4% of whom were HIV-infected[79]. These workers found that there was micro-biological cure by day 7 of therapy, but, although 99% of HIV seronegative patients were cured clinically, only 88% of sero-positive subjects had healing at that time.

Alternative treatment regimens have been described, and include

1. co-amoxiclav (amoxicillin 500 mg/ clavulanic acid 250 mg) given every 8 hours for 3 days[80]
2. spectinomycin given as a single intramuscular injection of 2 g[81].

Experience with these agents, however, is limited.

Treatment in pregnancy

Haemophilus ducreyi does not appear to influence adversely the course of pregnancy, and neonatal transmission is not known to occur. Ciprofloxacin and other fluoroquinolones are contraindicated in pregnancy, and the safety of azithromycin has not been established. Erythromycin and ceftriaxone are both safe and either can be used in the treatment of a pregnant woman.

Follow-up

Symptoms usually improve within 3 days of initiation of therapy, and ulcer healing becomes apparent within 3 to 7 days. The time taken to complete healing depends on the site and size of the ulcer, and may be more than 2 weeks. Healing is slower in the uncircumcised male. Failure to improve at 7 days may result from

- misdiagnosis
- concurrent infection with another STI such as HSV
- non-adherence to the treatment regimen
- resistance of *H. ducreyi* to the antimicrobial agent.

There has been some controversy surrounding the influence of HIV infection on treatment outcome. Until recently, lower rates of cure of HIV-infected patients were reported from Nairobi. However, when individuals with HSV infection are excluded from treatment trials, the cure rates between HIV-infected and non-infected patients are similar[77].

Local treatment

Local treatment of chancroid consists of frequently repeated applications of saline dressings to the ulcerated area to reduce the risk of development of secondary infection. A strip of gauze soaked in saline may be applied to separate inflamed surfaces. When a phimosis is present, and a balano-posthitis develops, the preputial sac should be gently irrigated with normal saline at hourly intervals. In more severe cases, to secure drainage and to prevent phagedenic ulceration of the glans, a slit should be made, extending dorsally along the prepuce from its orifice (dorsal slit) under general anesthesia. Such surgical procedures are preferably delayed until after ulcer healing to avoid secondary chancroidal ulcers at the line of incision.

Buboes should be aspirated before commencing treatment with antimicrobial drugs. The efficacy of antimicrobial therapy on the inguinal adenitis of chancroid has been equivocal, and buboes have been reported to develop during antimicrobial therapy despite ulcer healing[82]. Repeat aspiration of buboes may be required even after initiation of antimicrobial therapy to prevent the formation of sinuses.

Donovanosis (Granuloma inguinale)

Donovanosis (Granuloma inguinale) is a chronic granulomatous infection caused by the bacterium *Klebsiella granulomatis* (*Calymmatobacterium granulomatis*). The clinical effects are mainly in the anogenital region and less commonly elsewhere. Most cases occur in tropical and subtropical countries, but in the UK it may occasionally be seen in immigrants and merchant seamen.

The mode of transmission is not clear, although in many cases sexual intercourse, whether heterosexual or homosexual, probably plays a major role.

After a variable pre-patent period, an ulcer develops and slowly increases in size over the course of several months, or even years, until a considerable area of skin becomes affected. The duration of the untreated disease varies from about 1 month to over 30 years; healing generally occurs, however, within 2 to 3 years. Recurrences after apparent healing are common, and deformities of the anogenital region may result.

ETIOLOGY

In 1905, in India, Major Donovan noted the constant presence of intracellular bodies in smears from patients with granuloma inguinale. These bodies which he described as 'gigantic bacilli with rounded ends' are usually referred to as Donovan bodies. Following successful culture of the causative organism on chick yolk sac, it was evident that the Donovan bodies were bacterial in origin and the name *Donovania granulomatis* was proposed. In the 1970s, it was reclassified as *Calymmatobacterium granulomatis*, and recently it has been proposed that *C. granulomatis* should be reclassified as *Klebsiella granulomatis* comb. nov[83] for the following reasons.

1. The ultrastructure of the organism (see below) is similar to that of *Klebsiella* spp.
2. The capsule shares antigens with various members of the genus *Klebsiella*[84].
3. The similarity of its lesions to rhino-scleroma, caused by *K. rhinoscleromatis*. This disease is a chronic condition that occurs sporadically throughout the world and is endemic in certain countries, particularly where social and hygiene standards are low. It affects the upper respiratory tract where it produces an infiltrating granuloma with a marked tendency to sclerosis and subsequent obstruction[85].
4. Part of the chromosome of the organism has been amplified by PCR with primers for the 16S rRNA and *phoE* genes of *Klebsiella* spp. By sequencing 2089 base pairs of these genes, it was shown that *C. granulomatis* (Australian isolates) showed a high degree

of identity (99.7% to 99.8% homology in the *phoE* gene, and 98.8% to 99.8% in the 16s rRNA gene) with *K. pneumoniae* and *K. rhinoscleromatis*[83]. African isolates, however, have only shown 95% homology with *K. pneumoniae*[87].

Klebsiella granulomatis is a pleomorphic Gram-negative bacillus surrounded by a well-defined capsule that can be demonstrated by Wright's stain. The bacteria are intracellular parasites of the macrophages: occasionally they are found inside polymorphonuclear cells. In smears stained with Leishman or Giemsa stain the organisms usually appear as capsulate ovid or bean-shaped bodies varying in size from 1 μm to 1.5 μm in length and from 0.5 μm to 0.7 μm in thickness. A well-defined dense capsular material, pinkish in color, surrounds the body of the organism, which shows bipolar staining of chromatin material. The bipolar staining gives the organism the appearance of a closed 'safety pin'. Transmission electron microscopy[88] shows the characteristic trilaminar cell-wall structure of Gram-negative bacteria, surrounded by an electron-lucent layer that is thought to correspond to the capsule. The cytoplasm contains electron-dense material, especially at the periphery, and this probably causes the bipolar staining seen on light microscopy.

Klebsiella granulomatis has been cultured in peripheral blood mononuclear cells (PBMC)[89]. Specimens were treated with vancomycin and metronidazole to decontaminate them, and were then inoculated in a monocyte co-culture system with PBMC and fetal calf serum. Intra- and extracellular organisms were demonstrated in the culture by Giemsa staining or by indirect immunofluorescence. The ultrastructural characteristics confirmed that these organisms were *K. granulomatis*.

The successful culture of *K. granulomatis* in tissue culture has also been reported recently[86]. Specimens from lesions in three patients were inoculated on to cycloheximide-treated Hep-2 cell monolayers in RPMI 1640 medium, supplemented with vancomycin, benzylpenicillin, and fetal calf serum. Bacteria could be identified by 48 hours, and, using PCR to amplify gene products, it was shown that

DNA sequences from the cultured organisms were identical to those of the original lesion material.

PATHOGENICITY

Injection of material from pseudobuboes or suspensions of infected tissue can produce clinical disease in humans. However, disease cannot be produced in laboratory animals[90].

EPIDEMIOLOGY

Donovanosis is found in tropical and subtropical countries; in temperate climates its importation by immigrants and seafarers may occasionally occur. In 1954 it was considered to be endemic along the eastern seaboard of southern India, southern China, the East Indies, northern Australia, West and Central Africa, and the West Indies[91]. From 1958 to 1988, two peaks in the number of cases reported in Durban, South Africa were identified: one between 1969 and 1974, and the other in 1988[92]. The increased incidence was principally amongst men, and, although the explanation for this observation is uncertain, social change with increasing numbers of male migrant workers moving into the city from rural areas may have accounted for the 1988 peak.

The disease affects young men and women (aged 30 years and under) and exhibits a male:female ratio of approximately 2:1. Most studies have shown that donovanosis is related to low socioeconomic status and poor hygiene[92].

The popular view that donovanosis is usually sexually transmitted has been questioned[93]. The reported incidence of concomitant infection in sexual partners varies from infrequently[93] to over 50%[94]. The main points presented in favor of sexual transmission include

- history of sexual exposure before the appearance of the lesion
- increased incidence of the disease in age groups in which sexual activity is highest
- lesions found on internal genitalia, such as the cervix, without any other lesions
- lesions found only around the anus of men who have receptive anal intercourse

- the genital or perigenital location of lesions.

In contrast, the occurrence of the disease in very young children and sexually inactive persons and its rarity in the sexual partners of patients with open lesions are cited as evidence against sexual transmission[93].

As an alternative to sexual transmission it has been suggested that since *K. granulomatis* occurs in the intestine and in conditions of poor hygiene, then auto-inoculation of fecal material could establish it on skin made more susceptible by trauma or bacterial inflammation. An organism resembling *K. granulomatis* has been found in feces[95].

Klebsiella granulomatis can be transmitted to the neonate during vaginal delivery. This was shown clearly in the report of a 5-month-old child who had a polypoidal mass in the middle ear that showed histological features of donovanosis; the mother had biopsy-proven cervical infection[96].

Our lack of knowledge about the organism and its interaction with its host and the environment make it impossible to be certain about the way it is transmitted. Transmission could occur by both sexual and non-sexual means: perineal contamination with fecal organisms might precede transfer by a sexual route.

Association of donovanosis and HIV infection

Men with donovanosis seem to be at high risk for acquisition of HIV-1. O'Farrell et al.[97] observed that the probability of HIV-1 seropositivity increased as the duration of the lesions increased, from 0 of 43 men who had ulceration for less than 6 weeks to 5 of 18 men who had lesions for at least 3 months. Poor responses to treatment of granuloma inguinale in HIV-1 infected patients have been reported[98], and by increasing the duration of ulceration, transmission of HIV in the community may be facilitated.

CLINICAL FEATURES

As the mode of transmission is uncertain, the pre-patent period is not known. In cases considered to have been acquired sexually, the period between exposure to infection and the appearance of the initial lesion has varied from 3 days to 6 months, but it was acquired between 7 and 30 days in more than two-thirds of patients[94].

The disease has a predilection for the moist stratified epithelium of the skin and mucous membranes of the genital, anal, inguinal, and oral regions. In more than 90% of cases the initial lesion is reported to be in the anogenital area[91].

In the male the prepuce, frenum, and glans are the usual sites in which the initial lesions develop. In the female the labia minora, mons veneris, and the fourchette are the most commonly affected sites.

The earliest lesion may be a papule, a subcutaneous nodule, or an ulcer. Such lesions are often intensely pruritic. The 'papule' which is usually between 5 and 15 mm in diameter, is elevated above the surrounding skin, flat-topped, and covered by skin or mucous membrane; within a few days, ulceration occurs.

Less commonly the initial lesion may be nodular. This subcutaneous nodule, of varying size, is at first firm, but as the inflammatory process progresses, softening occurs with the production of an abscess. After several days the abscess ruptures through the skin, resulting in the formation of a granulomatous ulcer.

The lesion most frequently seen in clinical practice is the ulcer (Figures 16.3 and 16.4). It is of variable size, soft, velvety, bright red in color, and has a serpiginous edge. A serosanguineous exudate or a thin transparent membrane covers the base of the ulcer. The lesions bleed readily when abraded. Despite the appearance, the ulcer is generally painless unless there is secondary bacterial infection.

The disease spreads slowly along skin folds, taking months to involve a considerable area. In females the ulcerative process may progress posteriorly and downwards to involve the perineum and anal region. In Papua, New Guinea, Sengupta and Das[99] found that 10% of women with donovanosis had cervical involvement, with or without external anogenital lesions, that often resembled malignant disease. These authors also noted involvement of the endometrium and supporting structures of the uterus in the disease process. There is a

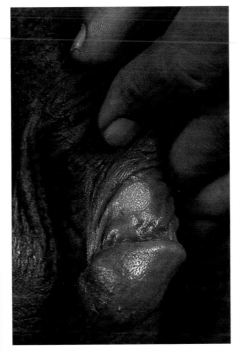

Figure 16.3 Donovanosis of the penis (reproduced from McMillan and Scott 2000[119])

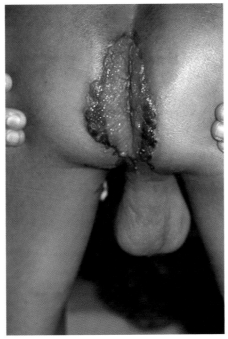

Figure 16.4 Donovanosis of the perianal region

tendency in the male for the disease to spread upwards and laterally to the inguinal region. Primary perianal lesions of donovanosis most commonly occur in homosexual men[100].

Extragenital lesions have been described, usually secondary to long-standing genital disease. Most commonly these lesions are found in or around the oral cavity, but they may occur anywhere in the body.

As the disease develops from the initial lesion, the base of the ulcer becomes elevated above the surface of the surrounding skin and the edge becomes thickened and grayish in color. This hypertrophic type of disease is slow to progress and may remain stationary for years.

In some patients, more commonly in females, there is a tendency early in the disease to extensive fibrous tissue formation. This often results in gross deformities.

Occasionally, in patients with long-standing disease, acute inflammation develops which results in necrosis and destruction of extensive areas of skin and subcutaneous tissue. This uncommon event may be fatal.

Even in extensive donovanosis, the regional lymph nodes are not enlarged, painful or tender. Histological examination of these glands shows only non-specific changes of endothelial hyperplasia and focal collections of mononuclear cells. Donovan bodies are not found[91]. Should the regional lymph nodes be enlarged, the possible co-existence of other diseases such as malignant metastases, syphilis, lymphogranuloma venereum, or secondary bacterial infection must be considered.

Systemic spread of infection from the primary site is said to be rare, although liver, spleen, subcutaneous tissue, and bone may be affected[91, 101].

Lesions of granuloma inguinale tend to proliferate in pregnancy, and fatal hematogenous spread of the organism can occur[102]. Bassa and colleagues[103] found that in both pregnant and non-pregnant women, the vulva was the most commonly infected anatomical site, but that the disease affected multiple sites (vulva, vagina, cervix) only in non-pregnant women.

The course of the disease is usually prolonged. Although in a few patients healing apparently takes place within a few weeks, the mean duration of the disease is about 18 months. There is a tendency for the disease to recur after apparent healing. Unless there is some concomitant disease such as pulmonary tuberculosis, the patient is otherwise generally well.

Complications

Edema of the genitalia may occur in 15% to 20% of patients following blockage of lymphatic vessels by the fibrotic changes associated with later manifestations of the disease. Females are more commonly affected than males. In long-standing cases genital deformities may occur; in the sclerotic forms of the disease there may be stenosis of the urethral, vaginal, and anal orifices.

Malignancy has been reported in association with granuloma inguinale[104, 100] and either basal cell or squamous cell carcinoma may occur. As the pseudoepitheliomatous hyperplasia associated with donovanosis may be difficult to differentiate from early carcinoma, care is required in interpreting histological reports[105].

The role of *K. granulomatis* as a predisposing factor in the etiology of carcinoma of the vulva and penis has long been suspected but not proven. The possibility of co-infection with certain HPV types, for example, cannot be ruled out.

DIAGNOSIS

The difficulties associated with the growth of the organism exclude culture as a routine diagnostic procedure. A diagnosis of donovanosis is based on the microscopic demonstration of the causative bacterium in tissue smears taken from the lesions. The lesions should be thoroughly and repeatedly cleansed with saline-soaked gauze, followed by gentle wiping with dry gauze. Since *K. granulomatis* is an intracellular parasite, granulation tissue must be examined: this is obtained either by punch biopsy from deep within the ulcer or from the edge of the lesion by means of a curette or scalpel. The tissue is spread between two slides and the resultant smear stained with Giemsa, Leishman, or Wright's stain. In 90% to 95% of lesions of donovanosis, organisms with intense polar staining, resembling closed safety pins, can be seen within mononuclear leukocytes (Figure 16.5)[91]. It may be difficult to demonstrate *K. granulomatis* in grossly

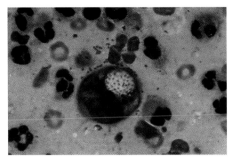

Figure 16.5 Donovan bodies in a tissue smear (Giemsa's stain, × 1000) (reproduced from McMillan and Scott 2000[119])

infected lesions contaminated by other organisms. Repeated examinations are often necessary.

In the diagnosis of donovanosis, biopsy of the ulcer may be helpful[106]. After infiltration of the base of the ulcer with lidocaine (lignocaine) hydrochloride (1% w/v), a wedge-shaped excision biopsy, which includes the margin of the lesion, is taken. Microscopically the deep layers of the dermis are densely infiltrated with plasma cells and macrophages with smaller numbers of polymorphonuclear leukocytes, including eosinophils. The superficial layers of the base of the ulcer may contain polymorphs. At the margins of the ulcer the epidermis may show marked acanthotic changes with elongation of the rete pegs, a pattern that may be mistaken for squamous cell carcinoma. This pseudoepitheliomatous appearance was found in 4 of 42 patients studied by Sehgal *et al.*[106].

In the deep layers of the dermis, large macrophages, up to 90 μm in diameter, with pyknotic nuclei and cyst-like vacuoles containing *K. granulomatis* (Greenblatt cells), are found. For the recognition of Donovan bodies in tissue sections, Giemsa-stained preparations are recommended[106]; the Warthin–Starry silver impregnation method can also be used to demonstrate the organisms in tissue sections[107].

Biopsy may be helpful in distinguishing the lesions from those of lymphogranuloma venereum; the ulcers of donovanosis show a more subacute type of inflammation[108]. Intradermal (Frei) testing and a complement fixation serological test have also been applied to the diagnosis of donovanosis, although their use is limited because of the lack of specificity and sensitivity and the

limited availability of suitable antigen[109]. An indirect immunofluorescence antibody test, using tissue sections of a lesion of donovanosis as substrate, was described by Freinkel *et al.*[110]. Although the test was reported as having a sensitivity of 100%, specificity of 98%, and positive and negative predictive values of 89% and 100% respectively, the relative scarcity of positive tissue sections precludes the use of this test as a standard diagnostic method.

A PCR for the detection of DNA in the *phoE* gene of *K. granulomatis* that may be of diagnostic value has been described recently[111], and the results of its use in clinical practice are awaited.

Since donovanosis may be associated with chancroid, syphilis, and lymphogranuloma venereum, either alone or in combination[91], it is important to undertake serological tests and to carry out dark ground or monoclonal antibody investigation of the lesions for *Treponema pallidum* to exclude syphilis, and to perform diagnostic tests for *Haemophilus ducreyi*. Bassa *et al.*[103] noted that 42% of 61 women with donovanosis were seropositive for syphilis. Donovanosis differs clinically from lymphogranuloma venereum; the latter diagnosis is usually supported by detection of *Chlamydia trachomatis* or serological tests for chlamydial infection.

TREATMENT

The *in vitro* susceptibility of *K. granulomatis* to antimicrobial agents is currently unknown, although its isolation in tissue culture should now make such testing possible. As there have been no controlled trials, the recommended treatment schedules are based on clinical experience (Table 16.2)[114].

Doxycycline

Evidence for the efficacy of tetracyclines in the treatment of donovanosis comes from early studies using older tetracyclines such as oxytetracycline. Greenblatt *et al.*[112] treated 36 patients with oxytetracycline given in a dosage of 2 g daily for 12.5 days. In 27 of these patients healing had occurred by the end of treatment or during

Table 16.2 Recommended treatment schedules for donovanosis

Antimicrobial agent	Dosage
Doxycycline[a]	100 mg by mouth every 12 h
Norfloxacin[b]	400 mg by mouth every 12 h
Ciprofloxacin[b]	750 mg by mouth every 12 h
Erythromycin[b]	500 mg by mouth every 6 h
Azithromycin[b]	1 g by mouth weekly *or* 500 mg by mouth daily
Cotrimoxazole[a]	960 mg by mouth every 12 h
Ceftriaxone	1 g by intramuscular injection once daily

[a] Denotes regimens recommended by the Centers for Disease Control and Prevention 2002[114]

[b] Denotes alternative regimens recommended by the Centers for Disease Control and Prevention 2002[114]

observation lasting from 1 to 18 months; 2 patients had relapse. It is presumed that doxycycline is as effective.

Fluoroquinolones

Good results in the treatment of donovanosis with norfloxacin were reported by Ramanan *et al.*[113]: in a small study (10 patients) the mean duration of treatment for complete healing was 7.3 days, the total oral dose of norfloxacin ranging from 1.6 to 8.8 g. In place of norfloxacin, the Centers for Disease Control and Prevention[114] recommend ciprofloxacin.

Azithromycin

The results of a pilot study of azithromycin in the treatment of granuloma inguinale were reported by Bowden *et al.*[115]. Two regimens of therapy were used

1. 1 g weekly for 4 weeks
2. 500 mg daily for 7 days

the drug being given orally. Of the 11 patients treated, the lesion re-epithelialized in all cases and there was no relapse during the observation period.

Erythromycin

Robinson and Cohen[116] who used different doses of the drug in 9 patients reported excellent results in the treatment of the condition: 8 of 9 patients had complete healing of the lesions with no relapse. Pregnant or lactating women should be treated with this regimen.

Cotrimoxazole (sulfamethoxazole-trimethoprim)

In a study on 116 patients (84 men and 32 women), Lal and Garg[117] reported healing in all cases after treatment for 7 to 22 days, with recurrence in only 2 of 45 patients who were followed up.

Ceftriaxone

Healing of lesions was found in each of 12 patients treated with ceftriaxone in a dosage of 1 g by intramuscular injection daily for up to 26 days[118].

Unlike other sexually acquired ulcerations, the lesions of donovanosis begin to heal from the periphery. Treatment should be continued until the lesions have completely epithelialized but, in any case, therapy should be for a minimum of 3 weeks. Gentamicin, given by intramuscular injection or by intravenous infusion in a dosage of 1 mg/kg every 8 hours, is recommended by the Centers for Disease Control and Prevention[114] if lesions have not responded within the first few days of therapy. Such adjuvant treatment is also recommended in HIV-seropositive patients in whom healing of lesions takes significantly longer with erythromycin treatment than in those with donovanosis who are HIV-seronegative[98].

Patients should be followed up until signs and symptoms have resolved. Patients whose lesions relapse will require retreatment. Plastic surgery may be required for genital deformities but this should be delayed until the active infection has been treated.

Treatment of donovanosis in pregnancy

Pregnant women should be treated with erythromycin. If cervical lesions are present at or shortly before the onset of labor in an untreated woman, or if there is doubt about the effectiveness of therapy, cesarean section is indicated[102]. Any infant who has been exposed to untreated infection as it passes down the birth canal should have careful cleaning of the ears, umbilicus, and genitalia, and should be treated with a course of erythromycin, given in an oral dose appropriate to the weight of the child[102].

References

1 Ducrey A. Recherches experimentales sur la nature intime du principle contagieux du chancre mou. *Ann Dermatol Syphiligraphie* 1890; **1**: 56–57.

2 Oberhofer TR, Back AE. Isolation and cultivation of *Haemophilus ducreyi*. *J Clin Microbiol* 1982; **15**: 625–629.

3 Kilian M. A taxonomic study of the genus Haemophilus, with the proposal of a new species. *J Gen Microbiol* 1976; **93**: 9–62.

4 Nobre GN. Isolation of *Haemophilus ducreyi* in the clinical laboratory. *J Med Microbiol* 1982; **15**: 243–246.

5 Sottnek FO, Biddle JW, Kraus SJ, Weaver RE, Stewart JA. Isolation and identification of *Haemophilus ducreyi* in a clinical study. *J Clin Microbiol* 1980; **12**: 170–174.

6 Hammond GW, Lian C-J, Wilt JC, Ronald AR. Antimicrobial susceptibility of *Haemophilus ducreyi*. *Antimicrob Agents Chemother* 1978; **13**: 608–612.

7 Hannah P, Greenwood JR. Isolation and rapid identification of Haemophilus ducreyi. *J Clin Microbiol* 1982; **16**: 861–864.

8 Spinola SM, Griffiths GE, Shanks KL, Blake MS. The major outer membrane protein of

Haemophilus ducreyi is a member of the OmpA family of proteins. *Infect Immun* 1993; **61**: 1346–1351.

9 Spinola SM, Castellazzo A, Shero M, Apicella MA. Characterization of pili expressed by *Haemophilus ducreyi. Microb Pathog* 1990; **9**: 417–426.

10 Totten PA, Norn DV, Stamm WE. Characterization of the hemolytic activity of *Haemophilus ducreyi. Infect Immun* 1995; **63**: 4409–4416.

11 Brunton JL, Maclean I, Ronald AR, Albritton WL. Plasmid-mediated ampicillin resistance in *Haemophilus ducreyi. Antimicrob Agents Chemother* 1979; **15**: 294–299.

12 MacLean IW, Bowden EHW, Albritton WL. TEM-type beta-lactamase production in *Haemophilus ducreyi. Antimicrob Agents Chemother* 1980; **17**: 897–900.

13 Deneer HG, Sloney L, Maclean FW, Albritton WL. Mobilization of non-conjugative antibiotic resistance plasmids in *Haemophilus ducreyi. J Bacteriol* 1982; **149**: 726–732.

14 Handsfield HH, Totten PA, Fennel CL, Falkow S, Holmes KK. Molecular epidemiology of *Haemophilus ducreyi* infections. *Ann Int Med* 1981; **95**: 315–318.

15 Brunton J, Meier M, Ehrman N, Maclean I, Sloney L, Albritton WL. Molecular epidemiology of betalactamase-specifying plasmids of *Haemophilus ducreyi. Antimicrob Agents Chemother* 1982; **21**: 857–862.

16 Anderson B, Albritton WL, Biddle J, Johnson SR. Common Beta-lactamase specifying plasmid in *Haemophilus ducreyi* and *Neisseria gonorrhoeae. Antimicrob Agents Chemother* 1984; **25**: 296–297.

17 Sng EH, Lim AL, Rajan VS, Goh AJ. Characteristics of *Haemophilus ducreyi. Br J Vener Dis* 1982; **58**: 239–242.

18 Mauff AG, Ballard RC, Bilgreri YR, Koomhof HJ. Isolation of *Haemophilus ducreyi* from genital ulcerations in white men in Johannesburg. *S Afr Med J* 1983; **63**: 236–237.

19 Fast M, Nsanze H, D'Costa L, *et al.* Treatment of chancroid by clavulanic acid with amoxycillin in patients with Betalactamase-positive *Haemophilus ducreyi* infection. *Lancet* 1982; **ii**: 509–511.

20 Lagergard T, Purven M, Fisk A. Evidence of *Haemophilus ducreyi* adherence to and cytotoxin destruction of human epithelial cells. *Microb Pathog* 1993; **14**: 417–431.

21 Purven M, Lagergard T. *Haemophilus ducreyi*, a cytotoxin-producing bacterium. *Infect Immun* 1992; **60**: 1156–1162.

21a Lagergard T, Purven M. Neutralizing antibodies to *Haemophilus ducreyi* cytotoxin. *Infect Immun* 1993; **61**: 1589–1592.

22 Lewis DA. The use of experimental animal and human models in the study of chancroid pathogenesis. *Int J STD AIDS* 1999; **10**: 71–79.

23 Spinola SM, Wild LM, Apicella MA, *et al.* Experimental human infection with *Haemophilus ducreyi. J Infect Dis* 1994; **169**: 1146–1150.

24 Al-Tawfiq JA, Harezlak J, Katz BP, Spinola SM. Cumulative experience with *Haemophilus ducreyi* 35000 in the human model of experimental infection. *Sex Transm Dis* 2000; **27**: 111–114.

25 Spinola SM, Orazi A, Arno JN, *et al. Haemophilus ducreyi* elicits a cutaneous infiltrate of CD4 cells during experimental human infection. *J Infect Dis* 1996; **173**: 394–402.

26 Palmer KL, Schnizlein Bick CT, Orazi A, *et al.* The immune response to *Haemophilus ducreyi* resembles a delayed-type hypersensitivity reaction throughout experimental infection of human subjects. *J Infect Dis* 1998; **178**: 1688–1697.

27 Abeck D, Freinkel AL, Korting HC, Szeimis R-M, Ballard RC. Immunochemical investigation of genital ulcers caused by *Haemophilus ducreyi. Int J STD AIDS* 1997; **8**: 585–588.

27a Abeck D, Johnson AP, Dangor Y, Ballard RC. Antibiotic susceptibilies and plasmid profiles of *Haemophilus ducreyi* isolated from Southern Africa. *J Antimicrob Chemother* 1988; **22**: 437–444.

28 Sheldon WH, Heyman A. Studies on chancroid I. Observations on the histology with an evaluation of biopsy as a diagnostic procedure. *Am J Pathol* 1946; **22**: 415–425.

29 King R, Gough J, Ronald A, *et al.* An immunochemical analysis of naturally occurring chancroid. *J Infect Dis* 1996; **174**: 427–430.

30 Pham-Kanter GBT, Steinberg MH, Ballard RC. Sexually transmitted diseases in South Africa. *Genitourin Med* 1996; **72**: 160–171.

31 Hammond GW, Slutchuk M, Scotliff J, Sherman E, Wilt JC, Ronald AR. Clinical, epidemiological, laboratory and therapeutic features of an urban outbreak of chancroid in North America. *Rev Infect Dis* 1980; **2**: 867–879.

32 Nayyar KC, Stolz E, Michel MF. Rising incidence of chancroid in Rotterdam. *Br J Vener Dis* 1979; **55**: 439–441.

33 Lykke-Oleson L, Larsen L, Pedersen TG, Gaarslev K. Epidemic of chancroid in Greenland 1977–1978. *Lancet* 1979; **i**: 654–665.

34 DiCarlo RP, Armentor BS, Martin DH. Chancroid epidemiology in New Orleans men. *J Infect Dis* 1995; **172**: 446–452.

35 Mertz KJ, Weiss JB, Webb RM, *et al.* An investigation of genital ulcers in Jackson, Mississipi, with the use of a multiplex polymerase chain reaction assay: high prevalence of chancroid and human immunodeficiency virus infection. *J Infect Dis* 1998; **178**: 1060–1066.

36 Mertz KJ, Trees D, Levine WC, *et al.* Etiology of genital ulcers and prevalence of human immunodeficiency virus coinfection in 10 US cities. The Genital Ulcer Disease Surveillance Group. *J Infect Dis* 1998; **178**: 1795–1798.

37 Asin J. Chancroid. *Am J Syphilis, Gonorrhea Vener Dis* 1952; **36**: 483–487.

38 Kerber RE, Rowe CE, Gilbert KR. Treatment of chancroid. A comparison of tetracycline and sulfisoxazole. *Arch Dermatol* 1969; **100**: 604–607.

39 Hart G. Venereal disease in a war environment. Incidence and management. *Med J Aust* 1975; **1**: 808–810.

40 Plummer FA, D'Costa LJ, Nsanze H, Dylewski J, Karasira P, Ronald AR. Epidemiology of chancroid and *Haemophilus ducreyi* in Nairobi, Kenya. *Lancet* 1983 **ii**: 1293–1295.

41 Hawkes S, West B, Wilson S, Whittle H, Mabey D. Asymptomatic carriage of *Haemophilus ducreyi* confirmed by the polymerase chain reaction. *Genitourin Med* 1995; **71**: 224–227.

42 Haydock AK, Martin DH, Morse SA, Cammarata C, Mertz KJ, Totten PA. Molecular characterization of *Haemophilus ducreyi* strains from Jackson, Mississippi, and New Orleans, Louisiana. *J Infect Dis* 1999; **179**: 1423–1432.

43 Wasserheit JN. Epidemiological synergy. Interrelationships between human immunodeficiency virus infection and other sexually transmitted diseases. *Sex Transm Dis* 1992; **19**: 61–77.

44 Cameron DW, Simonsen JN, D'Costa, *et al.* Female to male transmission of human immunodeficiency virus type 1: risk factors for seroconversion in men. *Lancet* 1989; **ii**: 403–407.

45 Plummer FA, Simonsen JN, Cameron DW, *et al.* Co-factors in male–female transmission of HIV. *J Infect Dis* 1991; **163**: 233–239.

46 Kreiss JK, Coombs R, Plummer F, *et al.* Isolation of human immunodeficiency virus from genital ulcers in Nairobi prostitutes. *J Infect Dis* 1989; **160**: 380–384.

47 Harkness AH. Chancroid. In: *Non-gonococcal Urethritis.* Edinburgh; Livingstone: 1950.

48 Chapel TA, Brown WJ, Jeffries C, Stewart JA. How reliable is the morphological diagnosis of penile ulcerations? *Sex Transm Dis* 1977; **4**: 150–152.

49 Dangor Y, Ballard RC, Exposto F da L, Fehler G, Miller SD, Koornhof HJ. Accuracy of clinical diagnosis of genital ulcer disease. *Sex Transm Dis* 1990; **17**: 184–189.

50 Nsanze H, Fast MV, D'Costa LJ, Tukei P, Curran J, Ronald A. Genital ulcers in Kenya: clinical and laboratory study. *Br J Vener Dis* 1981; **57**: 378–381.

51 Hammond GW, Lian F-J, Wilt JC, Albritton WL, Ronald AR. Determination of the hemin requirement of *Haemophilus ducreyi*: evaluation of the porphyrin test and media used in the satellite growth test. *J Clin Microbiol* 1978; **7**: 243–246.

52 Hammond GW, Lian C-J, Wilt JC, Ronald AR. Comparison of specimen collection and laboratory techniques for isolation of *Haemophilus ducreyi*. *J Clin Microbiol* 1978; **7**: 39–43.

53 Sottnek FO, Biddle JW, Kraus SJ, Weaver RE, Stewart JA. Isolation and identification of *Haemophilus ducreyi* in a clinical study. *J Clin Microbiol* 1980; **12**: 170–174.

53a Nsanze H, Plummer FA, Maggwa ABN, Maitha G, Dylewski J, Piot P, Ronald AR. Comparison of four media for the primary isolation of *Haemophilus ducreyi*. *Sex Transm Dis* 1984; **11**: 6–9.

54 Jones C, Rosen T, Clarridge J. *et al.* Chancroid: results from an outbreak in Houston, Texas. *South Med J* 1990; **83**: 1384–1389.

55 Karim QN, Finn GY, Easmon CSF, *et al.* Rapid detection of *Haemophilus ducreyi* in clinical and experimental infection using monoclonal antibody: a preliminary evaluation. *Genitourin Med* 1989; **65**: 361–365.

56 Ahmed HJ, Borrelli S, Jonasson J. *et al.* Monoclonal antibodies against *Haemophilus ducreyi* lipooligosaccharide and their diagnostic usefulness. *Eur J Clin Microbiol Infect Dis* 1995; **14**: 892–898.

57 Lewis DA. Diagnostic tests for chancroid. *Sex Transm Inf* 1999; **76**: 137–141.

58 Orle KA, Gates CA, Martin DH, *et al.* Simultaneous PCR detection of *Haemophilus ducreyi*, *Treponema pallidum* and herpes simplex virus types 1 and 2 from genital ulcers. *J Clin Microbiol* 1996; **34**: 49–54.

59 Morse SA, Trees DL, Htun Y, *et al.* Comparison of clinical diagnosis and standard laboratory and molecular methods for the diagnosis of genital ulcer disease in Lesotho: association with human immunodeficiency virus infection. *J Infect Dis* 1997; **175**: 583–589.

60 Chui L, Albritton W, Paster B, *et al.* Development of the polymerase chain reaction for diagnosis of chancroid. *J Clin Microbiol* 1993; **31**: 659–664.

61 Alfa MJ, Olson N, Degagne P, *et al.* Use of an adsorption enzyme immunoassay to evaluate the *Haemophilus ducreyi* specific and cross-reactive humoral immune response of humans. *Sex Transm Dis* 1992; **19**: 309–314.

62 Desjardins M, Thompson CE, Filion LG, *et al.* Standardization of an enzyme immunoassay for human antibody to *Haemophilus ducreyi*. *J Clin Microbiol* 1992; **30**: 2019–2024.

63 Muller F, Muller KH. Immunoglobulin M and G antibody response in rabbits after experimental *Haemophilus ducreyi* infection. *Zbl Bakt Hyg A* 1988; **268**: 238–244.

64 Elkins C, Yi K, Olsen B, Thomas C, Thomas K, Morse S. Development of a serological test for *Haemophilus ducreyi* for seroprevalence studies. *J Clin Microbiol* 2000; **38**: 1520–1526.

65 Chen CY, Mertz KJ, Spinola SM, Morse SA. Comparison of enzyme immunoassays for antibodies to *Haemophilus ducreyi* in a community outbreak of chancroid in the United States. *J Infect Dis* 1997; **175**: 1390–1395.

66 Bilgeri YR, Ballard RC, Duncan MO, Mauff AG. Antimicrobial susceptibility of 103 strains of *Haemophilus ducreyi* isolated in Johannesburg. *Antimicrob Agents Chemother* 1982; **22**: 686–688.

67 Fast MV, Nsanze H, Plummer FA, D'Costa LJ, Maclean IW, Ronald AR. Treatment of chancroid. A comparison of sulphamethoxazole and trimethoprim-sulphamethoxazole. *Br J Vener Dis* 1983; **59**: 320–324.

68 Slaney L, Chubb H, Ronald A, Brunham R. In-vitro activity of azithromycin, erythromycin, ciprofloxacin and norfloxacin against *Neisseria gonorrhoeae*, *Haemophilus ducreyi*, and *Chlamydia trachomatis*. *J Antimicrob Chemother* 1990; **25** (Suppl. A): 1–5.

69 Tyndall MW, Agoki E, Plummer FA, *et al.* Single dose azithromycin for treatment of chancroid: a randomised comparison with erythromycin. *Sex Transm Dis* 1994; **21**: 231–234.

70 Ballard RC, Ye H, Matta A, Dangor Y, Radebe F. Treatment of chancroid with azithromycin. *Int J STD AIDS* 1996; **7** (Suppl 1): 9–12.

71 Thornton AC, O'Mara EM, Sorensen SJ, *et al.* Prevention of experimental *Haemophilus ducreyi* infection: a randomized controlled clinical trial. *J Infect Dis* 1998; **177**: 1608–1613.

72 Knapp JS, Back AF, Babst AF, Taylor D, Rice RJ. In vitro susceptibilities of isolates of *Haemophilus ducreyi* from Thailand and the United States to currently recommended and newer agents for treatment of chancroid. *Antimicrob Agents Chemother* 1993; **37**: 1552–1555.

73 Martin DH, Sargent SJ, Wendel GD, McCormack WM, Spier NA, Johnson RB. Comparison of azithromycin and ceftriaxone for the treatment of chancroid. *Clin Infect Dis* 1995; **21**: 409–414.

74 Naamara W, Plummer FA, Greenblatt RM, D'Costa LJ, Ndinya Achola JO, Ronald AR. Treatment of chancroid with ciprofloxacin. A randomized controlled trial. *Am J Med* 1987; **82** (Suppl. 4A): 317–320.

75 D'Souza P, Pandhi RK, Khanna N, Rattan A, Misra RS. A comparative study of therapeutic response of patients with clinical chancroid to ciprofloxacin, erythromycin, and cotrimoxazole. *Sex Transm Dis* 1998; **25**: 293–295.

76 Bogaerts J, Kestens L, Martinez Tello W, *et al.* Failure of treatment for chancroid in Rwanda is not related to human immunodeficiency virus infection: in vitro resistance of *Haemophilus ducreyi* to trimethoprim-sulfamethoxazole. *Clin Infect Dis* 1995; **20**: 924–930.

77 Malonza IM, Tyndall MW, Ndinya-Achola JO, *et al.* A randomized, double-blind, placebo-controlled trial of single dose ciprofloxacin versus erythromycin for the treatment of chancroid in Nairobi, Kenya. *J Infect Dis* 1999; **180**: 1886–1893.

78 Behets FM, Liomba G, Lule G, *et al.* Sexually transmitted diseases and human immunodeficiency virus control in Malawi: a field study of genital ulcer disease. *J Infect Dis* 1995; **171**: 451–455.

79 Kimani J, Bwayo JJ, Anzala AO, *et al.* Low dose erythromycin regimen for the treatment of chancroid. *East Afr Med J* 1995; **72**: 645–648.

80 Ndinya-Achola JO, Nsanze H, Karasira P, *et al.* Three day oral course of Augmentin to treat chancroid. *Genitourin Med* 1986; **62**: 202–204.

81 Fransen L, Nsanze H, Plummer FA, *et al.* A comparison of single dose spectinomycin with five days of trimethoprim-sulfamethoxazole for the treatment of chancroid. *Sex Transm Dis* 1987; **14**: 98–101.

82 Marmar JL. The management of resistant chancroid in Vietnam. *J Urol* 1972; **107**: 807–808.

83 Carter JS, Bowden FJ, Bastian I, Myers GM, Sriprakash KS, Kemp DJ. Phylogenetic evidence for reclassification of *Calymmatobacterium granulomatis* as *Klebsiella granulomatis* comb. nov. *Int J System Bacteriol* 1999; **49**: 1695–1700.

84 Packer H, Goldberg J. Studies of the antigenic relationship of *D. granulomatis* to members of the tribe Escherichiae. *Am J Syphilis Gonorrhea Vener Dis* 1950; **34**: 342.

85 Hay RJ. Adrianns BM. Bacterial infections. In: Champion RH, Burton JL, Burns DA, Breathnach SM (eds) Rook/Wilkinson/Ebling. *Textbook of Dermatology* 6th edition. Oxford; Blackwell: 1998.

86 Carter J, Hutton S, Sriprakash KS, *et al.* Culture of the causative organism of donovanosis (*Calymmatobacterium granulomatis*) in Hep-2 cells. *J Clin Microbiol* 1997; **35**: 2915–2917.

87 Kharsany AB, Hoosen AA, Kiepiela P, Kirby R, Sturm AW. Phylogenetic analysis of *Calymmatobacterium granulomatis* based on 16S rRNA gene sequences. *J Med Microbiol* 1999; **48**: 841–847.

88 Kharsany ABM, Hoosen AA, Naicker T, Kiepiela P, Sturm AW. Ultrastructure of *Calymmatobacterium granulomatis*: comparison of culture with tissue biopsy specimens. *J Med Microbiol* 1998; **47**: 1069–1073.

89 Kharsany AB, Hoosen AA, Kiepiela P, Naicker T, Sturm AW. Growth and cultural characteristics of *Calymmatobacterium granulomatis* – the aetiological agent of granuloma inguinale (Donovanosis). *J Med Microbiol* 1997; **46**: 579–585.

90 Davis CM, Collins C. Granuloma inguinale: an ultrastructural study of *Calymmatobacterium granulomatis*. *J Invest Dermatol* 1969; **53**: 315–321.

91 Rajam RV, Rangiah PN. *Donovanosis (granuloma inguinale; granuloma venereum)*. World Health Organization, Monograph Series No 24; Geneva: 1954.

92 O'Farrell N. Trends in reported cases of donovanosis in Durban, South Africa. *Genitourin Med* 1992; **68**: 366–369.

93 Goldberg J. Studies on granuloma inguinale VII. Some epidemiological considerations of the disease. *Br J Vener Dis* 1964; **40**; 140–145.

94 Lal S, Nicholas C. Epidemiological and clinical features in 165 cases of granuloma inguinale. *Br J Vener Dis* 1970; **46**: 461–462.

95 Goldberg J. Studies on granuloma inguinale V. Isolation of a bacterium resembling *Donovania granulomatis* from the faeces of a patient with granuloma inguinale. *Br J Vener Dis* 1962; **38**: 99–102.

96 Govender D, Naidoo K, Chetty R. Granuloma inguinale (donovanosis): an unusual cause of otitis media and mastoiditis in children. *Am J Clin Pathol* 1997; **108**: 510–514.

97 O'Farrell N, Windsor I, Becker P. HIV-1 infection among heterosexual attenders at a sexually transmitted diseases clinic in Durban. *S Afr Med J* 1991; **80**: 17–20.

98 Jamkhedkar PP, Hira SK, Shroff HJ, Lanjewar DN. Clinico-epidemiologic features of granuloma inguinale in the era of acquired immune deficiency syndrome. *Sex Transm Dis* 1998; **25**: 196–200.

99 Sengupta SK, Das N. Donovanosis affecting cervix, uterus and adnexae. *Am J Trop Med Hyg* 1984; **33**: 632–636.

100 Davis CM. Granuloma inguinale. A clinical histological and ultrastructural study. *JAMA* 1970; **211**: 632–636.

101 Cliff S, Wilson A, Wansboroguh-Jones M, Ash S. Disseminated granuloma inguinale secondary to cervical infection. *J Infect* 1998; **36**: 129–130.

102 Richens J. The diagnosis and treatment of donovanosis (granuloma inguinale). *Genitourin Med* 1991; **67**: 441–452.

103 Bassa AG, Hoosen AA, Moodley J, Bramdev A. Granuloma inguinale (donovanosis) in women. An analysis of 61 cases from Durban, South Africa. *Sex Transm Dis* 1993; **20**: 164–167.

104 Goldberg J, Annamunthodo H. Studies on granuloma inguinale Viii. Serological reactivity of sera from patients with carcinoma of penis when tested with Donovania agents. *Br J Vener Dis* 1966; **42**: 205–209.

105 Beerman H, Snock CE. The epithelial changes in granuloma inguinale. *Am J Syphilis, Gonorrhea Vener Dis* 1952; **36**: 501–510.

106 Sehgal VN, Shyamprasad AL, Beohar R. The histopathological diagnosis of donovanosis. *Br J Vener Dis* 1984; **60**: 45–47.

107 Freinkel AL. Histological aspects of sexually transmitted genital lesions. *Histopathology* 1987; **11**: 819–831.

108 Stewart DB. The gynecological lesions of lymphogranuloma venereum and granuloma inguinale. *Med Clin North Am* 1964; **48**: 773–786.

109 Willcox RR. Granuloma inguinale (donovanosis). In: Morton RS, Harris JRW (eds) *Recent Advances in Sexually Transmitted Diseases*. Edinburgh; Churchill Livingstone: 1975.

110 Freinkel AL, Dangor Y, Koornhof HJ, Ballard RC. A serological test for granuloma inguinale. *Genitourin Med* 1992; **68**: 269–272.

111 Carter J, Bowden FJ, Sriprakash KS, Bastian I, Kemp DJ. Diagnostic polymerase chain reaction for donovanosis. *Clin Infect Dis* 1999; **28**: 1168–1169.

112 Greenblatt RB, Barfield WE, Dienst RB, *et al*. Terramycin in the treatment of granuloma inguinale. *J Vener Dis Information* 1951; **32**: 113–115.

113 Ramanan C, Sarma PSA, Ghorpade A, *et al*. Treatment of donovanosis with norfloxacin. *Int J Dermatol* 1990; **29**: 298–299.

114 Centers for Disease Control and Prevention. 2002 Guidelines for treatment of sexually transmitted diseases. *MMWR* 2002; **51**: RR–6.

115 Bowden FJ, Mein J, Plunkett C, Bastian I. Pilot study of azithromycin in the treatment of genital donovanosis. *Genitourin Med* 1996; **72**: 17–19.

116 Robinson HM, Cohen MM. Treatment of granuloma inguinale with erythromycin. *J Invest Dermatol* 1953; **20**; 407–409.

117 Lal S, Garg BR. Further evidence of the efficacy of cotrimoxazole in granuloma venereum. *Br J Vener Dis* 1980; **56**: 412–413.

118 Merianos A, Gilles M, Chuah J. Ceftriaxone in the treatment of chronic donovanosis in central Australia. *Genitourin Med* 1994; **70**: 84–89.

119 McMillan A, Scott GR. *Sexually Transmitted Infections, Colour Guide*. Churchill Livingstone; Edinburgh: 2000.

Chapter 17

Vaginal infections and vulvodynia
A McMillan

Trichomoniasis

Trichomoniasis in women is a common and sometimes distressing condition resulting from infection of the genitourinary tract with the protozoon, *Trichomonas vaginalis*. The parasite may be found in the vagina, urethra, bladder, paraurethral ducts, and occasionally in the ducts of the greater vestibular glands. Although many women are asymptomatic, vaginal discharge, vaginitis, dyspareunia, dysuria, and frequency are all common manifestations of infection with *T. vaginalis*.

Infection in men is often asymptomatic, but the protozoon may sometimes be found in men with signs of a urethritis or prostatitis. The ratio for cases of trichomoniasis in men and women respectively is difficult to determine, since in men the infection may be short lived and the organism difficult to detect. With few exceptions, transmission is by sexual intercourse when the incubation period is in the range of 4 days to 4 weeks. Neonates may occasionally develop a vulvovaginitis as a result of an infection acquired during passage through the birth canal.

ETIOLOGY

The causative organism, a flagellate protozoon of the urogenital tract, *Trichomonas vaginalis* was first described by Donne in 1836. Trichomonads vary in shape as a result of environmental conditions. When cultured *in vitro* the organism is approximately 10 μm in length (range 5 to 10 μm) and 7 μm in breadth (range 3 to 13 μm) and it tends to become ellipsoid or ovoid (Figure 17.1), whereas in the vagina the shape is very variable and the organism

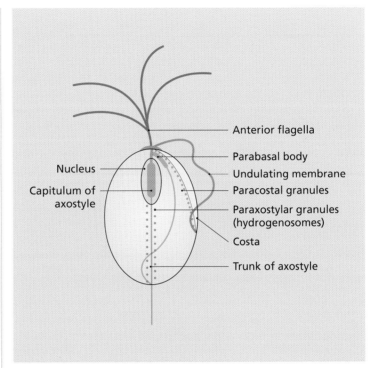

Figure 17.1 *Trichomonas vaginalis* showing its structure (modified from, and reproduced with the permission of the American Society of Parasitology, from Honigberg and King 1964[314])

Labels in figure: Nucleus; Capitulum of axostyle; Anterior flagella; Parabasal body; Undulating membrane; Paracostal granules; Paraxostylar granules (hydrogenosomes); Costa; Trunk of axostyle

is often elongated. Pseudopodia-like extensions from its surface allow for feeding and attachment to solid objects. There are four anterior flagella that are about the same length as the body. Movement of the undulating membrane is vigorous and is controlled by the posterior flagellum that passes along its upper margin. The undulating membrane is about two-thirds that of the body length of the organism. The flagella originate from, and are intimately related to, a kinetosomal complex situated at the anterior end of the cell. The costa, a slender chromatic basal rod, also originates from the kinetosomal complex, is uniform in diameter, tending to taper at its ends,

and is situated beneath the undulating membrane. A hyaline rod, the axostyle, is flattened into a capitulum closely applied to the nucleus, it passes down the center of the cell and appears to project posteriorly as a small spine. A single oval nucleus lies near the anterior end of the cell. Large granules – double membrane-bound organelles called hydrogenosomes – are found in the cytoplasm, and are involved in catabolic processes. From the evolutionary point of view hydrogenosomes themselves may be organelles derived from clostridia.

Trichomonads lack mitochondria. Multiplication is by longitudinal binary fission. Cysts are not formed[1].

Trichomonas vaginalis exhibits the characteristics of a micro-aerophile; in culture anaerobic conditions prolong the period of population increase. The principal mode of nutrition is by pinocytosis or, *sensu stricto*, macropinocytosis (namely 'cell drinking' or ingestion of large molecules and tiny particles by cells) and phagocytosis ('cell eating', a similar process to macropinocytosis except that particles are large enough to be seen in the light microscope), which may proceed in any part of the body. First, an invagination appears in the cytoplasm and gradually its edges are drawn together. The wall of the vesicle thickens and acquires a villous pattern. Micro-organisms and large particles are usually caught by pseudopodia; large and small particles including entire cells may be engulfed. Some, but not all entrapped organisms seem to be altered but it is impossible to say whether they have undergone changes after engulfment or have been phagocytosed in a poor condition. They are usually located in phagosomes but may lie freely in the cytoplasm with no evidence of a limiting membrane.

Two other species of trichomonads, *Trichomonas tenax* and *Pentatrichomonas hominis* occur in man. Apart from *P. hominis* with its five anterior flagella, these organisms are morphologically similar to *T. vaginalis*. *Trichomonas tenax* is generally considered to be a harmless commensal of the mouth and is commonly associated with poor oral hygiene. It does not survive passage through the intestinal tract and cannot be established in the vagina. *Pentatrichomonas hominis* is an inhabitant of the cecum and colon of humans, and a morphologically identical organism is found in primates. Although it is considered to be a harmless commensal, it is often found in association with true pathogenic protozoa, for example *Entamoeba histolytica*. *Pentatrichomonas hominis* does not survive in the mouth or vagina.

A sexually transmitted trichomonad, *Tritrichomonas fetus*, is seen in cattle, being found in the preputial sac and on the glans penis of bulls; the organism, transmitted to cows during sexual intercourse, may cause vaginitis, endometritis, and abortion.

PATHOLOGY

Trichomonads are gathered in small clusters on the stratified epithelium, but cover only a small area of the surface[2]. *Trichomonas vaginalis* invades the superficial epithelial cells but does not penetrate to the deeper layers of the epithelium. Epithelial damage is located under clusters of trichomonads, but an intense vaginitis is present whether or not *T. vaginalis* cells are present on the epithelial surface. Vaginal biopsies show a chronic non-specific inflammatory response in the lamina propria consisting of plasma cells, lymphocytes, and polymorphonuclear leukocytes. When there is mild inflammation, neutrophils are found in the superficial layers of the epithelium and in more severe cases, neutrophils are also found in the deeper layers. Sometimes there is superficial ulceration of the epithelium, and all layers of the cervical epithelium show some hyperchromasia and nuclear enlargement.

PATHOGENESIS

The subject of pathogenesis has been reviewed recently by Petrin and colleagues[3], and much of the following discussion is derived from their document. All isolates of *T. vaginalis* are capable of infection and disease production. Although the exact mechanism of the pathogenesis of *T. vaginalis* is unknown, contact dependent and contact independent mechanisms, and immune responses are probably all important. Adhesion of trichomonads to the vaginal epithelial cells is the first and most important step. A mosaic of adhesion molecules, receptors to host extracellular matrix proteins and carbohydrates, covers the trichomonad cell surface, and adhesion to the vaginal cell surface involves four adhesion proteins (adhesins) that act in a specific receptor-ligand fashion (a ligand is a linking or binding molecule)[4]. Gene expression is up regulated at the transcriptional level by iron[5]. Cysteine proteinases are also prerequisites for attachment to the host cell. Before adherence to the epithelial cells of the vagina, however, trichomonads must first traverse the mucin layer. The protozoon has been shown to bind to mucin (the principal glycoprotein of mucous secretions) possibly via a lectin-like adhesin; cysteine proteinases then degrade the mucin[6]. Motility is also needed to breach the mucin layer. On contact with the host cell, *T. vaginalis* undergoes amoeboid transformation with the production of pseudopodia and up regulation of adhesin synthesis[7]. Although adherence does not correlate with virulence, the presence of lectin-binding carbohydrates on the surface of *T. vaginalis* appears to[8], and these saccharides are involved in the hemolysis of erythrocytes and in phagocytosis. As *T. vaginalis* lacks the ability to synthesize lipids, erythrocytes may be an important source of fatty acids. Additionally, iron is an important nutrient for the protozoan, and the lysis erythrocytes may therefore provide this. *Trichomonas vaginalis* adheres to the surface of the erythrocyte by a specific ligand–receptor interaction, perforin-like proteins (possibly cysteine proteinases) that form pores in the cell, are released, the trichomonad then detaches itself from the erythrocyte, and lysis follows.

Contact-independent mechanisms are also important in the pathogenesis of *T. vaginalis* infection. When a cell-free filtrate (CDF) of *T. vaginalis* is applied to a cell culture monolayer, the cells of the monolayer detach, resembling the sloughing of vaginal cells during acute infection in women[9]. The cell-free filtrate (CDF) is a 200 kDa glycoprotein that is active within the pH range 5.0 to 8.5, and inactive at a pH under 4.5 (the pH of the normal vagina). The relatively high pH of the vagina in women with trichomoniasis (5.0 or above) may therefore contribute to the pathogenesis of the infection. Increasing production of CDF is associated with increasing severity of the disease. However, CDF is highly immunogenic and the appearance of local antibodies against the glycoprotein may ameliorate its effects. The concentration of sex hormones may also influence the concentration of CDF in the vagina: *in vitro* the production of CDF decreases in the presence of estrogen[10]. This may explain the worsening of symptoms at the time of menstruation when the estrogen levels are relatively low.

It is clear from clinical observation that any immune response elicited by the parasite is incapable of reliably eliminating it or of preventing re-infection. Although spontaneous eradication of the protozoan can occur, many women have chronic infection. Several mechanisms have been proposed to explain the parasite's ability to evade the immune system.

1. *In vitro* complement-mediated cyolysis by human serum has been observed but, in the vagina, there is little complement until menstruation and the organism has developed strategies to resist lysis. The high concentration of iron that is present in the vagina at the time of menses up up-regulates expression of cysteine proteinases which have been shown to degrade the C3 portion of complement on the protozoon's surface[11].

2. *Trichomonas vaginalis* induces a local immune response as shown by an increase in the number of IgA and IgM-bearing plasma cells in the cervices of women with trichomoniasis. However, many of the cysteine proteinases secreted by *T. vaginalis* degrade IgA, IgM, and IgG, allowing the organism to evade the antibody response[12].

3. A continuous release of soluble, immunogenic antigens may neutralize antibody or cytotoxic T cells[13].

4. The protozoon can coat itself with host plasma proteins so that the immune system does not recognize it[14].

5. Phenotypic variation is used by *T. vaginalis* as a means of evading the immune system. Only certain organisms that express the immunogenic glycoproteins (P270) can undergo phenotypic variation between cytoplasmic and cell surface expression of P270 (P270 positive)[15]. The positive phenotype protozoa lack adhesins and cannot adhere to host cells, but the negative phenotype organisms (which express adhesins) have the ability to do so. *In vivo*, there is an antigenic shift from positive to negative phenotype. Some P270-positive trichomonads are susceptible to antibody-mediated, complement-independent lysis[16] but, as adhesins are poorly immunogenic, negative phenotypes escape the effect of specific antibody.

6. An immunogen, P230, is present on the surface of *T. vaginalis*, but it undergoes conformational change, allowing it to evade antibody[17].

IMMUNITY

Trichomoniasis, like other mucosal infections, induces local production of secretory IgA in women[18], but this was seldom detected in men who harbored *T. vaginalis* or who were contacts of women who harbored the organism[18]. Antibodies of the IgG class reactive with cysteine proteinases, and specific IgG against P230 that become undetectable after treatment are found in the vaginas of women with trichomoniasis[19, 20].

Neutrophils are the predominant cell type in the inflammatory response elicited by *T. vaginalis*, and it has been suggested that the protozoon activates the alternative complement pathway and attracts neutrophils to the vagina[21]. These neutrophils, whose activity is oxygen-dependent, kill and ingest the organisms.

Using a whole-cell antigen, antibody to *T. vaginalis* has been assayed using an enzyme-linked immunosorbent assay (ELISA). Immunoglobulin G antibody was detected in sera of only 3% of children under 12 years of age. In contrast, IgG or IgM antibody or both were detected in about 80% of the women who had vaginal trichomoniasis and in about 14% of women considered to be uninfected on the basis of microscopy of wet or stained films. Antibodies of the IgG class reactive with cysteine proteinases of *T. vaginalis* are found in the serum of most women with vaginal trichomoniasis and become undetectable after successful treatment[22]. A recent study has shown that the IgG detected in the sera of women is also reactive against a common immunogenic protein of 115 kDa in size; all sera recognizing this antigen were reactive against *T. vaginalis* alpha-actinin[23].

EPIDEMIOLOGY

In adults infection with *T. vaginalis* is generally regarded as being sexually transmitted for the following reasons.

- Trichomoniasis is uncommon among children and virgins, but most common between the ages of 16 and 35 years (Figure 17.2), which is usually the period of greatest sexual activity.
- The relative risk of acquisition of *T. vaginalis* is increased in women who are more sexually active[24].
- In the past, trichomoniasis was commonly associated with other STIs: up to 40% of women attending STI clinics in the 1960s with this infection also had gonorrhea[25].
- In many instances cure of women with recurrent trichomoniasis has only resulted after the parasite has been eradicated from the genital tract of their partner(s). A varying proportion, even up to 60%, of male sex partners of infected women may harbor the parasite and many are asymptomatic. There is often difficulty, however, at a single examination, in demonstrating the parasite in male patients who are contacts of women with *T. vaginalis*.

Trichomonas vaginalis has been isolated from bath water, and viable organisms can be

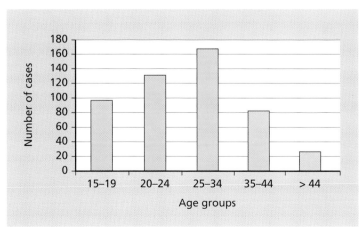

Figure 17.2 Age distribution of women with trichomoniasis in Scotland 1993 to 1997

found in washcloths several hours after contamination[26]. The protozoon can contaminate toilet seats, and indeed, after seeding toilet seats with vaginal exudate containing *T. vaginalis*, organisms have been shown to survive for between 10 and 45 minutes[27]. Despite these findings, nonsexual transmission of *T. vaginalis* is uncommon. Although direct female to female transmission, resulting from poor standards of sanitation and hygiene (for example contamination of baths or toilet seats) has been proposed as a means of acquiring the infection, there is little evidence to support this view. Neonatal infestation followed by a long and variable period of latency could account for nonsexually acquired infection. However, neonatal infection in female babies, although a recognized clinical entity, is rare. It has also been suggested that intestinal trichomonads could become adapted to the vagina. There is, however, no evidence that these trichomonads can be successfully established in the human vagina.

As studies are undertaken in various clinical settings, and have involved the use of tests of varying sensitivity and specificity, it is difficult to estimate the true prevalence of infection in the general population of a particular geographical area. However, temporal changes in the prevalence of infection may be obtained from STI clinic data. The number of women with trichomoniasis who attended STI clinics in the UK is shown in Figure 17.3, it is clear that the rates of infection have declined progressively since the 1980s. It also seems clear that infection is more common in some African countries than in western Europe. Amongst 249 women who attended a family planning clinic in a rural area of South Africa, 18% had trichomoniasis[28], and 22% of 549 pregnant women in Mali were infected[29]. In the USA, black women who attended an antenatal clinic were shown to have a rate of infection some four times that of white women[30]; this finding probably reflects the lower socioeconomic status of the former group of women. Similarly, the prevalence of infection amongst indigenous women in northern Australia greatly exceeds that of the general population[31]. A high prevalence of trichomoniasis has also been reported in female sex-industry workers in

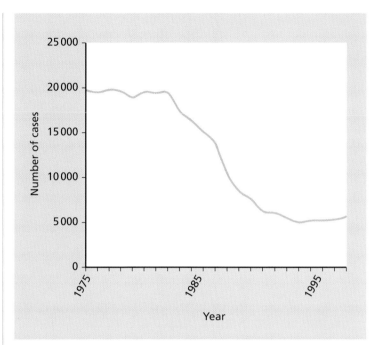

Figure 17.3 Number of cases of trichomoniasis in women reported from genitourinary medicine clinics in the UK 1975 to 1998

southern and western Africa: up to 45% of these women may be infected with *T. vaginalis*[32, 33].

As asymptomatic infections are common, and diagnosis is difficult, the prevalence of trichomoniasis in men is difficult to determine. Amongst men attending STI clinics in the USA, however, the prevalence appears to be high. For example, 12% of 204 men who attended a clinic in San Francisco were infected[34], and an extraordinarily high prevalence of 58% of 85 men was found amongst inner city youths in Washington DC[35]. Infection rates in some parts of Africa are also high. Hobbs *et al.*[36] found that 17% of men attending a STI clinic in Malawi were infected with *T. vaginalis*; the protozoon was identified in about 21% of men with urethritis and in 12% of asymptomatic individuals.

Epidemiological studies have shown an association between *T. vaginalis* and risk of transmission of HIV[37]. This increased risk may in part be explained by the following findings.

1. An increase in the number of CD4+ lymphocytes (the target cells for HIV) in the endocervix of women with trichomoniasis[38].
2. An increased HIV RNA concentration in the seminal plasma of HIV-infected men with urethritis caused by *T. vagin-*

alis compared with HIV-infected men without urethritis[36].

3. The degradation by the cysteine proteinases of *T. vaginalis* of secretory leukocyte protease inhibitor (SPLI), rendering it non-functional[39] (SPLI from saliva appears to prevent transmission of HIV by inhibiting virus entry into monocytic cells).

There is an association between cervical carcinoma and infestation with *T. vaginalis*[40] although a direct causal relationship has not been proved.

CLINICAL FEATURES

Clinical features in women

Trichomoniasis is not readily recognized, nor are clinical manifestations reliable diagnostic parameters; only a minority of women with trichomoniasis show classic signs[41]. The pre-patent period is difficult to determine although it has been estimated that clinical manifestations of the disease develop 4 to 28 days after sexual intercourse with an infected partner[42].

The clinical features of infection are very variable, the most common symptoms in those infected being vaginal discharge (56%) and dysuria (18%). Vulval soreness and an unpleasant odor may also be present. In many, sometimes in 40% of cases, there

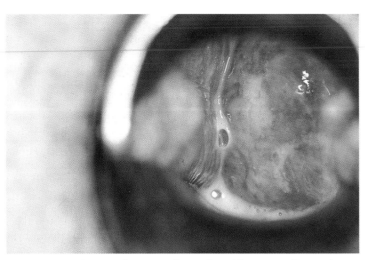

Figure 17.4 Trichomonal vaginitis (reproduced from McMillan and Scott 2000[315])

may be no complaint of vaginal discharge[40]. The concept that all women infected with *T. vaginalis* have vaginal discharge should be discarded. Clinical features appear to differ according to the population and possibly age group studied.

The most common sign, occurring in about 70% of cases of trichomoniasis, is a vaginal discharge (Figure 17.4), varying in consistency from thin and scanty to thick and profuse; the classic sign of a frothy yellow discharge is found in proportions varying between 10% and 30% of cases. Vulvitis and vaginitis are sometimes associated with trichomonal vaginal discharge and the cervix may be inflamed. On colposcopy, when inflammation due to *T. vaginalis* is severe, magnification shows patches of higher vascular density which, on naked-eye inspection, are usually described as forming a 'strawberry cervix'. The inflammation produces significant changes in the pattern of the original squamous epithelium as seen through the colposcope. The stromal papillae are higher and reach almost to the surface of the epithelium. In these papillae the vessels are clearly visible and form simple capillary loops running vertically to the surface, but at the top of the loop two or more crests may be found. The shape of the loops may be described as fork-like or antler-like. As the capillaries are separated from the surface by only a few layers of epithelial cells contact bleeding is common.

Urethritis is found in about a quarter of women. Bartholinitis is a rare complication and is perhaps produced by bacterial infec-tion rather than the protozoon. In about 5% of infected women there are no abnor-mal findings on clinical examination.

Clinical features in men

About 50% of men with trichomoniasis are asymptomatic. When there are symptoms, urethral discharge that is usually small to moderate in amount, is the most common feature[43]. Prostatitis, cystitis, and epididy-mitis have been given as manifestations of trichomoniasis, but the etiology of these con-ditions may be more related to the etiology of non-gonococcal urethritis and to pathogens, or potential pathogens, such as *Chlamydia trachomatis* and *Ureaplasma urealyticum*.

Trichomonas vaginalis may be isolated from the sub-preputial sac and may be associated with balanoposthitis which, rarely, may be ulcerative.

TRICHOMONIASIS AND PREGNANCY

Some studies have shown an association between trichomoniasis and prematurity. In the Vaginal Infections and Prematurity Study (VIP) reported by Cotch *et al.*[44], infection with *T. vaginalis* during the second trimester of pregnancy was associated with premature delivery (adjusted odds ratio (OR) = 1.3), low birth weight (OR = 1.3), and preterm delivery of a low birth weight infant (OR = 1.4). Amongst a group of Congolese women, an association between low birth weight and trichomoniasis was found[45]. Other studies, however, have shown no correlation between trichomonal

infection and preterm labor. In a multi-center study in which 2929 pregnant women were examined for the presence of vaginal pathogens at 24 and 28 weeks of gestation, there was no significant associa-tion between preterm birth and the detec-tion of *T. vaginalis*[46]. Similarly, a study from Lithuania showed that the prevalence of endocervical trichomonal infection was not significantly different in women in premature labor than in those delivering at term[47]. Further support for this lack of association between trichomonal infection and prematurity has come from a recent study in which 604 asymptomatic preg-nant women with vaginal trichomonal infection were treated with either metroni-dazole or placebo[47a]. It was shown that treatment did not prevent preterm delivery: delivery occurred before 37 weeks gestation in 19.0% of the 315 women in the metronidazole group and in 10.7% of the 289 women given placebo (relative risk 1.8; 95% confidence interval, 1.2 to 2.7). This difference was attributed to an increase in preterm delivery resulting from spontaneous preterm labour. The risk of prematurity, however, may be related to a synergistic effect between *T. vaginalis* and other genital tract infections. Although Minkoff and col-leagues[48] found an independent associa-tion between prematurity and infection with *T. vaginalis* (relative risk = 1.4) and with *Staphylococcus epidermidis* (relative risk = 1.57), the association was stronger in women who were co-infected (relative risk = 2.1). Similarly, McGregor *et al.*[49] found that the risk of preterm birth was 9.1% among women with trichomonal infection but not bacterial vaginosis, 17.8% among women with bacterial vaginosis but not trichomoniasis, and 27.8% among those with both bacterial vaginosis and trichomoniasis. Another factor that may contribute to the association between trichomonal infection and prematurity found in some studies is frequent sexual intercourse. Read *et al.*[50] observed that there was a correlation between preterm birth and the presence of *T. vaginalis* at 23 to 26 weeks gestation in those women who had frequent sexual intercourse (more than once per week) but not in women who had intercourse less often. Although not proven, it is possible that sexual intercourse leads to ascending infection with the protozoon.

Several mechanisms may be responsible for the premature rupture of the membranes associated with *T. vaginalis* infection

- lysis of the epithelial cells of the amniotic membrane through contact with the protozoon[51]
- elaboration of metabolites that stimulate prostaglandin synthesis, for example phospholipase A$_2$[52]
- erosion of the fetal membranes, for example, by cysteine proteases[53].

Trichomonas vaginalis can be transmitted to the neonate during vaginal delivery and cause a vulvovaginitis. In Trussel's study[54], 5% of 41 infants born to infected mothers were infected. It is thought that most neonatal infections are self-limiting and, unless the infant has severe signs, that treatment is unnecessary.

DIAGNOSIS

The diagnosis of trichomoniasis currently lies upon both microscopy and culture for the demonstration of *T. vaginalis* in secretions of patients. Repeated testing from a multiplicity of sites, especially in males, may be necessary to establish a diagnosis.

Specimens from women

Vaginal exudate is collected from the posterior fornix with a sterile cotton wool-tipped applicator stick or a 10 μL plastic inoculating loop. Although a larger volume of exudate can be collected from the vaginal fornices using small rectangles of polyester sponge[55], this method is seldom used in clinical practice.

Self-obtained vaginal specimens, obtained by inserting a cotton wool-tipped applicator stick into the vagina, rotating, and, after withdrawing, mixing with the medium in an InPouch™ TV test, yields results that are comparable to clinician-obtained specimens[56]. The improved sensitivity over conventional tests of the detection of trichomonal DNA by PCR in self-inserted tampons[57] suggests that these may be used for sampling.

Specimens from men

If a urethral discharge is present, this can be collected with a 10 μL inoculating loop, otherwise a scraping should be taken gently from the urethra before the patient passes the first morning urine. A centrifuged deposit (600 *g*) of a 20 mL urine sample taken preferably after the patient has held his urine overnight should also be examined. Krieger and colleagues[58] showed that culture of either urethral swabs or first-voided urine sediment identified 40 and 34 of 50 infected men respectively; not surprisingly, when both methods were used for the detection of the organism, 49 men were identified. Although material collected on Dacron swabs from the sub-preputial sac of uncircumcised men or from the coronal sulcus of circumcised men can be examined for *T. vaginalis*, the diagnostic yield is much lower than that of examination of urethral or urine specimens, and is probably unnecessary for routine diagnosis[58]. Trichomonads can also be found in expressed prostatic secretions, but this examination is seldom used routinely in the diagnosis of trichomoniasis. Similarly, although *T. vaginalis* can be detected in semen when culture of urethral material or urine sediment has yielded negative results[58], semen samples are not routinely examined.

The following diagnostic methods may be applied.

Examination of a wet smear

Although a fresh specimen of expressed prostatic secretion or the deposit from a centrifuged specimen of urine may be examined as a wet preparation directly, the density of polymorphonuclear leukocytes and epithelial cells in vaginal exudate may obscure the trichomonads and particularly the movement of the flagella. It is therefore preferable to examine vaginal discharge after suspension in a few drops of isotonic saline (0.154 M) or buffer. The actual method of microscopy varies from clinic to clinic, but dark ground illumination, phase contrast microscopy, and ordinary light microscopy with reduced illumination are all used routinely. *Trichomonas vaginalis*, which is larger than a polymorphonuclear leukocyte but smaller than an epithelial cell, is readily recognized by its usually rapidly moving flagella, the rippling movement of the undulating membrane, and the jerky movements of the organism. Ideally the specimen should be examined immediately, but if this is impracticable the swab should be placed preferably in Amies'

transport medium[59]; *T. vaginalis* does not survive well in Stuart's transport medium beyond 24 hours[60].

Compared with the results of culture, the reported sensitivity of wet smear microscopy by transmitted light, phase contrast, and dark field microscopy in the diagnosis of vaginal trichomoniasis has varied widely from as low as 38% to as high as 82%[61], with most workers considering that half of the cases may be missed if reliance is placed on examination of the wet smear alone[62]. This variation probably reflects the different culture media used in the studies and the variability in the number of organisms in the samples tested. When few organisms are present, a prolonged search may be necessary. Vaginal douching lowers the sensitivity of microscopy but not that of cultivation methods[62]. Although the specificity of wet smear microscopy is considered to be high, Robertson et al.[55] noted that the diagnosis of trichomoniasis could not be confirmed in 10 of 44 specimens that had been identified as infected on examination by immediate microscopy.

Examination of stained smears

In an attempt to improve the sensitivity of direct microscopy various stains have been added to the saline mount. Although trichomonads are not stained by dyes such as malachite green, safranin, and methylene blue, other cellular material takes up the dye and the organisms stand out against this colored background. This staining method, however, has not been shown convincingly to improve the detection rate of trichomonads in secretions and cannot be recommended for routine use.

Acridine orange is a fluorescent nucleic acid stain that has been used to differentiate DNA from RNA in cells. Under ultraviolet light, DNA and RNA-containing structures fluoresce yellow-green and brick-red respectively. In stained vaginal smears, *T. vaginalis* appears as a round or pear-shaped orange-red structure with a yellow-green nucleus. The results of acridine orange staining of vaginal material for trichomonads compare favorably with other methods. In reported series the sensitivity of this method has always exceeded that of direct wet smear microscopy, but

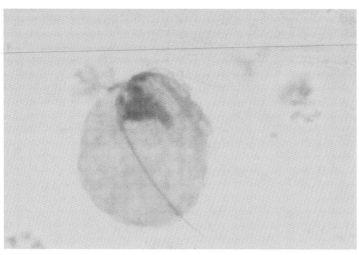

Figure 17.5 *Trichomonas vaginalis* (Giemsa's stain) (reproduced from McMillan and Scott 2000[315])

studies on sensitivity compared with culture have yielded conflicting results, with some workers finding the staining method to be superior and others finding it less sensitive[61]. The need for a fluorescence microscope has limited the use of this diagnostic method.

Fixed smears of vaginal discharge with Giemsa's or Leishman's stain have been used for many years in the diagnosis of trichomoniasis. The protozoa are stained bright blue with a dark-staining small eccentric nucleus; the axostyle and flagella may be seen (Figure 17.5). Although sensitivity is high approaching that of cultivation, the method is time consuming, requiring careful preparation and an experienced observer, and does not lend itself to routine use in a busy clinic.

Trichomonas vaginalis may be detected in Papanicolaou-stained cervical smears as an ovoid structure with gray-green cytoplasm containing eosinophilic granules, and a blue eccentric nucleus. Although the sensitivity of Pap smear microscopy in the diagnosis of trichomoniasis is said to be similar or superior to wet smear microscopy, serious doubts about specificity[63] should caution against its use in the routine diagnosis of vaginal trichomoniasis. Pap smear microscopy of cervical smears, however, may identify unsuspected trichomonal infection.

Although trichomonads may be detected in Gram-stained smears[64], inconsistency in the size and shape of the organism makes identification difficult, and few workers find the method useful in routine diagnosis.

Immunological techniques

Although *T. vaginalis* can be detected in secretions by direct immunofluorescence[65] and in fixed cervical cytology smears by immunoperoxidase methods[66], neither method is suitable for routine diagnosis. An enzyme-linked immunosorbent assay (EIA) for trichomonal antigen has been described[67]. Although the sensitivity and specificity of the test are high when compared with wet smear microscopy and culture, it is essentially a laboratory method requiring skilled technical support. A simple, latex agglutination test of comparable sensitivity and specificity to the EIA, and yielding results within a few minutes, has been described[68] but is not widely used.

Cultivation

Many culture media for the diagnosis of *T. vaginalis* infection have been described, they have in common nutrients (for example, liver extracts, peptone, trypticase), sera, essential salts, reducing agents, carbohydrates, and antibiotics to inhibit bacterial growth. Many diagnostic laboratories use liquid media, that is, media that do not contain agar. These undefined media include Feinberg–Whittington and Oxoid

No 2. Since *T. vaginalis* grows better when the medium is incubated under partial or complete anaerobic conditions, culture vessels should be filled as full as possible with liquid medium. Some laboratories routinely use semi-liquid media such as CPLM (cysteine–peptone–liver–maltose) or Diamond's TYM (trypticase–yeast extract–maltose) or, perhaps more sensitive, a modification[69]. The incorporation of agar into the medium reduces the diffusion of oxygen into the medium and allows better growth.

As expected, in the diagnosis of vaginal trichomoniasis, cultivation is a more sensitive diagnostic test than microscopy, particularly when there are low numbers of organisms in the secretions. In studies, the sensitivity of microscopical examination of cultured trichomonads has varied from just under 80% to about 95%[61]. Since vaginal exudate, or other secretions, may contain non-viable trichomonads, cultivation of that material may yield negative results. Under these circumstances microscopic methods (or PCR) are more sensitive than culture. On the other hand, when few but viable organisms are present, culture is more sensitive than microscopy. Not surprisingly then, the greatest diagnostic yield is obtained when a combination of methods is used[61].

As cultivation is regarded by many as expensive and time-consuming, it is not widely used for the diagnosis of trichomoniasis[70]. However, a novel method for the transport and cultivation of *T. vaginalis* – the InPouch™ TV test (BioMed Disgnostics) – has been developed and is suitable for routine use in the laboratory.

The InPouch™ TV test

Each pouch of the test system is divided into two chambers which are separated by a channel that allows fluid to flow between them. The lower chamber contains selective culture medium and, before specimen inoculation, a little fluid is squeezed from this reservoir into the upper chamber. The specimen obtained on a cotton wool-tipped applicator stick is mixed with the medium in the latter chamber in which, if desired, it can be examined microscopically. The inoculated medium is then squeezed into the bottom chamber that is then sealed.

After incubation at 37°C for 24 hours the pouch, held in a plastic viewer, is examined microscopically. A negative specimen should be re-incubated and examined at 48 hours and 5 days. The sensitivity of this method is higher than that of wet smear microscopy and of cultivation in other media[71, 72]. In geographical areas where the diagnostic laboratory is remote from the clinic, a clear advantage of this test system is that trichomonads remain viable for up to 7 days after specimen collection. The InPouch ™TV test has the additional advantage of a relatively long shelf life (6 months) at room temperature.

Methods based on the detection of *Trichomonas vaginalis* DNA

Fragments of *T. vaginalis* DNA have been used as probes in the molecular methods for the detection of infection. Although some have been used in oligonucleotide probing and fluorescent *in situ* hybridization[73, 74], cross-reactivity with *Pentatrichomonas hominis* and *Tritrichomonas foetus* has limited their usefulness. Various primer sets have been used in PCRs for the detection of *T. vaginalis* DNA, and a sensitivity in one method using nested primers was for DNA equivalent of one protozoan[75]. The detection of specific DNA by a PCR was shown by Heine *et al.*[76] to be more sensitive than wet smear microscopy and culture in the diagnosis of vaginal trichomoniasis, and this finding has been confirmed in subsequent studies. For example, in the study reported by Madico *et al.*[77] on the use of a PCR compared with wet smear microscopy and culture (InPouch ™TV culture system) to detect *T. vaginalis* in vaginal specimens from 350 women, the sensitivity and specificity of the PCR were 97% and 98% respectively, compared with a sensitivity of culture of 70% and of wet smear microscopy of 36%. Van der Schee and colleagues have compared the results of a PCR on urine with those on vaginal swabs, and have shown that the test on either sample can identify an equal number of infected women. They noted, however, that the results from the urine samples and from the vaginal swabs were not mutually confirmatory, possibly suggesting that some women had infection at only one anatomical

site. Recently, it has been shown that the rate of detection of *T. vaginalis* by PCR on DNA extracted from self-inserted tampons is significantly higher than that from urine[78]. *Trichomonas vaginalis* DNA can be detected in urine from infected men[79]. Because it is otherwise difficult to identify infection in men, this test may become the diagnostic method of choice.

Although PCR for the diagnosis of trichomoniasis is not used routinely at present, it is likely to become the method of choice where resources permit. It has the added advantage that it could be incorporated into a joint strategy for screening for multiple STIs by using molecular amplification methods[77].

TREATMENT

Treatment with 5-nitroimidazoles

The discovery in 1959 of the 5-nitroimidazole, metronidazole, as the first agent that is systemically active against trichomoniasis brought spectacular cure rates of 86% to 100% instead of the 10% to 20% of earlier treatments. Since 1969 the closely related 5-nitroimidazoles nimorazole, tinidazole, ornidazole, secnidazole, and carnidazole have been introduced into clinical practice, although not all of them are available in every country. In the USA only metronidazole is approved by the Federal Drugs Administration for the treatment of trichomoniasis. A review of the comparative data did not reveal a clear advantage for one compound over another and cure rates lie within the range of 85% to 95% with symptoms generally being relieved within a few days[80].

Metronidazole

Metronidazole is the most extensively used drug of the group and although the other 5-nitroimidazoles differ somewhat in their pharmacological properties, the mode of antimicrobial activity is similar for all.

Mode of action

The majority of clinically important anaerobe genera such as *Bacteroides*, *Fusobacterium*, and the spore-bearing *Clostridium*, and metronidazole-susceptible protozoa are inhibited by concentrations of approximately 3 µg/mL or less. Organisms such as

anaerobic Gram-positive cocci and non-sporing bacilli are usually inhibited by 6 µg/mL or less[81].

The action of the 5-nitroimidazoles in anaerobic micro-organisms is thought to consist of four successive steps[82, 83]
1. the entry of the drug into the cell
2. its reductive activation to short-lived cytotoxic intermediates, a process inhibited by aerobiosis
3. the toxic effect of these short-lived intermediates on intracellular components leading to cell death
4. the release of biologically inactive end products.

The main point of the hypothesis is the assumption that the nitro group of the drug has to be reduced in the target cell to form a toxic derivative; no cytotoxicity can be observed without such reduction.

The striking feature of the selectivity of metronidazole is that it affects anaerobic organisms, both prokaryotes and eukaryotes, where reduction of metronidazole, crucial to its action, appears to be achieved by redox mechanisms that are of great significance in the metabolism of anaerobes but have no, or only minor, significance for other organisms.

Cellular uptake of metronidazole appears to be passive and achieved by diffusion in both anaerobic and aerobic cells, but whereas in aerobic cells the drug remains unchanged, in anaerobic organisms it undergoes metabolic modification which decreases the intracellular concentration of unchanged drug and thus increases the concentration gradient across the cell membrane: this gradient promotes the continuous uptake of the drug and leads to an intracellular accumulation of its derivatives. The electrons necessary for the reduction of the nitro group of metronidazole origin and the direct donors of these electrons are thought to be ferredoxin-like electron transport proteins of low redox potential (doxins). Unstable intermediates in the process of reduction are thought to be cytotoxic, whereas end products such as acetamide and N-(2-hydroxyethyl)oxamic acid are not. The most significant competitor for available electrons is oxygen, as shown by diminished biological activity of metronidazole when susceptible organisms are present under aerobic conditions. Among other cytotoxic effects, metronidazole reduced in the presence of DNA binds to the nucleic acid and causes strand breakage with destabilization of the helix.

In vitro T. vaginalis stop cell division about 1 hour after to metronidazole, motility ceasing in 1 to 2 hours, and cell death is seen within 7 to 8 hours[84].

Resistance to metronidazole

Certain isolates of *T. vaginalis*, obtained from patients in whom several courses of metronidazole have failed, show normal susceptibility to metronidazole in *in vitro* assays performed under anaerobic conditions, but in certain aerobic *in vitro* assays their susceptibility is significantly lower than that of non-resistant isolates[85, 82]. There are marked differences in the effect of aerobiosis on metronidazole metabolism in various isolates of *T. vaginalis*. Aerobic conditions inhibit metronidazole uptake in resistant isolates to a greater extent than in susceptible ones, and changes in intracellular reduction may be responsible for relative resistance[83].

Under completely anaerobic conditions, metronidazole may be effective against all *T. vaginalis* stocks, but under partially aerobic conditions its effects may vary widely[86] and assays under aerobic conditions have been thought to give false results[87]. The crux of the matter seems to be that the activity of metronidazole *in vitro* under anaerobic conditions is little altered, but under aerobic conditions relative resistance is detected among ordinarily susceptible organisms and enhanced resistance among the resistant organisms. All the enzymes responsible for the cleavage of pyruvate to acetate, carbon dioxide and hydrogen appear to be located in the hyrogenosomes, which also enable the reduction of the 5-nitroimidazoles. The reduction products are unstable but their cytotoxic action appears to cause strand breakage in the DNA. This will only occur under anaerobic conditions and only with the reduced drug. There are data to suggest that in resistant trichomonads a low cytoplasmic nicotinamide adenine dinucleotide H oxidase may allow oxygen to permeate hydrogenosomes and interfere with their reductive action on the drug. The process is an example of selective toxicity, and intracellular concentration of drug metabolite is

50 to 100 times that of unchanged drug in body fluids.

The reduction of the nitro group of 5-nitroimidazoles and the production of cytotoxic intermediates is intimately connected with the functioning of the hydrogenosome, where the nitro group is reduced by electrons generated during hydrogenosomal pyruvate oxidation and donated to the drug by its doxins. Resistant strains show reduced levels of ferredoxin, ferredoxin mRNA, and ferredoxin gene transcription[88].

Mutagenicity and capacity to induce tumors in experimental animals

In some bacteria metronidazole can produce mutations, but a double-blind cross-over study showed that a daily dose of 0.8 g for 4 months did not induce an increase in the frequency of chromosomal aberrations in patients with Crohn's disease. Coulter[89] indicated that the connection between mutation, a heritable change in DNA sequence, and gross changes in chromosome anatomy is not, however, understood.

As a nitro compound in widespread therapeutic use, metronidazole has been investigated in regard to its capacity to induce tumors in some laboratory animals. In connection with the effect on tumor incidence in mice, Roe[90] writes that 'the effect involved the administration throughout the lives of the animals of total doses, on a mg/kg body weight basis, equivalent to between 350 to 1000 times that given to patients in the form of a 10-day course for the treatment of trichomoniasis'.

Metronidazole and another nitro compound, nitrofurantoin, have been in use for many years and so far no clinical evidence of carcinogenicity has been forthcoming. The cure of trichomoniasis and the control of secondary non-specific vaginal infection is highly desirable, and as a result may reduce the risk of cervical cancer itself[90]. The authors favor the use of metronidazole in the doses recommended for the treatment of trichomoniasis.

Absorption, distribution, and fate of metronidazole[91]

Peak serum concentrations of metronidazole after either oral or intravenous admin-

istration are quite similar and average approximately 10 μg/mL after a single 500 mg dose. After an oral dose the peak serum concentration is reached about 1 hour after administration. Food does not significantly affect absorption and bioavailability approaches 100%. Rectal administration of metronidazole by suppository results in peak concentrations approximately one half of those following equivalent oral doses and occurs 4 hours after administration; the bioavailability of a rectal suppository is about 80%. The systemic absorption of intravaginal metronidazole is very slow with peak serum concentrations of approximately 2 μg/mL being attained 8 to 24 hours after administration of a 500 mg dose.

The serum half-life of unchanged metronidazole (measured using high pressure liquid chromatography – HPLC) is about 8 hours. As less than 20% of the drug is protein bound and its molecular weight is low, metronidazole is widely distributed throughout the body with tissue levels, in most cases, approximating serum levels.

Metronidazole is metabolized in the liver by side chain oxidation and glucuronide conjugation. Hydroxymetronidazole and acetylmetronidazole are the major stable metabolites, the former having some biological activity (30% to 65% of the parent compound) against *T. vaginalis*[92], but having a longer elimination half-life than metronidazole. The majority of metronidazole and its metabolites are excreted in the urine and feces, with less than 12% being excreted unchanged[93]. By specific and sensitive methods such as HPLC in which unchanged metronidazole and the hydroxy and acetyl metabolites are measured separately, total excretion of these compounds after 48 hours is 30%, with the hydroxy metabolite being the primary excretion product.

Reductive metabolism of the nitro group of metronidazole occurs in humans, but to a very limited extent, probably by intestinal microflora and results in the formation of acetamide (a cause of hepatic cancer in rats) and N-(2-hydroxyethyl)oxamic acid. These compounds are detected in the urine and represent about 1% to 2% of the dose given.

Brown or reddish brown discoloration of the urine has been attributed to other

formation of azoxy compounds secondary to the reduction of the nitro group of metronidazole, probably by intestinal microflora possessing nitroreductors.

In lactating women, after a single 2 g oral dose, peak concentrations in breast milk of 45 to 48 µg/mL are found at 2 hours, with the elimination half-life in milk approximating that in serum. It has been estimated that an infant would consume about 25 mg of metronidazole in breast milk during the 48-hour period after the mother received a single 2 g dose. If breast-feeding were to be deferred for 24 hours, consumption of metronidazole would fall to about 4 mg.

Treatment with metronidazole

Dosage. In the treatment of trichomonal vaginitis the single 2.0 g oral dose of metronidazole is as effective as a 250 mg dose administered three times daily for 7 days, and for ease of administration, better patient compliance, and lower cost, and since it achieved a cure rate comparable with the 7-day course, it has been recommended, although some patients may experience nausea and/or vomiting[94]. A randomized double-blind comparison of 2.0 g in a single oral dose and 400 mg twice daily for 5 days led to a recommendation in favor of the single dose; nausea, vomiting and dizziness were reported by 1 of 96 patients treated with the single dose[95]. When used as single-dose therapy, the drug is usually prescribed in a dosage of 2.0 g (see below), but Spence *et al.*[96] found that a 1.5 g dose was just as efficacious.

Recommended treatment regimens for adults[97, 98] are

- metronidazole as a single oral dose of 2 g, given either in tablet form (five, 400 mg tablets) and taken during or after a meal, or in suspension taken at least 1 hour before a meal
- metronidazole 400 mg *or* 500 mg twice daily, during or after a meal, for 5 to 7 days.

The dosages in children are

- 1 to 3 years: 50 mg three times daily
- 4 to 7 years: 100 mg twice daily
- 8 to 10 years: 100 mg three times daily.

The elimination half-life of metronidazole is unaffected by renal failure, and dosage adjustment is unnecessary. As advanced liver disease, however, may result in decreased elimination of the drug, dose reduction is recommended: the daily dose should be reduced by one-third and may be given once daily (Hawgreen Ltd Data Sheet 2000).

Toxicity. At the dose generally used for trichomoniasis, metronidazole is well tolerated and during more than 35 years of its widespread use, it has earned a reputation of being remarkably safe. Occasional side effects at these doses include nausea, an unpleasant taste in the mouth, furring of the tongue, and gastro-intestinal upsets; headache, dizziness, anorexia, depression, and skin eruptions have been reported but rarely[90]. The single 2.0 g dose has been reported as producing nausea alone in 2% and with vomiting in 4% of patients. Peripheral neuropathy that is reversible when the drug is stopped or the dosage reduced, has been described in patients who received prolonged courses of metronidazole[99].

Metronidazole may produce a transient leukopenia in 4% of cases[100] but this appears to be caused by an accelerated disappearance of these elements from the blood, which temporarily exceeds bone marrow release, rather than to suppression of bone marrow[101]; no serious blood dyscrasias have been reported.

Metronidazole in pregnancy. The first trimester of pregnancy includes the stage of organogenesis in the embryo and it is during this stage that certain drugs are teratogenic and cause congenital malformations. The most critical period for gross congenital defects is the somite stage of embryonic development, which in humans occurs between the twenty-first and thirty-first days of intrauterine life (35 to 45 days after the start of the last menstrual period). The central nervous system, heart, gut, skeletal system, and muscle all begin to differentiate in the somite stage, and teratogenic drugs acting at this period may affect any of these systems. After the eighth to tenth week of intrauterine life the embryo is fully differentiated and drugs cannot, strictly speaking, be teratogenic although they can still cause disorders of growth and function. Thus, in the central nervous system particularly, damage after the first trimester can produce microcephaly and mental retardation. The total actual period for teratogenicity is usually believed to extend from about the third to the eighth or tenth week of intrauterine life, and during this time the mother may not know she is pregnant[102].

Metronidazole crosses the placenta, but there is no evidence that the drug is teratogenic in humans[103]. Although birth defects have been described in children born to mothers who had been exposed to the drug during the first trimester of pregnancy, two recent meta-analyses have found no relationship between metronidazole use in early pregnancy and birth defects[104, 105]. A population-based case-control study from Hungary also failed to show an association between oral metronidazole use and congenital abnormalities[106].

It has been pointed out[107], however, that like disulfiram metronidazole inhibits aldehyde dehydrogenase and might theoretically increase the risk of the fetal alcohol syndrome in the offspring of women who drink during pregnancy. Aldehyde, a breakdown product of alcohol, is cytotoxic and teratogenic at levels of over 35 mmol/L, levels, however, not ordinarily reached in most alcoholics. In women who drink, it is important therefore to avoid all drugs that inhibit aldehyde dehydrogenase, and therefore it is best to avoid metronidazole during pregnancy. If essential for symptomatic trichomoniasis, treatment with metronidazole should be postponed until after the sixteenth week of pregnancy and the strictest injunction given to avoid all alcohol[102].

Although metronidazole is excreted in breast milk, the drug appears to be safe for use in children, and mothers who are breast feeding can be given the drug. It is best to avoid the short, high-dosage regimens (Hawgreen Ltd Data Sheet 2000).

Drug interaction (alcohol and metronidazole). In a study of 53 alcoholic patients on metronidazole, in which one case in a male was described as representative of the results obtained in the others, a decreased tolerance for alcohol, a diminished compulsion to drink intoxicants, and an apparent aversion to ethanol were described[101]. Mild to moderate disulfiram-like effects were also described (for example facial flushing, headache, nausea, and sweating) with metronidazole, following alcohol ingestion. *In vitro* studies have shown that metronidazole can produce inhibition of aldehyde dehydrogenase and other alcohol-oxidizing enzymes, but a study in rats failed to substantiate the result of the *in vitro* studies[108].

In well-controlled clinical studies the disulfiram-like reaction has not been reported, nor have effects such as a decreased craving for alcohol, described as occurring within 1 or 2 weeks of commencing metronidazole treatment[109]. Adverse effects of concurrent metronidazole and alcohol are apparently infrequent but patients should be advised about these possibilities in the event of alcohol being ingested during metronidazole therapy and for at least 48 hours after its completion.

Anti-treponeme activity of metronidazole. Metronidazole has only weak anti-treponemal activity, and it seems unlikely that the small doses of metronidazole used in the treatment of trichomoniasis would delay diagnosis in a patient incubating syphilis.

Tinidazole

Tinidazole is used occasionally in the treatment of trichomoniasis in men and women. It has been shown to inhibit stocks of *T. vaginalis* at levels similar to those of metronidazole. After oral administration, the drug is rapidly and completely absorbed, and peak serum concentrations are achieved 2 hours later. The plasma levels then fall slowly and the drug can still be detected in plasma 72 hours after ingestion. It has a long elimination half-life (12 to 14 hours) when compared with metronidazole. It is widely distributed in the tissues, and vaginal concentrations are comparable to those achieved in the serum[110]. Tinidazole is not metabolized to any extent, and drug is excreted unchanged in the urine, and, to a lesser extent, in the feces.

The dose of tinidazole is 2 g (four tablets) as a single oral dose, during or after a meal.

Tinidazole crosses the placenta. As the effects on fetal development are unknown, the drug is contraindicated in the first trimester of pregnancy. Although the drug does not appear to be harmful in later pregnancy, its use should be avoided unless the benefits of treatment are likely to outweigh any risk.

Tinidazole is also excreted in breast milk and it is advised that women should not nurse until at least 3 days after completion of treatment (Pfizer Ltd Data Sheet 2000).

Toxic effects are similar to those of metronidazole and, as with metronidazole, alcohol consumption should be avoided, in the case of tinidazole for at least 72 hours after discontinuation of therapy.

Treatment failure in trichomonal vaginitis

Failure to cure trichomonal vaginitis with nitroimidazoles has distressing consequences because there is no certainly effective alternative treatment and palliatives are not satisfactory. With normal doses of metronidazole, namely 400 mg twice daily for 5 to 7 days, successful elimination of *T. vaginalis* is achieved in about 95% of infected women. In some women repeated failure to achieve this has been thought to result from a number of different factors

- poor absorption of the drug
- inability to produce trichomonicidal concentrations in vaginal tissue or contents
- inactivation of the drug by micro-organisms in the vagina
- non-adherence or failure to take the drug by the patient
- re-infection
- enhanced resistance of the organism.

Individual idiosyncrasies in absorption of metronidazole from the gut lumen or in its passage into the vagina are, however, unlikely to be the cause of treatment failure[111]. In this Edinburgh study of the concentrations of metronidazole in the plasma and vaginal content of 11 'treatment failure' patients on a dosage of 200 mg every 8 hours by mouth, given to the patient for 2 days in hospital under supervision, followed by high-dose metronidazole treatment (800 mg every 8 hours by mouth given subsequently under the same circumstances for 5 days), concurrent estimation by HPLC of the concentrations of metronidazole in plasma and vaginal content showed that the two levels are closely related to each other and to the dose. These patients showed a normal level of plasma metronidazole (mean 8.3 mg/L, standard error 0.7 mg/L) on the 200 mg dosage and on the high dosage a high plateau (mean 36.7 mg /L, standard error 2.0 mg/L) was quickly reached. The simultaneous collection of vaginal content gave metronidazole concentrations in vaginal content averaging 80% of the corresponding plasma levels. The hydroxy metabolite, which has a lower anti-trichomonal activity than metronidazole, was present in all plasma and vaginal content samples. When a single 2 g dose was administered to one 'treatment failure' patient no abnormality was detected in the metabolism of the drug. The plasma concentration of metronidazole fell exponentially from 58 mg/L at 75 minutes to 33 mg/L at 365 minutes giving an estimated half-life of 5.8 hours; concentrations of metronidazole in plasma at 184 and 305 minutes were 47 and 36 mg/L, similar to those in vaginal content of 47 and 31 mg/L respectively. The infection was not cleared in this patient.

Estimations of the *in vitro* sensitivity of *T. vaginalis* to metronidazole are not readily provided for clinical purposes, as methods are, as yet, of an experimental rather than a practical nature and show many variations in detail. The inocula are sometimes of organisms of unstated age or number; they are sometimes standardized in terms of the number inoculated; and the media are diverse in constitution, particularly with respect to the content of redox agents. Mostly no mention is made of the atmosphere superjacent to the cultures, which has an important influence on the metabolism and survival of the trichomonads[112]. Attempts have been made to control this feature[113] and Lumsden *et al.*[114] have made some progress in finding a way of controlling the oxygenation of the test medium at some precise level, less than that of air, and in determining the level at which best compromise could be reached between good growth conditions for the organism and optimum oxygen tension for detecting resistance to the drug. Under these conditions, although there were occasional discordant results, it was possible to distinguish between *T. vaginalis* from 'treatment failure' patients who are

Box 17.1 Factors to be considered when standard treatment of vaginal trichomoniasis has failed

Adherence to the treatment regimen, if multi-dosage
Vomiting after ingestion of the drug
Re-infection from an untreated sexual partner
Inactivation of metronidazole by aerobic or anaerobic vaginal bacteria
Low plasma zinc concentration (rare)

likely to be cured by enhanced dosage and those who are not; *T. vaginalis* isolates which were very sensitive to metronidazole could also be recognized.

In the management of a woman whose trichomoniasis has not been cured by standard therapy, several factors should be considered (Box 17.1), and the woman should be questioned about adherence, vomiting, and possible re-infection. As success is often achieved, patients who fail to respond to initial treatment should be re-treated with the same regimen[97], although one may wish to substitute single-dose therapy when adherence may be an issue. In those patients in whom vomiting, poor adherence, or re-infection have been excluded as causes of treatment failure, persistent infection may result from inactivation of metronidazole by vaginal anaerobic and aerobic bacteria, including β-hemolytic streptococci[115]. It is therefore worth giving the patient a 5 to 7-day course of amoxicillin, 250 mg three times per day by mouth or erythromycin 250 mg four times per day by mouth before re-treating with metronidazole. Although rarely a predisposing factor, low plasma zinc levels have been associated with treatment failure[116], and it is helpful to measure such concentrations and correct any deficiency. As metronidazole resistance seems to be relative rather than an all-or-none phenomenon, many women infected with resistant stocks of *T. vaginalis* can be cured with increasing doses of metronidazole[117]. Lossick and colleagues[118] found that there was some correlation between the minimum lethal concentration of metronidazole as measured in

an aerobic test system and the dose of drug required to cure the infection. These assays, however, are not generally available, and the clinician must be guided by treatment responses to increasing doses of metronidazole: up to 3 to 3.5 g of metronidazole per day for up to 14 days may be required to effect cure[117]. The dose-limiting factor is, of course, tolerability of the regimen and toxicity. When large doses are required, the drug may be given by the intravenous route. Although there is cross-resistance between the nitroimidazoles[119], this may be incomplete, and for some stocks of *T. vaginalis*, tinidazole may be more active than metronidazole[117]. In women with resistant trichomoniasis, therefore, it may be worth a trial of oral tinidazole. For example, Saurina *et al.*[120] cured a woman with metronidazole-resistant trichomoniasis by the use of tinidazole given orally in a dosage of 500 mg four times per day together with the insertion of a 500 mg tinidazole tablet intravaginally twice daily for 14 days. Anecdotal reports of other agents that have apparently been successful in the treatment of recalcitrant vaginal trichomoniasis include the topical application of paromomycin cream, zinc sulfate douches, and arsenic pessaries. The use of these and other preparations has been reviewed recently by Pattman[121], but in the absence of clear proof of efficacy under trial conditions, their role in patient management is uncertain.

Treatment of sexual partners of women with trichomoniasis

Trichomonal infection is readily found in the sexual partners of infected women, being demonstrable in 70% of the men who have had sexual contact within the past 48 hours; the percentage positive then appears to progressively decline, with 40% giving positive results if examined within 5 days and only 12% if examined after 21 days[122]. Often asymptomatic or with mild clinical features of non-gonococcal urethritis it is, however, often difficult to exclude the infection in the male, bearing in mind the variations in the efficiency of cultural methods and the difficulty in detecting trichomonads when few in number, of low infectivity to culture, or both. Using a 7-day standard course of metronidazole (250 mg three times daily) the

relapse rate may be very low (5%) even if the sexual partners are not treated[123]. Single-dose treatment of 2.0 g metronidazole, however, gave cure rates 6% to 12% lower than the 7-day standard regimen. The 7-day treatment may protect women from re-infection while the spontaneous reduction in numbers of *T. vaginalis* occurs in the infected male partner. The choice of treatment of the male partner of a woman with resistant trichomoniasis is unclear, but some physicians would use the same treatment regimen for both partners[24].

Genital candidiasis

Candidiasis (synonyms – candidosis, thrush) is a convenient generic term for infections caused by yeasts that are acting as opportunistic pathogens in individuals whose host defenses are impaired. Taxonomically the yeasts have been mostly assigned to a single genus *Candida*, but this 'genus' should be regarded as an artificial one comprised of non-sexually reproducing forms of members of a variety of other genera, some of which have now been identified. The most important member of the group, *Candida albicans*, is capable of causing the very common superficial infections of the mouth and vagina as well as widespread or more deep-seated disease, namely systemic candidiasis, an important hazard in modern medical procedures such as transplantation surgery, intravenous hyperalimentation, and immunosuppressive surgery as well as in symptomatic HIV infection (Chapter 7). Other species of *Candida*, particularly *C. glabrata*, may be associated with candidiasis; these species may be more resistant to therapy.

Although vulvovaginal candidiasis, characterized by pruritus with or without vaginal discharge, is often regarded as a minor condition in that it is transitory and its physical effects are not seriously damaging, it is a frequent cause of irritation and annoyance in women and – on account of its tendency to recur – an important cause of morbidity. Men tend to be less affected as the milieu of the glans and preputial sac is less favorable as a site for colonization by *Candida* spp.

ETIOLOGY

Morphology

Pathogenic yeast cells are typical of aerobic eukaryotes possessing intracellular organelles including mitochondria and ribosomes and a double-membraned nucleus containing chromosomes. All pathogenic *Candida* spp. multiply by the production of buds from a thin-walled ovoid *blastospore* or *blastoconidium* (yeast cell) 1.5 to 4.0 μm in diameter. The new growth or bud enlarges then stops as mitosis takes place and a septum is laid down between the parent and daughter cell unit. The blastoconidium is responsible for transmission of the yeasts.

A *hypha* is a long microscopic tube made up of multiple fungal cell units divided by *septa*. Hyphae arise as branches of existing hyphae or by the germination of spores. A *mycelium* is an entire fungal cellular aggregate including a hypha with all its branches. A *pseudohypha* arises by a budding process in which each generation of buds remains attached to its parent; the buds of the first and subsequent generations are narrow elongated cells that do not resemble the parent blastospore. The end-to-end aggregation of elongated blastoconidia or pseudohyphae are distinguished from true hyphae in that there are constrictions at the septal junctions. *Chlamydospores* are an *in vitro* form of a yeast pathogen induced by low temperature incubation under poor aeration and nutritional conditions and have thick double-layered cell walls.

The formation of so-called 'germ tubes' is accepted as a reliable property for identifying *C. albicans* and is used in medical laboratories because of its rapidity. The germ tube of *C. albicans* is a thin filamentous outgrowth from the cell without a constriction at its point of origin. Presumptive identifications based on the formation of germ tubes are 95% to 100% accurate when compared with stricter taxonomic methods, although their formation is influenced by temperature, amount of inoculum, composition of the medium, and strain. Cells from a 24-hour-old culture (10^5 to 10^6 cells/mL) are suspended in bovine serum and examined microscopically for germ tubes after 1 to 3 hours incubation at 37°C[124].

Taxonomy

Molecular studies have shown that the 'genus' *Candida* should be regarded as an artificial one in that its name does not imply descent from a common ancestor. The extreme diversity of its genetic material with base compositions (guaninine + cytosine) ranging from 30 to 64 molecules % suggest that the genus should be considered to be comprised of non-sexually reproducing forms of members of a variety of other genera, some of which have now been identified. Perfect forms of *C. pseudotropicalis* (*Kluyveromyces fragilis*) and *C. krusei* (*Issatchenkia orientalis*) have been established or confirmed by DNA hybridization methods[125]. Looking more closely at the base compositions of various species of medical interest, the ranges of guanine plus cytosine (G + C) content in the nuclear DNA have been recorded in molecules %: *C. albicans* 34.3 to 35.6; *C. tropicalis* 35.9 to 36.1; *C. parapsilosis* 40.5; *C. guillermondii* 44.1 to 44.4; *C. glabrata* 39.6 to 40.2. *Candida glabrata* was initially placed in the genus *Torulopsis* because of its lack of pseudohypha production. It is now clear, however, that the presence or absence of pseudohyphae is an inadequate basis for separating genera, and taxonomically *Torulopsis* spp. are included within the genus *Candida*[126].

DISTRIBUTION OF SPECIES

Yeasts that are the principal agents of human candidiasis are to be found in most warm-blooded animals and *C. albicans* has been recovered from a wider range of animal hosts than any other species[127]. Using terminology not yet modified by findings already described, Do Carmo-Sousa[128] considers that *C. albicans*, *C. stellatoidea*, and *C. glabrata* are obligatory animal saprophytes; that *C. guilliermondii*, *C. krusei*, *C. parapsilosis*, and *C. tropicalis* are facultative saprophytes, being species that, although recoverable from sources other than animal, are able to build up populations mainly in the digestive tract of animals; and that others are simple transients sometimes ingested but unable to grow inside the animal host.

Candida spp. are detected in the oral cavity of up to 55% of healthy individuals and *C. albicans* is the most commonly encountered of all species. More recently, however, an increasing proportion of isolates have been identified as *C. glabrata*, *C. tropicalis*, *C. parapsilosis*, and *C. krusei*[129]. Nosocomial colonization with *Candida* spp. has been shown to correlate well with the duration of hospital stay and frequency of antimicrobial use[130–132]. Patients may acquire *Candida* spp. from environmental surfaces contaminated with fungi derived from other patients, or from the hands of hospital personnel. In the feces *C. albicans* is the most commonly encountered fungus (48%) but it is less commonly isolated from feces than from the mouth. The most striking difference between fecal and oral isolates is the enormously higher proportion of *Rhodotorula* spp. (13%) in the feces than in the mouth (0.5%). In the vagina in those subjects without vaginitis the distribution of yeasts resembles the distribution in the feces but *C. glabrata* forms a much greater proportion (18%) than it does in oral or fecal isolates. In the vagina in individuals with vaginitis *C. albicans* has comprised a very high proportion of isolates (up to 90%); in none of the studies reported by Odds was the proportion less than 70%. The proportion of vaginal isolates of other species of *Candida* has been increasing, however, and Spinillo et al.[133] found *C. glabrata* in 90 (19%) of 472 cases of vulvovaginal candidiasis.

HOST DEFENSE AGAINST *CANDIDA ALBICANS* INFECTION

As evidenced by the high incidence of invasive candidiasis in neutropenic patients, polymorphonuclear leukocytes and macrophages play an important part in protecting against systemic spread of candidal infection. The observation that mucosal candidiasis is common in immunocompromised patients, including those with HIV infection, suggests that cell mediated immunity (CMI) is important in protecting against disease at these surfaces. Indeed, in individuals with reduced CMI, chronic mucocutaneous candidiasis is common. Through binding of specific IgG or IgA to candidal cells, adherence to epithelial cells may be impaired, preventing tissue invasion. In addition, mice immunized intravaginally with anti-*Candida* antibodies are protected against vaginal infection, and this is related to a rising vaginal titer of *Candida*-specific anti-idiotypic IgA antibodies that can passively transfer immunity to non-immunized mice[134].

In animal models, T_{H1}-type responses are associated with protection against *systemic C. albicans* infection. However, several lines of evidence suggest that systemic delayed-type hypersensitivity reactions (DTH) do not contribute to protection against *vaginal* infection. For example, DTH that has probably been elicited by candidal antigens permeating the vaginal wall and accessing regional lymph nodes, can be demonstrated systemically in mice with transient infection and in estrogenized mice (a state of constant estrus is required to establish vaginal infection in mice) with persistent vaginal infection with *C. albicans*[135, 136]. Cells from the draining lymph nodes respond to *Candida* antigens by the production of IL-2 and interferon-γ, that is a T_{H1}-type response. When mice that have developed a sustained systemic DTH after transient *C. albicans* infection are maintained in pseudo-estrus and rechallenged with viable *C. albicans*, however, there is partial protection against infection, concomitant with increased levels of DTH[137]. As this protection is not annulled when systemic DTH and the ability of lymph node cells to produce T_{H1}-type cytokines is reduced *in vivo* by *Candida*-specific suppressor T cells or by the depletion of CD4+ cells, it is likely that protection is the result of locally acquired mucosal immunity. It is proposed that asymptomatic colonization with small numbers of yeast cells is maintained through a T_{H1}-type dominated immune response, including the cytokines IL-2, IL-12, and interferon-γ, macrophages and polymorphonuclear leukocytes in the mucosa, and anti-*Candida* IgA antibodies[138].

PATHOGENESIS

In women *Candida* spp. are introduced into the vagina probably from the perianal area. Although the incidence of vulvovaginal candidiasis increases at the onset of sexual activity, and although yeasts identical to those found in the female can be detected on the male's penis[139], the role of sexual transmission in establishing colonization or infection is unclear.

Factors determining the virulence of *C. albicans* and *C. glabrata* have recently been reviewed by Fidel *et al.*[140] and several fungal factors were found to contribute to pathogenicity.

Colonization and adhesion

The most detailed studies of colonization and adherence of yeasts to cells have involved *C. albicans*; less is known about other fungi. Adherence of micro-organisms to epithelial cells is a critical step in the colonization of mucosal surfaces and their subsequent capacity to cause disease. In particular Kimura & Pearsal[141] demonstrated the capacity of *C. albicans* to adhere *in vitro* to human buccal epithelial cells and found that the adherence was significantly greater in human saliva than in phosphate-buffered saline. Enhanced adherence too was associated with germination of yeast cells (i.e. when germ tubes were formed) and under conditions conducive to germ-tube formation. Similarly Sobel *et al.*[142] showed that although the yeast form of *C. albicans* adheres to human buccal and vaginal epithelial cells, conditions conducive to germ-tube formation also increased the extent of adherence. The adherence of *C. albicans* to vaginal cells *in vitro* at pH 6 was considerably greater than at pH 3 to 4, a range corresponding to that of the normal vagina. Clinical observations have been correlated with the presence of filamentous forms with tissue invasion.

In the early stages of attachment to, and colonization of, mucosal surfaces it is the yeast form which is invariably found, and for this reason yeasts are used in adhesion assays. Similarly, since candidiasis of the mouth and vagina are the commonest clinical forms seen, *in vitro* adhesion to exfoliated buccal and vaginal epithelial cells is ordinarily measured. It has been found that adhesion of some strains of *C. albicans* is increased by growing the yeast in 'defined media' containing high concentrations of certain sugars (for example galactose, maltose, sucrose) and this enhancement appears to be related to the production of a fibrillar floccular layer on the yeast cell surface[143]. Such environ-

mental changes may be important, particularly in the mouth. Adherence of isolates of *C. glabrata* is less sensitive to changes in growth conditions[144].

The relative pathogenicity of the different *Candida* spp. is reflected in their individual ability to adhere to epithelial cells *in vitro*[145] as well as to a variety of other cell surfaces; *C. albicans* also shows strain differences in adhesion and virulence. It is thought that adhesion occurs because of specific binding molecules (adhesins) on yeast surfaces, possibly analagous to bacterial fimbriae, multiple rather than single. *Candida albicans* is the species best able to adhere to epithelial cells but others, such as *C. tropicalis* with respect to some denture material, are more adherent to inert materials[146]. *In vitro* studies of the adherence of yeasts to endothelial cells have shown that *C. albicans* was the most adherent and *C. glabrata* the least adherent[147]. The detection of β_2 integrins (adhesin receptors) on the surface of *C. albicans*, but failure to detect them on *C. glabrata*, suggests that these specific adhesins are not expressed on the latter yeast, limiting its adherence abilities[140]. Fibronectin, laminin receptors, fibrinogen-binding proteins and mannoprotein adhesins are important means of adhesion of *C. albicans* to epithelial and endothelial cells[148], but little is known about their role in the adhesion of other yeasts.

Yeast-to-mycelium conversion

Changes in the *in vitro* growth environment lead to changes in the growth form of *C. albicans*. Blastospore production is much more easily obtained in laboratory media, and filament formation is unusual, but serum at 37°C is a good stimulant to filament formation, a property commonly applied in the germ-tube test for *C. albicans*. Hyphal production *in vivo* is probably an indication of active growth but not necessarily of tissue invasion and therefore cannot be regarded as absolute diagnostic evidence for candidiasis[127]; the case for the connection of yeast-to-mycelium conversion to pathogenicity continues to be debated[149] (interestingly, *C. glabrata* that seems to be low in virulence does not form hyphae). Nevertheless, pseudohyphae penetrate intact epithelial cells and invade the superficial layers of the vaginal epithelium[150]. Blastoconidia, however, can also destroy epithelial cells by direct invasion.

Proteinase production

Isolates of *C. albicans* that produce aspartyl proteinase are more pathogenic in animal models than those that do not produce these proteinases[151]. The expression of genes for aspartyl proteinases only during the first week of infection of the rat vagina with virulent *C. albicans*, and the adherence of these strains to the epithelium, suggests that these proteinases are important in the establishment of infection. Expression of these genes was not detected in vaginal fluid from rats infected with avirulent strains of the yeast[152]. Further evidence of a role for proteinases in virulence comes from a study of candidal vaginitis in HIV-infected women: vaginal isolates of *C. albicans* from HIV-infected women with vaginitis produced higher levels of secretory aspartyl-proteinase than isolates from HIV-infected women with *C. albicans* colonization, or from non-HIV-infected women with vaginitis[153]. The probable function of these proteinases is to degrade proteins that are inhibitory for colonization and tissue invasion.

Phospholipase production

Phospholipase A and B and lyso-phospholipase-transacylase are produced by virulent, but not commensal, strains of *C. albicans*. These extracellular enzymes damage cell membranes and their production by clinical isolates correlates with pathogenicity[154].

Phenotypic switching

Specific phenotypic instability allows strains of *C. albicans* frequently to switch colony phenotype without affecting the genotype (phenotypic switching). There is some evidence of an association between phenotypic switching and virulence: switched phenotypes have been found in isolates from women with recurrent candidiasis[155]. Although the true importance to virulence of phenotypic switching is uncertain, it is the ability of some phenotypes to form

mycelia spontaneously and to produce other virulence factors that have proved this phenomenon to be an attractive hypothesis.

Antigenic modulation

Cell-surface expression of mannoproteins antigen is modulated during intravaginal growth and may be an important factor in determining virulence. Although an oligosaccharide epitope is readily identifiable on the cell surface of yeasts within 1 hour of experimental vaginal infection, this antigen becomes undetectable by 24 hours and on subsequent days during the development of germ tubes and the filamentous forms of the yeast[156].

Factors predisposing to candidiasis

Conditions that favor transition from saprophyte to pathogen, and are relevant to vaginal candidiasis particularly, include pregnancy, poorly controlled diabetes mellitus, damage or maceration of the tissue, the use of immunosuppressive drugs, and possibly also the oral contraceptive and oral antibiotics.

Pregnancy is an undisputed factor in pathogenicity – possibly by virtue of changes in cell-mediated immunity, in glucose metabolism, or by the provision of a glycogen-rich vaginal epithelium. In pregnancy there is a reduction of T-cell activity which may help to protect the fetus from rejection and there are changes in carbohydrate metabolism which may favor the growth of *Candida* spp. Through a cytosol receptor, estrogens can bind to *C. albicans* and enhance hyphal production and virulence[157]. Vaginal carriage of yeasts is highest in the third trimester, and an abrupt reduction in the incidence of *Candida* spp. in the vagina takes place in the post-partum period[158, 127].

Oral contraceptives containing an estrogen and a progestogen are the most effective preparations in general use and are called the 'combined' type of contraceptive. The estrogen content ranges from 20 to 50 μg, and the progestogen content is dependent upon the chemical nature and biological activity of the progestogens in

use. In respect to vaginal candidiasis, assembled evidence indicates that the use of the 'combined' type containing low-dose estrogen does not increase the risk[159]. Foxman also found no convincing evidence that the use of the diaphragm, condoms, or spermicides increased the risk of vulvovaginal candidiasis.

Antibiotics given orally appear to enhance the carriage of yeasts in the vagina but the evidence is more a matter of clinical consensus rather than from scientifically controlled trials[127]. The theory that anti-bacterial antibiotics may eliminate certain microbial elements in the microflora of the vagina, and that such alterations lead to yeast overgrowth because yeasts themselves are unaffected by antibacterial antibiotics, is difficult to substantiate. Contradictory evidence to the consensus view on the antibiotic–*Candida* relationship[127] suggests that other factors may be involved in the etiology. Certainly, it is clinical experience that most women given broad spectrum antibiotics do not develop vulvovaginal candidiasis.

Pathogenesis of recurrent vulvovaginal candidiasis

Recurrent vulvovaginal candidiasis (RVVC) may be defined as four episodes of mycologically proven candidiasis within 12 months and affects fewer than 5% of women. Although some women have recognizable factors that predispose to RVVC, the majority of affected individuals do not (idiopathic recurring vulvovaginitis). For many years it was proposed that the condition represented re-infection either from the gastrointestinal tract or from a sexual partner. This theory has now been abandoned in favor of one that suggests that organisms are not completely eliminated by treatment and that patients have relapsing vaginitis as a result of a change in the normal protective host defense mechanisms[138]. The finding that the identical strain type of *C. albicans* causes most sequential episodes, and that very high recolonization rates are found within 1 month of a short-term therapy supports this hypothesis.

Recurrent vulvovaginitis may be associated with the fungal virulence factors outlined above (page 487). Antifungal drug resistance, however, does not appear to play a role in RVVC in that the minimum inhibitory concentrations (MICs) of the azoles for 177 isolates collected sequentially does not appear to vary over time[160].

Corticosteroids depress cell-mediated immunity and as a result may predispose to candidiasis. Careful studies have shown that vaginal candidiasis is not more common amongst HIV-infected than in non-infected women[161]; when it does occur there is no relationship to the peripheral blood CD4+ cell count.

A possible role for female sex hormones in the pathogenesis of RVVC has been postulated, although there is no clear proof that they are important. The role of estrogen in predisposing to candidiasis is discussed above. Progesterone is immunosuppressive possibly by inhibiting monocyte function, and may also suppress the anti-candidal activity of polymorphonuclear leukocytes. The use of the combined oral contraceptive pill, by regulating the menstrual cycle, however, may offer some protection against vulvovaginal candidiasis.

The role of innate resistance in RVVC mediated by macrophages, natural killer cells, and polymorphonuclear leukocytes is uncertain. Reduced Candida-specific proliferation of peripheral blood lymphocytes from women with RVVC that could be partially restored by the addition of macrophages from healthy women has, however, been reported. It was shown that the inhibitory activity of macrophages from these women was related to increased production of the prostaglandin PGE$_2$ and could be reversed by prostaglandin inhibitors (PGE$_2$ is a down-regulatory biological response modifier)[162].

Adaptive immunity has been studied in women with RVVC. Although Candida-specific skin testing shows that most women with RVVC with acute vaginitis are anergic, this is transient and skin reactivity is restored after treatment of the acute episode[163]. This observation is probably explained by the release of candidal antigens into the systemic circulation during vaginal growth of the yeast, rather than a predisposing factor. In addition, the proliferative responses of peripheral blood lymphocytes to candidal antigens and T$_{H1}$-type lymphokine production (IL-2 and interferon-γ) did not differ between women with RVVC and controls. This situation is analogous to the mouse-model experiments described above (page 487), and implies that RVVC is not a consequence of impairment of the systemic immune response. Reductions in local immune responses, however, are more likely to be important in pathogenesis (see page 487).

There is some evidence that immediate type hypersensitivity reactions may contribute to RVVC. Anti-Candida IgE antibodies are often detected in vaginal secretions from women with RVVC but not from healthy women[164]. The apparent success in reducing the frequency of recurrent episodes by the subcutaneous vaccination with increasing doses of candidal extracts given over a one-year period supports this hypothesis[165]. Histamine and other mediators of allergic reaction released from vaginal mast cells may contribute to some of the clinical features of the condition such as pruritus. Prostaglandins may also contribute to the pathogenesis of RVVC. Histamine enhances the production of PGE$_2$, and mononuclear cells from women with RVVC but not from healthy women produce PGE$_2$ when incubated with C. albicans[166]. In addition, inhibitors of this prostaglandin reverse the macrophage-induced reduction in Candida-specific lymphocyte proliferation in RVVC patients. PGE$_2$ may also enhance germ-tube formation by C. albicans, thereby increasing virulence.

Fidel and Sobel[138] have proposed a possible mechanism for pathogenesis of RVVC. They postulate that an increase in antigenic load from increases in the vaginal population of C. albicans promotes the induction of T$_{H2}$-type responses, with increased expression of the cytokines IL-4, IL-5, and IL-10, and the production of PGE$_2$. This results in a continued down regulation of normal T$_{H1}$-type protective responses (support for this hypothesis comes from the observation in animal models that Candida-specific T$_{H1}$ and T$_{H2}$-type responses correlate with protection and susceptibility respectively to systemic infection). In the absence of such protection, and T$_{H1}$-type cytokines have been shown to inhibit germ-tube formation[167], and possibly influenced by PGE$_2$, C. albicans is converted from the blastoconidia form to the more pathogenic hyphal form.

Immediate-type hypersensitivity may be a consequence of the action of IL-4, enhancing the switch of B cells to IgE synthesis. Candidal antigen interacts with IgE bound to vaginal mast cells and histamine and other allergic mediators are released. Fidel and Sobel[138] also postulate that the small number of women who have large numbers of organisms but few, predominantly vaginal, symptoms, have reduced T$_{H1}$-type reactivity with little or no T$_{H2}$-type reactivity. Conversely, there is a small group of women who have few organisms but marked symptoms; this appears to represent predominance of immediate hypersensitivity in the presence of an intact local protective mechanism.

PATHOLOGY

Histological study of infected vulval and vaginal tissue is not part of routine clinical practice, and as a result reports are few. Gardner & Kaufman[168] noted mild to moderate inflammatory changes without invasion of vaginal tissue by the yeast. It has been shown, however, that in the mouth at least, in acute and chronic candidiasis there is invasion of the epithelium by hyphae, which grow downwards in more or less straight lines without respect for epithelial boundaries. In this site electron-microscopy examination confirmed that the growth of Candida spp. is intracellular and that the fine structure of the epithelial cytoplasm shows minimal change[169]. Certain changes in squamous cells such as radial clumping and emptiness of stained material in the cytoplasm, as well as increased nuclear activity and perinuclear haloes, have been described in cervical vaginal Papanicolaou smears[170].

CLINICAL FEATURES OF CANDIDIASIS

Symptoms and signs have diagnostic significance, and history taking and examination are therefore important.

Candidiasis of the female genitalia

Vulval pruritus which may vary from slight to intolerable is the cardinal symptom of candidiasis. When pruritus is intense vulval erythema is pronounced. Sometimes patients complain of pruritus or burning after intercourse. On occasions, however, even when plaques or pseudomembrane involve the vagina widely there are no subjective symptoms or even evidence of vulvitis.

Burning is a common complaint, particularly upon micturition and especially when there is also local excoriation because of scratching. Sometimes complaints of dysuria and frequency can be erroneously attributed to cystitis.

Dyspareunia, especially in the nulliparous, may be severe enough to make intercourse intolerable. Vulval edema may cause ill-defined vulval discomfort, and worry and apprehension may add to the patient's distress. A vaginal discharge is seldom the presenting complaint but the majority of patients have a discharge at some time and some may complain of dryness.

Erythema of the vulva is the commonest sign of candidiasis and tends to be limited to the mucocutaneous surfaces between the labia minora. Although often limited to the vestibule, erythema may extend to the labia majora, the perineum, the perianal skin, and occasionally to the mons veneris, the genitocrural folds, the inner thighs, and even buttocks.

Edema of the labia minora is commonly observed and is often more pronounced in candidiasis during pregnancy. Fissuring may occasionally be noted at the fourchette and at the anus. Traumatic excoriations from scratching are often found in patients with severe itching.

The vagina is abnormally reddened in about 20% of cases. If adherent patches or plaques of 'thrush' or pseudomembrane are removed the vaginal skin underneath appears erythematous, and superficial ulceration with bleeding may be seen. The vaginal contents may be apparently normal but a characteristic curdy material is found in 20% of non-pregnant and in 70% of pregnant patients (Figure 17.6). Although plaques may be small (1 mm) in size, larger (1 cm) with thick accumulations of exudate may be seen. A yeast odor is not thought to be characteristic in candidiasis. Vaginal discharge is noted less often by women with candidiasis caused by *C. glabrata* than by *C. albicans*, but burning may be more common than pruritus[171].

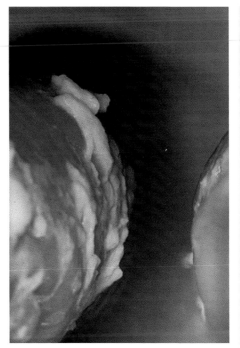

Figure 17.6 Candidal vaginitis (reproduced from McMillan and Scott 2000[315])

Infection by the former yeast is rarely associated with the curdy plaques that are so commonly seen in *C. albicans* infection. As few data are available, it is difficult to

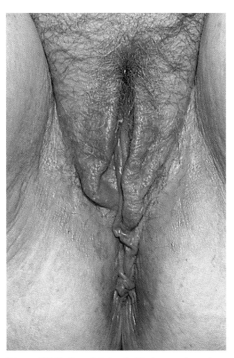

Figure 17.7 Candidal vulvitis (reproduced from McMillan and Scott 2000[315])

know whether infection with other species of *Candida* results in different clinical manifestations.

In contrast, primary cutaneous candidiasis involves the outer parts of the labia majora and the genitocrural fold, and not infrequently the mons veneris, the perianal region, and inner thighs. Vulval lesions tend to be reddened and moist with defined scalloped edges (Figure 17.7). Cutaneous lesions tend to begin as small papules on a red base with outlying small satellite vesicles or pustules and progress to form shallow ulcerated areas resulting from ruptured vesicopustules.

Candidiasis of the glans penis and prepuce

Characteristic symptoms of soreness and itching of the penis, accompanied sometimes by a discharge from under the prepuce, are seen in candidiasis of the penis. On examination there may be a balanoposthitis (Figure 17.8) with superficial erosions and sometimes eroded maculopapular lesions and preputial edema. *Candida albicans* may be isolated from the sub-preputial sac, but on occasions

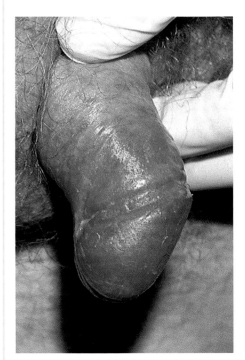

Figure 17.8 Candidal balanoposthitis (reproduced from McMillan and Scott 2000[315])

there may be a balanoposthitis, with erosions but without detectable yeasts, which appears to develop 6 to 24 hours after intercourse with a partner who has vaginal candidiasis. Such a balanitis may be caused by sensitivity to yeast-containing vaginal discharge. The balanoposthitis associated with diabetes has a similar appearance and *Candida* spp. may not always be isolated.

Neonatal candidiasis

Candidiasis in a neonate may involve the umbilicus, mouth, and napkin areas. The maternal vagina is only one source, as colonization may involve also the mouth and bowel. Attendants and environmental sources may also contribute to transmission. Systemic candidiasis in the neonate is being recognized with increasing frequency in very low birth weight infants who receive intensive care with prolonged antimicrobial therapy and parenteral nutrition.

DIAGNOSIS

Microscopy

Direct microscopy is essential as an 'on-the-spot' procedure in the diagnosis of candidiasis of the vagina and of the glans penis. In the case of the vagina, material is collected with a plastic loop or swab from the posterior fornix or from a characteristic plaque and smeared directly on a clean slide, as a dry preparation and as a wet preparation in a small quantity of saline, and covered with a glass cover-slip; alternatively, as a wet preparation, material is emulsified in 20% potassium hydroxide in water or in 20% potassium hydroxide dissolved in 40% aqueous dimethyl sulfoxide.

The smear is dried in air, fixed by heat, and then Gram stained; all yeasts, like all fungi, are Gram-positive (Figure 17.9), and detected using the oil immersion (× 100) objective. The wet saline mount is examined with the × 40 objective after racking down the condenser, or preferably with phase-contrast microscopy. In the case of the potassium hydroxide preparation, epithelial cells are cleared and the fungal elements revealed by direct or phase-contrast microscopy. Although budding yeasts may be found, hyphae are not seen

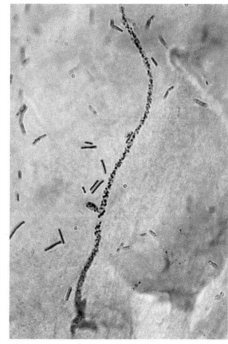

Figure 17.9 Hyphae of *Candida* spp. (reproduced from McMillan and Scott 2000[315])

in candidiasis associated with *C. glabrata*. Not infrequently, *C. glabrata* infection is found in association with bacterial vaginosis, perhaps because vaginitis caused by this fungus occurs at a somewhat higher vaginal pH than that caused by *C. albicans*.

Immunological tests

Although a slide latex agglutination test has been described for the diagnosis of vaginal candidiasis[172], it is seldom used in clinical practice.

Culture

In medical practice yeast isolates are not regularly identified to species level sufficiently well to satisfy taxonomists, although in deep-seated lesions particularly this is clearly desirable, and the characterization of isolates from superficial lesions would yield clinically and epidemiologically useful data. In recurrent candidiasis the resulting morbidity is a serious problem for the individual and research is desirable. Yeasts are eukaryotes and identification is a complex subject, and only a brief discussion based on Odds[127] is given here.

Candida spp. grow well in culture media such as malt extract or glucose-peptone agar at a lower pH than that required by bacteria[173]: the best known of the latter was first described by Sabouraud in 1894. The low pH (5.5) suppresses bacteria and the media can be made more inhibitory to bacteria by the incorporation of chloramphenicol (50 mg/L). The majority of clinical isolates from the genitalia will be *C. albicans*, for which two rapid specific tests are available.

1. *The germ-tube test.* *C. albicans* regularly produces hyphal shoots (germ tubes) after incubation in serum at 37°C for 3 hours. Occasional isolates of *C. stellatoidea* also produce germ tubes, but this is not surprising since its DNA is essentially identical to that of *C. albicans* and in present-day taxonomy *C. stellatoidea* is regarded as synonymous with *C. albicans*. *Candida dubliniensis* also produces germ tubes.

2. *Chlamydospore test.* Partially anaerobic conditions can be produced by the 'Dalmau' inoculation technique, by which the yeast isolate is partially scratched into the agar surface with the inoculation loop and glass cover-slips are pressed onto the inoculated surface. Incubation proceeds at 25°C. Chlamydospores are usually abundant under the edges of the cover-slips. The originally recommended media was corn-meal agar, but others are used and improved yields have been secured by incorporating the surfactant 'Tween 80'.

For the determination of species it is necessary to characterize isolates further by determining certain physiological properties, namely their abilities to assimilate and ferment individual carbon and nitrogen sources. Abbreviated tests are available which are sufficient as a means of making a presumptive rather than an absolute diagnosis[127].

Emphasis has been given to the fact that yeasts are complex eukaryotes and that accurate identification of species may have important prognostic and therapeutic implications. This is particularly the case in the management of an individual with refractory candidiasis. For example, *C. glabrata* rapidly mutates to full fluconazole resistance. New methods of characterization, such as the capacity of isolates to adhere to epithelial and other surfaces and DNA–DNA hybridization provide new methods for identification of *Candida* spp. and analysis of their genetic relationship[125]. The complex subject is provided for by the standard reference work edited by Kreger-van Rij[174].

TREATMENT OF VULVOVAGINAL CANDIDIASIS

In vaginal candidiasis treatment is indicated on the basis of the symptom of pruritus; the finding of vaginitis is based on the clinical appearance, and the detection of *C. albicans* or other yeast species. This mycotic infection can be an annoyance that is difficult to tolerate but it is not invasive. Its tendency to recur, however, necessitates on occasions fuller investigation as a cause of local irritation as well as disharmony in a personal sexual relationship. As the response to antifungal therapy does not appear to differ between HIV-infected and non-HIV-infected women with vulvovaginitis, the regimens detailed below are satisfactory for treatment. Preparations widely used in the treatment of vulvovaginal candidiasis include

1. the polyene antibiotic nystatin
2. the topical imidazoles clotrimazole, miconazole, econazole, fenticonazole, terconazole, butaconazole, and tioconazole
3. the triazoles ketoconazole, fluconazole, and itraconazole.

Terconazole, butaconazole and tioconazole are not available in the UK, and are not considered in detail here.

Polyene antifungals

Mode of action

The polyene antibiotics, nystatin and amphotericin B, are effective antifungal agents that bind to sterol components of cell membranes of susceptible fungi and act by increasing the permeability of the fungal membrane and causing a leakage of intracellular solutes. Cell death is secondary to the results of damage to the cell membrane.

Nystatin

Nystatin, discovered in 1950, was the first polyene to be used in the treatment of candidiasis. With respect to vaginal candidiasis it gradually replaced the topical use of 1% aqueous solution of gentian violet. Nystatin inhibits the *in vitro* growth of yeast pathogens at concentrations of 0.4 to 10 μg/mL, although higher MICs have been quoted[127].

The biological activity of nystatin is expressed in units, with the international standard for nystatin of 3000 units/mg and with the pure compound having activity in excess of 5500 units/mg. It is extremely toxic if given parentally and therefore never used thus, but it is not absorbed from the gut and may be safely given by mouth.

Nystatin is prescribed as vaginal tablets, each containing 100 000 units, with instructions to insert one at night for 14 nights, continuing during menstruation. The patient should wash her hands and vulva before bedtime, lie down on the bed and gently insert the tablet into the upper third of the vagina. Nystatin cream is also available and is dispensed in 60 g tube with a vaginal applicator. About 4 g is inserted high into the vagina for 14 consecutive nights. It should be explained that the nystatin is itself yellow in color and that the appearance of a yellow discharge is not a cause for worry. As the rubber may be damaged by the preparation, contact between the cream and contraceptive diaphragms and condoms should be avoided. Nystatin is also available as a cream, ointment, and gel for topical use. Each preparation contains 100 000 units/g, and it is applied two to four times per day. There is no evidence that nystatin is absorbed from the vagina, and there is no evidence for any adverse effects in pregnancy.

Antifungal imidazoles

Mode of action

The antifungal activity of the antifungal imidazoles differs from that of the polyenes (and 5-fluorocytosine) in that the imidazoles have a very broad spectrum of activity, affecting many filamentous fungi and dermatophytes as well as yeasts. In contrast to amphotericin, these drugs are fungistatic.

Azoles enter the fungal cells by an unknown mechanism, although, at least in the case of ketoconazole, active transport may be involved. The azoles in clinical use owe their antifungal effects to the inhibition of the synthesis of ergosterol or to an interaction with this sterol. Ergosterol is the principal component of the fungal cell membrane, and contributes to a variety of cellular functions. It is important for the fluidity and integrity of the membrane, and for the proper function of membrane-associated enzymes[175]. Integrity of cell membranes requires that the inserted sterols lack C-4 methyl groups. The primary target of the azoles is the heme protein which co-catalyzes cytochrome P450 dependent 14α-demethylation of lanosterol, and is encoded by the *ERG11* gene. Inhibition of 14α-demethylase leads to depletion of ergosterol and the accumulation of sterol precursors, including 14α-methylated sterols and resulting in a cell membrane with altered structure and function[176]. There is a heterogeneity of action among the triazoles and some of the earlier imidazole derivatives (miconazole, econazole, and ketoconazole) have a complex action, inhibiting membrane-associated enzymes in addition to their effect on sterol biosynthesis. Mammalian cholesterol synthesis can be blocked at the 14α-demethylation stage by azoles, but the inhibitory dose is very much higher than for fungi.

Topical imidazoles

Studies comparing the topical application of the imidazoles with nystatin are difficult to interpret because the two drugs would have to be used for the same duration; therefore one or other drug could have to be given for a period that is not recommended.

Clotrimazole

Clotrimazole concentrations in the vagina are very substantial; a mean value of 447 μg/mL has been obtained 6 to 9 hours after the first 100 mg tablet of a 12-day course of once-daily vaginal tablets had been inserted. Clotrimazole is supplied as a 1% w/w cream for topical use, as a 10%

w/w cream for intravaginal use, and as 100 mg, 200 mg, and 500 mg vaginal pessaries. One 100 mg vaginal tablet inserted every night for 6 nights is an effective alternative to nystatin and more pleasant to use; Masterton *et al.*[177] reported a cure rate of 93% when women were assessed 1 month after therapy. A shorter course of one 200 mg vaginal tablet inserted for 3 consecutive nights is also sufficient to cure most infections, with no significant difference in cure rate with the 6-day course. The insertion of a single 500 mg vaginal tablet at night is usually efficacious, with cure rates between the 3-day course and the single-dose therapy being identical[178]. About 5 g of the 10% vaginal cream is inserted into the vagina at night for 1 night, using the applicator provided by the manufacturer. In the treatment of candidal vulvitis, the cream is applied thinly and evenly to the vulval skin and introitus two to three times per day. Side effects are few, but include mild burning or irritation after insertion of the pessary or application of the cream, and hypersensitivity reactions have rarely been reported. In animal studies teratogenic effects have not been noted, but when given in high oral doses to rats, feto-toxicity has been observed. Clotrimazole has been used widely in the management of candidiasis in pregnant women without adverse effects.

Miconazole

Miconazole is not well absorbed after oral administration. Peak levels of miconazole are found in vaginal secretions within 1 hour of the insertion of a 100 mg pessary and remain high for long periods, the mean concentration (± standard error of the mean) of the drug being 1.2 (± 0.4) μg/mL at 48 hours[179]. Miconazole nitrate is supplied as a 2% w/w cream for topical use, as a 2% intravaginal cream, as vaginal pessaries each containing 100 mg, and as a soft gelatine capsule containing 1200 mg miconazole nitrate, for vaginal use. The intravaginal cream is effective when it is introduced into the vagina by means of an applicator, which is filled to contain the required 5 g of cream (equivalent to 100 mg miconazole nitrate). The pessary or cream, introduced into the vagina once a night for 14 consecutive nights, or twice a

day for 7 days is effective treatment, curing more than 80% of cases, and being as efficacious as nystatin and clotrimazole[180]. The 1200 mg capsule is inserted high into the vagina at night as a single dose. Occasionally irritation has developed during the use of miconazole, and rarely sensitization has been reported. As the emollient base of these preparations may damage latex condoms or diaphragms, contact between these should be avoided. As with the other imidazoles, feto-toxicity has been found in animals given large oral doses of miconazole, and it should be used in pregnancy only when considered necessary. Miconazole cream may be applied in a thin film to the vulval skin twice daily

Econazole

Econazole is poorly absorbed from the skin and vaginal mucosa, less than 0.1% of the applied dose being detected in the serum, and only about 2.5% of the dose is recovered from feces and urine during the 96 hours after a 5 g intravaginal dose[181]. The therapeutic properties of econazole, are as good as clotrimazole or miconazole. It is supplied as pessaries, the original formulation containing econazole nitrate 150 mg and being inserted high into the vagina nightly for 3 nights. A pessary containing 150 mg of econazole nitrate with a different base from the original pessary is available for single-dose use. The cream, containing econazole nitrate 1% w/w, can be applied to the vulval skin in a thin layer twice daily, or, using an applicator, about 5 g can be inserted into the vagina nightly for 14 days. The mycological success rate 2 weeks after treatment with econazole is about 90%[182]. Contact between the preparations and latex condoms and diaphragms should be avoided. Side effects, which are generally mild, include pruritus or stinging of the skin. Although the safety of systemic econazole in pregnancy has not been established, percutaneous absorption of the drug is low and it is likely to be safe.

Fenticonazole

Systemic absorption of fenticonazole nitrate from the skin and vaginal mucosa is minimal. Two formulations are available

1. a pessary containing 600 mg of fenticonazole nitrate and suitable for once only dosing
2. a pessary containing 200 mg of the drug, one pessary being inserted into the vagina nightly for 3 nights.

Slight transient burning may develop after insertion of a pessary. Interaction with latex condoms and contraceptive diaphragms is possible. The safety of fenticonazole in pregnancy remains to be established and, although likely to be safe, it is not currently recommended for use in pregnant women.

Oral triazoles

Fluconazole

Phamacokinetics. In healthy individuals more than 90% fluconazole is absorbed from the intestinal tract and plasma levels are almost as high as after intravenous administration; absorption of fluconazole is unaffected by food. Peak plasma concentrations occur 0.5 to 1.5 hours after ingestion, and the plasma elimination half-life is about 30 hours, allowing once daily dosing. It is well distributed throughout the body, including the CSF where levels are about 50% to 80% those in serum. Importantly, the peak concentration in vaginal secretions after a 150 mg single oral dose of fluconazole is high at 2.43 μg/mL[183]. After multiple daily dosing, 90% steady state levels occur by day 4 or 5.

Excretion. The drug is excreted unchanged in the urine by glomerular filtration, although some tubular re-absorption may occur; fluconazole clearance is proportional to creatinine clearance. There is no evidence of circulating metabolites.

Plasma protein binding. Only about 12% of the drug is protein bound.

Unwanted effects. Adverse effects are generally mild and predominantly gastrointestinal: nausea, abdominal discomfort, diarrhea, and flatulence. Skin rash is uncommon (in less than 1% of cases), but exfoliative dermatitis has been reported during fluconazole therapy, especially in HIV-infected patients with severe immunodeficiency. Epileptiform seizures, leukopenia and thrombocytopenia have also been recorded, but, as the patients had other medical conditions at the time of therapy, it is difficult to be certain that the drug was causative. Hepatic necrosis has been reported rarely, again in patients receiving other medication some of which was known to be hepatotoxic. As with other azoles, anaphylaxis has been reported rarely.

Fluconazole inhibits cytochrome P450 and can therefore interact with other drugs metabolized by this system. This is clearly important in individuals such as those with HIV infection who are being treated with various combinations of drugs. Levels of some drugs may be increased.

- *Phenytoin* Monitoring of plasma concentrations of phenytoin may be necessary in patients who are given courses of fluconazole.
- *Terfenadine* As serious dysrrythmias may develop in individuals given terfenadine with fluconazole in multiple doses of 400 mg/day, this combination of drugs must be avoided.
- *Rifabutin* Uveitis has been reported in individuals taking this drug combination.
- *Sulfonylureas* The possibility of hypoglycemic episodes should be considered if it is necessary to use fluconazole in diabetic patients receiving these agents.

In addition, other drugs such as rifampicin that are enzyme inducers, may lower plasma concentrations of fluconazole, necessitating an increase in dose.

Although there have been no drug interaction studies, cardiac events, including torsades de pointes, have been reported in patients receiving cisapride and fluconazole, and concomitant use of these drugs should be avoided.

Embryotoxic and feto-toxic effects have been described in pregnant rats, and it is recommended that the drug should be avoided in pregnancy, and given only to women who are using effective contraception. Nevertheless, compared with a comparable group of women who had not been given fluconazole, there was no increase in the prevalence of miscarriage, congenital abnormalities, or low birth weight amongst 226 Italian women given fluconazole during the first trimester of pregnancy[184]. Fluconazole is found in

breast milk at concentrations similar to those in plasma, and, as the effect on the infant is unknown, the drug should be avoided in nursing mothers

Formulations available. Fluconazole is available in 50 mg, 150 mg, and 200 mg capsules. A powder is also available that on reconstitution with water gives an oral suspension containing 50 mg or 200 mg per 5 mL. Parenteral therapy may be necessary for the treatment of invasive candidiasis and other fungal infections such as cryptococcosis (Chapter 7), and an intravenous infusion, containing 2 mg/mL in a saline solution is available. In the treatment of acute candidal vulvovaginitis, fluconazole is given in a single oral dose of 150 mg; dosage adjustment is unnecessary for single-dose use in patients with renal insufficiency. The drug is as effective as intravaginal, and clinical and mycological cure is achieved in more than 80% of cases[185, 186].

Itraconazole

Pharmacokinetics. Only about 55% of the orally administered drug given in capsule form is absorbed, although absorption is better when it is given with food. A reduction in gastric acidity further reduces absorption. Peak serum levels of about 1 μg/mL are found 2 to 4 hours after the oral administration of a 100 mg capsule of itraconazole; double the peak level is found 3 hours after the ingestion of the drug immediately after food (Janssen-Cilag Ltd Data Sheet 2000). When given as itraconazole solution, peak levels are found at 2 hours after administration in the fasting state, and at 5 hours when given with food. Steady state plasma levels fluctuate between 1 to 2 μg/mL when 200 mg itraconazole solution is given daily in the fasting state. The terminal half-life on repeated dosing is about 1.5 days. Peak concentrations in keratinized tissue, particularly skin, are up to three times higher than in plasma, and therapeutic concentrations are found in skin 2 to 4 weeks after cessation of drug therapy. Drug concentrations in other tissues such as bone, lung, and liver, are also significantly higher than in serum. There is by contrast very little penetration into the CSF.

Metabolism. Less than 0.03% of the oral dose of itraconazole is excreted unchanged in the urine, but between 3% to 18% of the parent drug is excreted in the feces. Itraconazole is extensively metabolized in the liver; the metabolites, most of which are inactive, are excreted in the urine and bile. One metabolite – hydroxy-itraconazole – is as active as the parent drug.

Plasma protein binding. Almost 99% of plasma itraconazole is bound to plasma proteins.

Unwanted effects. The most frequent side effects are nausea, abdominal pain, and constipation. Less frequently, skin rash, headache, and dizziness have been reported, and, rarely, peripheral neuropathy. Reversible and minor elevation in plasma enzyme tests of liver function may be found. As hepatitis and cholestatic jaundice have been reported rarely in patients treated with itraconazole for more than 1 month, monitoring of plasma enzymes in patients given prolonged treatment is recommended. If these tests become abnormal, or if there is clinical evidence of hepatitis, the drug should be discontinued. When itraconazole is given to some patients with hepatic cirrhosis, the elimination half-life is increased, and it is recommended that estimation of itraconazole plasma levels is undertaken in those who require prolonged therapy.

As itraconazole can inhibit cytochrome P450 CYP3A, concomitant use with terfenadine, astemizole, or cisapride can result in elevated plasma levels of these drugs causing cardiac arrythmias. Similarly, increases in plasma concentrations of oral anticoagulants midazolam and triazolam may occur, and caution should be exercised if concomitant therapy with itraconazole is necessary.

Enzyme inducers such as rifampicin and phenytoin can reduce plasma concentrations of itraconazole, and monitoring of plasma levels is recommended when the drugs are co-administered.

As feto-toxic effects have been observed in pregnant rats and mice given high oral doses of itraconazole, its use in pregnancy is contraindicated. Minimal concentrations of itraconazole are found in breast milk, and harm to the infant is unlikely to occur. The drug should, however, only be given to nursing mothers when the benefits of treatment outweigh any possible risk to the child.

Formulations available. Itraconazole is available as 100 mg capsules and as an oral solution containing 10 mg/mL, the latter formulation being used in the treatment of oropharyngeal candidiasis in HIV-infected patients (Chapter 7). In the treatment of vulvovaginal candidiasis, the capsules are given in an oral dosage of 200 mg twice daily, immediately after food, for 1 day. Itraconazole use has been shown to be as effective as intravaginal clotrimazole[187], and cure rates in excess of 95% have been reported[185].

Ketoconazole

Pharmacokinetics. The drug is incompletely absorbed orally and absorption is reduced when the gastric pH is increased, for example by antacids or H_2-receptor antagonists. Food delays absorption but does not affect peak plasma concentrations. Peak levels of ketoconazole are reached about 2 to 4 hours after administration, a 200 mg dose achieving a peak plasma level of 2 to 3 µg/mL. Higher peak concentrations can be reached by giving higher doses of ketoconazole. The elimination half-life, which appears to be dose dependent, varies between 6 and 10 hours. Ketoconazole penetrates the CSF poorly, although high doses (1200 mg) may achieve therapeutic concentrations.

Metabolism. Less than 1% of the drug is eliminated unchanged in the urine. Ketoconazole is metabolized in the liver and the metabolites, all of which are inactive, are excreted in the bile and urine.

Plasma protein binding. Ketoconazole is extensively bound to plasma proteins.

Unwanted effects. Nausea and vomiting are common, particularly when individual doses exceed 800 mg. Transient, minor elevations in plasma enzyme tests of liver function occur in up to 10% of patients, but if they persist or increase, the drug should be discontinued. Rash has also been described in treatment with ketoconazole.

In May 1982 the United States Federal Drugs Administration took regulatory action following the notification of three cases of fatal massive hepatic necrosis[188]. This serious hepatotoxicity, however, is idiosyncratic and rare, the incidence being between 1 in 10 000 to 1 in 15 000. Symptoms usually occurred within the first few months of treatment, and the median time of onset of icteric reactions was 6 weeks (extremes 1 and 20 weeks); and of anicteric reactions 11 weeks (extremes 3 and 24 weeks)[188]. In most cases, hepatic damage has been reversible on cessation of treatment. Advice has been given to the effect that because of the idiosyncratic hepatotoxicity, and because most data have been derived from uncontrolled trials and case reports, ketoconazole should be used cautiously, and it should be avoided particularly in patients with hepatic failure or an antecedent history of hepatic failure[188]. The risk of hepatotoxicity makes the oral use of ketoconazole unjustified in cases of superficial genital candidiasis, although it is valuable in some of the systemic mycoses such as certain forms of paracoccidiodomycosis and in histoplasmosis. The monitoring of the plasma bilirubin and liver-related enzyme tests are indicators of liver cell damage and should be performed 2 and 4 weeks after initiation of treatment, and monthly thereafter. Rollman & Loof[189], however, found that with serum 'liver function tests' (namely enzyme tests for hepatocellular damage and bilirubin) it is not possible to predict from the first observed abnormal result whether a progressive reaction has been initiated.

Gynecomastia and loss of libido and potency have occasionally been observed in men taking ketoconazole and may be related to a decrease in testosterone available to target organs[190]. Careful attention is advised as to the possible development of side effects secondary to diminished testicular, ovarian, or adrenal steroid synthesis, especially in patients being given higher doses of ketoconazole. Ketoconazole also has an inhibitory action on cortisol secretion both *in vitro* and *in vivo*, showing that patients with autonomous cortisol production caused by an adrenal tumor are prone to dangerous hypoadrenalism if treated with ketoconazole[191].

Ketoconazole is an inhibitor of certain P450 cytochrome enzymes (for example CYP3A4) and when used in combination with drugs metabolized by this system, such as the H_1 antihistamines, terfenadine and astemizole can increase plasma levels and possibly result in the emergence of serious arrythmias. The concomitant use of these drugs is therefore contraindicated. Other drug interactions of importance include phenytoin, anticoagulants, and rifampicin. Concomitant use of phenytoin and ketoconazole may alter the metabolism of either drug, and concomitant use of the antifungal and rifampicin may reduce the blood levels of both drugs. Isoniazid therapy reduces the plasma concentration of ketoconazole. A disulfiram-like reaction to alcohol characterized by transient flushing, nausea, headache, and peripheral edema has been described.

As with the other azoles, hypersensitivity reactions occur, albeit rarely.

Feto-toxic effects have been observed when ketoconazole has been administered orally in high doses to rats, and consequently, the drug should not be used in pregnancy. It is stated that ketoconazole may be excreted in breast milk, and, as the effects on the infant are unknown, its use in nursing mothers should be avoided (Janssen-Cilag Ltd Data Sheet 2000).

Formulations available. Ketoconazole is available in tablet form (200 mg) or as a suspension (20 mg/mL). In the treatment of vaginal candidiasis not responsive to other therapy, the drug is given in an oral dosage of 400 mg daily with food for 5 days.

Resistance to antifungal drugs

The subject of antifungal resistance is complex but has recently been well reviewed by White *et al.*[175] and Ghannoum & Rice[176], and much of the following description has been derived from these reviews. Only key references that the authors consider important are given here, and the reader is referred to the review articles for a complete list of references.

Acceptable testing methods for antifungal resistance have only recently been suggested. Suggested breakpoints were based on an examination of the *in vitro* MIC and clinical data from 729 patients (883 isolates), but these are limited to yeast (except *C. krusei* that is inherently resistant to azoles) and to fluconazole and itraconazole[192] (Table 17.1). A discussion of the technical methods used in the determination of the MIC is outwith the scope of this book, and the interested reader is referred to a recent review[193]. Although there is a reasonable correlation between the MIC of the antifungal and the treatment outcome, other factors are also important; for example, there is a weaker correlation between treatment success and MIC results in the severely immunocompromised host. It is not always possible to predict treatment failure from the MIC. Successful treatment has been described in patients whose isolates have had an MIC of 32 or 64 μg/mL[194], and 50% of patients with infection by strains of *C. albicans* with an MIC of 64 μg/mL have been cured with an increased oral dose of fluconazole. Fungal disease that is refractory to treatment with antifungal drugs is described as clinically drug resistant. Several factors may contribute to the presence of a resistant strain of *C. albicans* in a patient.

1. Intrinsic resistance of endogenous strains of the organism.
2. Replacement with a more resistant species such as *C. glabrata* or *C. krusei*. Most strains of the latter fungus are resistant to azoles, and strains of *C. glabrata* have MICs for azoles that are higher than for most isolates of *C. albicans*. These strains may have

been commensals until immunosuppression or azole therapy has led to the assumption of a pathogenic role. Alternatively they may have been acquired from the environment or from another individual. This superinfection would have been suppressed by endogenous species in the healthy host, but the selective pressure of antifungal therapy allows the infecting species to become established.

3. Replacement with a more resistant strain of *C. albicans*. Although this has been described in HIV-infected patients, the strain possibly having been acquired from another person, it is clear that strain replacement is less common than the development of resistance within the endogenous strain.
4. Genetic alterations that render a strain resistant. Drug therapy may select for growth of strains that are inherently more resistant than the majority of the fungal population (primary resistance). Specific random mutations in a population of cells under selective drug pressure may eventually result in these becoming the dominant strain in the population (secondary resistance); the mechanisms are discussed below.
5. Alteration in cell type. *Candida albicans* can be divided into two serotypes, A and B, on the basis of carbohydrate cell surface markers. Serotype B strains are more sensitive to azoles but more resistant to 5-flucytosine than serotype A strains. Differences in azole susceptibility have been described between switched phenotypes (see page 487).

Resistance to azoles

The occurrence of primary or secondary azole resistance is well documented in HIV-infected individuals and in other immunocompromised patients with oropharyngeal or disseminated candidiasis (Chapter 7). This emerging problem may be the result of the increased use of azoles that are fungistatic. Although azole-resistant *C. albicans* is a rare cause of recurrent vulvovaginitis, it is convenient to discuss mechanisms of resistance to antifungal agents here.

There is evidence that a modification of the quality or quantity of 14α-demethylase is an important mechanism in the development of resistance to the azoles. This alteration is probably caused by mutations that alter drug binding but not that of endogenous substrates. For example, a point mutation in the *ERG11* gene, resulting in a single amino acid substitution (the replacement of arginine with lysine at amino acid 467 to R467K), has been associated with reduced susceptibility to fluconazole of the target enzyme in *C. albicans*[195]. This mutation is thought to cause structural or functional alterations associated with the heme. The active site of 14α-demethylase represents a pocket on top of the heme cofactor and substrates enter the active site through a channel. Point mutations may therefore alter the ability of the drug to enter or bind to the active site of the enzyme, thereby resulting in drug resistance. Another mechanism of resistance that appears, however, to play a limited role in resistance, and has only been shown in *C. glabrata*[196] is the overexpression of 14α-demethylase. This results from gene amplification and causes an increase in ergosterol synthesis; this may contribute to cross-resistance between fluconazole and itraconazole. A mechanism for resistance that may be important in diploid cells such as *C. albicans* that have two alleles of each gene is loss of allelic variation. Clinical isolates of *C. albicans* contain several sequence variations between the two copies of a gene (allelic differences), but these differences are eliminated in isolates with the R467K mutation. A cell with two copies of the R467K mutation is more resistant to azoles than a cell containing only one allele with the mutation. Clearly this mechanism for

Table 17.1 Interpretative guidelines for susceptibility testing *in vitro* of *Candida* spp. (Rex *et al.* 1996[192])

Antifungal agent	MIC (μg/mL)		
	Susceptible strains	Susceptible (dose-dependent) strains	Resistant strains
Fluconazole	≤ 8	16–32	≥ 64
Itraconazole	≤ 0.125	0.25–0.5	≥ 1

resistance would not operate in haploid cells such as *C. glabrata*.

Alteration in the *ERG* genes encoding other enzymes in the biosynthesis of ergosterol may also contribute to azole resistance. Point mutations other than R467K have not been described in azole-resistant isolates, and no gene amplification has been noted for *C. albicans* genes. Alterations in the *ERG3* gene that encodes C-5 sterol desaturase may prevent the production of the diol that would cause growth arrest and result in resistance to azoles.

The active efflux of antifungal agents from cells may play an important role in azole resistance. For example, in a comparison of clinical isolates of *C. glabrata* that became resistant to fluconazole during treatment, there was no change in ergosterol biosynthesis between pre- and post-treatment isolates, but there was less accumulation of fluconazole in the resistant organism[197]. Fungi have at least two efflux pumps: major facilitators (MF) and ATP binding cassette (ABC) transporters (ABCT). A MF protein (BENʳ, encoded by the *MDR1* gene) associated with resistance specific for fluconazole has been described in *C. albicans*, over-expression being noted in resistant isolates[198]. The ABC proteins have transmembrane spanning domains and two nucleotide-binding domains that couple ATP hydrolysis to substrate transport. Much of the work that has been undertaken on efflux mechanisms has involved *Saccharomyces cerevisiae* in which 30 ABCTs have been identified. The ABCTs have been grouped into six families based on sequence similarities, and three, *PDR5*, *MRP/CFTR*, and *MDR* are known to cause drug resistance. In *C. albicans* ten members of the *PDR5* family have been described (the genes are named *CDR*) and have been implicated in azole resistance. Amongst some clinical isolates of azole-resistant *C. albicans*, an increase in *CDR1* mRNA has been found[198].

The major mechanisms of azole resistance are summarized in Figure 17.10.

A single mutation is unlikely to result in high-level antifungal resistance. During prolonged treatment, this is more likely to evolve as a result of several alterations resulting in continuous selective pressure

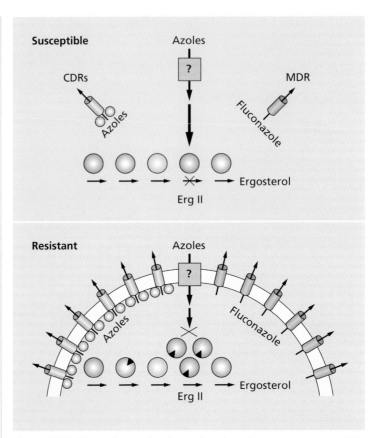

Figure 17.10 Molecular mechanisms of azole resistance. In a susceptible cell, azole drugs enter the cell through an unknown mechanism, perhaps by passive diffusion. The azoles then inhibit Erg11 (pink circles), blocking the formation of ergosterol. Two types of efflux pumps are expressed at low levels. The *CDR* proteins are ABCT with both a membrane pore (green tubes) and two ABC domains (green circles). The *MDR* protein is an MF with a membrane pore (red tubes). In a "model" resistant cell, the azoles also enter the cell through an unknown mechanism. The azole drugs are less effective against Erg11 for two reasons; the enzyme has been modified by specific point mutations (dark slice in pink circles) and the enzyme is over expressed. Modifications in other enzymes in the ergosterol biosynthetic pathway contribute to azole resistance (dark slice in blue sphere). The sterol components of the plasma membrane are modified (darker orange of membrane). Finally, the azoles are removed from the cell by over expression of the *CDR* genes (ABCT) and *MDR* (MF). The *CDR* genes are effective against many azole drugs, while *MDR* appears to be specific for fluconazole (reproduced from White *et al*. 1998[175] with permission of the author and the American Society for Microbiology)

from the drug. White[199] showed this in a unique study. The expression of several genes was examined in clinical isolates from patients with recurrent episodes of oropharyngeal candidiasis who required higher doses of fluconazole to control the infection. Early in the course of therapy, *MDR1* expression was increased, whereas *CDR1* mRNA levels were increased much later as the MIC of fluconazole increased markedly. *ERG16*, encoding 14α-demethylase increased fairly late in the course of treatment, and the increases in mRNA for

both *ERG16* and *CDR1* correlated with resistance to ketoconazole and itraconazole. These results also show that prolonged exposure to one azole may lead to over-expression of genes that result in cross-resistance to other azoles.

Resistance to polyenes

Resistance to the polyene antibiotics is rare but *in vitro* may develop by the selection of naturally occurring resistant cells that produce modified sterols with a low binding affinity for nystatin. Resistance to nystatin is lost after serial passage of yeasts in nystatin-free culture medium, suggesting repopulation by organisms producing sterols with a higher affinity for nystatin. It is also possible that resistance may result from mutation rather than selection. Amphotericin-resistant isolates may show a decreased ergosterol content and hence reduced susceptibility to polyenes. The reduced content of ergosterol and its substitution by other sterols with a lower affinity for polyenes such as amphotericin may result from blockage of the biosynthetic pathway leading to ergosterol. Resistant isolates showed slow growth, impaired pseudomycelia formation, and loss of pathogenicity, and therefore are unlikely to survive in nature[200, 201]. The use of the polyenes in the short-term therapy of vaginal candidiasis is not likely, therefore, to give rise to resistance in nature.

*Resistance to 5-fluorocytosine**

Resistance to 5-fluorocytosine may result from blocking the formation of 5-fluorouridylic acid (FUMP) by loss of cytosine deaminase activity or by loss of uracil phosphoribosyltransferase activity. Primary resistance of fungi to 5-fluorocytosine is common: only about 50% of clinical isolates were susceptible in a study reported by Stiller *et al.*[202]. Oral or parenteral drug is used then only in combination with other antifungal preparations, such as amphotericin B, in the treatment of systemic and refractory mucocutaneous infections.

---

* The fluorinated pyrimidine, 5-fluorocytosine, inhibits the *in vitro* growth of yeasts and many fungi. It is rarely used in the treatment of vaginal candidiasis but, when used in combination with amphotericin B, is valuable in the management of invasive candidiasis and other fungal infection. After entry into the cell, a process aided by a permease enzyme, 5-fluorocytosine is converted into 5-fluorouracil by the enzyme cytosine deaminase. 5-Fluorouracil is then phosphorylated by UMP pyrophosphorylase into 5-fluorouridylic acid (FUMP), which is phosphorylated further and incorporated into cellular RNA, thereby disrupting normal protein synthesis by the cell. 5-Fluorouracil also is converted to 5-fluorodeoxyuridine monophosphate, a potent inhibitor of thymidylate synthase, an enzyme involved in DNA synthesis.

Management of acute candidal vulvovaginitis

As the clinical features of candidal vulvovaginitis are not specific, it is desirable that the clinical diagnosis is confirmed by microscopy (page 490). With respect to efficacy, there is little difference between the various drugs and their route of administration. In selecting an antifungal

Table 17.2 Topical antifungal agents for use in acute vulvovaginitis

Antifungal agent	Formulation	Dosage
Nystatin	1. Vaginal tablet containing 100 000 units nystatin	One inserted nightly for 14 nights
	2. Vaginal cream, 4 g, containing 100 000 units nystatin	4 g inserted nightly for 14 nights
Clotrimazole	1. Vaginal pessary containing 500 mg clotrimazole	One inserted at night for 1 night
	2. Vaginal pessary containing 200 mg clotrimazole	One inserted at night for 3 nights
	3. Vaginal pessary containing 100 mg clotrimazole	One inserted at night for 6 nights
	4. Vaginal cream containing 10% clotrimazole	5 g , inserted at night for 1 night
Miconazole	1. Capsule containing 1200 mg miconazole	One inserted vaginally for 1 night
	2. Vaginal pessary containing 100 mg miconazole	One inserted at night for 14 days *or* twice daily for 7 days
	3. Cream containing miconazole 2% w/w	5 g inserted at night for 10–14 days *or* twice daily for 7 days
Econazole	1. Vaginal pessary for single-dose use, containing 150 mg econazole	One inserted at night for one night.
	2. Vaginal pessary containing 150 mg econazole	One inserted nightly for 3 nights.
	3. Cream containing econazole 1% w/w	5 g inserted nightly for 14 days.
Fenticonazole	1. Vaginal pessary containing 600 mg fenticonazole	One inserted at night for 1 night
	2. Vaginal pessary containing 200 mg fenticonazole	One inserted at night for 3 nights
Butoconzole[a]	1. 2% cream	5 g intravaginally for 3 days
Tioconazole[a]	1. 6.5% ointment	5 g intravaginally in a single application
Terconazole[a]	1. 0.4% cream	5 g intravaginally for 7 days
	2. 0.8% cream	5 g intravaginally for 3 days
	3. 80 mg	Vaginal suppository, one daily for 3 days

[a] Note these agents are not available in the UK.

Table 17.3 Oral antifungal agents for the treatment of acute vulvovaginal candidiasis

Drug	Dosage
Fluconazole	one 150 mg capsule as a single dose
Itraconazole	two 100 mg capsules twice daily for 1 day

agent, however, several factors should be taken into consideration

- patient choice between a topical or oral preparation
- pregnancy, or the possibility of pregnancy at the time of treatment
- in the case of topical preparations, the possibility of damage to latex condoms or contraceptive diaphragms
- in the case of oral antifungal drugs, the possibility of drug interactions, although the risk is small with single-dose therapy
- cost.

Tables 17.2 and 17.3 summarize the available agents. With the possible exception of clotrimazole preparations, for which data are lacking, the topical antifungal agents may alter the latex of condoms and contraceptive diaphragms, leading to failure. It is important that the patient is aware of this possibility. Although there is no evidence of any adverse effect in pregnancy, all topical agents should be used with caution and only when the benefits of treatment are likely to outweigh any potential risk. The patient should be fully involved in the discussions. The oral antifungal drugs should be avoided in the treatment of pregnant women with vulvovaginal candidiasis.

Management of recurrent vulvovaginal candidiasis

Good clinical trials of the treatment for this distressing condition are lacking, and guidelines are empirical[203]. Bingham[204] has published helpful suggestions for management of affected women.

Underlying conditions such as uncontrolled or poorly controlled diabetes mellitus should be identified and corrected. In the management of the woman who presents with recurrent vulvovaginitis, it is essential to make a definitive diagnosis of candidiasis as described on pp. 490–491. Although culture with speciation of the isolate is not generally undertaken in the management of women with acute candidal vulvovaginitis, recurrent disease may be associated with *Candida* spp. with reduced susceptibility to azoles, and in these cases, such testing is warranted. Antifungal susceptibility testing of *C. albicans* isolated from women with recurrent vulvovaginitis is rarely helpful (see above under Pathogenesis).

When the diagnosis is established, treatment is initiated with any of the antifungal preparations noted above. Either vaginal preparations or oral azoles may be used, but, as the response to single-dose therapy with the latter is sometimes unsatisfactory, a course of therapy lasting for 7 to 14 days should be given (fluconazole should be prescribed as a 50 mg capsule, given orally once daily). When vaginal pessaries or intravaginal cream are used, cream should also be applied to the vulval skin. Maintenance treatment is initiated immediately after resolution of symptoms. This may be with

1. vaginal pessaries, such as clotrimazole 500 mg used once weekly or 100 mg nightly for 6 nights, *or*
2. vaginal pessaries containing fenticonazole 600 mg once weekly or 200 mg nightly for 3 nights, *or*
3. oral fluconazole 150 mg given once weekly, *or*
4. oral ketoconazole 100 mg given once daily[205].

The length of treatment must be tailored to the individual patient, but is unlikely to be less than 6 months. At the end of this period it is worth discontinuing therapy to assess outcome. Further therapy may be necessary.

The clinical response of *C. glabrata*, the second most common isolate from women with recurrent vulvovaginal candidiasis, to topical or oral antifungal agents is unknown. The MICs of the available azoles are generally higher for *C. glabrata* than for *C. albicans*, and in many cases there is frank resistance to fluconazole. Itraconazole has moderate activity against *C. glabrata*, but the MIC for the isolate does not always predict therapeutic success. In the treatment of vulvovaginal candidiasis caused by *C. glabrata*, fluconazole should not be the drug of first choice; another azole should be selected and given for at least 7 days; shorter courses or single-dose therapy should be avoided. When azole treatment of recurrent vulvovaginitis caused by *C. glabrata* has failed, the intravaginal use of boric acid has resulted in mycological cure rates of about 75%[206]. A gelatin capsule, containing 600 mg boric acid powder, is inserted into the vagina twice daily for 14 days. If this treatment is successful, maintenance therapy in the form of nystatin pessaries, inserted into the vagina nightly, should be instituted. In the series of patients reported by Sobel & Chaim[206], patients received maintenance therapy in the form of capsules containing 600 mg boric acid inserted into the vagina twice weekly. As the safety of prolonged use of boric acid is unknown, and as there is the possibility of systemic toxicity, the present authors consider that maintenance therapy with this agent should be avoided. Prolonged absorption of boric acid causes anorexia, weight loss, diarrhea, skin rashes, epileptiform seizures, and anemia[207]. There are doubts about the safety of boric acid in pregnant women, and it has been suggested that its use should be discontinued 1 to 2 weeks before conception[208].

There is no evidence that treatment of the sexual partner influences recurrence.

Balanitis due to *Candida* spp.

Balanitis due to *Candida* spp. will generally settle with saline lavage (approximately 0.9% NaCl w/v being used) twice or three times daily; separation of the skin surfaces of the glans and inner surface of the prepuce is made by means of a strip of gauze (about 3.5 cm × 12 cm) soaked in saline which is renewed twice or three times daily. If such a measure fails, the topical application of nystatin, clotrimazole, miconazole, or econazole cream is effective. Alternatively, fluconazole may be given as a single oral dose of 150 mg: Stary *et al.*[209] reported that the clinical and mycological response to fluconazole was comparable to that from the topical application of clotrimazole cream.

As candidal balanoposthitis can be the presenting feature of diabetes mellitus, it is imperative to test the urine for glucose.

Vaginal infection with prokaryotes

Vaginal infection with prokaryotes consists of a number of etiologically separate clinical conditions of greatly differing clinical significance. The question of transmissibility by sexual intercourse as well as pathogenicity in the case of these organisms is a controversial subject although the principle applies that organismal flora of the genitals will bear some relationship to the degree of sexual mixing practised by the individual or the partner. Vaginal infections due to prokaryotes may be classified as follows

1. vaginal infection or colonization with *Streptococcus agalactiae*, more commonly referred to as the beta-hemolytic streptococcus, Lancefield Group B
2. bacterial vaginosis, an imperfect diagnosis based mainly on the bacterial flora, pH and amine content of the vaginal fluid
3. vaginal infection with *Actinomyces israelii* associated with the long-term use of chemically inert intrauterine contraceptive devices
4. the toxic shock syndrome in menstruating women associated with the continuous use of tampons during menstruation and vaginal infection with toxin-producing strains of *Staphylococcus aureus*.

Vaginal infection with Streptococcus agalactiae (Betahemolytic Lancefield Group B)

Streptococcus agalactiae is the name applied to human members of group B streptococci[210] although there are reasons to believe that they form a population group distinct from bovine Group B streptococci (classified by Lancefield on the basis of cell-wall carbohydrate antigens)[211].

In the last 25 years *S. agalactiae* has been a serious cause of bacteremia and other invasive infections in the neonate within the first few days of life. Dense vaginal colonization seems to make transmission more likely, and prematurity and a prolonged labor after rupture of the membranes are important risk factors. Vaginal colonization by group B streptococci has been defined as

1. light, when growth has only occurred in selective broth media
2. heavy, when growth has occurred on non-selective agar plate[212].

The rate of premature and low birth weight delivery in women with heavy vaginal colonization was reported as 7%, compared with 4.6% of women with no group B streptococci (odds ratio 1.6, 95% confidence interval 1.2–2.1)[212]. Light colonization by group B streptococci at 23 to 26 weeks gestation or at delivery, was not associated with adverse outcomes of pregnancy. Invasion of the chorioamnion by group B streptococci has been associated with histological evidence of chorioamnionitis[213], and heavy colonization may be associated with intra-amnion infection and postpartum endometritis[214].

Promiscuity in either the female or her male partner is one determinant of the organismal flora of the genital tract; in the case of Group B streptococci, carriage rates of about 12% to 36% have been noted in the case of women attending STI clinics[215, 216]. Carriage in adult women appears to be best detected by bacteriological examination of a urethral swab. Since the organism is also found on the penis, a presumptive case for its transmission sexually can be made out. Christensen *et al.*[217] found that prolonged urogenital carriage of group B streptococci in 88 women who used tampons during menstruation was twice that in women who did not (49% and 24% respectively), and thought that there was a causal relationship between the use of tampons and the persistence of Group B streptococci.

In relation to the problem of the newborn, however, positive cultures during pregnancy (6% to 28% recorded) may be less frequently found at delivery and a few patients may first acquire the organism at delivery. Invasive infections develop only in about 1% of colonized babies[218]. Children become infected by aspiration of infected amniotic fluid or as they pass through the birth canal[219].

Two clinical syndromes, 'early onset' and 'late onset', are recognized in the neonate. The early-onset disease, although septicemic in type, may also be meningitic, whereas the late-onset disease is almost always meningitic. Early-onset disease may occur within 5 days of birth, but usually within the first 24 to 36 hours. There is a close association between early-onset infection in the neonate and maternal complications, particularly premature labor and a prolonged period between rupture of the membranes and delivery. Infants of low birth weight tend to be affected. The late-onset disease presents usually after the tenth day of life as a purulent meningitis and can affect apparently healthy babies after a normal labor with a mortality rate of 15% to 20% (the mortality rate in early onset disease is more than 25%)[211].

Prevention of early-onset streptococcal infection seems possible. The Centers for Disease Control[219a], the American College of Obstetricians, and the American Academy of Pediatricians[220] recommended either antenatal screening with cultures of vaginal and rectal specimens or a risk-based strategy to identify those who would benefit from intrapartum antimicrobial prophylaxis. Risk assessment is performed at the time of labor: fever, prolonged rupture of the membranes, or imminent preterm delivery are the criteria on which to base a decision to initiate prophylaxis. As a result of the implementation of these recommendations, the incidence of disease caused by group B streptococci has fallen in the USA from 1.7 to 0.6 cases per 1000 live births[221].

Bacterial vaginosis

Bacterial vaginosis is recognized clinically by the presence of an often scanty but characteristic homogeneous gray discharge, vaginal fluid with a pH value of greater than 4.5, and commonly a complaint of a 'fishy odor', often noticed particularly after sexual intercourse. As an aid to recognition by the clinician, the 'fishy odor' can be intensified by the addition of 10% potassium hydroxide solution to a small sample of vaginal fluid from untreated patients. The odor released by the potassium hydroxide solution suggests the presence of amines, a finding confirmed by chemical analysis. Bacterial vaginosis is the preferred term to cover this clinical entity because

- it is associated with bacteria rather than fungi or protozoa
- no single bacterial agent can be recognized as solely responsible for the condition
- a true inflammatory response of 'vaginitis' is absent in most cases.

ETIOLOGY

Organisms associated with bacterial vaginosis.

Gardnerella vaginalis and the 'clue cell'

In 1954 Gardner and Dukes published a brief report that an organism, assigned the name *Haemophilus vaginalis*, had been isolated from 81 of 91 cases of non-specific vaginitis. Subsequent reports from independent and geographically diverse sources referred to this small Gram-negative bacillus, which could grow on blood agar and could be isolated from the urogenital tract. Initially classified as a species of *Haemophilus*, it was later shown, in conflict with the definition of the genus *Haemophilus*, that growth requirements did not include hemin (factor X), nicotinamide adenine dinucleotide (factor V), or other identifiable co-enzyme-like substances. Later, basing arguments on morphology, it was recommended that the organism should be reclassified in the genus *Corynebacterium* and the name *Corynebacterium vaginale* was suggested. In 1980 Greenwood and Picket[221a] studied 78 clinical isolates and found that although the cell-wall morphology is not that of a typical Gram-negative organism, for example *Escherichia coli*, it does resemble a Gram-negative organism more closely than a Gram-positive one. Chemical analysis of the cell wall supports this view. DNA hybridization showed that the organism had no genetic

relationship with other genera, and this and other detailed studies led them to propose that the organisms hitherto designated as *Haemophilus vaginalis* or *Corynebacterium vaginale* should be assigned to a new genus, *Gardnerella*, and given the name *Gardnerella vaginalis*. Because of the unusual cell wall of the organism the new genus could not be assigned to a particular family.

Gardner and Dukes[222] found that the microscopic appearance of epithelial cells in a wet preparation (vaginal fluid mixed with saline) gave a clue to the presence of the species now known as *G. vaginalis*. The cytoplasm was described as especially granular in appearance with small bacilli, uniform in size, regularly spaced upon the surface of the cells (see Figure 17.13). Not all cells were involved and some cells showed only partial involvement. Frampton and Lee[223] described particularly the Type I 'clue cell' with a dense layer of bacilli, uniform in size, covering the cell surface; when Type I 'clue cells' were found cultures were nearly always positive for *G. vaginalis*. In Type II 'clue cells', however, bacteria of variable size and shape were unevenly distributed over the cell surface. Although both Type I 'clue cells' and high concentrations of *G. vaginalis* are almost invariably found in the vaginal fluid in bacterial vaginosis, *G. vaginalis* has long been known to be present in the vaginal flora of normal women from geographically widely separated areas, and for this reason the significance of a positive culture for this organism in an individual patient is uncertain.

Studies on the morphology of the Gram-stained smear from vaginal fluid showed that there is an inverse relationship between the quantity of large Gram-positive rods (*Lactobacillus* morphotype) and the small Gram-negative rods (*Gardnerella* morphotype). When the *Lactobacillus* morphotype is absent or present in low numbers, the *Gardnerella* morphotype may be numerous but is not used as a basis for diagnosis. When other forms of Gram-negative rods (possibly *Bacteroides* spp.) Gram-positive cocci (possibly peptostreptococci), and Gram-negative or Gram-variable curved rods (possibly the motile *Mobiluncus* spp.) are present, then the diagnosis is consistent with bacterial vaginosis[224, 225].

Anaerobic bacteria

In bacterial vaginosis the anaerobic bacterium that is frequently detected in bacterial vaginosis and often present in highest concentrations is *Mobiluncus mulieris*[224]; the other species of *Mobiluncus*, *M. curtisii* is more frequently isolated from the vagina of apparently normal women[226]. These curved motile Gram-negative to Gram-variable rod-shaped bacteria are characteristically more resistant to alkaline solutions than most bacteria in vaginal discharge. High concentrations of other anaerobic non-hemolytic peptostreptococci (for example *Streptococcus intermedius*), *Prevotella* spp. (for example *P. bivia*), *Porphyromonas* spp., *Bacteroides ureolyticus*, and *Fusobacterium nucleatum* are also found[227, 228].

Other organisms include aerobes such as alpha-hemolytic streptococci (for example *Streptococcus acidominimus*), and occasionally coliforms. *Mycoplasma hominis* and *Ureaplasma urealyticum* are also often present, *M. hominis* having been detected in about two-thirds of women studied by Pheifer *et al.*[229]. In bacterial vaginosis, the concentrations of *G. vaginalis*, *Prevotella* spp., *Bacteroides* spp., and *M. hominis* increase by almost a thousandfold. After a 7-day course of treatment with metronidazole the vaginal flora changes radically, anaerobes diminish and lactobacilli become the predominant organism[230], but the previous pattern of bacterial flora may return in a high proportion of patients.

Diamines and polyamines in the vaginal fluid of bacterial vaginosis

The 'fishy' odor associated with bacterial vaginosis and recognized by the addition of 10% potassium hydroxide to a sample of vaginal fluid[229], suggests the presence of amines. Their presence has been confirmed by qualitative analysis and, after dansylation (the addition of dansyl chloride to the vaginal washings) a number of amines have been identified by chromatography, of which putrescine, cadaverine, and trimethylamine are the most abundant[231, 232]; trimethylamine in particular may be partly responsible for the 'fishy' odor. These diamines and polyamines are to be found in trichomonal vaginitis as well as in bacterial vaginosis[231]. The presence of putrescine and cadaverine in the vaginal fluid have a predictive value (percentage of women with a positive result who have been diagnosed on clinical examination as having bacterial vaginosis or trichomonal vaginitis) found in one study to be 84%[231]. In the case of a negative result for the two diamines, the predictive value (percentage of women with a negative result who did not have bacterial vaginosis or trichomonal vaginitis) was estimated by the same group as 92%. The presence of another substance frequently found (gamma-amino-butyric acid, GABA) gave a less secure value (73%).

In vitro studies have shown that the amines, putrescine and cadaverine, can be produced by metronidazole-sensitive organisms isolated anaerobically from patients with bacterial vaginosis, presumably through the decarboxylation of ornithine and lysine, but diamines are not produced by *G. vaginalis* isolated in this way. Similarly, GABA, produced *in vitro* by the mixed anaerobic growth of organisms from bacterial vaginosis, is not so produced by *G. vaginalis*.

The pH value of vaginal fluid in bacterial vaginosis

In bacterial vaginosis the pH range of vaginal washings is from 4.7 to 6.5. Any amines in this range exist in the protonated form (salt) and are not volatile. After addition of 10% potassium hydroxide, the amines are converted to an unprotonated form (free base), become volatile and give a characteristic odor. It is possible that during and after intercourse the alkaline prostatic fluid may convert part of the amines to the unprotonated form and thus cause the characteristic odor[233].

Conclusion

After a 7-day course of treatment with metronidazole there is clinical improvement, and the organisms (*Gardnerella vaginalis*, anaerobes such as *Mobiluncus* spp., *Prevotella* spp., and peptostreptococci), the 'fishy' odor, and the amines such as putrescine and cadaverine, and gamma-amino-butyric acid, diminish or disappear, at least in the short term. The pH of the vaginal fluid is reduced

to below 4.5 and *Lactobacillus* spp. regain their predominance[229, 230, 234]. In bacterial vaginosis before treatment, vaginal flora contains large numbers of *G. vaginalis* (>10⁶/mL) and anaerobes (> 10⁶/mL) in virtually all patients, whereas afterwards these organisms are markedly reduced or absent and the lactobacilli predominate[230]. The inverse relationship between the quantities of the *Lactobacillus* morphotype and the *Gardnerella* morphotype observed on microscopic examination of Gram-stained vaginal smears by Spiegel *et al.*[224, 225], suggests an inter-relationship between the populations of these organisms. Diagnosis of bacterial vaginosis, in their view, depends more on a microscopically detectable change in the vaginal microflora from the *Lactobacillus* morphotype, with or without *Gardnerella* morphotype (normal), to a mixed flora with few or no *Lactobacillus* morphotypes.

PATHOGENESIS

Organisms found in the vagina have a complex and dynamic inter-relationship and the degree of sexual mixing by the individual patient will play its role. The majority of women without evidence of vaginal infection have significant but transient changes in their vaginal flora[235]. Factors associated with an unstable flora, as identified in a prospective study of 51 women and compared with those with stable flora, included a previous history of bacterial vaginosis, a greater number of sexual partners, and more frequent episodes of receptive oral–genital sexual contact[235]. Bacterial vaginosis is significantly less prevalent amongst women who have not had any sexual contact than amongst sexually experienced women[236]. This finding, and the production of vaginal discharge following the intravaginal inoculation of grivet monkeys with both *Gardnerella vaginalis* and *Mobiluncus* spp. (but not with *G. vaginalis* alone)[237], suggests that bacterial vaginosis is initiated by organisms introduced during sexual intercourse.

It has been known for some time that lactobacilli inhibit many of the species of bacteria associated with the condition[238], and it has been proposed that this results from the production of hydrogen peroxide. Some strains of *Lactobacillus* spp. produce

hydrogen peroxide, and these strains are isolated more frequently from the vagina of normal women than from those with bacterial vaginosis[239]. The importance of these strains was shown in a prospective study of a group of women who attended an STI clinic in Seattle, USA[240]. During a 2-year follow-up, 50 women acquired bacterial vaginosis, and there was a clear relationship between the acquisition of the condition and lack of hydrogen peroxide-producing lactobacilli. As there was no relationship between the acquisition of bacterial vaginosis and the presence of non-hydrogen peroxide-producing strains of lactobacilli, this study supports the hypothesis that hydrogen peroxide-producing strains are protective. *In vitro* studies provide further evidence for the importance of hydrogen peroxide in controlling the vaginal microflora. In culture, a high concentration of hydrogen peroxide-producing lactobacilli caused lysis of *G. vaginalis*. When the concentration of lactobacilli in the medium was reduced to a level where they were ineffective alone, toxicity could be restored by the addition of myeloperoxidase and chloride[241]. Toxicity could be inhibited by catalase, an enzyme that degrades hydrogen peroxide. However, bacterial vaginosis can develop in women despite the presence of hydrogen peroxide-producing lactobacilli[242], and it is probable that other, as yet unidentified, factors may predispose to colonization with abnormal bacterial flora and progression to bacterial vaginosis.

A significant polymorphonuclear cell inflammatory reaction is not a feature of bacterial vaginosis. A possible explanation for this may be the production of organic acids, such as succinic acid, which is present in high concentration in the vaginal fluid of patients with bacterial vaginosis[243]. Sturm[244] showed that chemotaxis of polymorphs was inhibited by the products of vaginal anaerobes, particularly those that produced succinate.

Sialidases produced by bacterial vaginosis-associated bacteria[245, 246] may play a role in ascending infection (Chapter 12). In addition to the mucolytic effect on the cervical mucus, these proteases may also degrade secretory IgA or IgM with resultant loss of immunity to other infections[247].

EPIDEMIOLOGY

Prevalence studies

As different diagnostic criteria have been used in many studies, it is often difficult to compare the results from center to center. Published studies, however, have given some indication as to the extent of the condition. Bacterial vaginosis is a common cause of vaginal discharge amongst women attending STI clinics. For example, during 1998, 46 910 cases were reported from clinics in England[248], and at an STI clinic in Copenhagen in 1997, bacterial vaginosis was the leading cause of vaginal discharge[249]. It is also a common condition in other groups of women, but the prevalence may vary geographically: bacterial vaginosis was identified in 70 (4.9%) of 1441 asymptomatic pregnant Italian women[250] and a similar proportion (4.5%) of 492 pregnant Spanish women[251], and in 14% and 16% of pregnant Japanese and Thai women respectively[252].

Sexual transmission of the organisms of bacterial vaginosis?

The question as to whether or not bacterial vaginosis is sexually transmissible has not been fully answered. Larsson et al.[253] found that the mean age at first coitus was significantly lower in women with bacterial vaginosis than in unaffected women, and that the former had a greater number of life-time sexual partners. Holst[254] proffered evidence that the organisms of bacterial vaginosis were not sexually transmitted. He examined the occurrence of four species of bacteria that are associated with the condition, namely *Mobiluncus mulieris*, *Mobiluncus curtisii*, *Mycoplasma hominis*, and *Gardnerella vaginalis*, in sexual partners of women with bacterial vaginosis. Organisms were recovered from the urethra and/or coronal sulcus of 10 of 44 male contacts, but, after 2 weeks of condom use for sexual intercourse, only *Mycoplasma hominis* was recovered from the urethra of one man. He argued that the organisms associated with bacterial vaginosis were not spread sexually but colonized the vagina from an endogenous intestinal tract reservoir. Bacterial vaginosis has been reported in young women who have not had any sexual contact, and the condition has been

identified in 15% of 68 sexually active adolescents and 12% of 52 virginal adolescents[255]. Further evidence against sexual transmission comes from studies involving the treatment of sexual partners: the cure or recurrence rate is not influenced by simultaneous treatment of both partners[256]. If the organisms of bacterial vaginosis are sexually transmitted, it is likely that the condition would be more prevalent amongst the partners of uncircumcised men; this, however, is not the case[257]. There is a high prevalence of bacterial vaginosis amongst lesbians: in a recent study 29% of 101 women who attended clinics in New York City were found to have the condition[258]. The authors of that report concluded that, as 8 of 11 monogamous sexual partners of women with bacterial vaginosis were also affected, sexual transmission of the associated micro-organisms was possible. In a detailed study from London[259], bacterial vaginosis was diagnosed in 52% of 91 lesbians, but there was no association between the infection and having had a male sexual partner in the preceding 12 months, and the authors concluded that this was evidence for lack of heterosexual transmission. These authors also failed to identify any sexual practice, including anal penetration with fingers or dildoes that would have the propensity to transmit the micro-organisms. This finding suggested that the intestinal tract might not be the reservoir of infection of these bacteria.

HIV and bacterial vaginosis

An association between HIV infection and bacterial vaginosis was shown in a cross-sectional study amongst female sex-industry workers in the north of Thailand[260]. Using clinical criteria for the diagnosis of bacterial vaginosis, 33% of 144 women had bacterial vaginosis and 43% of the 144 women were seropositive for HIV, an association that was significant (odds ratio 2.7, 95% confidence interval 1.3–5.0). This association was confirmed in another cross-sectional study from Malawi[261] which showed that amongst 2617 women, 820 of whom had normal vaginal flora, the risk ratio for HIV amongst those with any abnormal vaginal flora was 1.49 (95% confidence interval 1.32–1.68). They

showed further that the prevalence of HIV antibody increased as the severity of the disturbance of vaginal flora increased. The association between bacterial vaginosis and HIV infection was independent of the association of bacterial vaginosis and an increasing number of sexual partners.

The possibility that a disturbance of vaginal flora might predispose to HIV seroconversion was suggested by the findings of Taha et al.[262] in a prospective study of 1169 pregnant women in Malawi who were HIV-seronegative at their first antenatal visit. Seroconversion to HIV was found by the time of delivery in 27 women, and a further 97 women who were followed-up for a median of 2.5 years seroconverted postnatally. Bacterial vaginosis was significantly associated with both antenatal and postnatal seroconversion (odds ratios 3.7 and 2.3 respectively). Similarly, in a prospective study, Martin et al.[263] found a significant relationship between absence of vaginal lactobacilli and increased risk of acquisition of HIV-1 by sex-industry workers in Mombasa, Kenya.

The mechanisms that contribute to this increased risk of infection with HIV-1 in the presence of an abnormal vaginal flora are uncertain. Some time ago it was shown that hydrogen peroxide-producing lactobacilli are cidal to HIV-1[264]. The loss of protection from the reduction in the numbers of these organisms that accompanies bacterial vaginosis may contribute to HIV-1 infection. Another possible mechanism has been postulated. A heat-stable protein produced by *G. vaginalis* increases production of HIV by HIV-infected cells by up to 77-fold[265], and a soluble HIV-inducing factor has been found in cervicovaginal washings. This factor can activate HIV-1 gene expression in monocytes and T cells through activation of the κB enhancer sites[266]. There is a significant association between the presence of this factor and bacterial vaginosis[267], and it is probable that the main source of this factor is *Mycoplasma hominis*[266], a component of the microflora associated with bacterial vaginosis. Interleukin-10 concentrations are elevated in the vaginal fluid of women with bacterial vaginosis, and because IL-10 is known to increase susceptibility of macrophages to HIV infection[268], this may be another mechanism by which bacterial vaginosis increases the risk of HIV infection.

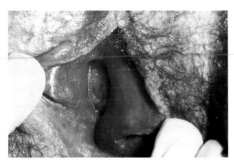

Figure 17.11 Bacterial vaginosis showing white vaginal discharge at the introitus

CLINICAL FEATURES

The woman complains of an increased vaginal discharge that is often described as gray or milky, and she may have noted a 'fishy' odor during or after sexual intercourse. In the absence of concurrent infection with, say, *Candida* spp., pruritus vulvae is not a feature.

On examination, a gray-white discharge may be seen pooling at the introitus (Figure 17.11). A similar homogeneous discharge may be seen to coat the walls of the vagina (Figure 17.12), which are normal or slightly pale in color.

DIAGNOSIS

Before considering the diagnosis of bacterial vaginosis it is necessary to screen patients to exclude *Neisseria gonorrhoeae*, *Chlamydia trachomatis*, *Candida* spp., and *Trichomonas vaginalis*, and to examine the patient vaginally to exclude physical signs of pelvic inflammatory disease. Diagnosis of bacterial vaginosis does not rest upon the detection of any single specific organism. Essentially it is an imperfect diagnosis based on the state of the vaginal fluid, its complex bacterial flora, and its amine products.

Symptom

A complaint of an unpleasant 'fishy' odor often noticed during or after sexual intercourse.

Range in pH of vaginal fluid

Vaginal fluid in bacterial vaginosis is alkaline with a pH in the range of 4.7 to 6.5 (tests are invalid if made in the presence of blood, seminal fluid, or an excess of cervical mucus), for practical purposes the pH tends to be more than 5.0.

Release of volatile amines by potassium hydroxide

The characteristic smell can be recognized if a drop of potassium hydroxide solution (10% w/w) is added to a drop of vaginal discharge. This is a subjective test and not recommended as a practice in the clinic or laboratory.

Biochemical diagnosis of bacterial vaginosis

An objective biochemical diagnosis of bacterial vaginosis is generally not available on account of its cost, namely thin layer chromatography or gas chromatography for the determination of the amines. A new test that yields results within 1 minute is based on the reaction of diamine oxidases with diamines present in vaginal fluid: the reaction causes a color change in a chromogenic system[269]. Published results of this test have been promising, the sensitivity and specificity compared with the microscopical detection of clue cells being 94% and 84% respectively. Further experience, however, is needed before firm recommendations about its use can be made.

Microscopy of the wet vaginal film

Epithelial cells in wet preparations give a 'clue' to the presence of bacterial vaginosis. The cytoplasm of the clue cell is especially granular in appearance with small bacilli, uniform in size, regularly spaced on the surface of the cell. The clue cell is best recognized by the addition of 0.1% w/w methylene blue in saline to wet smear preparations. The bacteria are stained deep blue and can be distinguished from the normal flora (lactobacilli). Wet-smear microscopy, however, is a subjective test that requires considerable experience.

Microscopy of a Gram-stained vaginal smear

The morphological basis for microscopic diagnosis of bacterial vaginosis from a Gram-stained smear has been discussed and a 'clue cell' is shown in Figure 17.13. As a method it was derived from early experience and reports, but it has been more fully studied and developed by Spiegel *et al.*[224, 225], and more recently by Nugent and colleagues[270]. The latter authors described a scoring system for the evaluation of Gram-stained smears that has shown good inter-center reproducibility (Table 17.4). In this system, note is made of the number of morphotypes per

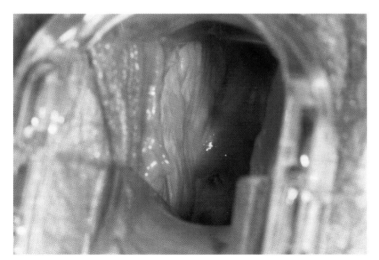

Figure 17.12 Thin, milky-white, homogeneous vaginal discharge in bacterial vaginosis (reproduced from Rein 1996[316])

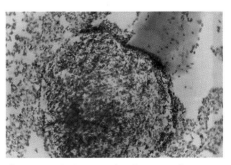

Figure 17.13 Gram-stained smear of bacterial vaginosis, showing clue cells (× 1000)

Table 17.4 Scoring system (1 to 10) for Gram-stained vaginal smears[a] (Nugent et al. 1991[270], with permission of the American Society for Microbiology)

Score[b]	Lactobacillus morphotypes	Gardneralla and Bacteroides spp. morphotypes	Curved Gram-variable rods
0	4+	0	0
1	3+	1+	1+ or 2+
2	2+	2+	3+ or 4+
3	1+	3+	
4	0	4+	

[a] Morphotypes are scored as the average number seen per oil immersion field. Note that less weight is given to curved Gram-variable rods. Total score = lactobacilli + G. vaginalis and Bacterioides spp. + curved rods.

[b] 0 = no morphotypes present; 1 = less than 1 morphotype present; 2 = 1–4 morphotypes present; 3 = 5–30 morphotypes present; 4 = 30 or more morphotypes present.

× 1000 microscope field. The lower the score, the greater the proportion of *Lactobacillus* morphotypes, and the higher the score, the greater proportion of *Gardnerella* and *Bacteroides* morphotypes. Compared with the Amsel criteria* that had until the early 1990s been used widely for the diagnosis of bacterial vaginosis, Gram-smear microscopy, using Nugent's criteria, had a sensitivity of 89% and a specificity of 83% in a study of 617 women, 192 of whom had bacterial vaginosis[271]. Thomason et al.[272] also showed that the specificity of Nugent's method was higher than that of the older Spiegel's method (96% versus 89%). This is a useful method for research studies, but for routine clinical purposes a simplified method for the diagnosis of bacterial vaginosis has been devised by Thomason et al.[272]. This system, which has been found to be comparable to Nugent's interpretative method in terms of sensitivity, does not require enumeration of morphotypes. Bacteria in each field are evaluated as to whether lactobacilli morphotypes exceed other morphotypes, and if 'clue cells' are seen in at least two of twenty fields.

---

* Criteria for the diagnosis of bacterial vaginosis were introduced by Amsel et al.[236]. For correct diagnosis, 3 of 4 criteria had to be fulfilled
1. typical homogeneous vaginal discharge
2. positive amine test
3. pH greater than 4.5
4. 'clue cells' in a wet-mount preparation.

TREATMENT

Clinical evidence shows that metronidazole is effective in the short term treatment of bacterial vaginosis[229, 230, 274] although relapse is common (14% to 39%). The therapeutic effect of metronidazole is, however, difficult to evaluate and account for in specific terms, but its efficacy is more related to its effect on obligate anaerobes rather than on the facultative organism, *Gardnerella vaginalis*[234].

Although *G. vaginalis* is not an anaerobe its growth in the laboratory is inhibited by metronidazole[275], however, the organism is less susceptible than most anaerobes. The hydroxy-metabolite of metronidazole (1-[2-hydroxyethyl]-2-hydroxymethyl-5-nitroimidazole) is more active against *G. vaginalis* than is metronidazole itself[276].

Obligate anaerobes against which metronidazole has been shown to be effective experimentally and clinically[277] were isolated in the majority of cases in the study by Pheifer et al.[229].

Clindamycin, given either orally or intravaginally, is also effective in the treatment of bacterial vaginosis. The majority of organisms associated with the condition are susceptible to this antimicrobial drug[273].

Metronidazole

The mechanism of action, pharmacology, unwanted effects, and use in pregnancy of metronidazole are discussed earlier in this chapter in the section on trichomoniasis.

Treatment regimens with metronidazole

The following regimens have all been shown to be effective in the treatment of bacterial vaginosis.

- Metronidazole 400 to 500 mg by mouth every 12 hours for 5 to 7 days. In reported open or open-randomized studies the cumulative cure rate after 4 weeks is 81.3%[278].
- Metronidazole 2 g as a single oral dose. Compared with a 7-day regimen of therapy, the cure rate at 4 weeks after treatment with a single oral dose of metronidazole is significantly lower: in an analysis of double-blind studies[278] the single-dose cumulative cure rate was 54% compared with 88% amongst women given a 7-day course of treatment.
- Metronidazole gel 0.75% w/w, one 5 g application inserted into the vagina once daily for 5 days. This has been shown to be as effective as a 7-day course of oral metronidazole: up to 85% of women have short-term cure[279]. Mean peak serum concentrations of metronidazole gel are less than 2% of the standard 500 mg oral dose[280].

Clindamycin

Clindamycin is a chlorine-substituted derivative of lincomycin.

Mechanism of action

Clindamycin inhibits protein synthesis by interfering with the formation of initiation complexes and with aminoacyl translocation reactions. The receptor for lincomycins on the 50S subunit of the bacterial ribosome is a 23S rRNA, thought to be identical to the receptor for erythromycins. The action is predominantly bacteriostatic, but at higher concentrations, bactericidal activity against certain sensitive strains may be found.

Pharmacokinetics (Pharmacia and Upjohn Data Sheet 2000)

About 90% of the *oral* dose of clindamycin is absorbed from the gastrointestinal tract, a peak serum level of 2 to 3 mg/mL being reached within 1 hour of administration of a 150 mg dose. When given by the vaginal route to normal women, about 3% (range 0.1% to 7%) of the 100 mg dose of clindamycin is absorbed systemically, the peak serum level averaging about 20 ng/mL (range 3 to 93 ng/mL). The systemic absorption of the drug is similar when used in women with bacterial vaginosis.

The drug is widely distributed throughout the body, although little appears to enter the central nervous system. Clindamycin crosses the placenta and is found in breast milk. About 90% of the drug is protein bound. It is said to accumulate in macrophages. The plasma half-life is 2 to 3 hours.

Excretion

Clindamycin is metabolized in the liver to the active N-demethyl and sulfoxide metabolites. About 10% of the administered dose is excreted in urine as active drug or metabolites; less than 5% is excreted in the feces.

Unwanted effects

The most common side effects of orally administered clindamycin are nausea, vomiting, abdominal pain, and diarrhea. Antibiotic-associated colitis is a well-recognized complication of oral clindamycin treatment: toxigenic *Clostridium difficile* is selected out under pressure from the antibiotic. Transient leukopenia, thrombocytopenia, and eosinophilia have been reported, and abnormalities of plasma enzyme tests of liver function, sometimes with jaundice, have been described. Generalized pruritus and skin rashes, including, rarely, erythema multiforme exudativum, may occasionally develop. Intravaginal application of clindamycin cream may cause pruritus vulvae, and sometimes (about 14%), vaginitis or cervicitis.

Use in pregnancy and lactation

In animal studies, clindamycin has not shown feto-toxicity or evidence of impaired fertility. The safety of clindamycin in human pregnancy, however, has not been established, and, as with all such drugs, it should be used only when the benefits outweigh any possible risk. Although the drug is found in breast milk, it is stated that the infant is unlikely to absorb significant amounts of the drug from its intestinal tract (Pharmacia & Upjohn Data Sheet 2000).

Preparations available

Clindamycin is available as capsules containing either 75 mg or 150 mg of clindamycin hydrochloride equivalent to 75 mg or 150 mg of clindamycin. It is also available as a cream suitable for intravaginal use: each gram of cream contains clindamycin phosphate equivalent to 2 mg clindamycin. NB as the cream contains oil-based components, latex condoms may be damaged.

Treatment regimens with clindamycin

The following regimens are effective in the treatment of bacterial vaginosis.

1. Clindamycin 300 mg by mouth every 12 hours for 7 days. In a comparison of the efficacy of clindamycin and metronidazole in the treatment of bacterial vaginosis, Greaves et al.[281] found that 7 to 10 days after initiation of therapy, 94% of 49 women treated with clindamycin were cured (as defined by resolution of vaginal discharge, and failure to satisfy entry criteria for the study), compared with 96% of 50 women who had received metronidazole. Mild side effects were noted in 16% of the former and in 22% of the latter groups.
2. Clindamycin cream (2%), one applicator full (about 5 g), inserted into the vagina at bedtime for 7 consecutive days; lower concentrations of cream appear to be less efficacious[282]. The cumulative cure rate for clindamycin cream 4 to 10 days after completion of therapy is 80%, and 25 to 39 days after treatment is 82%[283].
3. Clindamycin ovules 100 mg intravaginally once at bedtime for 3 days

Treatment of sexual partners

There is no evidence that treatment of sexual partners reduces the risk of recurrence, and there is no clear indication for their treatment.

BACTERIAL VAGINOSIS AND PREGNANCY

There have now been several good studies that have shown an association between bacterial vaginosis and pre-term birth and low birth weight delivery, the relative risk being 1.5 to 2.3[284]. Infection of the amniotic fluid and chorioamnion are related to premature birth, and bacterial vaginosis is associated with an increased risk of amniotic fluid or chorioamniotic infection, and histological evidence of chorioamnionitis[285, 286]. Furthermore, the organisms found in bacterial vaginosis have been isolated from the upper genital tract of women in premature labor[284].

It is thought that pre-term labor is triggered by the cytokines and prostaglandins produced as a result of bacterial infection. Certainly, elevated levels of tumor necrosis factor, interleukin-1α, interleukin-6, interleukin-8, and prostaglandin E_2 are found in the amniotic fluid of most women with amniotic infection but intact membranes[284]. The mechanisms underlying upper genital tract infection in pregnant women are unknown but it is possible that enzymes such as sialidases may have a mucolytic effect on the cervical mucus, permitting ascent of bacteria from the vagina. The time of infection of the amniotic fluid or chorioamnion is also uncertain, but the frequency of upper genital tract infection decreases with increasing gestational age at delivery[287]. The proportion of premature deliveries with evidence of infection is high when delivery occurs from 23 to 30 weeks, intermediate in deliveries from 30 to 34 weeks, and low beyond 34 weeks gestation[284].

Bacterial vaginosis has also been implicated as a cause of endometritis following cesarean section. In the study by Watts et al.[288], the odds ratio for the development of post-operative endometritis in women with bacterial vaginosis was 5.8 (95% confidence interval 3.0–10.9), and the bacteria associated with bacterial vaginosis were cultured from the endometrium. Bacterial vaginosis is also associated with intra-amniotic infection during vaginal delivery. Newton et al.[289] showed that in the population of 936 women studied, there was a significant relationship between infection and the presence of abnormal vaginal flora, including the pattern associated with bacterial vaginosis. They also noted an independent relationship between the duration of use of fetal electrodes and number of vaginal examinations, and concluded that abnormal vaginal flora combine with clinical variables to increase the risk of intra-amniotic infection.

As there is little doubt that bacterial vaginosis predisposes to pre-term delivery, studies have addressed the issue of treating affected pregnant women to reduce the risk. Although one study showed that treatment with metronidazole and erythromycin reduced the rates of premature delivery in women with bacterial vaginosis who had had a previous pre-term or low birth weight delivery[290], this finding has not been confirmed in a recent report. This concerned a placebo-controlled trial of metronidazole in the treatment of asymptomatic women with bacterial vaginosis who were between 16 weeks and less than 24 weeks pregnant[291]. The primary outcome was the rate of delivery before 37 weeks gestation. Despite resolution of infection in 78% of women, treatment did not reduce the occurrence of pre-term labor, intra-amniotic or post-partum infection, or neonatal sepsis, either in women who had had previous premature deliveries or in those who were not considered to be at risk. As the results of this and a previous study[292] showed no benefit from treatment with metronidazole, routine screening for, and treatment of bacterial vaginosis in asymptomatic pregnant women does not appear to be justified.

A recent study has shown that amongst women undergoing assisted conception, there is an increased risk of miscarriage in the first trimester if the woman has bacterial vaginosis[293]. After adjusting for other factors known to increase the risk of spontaneous abortion, the odds ratio was 2.67 (95% confidence interval 1.26–5.63). Neither bacterial vaginosis nor intermediate vaginal flora, however, have an adverse effect on fertilization rates in women undergoing *in vitro* fertilization treatment[294, 293].

Treatment of bacterial vaginosis in pregnancy

Pregnant women who are symptomatic and in whom examination confirms bacterial vaginosis should be treated. The results of several studies have also suggested that women who have previously had a preterm birth or a second trimester loss should be screened and treated if found to have bacterial vaginosis[290, 292, 295]. Treatment should be instituted early in the second trimester of pregnancy, and should be systemic with either metronidazole or clindamycin. Studies using intravaginal clindamycin cream have not shown a reduction in the preterm birth rate[296, 297]. As a 5-day course of metronidazole has been shown to be more effective than single high-dose therapy, this should be the regimen of choice. One month after treatment, Gram-stained vaginal smears should be examined to ensure resolution of infection. It may also be worth screening the woman prior to delivery because of the risk of ascending infection at the time of delivery.

BACTERIAL VAGINOSIS AND POST-OPERATIVE COMPLICATIONS

In women who have had abdominal hysterectomy, vaginal cuff infection has been associated with bacterial vaginosis. Seven of 20 women with 'clue cells' in vaginal smears developed wound infections, compared with only 4 of 50 women who had no evidence of bacterial vaginosis. Postoperative fever is more common amongst women with bacterial vaginosis undergoing other forms of gynecological surgery[298]. There is also an increased incidence of pelvic inflammatory disease amongst women with bacterial vaginosis who undergo first trimester termination of pregnancy[299]. Treatment with metronidazole significantly reduces the risk of this complication: amongst a group of 174 women randomized to receive either placebo or oral metronidazole, pelvic inflammatory disease developed in 3 women (3.8%) who were given metronidazole, but in 11 (12.2%) placebo recipients[300].

Colonization of the uterine tract and vagina with Actinomyces israelii (associated particularly with the use of the chemically inert intrauterine contraceptive device)

In the vagina or endocervix, *Actinomyces* spp. do not proliferate to form recognizable colonies in the absence of a foreign body, particularly an intrauterine contraceptive device (IUD). The most commonly found species, *Actinomyces israelii*, was isolated from patients in the Dundee area in Scotland during the years 1978 to 1981 and was always associated with the long-term (more than 2 years) use of a chemically inert IUD. Patients with copper-containing devices had a low prevalence, 2% (209 patients examined), compared with 42% (197 patients examined) of those using a plastic (inert) device. It was considered that this was related to the known bacteriostatic action of copper or to the practice of replacing devices containing copper at regular, usually 2-yearly, intervals[301–303]. Bacteriostasis, however, in cases of copper-containing IUDs, is not likely to be absolute since the organism *Eikenella corrodens* may be found and act as a conditional or opportunistic pathogen in association with such an IUD.

Actinomyces spp. and organisms of the related genus *Arachnia* produce masses of interwoven filaments sufficient to erode but not invade surface membranes and the mere finding of these organisms may have no clinical significance. The organism rarely spreads to involve the upper genital tract but when it does it causes a chronic suppurative condition known as actinomycosis, a cause of serious morbidity. This condition is rare, and it has been estimated that the incidence of pelvic actinomycosis is about 1 in 209 070 women[304].

Detectable in wet mounts or Gram-stained smears, it may be identified by staining with fluorescein isothiocyanate (FITC)-labeled species-specific antiserum. The examination of a Papanicolaou-stained smear lacks specificity: 18% of slides initially considered showing *Actinomyces*-like organisms were not confirmed in the study reported by Petitti *et al.*[305]. Microscopical examination of hematoxylin and eosin-stained sections of endometrial curettings also lacks specificity: O'Brien *et al.*[306] confirmed the presence of *Actinomyces* spp. by Gram-smear microscopy in only 1 of 16 specimens thought to contain sulfur granules. Immunoassays are available and initial electrophoretic separation by SDS-PAGE (polyacrylamide gel electrophoresis) followed by electrophoretic transfer of separated antigens in the gel matrix to a nitrocellulose membrane is a method[307].

The presence of *Actinomyces* spp. in the vagina has no significance in an *asymptomatic* woman, and neither antibiotic treatment nor removal of an IUD, if present, is warranted[304]. When *Actinomyces*-like organisms are found in the vagina or cervix of a woman with intermenstrual bleeding, pelvic pain, deep dyspareunia, or dysuria, or who has a pelvic infection and/or pelvic mass not caused by another cause, the IUD should be removed[308]. The threads from the coil should be cultured, and erthromycin, tetracycline, or phenoxymethylpenicillin should be prescribed for 14 days.

Toxic shock syndrome

The toxic shock syndrome was first described in 1978 in children, and toxin-producing strains of *Staphylococcus aureus*, phage group 1 were recovered in most cases from various anatomical sites. Later, most cases of the toxic shock syndrome were found to occur in women of reproductive age and there was a striking association with the menstrual period. The syndrome has been described in women who are not menstruating and, occasionally, in men. The clinical picture was described fully in 1980 by the United States Public Health Services Center for Disease Control[309].

The risk of acquiring the disease appeared mainly to be associated with the use of a brand of highly absorbent tampons which contained a form of carboxymethylcellulose liable to enzymic degradation by vaginal organisms to yield glucose. The tampon may obstruct menstrual flow and, when digested, provide nutrient for the rapid growth of staphylococci. Toxic shock syndrome in menstruating women is caused by an exotoxin (toxic shock syndrome toxin (TSST-1)) produced by phage group 1 *S. aureus*. Only about half of the strains of the organism recovered from non-menstruating women produce TSST-1; in some of these cases, phage group V *S. aureus* strains that produce enterotoxin B have been identified.

CLINICAL FEATURES

The toxic shock syndrome typically, and in almost all patients, begins abruptly with fever, vomiting, diarrhea, and sometimes rigors (25%). The temperature is frequently (in 85% of cases) above 40°C and patients may have abdominal pain. Hypotension develops within 72 hours and the fall in blood pressure may occur abruptly. A diffuse macular erythematous rash may go unnoticed or evolve into a more discrete macular rash. Headache and sore throat may be a presenting symptom or may develop in the course of the illness. A vaginal discharge, perhaps obscured by menstruation, may be observed (28% of cases). On removal tampons often emit a foul odor. Diffuse myalgia is almost always present, and many complain of skin or muscular tenderness when touched or moved. Recovery in the majority of patients occurs in 7 to 10 days although individuals may require 8 to 12 liters of fluid parenterally per 24 hours to maintain perfusion, and many become edematous.

Desquamation occurs within 1 to 2 weeks, particularly on the palms of the hands and the soles of the feet and sometimes also on the face, trunk, and tongue. Peeling of the skin may be extensive and the denuded finger tips may be sensitive as a result. Hair and nail loss may be seen in some patients.

The serum creatinine is typically (69%) elevated. Thrombocytopenia, hypocalcemia, raised plasma bilirubin, and elevated plasma enzymes are seen in 60% of cases. Creatine kinase is elevated in about 40% of cases[309].

TREATMENT

General supportive measures to combat shock are necessary; details lie outwith the scope of this text. Clearly, the tampon or its debris should be removed, if present. Recovery occurs in the majority of patients within 7 to 10 days. Desquamations occur within 1 to 2 weeks, most prominently on the palms and soles, but also on the face, trunk, and tongue. The skin may peel in large sheets and there may be loss of nails and hair.

PREVENTION

The toxic shock syndrome is associated with continuous use of tampons throughout the menstrual period. Women who have had the toxic shock syndrome may have recurrences and should not use tampons until *Staphylococcus aureus* has been eradicated from the vagina. Recurrences, if multiple, tend to have progressively less intense episodes. Toxin-producing staphylococci might be carried in the flares. Women who have not had the toxic shock syndrome have a low risk of its development (6.2 cases per 100 000 menstruating women). Since risk can be reduced further by using tampons for only part of the day or night, or part of the menstrual cycle, individuals who have had the toxic shock syndrome should be advised accordingly[310].

Vulvodynia

Vulvodynia distinguishes chronic painful vulval discomfort such as burning, rawness, and stinging, from pruritus vulvae, although there is undoubtedly some overlap between these features[311]. Previously regarded by many as a psychogenic condition, vulvodynia is an organic disease that presents with surface changes or as an aberration of sensory function in which surface changes may be absent[311].

Four categories of vulvodynia can be distinguished[311].

1. Vulval vestibulitis

The principal feature of this condition that usually presents in women of reproductive age is severe pain on touching the vestibule. The most common symptom is of introital dyspareunia, although discomfort at rest with or without dyspareunia may occur. Vulval vestibulitis may be primary, developing at the time of initiation of sexual activity, and possibly representing a developmental hymenal disorder, or secondary. In the latter case, the onset is usually insidious. On touching the vestibule with a cotton wool-tipped applicator stick, there is pain of variable severity in localized areas. When the introitus is examined with the naked eye, erythema of varying severity is the only abnormal clinical sign. After the application of acetic acid and examination with the colposcope, dense inflammatory-type acetowhite areas are seen, and metaplasia around the orifices of the ducts of Bartholin's glands is found. It is these areas that show tenderness to touch. Histological examination of these areas shows a mixed lymphocytic and plasma cell infiltration around the minor vestibular glands and the ducts of Bartholin's glands[312]. The etiology of vulval vestibulitis is unknown, but, as HPV DNA is found in biopsies from only a minority of women, it is not considered causative. Infective conditions that can cause vulvodynia, for example candidiasis or trichomoniasis, should be excluded by undertaking the appropriate investigation (see pp. 478–480 and 490–491). Treatment should be as conservative as possible, the patient being advised to avoid possible irritants such as soaps. Pure water should be used for bathing the affected areas and mild emollients may provide some symptomatic relief. Some physicians have found the topical application of zinc oxide cream to be efficacious. Surgery, in the form of simple excision, or vestibulectomy achieves cure rates of about 80%, but should be reserved for those women whose symp-toms fail to be relieved by conservative treatment.

2. Dysesthetic vulvodynia

This condition is defined as genital burning or pain that is not limited to the vestibule: it is often a component of vulval vestibulitis. Unlike the latter disorder, introital dyspareunia is not a feature and clinical examination does not usually cause discomfort. The pain may be well localized or difficult to localize, and there may be associated backache and lower urinary tract symptoms. There may be areas of hyperesthesia, or a different sensation may be perceived from that applied (allodynia). There are variable degrees of vulval erythema. The etiology is obscure, but causalgia has been suggested as a possible mechanism for the discomfort. Dysesthetic vulvodynia may also present as pudendal neuralgia, a hyperesthesia following the S2–S4 distribution of the pudendal nerve. Post-herpetic neuralgia should also be considered in the differential diagnosis. Treatment is with amitriptyline in increasing doses from 10 mg daily by mouth.

3. Vulval dermatoses

Such conditions, including lichen sclerosus and lichen planus, and discussed in Chapter 20, may be associated with vulvodynia.

4. Vaginismus

This condition may present as vulvodynia and, if suspected, the patient should be referred to a specialist in psychosexual medicine.

The condition of *cyclic vulvitis* is diagnosed when symptoms are not limited to the vestibule, and exacerbation and remission are related to the menstrual cycle[313]. Symptoms are usually worse after intercourse. There are often few clinical abnormalities, although mild erythema may be noted on careful examination. The etiolgy is uncertain, but hypersensitivity to *Candida* spp. antigens may play a role, and prolonged treatment with topical or oral antifungal agents is often effective.

References

1 Honigberg BM. Trichomonads of importance in human medicine. In: Kreier JP (ed.) *Parasitic Protozoa*, vol. II. Academic Press; New York: 1978.

2 Nielsen MH, Nielsen R. Electron microscopy of *Trichomonas vaginalis* Donne: interaction with vaginal epithelium in human trichomoniasis. *Acta Pathol Microbiol Scand, Section B* 1975; **83**: 305–320.

3 Petrin D, Delgaty K, Bhatt R, Garber G. Clinical and microbiological aspects of *Trichomonas vaginalis*. *Clin Microbiol Rev* 1998; **11**: 300–317.

4 Bonihla VL, Ciavaglia M, de Souza W, Costa e Silva Filho F. The involvement of terminal carbohydrates of the mammalian cell surface in the cytoadhesion of trichomonads. *Parasitol Res* 1995; **81**: 121–126.

5 Lehker MW, Arroyo R, Alderete JF. The regulation by iron of the synthesis of adhesins and cytadherence levels in the protozoan *Trichomonas vaginalis*. *J Exp Med* 1991; **174**: 311–318.

6 Lehker MW, Sweeney D. Trichomonad invasion of the mucous layer requires adhesins, mucinases, and motility. *Sex Transm Infect* 1999; **75**: 231–238.

7 Arroyo R, Gonzales-Robles A, Martinez-Palomo A, Alderete JF. Signalling of *Trichomonas vaginalis* for amoeboid transformation and adhesion synthesis follows cytoadherence. *Mol Microbiol* 1993; **7**: 299–309.

8 Kon VB, Papadimitriou JM, Robertson TA, Warton A. Quantitation of concanavalin A and wheat germ agglutinin binding by two strains of *Trichomonas vaginalis* of differing pathogenicity using gold particle-conjugated lectins. *Parasitol Res* 1988; **75**: 7–13.

9 Garber GE, Lemchuk-Favel LT, Bowie WR. Isolation of a cell-detaching factor of *Trichomonas vaginalis*. *J Clin Microbiol* 1989; **27**: 1548–1553.

10 Garber GE, Lemchuk-Favel LT, Rousseau G. Effect of beta-estradiol on production of the cell-detaching factor of *Trichomonas vaginalis*. *J Clin Microbiol* 1991; **29**: 1847–1849.

11 Alderete JF, Provenzano D, Lehker W. Iron mediates *Trichomonas vaginalis* resistance to complement lysis. *Microb Pathog* 1995; **19**: 93–103.

12 Provenzano D, Alderete JF. Analysis of human immunoglobulin-degrading cysteine proteinases of *Trichomonas vaginalis*. *Infect Immun* 1995; **63**: 3388–3395.

13 Alderete JF, Garza GE. Soluble *Trichomonas vaginalis* antigens in cell-free culture supernatants. *Mol Biochem Parasitol* 1984; **13**: 147–158.

14 Peterson KM, Alderete JF. Host plasma proteins on the surface of pathogenic *Trichomonas vaginalis*. *Infect Immun* 1982; **37**: 755–762.

15 Alderete JF. Alternating phenotypic expression of two classes of *Trichomonas vaginalis* surface markers. *Rev Infect Dis* 1988; **10** (Suppl. 2): S408–S412.

16 Alderete JF, Kasmala L. Monoclonal antibody to a major glycoprotein immunogen mediates differential complement-independent lysis of *Trichomonas vaginalis*. *Infect Immun* 1986; **56**: 697–699.

17 Alderete JF, Demes P, Gombosova A, *et al*. Phenotypes and protein-epitope phenotypic variation among fresh isolates of *Trichomonas vaginalis*. *Infect Immun* 1987; **55**: 1037–1041.

18 Ackers JP, Lumsden WHR, Catterall RD, Coyle R. Antitrichomonal antibody in the vaginal secretions of women infected with *T vaginalis*. *Br J Vener Dis* 1975; **51**: 319–323.

19 Alderete JF, Newton E, Dennis C, Neale KA. The vagina of women infected with *Trichomonas vaginalis* has numerous proteinases and antibody to trichomonad proteinases. *Genitourin Med* 1991; **67**: 469–474.

20 Alderete JF, Newton E, Dennis C, Engbring J, Neale KA. Vaginal antibody of patients with trichomoniasis is to a prominent surface immunogen of *Trichomonas vaginalis*. *Genitourin Med* 1991; **67**: 220–225.

21 Rein MF, Sullivan JA, Mandell GL. Trichomonacidal activity of human polymorphonuclear neutrophils: killing by disruption. *J Infect Dis* 1980; **142**: 575–585.

22 Alderete JF, Newton E, Dennis C, Neale KA. Antibody in sera of patients infected with *Trichomonas vaginalis* is to trichomonad proteinases. *Genitourin Med* 1991; **67**: 331–334.

23 Addis MF, Rappelli P, Pinto de Andrade AM, *et al*. Identification of *Trichomonas vaginalis* alpha-actinin as the most common immunogen recognized by sera of women exposed to the parasite. *J Infect Dis* 1999; **180**: 1727–1730.

24 Lossick JG. Epidemiology of urogenital trichomoniasis. In: *Trichomonads Parasitic in Humans*. Honigberg BM (ed.) Springer-Verlag; New York: 1989, pp. 311–323.

25 Tsao W. Trichomoniasis and gonorrhoea. *Br Med J* 1969; **1**: 632–643.

26 Burch TA, Rees CW, Reardon LV. Epidemiological studies on human trichomoniasis. *Am J Trop Med Hyg* 1959; **8**: 312–318.

27 Whittington JM. Epidemiology of infections with *Trichomonas vaginalis* in the light of improved diagnostic methods. *Br J Vener Dis* 1957; **33**: 80–91.

28 Schneider H, Coetzee DJ, Fehler HG, *et al*. Screening for sexually transmitted diseases in rural South African women. *Sex Transm Infect* 1998; **74**: S147–S152.

29 Mulanga-Kabeya C, Morel E, Patrel D, *et al*. Prevalence and risk assessment for sexually transmitted infections in pregnant women and female sex workers in Mali: is syndromic approach suitable for screening? *Sex Transm Infect* 1999; **75**: 358–360.

30 Cotch MF, Pastorek JG, Nugent RP, *et al*. *Trichomonas vaginalis* associated with low birth weight and preterm delivery. The Vaginal Infection and Prematurity Study Group. *Sex Transm Dis* 1997; **24**: 361–362.

31 Tabrizi SN, Paterson B, Fairley CK, Bowden FJ, Garland SM. A self-administered technique for the detection of sexually transmitted diseases in remote communities. *J Infect Dis* 1997; **176**: 289–292.

32 Ndoye I, Mboup S, de Schryver A, *et al*. Diagnosis of sexually transmitted infections in female prostitutes in Dakar, Senegal. *Sex Transm Infect* 1998; **74**: S112–S117.

33 Ramjee G, Karim SS, Sturm AW. Sexually transmitted infections among sex workers in KwaZulu-Natal, South Africa. *Sex Transm Dis* 1998; **25**: 346–349.

34 Borchardt KA, Al-Haraci S, Maida N. Prevalence of *Trichomonas vaginalis* in a male sexually transmitted disease clinic population by interview, wet mount microscopy, and the InPouch™ TV test. *Genitourin Med* 1995; **71**: 405–406.

35 Saxena SB, Jenkins RR. Prevalence of *Trichomonas vaginalis* in men at high risk of sexually transmitted diseases. *Sex Transm Dis* 1991; **18**: 138–142.

36 Hobbs MM, Kazembe P, Reed AW, *et al*. *Trichomonas vaginalis* as a case of urethritis in Malawian men. *Sex Transm Dis* 1999; **26**: 381–387.

37 Laga M, Manoka A, Kivuvu M, *et al*. Non-ulcerative sexually transmitted diseases as risk factors for HIV-1 transmission in women: results from a cohort study. *AIDS* 1993; **7**: 95–102.

38 Levine WC, Pope V, Bhoomkar A, *et al*. Increase in endocervical CD4 lymphocytes among women with nonulcerative sexually transmitted diseases. *J Infect Dis* 1998; **177**: 167–174.

39 Draper D, Donohoe W, Mortimer L, Heine RP. Cysteine proteases of *Trichomonas vaginalis* degrade secretory leucocyte protease inhibitor. *J Infect Dis* 1998; **178**: 815–819.

40 Berggren O. Association of carcinoma of the uterine cervix and *Trichomonas vaginalis* infestations. *Am J Obstet Gynecol* 1969; **105**: 166–168.

41 Fouts AC, Kraus SJ. *Trichomonas vaginalis*: reevaluation of its clinical presentation and laboratory diagnosis. *J Infect Dis* 1980; **141**: 137–143.

42 Catterall RD. Trichomonal infections of the genital tract. *Med Clin N Am* 1972; **56**: 1203–1209.

43 Krieger JN, Jenny C, Verdon M, *et al*. Clinical manifestations of trichomoniasis in men. *Ann Int Med* 1993; **118**: 844–849.

44 Cotch MF, Pastorek JG, Nugent RP, *et al*. *Trichomonas vaginalis* associated with low birth weight and preterm delivery. The Vaginal Infection and Prematurity Study Group. *Sex Transm Dis* 1997; **24**: 361–362.

45 Sutton MY, Sternberg M, Nsuami M, Behets F, Nelso AM, St Louis ME. Trichomoniasis in pregnant human immunodeficiency virus-infected and human immunodeficiency virus-uninfected Congolese women: prevalence, risk factors, and association with low birth weight. *Am J Obstet Gynecol* 1999; **181**: 656–662.

46 Meis PJ, Goldenberg RL, Mercer B, *et al*. The preterm prediction study: significance of vaginal infections. National Institute of Child Health and Human Development Maternal-Fetal Units Network. *Am J Obstet Gynecol* 1995; **173**: 1231–1235.

47 Nadisauskiene R, Bergstrom S, Stankeviciene I, Spukaite T. Endocervical pathogens in women with preterm and term labour. *Gynecol Obstet Invest* 1995; **40**: 179–182.

47a Klebanoff MA, Carey JC, Hauth JC, *et al*. Failure of metronidazole to prevent preterm delivery among pregnant women with asymptomatic *Trichomonas vaginalis* infection. *N Engl J Med* 2001; **345**: 487–493.

48 Minkoff H, Grunebaum RL, Schwarz RH, *et al*. Risk factors for prematurity and premature rupture of membranes: a prospective study of the vaginal flora in pregnancy. *Am J Obstet Gynecol* 1984; **150**: 965–972.

49 McGregor JA, French JI, Jones W, *et al*. Prevention of premature birth by screening and treatment for common genital tract infections: results of a prospective controlled evaluation. *Am J Obstet Gynecol* 1995; **173**: 157–167.

50 Read JS, Klebanoff MA for the Vaginal Infections and Prematurity Study Group. Sexual intercourse during pregnancy and preterm delivery: effects of vaginal microorganisms. *Am J Obstet Gynecol* 1993; **168**: 514–519.

51 Mirhaghani A, Warton A. An electron microscope study of the interaction between *Trichomonas vaginalis* and epithelial cells of the human amnion membrane. *Parasitol Res* 1996; **82**: 43–47.

52 McGregor JA, French JI, Jones W, Parker R, Patterson E, Draper D. Association of

cervicovaginal infections with increased vaginal fluid phospholipase A$_2$ activity. *Am J Obstet Gynecol* 1992; **167**: 1588–1594.

53 Alderete JF, Newton E, Dennis C, Neale KA. The vagina of women infected with *Trichomonas vaginalis* has numerous proteinases and antibody to trichomonad proteinases. *Genitourin Med* 1991; **67**: 469–474.

54 Trussell RE, Wilson ME, Longwell FH, Laughlin KA. Vaginal trichomoniasis. *Am J Obstet Gynecol* 1942; **44**: 292–295.

55 Robertson DHH, Lumsden WHR, Frasere KF, Hosie DD, Moore DM. Simultaneous isolation of *Trichomonas vaginalis* and collection of vaginal exudate. *Br J Vener Dis* 1969; **45**: 42–43.

56 Schwebke JR, Morgan SC, Pinson GB. Validity of self-obtained vaginal specimens for diagnosis of trichomoniasis. *J Clin Microbiol* 1997; **35**: 1618–1619.

57 Paterson BA, Tabrizi SN, Garland SM, Fairley CK, Bowden FJ. The tampon test for trichomoniasis: a comparison between conventional methods and a polymerase chain reaction for *Trichomonas vaginalis* in women. *Sex Transm Dis* 1998; **74**: 136–139.

58 Krieger JN, Viridans M, Siegel N, *et al.* Risk assessment and laboratory diagnosis of trichomoniasis in men. *J Infect Dis* 1992; **166**: 1362–1366.

59 Beverly AL, Venglarik M, Cotton B, Scwebke JR. Viability of *Trichomonas vaginalis* in transport medium. *J Clin Microbiol* 1999; **37**: 3749–3750.

60 Nielsen R. *Trichomonas vaginalis* 1. Survival in solid Stuart's medium. *Br J Vener Dis* 1969; **45**: 328–331.

61 McMillan A. Laboratory diagnostic methods and cryopreservation of trichomonads. In: Honigberg BM (ed.) *Trichomonads Parasitic in Humans.* Springer-Verlag; New York: 1989, pp. 297–310.

62 Fouts AC, Kraus SJ. *Trichomonas vaginalis*: reevaluation of its clinical presentation and laboratory diagnosis. *J Infect Dis* 1980; **141**: 137–143.

63 Pert G. Errors in the diagnosis of *Trichomonas vaginalis* infection as observed among 1199 patients. *Obstet Gynecol* 1972; **39**: 7–9.

64 Sobrepena RL. Identification of *Trichomonas vaginalis* in Gram-stained smears. *Lab Med* 1980; **11**: 558–560.

65 Chang TH, Tsing SY, Tzeng S. Monoclonal antibodies against *Trichomonas vaginalis*. *Hybridoma* 1986; **5**: 43–51.

66 O'Hara CM, Gardner WA, Bennett BD. Immunoperoxidase staining of *Trichomonas vaginalis* in cytologic material. *Acta Cytol* 1980; **24**: 448–451.

67 Yule A, Gellan MCA, Oriel JD, Ackers JP. Detection of *Trichomonas vaginalis* antigen in women by enzyme immunoassay. *J Clin Pathol* 1987; **40**: 566–568.

68 Carney JA, Unadkat P, Yule A, Rajakumar R, Lacey CJN, Ackers JP. New rapid latex agglutination test for diagnosing *Trichomonas vaginalis* infection. *J Clin Pathol* 1988; **41**: 806–808.

69 Linstead D. Cultivation. In: Honigberg BM, (ed.) *Trichomonads Parasitic in Humans.* Springer-Verlag; New York: 1989, pp. 91–111.

70 Smith RF. Incubation time, second blind passage and cost considerations in the isolation of *Trichomonas vaginalis*. *J Clin Microbiol* 1986; **24**: 139–140.

71 Borchardt KA, Smith RF. An evaluation of an InPouch™ TV culture method for diagnosing *Trichomonas vaginalis* infection. *Genitourin Med* 1991; **67**: 149–152.

72 Borchardt KA, Zhang MZ, Shing H, Flink K. A comparison of the sensitivity of the InPouch TV, Diamond's, and Trichosel media for detection of *Trichomonas vaginalis*. *Genitourin Med* 1997; **73**: 297–298.

73 Rubino S, Muresu R, Rapelli P, *et al.* Molecular probe for identification of *Trichomonas vaginalis* DNA. *J Clin Microbiol* 1991; **29**: 465–472.

74 Muresu R, Rubino S, Rizzu P, Baldini A, Colombo M, Cappuccinelli P. A new method for identification of *Trichomonas vaginalis* by fluorescent DNA in situ hybridization. *J Clin Microbiol* 1994; **32**: 1018–1022.

75 Shaio M-F, Lin P-R, Liu J-Y. Colorimetric one-tube nested PCR for detection of *Trichomonas vaginalis* in vaginal discharge. *J Clin Micobiol* 1997; **35**: 132–138.

76 Heine RP, Wiesenfeld HC, Sweet RL, Witkin SS. Polymerase chain reaction analysis of distal vaginal specimens: a less invasive strategy for detection of *Trichomonas vaginalis*. *Clin Infect Dis* 1997; **24**: 985–987.

77 Madico G, Quinn TC, Rompalo A, McKee KT, Gaydos CA. Diagnosis of *Trichomonas vaginalis* infection by PCR using vaginal swab samples. *J Clin Microbiol* 1998; **36**: 3205–3210.

78 Tabrizi SN Paterson BA, Fairley CK, Bowden FJ, Garland SM. Comparison of tampon and urine as self-administered methods of specimen collection in the detection of *Chlamydia trachomatis*, *Neisseria gonorrhoeae* and *Trichomonas vaginalis* in women. *Int J STD AIDS* 1998; **9**: 347–349.

79 Van der Schee C, van Belkum A, Zwijgers L, *et al.* Improved diagnosis of *Trichomonas vaginalis* infection by PCR using vaginal swabs and urine specimens compared to diagnosis by wet mount microscopy, culture, and fluorescent staining. *J Clin Microbiol* 1999; **37**: 4127–4130.

80 Meingassner JG, Stockinger K. In vitro studies on the identification of metronidazole-resistant strains of *T. vaginalis. Z Haut Krankheiten* 1981; **56**: 7–15.

81 Ralph ED. Clinical pharmacokinetics of metronidazole. *Clin Parmacokinet* 1983; **8**: 43–62.

82 Muller M. Mode of action of metronidazole on anaerobic bacteria and protozoa. *Surgery* 1983; **93**: 165–171.

83 Muller M, Gorrell TE. Metabolism and metronidazole uptake in *Trichomonas vaginalis* isolates with different metronidazole susceptibilities. *Antimicrob Agents Chemother* 1983; **24**: 667–673.

84 Nielsen MH. *In vitro* effect of metronidazole on the ultrastructure of *Trichomonas vaginalis* Donne. *Acta Pathol Microbiol Scand (B)* 1976; **84**: 93–100.

85 Meingassner JG, Heyworth PG. Intestinal and urogenital flagellates. *Antibiot Chemother* 1981; **30**: 163–202.

86 Muller M. Mode of action of metronidazole on anaerobic micro-organisms. In: Phillips I, Collier J (eds) *Metronidazole*. Academic Press; London: 1979; pp. 224–228.

87 Edwards DI, Shanson D. Metronidazole inactivity in aerobes. *J Antimicrob Chemother* 1980; **6**: 402–403.

88 Quon DV, d'Oliveira CE, Johnson PJ. Reduced transcription of the ferredoxin gene in metronidazole-resistant *Trichomonas vaginalis. Proc Natl Acad Sci USA* 1992; **89**: 4402–4406.

89 Coulter JR. Mutagenicity of metronidazole. *Lancet* 1979; **I**: 609.

90 Roe FJC. Metronidazole: review of uses and toxicity. *J Antimicrob Chemother* 1977; **3**: 205–212.

91 Ralph ED. Clinical pharmacokinetics of metronidazole. *Clin Parmacokinet* 1983; **8**: 43–62.

92 Lindmark DG, Muller M. Antitrichomonad action, mutagenicity and reduction of metronidazole and other nitroimidazoles. *Antimicrob Chemother* 1976; **10**: 476–482.

93 Lamp KC, Freeman CD, Klutman NE, Lacy MK. Phamacokinetics and pharmacodynamics of the nitroimidazole antimicrobials. *Clin Pharmacokinetics* 1999; **36**: 353–373.

94 Aubert JM, Sesta HJ. Treatment of vaginal trichomoniasis. *J Repro Med* 1982; **27**: 742–745.

95 Thin RN, Symonds MAE, Booker R, Cook S, Langlet F. Double blind comparison of a single dose and a five day course of metronidazole in the treatment of trichomoniasis. *Br J Vener Dis* 1979; **55**: 354–356.

96 Spence MR, Harwell TS, Davies MC, Smith JL. The minimum single oral metronidazole dose for treating trichomoniasis: a randomized, blinded study. *Obstet Gynecol* 1997; **89**: 699–703.

97 UK National guideline for the management of *Trichomonas vaginalis*. www.mssvd.org.uk/ceg.htm

98 Centers for Disease Control and Prevention. 2002 Guidelines for treatment of sexually

transmitted diseases. *MMWR* 2002; **51**: RR–6.

99 Duffy LF, Daum F, Fisher SE, *et al.* Peripheral neuropathy in Crohn's disease patients treated with metronidazole. *Gastroenterol* 1985; **88**: 681–684.

100 Lefebre Y, Heseltine HC. The peripheral white blood cells and metronidazole. *JAMA* 1965; **194**: 127–130.

101 Taylor JAT. Metronidazole and transient leukopenia. *JAMA* 1965; **194**: 1331–1332.

102 Davies DM (ed.). Disorders of the foetus and infant. In: *Textbook of Adverse Drug Reactions.* Oxford University Press; Oxford: 1981, pp. 71–113.

103 Hawkins DF. Effects of drugs taken in pregnancy on the foetus. *J Matern Child Health* 1976; 24.

104 Burtin P, Taddio A, Ariburnu O, Einarson TR, Koren G. Safety of metronidazole in pregnancy: a meta-analysis. *Obstet Gynecol* 1995; **172**: 525–529.

105 Caro-Paton D, Carvajal A, de Diego IM, Martin-Arias LH, Requejo A, Pinilla ER. Is metronidazole teratogenic? A meta-analysis. *Br J Clin Pharmacol* 1997; **44**: 179–182.

106 Czeizel AE, Rockenbauer M. A population based case-control teratological study of oral metronidazole treatment during pregnancy. *Br J Obstet Gynaecol* 1998; **105**: 322–327.

107 Dunn PM, Stewart-Brown S, Peel R. Metronidazole and the fetal alcohol syndrome. *Lancet* 1979; **ii**: 144.

108 American Pharmaceutical Association. In: *Evaluations of Drug Interactions* 2nd edition. Washington DC; American Pharmaceutical Association: 1976, p. 158.

109 Semer JM, Friedland P, Vaisberg M, Greenberg A. The use of metronidazole in the treatment of alcoholism. *Am J Psychiatr* 1966; **123**: 722–724.

110 Ripa T, Westrom L, Mardh PA, Anderson KE. Concentrations of tinidazole in body fluids and tissues in gynaecological patients. *Chemotherapy* 1977; **23**: 227–235.

111 Robertson DHH, Heyworth R, Harrison C, Lumsden WHR. Treatment failure in *Trichomonas vaginalis* infections in females. 2. Concentrations of metronidazole in plasma and vaginal content during normal and high dosage. *J Antimicrob Chemother* 1988; **21**: 373–378.

112 Meingassner JG, Mieth H, Lindmark DG, Muller M. Assay conditions and demonstration of nitroimidazole resistance to *Trichomonas foetus. Antimicrob Agents Chemother* 1978; **13**: 1–3.

113 Meingassner JG, Stockinger K. In vitro studies on the identification of metronidazole-resistant strains of *T. vaginalis. Z Haut Krankheiten* 1981; **56**: 7–15.

114 Lumsden WHR, Harrison C, Robertson DHH. Treatment failure in *Trichomonas vaginalis* in females. 2. In vitro estimation of the sensitivity of the organism to metronidazole. *J Antimicrob Chemother* 1988; **21**: 555–564.

115 Ralph ED, Clarke DA. Inactivation of metronidazole by anaerobic and aerobic bacteria. *Antimicrob Agents Chemother* 1978; **14**: 377–383.

116 Willmott F, Say J, Downey D, *et al.* Zinc and recalcitrant trichomoniasis. *Lancet* 1983; **I**: 1053.

117 Lossick JG. Epidemiology of urogenital trichomoniasis. In: Honigberg BM (ed.) *Trichomonads Parasitic in Humans.* Springer-Verlag; New York: 1989, pp. 311–323.

118 Lossick JG, Muller M, Gorrell RE. *In vitro* drug susceptibility and doses required for sure in metronidazole resistant vaginal trichomoniasis. *J Infect Dis* 1986; **153**; 948–955.

119 Narcisi EM, Secor WE. In vitro effect of tinidazole and furazolidone on metronidazole-resistant *Trichomonas vaginalis. Antimicrob Agents Chemother* 1996; **40**: 1121–1125.

120 Saurina G, DeMeo L, McCormack WM. Cure of metronidazole- and tinidazole-resistant trichomoniasis with use of high-dose oral and intravaginal tinidazole. *Clin Infect Dis* 1998; **26**: 1238–1239.

121 Pattman RS. Recalcitrant vaginal trichomoniasis. *Sex Transm Infect* 1999; **75**: 127–128.

122 Weston TET, Nicol CS. Natural history of trichomonal infection in males. *Br J Vener Dis* 1963; **39**: 251–257.

123 Rein MF. Current therapy of vulvovaginitis. *Sex Transm Dis* 1981; **8**: 316–320.

124 van der Walt JP, Yarrow D. Methods for the isolation, maintenance, classification and identification of yeasts. In: Kreger-van Rij NJW (ed.) *The Yeasts a Taxonomic Study* 3rd edition. Elsevier; Amsterdam: 1984, pp. 45–104.

125 Riggsby WS. Some recent developments in the molecular biology of medically important *Candida. Microbiol Sci* 1985; **2**: 257–263.

126 Meyer SA, Ahearn DG, Yarrow D. Genus 34 *Candida Berkhout.* In: Kreger-van Rij NJW (ed.) *The Yeasts a Taxonomic Study* 3rd edition. Elsevier; Amsterdam: 1984 pp. 841–843.

127 Odds FC. *Candida and Candidosis.* Leicester University Press; Leicester: 1979.

128 Do Carmo-Sousa L. Distribution of yeasts in nature. In: Rose AH, Harrison JS (eds) *The Yeasts, vol. 1, Biology of Yeasts.* Academic Press; London: 1969, pp. 79–105.

129 Beck-Sague CM, Jarvis TR. Secular trends in the epidemiology of nosocomial fungal infections in the United States. *J Infect Dis* 1993; **167**: 1247–1251.

130 Sanchez VT, Vazquez JA, Jones D, Dembry LM, Sobel JD, Zervos MJ. Epidemiology of nosocomial infection with *Candida lusitaniae. J Clin Microbiol* 1992; **30**: 3005–3008.

131 Sanchez VT, Vazquez JA, Barth-Jones D, Sobel JD, Zervos MJ. Nosocomial acquisitions of *Candida parapsilosis*: an epidemiological study. *Am J Med* 1993; **94**: 577–582.

132 Vazquez JA, Sanchez C, Dmuchowski C, Dembry L, Sobel JD, Zervos MJ. Nosocomial acquisition of *Candida albicans*: an epidemiological study. *J Infect Dis* 1993; **168**: 195–201.

133 Spinillo A, Nicola S, Colonna L, Maragoni E, Cavanna C, Michelone G. Frequency and significance of drug resistance in vulvovaginal candidiasis. *Obstet Gynecol Invest* 1994; **38**: 130–133.

134 Polonelli L, de Bernardi F, Conti M, *et al.* Idiotypic intravaginal vaccination to protect against candidal vaginitis by secretory, yeast killer toxin-like anti-idiotypic antibodies. *J Immunol* 1994; **152**: 3175–3182.

135 Fidel PL, Lynch ME, Sobel JD. *Candida*-specific cell-mediated immunity is demonstrable in mice with experimental vaginal candidiasis. *Infect Immun* 1993; **61**: 1990–1995

136 Fidel PL, Lynch ME, Sobel JD. *Candida*-specific Th1-type responsiveness in mice with experimental vaginal candidiasis. *Infect Immun* 1993; **61**: 4202–4207.

137 Fidel PL, Lynch ME, Sobel JD. Circulating CD4 and CD8 cells have little impact on host defense against experimental vaginal candidiasis. *Infect Immun* 1995; **63**: 2403–2408.

138 Fidel PL, Sobel JD. Immunopathogenesis of recurrent vulvovaginal candidiasis. *Clin Microbiol Rev* 1996; **9**: 335–348.

139 O'Connor MI, Sobel JD. Epidemiology of recurrent vulvovaginal candidiasis: identification and strain differences. *J Infect Dis* 1986; **154**: 358–363.

140 Fidel PL, Vazquez JA, Sobel JD. *Candida glabrata*: review of epidemiology, pathogenesis, and clinical disease with comparison to *C. albicans. Clin Microbiol Rev* 1999; **12**: 80–96.

141 Kimura LH, Pearsall NN. Adherence of *Candida albicans* to human buccal epithelial cells. *Infect Immun* 1978; **21**: 64–68.

142 Sobel JD, Myers PG, Kaye D, Levison ME. Adherence of *Candida albicans* to human vaginal and buccal epithelial cells. *J Infect Dis* 1981; **143**: 76–82.

143 McCourtie J, Douglas LJ. Relationship between cell surface composition of *Candida albicans* and adherence to acrylic after growth on different carbon sources. *Infect Immun* 1984; **45**: 6–12.

144 Hazen KC, Plotkin BJ, Klima DM. Influence of growth conditions on cell surface hydrophobicity of *Candida albicans* and

Candida glabrata. Infect Immun 1986; **54**: 269–271.

145 King RD, Lee JC, Morris AL. Adherence of *Candida albicans* and other *Candida* species to mucosal epithelial cells. *Infect Immun* 1980; **27**: 667–674.

146 Douglas LJ. Adhesion of pathogenic *Candida* species to host surfaces. *Microbiological Sciences* 1985; **2**: 243–247.

147 Klotz SA, Drutz AD, Harrison JL, Huppert M. Adherence and penetration of vascular endothelium by *Candida* yeasts. *Infect Immun* 1983; **42**: 374–384.

148 Kostetter MK. Adhesins and ligands involved in the interaction of *Candida* spp. With epithelial and endothelial surfaces. *Clin Microbiol Rev* 1994; **7**: 29–42.

149 Sobel JD, Muller G, Buckley HR. Critical role of germ tube formation in the pathogenesis of candidal vaginitis. *Infect Immun* 1984; **44**: 576–580.

150 Sobel JD, Muller G, McCormick JF. Experimental chronic vaginal candidosis in rats. *Sabouraudia* 1985; **23**: 199–206.

151 De Bernardis F, Agatensi L, Ross IK, et al. Evidence for a role for secreted aspartate proteinase of *Candida albicans* in vulvovaginal candidiasis. *J Infect Dis* 1990; **161**: 1276–1283.

152 De Bernardis F, Cassone A, Sturtevant J, Calderone R. Expression of *Candida albicans* SAP1 and SAP2 in experimental vaginitis. *Infect Immun* 1995; **63**: 1887–1892.

153 De Bernardis F, Mondello F, Scaravelli G, et al. High aspartyl proteinase production and vaginitis in human immunodeficiency virus-infected women. *J Clin Microbiol* 1999; **37**: 1376–1380.

154 Ibrahim AS, Mirbod F, Filler SG, et al. Evidence implicating phospholipase as a virulence factor of *Candida albicans*. *Infect Immun* 1995; **63**: 1993–1998.

155 Soll DR, Galask R, Isley S, et al. Switching of *Candida albicans* during successive episodes of recurrent vaginitis. *J Clin Microbiol* 1989; **27**: 681–690.

156 De Bernardis F, Molinari A, Boccanera M, et al. Modulation of cell surface-associated mannoprotein antigen expression in experimental candidal vaginitis. *Infect Immun* 1994; **62**: 509–519.

157 Madani ND, Malloy PJ, Roriguez-Pombo P, Krishnan AV, Feldman D. *Candida albicans* estrogen-binding protein gene encodes an oxidoreductase that is inhibited by estradiol. *Proc Natl Acad Sci* 1994; **91**: 922–926.

158 Spellacy WN, Zaias N, Buhi WC, Birk SA. Vaginal yeast growth and contraceptive practice. *Obstet Gynecol* 1971; **38**: 343–349.

159 Foxman B. The epidemiology of vulvovaginal candidiasis: risk factors. *Am J Public Health* 1990; **80**: 329–331.

160 Lynch ME, Sobel JD, Fidel PL. Role of antifungal resistance in the pathogenesis of recurrent vulvovaginal candidiasis. *J Med Vet Mycol* 1996; **34**: 337–339.

161 White MH. Is vulvovaginal candidiasis an AIDS-related illness? *Clin Infect Dis* 1996; **22** (Suppl. 2): S124–S127.

162 Witkin SS, Kalo-Klein A, Galland L, Teich M, Ledger WJ. A macrophage defect in women with recurrent *Candida* vaginitis and its reversal in vitro by prostaglandin inhibitors. *Am J Obstet Gynecol* 1986; **155**: 790–795.

163 Fidel PL, Lynch ME, Redondo-Lopez V, Sobel JD, Robinson R. Systemic cell-mediated immune reactivity in women with recurrent vulvovaginal candidiasis (RVVC). *J Infect Dis* 1993; **168**: 1458–1465.

164 Regulez P, Garcia Fernandez JF, Moragues MD, Schneider J, Quindos G, Ponton J. Detection of anti-*Candida albicans* IgE antibodies in vaginal washes from patients with acute vulvovaginal candidiasis. *Gynecol Obstet Invest* 1994; **37**: 110–114.

165 Rigg D, Miller MM, Metzger WJ. Recurrent allergic vulvovaginitis: treatment with *Candida albicans* allergen immunotherapy. *Am J Obstet Gynecol* 1990; **162**: 332–336.

166 Witkin SS, Jeremias J, Ledger WJ. Effect of *Candida albicans* plus histamine on prostaglandin E2 production by peripheral blood mononuclear cells from healthy women and women with recurrent candidal vaginitis. *J Infect Dis* 1991; **164**: 396–399.

167 Lynch ME, Fidel PL, Sobel JD. Characterization of a *Candida albicans* germ tube inhibitor in culture supernatants from stimulated peripheral blood mononuclear cells. In: *Abstracts of the 94th General Meeting of the American Society for Microbiology*. Washington DC; American Society for Microbiology: 1994, Abstract F-22.

168 Gardner HL, Kaufman RH. *Benign Diseases of the Vulva and Vagina*. Mosby; St Louis: 1969, pp. 149–167.

169 Cawson RA, Rajasingham KC. Ultrastructural features of the invasive phase of *Candida albicans*. *Br J Dermatol* 1972; **87**: 435–443.

170 Heller C, Hoyt V. Squamous cell changes associated with the presence of *Candida* sp. in cervical-vaginal Papanicalaou smear. *Acta Cytol* 1971; **15**: 379–384.

171 Geiger AM, Foxman B, Sobel JD. Chronic vulvovaginal candidiasis: characteristics of women with *Candida albicans*, *Candida glabrata*, and no *Candida*. *Genitourin Med* 1995; **71**: 304–307.

172 Hopwood V, Evans EGV, Carney JA. Rapid diagnosis of vaginal candidosis by latex particle agglutination. *J Clin Pathol* 1985; **38**: 455–458.

173 Gentles JC, La Touche CJ. Yeasts as human and animal pathogens. In: Rose AH, Harrison JS (eds) *The Yeasts, vol. 1, Biology of Yeasts*. Academic Press; London: 1969, pp. 107–182.

174 Kreger-van Rij NJW (ed.). *The Yeasts, a Taxonomic Study* 3rd edition. Elsevier; Amsterdam: 1984.

175 White TC, Marr KA, Bowden RA. Clinical, cellular, and molecular factors that contribute to antifungal resistance. *Clin Microbiol Rev* 1998; **11**: 382–402.

176 Ghannoum MA, Rice LB. Antifungal agents: mode of action, mechanisms of resistance, and correlation of these mechanisms with bacterial resistance. *Clin Microbiol Rev* 1999; **12**: 501–517.

177 Masterton G, Henderson J, Napier IR, Moffet M. Six-day clotrimazole therapy in vaginal candidiasis. *Curr Med Res* 1975; **3**: 83–88.

178 Milsom I, Forssman L. Treatment of vaginal candidosis with a single 500-mg clotrimazole pessary. *Br J Vener Dis* 1982; **58**: 124–126.

179 Odds FC, MacDonald F. Persistence of miconazole in vaginal secretions after single applications. *Br J Vener Dis* 1981; **57**: 400–401.

180 Eliot BW, Howat RC, Mack AE. A comparison between the effects of nystatin, clotrimazole and miconazole on vaginal candidiasis. *Br J Obstet Gynaecol* 1979; **86**: 572–577.

181 Vukovich RA, Heald A, Darragh A. Vaginal absorption of two imidazole antifungal agents, econazole and miconazole. *Clin Pharmacol Ther* 1977; **21**: 121.

182 Gabriel G, Thin RNT. Clotrimazole and econazole in the treatment of vaginal candidosis. *Br J Vener Dis* 1983; **59**: 56–58.

183 Houang ET, Chappatte O, Byrne D, Macrae PV, Thorpe JE. Fluconazole levels in plasma and vaginal secretions of patients after a 150-milligram single oral dose and rate of eradication of infection in vaginal candidiasis. *Antimicrob Agents Chemother* 1990; **34**: 909–910.

184 Mastroiacovo P, Mazzone T, Botto LD, et al. Prospective assessment of pregnancy outcomes after first-trimester exposure to fluconazole. *Am J Obstet Gynecol* 1996; **175**: 1645–1650.

185 Woolley PD, Higgins SP. Comparison of clotrimazole, fluconazole and itraconazole in vaginal candidiasis. *Br J Clin Pract* 1995; **49**: 65–69.

186 Prasertsawat O, Bourlert A. Comparative study of fluconazole and clotrimazole for the treatment of vulvovaginal candidiasis. *Sex Transm Dis* 1995; **22**: 228–230.

187 Stein GE, Mummaw N. Placebo-controlled trial of itraconazole for treatment of acute vaginal candidiasis. *Antimicrob Agents Chemother* 1993; **37**: 89–92.

188 Astahova AV. Drugs; ketoconazole and the liver. In: Dukes MNG (ed.) *Side Effects of Drugs* Annual 7, Ch. 8. Excerpta Medica; Amsterdam: 1983, pp. 287–293.

189 Rollman O, Loof L. Hepatic toxicity of ketoconazole. *Br J Dermatol* 1983; **108**: 376–378.

190 Schurmeyer TH, Nieschlag E. Ketoconazole-induced drop in serum and saliva testosterone. *Lancet* 1982; **ii**: 1098.

191 Astahova AV. Antifungal agents. In: Dukes MNG (ed.) *Side Effects of Drugs* Annual 9, Ch. 28. Excerpta Medica; Amsterdam: 1985, 246–250.

192 Rex JH, Pfaller MA, Galgiani JN, *et al.* Development of interpretive breakpoints for antifungal susceptibility testing: conceptual framework and analysis of in vitro-in vivo correlation data for fluconazole, itraconazole, and *Candida* infections. *Clin Infect Dis* 1996; **24**: 235–247.

193 Pfaller MA, Rex JH, Rinaldi MG. Antifungal susceptibility testing: technical advances and potential clinical applications. *Clin Infect Dis* 1997; **24**: 776–784.

194 Revankar SG, Kirkpatrick WR, McAtee RK, *et al.* Detection and significance of fluconazole resistance in oropharyngeal candidiasis in Human Immunodeficiency Virus-infected patients. *J Infect Dis* 1996; **174**: 821–827.

195 White TC. Antifungal drug resistance in *Candida albicans*. *ASM News* 1997; **63**: 427–433.

196 Vanden Bossche H, Marichai P, Odds FC, Le Jeune L, Coene MC. Characterization of an azole-resistant *Candida glabrata* isolate. *Antimicrob Agents Chemother* 1992; **36**: 2602–2610.

197 Parkinson T, Falconer DJ, Hitchcock C. Fluconazole resistance due to energy-dependent drug efflux in *Candida glabrata*. *Antimicrob Agents Chemother* 1995; **39**: 1696–1699.

198 Sanglard D, Kuchler K, Ischer F, Pagani JL, Monod M, Bille J. Mechanisms of resistance to azole antifungal agents in *Candida albicans* isolates from AIDS patients involve specific multidrug transporters. *Antimicrob Agents Chemother* 1995; **39**: 2378–2386.

199 White TC. Increased mRNA levels of *ERG16*, *CDR*, and *MDR1* correlate with increases in azole resistance in *Candida albicans* isolates from a patient infected with human immunodeficiency virus. *Antimicrob Agents Chemother* 1997; **41**: 1482–1487.

200 Drutz DJ, Wood RA. Development of ergosterol-deficient amphotericin B resistant *Candida tropicalis* during therapy of *Candida* pyelonephritis. *Clin Res* 1973; **21**: 270.

201 Woods RA, Bard M, Jackson M, Drutz DJ. Resistance to polyene antibiotics and correlated sterol changes in two isolates of *Candida tropicalis* from a patient with an amphotericin B-resistant funguria. *J Infect Dis* 1974; **129**: 53–58.

202 Stiller R, Bennet J, Scholer J, Wall M, Polak A, Stevens DA. Susceptibility to 5-flucytosine and prevalence of serotype in 402 *Candida albicans* isolates from the United States. *Antimicrob Agents Chemother* 1982; **22**: 482–487.

203 Clinical Effectiveness Group. National guideline for the management of vulvovaginal candidiasis. *Sex Transm Inf* 1999; **75** (Suppl. 1): S19–S20.

204 Bingham JS. What to do with the patient with recurrent vulvovaginal candidiasis. *Sex Transm Inf* 1999; **75**: 225–227.

205 Centers for Disease Control and Prevention. 2002 Guidelines for treatment of sexually transmitted diseases. *MMWR* 2002; **51**: RR-6.

206 Sobel JD, Chaim W. Treatment of *Torulopsis glabrata* vaginitis: retrospective review of boric acid therapy. *Clin Infect Dis* 1997; **24**: 649–652.

207 Dukes MNG. Meyler's side effects of drugs. Amsterdam; Elsevier Science: 1996.

208 Culver BD. Vaginitis. *N Engl J Med* 1998; **338**: 1548–1549.

209 Stary A, Soeltz-Szoets J, Ziegler C, Kinghorn GR, Roy RB. Comparison of the efficacy and safety of oral fluconazole and topical clotrimazole in patients with candidal balanitis. *Genitourin Med* 1996; **72**: 98–102.

210 Parker MT. The pattern of streptococcal disease in man. In: Skinner FA, Quesnel LB (eds) *Streptococci*. London; Academic Press: 1978.

211 Ross PW. Ecology of group B streptococci. In: Skinner FA, Quesnel LB (eds) *Streptococci*. London; Academic Press: 1978.

212 Regan JA, Klebanoff MA, Nugent RP, *et al.* Colonization with group B streptococci in pregnancy and adverse outcome. *Am J Obstet Gynecol* 1996; **174**: 1354–1360.

213 Hillier SL, Krohn MA, Kiviat NB, Watts DH, Eschenbach DA. Microbial etiology and neonatal outcomes associated with chorioamnion infection. *Am J Obstet Gynecol* 1991; **165**: 955–960.

214 Krohn MA, Hillier SL, Baker CJ. Maternal peripartum complications associated with vaginal group B streptococci colonization. *J Infect Dis* 1999; **179**: 1410–1415.

215 Christensen KK, Christensen P, Flamhole L, Ripa T. Frequencies of streptococci in groups A, B, C, D and G in urethra and cervix swab specimens from patients with suspected gonococcal infection. *Acta Pathol Microbiol Scand Section B* 1974; **82**: 470–474.

216 Finch RG, French GL, Phillips I. Group B streptococci in the female genital tract. *Br Med J* 1976; **1**: 1245–1247.

217 Christensen KK, Dykes A-K, Christensen P. Relation between the use of tampons and urogenital carriage of group B streptococci. *Br Med J* 1984; **289**: 731–732.

218 Editorial. Prevention of early onset group B streptococcal infection in the newborn. *Lancet* 1984; **i**: 1056–1057.

219 Schuchat A. Epidemiology of group B streptococcal disease in the United States: shifting paradigms. *Clin Microbiol Rev* 1999; **11**: 497–513.

219a Anonymous. Prevention of perinatal group B streptococcal disease: a public health perspective. *MMWR* 1996; **45** (RR-7): 1–24.

220 Anonymous. Revised guidelines for prevention of early-onset group B streptococcal (GBS) infection. American Academy of Pediatrics Committee on Infectious Diseases and Committee on Fetus and Newborn. *Pediatrics* 1997; **99**: 489–496.

221 Schrag SJ, Zywicki S, Farley MM, *et al.* Group B streptococcal disease in the era of intrapartum antibiotic prophylaxis. *N Engl J Med* 2000; **342**: 15–20.

221a Greenwood JR, Picket MJ. Transfer of *Haemophilus vaginalis* Gardner and Dukes to a new genus, *Gardnerella*: G vaginalis (Gardner and Dukes) comb nov. *Int J System Bacteriol* 1980; **30**: 170–178.

222 Gardner HL, Dukes CD. *Haemophilus vaginalis* vaginitis. *Am J Obstet Gynecol* 1955; **69**: 962–976.

223 Frampton J, Lee Y. Is *Haemophilus vaginalis* a pathogen in the female genital tract? *J Obstet Gynaecol Br Commonw* 1964; **71**: 436–442.

224 Spiegel CA, Escenbach DA, Amsel R, Holmes KK. Curved anaerobic bacteria in bacterial (nonspecific) vaginosis and their response to antimicrobial therapy. *J Infect Dis* 1983; **148**: 817–822.

225 Spiegel CA, Amsel R, Holmes KK. Diagnosis of bacterial vaginosis by direct gram stain of vaginal fluid. *J Clin Microbiol* 1983; **18**: 170–177.

226 Schwebke JR, Lukehart SA, Roberts MC, Hillier SL. Identification of two new antigenic subgroups within the genus *Mobiluncus*. *J Clin Microbiol* 1991; **29**: 2204–2208.

227 Spiegel CA, Amsel R, Eschenbach D, Schoenknecht F, Holmes KK. Anaerobic bacteria in nonspecific vaginitis. *N Engl J Med* 1980; **303**: 601–607.

228 Hillier SL, Krohn MA, Rabe LK, Klebanoff SJ, Eschnebach DA. Normal vaginal flora, H_2O_2-producing lactobacilli and bacterial vaginosis in pregnant women. *Clin Infect Dis* 1993a; **16** (Suppl. 4): S273–S281.

229 Pheifer TA, Forsyth PS, Durfee MA, Pollock HM, Holmes KK. Nonspecific vaginitis – role of *Haemophilus vaginalis* and treatment with metronidazole. *N Engl J Med* 1978; **298**: 1429–1434.

230 Blackwell AL, Fox AR, Phillips I, Barlow D. Anaerobic vaginosis (non-specific vaginitis): clinical, microbiological and therapeutic findings. *Lancet* 1983; **ii**: 1379–1382.

231 Chen KCS, Amsel R, Eschenbach DA, Holmes KK. Biochemical diagnosis of vaginitis: determination of diamines in vaginal fluid. *J Infect Dis* 1982; **145**: 337–345.

232 Brand JM, Galask RP. Trimethylamine: the substance mainly responsible for the fishy odor often associated with bacterial vaginosis. *Obstet Gynecol* 1986; **68**: 682–685.

233 Chen KCS, Forsyth PS, Buchanan TM, Holmes KK. Amine content of vaginal fluid from untreated and treated patients with nonspecific vaginitis. *J Clin Invest* 1978; **63**: 828–835.

234 Spiegel CA, Amsel R, Eschenbach D, Schoenknecht F, Holmes KK. Anaerobic bacteria in nonspecific vaginitis. *N Engl J Med* 1980; **303**: 601–607.

235 Schwebke JR, Richey CM, Weiss HL. Correlation of behaviors with microbiological changes in vaginal flora. *J Infect Dis* 1999; **180**: 1632–1636.

236 Amsel R, Totten PA, Spiegel CA, Chen KCS, Eschenbach DA, Holmes KK. Nonspecific vaginitis: diagnostic criteria and microbial and epidemiologic associations. *Am J Med* 1983; **74**: 14–22.

237 Mardh P-A, Holst E, Moller BR. The grivet monkey as a model for study of vaginitis. Challenge with anaerobic curved rods and *Gardnerella vaginalis. Scand J Urol Nephrol* 1984; **86** (Suppl.): 201–205.

238 Skarin A, Sylwan J. Vaginal lactobacilli inhibiting growth of *Gardnerella vaginalis, Mobiluncus* and other bacterial species cultured from vaginal content of women with bacterial vaginosis. *Acta Pathol Microbiol Immunol Scand. Sect B* 1986; **94**: 399–403.

239 Hillier SL, Krohn MA, Klebanoff SJ, Eschenbach DA. The relationship of hydrogen peroxide-producing lactobacilli to bacterial vaginosis and genital microflora in pregnant women. *Obstet Gynecol* 1992; **79**: 369–373.

240 Hawes SE, Hillier SL, Benedetti J, *et al.* Hydrogen peroxide-producing lactobacilli and acquisition of vaginal infections. *J Infect Dis* 1996; **174**: 1058–1063.

241 Klebanoff SJ, Hillier SL, Eschenbach DA, Waltersdorph AM. Control of the microbial flora of the vagina by H$_2$O$_2$-generating lactobacilli. *J Infect Dis* 1991; **164**: 94–100.

242 Rosenstein IJ, Fontaine EA, Morgan DJ, Sheehan M, Lamont RF, Taylor-Robinson D. Relationship between hydrogen peroxide-producing strains of lactobacilli and vaginosis-associated bacterial species in pregnant women. *Eur J Clin Microbiol Inf Dis* 1997; **16**: 517–522.

243 Ison C, Easmon CSF, Dawson SG, Southerton G, Harris JRW. Non-volatile fatty acids in the diagnosis of non-specific vaginitis. *J Clin Pathol* 1983; **36**: 1367–1370.

244 Sturm AW. Chemotaxis inhibition by *Gardnerella vaginalis* and succinate producing vaginal anaerobes: composition of vaginal discharge associated with *G. vaginalis. Genitourin Med* 1989; **65**: 109–112.

245 Briselden AM, Moncla BJ, Stevens CE, Hillier SL. Sialidases (neuraminidases) in bacterial vaginosis and bacterial vaginosis-associated microflora. *J Clin Microbiol* 1992; **30**: 663–666.

246 Howe L, Wiggins R, Soothill PW, Millar MR, Horner PJ, Corfield AP. Mucinase and sialidase activity of the vaginal microflora: implications for the pathogenesis of preterm labour. *Int J STD AIDS* 1999; **10**: 442–447.

247 Cauci S, Monte R, Driussi S, Lanzafame P, Quadrifoglio F. Impairment of the mucosal immune system: IgA and IgM cleavage detected in vaginal washings of a subgroup of patients with bacterial vaginosis. *J Infect Dis* 1998; **178**: 1698–1706.

248 Lamagni TL, Hughes G, Rogers PA, Paine T, Catchpole M. New cases seen at genitourinary medicine clinics: England 1998. *Commun Dis Rep* 1999; **9** (Suppl. 6): S2–S12.

249 Petersen CS, Danielsen AG, Renneberg J. Bacterial vaginosis: the leading cause of vaginal discharge in women attending an STD clinic in Copenhagen. *Acta Derm Venereol* 1999; **79**: 414–415.

250 Cristiano L, Rampello S, Noris C, Valota V. Bacterial vaginosis: prevalence in an Italian population of asymptomatic pregnant women and diagnostic aspects. *Eur J Epidemiol* 1996; **12**: 383–390.

251 Gratacos E, Figueras F, Barranco M, *et al.* Prevalence of bacterial vaginosis and correlation of clinical to Gram stain diagnostic criteria in low risk pregnant women. *Eur J Epidemiol* 1999; **15**: 913–916.

252 Puapermpoonsiri S, Kato N, Watanabe K, Ueno K, Chongsomchai C, Lumbiganon P. Vaginal microflora associated with bacterial vaginosis in Japanese and Thai pregnant women. *Clin Infect Dis* 1996; **23**: 748–752.

253 Larsson PG, Platz-Christensen JJ, Sundstrom E. Is bacterial vaginosis a sexually transmitted disease? *Int J STD AIDS* 1991; **2**: 362–364.

254 Holst E. Reservoir of four organisms associated with bacterial vaginosis suggests lack of sexual transmission. *J Clin Microbiol* 1990; **28**: 2035–2039.

255 Bump RC, Buesching WJ. Bacterial vaginosis in virginal and sexually active females: evidence against exclusive sexual transmission. *Am J Obstet Gynecol* 1988; **158**: 935–939.

256 Moi H, Erkkola R, Jerve F, *et al.* Should male consorts of women with bacterial vaginosis be treated? *Genitourin Med* 1989; **65**: 263–268.

257 Zenilman JM, Fresia A, Berger B, McCormack WM. Bacterial vaginosis is not associated with circumcision status of the current male partner. *Sex Transm Inf* 1999; **75**: 347–348.

258 Berger BJ, Kolton S, Zenilman JM, Cummings MC, Feldman J, McCormack WM. Bacterial vaginosis in lesbians: a sexually transmitted disease. *Clin Infect Dis* 1995; **21**: 1402–1405.

259 McCaffrey M, Varney P, Evans B, Taylor-Robinson D. Bacterial vaginosis in lesbians: evidence for lack of sexual transmission. *Int J STD AIDS* 1999; **10**: 305–308.

260 Cohen CR, Duerr A, Pruithithada N, *et al.* Bacterial vaginosis and HIV seroprevalence among female commercial sex industry workers in Chiang Mai, Thailand. *AIDS* 1995; **9**: 1093–1097.

261 Sewankambo N, Gray RH, Wawer MJ, *et al.* HIV-1 infection associated with abnormal vaginal flora morphology and bacterial vaginosis. *Lancet* 1997; **350**: 546–550.

262 Taha TE, Hoover DR, Dallabetta GA, *et al.* Bacterial vaginosis and disturbances of vaginal flora: association with increased acquisition of HIV. *AIDS* 1998; **12**: 1699–1706.

263 Martin HL, Richardson BA, Nyange PM, *et al.* Vaginal lactobacilli, microbial flora, and risk of human immunodeficiency virus type 1 and sexually transmitted disease acquisition. *J Infect Dis* 1999; **180**: 1863–1868.

264 Klebanoff SL, Coombs RW. Viricidal effect of *Lactobacillus acidophilus* on human immunodeficiency virus type 1: possible role in heterosexual transmission. *J Exp Med* 1991; **174**: 289–292.

265 Hashemi F, Ghassemi M, Roebuck KA, *et al.* Activation of human immunodeficiency virus type 1 expression by *Gardnerella vaginalis. J Infect Dis* 1999; **179**: 924–930.

266 Al-Harti L, Roebuck KA, Olinger GG, *et al.* Bacterial vaginosis-associated microflora isolated from the female genital tract activates HIV-1 expression. *J Acquir Immune Defic Syndr Hum Retrovirol* 1999; **21**: 194–202.

267 Olinger GG, Hashemi FB, Sha BE, Spear GT. Association if indicators of bacterial vaginosis with a female genital tract factor that induces expression of HIV-1. *AIDS* 1999; **13**: 1905–1912.

268 Cohen CR, Plummer FA, Mugo N, *et al.* Increased interleukin-10 in the endocervical secretions of women with non-ulcerative sexually transmitted diseases: a mechanism for enhanced HIV-1 transmission? *AIDS* 1999; **13**: 827–832.

269 O'Dowd TC, West RR, Winterburn PJ, Hewlins MJ. Evaluation of a rapid diagnostic test for bacterial vaginosis. *Br J Obstet Gynaecol* 1996; **103**: 366–370.

270 Nugent RP, Krohn MA, Hillier SL. Reliability of diagnosing bacterial vaginosis is improved by a standardized method of

Gram stain interpretation. *J Clin Microbiol* 1991; **29**: 297–301.

271 Schwebke JR, Hillier SL, Sobel JD, McGregor JA, Sweet RL. Validity of the vaginal gram stain for the diagnosis of bacterial vaginosis. *Obstet Gynecol* 1996; **88**: 573–576.

272 Thomason JL, Anderson RJ, Gelbart SM, *et al*. Simplified Gram stain interpretive method for diagnosis of bacterial vaginosis. *Am J Obstet Gynecol* 1992; **167**: 16–19.

273 Hillier SL. Clindamycin treatment of bacterial vaginosis. *Rev Contemp Pharmacother* 1992; **3**: 263–268.

274 Balsdon J, Taylor GE, Pead L, Maskell R. *Corynebacterium vaginale* and vaginitis: a controlled trial of treatment. *Lancet* 1980; **i**: 501–504.

275 Ralph ED, Austin TW, Pattison FL, Schieven BC. Inhibition of *Haemophilus vaginalis* (*Corynebacterium vaginale*) by metronidazole, tetracycline and ampicillin. *Sex Transm Dis* 1979; **6**: 199–202.

276 Easmon CSF, Ison CA, Kaye CM, Timewell RM, Dawson SG. Pharmacokinetics of metronidazole and its principal metabolites and their activity against *Gardnerella vaginalis*. *Br J Vener Dis* 1982; **58**: 246–249.

277 May and Baker. *Anaerobicidal-agent, Flagyl (metronidazole)* 2nd edition. Essex; May and Baker; 1980: pp. 1–15.

278 Larsson PG. Treatment of bacterial vaginosis. *Int J STD AIDS* 1992; **3**: 239–247.

279 Hillier SL, Lipinski C, Briselden AM, Eschenbach DA. Efficacy of intra-vaginal 0.75% metronidazole gel for the treatment of bacterial vaginosis. *Obstet Gynecol* 1993; **81**: 963–967.

280 Centers for Disease Control and Prevention. 2002 Guidelines for treatment of sexually transmitted diseases. *MMWR* 2002; **51**: RR-6.

281 Greaves WL, Chungafung J, Morris B, Haile A, Townsend JL. Clindamycin versus metronidazole in the treatment of bacterial vaginosis. *Obstet Gynecol* 1988; **72**: 799–802.

282 Hillier SL, Krohn MA, Watts DH, Wolner-Hanssen P, Eschenbach DA. Microbiologic efficacy of intravaginal clindamycin cream for the treatment of bacterial vaginosis. *Obstet Gynecol* 1990; **76**: 407–413.

283 Joesoef MR, Schmid GP, Hillier SL. Bacterial vaginosis: review of treatment options and potential clinical indications for therapy. *Clin Infect Dis* 1999; **28** (Suppl. 1): S57–S65.

284 Eschenbach DA. Bacterial vaginosis. In: Hitchcock PJ, MacKay HT, Wasserheit JN (eds) *Sexually Transmitted Diseases and Adverse Outcomes of Pregnancy*. Washington DC; ASM Press; 1999.

285 Gravett MG, Hummel D, Eschenbach DA, Holmes KK. Preterm labor associated with

subclinical amniotic fluid infection and with bacterial vaginosis. *Obstet Gynecol* 1986; **67**: 229–237.

286 Hillier SL, Martius J, Krohn MA, Kiviat NB, Holmes KK, Eschenbach DA. A case-control study of chorioamniotic infection and chorioamnionitis in prematurity. *N Engl J Med* 1988; **319**: 972–978.

287 Simpson JL. Fetal wastage. In: Gabbe S, Niebyl JR, Simpson JL (eds) *Obstetrics: Normal and Problem Pregnancies*. New York; Churchill Livingstone; 1996.

288 Watts DH, Krohn MA, Hillier SL, Eschenbach DA. Bacterial vaginosis as a risk factor for postcesarean endometritis. *Obstet Gynecol* 1990; **75**: 52–58.

289 Newton ER, Piper J, Peairs W. Bacterial vaginosis and intraamniotic infection. *Am J Obstet Gynecol* 1997; **176**: 672–677.

290 Hauth JC, Goldenberg RL, Andrews WW, DuBard MB, Copper RL. Reduced incidence of preterm delivery with metronidazole and erythromycin in women with bacterial vaginosis. *N Engl J Med* 1995; **333**: 1732–1736.

291 Carey JC, Klebanoff MA, Hauth JC, *et al*. Metronidazole to prevent preterm delivery in pregnant women with asymptomatic bacterial vaginosis. *N Engl J Med* 2000; **342**: 534–540.

292 McDonald HM, O'Loughlin JA, Vigneswaran R, *et al*. Impact of metronidazole therapy on preterm birth in women with bacterial vaginosis flora (*Gardnerella vaginalis*): a randomised, placebo-controlled trial. *Br J Obstet Gynaecol* 1997; **104**: 1391–1397.

293 Ralph SG, Rutherford AJ, Wilson JD. Influence of bacterial vaginosis on conception and miscarriage in the first trimester: cohort study. *Br Med J* 1999; **319**: 220–223.

294 Liversedge NH, Turner A, Horner PJ, Keay SD, Jenkins JM, Hull MG. The influence of bacterial vaginosis on in-vitro fertilization and embryo implantation during assisted reproduction treatment. *Hum Reprod* 1999; **14**: 2411–2415.

295 Morales WJ, Schorr S, Albritton J. Effect of metronidazole in patients with preterm birth in preceding pregnancy and bacterial vaginosis: a placebo-controlled, double blind study. *Am J Obstet Gynecol* 1994; **171**: 345–347.

296 McGregor JA, French JL, Jones W, *et al*. Bacterial vaginosis is associated with prematurity and vaginal fluid mucinase and sialidase: results of a controlled trial of topical clindamycin cream. *Am J Obstet Gynecol* 1994; **170**: 1048–1059.

297 Joesoef MR, Hillier SL, Wiknjosastro G, *et al*. Intravaginal clindamycin cream for bacterial vaginosis: effects on preterm delivery and low birth weight. *Am J Obstet Gynecol* 1995; **173**: 1527–1531.

298 Lin L, Song J, Kimber N, *et al*. The role of bacterial vaginosis in infection after major

gynecologic surgery. *Inf Dis Obstet Gynecol* 1999; **7**: 169–174.

299 Larsson PG, Bergman B, Forsum U, Platz-Christensen JJ, Pahlson C. Mobiluncus and clue cells as predictors of PID after first-trimester abortion. *Acta Obstet Gynecol Scand* 1989; **68**: 217–220.

300 Larsson PG, Platz-Christensen JJ, Thejls H, Forsum U, Pahlson C. Incidence of pelvic inflammatory disease after first-trimester legal abortion in women with bacterial vaginosis after treatment with metronidazole: a double-blind, randomized study. *Am J Obstet Gynecol* 1992; **166**: 100–103.

301 Duguid HLD, Parratt D, Traynor R, *et al*. Studies on uterine tract infections and the IUCD with special reference to actinomycetes. IUCD Workshop, London, 1982. *Br J Obstet Gynaecol* 1982; Suppl. 4: 32–40.

302 Duguid H, Duncan I, Parratt D, Traynor R. Actinomyces and intrauterine devices. *JAMA* 1982; **248**: 1379.

303 Duguid HLD, Duncan ID, Parratt D, Taylor D. Risk of intrauterine devices. *Br Med J* 1984; **289**: 767.

304 Lippes J. Pelvic actinomycosis: a review and preliminary look at prevalence. *Am J Obstet Gynecol* 1999; **180**: 265–269.

305 Petitti DB, Yamamoto D, Morgenstern N. Factors associated with actinomyces-like organisms on Papanicolaou smear in users of intrauterine contraceptive devices. *Am J Obstet Gynecol* 1983; **145**: 338–341.

306 O'Brien PK, Roth-Mayo LA, Davis BA. Pseudo-sulfur granules associated with intrauterine contraceptive devices. *Am J Clin Pathol* 1981; **75**: 822–825.

307 Holmberg L. Diagnostic methods for human actinomycosis. *Microbiol Sci* 1987; **4**: 72–78.

308 Cayley J, Fotherby K, Guillebaud J, *et al*. Recommendations for clinical practice: actinomyces like organisms and intrauterine contraceptives. The Clinical and Scientific Committee. *Br J Fam Plann* 1998; **23**: 137–138.

309 Shands KN, Schmid GP, Dan BB, *et al*. Toxic-shock syndrome in menstruating women. Association with tampon use and *Staphylococcus aureus* and clinical features in 52 cases. *N Engl J Med* 1980; **303**: 1436–1442.

310 Davis JP, Chesney PJ, Wand PJ, La Venturi M, and the Investigation and Laboratory Team. Toxic shock syndrome: epidemiologic features, recurring risk factors and prevention. *N Engl J Med* 1980; **303**: 1429–1435.

311 Davis GD, Hutchison CV. Clinical management of vulvodynia. *Clin Obstet Gynecol* 1999; **42**: 221–233.

312 Chadha S, Gianotten WL, Drogendijk AC, Weijmar Schultz WC, Blindeman LA, van

der Meijden WI. Histopathologic features of vulvar vestibulitis. *Int J Gynecol Pathol* 1998; **17**: 7–11.

313 McKay M. Vulvodynia: diagnostic patterns. *Dermatol Clin* 1992; **10**: 423–433.

314 Honigberg BM, King VM Structure of *Trichomonas vaginalis* Donne. *J Parasitol* 1964; **50**: 345–364.

315 McMillan A, Scott GR. *Sexually Transmitted Infections, Colour Guide*. Churchill Livingstone; Edinburgh: 2000.

316 Rein MF (ed.). *Atlas of Infectious Diseases, Volume V, Sexually Transmitted Diseases*. Churchill Livingstone; Philadelphia: 1996.

Chapter 18

Intestinal and anorectal disorders in homosexual men
A McMillan

Infections

During sexual contact amongst men who have sex with men, the transmission of organisms that infect the intestinal tract, i.e. viruses, bacteria, protozoa, and nematodes, may take place and is well-recognized as important. Although these infections can also affect women, there is little evidence that they are as prevalent in women as in homosexual men. In the case of certain infective agents or organisms, these are acquired directly as a result of penetration of the rectum in anorectal intercourse, but in the case of others, their habitat is intestinal and transmission occurs by ingestion of fecal material during oral–anal or oral–genital contact. Extensive fecal contamination of the skin surface that occurs during anal sexual intercourse facilitates transmission of enteric organisms. With respect to intestinal protozoa, in geographical localities where the overall prevalence is high, prevalence of intestinal protozoa among homosexual males may be expected to be very high; in areas of low prevalence, the prevalence among homosexual males will be higher than in the general population.

PROCTOCOLITIS

This is a common disorder amongst men who have had homosexual contact. Although proctitis can result from a wide variety of insults including irradiation, chemicals, and drug therapy, most cases amongst homosexual men are associated with infection. It should be remembered, however, that men with idiopathic inflammatory bowel disease may present to an STI clinic in the belief that their symptoms are related to anal intercourse.

Etiology

Proctitis may result from infection with organisms or agents acquired either by mucosa–skin contact (through anal intercourse) or through the fecal–oral route. The first group includes *Treponema pallidum*, *Neisseria gonorrhoeae*, *Chlamydia trachomatis*, and herpes simplex virus (HSV). The second group consists of enteric organisms such as *Entamoeba histolytica*, *Shigella* spp., *Campylobacter* spp., and *Cryptosporidium* spp. Infection with two or more organisms is common; in a study by Quinn *et al.*[1] 22 out of 119 men with proctitis were infected with two or more organisms or agents. The characteristics of intestinal infection with these organisms, their role in the etiology of proctitis, and their diagnosis and treatment are discussed in separate sections in this chapter. There is also a group of patients with clinical features of proctitis but in whom no specific cause can be identified (non-specific proctitis). In some cases an infective cause may not have been identified and in others repeated rectal trauma may be the cause. Irrespective of the cause of non-specific proctitis, there is a strong relationship between this condition and seropositivity for HIV: the adjusted odds ratio for the association of histologically confirmed proctitis with HIV infection was 8.2 (95% confidence interval 2.1–31.8) in the study reported by Law *et al.*[2].

Pathology

In the early stages (0 to 4 days after the onset of symptoms) of *acute infective proctitis*[3] there is mucosal edema, with infiltration of the lamina propria with neutrophils and, to a much lesser extent, with lymphocytes and plasma cells. Polymorphs migrating between the epithelial cells of the mucosal surface and crypts, which may be eroded (Figure 18.1), hemorrhages are common and crypt abscesses may be a feature.

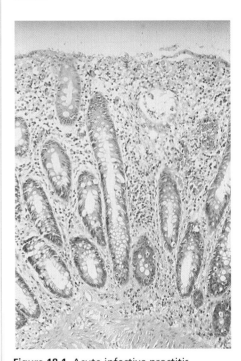

Figure 18.1 Acute infective proctitis showing mucosal erosion, vasodilatation of the vessels of the lamina propria with a polymorphonuclear infiltrate, and hemorrhage (hematoxylin and eosin, × 60)

As the acute inflammatory response resolves, the mucosal edema becomes less pronounced and there is regeneration of the surface and crypt epithelium, the goblet cells of which show mucus depletion. The neutrophil content of the lamina propria is less pronounced, but there is a moderate increase in the numbers of lymphocytes, plasma cells, and eosinophils.

Generally these histological findings are not specific for any particular organism, but in both syphilis and chlamydial infections with lymphogranuloma venereum serovars granulomas may be formed, and in herpetic proctitis intranuclear inclusions are to be seen.

Certain histological features usually help to differentiate an acute, self-limiting proctocolitis from ulcerative colitis and Crohn's disease

1. a lack of distortion of the crypt architecture
2. a lack of marked mucus depletion of the goblet cells in the acute stage
3. only a moderate increase in the numbers of mononuclear cells in the lamina propria[4].

Occasionally, however, differentiation between the two conditions is not possible.

Clinical features

The most common clinical features of *acute proctocolitis* are mucopurulent anal discharge (in mild cases mucus streaking of the stool) diarrhea, anorectal bleeding, perianal pain, and a sensation of incomplete defecation. Lower abdominal pain and tenderness over

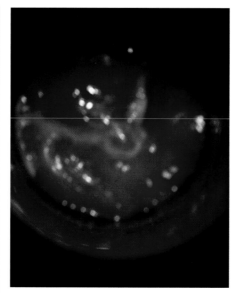

Figure 18.2 Gonococcal proctitis showing mucopus in the lumen of rectum

the colon are features more characteristic of colitis. At sigmoidoscopy there is often mucopus on the mucosa (Figure 18.2), which usually shows loss of the normal ramifying vascular pattern, edema, contact bleeding, and sometimes ulceration. It should be noted that the vascular pattern is often absent from the distal 10 cm of the normal rectum. Sometimes, in the presence of gross microscopic disease, the rectal mucosa appears normal to the naked eye[5].

Generally, in patients with gonococcal, chlamydial, herpetic and early-stage syphilitic infection, the inflammation is principally restricted to the rectum, but in amoebic and bacterial dysentery the inflammatory process is seen to extend beyond the rectosigmoid junction. Double-contrast barium enema examination in patients with proctitis shows nodularity and ulceration of the mucosa[6].

In patients with *chronic proctitis* symptoms are usually mild and consist of intermittent anal discharge or mucus streaking of the stool and anorectal bleeding. The sigmoidoscopic appearance of the mucosa is usually normal[7].

Diagnosis

The enumeration of polymorphs in a smear of rectal exudate, obtained by rolling a cotton-wool-tipped applicator stick over the mucosa, is an unreliable and unnecessary investigation when the proctoscopic and sigmoidoscopic appearance is consistent with acute proctitis. There is little correlation between the numbers of cells and the histology. Although McMillan *et al.*[7], using impression smears, found good correlation between the cytological and histological findings in patients with acute infective proctitis, the method is inconvenient and does not lend itself to use in a busy clinic. In most cases a diagnosis can be made on the basis of the symptoms and proctoscopic findings. Cytology is of little value in the detection of chronic proctitis.

The appropriate specimens for microbiological examination should be obtained as detailed on pp. 54–55. When these investigations are unhelpful and the patient's symptoms persist sigmoidoscopy, plus rectal biopsy and radiological examination of the colon, are indicated to exclude ulcerative proctocolitis and Crohn's disease.

Table 18.1 Prevalence of intestinal protozoa in homosexual men. References: 1. William *et al.*[120]; 2. Phillips *et al.*[61]; 3. Markell *et al.*[8]; 4. Keystone *et al.*[121]; 5. McMillan (1982, unpublished data); 6. McMillan[122]; 7. Chin & Gerken[123]

Organism	Studies on prevalence (numbers examined)						
	New York City[1] (89)	New York City[2] (99)	San Francisco[3] (508)	Toronto[4] (200)	Edinburgh[5] (310)	Glasgow[6] (118)	London[7] (83)
Entamoeba histolytica	20	11	29	27	10	3	12
Entamoeba hartmanni	–	–	25	–	1	–	5
Entamoeba coli	13	–	21	–	10	–	25
Endolimax nana	11	–	38	–	5	–	22
Iodamoeba butschlii	5	–	13	–	2	1	4
Giardia duodenalis	12	4	6	13	6	2	8
Dientamoeba fragilis	1	–	1	–	0	–	–
Chilomastix mesnili	–	–	1	–	1	–	–

Table 18.2 Microscopic features of the intestinal flagellates and ciliates

Protozoon	Shape and size	Nuclear characteristics (stained smear)	Number and position of flagella	Other features
TROPHOZOITES **Flagellates**				
Retortamonas intestinalis	Pear shaped 4–9 μm × 3–4 μm	Spherical nucleus anterior end of organisms.	1 anterior, 1 recurrent	Ventral cytostome extending half-way down body.
Enteromonas hominis	Pear shaped 4–10 μm × 306 μm	Anterior oval nucleus with eccentric endosome.	3 anterior long posterior	Narrow cytostome, prominent funis on left of cytostome extending for two-thirds of body length.
Chilomastix mesnili	Pear shaped, Rounded anteriorly, tail-like posterior projection 6–20 μm × 4–7 μm	Round anterior nucleus with several peripheral deeply staining plaques.	3 anterior short recurrent	Prominent cytostomal groove with long posteriorly curved right cytostomal fiber.
Giardia intestinalis	Pear shaped 10–20 μm × 5–15 μm	2 with large endosomes	2 ventral, 2 anterolateral, 2 posterolateral, 2 caudal	
Dientamoeba fragilis	3.5 × 22 μm Moves by extension of broad hyaline pseudopodia	Usually 2 nuclei but not uncommonly 1 only, large central endosome; no peripheral chromatin.	–	–
Ciliate				
Balantidium coli	Elongated or ovoid 30–300 μm × 30–300 μm	Kidney shaped, macronucleus enclosing micronucleus.	–	Ciliated, peristome at anterior end, two contractile vacuoles.
CYSTS **Flagellates**				
Retortamonas intestinalis	Thick-walled, oval Single nucleus or lemon shaped 4.5–7 μm × 3–4.5 μm		–	Internal flagella and cytostomal fibers seen in stained preparations.
Enteromonas hominis	Oval. 6–8 μm × 4–6 μm	1–4 nuclei	–	–
Chilomastix mesnili	Pear or lemon shaped with hyaline anterior protuberance 7–10 μm × 4.5 μm	1 nucleus	–	Cytostomal fibers visible in unstained cysts.
Giardia duodenalis	Oval or round 8–20 μm.	4 nuclei	–	Longitudinal fibers within cyst.
Ciliate				
Balantidium coli	Spherical or ovoid 40–60 μm, thick hyaline wall	1 nucleus	–	–

Treatment

Treatment of infective proctitis is discussed in relation to the individual infecting organism. In patients with so-called non-specific proctitis every effort should be made to exclude inflammatory bowel disease and to identify any possible etiological factor. Treatment with broad spectrum antibiotics such as tetracycline usually does not prove useful, and the use of steroids and sulfasalazine has not been studied adequately to allow firm conclusions to be obtained regarding their efficacy and safety.

PROCTOCOLITIC INFECTIONS ACQUIRED BY THE FECAL–ORAL ROUTE

Eukaryotes – protozoa

Table 18.1 gives the results of studies on the prevalence of intestinal protozoa amongst homosexual men who have attended STI specialists in developed countries or, in the series reported by Markell et al.[8], who were recruited for investigation through gay organizations. The prevalence of infection amongst heterosexuals of the western world (in countries of low incidence) is much lower, with less than 3% of heterosexuals infected with Giardia duodenalis. As most studies have involved some form of selection, the true prevalence of enteric protozoal infections amongst homosexual men cannot readily be determined; prevalence is likely to be lower in close-coupled or asexual homosexual men than among open-coupled or functional homosexual men.

Giardia duodenalis

Giardia duodenalis (intestinalis or lamblia) is a protozoal flagellate found in its trophozoite form in the upper small intestine. Transmission occurs by ingestion of cysts, formed in the small intestine and excreted in the feces. The microscopic features of Giardia are given with those of other intestinal flagellates and ciliates in Table 18.2.

Epidemiology

Giardiasis is an infection found in both temperate and tropical countries especially where sanitation is poor. Although the protozoon is acquired mainly through the ingestion of viable cysts in water or food contaminated with feces, person-to-person transmission of the parasite also occurs by the fecal–oral route[9]. The inoculum required for infection in humans is between 10 and 100 cysts[10]. During outbreaks of infection, many of those infected have no symptoms. The homosexual transmission of G. duodenalis was first recognized by Meyers et al.[11] in Seattle and later supported by Schmerin et al.[12] in New York City.

Giardia duodenalis is more likely to produce disease in patients with immunodeficiency syndromes, including selective IgA deficiency. Individuals with HIV infection, however, do not appear to be at increased risk for giardiasis[13].

Pathology

In many patients with no underlying immunodeficiency, the histology of the jejunum is normal. The histological changes, which have been described in association with Giardia infection, are generally mild and include villous blunting and lymphocytic infiltration of the lamina propria. The crypt epithelium is sometimes infiltrated with neutrophils and lymphocytes[14, 15]. More severe changes are found, however, in patients with underlying immunodeficiency. Trophozoites of G. duodenalis appear in hematoxylin and eosin or Giemsa-stained tissue sections as pear or sickle-shaped organisms with two nuclei, in the lumen of the intestine or attached to the epithelial surface.

Clinical features

Many, if not most, infections with G. duodenalis are asymptomatic, with the parasite being detected by chance on routine stool examination. After a pre-patent period of between 12 and 19 days the onset of foul-smelling diarrhea is sudden. Characteristically the stools tend to float on the surface of the water and the patient complains of increased flatulence, abdominal distention, cramping abdominal pain, anorexia, nausea, and weight loss. Blood and pus are not present in the feces. Untreated, symptoms usually resolve after a variable interval of up to 3 months. In patients with underlying immunodeficiency the illness is more prolonged with intermittent diarrhea or steatorrhea, increased flatulence, nausea, and weight loss.

In about half of symptomatic patients, there is biochemical evidence of malabsorption[16]. On radiological examination after ingestion of contrast media, characteristic features, found in about 70% of cases, include thickening of the mucosal folds, particularly of the duodenum and proximal jejunum, and, as a result of excessive secretions in the gut lumen,

fragmentation of the column of barium sulfate can be seen.

Diagnosis of giardiasis

1. *Examination of feces.* In diarrheal stools, trophozoites may be seen in saline mount or in trichrome-stained preparations of fresh or preserved specimens (Figure 18.3). Cysts may be found in formed stools (Figure 18.4) but, as the numbers may be too small to detect by direct microscopy, concentration by the formol-ether method[17] is recommended. Giardia spp. cannot be cultivated satisfactorily from the feces. As cyst excretion is often intermittent, at least three stool samples, obtained on alternate days, should be examined. The ingestion of antidiarrhea agents, antacids, antimicrobials, and barium sulfate interferes with the excretion of Giardia cysts, so these preparations should be avoided while attempts at diagnosis are being made.

As the detection of Giardia cysts by microscopy can be difficult, immunological methods for the identification of the antigen in feces have been developed[18]. An enzyme-linked immunosorbent assay, using

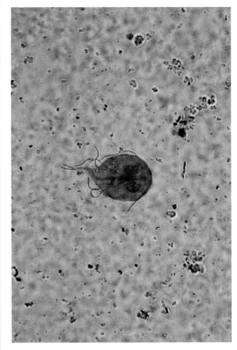

Figure 18.3 Trophozoite of *Giardia duodenalis* (trichrome stain, × 1000) (courtesy of Prof. JP Ackers, reproduced from McMillan and Scott 2000[124])

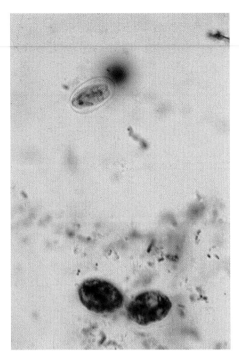

Figure 18.4 Cysts of *Giardia duodenalis* (iron hematoxylin stain, × 1000) (reproduced from McMillan and Scott 2000[124])

antibody against a *G. duodenalis* antigen (GSA) of approximate molecular weight 65 kDa, is available commercially and has a sensitivity of between 95% to 100%, and a specificity of 100%. It has greater sensitivity than examination of a single stool sample, and the test has been reported as detecting about one-third more infections than microscopy[19].

2. Detection of Giardia trophozoites in jejunal samples. When neither trophozoites or cysts are seen in the feces, but giardiasis is suspected clinically, jejunal intubation with aspiration of the secretions and/or biopsy may be necessary if it is important to make an organismal diagnosis. Biopsy seems to be the most sensitive technique for the diagnosis of *Giardia* infections[20]. Trophozoites may be seen by direct microscopy of the jejunal aspirate or cultured from this source in Diamond's medium[21]. Tissue impression smears, fixed in methanol and stained by Giemsa's method, should also be prepared for microscopy[20]. In Giemsa-stained tissue sections the trophozoites are found in the lumen of the intestine or attached to the epithelial cells of the villi or crypts.

As an alternative to duodenal or jejunal intubation and biopsy, the so-called 'string test' or Enterotest* has been advocated[22]. The patient swallows a length of prepared thread, and after about 4 hours this is withdrawn and the retained secretion examined microscopically for trophozoites.

Although specific antibodies can be detected by immunofluorescence, ELISA, immunodiffusion, or western blot in the sera of the majority of patients with symptomatic giardiasis[18], serological tests are of limited value in diagnosis. Antibodies remain detectable for many months after successful treatment and their prevalence is high in currently non-infected groups.

Treatment

Metronidazole (Chapter 17) given in a single oral dose of 2 g daily for 3 days is often successful: 20 (91%) of 22 patients treated by Wright *et al.*[16] had protozoological cure.

Mepacrine hydrochloride taken orally in a dosage of 100 mg 3 times a day for 7 days gives a cure rate of about 95% in giardiasis[23]. Side effects include gastrointestinal upsets and, on very rare occasions, exfoliative dermatitis and toxic psychosis; it should not be used in patients with psychotic illness or with psoriasis.

Entamoeba histolytica

Amoebiasis is caused by the protozoon *Entamoeba histolytica*. After ingestion by the host, those cysts which escape the gastric juices, pass into the small intestine where they excyst to form trophozoites, which colonize the large intestine. Trophozoites may remain free-living in the intestinal lumen and in turn encyst to be excreted in the feces. Alternatively they may invade the mucous membrane of the intestinal wall, cause ulceration and sometimes produce

the clinical features of amoebic dysentery. The amoebae may be carried from the intestine to the liver or, less commonly, to other organs where abscesses may develop. The microscopic features of *E. histolytica* and of the four non-pathogenic intestinal amoebae are given in Table 18.3.

Pathogenicity of Entamoeba histolytica *and the occurrence of* Entamoeba spp. *in homosexual men*

For decades, controversy has existed regarding the pathogenicity of *E. histolytica*. It is known that many asymptomatic individuals excrete amoebic cysts in their feces and that comparatively few people develop serious disease as a result of the infection. Such observations prompted numerous authorities to postulate the existence of pathogenic and non-pathogenic strains of *E. histolytica*. Differences in the isoenzyme profiles for four enzymes (glucose phosphate isomerase, phosphoglucomutase, L-malate: $NADP^+$ oxidoreductase, and hexokinase) have been used as the basis for classifying stocks of *E. histolytica*. Certain of these stocks, classified in this way and termed zymodemes, have been found to be associated with invasive amoebiasis[24–26]. The non-pathogenic stocks have been reclassified *Entamoaeba dispar*[27].

In a study of 52 stocks of *E. histolytica* obtained from the feces of 470 homosexual men who attended STI clinics in Edinburgh and London, Sargeaunt *et al.*[28] found zymodemes which he recognized as 'non-pathogenic'. The non-invasive nature of *E. histolytica* in homosexual men in Edinburgh was confirmed by the clinical and histopathological studies undertaken by McMillan *et al.*[29] and Goldmeier *et al.*[30]. *Entamoeba dispar* is found frequently in the feces of homosexual men who attend STI clinics. In a recent study, Pakianathan and McMillan[31] identified the protozoan in 9% of 175 men who attended the Edinburgh clinic.

Invasive amoebiasis in homosexual men appears to be rare. Burnham *et al.*[32] reported acute proctitis with tissue invasion with amoebic trophozoites in a young homosexual man, and Thompson *et al.*[33] described a case of a hepatic amoebic abscess in a homosexual. In neither case was the zymodeme determined.

---

* Enterotest in giardiasis. In the enterotest a long thread is packed in a gelatin pharmaceutical capsule. The free end of the thread protruding from the capsule is fixed with adhesive tape to the corner of the mouth and the capsule swallowed. Within 3 to 4 hours much of the line is extended to the duodenum or jejunum. It is then withdrawn and the bile-stained mucus is scraped off and immediately examined microscopically[9].

Table 18.3 Microscopic features of *Entamoeba histolytica* and of four non-pathogenic intestinal amoebae

| Organism | Size (μm) | TROPHOZOITES | | | |
| | | Nucleus | | Cytoplasm | |
		Peripheral chromatin	Endosome	Appearance	Inclusions
Entamoeba histolytica/ dispar	15–50 (usually 15–20)	fine granules, beaded	small central	granular ectoplasm and endoplasm clearly differentiated	bacteria, may have erythrocytes
Entamoeba coli	15–50 (usually 20–25)	clumped unevenly, arranged on membrane or as solid ring	large, often eccentric	granular, no differentiation into ecto- and endoplasm	bacteria, debris
Entamoeba hartmanni	5–12 (usually 8–10)	similar to *E. histolytica*	small, compact, often central	fine, granular	bacteria
Endolimax nana	6–18 (usually 8–10)	absent	large, irregular, usually central	granular vacuolated	bacteria
Iodamoeba butschlii	8–20 (usually 12–15)	absent	large, rounded; surrounded by achromatic granules	coarse granular vacuolated	bacteria, debris

| Organism | Size (μm) and shape | CYSTS | | | | |
| | | Nucleus or nuclei | | | Cytoplasm | |
		Number	Peripheral chromatin	Endosome	Chromatoidal bodies	Glycogen iodine-stained
Entamoeba histolytica/ E. dispar	10–20 spherical	1–4	as trophozoite	as trophozoite	common, blunt ends	ill-defined glycogen vacuole
Entamoeba coli	10–30 Usually spherical	1–8, seldom 2, occasionally 16	coarse, granular, may be clumped on membrane	large, eccentric	infrequent, splinter-like ends	well-defined mass lying between nuclei in binucleate cysts
Entamoeba hartmanni	5–9 spherical	1–4, often 2	fine granules on membrane	small, central	common, blunt smooth ends	diffuse or absent
Endolimax nana	5–12 ovoid	1–4	absent	large, central	absent	diffuse if present
Iodamoeba butschlii	6–15 very irregular, ovoid spherical	1, rarely 2	absent	large, eccentric	absent	large, well-defined

Histopathology

Intestinal amoebiasis. A common finding in intestinal amoebiasis is an acute inflammatory cell infiltration of varying degrees of the lamina propria, with migration of polymorphs through the surface epithelium and lymphoid hyperplasia[34, 35], but the nature of this mucosal response is non-specific. In early invasive lesions there are foci of interglandular epithelial cell and basement membrane destruction with invasion by amoebae of the superficial lamina propria. A mild polymorph infiltration is found in the tissues adjacent to the site of amoebic infiltration. As invasion progresses, there is further necrosis with involvement of the submucosa, and the ulcer assumes the typical flask-shaped appearance.

Cutaneous amoebiasis. The floor of the ulcer consists of necrotic tissue containing trophozoites which overlies granulation tissue. At the edge of the ulcer the epidermis shows acanthosis and papillomatosis[36].

Clinical features

About 90% of patients with amoebiasis are asymptomatic; in the remainder the severity of the illness varies greatly. In symptomatic intestinal amoebiasis the patient has diarrhea, abdominal discomfort, flatulence, and blood and mucus in the stool, and may also complain of anorexia and weight loss. Sigmoidoscopy may reveal a normal rectal mucosal pattern or a mucous membrane which is red, edematous, and friable. The inflammatory reaction extends beyond the rectosigmoid junction. The appearance may, however, be identical to that of non-specific ulcerative procto-colitis[35] when there may be multiple areas of ulceration, with individual ulcers reaching up to a few millimeters in diameter, with a yellow base and an erythematous margin.

The development of hepatic abscess is associated with tenderness in the right hypochondrium, fever, and weight loss. Aspiration of the abscess produces a red-brown thick fluid, in which amoebae are rarely demonstrable. Cutaneous amoebiasis may rarely produce perianal or genital ulceration. The ulcers, which are exquisitely tender, are irregularly shaped with an undermined edge and blood-encrusted necrotic base[36]. The inguinal lymph nodes are usually enlarged. Untreated, the lesions progress at a variable rate and can produce large areas of ulceration.

Diagnosis of amoebiasis

The diagnosis of intestinal amoebiasis rests on the detection of cysts and/or trophozoites of *E. histolytica* in the feces or material obtained from rectal ulcers (Table 18.3).

Detection by microscopy of trophozoites and cysts

It is useful to examine saline mounts of feces, rectal exudate, or material scraped from a rectal ulcer for the presence of trophozoites. These are 15 to 25 μm in diameter and exhibit unidirectional movement with the often explosive protrusion of finger-like pseudopodia (lobopodia). The presence of erythrocytes in the cytoplasm is pathognomonic of *E. histolytica*. Differentiation of *E. histolytica* trophozoites from other non-pathogenic species of intestinal amoebae is important but, except for finding erythrocyte-containing organisms, is not possible from examination of unstained fecal preparations.

It must be emphasized that microscopy *cannot* differentiate *E. histolytica* from *E. dispar* (these amoebae can only be identified correctly by isoenzyme electrophoresis or by PCR, Britten *et al.*[37]).

Smears of feces, rectal exudate, and ulcer material, fixed in Schaudinn's fluid, and stained with modified Gomori's stain (Figure 18.5)[38], however, enable differentiation of *E. histolytica/dispar* from other amoebae, but care and experience are required. Microscopic features helpful in the differentiation of *E. histolytica/dispar* from other amoebae are summarized in Table 18.3.

Trophozoites are not commonly found in formed stools, which should routinely be examined for cysts of *E. histolytica* when amoebiasis is suspected. As the number of cysts in a given sample may be small, it is helpful to examine the feces after cyst concentration by the formol-ether method[17]. The characteristics that distinguish cysts of *E. histolytica* from those of the non-pathogenic amoebae (except *E. dispar*) are

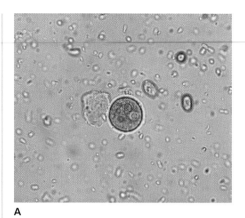

A

Figure 18.6A Cysts of *Entamoeba histolytica/dispar* (in iodine solution, × 160)

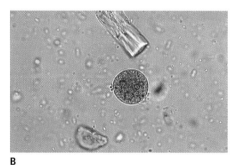

B

Figure 18.6B Cysts of *Entamoeba coli* (in iodine solution, × 160)

1. size
2. number of nuclei
3. presence in the cyst of blunt-ended chromatoidal bodies (Table 18.2 and Figure 18.6).

As the identification of amoebic cysts may be difficult, in cases of doubt, samples should be sent fresh or in preservative to a reference laboratory.

Detection by culture. Cultivation of intestinal amoebae is desirable from the clinical point of view. Cultured trophozoites are required for zymodeme analysis.

Detection by immunological tests. The accurate diagnosis of *E. histolytica* trophozoites and cysts is often difficult, time consuming and requires experience. More objective methods for the identification of amoebic infection have been described. Root *et al.*[41] developed an ELISA method for the detection of *E. histolytica* antigens in feces but it did not gain general acceptance as a diagnostic test. A double antibody indirect ELISA method using a

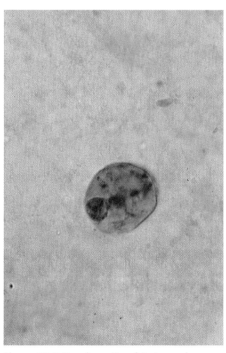

Figure 18.5 Trophozoite of *Entamoeba histolytica/dispar* (modified Gomori's stain, × 1000) (reproduced from McMillan and Scott 2000[124])

Technique for preserving feces for later microscopy

Polyvinyl alcohol (PVA)/fixative[39] has been used most often:

mercuric chloride saturated solution in water (2 parts)/95% ethanol (1 part) 93.5 mL

glycerol 1.5 mL

glacial acetic acid 5.0 mL

polyvinyl alcohol (Sigmal Type II low MW) 5.0 g

PVA is added with continuous stirring to the rest of the ingredients and heated slowly to about 75°C; when as clear as water, 5 mL quantities are dispensed in wide-mouthed screw-capped containers. These will remain effective for about 6 months if stored at room temperatures. With an applicator stick, about 1 mL of feces is mixed with the 5 mL of PVA/fixative in the container; this preparation will remain satisfactory for microscopy for several months. When convenient, a little of the suspension is pipetted on to a clean paper towel and, after a few minutes when most of the fluid has been absorbed, smears are made on slides using an applicator stick. After drying the smears overnight at 37°C, they are stained with Giemsa or with a trichrome stain.

There are concerns, however, about the safety of this preservative. Other preservatives evaluated by Jensen et al.[40], that do not contain mercuric salts, have been shown to be almost as satisfactory.

combination of monoclonal and polyclonal antibodies, however, has given encouraging results[42]. Further studies are required before conclusions can be drawn regarding the value of this test in diagnosis.

Serological tests for antibodies against E. histolytica, using indirect hemagglutination assays, complement fixation tests, or indirect immunofluorescence are of value only in the diagnosis of invasive disease[43–45], in the majority of individuals with hepatic amoebic abscesses there are high titers of antibody against the protozoa. Although the indirect hemagglutination test is sensitive, the antibodies

detected persist for many years, even after successful treatment and for this reason the value of the test in the assessment of cure is limited. It is, however, of some value in epidemiological studies. The indirect immunofluorescent antibody test is better in determining the cure of extra-intestinal disease. When treatment has been successful the titers of antibodies detected in the test fall significantly within 2 months.

Treatment

In acute invasive amoebiasis immediate treatment is necessary. Metronidazole is the drug of choice for it is very effective against the trophozoites in ulcers at a dosage of 800 mg 3 times a day for 5 days. It is also effective against amoebae which may have migrated to the liver. Metronidazole is given either for 5 days or for 10 days, followed by a 10-day course of diloxanide furoate 500 mg every 8 hours by mouth which is effective against the cysts of E. histolytica. Large hepatic abscesses may require aspiration. After completion of treatment, stool samples should be examined at intervals, say monthly, for 3 months, for cysts and trophozoites of E. histolytica.

The efficacy of treatment of hepatic abscesses is assessed by clinical or radiological examination, possibly supplemented by serological testing. In most cases treated successfully, titers of amoebic antibodies detected by immunofluorescence fall significantly within 2 months of completion of therapy.

Chloroquine is effective in the treatment of liver abscess but is ineffective against other forms of amoebiasis. It is given in a dose for adults of 600 mg (base) daily by mouth for 5 days and then reduced to 300 mg (base) daily for 14 to 21 days. This may be followed by a course of metronidazole. For abscesses containing more than 100 mL pus (i.e. approximately 60 to 100 mm in diameter) aspiration carried out in conjunction with drug therapy will greatly reduce the period of disability. A 10-day course of diloxanide furoate should be given on completion of chloroquine treatment.

Cryptosporidium species

Cryptosporidium spp. are coccidian protozoal parasites of the suborder Eimeriina

which are not species-specific and can infect mammals including man, reptiles, and birds. Most human infections are caused by C. parvum[46].

Epidemiology

On the basis of occasional case reports[47, 48] human cryptosporidiosis was recognized initially as a cause of severe protracted diarrhea in immunodeficient patients. With the occurrence of AIDS and its frequent association with it, Cryptosporidium spp. are now recognized as an important cause of morbidity in this condition. Cryptosporidiosis is now also being recognized, however, as an important cause of self-limiting diarrhea in immunocompetent individuals in both developed and developing countries. All age groups can be infected, but mostly there is an increased prevalence amongst children, particularly those living in poor and unhygienic urban areas[49]. Although the coccidian can infect domestic animals and transmission to man from them has been described[50, 51], human-to-human spread by the fecal–oral route is probably more important. Oocyst excretion has been found both in symptomatic and asymptomatic family contacts of patients with cryptosporidiosis[52, 53]. The observation by Jokipii et al.[54] that 12 of 14 patients had visited Leningrad, a city where individuals have previously acquired giardiasis, suggested that the protozoon may be spread in the water supply.

The probable transmission of Cryptosporidium spp. by the fecal–oral route suggests that homosexual men might be at risk. Although sporadic cases of cryptosporidiosis have been described in homosexual men who did not have AIDS[55] it has not yet been found in such patients attending the Department of Genitourinary Medicine in Edinburgh[31].

Pathology

Cryptosporidium spp. can infect the epithelial cells of the entire gastrointestinal tract, the biliary and pancreatic ducts, the gall bladder, and the respiratory tract. Jejunal and ileal biopsies from infected patients show hyperplasia of the crypts, blunting and loss of villi, and degenerating

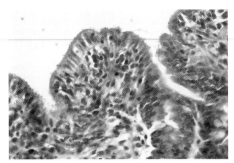

Figure 18.7 Oocysts of *Cryptosporidium* spp. in the jejunum (hematoxylin and eosin, × 160)

surface cells. There is a mild to moderate increase in the numbers of polymorphonuclear leukocytes, plasma cells, and lymphocytes within the lamina propria[47]. Rectal biopsies show the pattern of nonspecific proctitis: there is infiltration of the lamina propria with acute and chronic inflammatory cells, the goblet cells show some mucin depletion and the columnar epithelial cells may be replaced by abnormal cuboidal cells[56].

In tissue sections cryptosporidia appear as small (2 to 3 μm) round or oval nucleate bodies on the microvillous surface of epithelial cells (Figure 18.7). They are most numerous in the jejunum and ileum, and less common in the colon. Electronmicroscopy shows various stages in the life cycle of the parasite[57].

Clinical features

In the *immunocompetent* individual cryptosporidial infection is associated with a self-limiting diarrhea. The diarrhea may be intermittent or continuous and the stools are often watery and offensive, but they do not contain blood or mucus. Abdominal pain before defecation, anorexia, and vomiting are common additional features, and fever may be found in about one-fifth of patients. Unless there is concomitant infection, white blood cells are usually not detected in the feces. The diarrhea usually ceases in 2 to 3 weeks, but excretion of oocysts may continue for up to 2 weeks afterwards[53].

In the *immunodeficient* individual the diarrhea – which is often profuse with up to 10 liters of fluid stool being passed daily – is prolonged with weight loss and general

debility. Many AIDS patients with cryptosporidiosis die from other opportunistic infections. In the few non-AIDS cases with cryptosporidiosis associated with immunosuppression, discontinuation of the drug(s) has resulted in spontaneous resolution of the infection[47].

Diagnosis

The diagnosis of cryptosporidiosis relies on the detection of oocysts in the feces or on the discovery of the various stages of its life cycle within enterocytes on histological examination of jejunal, ileal, colonic, or rectal biopsies. In fecal smears stained by a modified Ziehl–Neelsen method[58], oocysts of *Cryptosporidium* spp. appear as round or oval red structures, 5 to 6 μm in diameter, containing a single deeply stained red 'dot' which stands out clearly against a green background (Figure 18.8). With experience the oocysts are readily distinguishable from yeasts, but for confirmation Giemsa-stained smears should be examined also. Oocysts appear as pale blue, semitranslucent structures containing eccentrically placed pink-staining granules. Enzyme immunoassays and direct immunofluorescence tests are

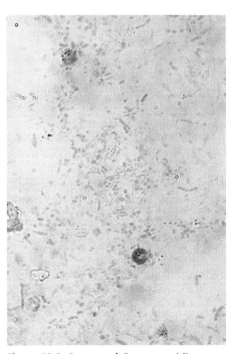

Figure 18.8 Oocysts of *Cryptosporidium* spp. in feces (modified Ziehl–Neelsen stain, × 1000) (reproduced from McMillan and Scott 2000[124])

available commercially; they have high sensitivity (94.5% to 96.4%) when compared with an acid-fast stain, but are more expensive[59].

Although a sugar flotation method for the concentration of oocysts is available, the HIV risks involved in its use do not justify its routine application.

Treatment

Unfortunately there is no specific treatment for cryptosporidiosis.

Other protozoa

With the possible exception of *Dientamoeba fragilis* the other protozoa which have been found at increased frequency in the feces from homosexual men are not pathogenic. The increasing prevalence is probably a result of sexual activity associated with fecal contamination among a promiscuous but relatively closed population.

Nematodes

Enterobius vermicularis

Enterobius vermicularis is an intestinal parasite, usually transmitted by food or fomites contaminated by ova, and is most commonly found in children. After ingestion the ova hatch and develop within 6 weeks into adult worms, which inhabit the cecum and adjacent regions of the small and large intestines. The male worms are small, 2 to 5 mm in length, while the females are larger, 8 to 13 mm long. When fully mature, the females emerge from the anus and deposit eggs on the perianal skin. It is this activity which produces pruritus ani, particularly at night. Uncommonly, threadworms enter the vagina and produce vulvovaginitis in young girls. On rare occasions ova may be found in cervical smears.

Reports of threadworms in homosexual males[60], probably indicate oral–anal contact, a common practice in some homosexual men. Threadworms should therefore be excluded as a cause of pruritus ani.

Diagnosis

Adult worms may be seen in the feces, or in the anal canal or rectum, or ova may be found on the perianal skin. Alternatively, to

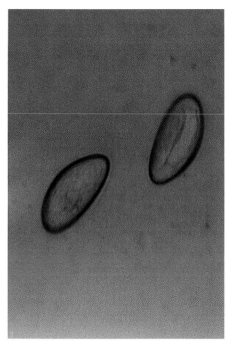

Figure 18.9 Ova of *Enterobius vermicularis* (× 60) (reproduced from McMillan and Scott 2000[124])

make a diagnosis, transparent adhesive tape (Sellotape) sticky side down, is applied to the perianal skin, preferably in the morning before the patient has defecated. The tape is then applied to a slide for examination by microscopy for ova. Threadworm ova are oval and flattened on one side (50 to 60 μm × 10 to 30 μm) (Figure 18.9).

Treatment

Piperazine is the most widely used drug in the treatment of enterobiasis, most conveniently being given to adults and children over 6 years of age as a single sachet containing 4 g of piperazine phosphate with standardized senna – stirred into a small glass of milk and drunk immediately. It should be repeated as a follow-up dose after 14 days. Side effects include dizziness and ataxia, but are rare. It should not be used in patients with severe bilateral renal dysfunction and its use in the first trimester of pregnancy is not advised (ABPI Data Sheet Compendium 1999–2000).

Mebendazole in a single oral dose of 100 mg is satisfactory for patients of all ages. It may be given as a single tablet or as 5 mL of a 2% w/v suspension. Side effects are rare and include diarrhea and abdom-

inal pain. As it has been shown to be toxic in animal studies the drug is not advised in pregnancy (ABPI Data Sheet Compendium 1999–2000).

Strongyloides stercoralis

In the case of the nematode *Strongyloides stercoralis*, non-infective rhabitiform larvae may develop into infective filariform larvae before leaving the colon. Hence, during homosexual intercourse between males, the ingestion of feces containing these infective filariform larvae, during oral–anal contact, will enable transmission to occur. Alternatively penetration of the mucosa or skin of the penis or elsewhere by infective larvae and the acquisition of *Strongyloides* infection will be possible by direct fecal contact during or following anal intercourse.

Phillips *et al.*[61] detected *Strongyloides* spp. in the feces of 2 of 51 homosexual men who attended an STI clinic in New York City, and Sorvillo *et al.*[62], in San Francisco, reported the probable sexual transmission of the helminth. Although the larvae most commonly infect the upper intestine, the rectum may be involved. The larvae penetrate the submucosa and induce a chronic inflammatory cell reaction with eosinophilic infiltration[63].

Since overwhelming infection may occur in immunocompromised individuals, producing massive re-invasion of the ileum or colon with hemorrhage, it is very important to exclude strongyloidiasis by examination of the stool in patients who are to be immunosuppressed.

The diagnosis of strongyloidiasis is made by the detection of larvae in stool samples by microscopy after concentration or by culture[64]. Treatment is with thrabendazole.

Prokaryotes

Shigella species

Most cases of bacillary dysentery occur in children of either pre-school or school age, and in boys more often than girls. Generally, in adults, the sexes are affected almost equally, with a slight preponderance of cases in females. Transmission of the organism is usually by hand-to-mouth contact; the infected individual contam-

inates toilet fixtures, which are then handled and the organism is transferred to the mouth of the new host. Occasionally, infection results from contaminated water, food, or fomites. In several outbreaks of the disease in the USA, more than two-thirds of adult cases were in young men, many of whom were homosexual; transmission occurred possibly as a result of oral–anal and oral–genital sexual contact[65]. Infectivity persists throughout the acute phase of the illness, and for a variable time, usually 3 to 4 weeks thereafter. It is important to note that *Shigella* dysentery in homosexual males may be accompanied by infection with other intestinal pathogens such as *Giardia duodenalis*, and with other STIs.

Clinical features

In the majority of cases bacillary dysentery is mild. After a pre-patent period of 2 to 7 days, the patient suffers from the frequent passage of loose stools. The following day the passage of stools becomes more frequent, but less copious, and symptoms subside after a few days; there is usually no pyrexia, and only small quantities of mucus and blood may be passed.

In some cases the disease is more severe, beginning abruptly with the frequent passage of loose stools that contain blood and mucus; there is also fever, tenesmus, and abdominal tenderness. Symptoms persist for about a week and then subside, the illness occasionally passing into a chronic phase. As the disease process is not confined to the rectum, at sigmoidoscopy the inflammatory changes in the rectum are seen to extend into the sigmoid colon.

Fulminating dysentery, with dehydration and electrolyte imbalance, is rarely seen in adults in developed countries.

Uncommon complications of bacillary dysentery include acute pyelonephritis, conjunctivitis, and arthritis.

Diagnosis

Shigella spp. can readily be cultured from stool specimens plated on to medium such as MacConkey agar, deoxycholate citrate agar, or xylose lysine decarboxylase agar. The groups within the genus Shigella (e.g. *Sh. dysenteriae*, *Sh. flexneri*, *Sh. boydii*, and

Sh. sonnei) are identified by appropriate biochemical and serological tests.

Treatment

In management of the patient, bed rest and adequate fluid intake are necessary, and careful attention to hygiene is important to prevent further transmission. Antibiotic therapy should not be given unless the illness is severe; the laboratory should confirm that the drug selected is active *in vitro* against the patient's isolate. In the past, antibiotic treatment has resulted in the emergence of resistant strains of the organism and clearance of the pathogen may not occur significantly earlier than when non-specific treatment has been given.

Diarrhea may be controlled by the use of agents such as kaolin and morphine mixture, BNF, 10 mL given orally every 6 hours.

Campylobacter species

Campylobacter jejuni is an important cause of enteritis worldwide, and *C. fetus* subsp. *intestinalis* is associated with enteritis in debilitated individuals. The organism is present in the feces of wild or domestic animals, and contaminated water has been the source of outbreaks of disease[66]. Other means of acquiring the infection include the ingestion of contaminated food or milk[67, 68] and the handling of infected animal carcasses[69]. Person-to-person transfer seems to be uncommon.

Sporadic cases of infection with *C. jejuni* in homosexual men have been reported. The infection does not appear to be widespread, nor is it always a problem of homosexual males. In London, Simmons and Tabaqchali[70] did not isolate *Campylobacter* spp. from the rectal material of 50 homosexual men who attended an STI clinic. McMillan *et al.*[71] found a similar prevalence of serum IgG antibodies against *Campylobacter* spp. in both homosexual and heterosexual men. However Quinn *et al.*[72], in Seattle, isolated *C. jejuni* from the feces of 6% of 158 homosexual men with proctocolitis, and from 3% of 75 asymptomatic homosexuals; *C. fetus* was cultured from the feces of 1 patient with proctitis. The Seattle group did not culture *Campylobacter*

spp. from the feces of 150 heterosexual men and women.

Quinn *et al.*[72] cultured groups of *Campylobacter*-like organisms from rectal material from 16% of 158 homosexual men with proctocolitis and from 8% of 75 asymptomatic homosexuals. These organisms differed from other species of *Campylobacter* in several respects, but their association with symptoms and signs of proctitis suggested that they were pathogenic. *Campylobacter cinaedi* and *C. fenelliae* were the species most frequently isolated from symptomatic men[73, 74]. The occurrence of *Campylobacter*-like organisms in a group at risk of acquiring enteric infection suggests their transmission by the fecal–oral route as a result of homosexual practices.

Clinical features

Although asymptomatic infections are known to occur, infection with *Campylobacter* spp. is often associated with a self-limiting diarrheal illness[75]. After a pre-patent period of up to 10 days there is sudden diarrhea with bile-stained stools, which later become mucoid and sometimes blood stained. There is often anorexia (but not vomiting), malaise, pyrexia, headache, cramping lower abdominal pain, myalgia, arthralgia, and backache.

Reactive arthritis is a rare complication. These constitutional features are usually noted during the early stage of the illness. On sigmoidoscopy a marked proctitis is seen to extend beyond the rectosigmoid junction. Radiological examination shows a pancolitis with no distinguishing features[76]. During the acute phase of the disease, rectal biopsy specimens show a non-specific acute infective proctitis pattern (see pp. 517–518)[76].

Untreated, the illness generally lasts for less than 10 days, the organism is eliminated within 2 months and radiological abnormalities resolve within 6 months.

Diagnosis

A diagnosis based on clinical features is confirmed by culture of *Campylobacter* spp. on selective media, and serologically by the detection of specific IgM or by rising titers of IgG antibodies[77].

Treatment

As the illness is self-limiting in mild cases, treatment is not necessary unless the patient is a food handler and likely to infect others. If symptoms are more severe, erythromycin in a dosage of 500 mg twice a day by mouth for 5 days has proved useful, but resistance to this drug has been reported from Sweden[78].

Viruses

Hepatitis A virus is acquired by the fecal–oral route and can be spread amongst homosexual men during sexual activity (Chapter 8).

PROCTOCOLITIC INFECTIONS SPREAD BY MUCOSAL–SKIN CONTACT DURING ANAL INTERCOURSE

Prokaryotes

Neisseria gonorrhoeae

This organism, perhaps the most common pathogen, actual or potential, acquired by anal intercourse is considered in detail in Chapter 11.

Neisseria meningitidis

The significance of rectal infection with *Neisseria meningitidis* of differing serogroups is uncertain. In the authors' experience and that of Judson *et al.*[79], the organism can be isolated from the rectums of about 2% of homosexual men who attend STI clinics. Janda *et al.*[80] did not show any correlation between the presence of the organisms and clinical features. The importance of the organism lies in its possible confusion with *N. gonorrhoeae* on culture.

Treponema pallidum

Primary syphilis of the anal margin presents often as a painful, tender, non-indurated ulcer which sometimes bleeds easily on palpation. As the clinical features, unlike those of primary genital lesions, closely resemble those of a traumatic anal fissure, it is important to examine by dark ground microscope – or by a method based on monoclonal antibody (Chapter 15) – material from any anal ulcer in men who have had receptive anal intercourse.

As many homosexual men with secondary syphilis give no history suggestive of a primary lesion, it is probable that the majority of rectal primary lesions do not produce symptoms. Occasionally patients with serological evidence of primary syphilis present with symptoms of proctitis and single or multiple indurated rectal masses, some of which may be ulcerated and are palpable and visible at proctoscopy[81, 82]. A diffuse distal proctitis may be part of the secondary stage of the disease[83].

Biopsy specimens of these lesions show a dense infiltration of the lamina propria and submucosa with plasma cells, lymphocytes, and histocytes. There is proliferation of the endothelial cells of the capillaries, and crypt abscesses may be a feature. Spirochetes can sometimes be demonstrated in the lesions by silver staining or immunofluorescence[72a].

The diagnosis of syphilitic proctitis is best made by proctoscopy backed by the results of serological testing. As profuse hemorrhage may result, biopsy of the lesions is not recommended in clinical practice.

Rectal spirochetosis

On the epithelial surfaces of the large intestine of humans and other animals such as monkeys, treponemes of the genus *Brachyspira*[84] (Figure 18.10) and flagellated bacteria (family Spirillaceae) may be found; this situation has been referred to as intestinal spirochetosis[85, 86]. Although electron microscopy is necessary to distinguish these organisms, their presence in hematoxylin and eosin-stained sections is indicated by a basophilic zone about 3 μm in width on the surface of the epithelium (Figure 18.11). As it is uncertain whether the entire mucosal surface of the intestine is occupied by these organisms, a more appropriate term may be rectal spirochetosis. Although the condition is found in about 7% of unselected rectal biopsies[87], McMillan and Lee[88] detected rectal spirochetosis in 36% of 100 biopsies from homosexual men who attended an STI clinic in Glasgow; a similarly increased prevalence amongst a similar homosexual group was also found in Edinburgh. The source and significance of these organisms is unknown, but the increased prevalence in men who have had receptive anal inter-

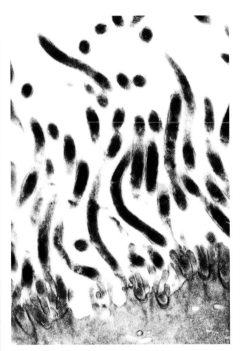

Figure 18.10 Transmission electron micrograph of *Brachyspira* spp. on the epithelial surface of the rectum

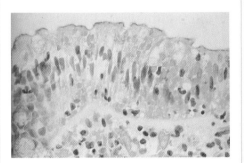

Figure 18.11 Rectal spirochetosis as indicated by the hematoxyphil zone on the surface of epithelial cells (hematoxylin and eosin, × 160)

course suggests that they can be sexually transmitted.

Although there have been sporadic case reports of diarrhea and rectal bleeding in patients with rectal spirochetosis[89, 90], other causes for these symptoms had not been excluded. In an unpublished series from Edinburgh, McMillan and Gilmour found no correlation between the presence of the condition and gastrointestinal symptoms.

Chlamydia trachomatis

Infection due to *Chlamydia trachomatis* is discussed in detail in Chapter 10.

Mycoplasma hominis, Mycoplasma genitalium and Ureaplasma urealyticum

The role of these organisms in the etiology of non-specific urethritis is uncertain (Chapter 10). Few studies comment on differences in isolation rates between homo- and heterosexual men. Bowie *et al.*[91] isolated *Ureaplasma urealyticum* from the urethra in 7 of 18 homosexual and 35 of 95 heterosexual men with untreated urethral gonorrhea. Munday *et al.*[92] cultured *U. urealyticum* and *Mycoplasma hominis* from rectal material about equally often (41% and 39% respectively in 49 men with non-gonococcal proctitis and equally often (28%) in each infection in men without evidence of proctitis. Similarly Quinn *et al.*[11] found no difference in the isolation rates of *M. hominis* and *U. urealyticum* between men with proctitis and asymptomatic patients. It is difficult to believe that these organisms play any prominent role in the etiology of proctitis.

Mycoplasma genitalium was detected more frequently in the urethra of homosexual men than of heterosexual men, irrespective of whether or not they had urethritis[93]: 11 (30%) of 37 homosexual men versus 19 (11%) of 166 heterosexual men. The significance of this finding is still uncertain, and the source of the *Mycoplasma* organisms is unknown. *Mycoplasma genitalium* was not detected in any of the 99 men, including 6 homosexual men, who were studied by Jensen *et al.*[94].

VIRUSES

Herpes simplex virus

Although the lesions of primary herpetic infection of the perianal region are usually multiple, a single primary tender ulcer of the anal canal may be the only visible sign of infection and will require differentiation from a traumatic anal fissure or primary syphilis. Sacral radiculomyelitis is a common feature of primary perianal herpes, and proper appreciation of the clinical features associated with it (Table 18.4) should assist in diagnosis. Unnecessary and possibly harmful surgical procedures, such as anal dilatation and sphincterotomy, can be avoided and aciclovir therapy initiated as

Table 18.4 Characteristics of patients with traumatic and herpetic anal ulceration (McMillan and Smith[101])

	Data for group with anal ulceration due to			
	Trauma (21 cases) mean	range	Herpes simplex virus (14 cases) mean	range
Age	24.2 years	(18–34 years)	25.7 years	(19–32 years)
Duration of ulceration	2.2 days	(1–5 days)	3.2 days	(1–7 days)
Interval between most recent sexual intercourse and development of ulceration	1.6 days	(0.5–4 days)	9.9 days	(5–16 days)
Presenting clinical features	**Number of cases**	**%**	**Number of cases**	**%**
Fever	2	(10)	12	(86)[a]
Constipation	18	(86)	12	(86)
Anorectal bleeding	17	(81)	5	(36)
Paraesthesiae	0	(0)	8	(57)[a]
Difficulty in urination	0	(0)	11	(79)[a,b]
Perianal lesions in addition to that in the anal canal	0	(0)	3	(21)
Multiple lesions in anal canal	0	(0)	4	(29)[c]
Proctitis	1	(5)	3	(21)
Rectal ulceration	0	(0)	1	(7)
Inguinal lymphadenitis	1	(5)	6	(43)[c]

[a] $P < 0.01$ (Fisher's exact test). [b] Including two men with acute urinary retention. [c] $P < 0.02$ (Fisher's exact test).

soon as possible. In all cases, the clinical diagnosis should be supported by obtaining material for diagnosis by PCR culture or immunofluorescence (Chapter 6). As the two diseases may co-exist, syphilis should be excluded by dark ground microscopy of ulcer material and repeated serological testing.

When external lesions of herpes are present in primary anal herpes there is often also an acute distal proctitis, sometimes with multiple ulceration of the mucosa. In the absence of external lesions HSV seems to be an uncommon cause of proctitis[95, 96] but the diagnosis may be suspected by the associated neurological features (Table 18.4)[97]. Although multinucleated cells with intranuclear inclusions are characteristic of all herpes lesions and may also be seen in sections of affected rectal mucosa, the histology is usually that of a non-specific proctitis[98] and a definitive diagnosis relies on detection of the virus.

Other viruses

Hepatitis B virus, HIV, and cytomegalovirus are present in semen, and homosexual transmission of these viruses is well recognized (Chapters 7, 8, 9). Anal warts are described in Chapter 5, but it is important to note that there may be concomitant anorectal infection. Echovirus 11 was demonstrated in the feces of 119 homosexual men with proctitis and of 1 of 75 asymptomatic homosexuals[1]. The significance of this finding is not clear.

Traumatic, neoplastic, and other non-infective conditions

ANAL FISSURE

Anal fissures are common in the general population and it is uncertain whether their incidence is higher amongst men who have receptive anal intercourse. Nevertheless, anal fissures may indeed result from this form of sexual activity. Rarely partial tears of the internal anal sphincter have been described following fisting[99]. There is a relative deficiency of blood vessels in the posterior commissure of the anal canal, and there is hypoperfusion of this area[100]. The anal resting pressure, which is mostly a function of the internal sphincter, of the patient with anal fissures is unusually high, and as the blood supply to the anal canal passes through this sphincter, these pressures can impede blood flow.

When *acute*, the patient complains of perianal pain, especially during and immediately after defecation, bleeding during defecation and, as a result of the pain, he tends to become constipated. The fissure, which is usually situated at the exterior anal margin, appears as a single ulcer, almost triangular in shape. As a chancre may also be painful, it is important to exclude primary syphilis in any homosexual patients with anal fissuring or ulceration (Chapter 15). Furthermore the clinical features of primary and, less frequently, recrudescent anorectal HSV infection may resemble those of acute traumatic anal fissure. Features which assist the physician in reaching a correct diagnosis are summarized in Table 18.4[101]. In tropical countries, donovanosis (Chapter 16) and tuberculous ulceration have to be considered in the differential diagnosis.

Chronic anal fissure produces similar but less severe symptoms. There is usually a single elongated, somewhat indurated ulcer at the posterior anal margin and frequently a skin tag ('sentinel pile') is to be seen at the distal end of the ulcer.

Biopsy of the fissure is indicated only if there is doubt about the nature of the anal ulcer. Histologically, there is ulceration of the squamous epithelium with edema and dense infiltration of the surrounding tissues with lymphocytes and plasma cells.

The treatment of anal fissure falls within the province of the surgeon, and methods used in management include anal dilatation and sphincterotomy. Relaxation of the internal sphincter is mediated by nitric oxide[102], and healing of fissures has been reported following the topical application of the organic nitrates glyceryl trinitrate (0.2%) or isosorbide dinitrate (1%)[103, 104]. The injection into the internal sphincter of botulinum toxin, that prevents the release of acetylcholine from presynaptic nerve endings, thereby reducing resting anal pressure, has produced good results in the experience of Maria et al.[105].

OTHER TRAUMATIC CONDITIONS

Lacerations of the rectal mucosa and perforation of the rectosigmoid junction may occur as a result of traumatic forms of anal intercourse, including fisting and the insertion of foreign bodies[106, 99]. Bleeding is the cardinal symptom of mucosal lacerations, which may occur at any site within the rectum. Systemic disturbance and abdominal tenderness are not features of tears in the mucosa. However, when there is transmural laceration into the peritoneal cavity, there is usually a sudden onset of abdominal pain which may radiate to the shoulders, rectal bleeding of varying severity, and pyrexia. The abdomen does not move with respiration, there is generalized tenderness with guarding, and bowel sounds are absent. Radiographs of the abdomen with the patient in the erect position may show air below the diaphragm (Figure 18.12).

Pelvic cellulitis may occur as a complication of fisting[107]. The three patients described complained of anorectal pain, abdominal pain and fever which developed 1 to 7 days after the fisting episode. Although rectal tears were not visible during sigmoidoscopy there was a marked proctitis extending from 7 to 15 cm from the anal margin. Induration of the tissue between the rectal mucosa and pelvis was also noted in

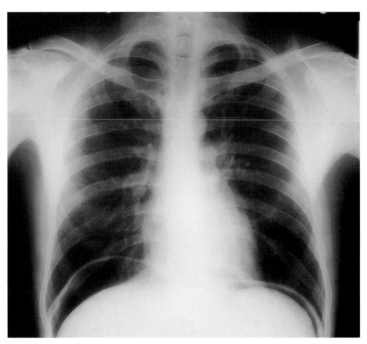

Figure 18.12 Radiograph of the abdomen showing air under the diaphragm in a young man with a rupture at the rectosigmoid junction following 'fisting'

each case. The salient feature at laparotomy, undertaken in one case, was retroperitoneal edema, particularly around the rectum. It was postulated that the cellulitis may have resulted from extraperitoneal microperforation of the rectum during fisting.

Patients with rectal tears and/or pelvic cellulitis should be treated in hospital in co-operation with surgical colleagues. If the laceration involves the rectal mucosa only, the patient does not usually require surgical treatment other than suture of the tear and blood replacement if needed. He should be observed for signs of further bleeding or intraperitoneal rupture of the rectum. Immediate laparotomy is indicated in patients with transmural laceration with signs of peritonitis. Repair of the tear, proximal colostomy, and broad spectrum antibiotics are required. In cases of pelvic cellulitis, broad spectrum antibiotics should be given, but should there be signs of continuing peritonitis, laparotomy is necessary.

CHANGES IN THE ANAL CANAL AS A CONSEQUENCE OF RECEPTIVE ANAL INTERCOURSE

The maximum anal resting pressures of men who have had receptive anal inter-

course are lower than those of heterosexual subjects, although the voluntary anal squeeze pressures are normal in continent homosexual men[108]. Reduction in anal sensitivity is not a feature in men who have had anal sex, and, other than in those who have had brachioproctic intercourse ('fisting'), the threshold of rectal sensation to filling is unaffected. Perineal descent is also not excessive in homosexual men, and the rectoanal inhibitory reflex that is dependent on intact local reflexes in the myenteric and submucosal nerve plexuses is not permanently disrupted[108]. In an unpublished study of 143 homosexual men, 113 of whom had had receptive anal intercourse, and 81 heterosexual men, McMillan noted that the prevalence of fecal incontinence was identical in both groups (1%).

SOLITARY ULCER SYNDROME OF THE RECTUM

This is a condition of young patients, with men and women being affected equally often, the etiology of which is uncertain. The most common symptom is that of anorectal bleeding which may be severe, perineal, sacral, or iliac fossa pain, tenesmus, and a feeling of incomplete defecation are less common symptoms. At sigmoidoscopy, the characteristic sign is ulceration, which, despite the name of the syndrome, is often multiple. Rounded oval ulcers, usually about 2 cm in diameter (range 2 to 5 cm), are generally found within 7 to 10 cm of the anal margin on the anterior or anterolateral wall of the rectum[109]. Typically, the ulcer is only slightly depressed below the surrounding mucosa and the base is covered with a whitish-gray or yellow slough. At the margin is a thin area of hyperemia. Occasionally the base of the ulcer is granular and the surrounding mucosa is heaped up. A non-ulcerating syndrome is also well recognized, the mucosa appearing nodular at the site of the lesion.

Histologically, the lamina propria is replaced by fibroblasts and fibrous tissue, and smooth muscle fibers that emanate from a thickened muscularis mucosae and stream towards the surface of the mucosa. The mucosal surface shows goblet cell depletion and reactive hyperplasia, and the crypts sometimes show cystic dilatation. When the biopsy is taken from the center of an ulcer, dense fibrosis of the submucosa is seen with overlying granulation tissue and necrotic cells.

The solitary ulcer syndrome is chronic and ulcers may persist unchanged for many years.

Etiology

The etiology of the solitary ulcer syndrome is uncertain. In some patients[110] there is electromyographic evidence of hyperactivity of the puborectalis muscle as is seen in the descending perineum syndrome[111], and it has been suggested that during defecation high intra-abdominal pressure forces the anterior wall of the rectum on to the contracted puborectalis. The anterior wall of the rectum may also be forced towards the anal canal with resulting ischemia. Direct trauma to the rectal mucosa by insertion of the patient's finger into the rectum (self digitation) or the insertion of foreign bodies into the rectum has been suggested as a possible cause of the rectal ulceration[112]. In this respect it is interesting to note that 8 of 234 homosexual men who consecutively attended an STI clinic in Edinburgh had histological changes suggestive of the syndrome, namely thickened muscularis mucosae, streaming of muscle fibers between the crypts, and fibrosis of the lamina propria. In only one of these men was there rectal ulceration.

Treatment

Treatment consists of reassurance about the benign nature of the syndrome and symptomatic therapy if severe bleeding occurs. Exclusion of STIs remains a constant medical duty in the case of those at risk.

PERIANAL HEMATOMA ('THROMBOSED EXTERNAL PILE')

A perianal hematoma is a common problem amongst homosexual men. It presents as a painful swelling of the anal margin often following, or soon after, traumatic receptive anal intercourse. On examination there is a tender dark blue-purple swelling about 2 to 4 cm in diameter at the anal margin. Although it has been suggested that such lesions arise from rupture of small blood vessels, it seems more likely that it results from clotting within a vein under the non-hairy anal skin[113].

Although the lesion will burst or regress spontaneously, rapid relief can be achieved by opening the vein through a small incision.

PROCTALGIA FUGAX

This condition, whose symptoms may be mistaken for organic disease of the anorectum or prostate, is characterized by episodes of sudden onset pain apparently rising deeply within the rectum and lasting a few seconds to several minutes. The pain may occur at any time, but often at night when it awakens the sufferer. There are no abnormal clinical signs and investigation of the bowel shows no evidence of organic disease.

The etiology is unknown, but the condition may be a variant of the irritable colon syndrome[114].

Treatment consists of reassurance about the benign nature of proctalgia fugax.

ANORECTAL MALIGNANCY IN HOMOSEXUAL MEN

Anal intra-epithelial neoplasia and its association with HPV and HIV infection is discussed in Chapter 5.

Neoplasms may arise from
1. the columnar epithelium of the rectum
2. the stratified squamous epithelium of the anal canal and anal skin
3. the modified stratified epithelium which lies between the columnar epithelium of the rectum and the stratified squamous epithelium of the anal canal, namely the transitional zone, a segment of about 0.5 cm in length.

The majority (about 95%) of carcinomas of the rectum are adenocarcinomas, the others being undifferentiated anaplastic tumors and anaplastic mucus-secreting tumors ('signet-ring' cell carcinoma). Endocrine tumors, secondary tumors, leiomyosarcomas, and malignant lymphomas are less commonly found in the rectum.

Squamous cell carcinomas of the anal canal (that is those at the dentate line or above) arise from the transitional zone (cloagenic carcinoma). These carcinomas may be
1. of the basaloid type whose morphology, but not behavior, resembles that of basal cell carcinoma of the skin
2. the transitional cell type
3. squamous cell carcinomas of the ordinary type, with considerable variation in their differentiation.

Often there is an admixture of the various cell types. Mucoepidermoid carcinomas of the anal canal also arise from the transitional epithelium, but are rare. The carcinomas of the anal margin (that is those situated below the dentate line) are almost invariably well differentiated squamous cell carcinomas. Intra-epidermal squamous cell carcinoma (Bowen's disease) of the skin of the anal region may also be found.

In a study of colonic and rectal diseases in 260 homosexual men, Sohn and Robilotti[115] noted one case of Bowen's disease and another of squamous cell carcinoma of the anal region. Subsequently, other cases of cloagenic and squamous carcinoma of the anorectum have been reported[116–118].

Clinical features of anorectal neoplasia

Patients with anal neoplasm often complain of pain in the anal region, bleeding, and anal discharge. Rectal neoplasms often produce painless bleeding, a sensation of incomplete defecation if the lesion is in the lower part of the rectum, and alteration in bowel habit. Unless seen early, anal neoplasms may first be recognized as deeply ulcerated lesions. The appearance at sigmoidoscopy of rectal carcinomas varies considerably but in general they present as an ulcerated or polypoidal lesions. In all cases of anorectal ulceration for which there is no readily identifiable cause, a referral should be made to a surgical colleague for biopsy.

Treatment

The treatment of anorectal neoplasm falls outside the scope of this book and interested readers are referred to text books of anorectal surgery.

PERIANAL ABSCESSES, ANAL FISSURES, AND HEMORRHOIDS

The prevalence of these conditions in homosexual and heterosexual men is similar. Abscesses present as painful, tender, perianal swellings which, unless small, require surgical drainage. Anal fistulae result from internal and external rupture of anal abscesses. Their internal orifice is often difficult to locate, but sometimes the fistulous tract can be palpated. The treatment of anal fistulae, which is often difficult, falls within the province of the surgeon. Similarly symptomatic hemorrhoids warrant surgical referral. It should be noted that the hemorrhoids may not be the cause of the patient's anorectal symptoms and that a careful rectal examination is necessary.

METAPLASTIC POLYPS

A common sigmoidoscopic finding in men and women of all ages is the presence of discoid nodules of only a few millimeters in size projecting from the mucosa. They are of the same color as the surrounding mucosa and are seldom pedunculated. Histologically there is lengthening of the crypts which are dilated and their epithelium becomes flattened or papillary. The number of goblet cells is diminished[119].

Metaplastic polyps should be regarded as benign lesions which do not produce symptoms, and removal is not indicated. The management of other polyps, which may occasionally be found in homosexual men[115], falls outside the scope of the physician and referral to a surgeon is indicated.

References

1 Quinn TC, Stamm WE, Goodell SE *et al.* The polymicrobial origin of intestinal infections in homosexual men. *N Engl J Med* 1983; **309**: 576–582.

2 Law CLH, Qassim M, Cunningham AL, Mulhall B, Grierson JM. Nonspecific proctitis: association with human immunodeficiency virus infection in homosexual men. *J Infect Dis* 1992; **165**: 150–154.

3 Kumar NB, Nostrant TT, Appelman HD. The histopathologic spectrum of acute self-limited colitis (acute infectious-type colitis). *Am J Surg Pathol* 1982; **6**: 523–529.

4 Mandal BK, Schofield PF, Morson BC. A clinicopathological study of acute colitis: the dilemma of transient colitis syndrome. *Scand J Gastroenterol* 1982 **17**: 865–869.

5 Watts JMcK, Thompson H, Goligher JC. Sigmoidoscopy and cytology in the detection of microscopic disease of the rectal mucosa in ulcerative colitis. *Gut* 1966; **7**: 288–294.

6 Sider L, Mintzer RA, Mendelson EB, Rogers LF, Degesys GE. Radiographic findings of infectious proctitis in homosexual men. *Am J Roentgenol* 1982; **139**: 667–671.

7 McMillan A, Gilmour HM, Slatford K, McNeillage GJC. Proctitis in homosexual men. A diagnostic problem. *Br J Vener Dis* 1983; **59**: 260–264.

8 Markell EK, Havens RF, Kuritsubo RA, Wingerd J. Intestinal protozoa in homosexual men of the San Francisco Bay Area: prevalence and correlates of infection. *Am J Trop Med Hyg* 1984; **33**: 239–245.

9 Kulda J, Nohynkova E. Intestinal flagellates. In: Kreir J (ed) *Parasitic Protozoa* vol. II. London; Academic Press: 1978.

10 Rendtorff RC. The experimental transmission of *Giardia lamblia* among volunteer subjects. In: Jacubowski W, Hoff JC (eds) *Waterborne Transmission of Giardiasis*. Washington DC; US Environmental Protection Agency 600/9-79-001: 1978.

11 Meyers JD, Kuharic HA, Holmes KK. *Giardia lamblia* infection in homosexual men. *Br J Vener Dis* 1977; **53**: 54–55.

12 Schmerin MJ, Jones TC, Klein H. Giardiasis association with homosexuality. *Ann Int Med* 1978; **88**: 801–803.

13 Smith PD, Lane HV, Gill JF, *et al.* Intestinal infections in patients with acquired immunodeficiency syndrome (AIDS). *Ann Intern Med* 1988; **108**: 328–333.

14 Ridley MJ, Ridley DS. Serum antibodies and jejunal histology in giardiasis associated with malabsorption. *J Clin Pathol* 1976; **29**: 30–34.

15 Hartong WA, Gourley WK, Arvanitakis C. Giardiasis: clinical spectrum and functional-structural abnormalities of the small intestinal mucosa. *Gastroenterology* 1979; **77**: 61–69.

16 Wright SG, Tomkins AM, Ridley DS. Giardiasis: clinical and therapeutic aspects. *Gut* 1977; **18**: 343–350.

17 Ridley DS, Hagwood BC. The value of formol-ether concentration of faecal cysts and ova. *J Clin Pathol* 1956; **9**: 74–76.

18 Faubert G. Immune response to *Giardia duodenalis. Clin Microbiol Rev* 2000; **13**: 35–54.

19 Rosoff JD, Sanders CA, Seema SS, *et al.* Stool diagnosis of giardiasis using a commercially available enzyme immunoassay to detect *Giardia*-specific antigen (GSA 65). *J Clin Microbiol* 1989; **27**: 1997–2002.

20 Kamath KR, Murugasu RA. A comparative study of four methods for detecting *Giardia lamblia* in children with diarrheal disease and malabsorption. *Gastroenterology* 1974; **66**: 16–21.

21 Diamond LS, Harlow DR, Cunnick CC. A new medium for the axenic cultivation of *Entamoeba histolytica* and other *Entamoeba. Trans R Soc Trop Med Hyg* 1978; **72**: 431–432.

22 Beal CB, Viens P, Grant RGL, Hughes JMA. A new technique for sampling duodenal contents. Demonstration of upper

small-bowel pathogens. *Am J Trop Med Hyg* 1970; **19**: 349–352.

23 Wolfe M S. Giardiasis. *JAMA* 1975; **233**: 1362–1365.

24 Sargeaunt PG, Jackson TFHG, Simjee A. Biochemical homogeneity of *Entamoeba histolytica* isolates especially those from liver abscess. *Lancet* 1982; **i**: 1386–1388.

25 Sargeaunt PG, Baveja VK, Nanda R, Anand BS. Influence of geographical factors in the distribution of pathogenic zymodemes of *Entamoeba histolytica*: identification of zymodeme XIV in India. *Trans R Soc Trop Med Hyg* 1984; **78**: 96–101.

26 Gathiram V, Jackson TFHG. Frequency distribution of *Entamoeba histolytica* zymodemes in a rural South African population. *Lancet* 1985; **i**: 719–721.

27 Diamond LS, Clark CG. A redescription of *Entamoeba histolytica* Schaudinn 1903 (amended Walker 1911) separating it from *Entamoeba dispar* (Brumpt 1925). *J Eukaryot Microbiol* 1993; **40**: 340–344.

28 Sargeaunt PG, Oates JK, MacLennan I, Oriel JD, Goldmeier D. *Entamoeba histolytica* in male homosexuals. *Br J Vener Dis* 1983; **59**: 193–195.

29 McMillan A, Gilmour HM, McNeillage Gillian, Scott G R. Amoebiasis in homosexual men. *Gut* 1984; **25**: 356–360.

30 Goldmeier D, Sargeaunt PG, Price AJ, *et al.* Is *Entamoeba histolytica* in homosexual men a pathogen? *Lancet* 1986; **i**: 641–644.

31 Pakianathan MR, McMillan A. Intestinal protozoa in homosexual men in Edinburgh. *Int J STD AIDS* 1999; **10**: 780–784.

32 Burnham WR, Reeve RS, Finch RG. *Entamoeba histolytica* infection in male homosexuals. *Gut* 1980; **21**: 1097–1099.

33 Thompson JE, Freischlag J, Thomas DS. Amebic liver abscess in a homosexual man. *Sex Transm Dis* 1983; **10**: 153–155.

34 Prathap K, Gilman R. The histopathology of acute intestinal amebiasis. A rectal biopsy study. *Am J Pathol* 1970; **60**: 229–246.

35 Pittman FE, Hennigar GR, Charleston SC. Sigmoidoscopic and colonic mucosal biopsy findings in amebic colitis. *Arch Pathol* 1974; **97**: 155–158.

36 Purpon I, Jimenez D, Engelking RL. Amebiasis of the penis. *J Urol* 1967; **98**: 372–374.

37 Britten D, Wilson SM, McNerney R, Moody AH, Chiodini PL, Ackers JP. An improved colorimetric PCR-based method for detection and differentiation of *Entamoeba histolytica* and *Entamoeba dispar* in feces. *J Clin Microbiol* 1997; **35**: 1108–1111.

38 Wheatley WB. A rapid staining procedure for intestinal amoebae and flagellates. *Am J Clin Pathol* 1951; **21**: 990–991.

39 Brooke MM, Goldman M. Polyvinyl alcohol-fixative as a preservative and adhesive for protozoa in dysenteric stools and other liquid materials. *J Lab Clin Med* 1949; **34**: 1554–1560.

40 Jensen JB, Kepley W, Guarner J, *et al.* Comparison of polyvinyl alcohol fixative with three less hazardous fixatives for detection and identification of intestinal parasites. *J Clin Microbiol* 2000; **38**: 1592–1598.

41 Root DM, Cole FX, Williamson J A. The development and standardization of an Elisa method for the detection of *Entamoeba histolytica* antigens in fecal samples. *Archivos de Investigacion Medica* 1978; **9**: 203–210.

42 Ungar BLP, Yolken RH, Quinn TC. Use of a monoclonal antibody in an enzyme immunoassay for the detection of *Entamoeba histolytica* in fecal specimens. *Am J Trop Med Hyg* 1985; **34**: 465–472.

43 Juniper K, Worrell CL, Minshew MC, Roth LS, Cypert H, Lloyd RE. Serologic diagnosis of amebiasis. *Am J Trop Med Hyg* 1972; **21**: 157–168.

44 Kessel JF, Lewis WP, Pasquel CM, Turner JA. Indirect hemagglutination and complement fixation tests in amebiasis. *Am J Trop Med Hyg* 1965; **14**: 540–550.

45 Jeanes A. Evaluation in clinical practice of the fluorescent amoebic antibody test. *J Clin Pathol* 1969; **22**: 427–429.

46 Upton SJ, Current WL. The species of *Cryptosporidium* (Apicomplexa: Cryptosporidiidae) infecting mammals. *J Parasitol* 1985; **71**: 625–629.

47 Meisel JL, Perera DR, Meligro C, Rubin CE. Overwhelming watery diarrhea associated with a Cryptosporidium in an immunosuppressed patient. *Gastroenterology* 1976; **70**: 1156–1160.

48 Lasser KH, Lewin KJ, Ryning FW. Cryptosporidial enteritis in a patient with congenital hypogammaglobulinemia. *Hum Pathol* 1979; **10**: 234–240.

49 Hojlying N, Molbak K, Jepsen S, Hansson AP. Cryptosporidiosis in Liberian children. *Lancet* 1984; **i**: 734.

50 Anderson BC, Donndelinger T, Wilkins RM, Smith J. Cryptosporidiosis in a veterinary student. *J Am Vet Med Assoc* 1982; **180**: 408–409.

51 Current WL, Reese NC, Ernst JV, Bailey WS, Hevman MB, Weinstein WM. Human cryptosporidiosis in immunocompetent and immunodeficient persons. Studies of an outbreak and experimental transmission. *N Engl J Med* 1983; **308**: 1252–1257.

52 Casemore DP, Jackson FB. Hypothesis: cryptosporidiosis in human beings is not primarily a zoonosis. *J Infect* 1984; **9**: 153–156.

53 Hart CA, Baxby D, Blundell N. Gastro-enteritis due to Cryptosporidium: a

prospective survey in a children's hospital. *J Infect* 1984; **9**: 264–270.

54 Jokipii L, Pohjola S, Jokipii AMM. Cryptosporidium: a frequent finding in patients with gastro-intestinal symptoms. *Lancet* 1983; **ii**: 358–361.

55 Soave P, Danner RL, Honig CL, Ma P, Hart CC, Nash T, Roberts RB. Cryptosporidiosis in homosexual men. *Ann Int Med* 1984; **100**: 504–511.

56 Nime FA, Burek JD, Page DL, Holscher MA, Yardley JH. Acute enterocolitis in a human being infected with the protozoan Cryptosporidium. *Gastroenterology* 1976; **70**: 592–598.

57 Bird RG, Smith MD. Cryptosporidiosis in man: parasite life cycle and fine structural pathology. *J Pathol* 1980; **132**: 217–233.

58 Henriksen Sv Aa, Pohlenz JEL. Staining of Cryptosporidia by a modified Ziehl-Neelsen technique. *Acta Vet Scand* 1981; **22**: 594–596.

59 Kehl KS, Cicirello H, Havens PL. Comparison of four different methods for the detection of *Cryptosporidium* species. *J Clin Microbiol* 1995; **33**: 416–418.

60 Waugh MA. Threadworm infestation in homosexuals. *Transactions of the St Johns' Hospital Dermatological Society* 1972; **58**: 224–225.

61 Phillips SC, Mildvan D, Williams DC, Gelb AM, White MC. Sexual transmission of enteric protozoa and helminths in a venereal-disease-clinic population. *N Engl J Med* 1981; **305**: 603–606.

62 Sorvilloi F, Mori K, Sewake W, Fishman L. Sexual transmission of *Strongyloides stercoralis* among homosexual men. *Br J Vener Dis* 1983; **59**: 342.

63 Carvalho-Filho E. Strongyloidiasis. *Clinics in Gastroenterology* 1978; **7/1**: 179–200.

64 Garcia LS, Ash LC. *Diagnostic Parasitology, Clinical Laboratory Manual.* CV Mosby Company; St Louis: 1979.

65 Dritz SK, Ainsworth TE, Garrard WF, Back A, Palmer RD, Boucher LA, River E. Patterns of sexually transmitted enteric diseases in a city. *Lancet* 1977; **ii**: 3–4.

66 Mentzing L-O. Waterborne outbreaks of *Campylobacter* enteritis in Central Sweden. *Lancet* 1981; **ii**: 352–354.

67 Robinson DA, Jones DM. Milk-borne campylobacter infection. *Br Med J* 1981; **282**: 1374–1376.

68 Blaser MJ, Checko P, Bopp C, Bruce A, Hughes JM. *Campylobacter* enteritis associated with foodborne transmission. *Am J Epidemiol* 1982; **116**: 886–894.

69 Jones DM, Robinson DA. Occupational exposure to *Campylobacter jejuni* infection. *Lancet* 1981; **i**: 440–441.

70 Simmons PD, Tabaqchali S. Campylobacter species in male homosexuals. *Br J Vener Dis* 1979; **55**: 66.

71 McMillan A, McNeillage GJC, Watson KC. The prevalence of antibodies reactive with

Campylobacter jejuni in the serum of homosexual men. *J Infect* 1984; **9**: 63–68.

72 Quinn TC, Goodell SE, Fennell C, *et al.* Infections with *Campylobacter jejuni* or *Campylobacter*-like organisms in homosexual men. *Ann Int Med* 1984; **101**: 187–192.

72a Quinn TC, Lukehart SA, Goodell S, Mkrtichian E, Schuffler MD, Holmes KK. Rectal mass caused by *Treponema pallidum*: confirmation by immunofluorescent staining. *Gastroenterology* 1982; **82**: 135–139.

73 Totten PA, Fennell CL, Tenover FC, *et al.* *Campylobacter cinaedi* (sp. nov.) and *Campylobacter fennelliae* (sp. nov.): two new *Campylobacter* species associated with enteric disease in homosexual men. *J Infect Dis* 1985; **151**: 131–139.

74 Laughon BE, Vernon AA, Druckman DA, *et al.* Recovery of *Campylobacter* species from homosexual men. *J Infect Dis* 1988; **158**: 464–467.

75 Blaser MJ, Berkowitz ID, LaForce FM, Cravens J, Reller LB. Wang W-LL. Campylobacter enteritis: clinical and epidemiological features. *Ann Int Med* 1979; **91**: 179–185.

76 Lambert ME, Schofield PF, Ironside AG, Mandal BK. Campylobacter colitis. *B Med J* 1979; **i**: 857–859.

77 Watson KC, Kerr EJC, McFadzean SM. Serology of human campylobacter infections. *J Infect* 1979; **1**: 151–158.

78 Taylor DE, DeGrandis SA, Karmali MA, *et al.* Erythromycin resistance in *Campylobacter jejuni.* In: Newell DG (ed.) *Campylobacter Epidemiology Pathogenesis and Biochemistry.* Baltimore; MTP Press: 1982.

79 Judson FN, Ehret JM, Eickhoff TC. Anogenital infection with *Neisseria meningitidis* in homosexual men. *J Infect Dis* 1978; **137**: 458–463.

80 Janda WM, Bohnhoff M, Morello JA, Lerner SA. Prevalence and site-pathogen studies of *Neisseria meningitidis* and *N. gonorrhoeae* in homosexual men. *JAMA* 1980; **244**: 2060–2064.

81 Nazemi MM, Musher DM, Schell RF, Milo S. Syphilitic proctitis in a homosexual. *JAMA* 1975; **231**: 389.

82 Voinchet O, Quivarc'h M. Chancre syphilitique simulant un cancer du rectum. *Gastroenterologie Clinique et Biologique* 1980; **4**: 134–136.

83 Akdamar K, Martin RJ, Ichinose H. Syphilitic proctitis. *Dig Dis* 1977; **22**: 701–704.

84 Hovind-Hougen K, Birch-Andersen A, Henrik-Nielsen R, *et al.* Intestinal spirochaetosis: morphological characterization and cultivation of the spirochaete *Brachyspira aalborgi* gen. nov. sp. nov. *J Clin Microbiol* 1982; **16**: 1127–1136.

85 Harland WA, Lee FD. Intestinal spirochaetosis. *Br Med J* 1967; **iii**: 718–719, plate between pages 708 and 709.

86 Takeuchi A, Jarvis HR, Nakazawa H, Robinson DM. Spiral-shaped organisms on the surface colonic epithelium of the monkey and man. *Am J Clin Nutr* 1974; **27**: 1287–1296.

87 Lee FD, Krazewski A, Gordon J, Howie JGR, McSeveney D, Harland WA. Intestinal spirochaetosis. *Gut* 1971; **12**: 126–133.

88 McMillan A, Lee FD. Sigmoidoscopic and microscopic appearance of the rectal mucosa in homosexual men. *Gut* 1981; **22**: 1035–1041.

89 Douglas JG, Crucioli V. Spirochaetosis: a remediable cause of diarrhoea and rectal bleeding. *Br Med J* 1981; **283**: 1362.

90 Cotton DWK, Kirkham N, Hicks DA. Rectal spirochaetosis. *Br J Vener Dis* 1984; **60**: 106–109.

91 Bowie WR, Alexander ER, Holmes KK. Etiologies of post gonococcal urethritis in homosexual and heterosexual men: roles of *Chlamydia trachomatis* and *Ureaplasma urealyticum. Sex Transm Dis* 1978; **5**: 151–154.

92 Munday PE, Dawson SG, Johnson AP, *et al.* A microbiological study of non-gonococcal proctitis in passive male homosexuals. *Postgrad Med J* 1981; **57**: 705–711.

93 Hooton TM, Roberts MC, Roberts PL, Holmes KK, Stamm WE, Kenny GE. Prevalence of *Mycoplasma genitalium* determined by DNA probe in men with urethritis. *Lancet* 1988; **i**: 266–268.

94 Jensen JS, Orsum R, Dohn B, Uldum S, Worm A-M, Lind K. *Mycoplasma genitalium*: a cause of male urethritis? *Genitourin Med* 1993; **69**: 265–269.

95 Goldmeier D. Proctitis and herpes simplex virus in homosexual men. *Br J Vener Dis* 1980; **56**: 111–114.

96 Munday PE, Dawson SG, Johnson AP, *et al.* A microbiological study of non-gonococcal proctitis in passive male homosexuals. *Postgrad Med J* 1981; **57**: 705–711.

97 Goodell SE, Quinn TC, Mkrtichian E, Schuffler MD, Holmes KK, Corey L. Herpes simplex virus proctitis in homosexual men. Clinical, sigmoidoscopic and histopathologic features. *N Engl J Med* 1983; **308**: 868–871.

98 Curry JP, Embil JA, Williams CN. Manuel FR. Proctitis associated with *Herpesvirus hominis* type 2 infection. *Can Med Assoc J* 1978; **119**: 485–486.

99 Barone JE, Yee J, Nealon TF. Management of foreign bodies and trauma of the rectum. *Surgery, Gynecology and Obstetrics* 1983; **156**: 453–457.

100 Schouten WR, Briel JW, Auwerda JJ. Relationship between anal pressure and anodermal blood flow: the vascular

pathogenesis of anal fissures. *Dis Colon Rectum* 1994; **37**: 664–669.

101 McMillan A, Smith IW. Painful anal ulceration in homosexual men. *Br J Surg* 1984; **71**: 215–216.

102 O'Kelly T, Brading A, Mortensen N. Nerve mediated relaxation of the human internal anal sphincter: the role of nitric oxide. *Gut* 1993; **34**: 689–693.

103 Lund JN, Scholefield JH. A randomised, prospective, double-blind, placebo-controlled trial of glyceryl trinitrate ointment in treatment of anal fissure. *Lancet* 1997; **349**: 11–14.

104 Schouten WR, Briel JW, Boerma MO, Auwerda JJA, Wilms EB, Graatsma BH. Pathophysiological aspects and clinical outcome of intra-anal application of isosorbide dinitrate in patients with chronic anal fissure. *Gut* 1996; **39**: 465–469.

105 Maria G, Cassetta E, Gui D, Brisinda G, Bentivoglio AR, Albanese A. A comparison of botulinum toxin and saline for the treatment of chronic anal fissure. *N Engl J Med* 1998; **338**: 217–220.

106 Sohn N, Weinstein M A, Gonchar J. Social injuries of the rectum. *Am J Surg* 1977; **134**: 611–612.

107 Weinstein MA, Sohn N, Robbins RD. Syndrome of pelvic cellulitis following rectal sexual trauma. *Am J Gastroenterol* 1981; **75**: 380–381.

108 Miles AJG. Pathophysiology of anoreceptive intercourse. In: Allen-Mersh TG, Gottesman L (eds) *Anorectal Disease in AIDS.* London; Edward Arnold: 1991.

109 Madigan MR, Morson BC. Solitary ulcer of the rectum. *Gut* 1969; **10**: 871–881

110 Rutter KRP. Solitary rectal ulcer syndrome. *Proc R Soc Med* 1975; **68**: 22–26.

111 Parks AG, Porter NH, Hardcastle J. The syndrome of the descending perineum. *Proc Roy Soc Med* 1966; **59**: 477–482.

112 Thomson H, Hill D. Solitary rectal ulcer: always a self-induced condition? *Br J Surg* 1980; **67**: 784–785.

113 Thomson H. The real nature of 'perianal haematoma'. *Lancet* 1982; **ii**: 467–468.

114 Harvey RF. Colonic motility in proctalgia fugax. *Lancet* 1979; **ii**: 713–714.

115 Sohn N, Robilotti JG. The gay bowel syndrome. A review of colonic and rectal conditions in 200 male homosexuals. *Am J Gastroenterol* 1977; **67**: 478–484

116 Cooper HS, Patchefsky AS, Marks G. Cloagenic carcinoma of the anorectum in homosexual men: an observation of four cases. *Dis Colon Rectum* 1979; **22**: 557–558.

117 Leach RD, Ellis H. Carcinoma of the rectum in male homosexuals. *J R Soc Med* 1981; **74**: 490–491.

118 Li FP, Osborn D, Cronin CM. Anorectal squamous carcinoma in two homosexual men. *Lancet* 1982; **ii**: 391.

119 Morson BC. The large intestine. In: Symmers HSTC (ed.) *Systemic Pathology* 2nd edition. Edinburgh; Churchill Livingstone: 1978.

120 William DC, Shookhoff HB, Felman YM, DeRamos SW. High rates of enteric protozoal infections in selected homosexual men attending a venereal disease clinic. *Sex Transm Dis* 1978; **5**: 155–157.

121 Keystone JS, Keystone DL, Proctor EM. Intestinal parasitic infections in homosexual men: prevalence, symptoms and factors in transmission. *Can Med Assoc J* 1980; **123**: 512–514.

122 McMillan A. Intestinal parasites in homosexual men. *Scott Med J* 1980; **25**: 33–35.

123 Chin ATL, Gerken A. Carriage of intestinal protozoal cysts in homosexuals. *Br J Vener Dis* 1984; **60**: 193–195.

124 McMillan A, Scott GR. *Sexually Transmitted Infections, Colour Guide*. Churchill Livingstone; Edinburgh: 2000.

125 Robertson DHH., McMillan A, Young H. *Clinical Practice in Sexually Transmissible Diseases* 2nd edition. Edinburgh; Churchill Livingstone: 1989.

Chapter 19

Arthropod infestations
A McMillan

Scabies

The condition known as scabies or 'the itch' is caused by the invasion of the stratum corneum of man by the mite *Sarcoptes scabiei* var. *hominis*. Although promiscuous sexual behavior may contribute to its spread among adolescents and young adults, in most cases it is not spread by this means and, in this regard, domestic outbreaks within a household or family are more important within the community. Control may be achieved by early diagnosis and correct treatment of the patient and all members of the household, whether sharing beds or not. Individuals harboring very large numbers of *Sarcoptes* mites may play an important part in the maintenance and spread of the disease in the community, and waxing and waning of herd immunity may contribute to fluctuations in its incidence.

ETIOLOGY

The mite, *Sarcoptes scabiei* var. *hominis*, the cause of scabies, is translucent and hemispherical, the female mite measures 0.4 × 0.3 mm (Figure 19.1) and the male is about half this size. The adult mite has eight legs, there are transverse corrugations on its body, and spines and bristles on its dorsal surface. Fuller morphological details are given by Mellanby in the important monograph on his original work[1], and fine anatomical detail is provided beautifully by Heilesen[2].

Mites can move rapidly on the warm skin (at a rate of about 2.5 cm/min). The female, when fertilized, reaches its adult size and exercises some selection of the site on the stratum corneum into which to

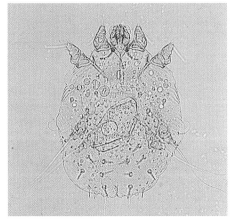

Figure 19.1 Mite of *Sarcoptes scabiei* (× 40) (reproduced from McMillan and Scott 2000[64])

excavate a burrow. The capitulum ('head') dips into the nucleated cellular layer of the stratum granulosum to obtain nourishment and fluids[3]. The mite extends its burrow daily by 2 mm, lays 1 to 3 eggs each day, and dies after 25 or more eggs have been laid. Six-legged larvae emerge after 3 to 4 days and shelter in hair follicles where they undergo a molt to form an eight-legged nymph, which possibly molts again to form a second nymph. After another molt a mature adult male or an immature female is formed.

Mites are to be found in burrows at certain anatomical sites not influenced by the site of the initial infestation. The majority of mites (63%) are found on the hands and wrists; the next most favored site is the extensor aspect of the elbow, where about 11% of the acari are found, the feet and genitals each may harbor about 9%, the buttocks 4%, the axillae 2%, and on the whole remaining surface of the body only 2% of the mite population can be found[1]. The total population of mites is generally

only about a dozen, but in 3% of patients there may be over 500. In the case of crusted scabies (Norwegian scabies) there may be very high counts, both on the patient and in the scale from the skin; in one such patient, washings from pajamas and bed linen over a 48-hour period yielded 7640 mites[4].

EPIDEMIOLOGY

Scabies occurs in cyclical epidemics. From a study in Sheffield, where notification had been introduced in 1975, it was concluded that spread by sexual contact plays only a small part in the spread of the disease[5]. Infestation is introduced to households mainly by schoolchildren and teenagers, especially girls. The commonest sources are friends and relatives outside the home, and schools do not play an appreciable part in the spread. The high incidence in teenage girls is attributed to their greater contact with younger children and their habit of holding hands; girls also may share a bed more often than boys[6]. In Sheffield, notification and contact tracing led to the detection of cases of scabies in 17% of the 873 contacts examined; despite these efforts in contact tracing however, the incidence of the disease in the community was not reduced[5].

It is thought that about 15 years of widespread infestation is followed by a similar period when the disease becomes rare, although the cycle does not appear to be clear-cut[7]. Some degree of immunity is induced by *S. scabiei* and epidemics may be related to resurgence of the disease when 'herd immunity' had declined during a period of low incidence[1]. An increased frequency of human leukocyte antigen (HLA) A11 (36.7%) was found in a non-atopic group of patients with scabies, compared to a frequency of 10.4% in a healthy Norwegian population; the relative risk (RR) for scabies in those who carry HLA-A11 is about 4. If this tendency holds true for other populations it would support the view that genetic differences in hosts may play some role in defense[8]. Normally in scabies there is an immune response up to the third month, in which there is a marked reduction in parasite numbers. This is a delayed hypersensitivity caused by a cell-mediated immunity response, probably with some skin IgE[9]. The persistence of the acarus in asymptomatic patients and in cases of undiagnosed Norwegian scabies will form important sources of infection. Within hospital ward epidemics, isolation of the individual with crusted scabies (Norwegian scabies) may require environmental followed by personal disinfestation, because cuticular fragments containing mites are abundant in the surrounding environment in such cases[4]. In scabies treated with topical steroids or immunosuppressants, patients sometimes carry large numbers of acari[10].

Although family outbreaks are important in most communities, it is important to take a sexual history and exclude other STIs when scabies is found in an adolescent or young adult. Scabies is seen not uncommonly in STI clinics: for example, in the year ending March 1998, scabies was diagnosed in 131 patients who attended STI clinics in Scotland.

IMMUNOLOGY OF SCABIES

The morbidity of scabies depends to a very large extent on the inflammation and intense itch that accompanies the host response. Although the attribution of individual immunological responses to specific antigens in or on the surface of the mite is not yet possible, it is useful to consider briefly some of the assembled evidence[11] for the 'classical' types of reaction by which an individual 'sensitized' by previous experiences of the antigen(s) may react and, if the reaction is intense enough, suffer as a result of the allergic state[12].

Type I reactions are 'wheal and flare' responses – with the development of burrows, antigen probably diffuses down gradually through the epidermis and pro-

duces interaction with specific IgE on the mast cell surface in a way so insidious or sporadic that sudden whealing does not occur. Although anaphylaxis has not been reported, sometimes there is a generalized urticaria. Among the changes seen in a Type I reaction the following have been noted

1. IgE antibody levels are elevated in infected patients and fall after successful treatment
2. intracutaneous tests with extract of adult female mites cause wheal reactions in those who have had scabies but not in those who have not had it
3. this reaction can be passively transferred by a factor in the serum (Prausnitz–Küstner)
4. serum from a patient with crusted scabies caused histamine release using a basophil degranulation test
5. in crusted scabies serum IgE levels may be very high
6. antigen-specific IgE in serum is elevated using crude scabies antigens
7. IgE antibodies cross-react with antigens from a common house mite, *Dermatophagoides pteronyssinus*[11].

Type II reactions are cytotoxic reactions generated by a combination of IgG or IgM antibodies with antigens. High levels of IgG or IgM are sometimes present in some patients with scabies, but it is not known if these are specific or non-specific or are caused by the associated pyogenic infection.

Serum levels of IgA are sometimes decreased during infestation and rise after treatment. The reason for the decreased levels is not known.

Levels of complement components C3 and C4 are usually normal. Immunoglobulin M and C3 have been found at the dermal and epidermal junction of affected skin by direct immunofluorescence techniques, but this could be secondary to inflammation or non-specific.

Type III reactions are caused by immune complexes which have been found in the serum of patients with crusted scabies and ordinary scabies before and after treatment. Generalized cutaneous vasculitis has been associated with scabies infections[13] and vasculitis with blood-vessel necrosis has been seen in biopsy specimens[14].

Type IV reactions are cell-mediated immune reactions. Cell-mediated immunity is the probable explanation for the production of itchy papules. The evidence for this includes

1. non-reactivity in the unexposed individual
2. the latent period between infestation and rash
3. the clinical appearance of the papules
4. the life of the papules from 2 days to 2 weeks.

The histopathology of the papules shows a superficial and deep perivascular mixed inflammatory cell infiltrate composed of lymphocytes (mostly T cells), histiocytes and eosinophils, and is compatible with cell-mediated immune reactions.

In the patient the pattern seen is complex and may involve not one but several of the pathways. Patients with sensory defects do not sense itch and so do not scratch, thus mites may be allowed to reproduce *ad libidum*. In the immunodeficient and in those applying topical corticosteroids, crusted scabies has occurred; such evidence supports an immunological basis for this form of scabies, at least in some patients.

CLINICAL FEATURES

The presenting symptom is itching which is worse at night. This appears to be because of sensitization and tends to develop about 5 weeks after a first infection, but earlier in the second and subsequent attacks. The reaction tends to be most intense on the genitals and buttocks where the acari may be destroyed by scratching.

Burrows and vesicles associated directly with the presence of the mite

The pathognomonic lesions are the burrows, appearing as serpiginous grayish ridges, 5 to 15 mm in length, which may be difficult to find if hygiene is good. The mite is visible in the burrow as a raised whitish oval with dark pigmentation anteriorly.

Sarcoptes scabiei can be found mainly in burrows at specific sites, namely, on the anterior aspect of the wrist (Figure 19.2), along the ulnar border of the hand, between the fingers, on the extensor aspects

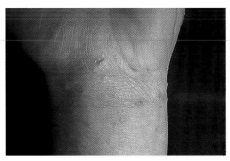

Figure 19.2 Scabetic burrows (reproduced from McMillan and Scott 2000[64])

of the elbows, around the nipples in the female, and in the natal cleft. Mellanby[15] lists the frequency with which the different sites were affected in 886 cases (given as percentages): hands and wrists 85%, extensor aspect of the elbows 41%, feet and ankles 37%, penis and scrotum 36%, buttocks 16%, axillae 15%, knee 6%, umbilicus 3%, and hip, thigh, abdomen, arm, chest, nipples, back, and neck were other sites less commonly affected.

Vesicles occur at the end of burrows and also separately from them, especially at the sides of the fingers. In infants bullae may form, particularly on the palms and soles[16].

Urticarial papules not associated directly with the presence of the mite

Although papular lesions occur near the mite, an erythematous rash with urticarial papules is often most prominent in areas where mites are not necessarily found. Mellanby[1] has mapped these areas (Figure 19.3). Scratch marks, often with pin-point blood crusts at the apices of follicles, may be numerous. Papules may ulcerate as a result of scratching but could be caused by a Type III reaction with local formation of immune complexes (Arthus reaction)[11]. In 30% of patients there are penile and scrotal lesions[16].

Indurated nodules

In about 7% of cases itchy indurated nodules may be found. The commonest sites have been recorded as axillae 50%, scrotum 40% (Figure 19.4), abdomen, sides of chest, and groins, each about 30%, and on the penis about 20%. The nodules may persist after

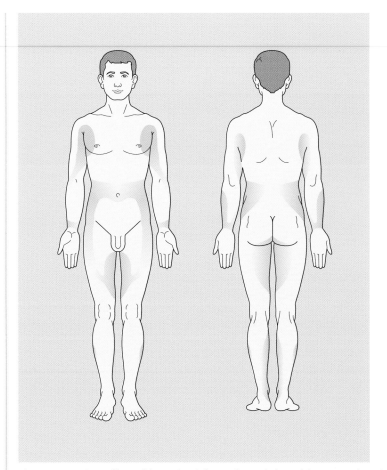

Figure 19.3 Sites affected by urticarial papular rash in scabies. Note that the rash does not correspond with the sites of election of the acari – see text (reproduced from Mellanby 1972[1])

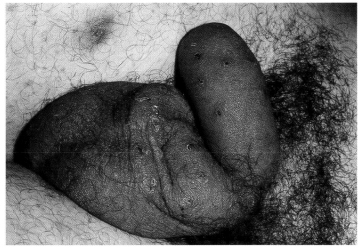

Figure 19.4 Scabetic nodules on the scrotum and penis

treatment, but in only 20% of cases do they persist for longer than 3 months[17]. Nodules may result from persisting antigen although parts of the mite are not usually to be seen after the first month[11].

Other changes seen in scabies

Eczematous changes may follow scratching, and secondary bacterial infection may cause pustular lesions or even pyoderma.

Colonization of scabetic lesions with alpha-hemolytic streptococci is common; when these are nephritogenic acute glomerulonephritis may result, as in Trinidad in 1971 where the attack rate for acute glomerulonephritis reached 5.2 per 1000 children of 5 to 9 years of age[18].

Crusted scabies or Norwegian scabies, associated with vast numbers of mites, tends to be seen in people with learning difficulties and in immunocompromised individuals, including those with HIV infection[19] and in cases where there is lack of cutaneous sensibility as in leprosy, syringomyelia, and tabes dorsalis. Crusted scabies occurs also when there is a lack of hypersensitivity as may occur because of a failure of sensitization to mite antigens, acquisition of immune tolerance, or during treatment with corticosteroid or immunosuppressive drugs[20, 21]. It has also been suggested that low IgE levels may predispose to scabies[22]. Crusted scabies affects the hands and feet where it appears psoriasiform with hyperkeratosis of the nails, and the face, neck, scalp, and trunk where there is an erythematous, scaling eruption[23]. The condition may be localized, for example, to the scalp. The itch is often mild. The differential diagnosis includes psoriasis, hyperkeratotic eczema, and Darier's disease.

DIAGNOSIS

The mite can best be found by means of an illuminated magnifier and can be secured from a burrow on the point of a needle; it may be examined on a dry slide without mounting fluid. The burrows are pathognomonic lesions of scabies, but identification of the mite is desirable to secure accuracy in diagnosis. If scrapings are to be examined because an individual mite cannot be found, it has been suggested that a drop of liquid paraffin should be placed over the suspected site and the lesion scraped with a scalpel blade. The suspended material can then be examined microscopically as an oily film covered by a cover-slip[24].

In scabies of animal origin the clinical presentation is 'scabies without burrows'. Irritable papules or papulovesicles, appearing at sites of close contact with the family pet, may be due to Sarcoptes scabiei var. canis. Its feline counterpart, Notoedres cati, is rare in Britain but not uncommon in Czechoslovakia and Japan[17].

TREATMENT

Several agents (Table 19.1) are available for the topical treatment of scabies, but permethrin has several advantages over the others and it is the authors' treatment of choice.

Permethrin cream

Permethrin [(±)-3-phenoxybenzyl 3-(2,2-dichlorovinyl)-2,2-dimethylcyclo-propanecarboxylate] is a synthetic pyrethroid with potent insecticide activity[25] that, in clinical trials, has been found to be as efficacious as lindane[26]. Several studies have shown that it is poorly absorbed from the human skin: only about 0.7% of the applied chemical is absorbed[27]. After its application permethrin is metabolized by esterases in the skin into inactive metabolites that are excreted in the urine; only very small quantities of unchanged drug are found in plasma. Adverse events with permethrin are uncommon (2.5 per 1000 applications)[28] and include localized burning, irritation, or tingling sensations, usually of short duration. The incidence of burning sensations appears to be higher in individuals with symptomatic HIV infection[25].

Instructions for use (British National Formulary, Number 42, 2001)

1. Apply permethrin dermal cream, 5% w/w, over the whole body, including the face, neck, scalp, and ears. Particular attention should be paid to the webs of the fingers and toes, and brushing the cream under the ends of the nails.
2. Wash off 8 to 12 hours later. If the hands are washed within 8 hours of the application, cream should be re-applied (the same advice is given for all the topical scabicides).

Lindane (gamma benzene hexachloride)

Since the successful use of a 1% gamma benzene hexachloride (lindane) cream in the treatment of scabies, recorded by Wooldridge[29], this insecticide has been regarded as the most effective, safest, and least irritant form of treatment. The preferred preparation is lindane 1% in a water-dispersible base. Although ill effects are seldom reported with the one or two applications required in treatment of the individual case, and although such treatment cannot be equated with risks in more intense or prolonged exposure, theoretical considerations of toxicity have led to the advocacy of more caution in its use[30]. These concerns about safety have led to the withdrawal of lindane from the markets of some countries, including the UK.

In the treatment of scabies with lindane lotion, according to Solomon et al.[30] there are 'rare anecdotal communications' of toxicity (headache, nausea, transient seizures) which resemble the more serious effects of exposure to a very high dosage. Brief consideration of the subject of toxicity is therefore justified here. Lindane can be absorbed percutaneously, and the scrotal skin, for example, poses virtually no barrier

Table 19.1 Topical agents used in the treatment of scabies

Scabicide	Frequency of application	Toxicity
Permethrin 5% cream	One application left on over 8–12 hours	Low
Malathion liquid emulsion	One application left on over 4 hours	Low
Benzyl benzoate	Two applications over 48 hours	Low
Lindane	Two applications 72 hours apart	Medium
Sulfur ointment	Each night for 3 nights	Low

to its penetration[31]. Early experimental work showed that, although metabolized by the liver and stored in depot fat and other lipophilic tissues, the gamma isomer of benzene hexachloride (lindane) was eliminated very rapidly and disappeared from fat depots in rats, for example, within 3 weeks[32]; there are, however, no data of this kind for man.

A study of pesticide workers in Hungary[33] showed a correlation between blood concentrations about 0.02 parts per million and EEG abnormalities in 15 of 17 subjects; additional toxic effects such as depressed liver function and cardiac arrhythmia have been referred to by Solomon et al.[30] in those suffering from chronic exposure. Although ill effects of a systemic nature resulting from the topical application of the 1% lindane lotion in the limited manner used in the treatment of scabies, have not been recorded in the literature, Solomon et al.[30] make certain observations regarding its use. Because percutaneous absorption may well be greater in those whose skin has been damaged by excoriation, or in infants, it is suggested that it might be better to apply the agent to the dry cool skin, or to allow the skin to dry and cool after any cleansing bath is taken, rather than to prescribe the bath with hot soapy water originally advised by Wooldridge[29]. Cannon and McRae[34] found the application to be quite effective without bathing. Other suggestions of Solomon et al.[30] included a view that to leave the application on the skin for 24 hours before washing it off may be unnecessarily long, and that a shorter contact time might be as effective; similarly the 1% concentration might also be more than required. The substance should be avoided, Solomon et al.[30] suggest, in pregnancy, in very small infants, and in those with marked excoriation. They also advise that retreatment should not take place before 8 days and only if living acari are found.

Although the minimum dose needed to effect a cure in scabies has not been found, extensive clinical experience has shown that lindane 1% is an effective sarcopticide, even when as many as 10% of cases may also be secondarily infected[35]. Lindane-resistant scabies has now been reported from several geographical areas in the Americas and Asia[23].

The authors consider that lindane should be avoided in pregnant and lactating women, and it is better avoided in children under the age of 2 years[36]. Hospital staff should avoid regular contact with the substance.

Instructions for use*

1. Apply the lotion to all the skin from below the neck to, and including, the soles of the feet, and allow it to dry.
2. Dress in the clothing worn before the application of lindane.
3. After 12 hours wash with soap and water.
4. After an interval of 3 days apply the lotion again to all the skin from below the neck to the soles of the feet for the second and last time and allow to dry.
5. Change clothing and bed linen.
6. After 12 hours wash thoroughly with soap and water.

Benzyl benzoate application

Benzyl Benzoate Application BP, a 25% w/v emulsion (British National Formulary 2001, Number 42), is effective and suitable for adolescents or adults when there is little excoriation (it should not be used on broken or excoriated skin). It is rather sticky to use and irritant to excoriated skins, and it can cause eczematous lesions. It should not be used for children as it causes stinging in children. The safety of benzyl benzoate in pregnancy has not been established and its use should be avoided in pregnant women. Breast feeding should be suspended during treatment, but it may be restarted after the application has been washed off.

Instructions for use*

1. Apply the emulsion over the whole body, avoiding the eyes and mucous membranes.
2. The following day repeat the application without bathing.
3. Wash off with soap and water after 24 hours.

---

* Although different treatment regimens have been proposed[23], this is the schedule that the authors have used successfully for some years.

Malathion

Malathion is an organophosphate that, although data on efficacy are lacking, has been used widely in the treatment of scabies. It is available as a 0.5% w/w liquid emulsion (Quellada-M liquid, Stafford Miller Ltd). In plasma malathion is rapidly hydrolyzed into non-toxic compounds, and is considered safe for use in humans[37]. Although epidemiological studies suggested that individuals with chronic occupational exposure to malathion have an increased risk of hematological malignancies, the chemical has a low potential to cause chromosome damage in vitro, and corresponding doses are much higher than those that aerial sprayers are likely to be exposed to[38]. The risk of chromosome damage from the use of the insecticide in clinical practice must therefore be exceedingly low. Rarely, malathion application causes skin irritation, but prolonged use should be avoided; it should be used not more than once per week or for not more than three consecutive weeks. Its use should also be avoided in children under the age of 6 months. As data on safety in pregnant or lactating mothers are lacking, malathion should be used only after careful consideration of the possible risk; the authors prefer to use permethrin in these situations.

Instructions for the use of malathion (Stafford Miller Ltd Data Sheet 2000, Seton Scholl Healthcare plc Data Sheet 2000)

1. Apply the emulsion to the entire skin surface avoiding the eyes and mucous membranes.
2. Wash off after 24 hours.

Sulfur

Although not widely used in the UK, sulfur is an alternative to permethrin in the treatment of scabies[36]. Precipitated sulfur (6% w/w) in simple ointment* is applied thinly to all areas nightly for 3 nights. Previous applications should be washed off before the new application.

---

* Simple ointment BP:
       Wool fat, 5 parts
       Cetostearyl alcohol, 5 parts
       Hard paraffin, 5 parts
       White soft paraffin, 85 parts.

Ivermectin

Ivermectin is the first drug to be developed that can be given orally for the treatment of scabies (and head lice). It is not yet licensed for use in ectoparasitic infections.

Ivermectin is a semi-synthetic derivative of a family of macrocyclic lactones – the avermectins – that has been used extensively in the control of onchocerciasis in Africa and Latin America, and has been shown to be active against *S. scabiei*. The avermectins induce paralysis in nematodes and arthropods by interrupting γ-aminobutyric acid-mediated neurotransmission[39].

When given by mouth, the drug is rapidly absorbed, reaching peak plasma concentrations 4 hours after a 12 mg dose[40]. The drug is widely distributed but little crosses the blood–brain barrier. It is excreted almost entirely in the feces and its half-life is about 28 hours. In humans adverse events are rare. As teratogenic effects and maternal deaths have been reported in mice, its use should be avoided in pregnancy.

The efficacy of ivermectin in common scabies was shown in a placebo-controlled trial[41]. Although studies have shown that a single dose of the drug is as effective as the topical application of lindane or benzyl benzoate[42, 43], the numbers of patients studied were small, and it is difficult to draw meaningful conclusions. A single dose of ivermectin (200 μg/kg body weight) appears to be less effective than a single application of permethrin cream[44]. Scabies in HIV-infected individuals can be difficult to treat and Meinking *et al.*[45] reported cure of 8 of 11 patients using ivermectin.

Treatment of crusted scabies

Patients with crusted scabies should be admitted to hospital for treatment, and must be nursed in isolation to prevent dissemination of infection. Repeated applications of scabicide, preferably permethrin, should be used, and the crusts should be treated with a keratotolytic agent such as salicylic acid 10% w/w in white soft paraffin. Oral ivermectin given alone or combined with topical treatment has been useful in the management of patients with crusted scabies. Although some individuals are cured after a single oral dose of ivermectin (200 μg/kg), two or three

repeated doses at 1 or 2 weekly intervals are usually required[46]. Huffam and Currie[47] treated their patients with crusted scabies with oral ivermectin (200 μg/kg) combined with topical permethrin (5%), and reported complete response in 8 of 20 individuals; recurrence or re-infestation occurred in 4 patients. The rationale for the use of topical scabicide and keratolytics is that ivermectin may not penetrate the crust. Cure is usually effected in a mean of 3 weeks from initiation of therapy.

Treatment of scabies in pregnancy

There is little information on the safety of the available scabicides in pregnancy. Permethrin, however, is poorly absorbed from the skin and would appear to be safe for use in pregnant and lactating women. The topical application of lindane is not recommended, and, although there is no clear evidence that they are harmful to pregnant women, benzyl benzoate and malathion are probably better avoided. Ivermectin should not be used in pregnancy. If there are concerns about the safety of permethrin, sulfur in soft paraffin is a safe alternative.

Treatment of scabies in children

Permethrin is the treatment of choice. Lindane should not be used on children under the age of 2 years, and the use of malathion is best avoided in those aged 6 months and less. As stinging can occur in children treated with benzyl benzoate, its use cannot be recommended, but, if there is no suitable alternative, it can be used diluted twice to three times with water.

Other aspects of the treatment of scabies

It is helpful to give the patient a careful explanation of the condition together with written instructions for its treatment.

The patient should be told that although itching will diminish rapidly, it may not be completely relieved for some days or weeks. Although crotamiton cream, 10% w/w (Eurax cream, Novartis Consumer Health), applied twice or three times per day may be used to relieve the itch, it can cause contact allergy or irritation of the skin, particularly if there is excoriation. A sedating antihistamine such as chlorphenamine (chlorpheniramine) 10 mg taken at night may be useful. There are several possible causes of itching after treatment (Table 19.2).

All members of the household, irrespective of symptoms of infection, should be treated as well as any sexual contacts and an attempt should be made to find the primary or source case. When scabies has been acquired through sexual contact, screening for other STIs should be offered.

Ordinary laundering at 60°C of clothes and bed linen will destroy the mites.

Table 19.2 Causes and management of itching after treatment of scabies (after Chosidow 2000[23])

Cause	Management
Over-treatment or severe eczematous scabies	emollients with or without topical steroids
Contact dermatitis	topical steroid
Treatment failure	
poor adherence	further application of scabicide
resistance	change scabicide
relapse	further application of scabicide, consider re-infection or inadequate application of initial agent
Delusions of parasitosis	psychiatric referral
Misdiagnosis	treat appropriately, consider referral to a dermatologist

Pediculosis

The human louse, *Pediculus humanus*, is found in two forms, the head louse and the body louse, which can be considered as unstable environmental subspecies of the one species. The morphological differences between them are slight and variable and many specimens cannot be assigned to one or other type. The two forms are interfertile, with no evidence of type-specific mating choice[48]. The pubic louse is a different species, *Phthirus pubis*. All are obligate parasites of man and have mouth parts adapted for piercing the skin and sucking blood[49].

PEDICULUS HUMANUS AS THE BODY LOUSE

The adult female is a grayish-white insect 3 to 4 mm long, and the male a little smaller. The legs are adapted for grasping hairs. Both sexes suck blood and inject saliva while doing so. During a life-span of about a month the female lays 7 to 10 eggs per day. Eggs hatch in 8 days and the nymphs require a further 8 days to reach maturity. The eggs are oval-lidded capsules, firmly cemented to a hair or to a thread, particularly along the inside of seams. Lice survive more than 10 days away from their hosts, but eggs may survive in garments for a month.

Epidemiology

The infestation is occasionally seen in the homeless or mentally handicapped individuals who may attend clinics. The insects are spread by clothing or bedding, but the lice can travel short distances from the host.

The dimension to be faced in areas where a high proportion of the population carry *P. humanus* and where louse-borne typhus is endemic or epidemic, is quite different to that faced by doctors treating a single patient[50].

Clinical features

In previously unexposed individuals the bite provokes only pin-point red macules. After 7 days small wheals or more persistent papules develop as pruritus becomes more troublesome.

Treatment

The resistance of body lice to insecticides has been widely reported and may be determined by the use of the WHO standard test method. Where resistance has been found, various alternative dusting powders may have to be used (for example 1% malathion, 2% temephos, 5% carbaryl, and 1% propoxur)[50]. Malathion-resistant body lice have occurred in Africa, and resistance ultimately threatens all types of control by conventional insecticides.

When a vacuum steam disinfestor is not available, as in overcrowded camps, the infested clothing may be treated with a fumigant, such as ethyl formate, by personnel trained in its use[51, 50]. In hospitals, or where a large number of clothes have to be disinfested, the clothes are placed in a cotton bag and disinfested by a vacuum steam method. An ordinary tumble dryer is effective and kills the lice and eggs on dry clothing, after which they may be sent quite safely to a conventional laundry, if desired.

PEDICULUS HUMANUS AS THE HEAD LOUSE

Head lice are almost confined to the scalp, but may be found on hairs in other parts of the body. Long fine hair and infrequent washing increase the chance of infestation.

Epidemiology

The incidence of head louse infestation in the UK was high in school children before 1939, by 1960 it had been greatly reduced until in 1969 it was again found that in some cities 10% of school entrants were infested[17]. Sales by pharmacists in England and Wales of licensed insecticides increased 3.7-fold between 1990 and 1995[52]. Although head lice can be found at any time of year, the incidence appears to be higher in the warmer months[53]. It is occasionally seen in clinics in female patients, although long-haired men may also be infested. Morley[54] noted that in Teesside 23% of children in areas of poor and overcrowded housing were infested, compared with 0.4% in suburban areas; areas of local authority housing occupied an intermediate position with infestation rates of 13.4%. The lowest infestation rates were in children under 5 years of age, and the highest were in teenagers.

Clinical features

Pruritus is most severe around the back and sides of the scalp. Pruritus depends on hypersensitivity to the salivary antigens of the louse, and in heavy infestation there may be no itching. Later the hair may become matted with pus. Impetigo of the scalp of the nape of the neck may accompany the infection.

Treatment

As lice resistant to lindane are common, the treatments of choice in this infestation have been permethrin, malathion, and carbaryl.

Permethrin

Permethrin cream rinse 1% w/w permethrin with 20% w/w isopropanol in a cream base (Lyclear Crème Rinse, Warner-Lambert). It is applied liberally to hair and scalp that has just been washed and towel-dried. After leaving the cream on for 10 minutes, the hair is washed thoroughly with water. It is unnecessary to remove the egg cases.

Malathion

Malathion lotion 0.5% w/v in an alcoholic base (flammable) (Prioderm, Napp Laboratories), 55 mL is enough for five treatments. Sufficient lotion should be rubbed well into dry hair, *avoiding the eyes*. It is allowed to dry and to remain untouched for 12 hours. After a shampoo the hair should be combed with a fine comb to remove the dead lice and egg cases.

Carbaryl

Carbaryl lotion 0.5% w/v in an alcoholic base (flammable) (Carylderm, Seton Scholl) is applied in the same manner as malathion lotion. Ideally the insecticide should be active against both the louse and the egg. Unfortunately, there is variation in the ovicidal activity of the available preparations and, as none is thought to be 100% effective in this regard[55], it is recommended that the treatment is repeated after 7 days. If there is doubt about a patient's capacity to carry out instructions, treatment should be given by a nurse who should wear rubber gloves when applying malathion. Aqueous preparations of malathion, 0.5% as a liquid emulsion (Derbac-M, Seton Scholl) and carbaryl liquid, 1.0% (Carylderm Lotion, Seton Scholl) are available, and are preferable to alcoholic solutions in the treatment of patients with asthma or eczema; they are used in the same manner as the alcohol-based forms. As the contact time is short and the drug concentration is low, insecticide-containing shampoos should be avoided.

Insecticide resistance in head lice

There is increasing evidence that head lice are becoming resistant to both permethrin and malathion. Downs *et al.*[52] showed that head lice from schoolchildren in the west of England had high survival rates on insecticide-impregnated filter papers, and that treatment failure was high. Resistance has been attributed to the excessive chronic application of over-the-counter preparations, and it is interesting that the head lice studied by Downs remained sensitive to carbaryl, an agent whose sale in the UK is restricted.

Synthetic pyrethroids have two effects on insect tissue[52]

1. type I effects cause hyperexcitability and uncoordinated movements, and are not related to mortality
2. type II effects cause convulsions and paralysis and are related to mortality.

At low concentrations, permethrin shows type I effects, but at higher concentrations, type II effects are seen. Pyrethroids and DDT bind to sodium channel membrane proteins and block nerve conduction, or induce tetanus by delaying signal inactivation[56]. An altered insecticide-binding site within the insect nerves – the knockdown resistance (kdr) mechanism – caused by an amino acid substitution results in pyrethroid and DDT resistance.

Malathion (an organophosphate) and carbaryl (a carbamate) bind irreversibly to acetylcholinesterase at the same binding site, preventing its function[57]. As head lice remain fully sensitive to carbaryl, it is unlikely that resistance is associated with an altered acetylcholinesterase-binding site.

It is possible that there is a specific malathion-resistance mechanism, and if this is so, lice may not show cross resistance with other organophosphates[52].

As the geographical extent of resistance of head lice to insecticides is unknown, it is reasonable to use permethrin first, and should this fail to eradicate the infestation, carbaryl should be prescribed[58]. All members of the affected individual's family and close contacts should be examined.

THE CRAB LOUSE, *PHTHIRUS PUBIS*

The crab louse (*Phthirus pubis*) is grayish-white and measures about 1.2 to 2 mm in length and is nearly as broad as it is long (Figure 19.5). There are three spiracles on its first abdominal segment[49]. It remains almost immobile on its host, the hind legs grasping two hairs. In this position it continues to feed intermittently for hours or days, rarely removing its mouth parts from their positions in the host. The claws on the last two pairs of legs are adapted for grasping the widely spaced pubic hairs[48]. As it feeds it defecates frequently, voiding intermixed blood and feces. Defecation is frequent and much more localized on the skin than in *P. corporis* and since feeding is virtually continuous, there is more obvious 'dirtiness'[59].

Mating takes place on the host and some 26 eggs (Figure 19.6) may be laid in 12 days. After a week the eggs hatch and the nymph attaches within a few hours. Three

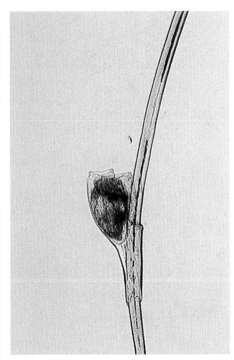

Figure 19.6 *Phthirus pubis* egg, nymph about to hatch (× 10) (reproduced from McMillan and Scott 2000[64])

molts occur within 17 days. The nymphs and adults cannot survive more than 2 days when removed from their host[60].

The blue 'spots' induced by the bites of *P. pubis* in the skin are known as *maculae coeruleae* and are caused by an enzyme from its salivary glands. These consist of *bean-shaped* and *horse-shoe-shaped* glands and it was established by Pavlovsky and Stein[61], working in Petrograd, that it is the

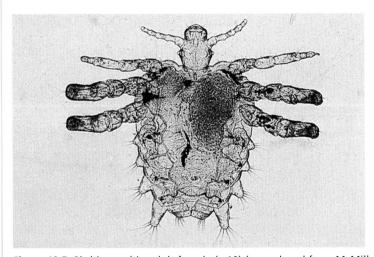

Figure 19.5 *Phthirus pubis*, adult female (× 10) (reproduced from McMillan and Scott 2000[64])

enzyme specifically from the bean-shaped glands, apparently acting on the hemoglobin, which causes the diffuse bluish discoloration.

Epidemiology

This louse is usually transferred by close body contact, but it can be spread by clothing. Pubic lice are a common infestation seen in patients attending clinics[62].

Clinical features

Intense irritation is often the only symptom. The blue-gray macules (*maculae coeruleae*) induced by the bite of the insect may be seen sometimes on the patient's abdominal wall and upper thighs. In some patients irritation is minimal and the numbers of lice or eggs to be found are few.

The louse is mainly confined to the hairs of the pubic (Figure 19.7) and perianal regions, but they may be found attached to the hairs of the abdomen, thighs, and axillae. Very rarely they may be seen on the margin of the scalp, the eyebrows and eyelashes. In infants they may have reached such sites from the breast hairs of the mother.

Treatment

In the treatment of pubic lice (Table 19.3), malathion or carbaryl are effective but, as the alcoholic solutions irritate the genital skin, only the aqueous preparations should be used. It is important to apply the lotion directly to the pubic hair, the hair of the axilla, and between the legs and around the anus; body hair elsewhere below the neck should also be treated as should the beard and moustache, if necessary. Permethrin is safe for use in pregnancy and in breast-feeding women.

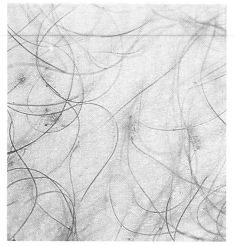

Figure 19.7 Phthiriasis of pubic hair (reproduced from McMillan and Scott 2000[64])

In eyelash infestations individual lice may be removed with forceps; an application of yellow soft paraffin may kill the lice by occlusion of its spiracles. The anticholinesterase effect of physostigmine is toxic to *P. pubis*, and the ophthalmic solution (0.25% w/v), applied three times per day for 5 days, has been used successfully[63]. Other sites should be treated simultaneously with carbaryl or malathion.

Sexual partners should be treated, and all clothes and bed linen should be machine washed. It is important to offer screening for other STIs.

There are no reports of insecticide resistance in *P. pubis*, but in view of the increased use of malathion and carbaryl, the future development of resistance cannot be excluded. Box 19.1 shows the possible reasons for treatment failure[23].

> **Box 19.1 Possible causes of treatment failure in phthiriasis**
>
> Non-adherence to the treatment regimen
>
> Misunderstanding of instructions
>
> Incomplete ovicidal activity
>
> Inappropriate insecticide preparation (e.g. shampoo)
>
> Insufficient dose time or quantity of agent
>
> Re-infestation
>
> Live eggs not removed
>
> Misdiagnosis

Table 19.3 Treatment of *Phthirus pubis* infestation

Agent	Frequency of application
Malathion 0.5% as liquid emulsion	one application[a] left on over 12 hours
Carbaryl 1% liquid	one application[a] left on over 12 hours
Permethrin 1% cream	apply and wash off in 10 minutes
Lindane 1% shampoo	apply for 4 minutes, then wash off
Pyrethrins with piperonyl butoxide	apply and wash off in 10 minutes

[a] A further application after 7 days is recommended.

References

1 Mellanby K. Scabies. Classey; Faringdon: 1972.

2 Heilesen B. Studies on *Acarus scabiei* and scabies. *Acta Dermatol* 1946; Suppl. 14: 86–138.

3 Shelley WB, Shelley D. Scanning electron microscopy of the scabies burrow and its contents with special reference to the *Sarcoptes scabiei* egg. *J Am Acad Dermatol* 1983; **9**: 673–679.

4 Carslaw EW, Dobson RM, Hood AJK, Taylor RN. Mites in the environment of cases of Norwegian scabies. *Br J Dermatol* 1975; **92**: 333–337.

5 Church RE, Knowelden J. Scabies in Sheffield, a family infestation. *Br Med J* 1978; **i**: 761–763.

6 Christophersen J. The epidemiology of scabies in Denmark, 1900–1975. *Arch Dermatol* 1978; **114**: 747–750.

7 Orkin M. Resurgence of scabies. *JAMA* 1971; **217**: 593–597.

8 Falk ES, Thorsby E. HLA antigens in patients with scabies. *Br J Dermatol* 1981; **104**: 317–320.

9 Burgess I. Unusual features of scabies associated with topical fluorinated steroids. *Br J Dermatol* 1973; **87**: 519–520.

10 MacMillan AL. Unusual features of scabies associated with topical fluorinated steroids. *Br J Dermatol* 1972; **87**: 496–497.

11 Dahl MV. Immunology of scabies: a review. *Ann Allergy* 1983; **51**: 560–565.

12 Coombs RRA, Gell PGH. Classification of allergic reactions responsible for clinical hypersensitivity and disease. In: Gell PGH, Coombs RRA (eds) *Clinical Aspects of Immunology* 3rd edition. Blackwell Scientific Publications; Oxford: 1976, p. 761.

13 Hay RJ. Norwegian scabies in a patient with cutaneous vasculitis. *Guy's Hospital Reports* 1974; **123**: 77.

14 Ackerman AB. Histopathology of human scabies. In: Orkin M, Maibach HI, Parish LC, Schwartzman RM, (eds) *Scabies and Pediculosis*. JB Lippincott; Philadelphia: 1977, pp. 88–89.

15 Mellanby K. Biology of the parasite (*Sarcoptes scabiei*). In: Orkin M, Maibach HI, Parish LC, Schwartzman RM, (eds) *Scabies and Pediculosis*. JB Lippincott; Philadelphia: 1977, p. 8–14.

16 Burns DA. Human scabies. In: Champion RH, Burton JL, Burns DA, Breatnach SM. Textbook of Dermatology, 6th edition. Blackwell Science; Oxford: 1998.

17 Bagnal B, Rook A. Arthropods and the skin. In: Rook A (ed.) *Recent Advances in Dermatology*. Churchill Livingstone; Edinburgh: 1977, pp. 59–90.

18 Potter EV, Mayon-White R, Svartman M, Abidh S, Poon-King T, Earle DT. Secondary infections in scabies and their complications. In: Orkin M, Maibach HI, Parish LC, Schwartzman RM (eds) *Scabies and Pediculosis*. JB Lippincott; Philadelphia: 1977, pp. 39–50.

19 Portu JJ, Santamaria JM, Zubero Z, Almeida-Llamas MV, San Sebastian MA-E, Gutierrez AR. Atypical scabies in HIV-positive patients. *J Am Acad Dermatol* 1996; **34**: 915–917.

20 Paterson WD, Allen BR, Beveridge GW. Norwegian scabies during immunosuppressive therapy. *Br Med J* 1973; **4**: 211–212.

21 Epsy PD, Jolly HW. Norwegian scabies, occurrence in a patient undergoing immunosuppression. *Arch Dermatol* 1976; **112**: 193–196.

22 Hancock BW, Ward AN. Serum immunoglobulins in scabies. *J Invest Dermatol* 1974; **63**: 482–484.

23 Chosidow O. Scabies and pediculosis. *Lancet* 2000; **355**: 819–826.

24 Muller GH. 1977 Laboratory diagnosis of scabies. In: Orkin M, Maibach HI, Parish LC, Schwartzman RM (eds) *Scabies and Pediculosis*. JB Lippincott; Philadelphia: 1977, pp. 99–104.

25 Meinking TL, Taplin D. Safety of permethrin vs lindane for the treatment of scabies. *Arch Dermatol* 1996; **132**: 959–962.

26 Schultz MW, Gomez M, Hansen RC, *et al.* Comparative study of 5% permethrin cream and 1% lindane lotion for the treatment of scabies. *Arch Dermatol* 1990; **126**: 167–170.

27 Franz TJ, Lehman PA, Franz SF, Guin JD. Comparative percutaneous absorption of lindane and permethrin. *Arch Dermatol* 1996; **132**: 901–905.

28 Andrews EB, Joseph MC, Magenheim MJ, Tilson HH, Toi PA, Schultz MW. Postmarketing surveillance of permethrin crème rinse. *Am J Public Health* 1992; **82**: 857–861.

29 Wooldridge WE. Gamma isomer of hexachloro cyclohexone in the treatment of scabies. *J Invest Dermatol* 1948; **10**: 363–366.

30 Solomon LM, Fahrner L, West DP. Gamma benzene hexachloride toxicity. *Arch Dermatol* 1977; **113**: 353–357.

31 Feldman RJ, Maibach HI. Percutaneous penetration of some pesticides and herbicides in man. *Toxicol Appl Pharmacol* 1974; **28**: 126–132.

32 Davidow B, Frawley JP. Tissue distribution, accumulation and elimination of the isomers of benzene hexachloride. *Proc Soc Exp Biol Med* 1951; **776**: 780–783.

33 Czegledi-Janko G, Avar P. Occupational exposure to lindane – clinical and laboratory findings. *Br J Industr Med* 1970; **27**: 283–286.

34 Cannon AB, McRae ME. Treatment of scabies. *JAMA* 1948; **138**: 557–560.

35 James BHE. Gamma benzene hexachloride as a scabicide. *Br Med J* 1972; **i**: 178–179.

36 Centers for Disease Control and Prevention. 2002 Guidelines for treatment and prevention of sexually transmitted diseases. *MMWR* 2002; **51**: RR–6.

37 Abramowicz M. Malathion for treatment of head lice. *Med Lett Drugs Ther* 1999; **41**: 73–74.

38 Titenko-Holland N, Windham G, Kolachana P, *et al.* Genotoxicity of malathion in human lymphocytes assessed using the micronucleus assay in vitro and in vivo: a study of malathion-exposed workers. *Mutat Res* 1997; **388**: 85–95.

39 Jackson HC. Ivermectin as a systemic insecticide. *Parasitol Today* 1989; **5**: 146–156.

40 Goa KL, McTavish D, Clissold SP. Ivermectin. A review of its antifilarial activity, pharmacokinetic properties and clinical efficacy in onchocerciasis. *Drugs* 1991; **42**: 640–650.

41 Macotela-Ruiz E, Pena-Gonzalez G. Tratamiento de la escabiasis con ivermectina por via oral. *Gac Med Mex* 1993; **129**: 201–205.

42 Glaziou P, Cartel JL, Alzieu P, Briot C, Moulia-Pelat JP, Martin PMV. Comparison of ivermectin and benzyl benzoate for treatment of scabies. *Trop Med Parasitol* 1993; **44**: 331–332.

43 Chouela EN, Abeldano AM, Pellerano G, *et al.* Equivalent therapeutic efficacy and safety of ivermectin and lindane in the treatment of human scabies. *Arch Dermatol* 1999; **135**: 651–655.

44 Usha V, Gopalakrishnan Nair TV. A comparative study of oral ivermectin and topical permethrin cream in the treatment of scabies. *J Am Acad Dermatol* 2000; **42**: 236–240.

45 Meinking TL, Taplin D, Hermida JL, Pardo R, Kerdel FA. The treatment of scabies with ivermectin. *N Engl J Med* 1995; **333**: 26–30.

46 Del Giudice P, Marty P. Ivermectin. A new therapeutic weapon in dermatology? *Arch Dermatol* 1999; **135**: 705–706.

47 Huffam SE, Currie BJ. Ivermectin for *Sarcoptes scabiei* hyperinfestation. *Int J Infect Dis* 1998; **2**: 152–154.

48 Busvine JR. Pediculosis: biology of the parasites. In: Orkin M, Maibach HI, Parish LC, Schwartzman RM (eds) *Scabies and Pediculosis*. JB Lippincott; Philadelphia: 1977, pp. 143–152.

49 Clay T. In: Smith KGV (ed.) *Insects and Other Arthropods of Medical Importance*. British Museum; London: 1973, p 9.

50 Gratz N. In: Orkin M, Maibach HI, Parish LC, Schwartzman RM (eds) *Scabies and Pediculosis*. JB Lippincott; Philadelphia: 1977, pp. 179–190.

51 Davies FG, Bassett WH. *Clay's Public Health Inspectors Handbook* 14th edition. Lewis; London: 1977, p. 493.

52 Downs AMR, Stafford KA, Harvey I, Coles GC. Evidence for double resistance to permethrin and malathion in head lice. *Br J Dermatol* 1999; **141**: 508–511.

53 Gillis D, Slepon R, Karsenty E, Green M. Seasonality and long-term trends of pediculosis capitis and pubis in a young adult population. *Arch Dermatol* 1990; **126**: 638–641.

54 Morley WN. Body infestations. *Scott Med J* 1977; **22**: 211–216.

55 Clore ER, Longyear LA. A comparative study of seven pediculicides and their packaged nit removal combs. *J Pediatr Health Care* 1993; **7**: 55–60.

56 Pauron D, Barhanin J, Amichot M, Pravaloriio M, Berge JB, Ladzunski M. Pyrethroid receptor in the insect Na⁺ channel: alteration of its properties in pyrethroid-resistant flies. *Biochemistry* 1989; **28**: 1673–1677.

57 Mutero A, Praalavorio M, Bride JM, *et al.* Resistance-associated point mutations in insecticide-insensitive acetylcholinesterase. *Proc Natl Acad Sci USA* 1994; **91**: 5922–5926.

58 Dawes M, Hicks NR, Fleminger M, Goldman D, Hamling J, Hicks LJ. Treatment for head lice. *Br Med J* 1999; **318**: 385–386.

59 Nuttall GHF. The biology of *Phthirus pubis*. *Parasitol* 1918; **10**: 383–405.

60 Matheson R. *Medical Entomology*. Constable; London: 1950, pp. 194–217.

61 Pavlovsky EN, Stein AK. *Maculae coeruleae* and *Phthirus pubis*. *Parasitol* 1924; **16**: 145–149.

62 Fisher I, Morton RS. *Pthirus pubis* infestation. *Br J Vener Dis* 1970; **46**: 326–329.

63 Skinner CJ, Viswalingam ND, Goh BT. *Phthirus pubis* infestation of the eyelids: a marker for sexually transmitted diseases. *Int J STD AIDS* 1995; **6**: 451–452.

64 McMillan A, Scott GR. *Sexually Transmitted Infections, Colour Guide*. Churchill Livingstone; Edinburgh: 2000.

Chapter 20

Ulcers and other conditions of the external genitalia
A McMillan

In this chapter it is necessary to include a number of clinical topics related only on account of the anatomical site involved.

1. Ulcers of the external genitalia.
2. The prepuce and the development of the preputial sac.
3. Balanoposthitis.
4. Some non-infective conditions: erythema multiforme, psoriasis, lichen simplex and lichen planus. Minor conditions sometimes causing anxiety: trichomycosis axillaris, coronal papillae, sebaceous glands (Fordyce's spots).
5. Tinea cruris.
6. Erythrasma.
7. Lichen sclerosus.
8. Erythroplasia of Queyrat.
9. Peyronie's disease.
10. Lymphocele and localized edema of the penis.
11. Behçet's disease.
12. Pyoderma gangrenosum.

1. Ulcers of the external genitalia

ACUTE ULCERS

In the differential diagnosis of an acute genital ulcer, the first cause to be considered must be a sexually transmissible agent, particularly *Treponema pallidum*: within this group ulcers found elsewhere, particularly in the oral and anal regions, must be included also for consideration. In the context of general practice patients should be referred to clinics where facilities for the necessary procedures are at hand. Antibiotics, which may obscure an important diagnosis, should not be prescribed blindly.

In all cases of a genital ulcer the first objective will be to diagnose or exclude early-stage contagious syphilis and to take steps to trace sexual contacts. Exclusion of other STIs, particularly gonorrhea and herpes genitalis, is also necessary. In warmer climates, or in patients returning from them, possibilities of lymphogranuloma venereum, chancroid, and, rarely, donovanosis will require consideration, although in lymphogranuloma venereum the ulcer itself tends to be transitory and herpetiform.

The chancre of primary syphilis may often be a painless indurated ulcer with enlarged indurated non-tender lymph nodes, but its tendency to heal and to be modified by injudicious (for example topical steroid applications) and inadequate treatments makes it improper to base a diagnosis on clinical appearance alone. The importance of repeating serological tests for syphilis for a 3-month follow-up period has been discussed (Chapter 15).

In secondary syphilis moist eroded papules are seen in the mouth, on the genitalia, or around the anus, but the larger hypertrophic papules (condylomata lata) tend to be most obvious on the vulva in the female and in the anal region of both sexes.

Although chancroid (soft sore) is rare in the UK and western Europe, but common in the tropics and subtropics, it is important to exclude syphilis by dark-ground or monoclonal antibody examinations and serological tests over a period of 3 months, and to treat with a sulfonamide (for example sulfadimidine) to avoid masking the treponemal infection if it is present.

In the diagnosis of donovanosis (Chapter 16) a small biopsy should be taken from the edge of the lesion and a tissue smear prepared and stained with Giemsa's or Leishman's stains to demonstrate the capsulate pleomorphic bacillus with bipolar staining.

Among other ulcers caused by infective agents are superficial herpetiform erosions at the introitus, associated with *Trichomonas vaginalis* vaginitis. Some erosions, particularly at the frenum in the male and at the fourchette in the female, may be traumatic from intercourse.

In *Candida* spp. infection there may be erosions under the exudate in the vagina and fissuring, particularly of the fourchette (Chapter 17). In the male contact a small proportion may show balanoposthitis with superficial ulceration of the glans and occasionally with fissures at the preputial orifice and a phimosis. Whenever there is a pruritus a search should also be made for pubic lice on the vulva, tinea in the groin in the male, and threadworms (*Enterobius vermicularis*) or their ova if the itch is perianal (Chapter 18).

Herpes zoster affecting the lumbar or sacral roots may cause vesicles and tender ulcers on the genitalia. There is consider-

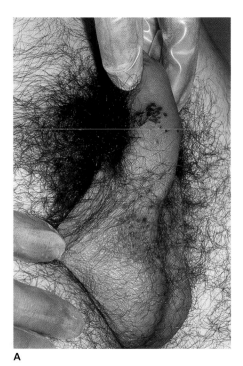

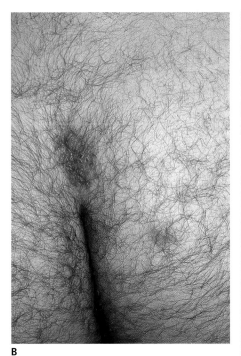

A   **B**

Figure 20.1 (A) Herpes zoster on the penis and scrotum, and (B) on the buttock

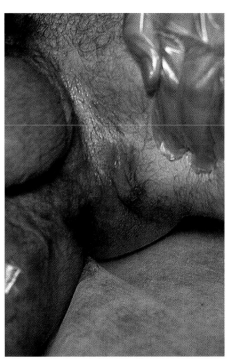

Figure 20.2 Perianal Crohn's disease showing sinuses (reproduced from McMillan and Scott 2000[82])

able variation in the severity of the eruption, and, when only a few lesions are present, the condition may resemble herpes simplex virus infection. The clue is the unilateral distribution of the lesions and the presence of vesicles or cursts elsewhere within the same dermatome (Figure 20.1)

Non-specific urethritis, and the perhaps equivalent non-specific genital infection in the female, is another possibility. In the male with non-specific urethritis, superficial fissuring is sometimes seen in the frenal and orifice portions of the prepuce. In sexually acquired reactive arthritis or Reiter's disease (Chapter 14) there is psoriasis (circinate balanitis) in 21% to 43% of cases, and in the uncircumcised individual these lesions on the glans may show maceration.

Condylomata acuminata are very common (Chapter 5) and neglect, co-existent vaginitis, urethritis, or herpes infection may cause genital ulceration.

In scabies (Chapter 19), indurated papules, sometimes with pustulation and impetiginization, are common on the shaft of the penis. The diagnosis rests on the history of pruritus, finding burrows, and the recognition of *Sarcoptes scabiei*.

Even when furuncles and other pyogenic lesions are recognized, exclusion of syphilis remains a first consideration.

CHRONIC ULCERS

Patients with oral aphthous ulcers have a 1 in 5 chance of having some hematological deficiency or malabsorption syndrome[1], it is therefore wise to extend the investigations in cases with recurrent genital or orogenital aphthous ulcers to include serum ferritin, serum folate, whole blood folate, and vitamin B_{12}.

In lichen sclerosus et atrophicus, described later in this chapter, fibrotic, ivory-white areas are found on the margin of the prepuce, which shows fissuring and adhesion to the glans. This condition may affect the urethral meatus and lead to stenosis with a distinctive white periurethral collar. In women, lichen sclerosus et atrophicus causes ivory papules and violaceous tissue-paper skin in the anogenital area. In the rare Behçet's disease, considered also in this chapter, there is also recurrent orogenital ulceration associated with uveitis. Tuberculosis is now a rare cause of genital ulceration.

Crohn's disease (regional enteritis) can involve the anal region alone without apparent involvement of other parts of the gastrointestinal tract, presenting clinically as anal ulceration, anorectal sinuses or fistulae (Figure 20.2) or edematous anal

skin tags. Ulceration of the skin, separated from other areas of ulceration by normal skin, can occur and has been seen on the penis and on the vulva, as well as elsewhere. Spreading ulceration of the skin of the perineum with linear extension into the groins and genitalia may occur after surgical treatment of an anal lesion[2]. Pyoderma gangrenosum, which may be associated with inflammatory bowel disease or rheumatoid arthritis, can produce extensive ulceration of the vulva. A rare cause of granulomatous ulceration is eosinophilic granuloma. In this condition there is diffuse nodulation and superficial ulceration. Biopsy is essential for diagnosis.

In cases of chronic ulceration, premalignant and malignant disease must also be excluded – particularly in erythroplasia of Queyrat in which there is a raised bright-red, well-demarcated plaque with a velvety surface to be seen on the glans, and in which a biopsy is necessary (see page 559). Squamous cell carcinoma of the penis is uncommon and, in the circumcised male, extremely rare. The neoplasm develops within the preputial sac and it is usually wart-like rather than ulcerative (Figure 20.3). Other malignant tumors are very rare. Squamous cell carcinoma of the

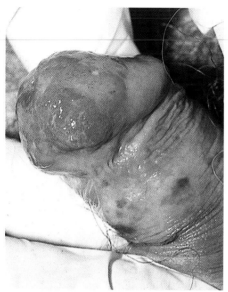

Figure 20.3 Squamous cell carcinoma of the penis (reproduced from McMillan and Scott 2000[82])

scrotum is associated with contamination of the skin with mineral oil and other carcinogens.

The characteristic symptom of vulvar squamous intraepithelial lesions considered in Chapter 5, is intense and persistent itch. Thickened white plaques tend to develop on the vulva, particularly around the clitoris,

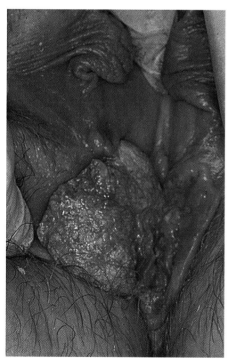

Figure 20.4 Squamous cell carcinoma of the vulva (reproduced from McMillan and Scott 2000[82])

sometimes extending back to the anus, they do not encroach on the vestibule or vagina. The condition has a tendency to occur in middle age, but an increasing number of younger women are being affected. Squamous carcinoma appears as a hard indurated swelling or an ulcerating lesion (Figure 20.4) in the vulva with lymph node enlargement. In cases with pre-existing leukoplakia there is a long history of vulval irritation.

2. The prepuce and the development of the preputial sac

The prepuce is composed of five layers[3]
  1. *mucosal epithelium* (the inner surface of the prepuce) composed of squamous epithelium containing Langerhans cells
  2. *lamina propria* consisting of loose collagen tissue
  3. *dartos muscle* consisting of smooth muscle and elastic fibers
  4. *dermis* consisting of connective tissue, blood vessels, nerve trunks, Meissner corpuscles and sebaceous glands.
  5. *outer epithelium* composed of stratified keratinized squamous cells, and containing melanocytes in the basal layers, Langerhans cells are also present.

The development of the prepuce starts when the human embryo is about 65 mm (13 weeks) and it covers the glans when the fetus is 100 mm (end of the fourth month – 50 g). The inner surface of the prepuce and the surface of the glans receive a common squamous epithelium which separates at about the time of birth gradually and spontaneously as a normal biological process.

Separation of the epithelium common to the glans and prepuce occurs by a process of desquamation. In places the squamous cells arrange themselves into whorls, forming epithelial cell nests, or epithelial 'pearls', which contain a laminated mass of keratin. The centers of these nests degenerate to form spaces which increase in size and link up and finally form a continuous preputial sac[4]. The prepuce is in the course of developing at the time of birth, and by the age of 3 years the prepuce is still non-retractable in 10% of boys. Spontaneous retractability of the prepuce appeared in Gairdner's study[5] to be possible by the age of 3 years (Figure 20.5a) in 90% of boys but Oster[6] showed in a study of an unselected group of Danish schoolboys that complete separation of the preputial sac may not in fact be completed until the age of 17 years (Figure 20.5b); so called 'adhesions' (non-separation) diminish with age gradually and spontaneously. This normal biological process is probably androgen-dependent[7] and the process is known to be arrested by castration.

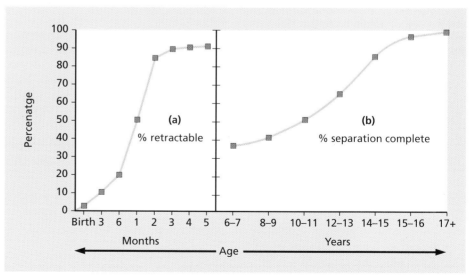

Figure 20.5 (a) Proportion of boys from birth to 5 years in whom the prepuce has become spontaneously retractable (Gairdner 1949[5]), (b) Proportion of boys from 6 to 17 years in whom separation of the prepuce and glans was complete (Oster 1968[6])

In mice the glans penis and prepuce are not separable until about 46 days after birth, and this process is prevented by the removal of the testes. Separation of the adherent prepuce, whether brought about naturally through testicular activity or artificially by the administration of androgen in the castrated animal, is caused by keratinization of the hitherto embryonic cells composing the adherent epithelia[7].

Forcible retraction of the prepuce in boys is painful and may lead to overstretching of the preputial orifice and consequent phimosis. The procedure can also cause paraphimosis, and bleeding points may also be seen where the stretching has damaged areas where separation has been incomplete. Very gentle retraction and washing is all that is generally required. Retraction under anesthesia, whether general[8] or local[9], should rarely be necessary[10, 11].

The predicted lifetime risk for cancer of the penis in the uncircumcised male in the USA is 166 per 100 000, or one in 600, and the estimated median age is 67 years. Since this neoplasm is virtually unknown in those who have undergone circumcision at an early age, the issue has been put forward as a factor to be considered in discussions on the advisability or otherwise of neonatal circumcision[12]. Even in an uncircumcised population (Denmark), however, the incidence of cancer of the penis has been declining since the mid-1940s. This decline has been attributed to better penile hygiene[13]. Although Kochen[12] thought that mortality in the USA from circumcision was rare and found only two reports of this in the literature since 1953, adequate statistical records on mortality from this cause did not seem to be available. In Gairdner's paper[5] 10 to 19 deaths in those under 5 years of age were recorded annually between 1942 and 1947 in England and Wales.

The origins of male circumcision are unknown; it is a very ancient practice, with evidence of it in some of the earliest Egyptian mummies. Even in recent years there have been many attempts to justify the operation in western countries on medical grounds, particularly to protect against HIV infection[14].

CIRCUMCISION IN MEN AND THE RISK OF HIV INFECTION

Since the first suggestion of an association between having a foreskin and a greater risk of acquiring HIV, there has been much debate on the role of circumcision in the prevention of HIV transmission. Although HIV seroprevalence is apparently lower in areas of Africa where circumcision is practised than where it is not, other risk factors were not considered in these early studies, and the conclusion that circumcision is protective has been questioned[15]. As reviewed by Van Howe[15], other studies that examined the association between cicumcision status and HIV infection amongst high-risk individuals yielded conflicting results. A meta-analysis of thirty-three published studies was reported by O'Farrell and Egger[16]. They chose the odds ratio as the only measure of association, and found that the combined estimates from both fixed and random effect models* indicated that lack of circumcision was associated with an increased risk of HIV infection. This association was particularly strong in studies from high-risk populations such as long-distance lorry drivers in Africa and attendees at STI clinics. Further support for this finding has come from two recently reported studies from Africa. In a prospective study from Kenya, the uncircumcised state was an independent risk factor for HIV infection and genital ulcer disease[17], and in Uganda, the prevalence of HIV infection was lower in men circumcised before puberty than those circumcised after the age of 20 years[18]. The mechanism by which circumcision protects against HIV infection is uncertain. It is well recognized, however, that genital ulcer disease facilitates transmission of HIV (Chapters 15 and 16), and, as already discussed, that being uncircumcised is a risk factor for genital ulceration. This observation may also explain the heterogeneity in the results of the protective effect of circumcision between different studies. Circumcision may be protective in some populations where genital ulcer disease and other STIs are closely associated with transmission of HIV but not in populations where these infections play a minor role[16]. Another possible explanation for the protective value of circumcision is that the operation removes the abundance of Langerhans cells that are found in the mucosal epithelium lining the inner surface of the prepuce and that may be important in acquisition of HIV (Chapter 7).

3. Balanoposthitis

The terms balanitis and posthitis refer respectively to inflammation of the glans and mucosal surface of the prepuce. As these conditions will ordinarily co-exist, the term balanoposthitis is strictly more correct than the commonly used shorter word balanitis. Balanoposthitis, however, is a descriptive term that encompasses a variety of conditions, the appearance of some of which is characteristic for this disease.

ETIOLOGY
Irritant dermatitis

Within the moist preputial sac an accumulation of smegma resulting from poor hygiene is an obvious predisposing factor in the etiology of balanoposthitis. Irritation may also be caused by friction of clothes, the unwise application of antiseptics, or previous contact during sexual intercourse with pathogenic or opportunistic organisms within the vagina. Allergy to spermicidal lubricants is a well-recognized cause of balanoposthitis[20]. In one study a history of atopy and frequent washing with soap of the genitalia has been associated with recurrent balanoposthitis[21]. The histology of the mucosa from such patients shows non-specific changes with a patchy, perivascular infiltrate in the dermis, and edema and spongiosis of the epidermis.

---

* Meta-analysis is the combination of data from several studies to produce a single estimate. Two models that are often used in meta-analysis are (a) the 'fixed-effect' model, in which variability of results between studies is considered as exclusively resulting from random variation, and (b) the 'random-effect' model in which a different underlying effect is assumed for each study and this is taken into consideration as an additional source of variation[19].

Infective causes

Bacteria, yeasts, or trichomonads may flourish in the moist environment, but sometimes balanitis may develop after intercourse, possibly as a result of sensitivity to a vaginal discharge containing yeasts such as *Candida albicans*, or substances derived from it, or from soap washing after intercourse. With the restricting effect of phimosis, whether primary or secondary and caused by inflammation, discharge may accumulate under pressure and, if neglected, may be associated with a necrotizing ulceration of the glans (phagedena). Under these circumstances anaerobes may be secondary invaders. Although anaerobes are isolated infrequently from the sub-preputial sac of healthy men, at least three-quarters of patients with balanoposthitis are infected at that site with anaerobic bacteria, especially *Bacteroides* spp.[22]. In one study[23] *Gardnerella vaginalis*, usually in association with anaerobes, was cultured from the sub-preputial sac of 9 of 39 men with balanoposthitis. Group B β-hemolytic streptococci can cause balanitis whose severity ranges from mild erythema to cellulitis[24], and pyoderma caused by Group A hemolytic streptococci has followed fellatio[25].

Herpes simplex virus (HSV) may be isolated from erosions and, rarely, causes a necrotizing balanitis[26]. Chronic or recurrent balanoposthitis has been associated with HPV infection.[27].

In addition to possible hypersensitivity to fungal antigens, *Candida* spp. can cause balanoposthitis by tissue invasion. Balanoposthitis can be caused by *Trichomonas vaginalis*[28] and, rarely, by *Entamoeba histolytica*[29].

Balanoposthitis as part of a dermatological or systemic disease

Balanoposthitis may be a component of a generalized skin disease such as fixed drug eruption or erythema multiforme exudativum, and may be associated with diabetes or debilitating disease, particularly in the elderly.

CLINICAL FEATURES

In infective balanoposthitis there is erythema of the glans, coronal sulcus, and

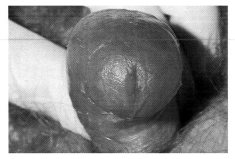

Figure 20.6 Anaerobic balanoposthitis (reproduced from McMillan and Scott 2000[82])

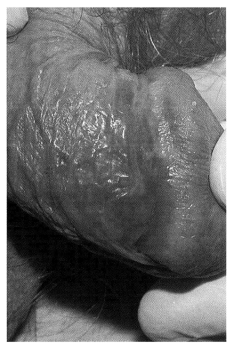

Figure 20.7 Streptococcal balanoposthitis (reproduced from McMillan and Scott 2000[82])

inner surface of the prepuce (Figures 20.6 and 20.7). It can be insidious in onset and pass unnoticed but sometimes, particularly in infective cases, erythema and edema are pronounced and a resulting phimosis may make inspection of the glans difficult or impossible. In the uncircumcised male the affected surfaces become macerated and a purulent exudate accumulates rapidly becoming malodorous. Erosion and ulceration may be painful.

In balanitis either associated with or caused by diabetes or candidiasis, there may be fissuring of the prepuce particularly at its orifice. The clinical appearance

of irritant balanitis is variable. In some patients there is mild erythema but in others penile edema can be pronounced. In sexually acquired reactive arthritis or Reiter's disease a recurring circinate balanitis (psoriasis) develops in 25% of cases on the glans penis and mucous surface of the prepuce. In middle-aged or elderly men a chronic localized balanitis may develop and, as there is a marked plasma cell infiltration of the dermis, this is referred to as plasma cell balanitis of Zoon[30]. The surface of the plaque of balanitis is moist, shiny, and often finely speckled. Biopsy is essential to distinguish this condition from erythroplasia of Queyrat.

All forms of balanitis may become chronic or relapse frequently, particularly in the elderly, when the fibrotic changes are those seen in lichen sclerosus.

INVESTIGATIONS

Generally few investigations are required in the management of the man with acute balanoposthitis. Culture for eubacteria can exclude an infective etiology and is sometimes diagnostic (it is important to note that the detection of aerobic or anaerobic bacteria does not always imply an etiological role for these organisms). It is also helpful to look for *Candida* spp., this is best performed using an 'adhesive tape' method[31]. A strip of double-sided transparent adhesive tape is attached to a microscope slide, the other side of the tape is pressed against the affected epithelium, the slide is passed quickly through a flame, and then stained by Gram's method before microscopic examination. This is more sensitive than using material collected on a cotton wool-tipped applicator stick. As balanoposthitis, particularly candidal, can be the presenting feature of diabetes mellitus, the urine should always be tested for glucose. Culture of HSV from ulcers or erosions should be attempted. When trichomonal infection is suspected, material from the sub-preputial sac should be examined microscopically and by culture (Chapter 17).

In the case of recurrent or chronic balanoposthitis, histological examination of a punch biopsy can be helpful in the diagnosis of unsuspected conditions such as lichen planus, lichen sclerosus, and penile squamous intraepithelial lesions[32]. Excision biopsy is necessary when malignant disease is suspected.

Patch tests are really only useful in the small number of patients with true allergy.

TREATMENT

Mild forms of infective balanitis are cleared readily by retracting the prepuce and bathing with physiological saline. This treatment should be repeated two or three times daily and, if inflammation is more than trivial, a strip of gauze (2.5 × 15 cm) soaked in saline should be applied to the glans and coronal sulcus in such a way that, on bringing the prepuce forward, the skin surfaces of the glans and the inner aspect of the prepuce are separated by gauze. The prescription of metronidazole in an oral dosage of 200 mg every 8 hours for 7 days is useful when inflammation is pronounced and when local wide-spectrum antibacterial agents are to be avoided, particularly when the diagnosis of early syphilis is to be considered.

When phimosis is present, sub-preputial lavage with saline 3 to 6 hourly is often sufficient to promote drainage and healing. As inflammation subsides the prepuce may become retractable and any ulcer inspected. When a necrotizing ulceration of the glans develops, rapid local destruction can occur. A swab of the sub-preputial discharge should be examined microbiologically, and if anaerobes are discovered antibacterial agents, such as metronidazole, may be prescribed. Sub-preputial lavage with 0.9% saline may be carried out with a disposable hypodermic syringe. Should this be unsuccessful in securing resolution the antibiotic or chemotherapeutic agent, effective against the organism isolated, may be given. When there is a dusky erythema of the penile skin with persistent phimosis and the inflammation is unrelieved by the saline lavage described and supplemented by the antibiotic, surgical exposure of the glans by a dorsal slit is necessary to secure the drainage of a necrotizing ulcer.

Candidal balanoposthitis is treated with a topical imidazole, or with fluconazole given in a single dose of 150 mg by mouth (Chapter 17). The use of an imidazole cream containing 1% hydrocortisone is often used in patients with marked inflammation and preputial edema.

Sensitizing agents such as soaps should not be used during acute inflammation. Patients with non-specific dermatitis benefit from the use of emollients such as E45 cream applied topically twice daily. These emollients can also be used as soap substitutes. Topical hydrocortisone cream 1% w/w applied three times per day for 7 days is often successful in those patients whose non-specific balanitis fails to resolve with emollients. When spermicides have been implicated as the cause of the balanoposthitis in the individual, they should be avoided subsequently.

Plasma cell balanitis often responds poorly to topical treatments but circumcision has been effective[30].

4. Some non-infective conditions[33]

ERYTHEMA MULTIFORME

Erythema multiforme is a condition of unknown etiology that can be precipitated by many agents including viruses, particularly HSV; bacteria, especially mycoplasmas; fungi, especially *Histoplasma capsulatum*; drugs, especially sulfonamides; sarcoidosis; polyarteritis nodosa; and malignant neoplasms. In almost 50% of cases, however, precipitating factors cannot be identified.

The skin lesions are dull red, flat maculopapules that often reach 1 to 2 cm in diameter. As the lesion increases in size the center becomes purplish and the periphery remains red. Cropping of lesions occurs over a few days and generally the lesions fade within 2 weeks. Classically the affected sites are the dorsa of the hands, palms, wrists, forearms and feet, elbows and knees.

In the severe bullous form of the disease (erythema multiforme exudativum; Stevens–Johnson syndrome) there is a sudden onset of a bullous eruption of the mouth and lips; these bullae rupture to show the floor of the erosion covered by a grayish-white membrane. Hemorrhagic crusting is characteristic (Figure 20.8). Severe conjunctivitis is often associated with corneal ulceration, genital ulceration (Figure 20.9) and, in about 80% of cases, skin lesions that are similar to those described above or bullous. New crops of lesions develop over a period of about 10 days. Systemic features including fever, malaise, and anorexia present for 2 to 3 weeks. Renal failure has been reported rarely.

In mild cases of localized bullous erythema multiforme symptomatic treatment is all that is required, but in severe illness, steroids such as prednisolone may be indicated. When there is severe ocular involvement, the advice of an ophthalmologist should be sought.

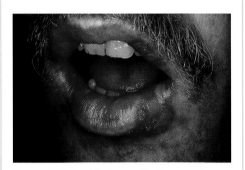

Figure 20.8 Oral lesions of bullous erythema multiforme

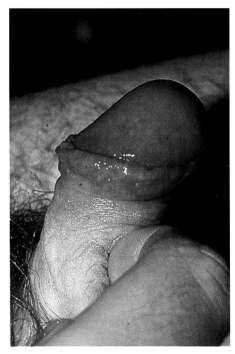

Figure 20.9 Penile lesions of bullous erythema multiforme (reproduced from McMillan and Scott 2000[82])

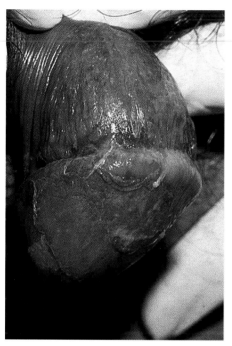

Figure 20.10 Fixed drug eruption of the penis, caused by sulfonamides (reproduced from McMillan and Scott 2000[82])

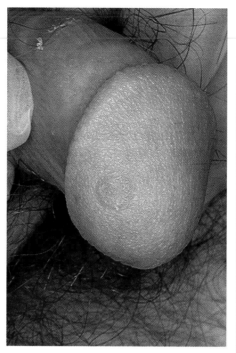

Figure 20.11 Psoriasis of the glans penis in a circumcised male (reproduced from McMillan and Scott 2000[82])

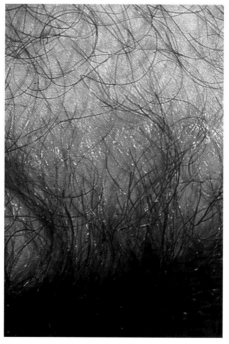

Figure 20.12 Psoriasis of the perianal region (reproduced from McMillan and Scott 2000[82])

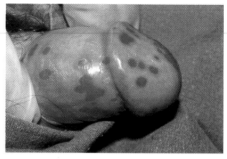

Figure 20.13 Psoriasis of the glans penis in an uncircumcised man

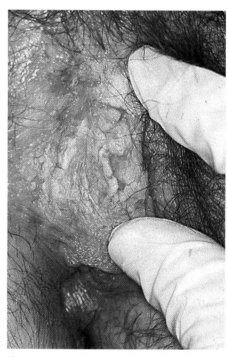

Figure 20.14 Lichen simplex of the labium minus (reproduced from McMillan and Scott 2000[82])

FIXED DRUG ERUPTION

These are lesions that tend to recur in the same site each time the particular drug is given. The glans penis is a common site (Figure 20.10). There is an erythematous plaque that later darkens and is often surmounted by a bulla. Healing is accomplished by crusting and scaling. Residual pigmentation is common. Drugs that may be responsible include tetracyclines, sulfonamides, and barbiturates.

GENITAL ULCERATION CAUSED BY DRUGS

Genital ulceration can be caused by drugs such as foscarnet[34]. The mechanism by which the ulcers are produced is unknown.

PSORIASIS, LICHEN SIMPLEX, LICHEN PLANUS

Psoriasis produces scaly lesions on the penis (Figure 20.11), perianal region (Figure 20.12), or vulva. On the glans of the uncircumcised male, the lesions are bright red and sharply marginated (Figure 20.13). Psoriatic lesions will occur elsewhere and pits may be found in the finger nails. Psoriatic

lesions of the penis may be a feature of sexually acquired reactive arthritis or Reiter's disease (Chapter 14). Lichen simplex with erythema, lichenification, and fissuring in the

anogenital lesions (Figure 20.14) is associated with pruritus and affects a 'trigger-zone'. Lichen planus produces annular papular lesions which are pink or violet in color and sometimes restricted to the genitals (Figure 20.15) and mouth in young men. The surface of the lesions shows a network of fine lines.

MINOR CONDITIONS SOMETIMES CAUSING ANXIETY IN PATIENTS

Trichomycosis axillaris

Trichomycosis axillaris is a superficial infection of the axillary and pubic hairs with

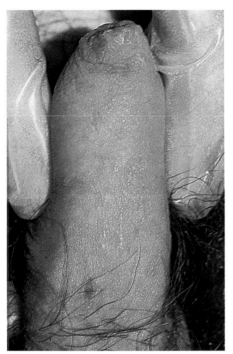

Figure 20.15 Lichen planus of the shaft of the penis (reproduced from McMillan and Scott 2000[82])

the formation of adherent yellow, black, or red nodules on the hair shaft. These concretions consist of tightly packed bacteria, which may grow within the cells of the cuticle; the organism is named *Corynebacterium tenuis*.

Coronal papillae

Coronal papillae are dome-shaped or hair-like papules involving the corona of the penis (Figure 20.16), that may be mistaken for warts. The papillae are a normal variant. When histological examination of a papule has been undertaken[35], it is seen to be covered by normal epithelium. The stratum corneum and the stratum granulosum are thin and pigment is present in the basal layer. Mild exocytosis is occasionally seen. The lamina propria is composed of connective tissue containing many capillary sized blood vessels and numerous fibroblasts. Nests of non-myelinated nerve fibers are found in the upper layer of the lamina propria.

Sebaceous glands

Small yellow papules (about 0.2 mm) may be seen sometimes in clusters on the inner surface of the prepuce; these are seen also on the buccal mucosa and consist of sebaceous glands. Sometimes referred to as Fordyce's spots, they are normal sebaceous glands which increase in number at puberty and continue to do so in adult life.

5. *Tinea cruris*

Tinea cruris is an infection of the groins by filamentous fungi known as dermatophytes, which live only in the fully keratinized layers of the skin and, when established, may cause only minimal disturbance to their host. Although a variety of lesions occur, dermatophytes have been found in apparently healthy skin[36].

ETIOLOGY

In groin infections *Trichophyton rubrum* and *Epidermophyton floccosum* are usually implicated, although *T. mentagrophytes* var. *interdigitale* may be detected on occasions. In Denmark it was found that in 17% of *T. rubrum* infections in men, both the groin and feet were involved: this fungus species has become the most common dermatophyte in western Europe since the Second World War[37].

Transmission takes place as a result of sharing towels and communal facilities. Autoinoculation from the foot is not uncommon. Tinea cruris is rare in females.

CLINICAL FEATURES

Itching is a predominant feature whatever species of fungus is involved. Initially the lesions are erythematous plaques, arciform with sharp margins, they extend from the groin towards the thighs (Figure 20.17). There is little tendency to central clearing and the surface is scaly, sometimes sufficient to mask the underlying erythema. Vesiculation is rare but dermal nodules may be found in older lesions. Lesions due to *E. floccosum* are typically acute in onset and

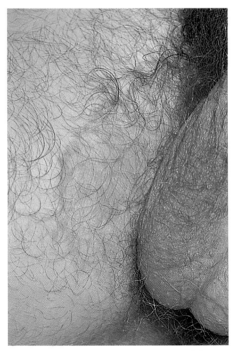

Figure 20.17 Tinea cruris (reproduced from McMillan and Scott 2000[82])

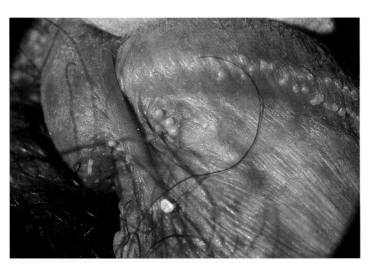

Figure 20.16 Coronal papillae

inflammatory. In *T. rubrum* infections, lesions are classically chronic and perhaps more nodular; the rare *T. mentagrophytes* var. *interdigitale* infections may be vesicular and inflammatory[38]. Involvement of the scrotal skin by the dermatophyte is common, but the cutaneous reaction is often inconspicuous[39]. In one survey of Air Force recruits in the USA, 9% yielded dermatophytes from the inguinal region or natal cleft[40], although the skin was apparently normal.

DIAGNOSIS

The differential diagnosis includes psoriasis, erythrasma, seborrheic dermatitis, and *Candida* spp. and bacterial intertrigo. For that reason, mycological confirmation of the diagnosis is advisable. Material for mycological study may be taken by scraping outwards from the edge of the lesions; for the laboratory it is best to collect the specimens on to a folded slip of black paper. Alternatively, particles of keratin may be stripped from the skin with a vinyl adhesive tape, affixed to a microscope slide for transfer to the laboratory for culture[41].

For routine diagnosis, microscopic examination is most easily carried out by mounting skin scrapings in potassium hydroxide fluid (distilled water 80 mL, potassium hydroxide 20 g, glycerine 10 mL). The process may be hastened by gentle heating. Alternatively the mounting fluid may be prepared with dimethylsulfoxide (40 mL), potassium hydroxide (20 g), and distilled water (60 mL). Fungal elements can then be detected by microscopic examination of the unstained potassium hydroxide preparation covered by a cover-slip[42].

Dermatophytes grow well on Sabouraud's medium and are distinguished principally by the nature of the spores. In addition to the species already named, *Microsporum gypseum* is a cause of tinea cruris worldwide and *M. (Trichophyton) simiae* is a cause in Brazil, Guinea, and India[43]. Keys to their identification may be found in Rebell and Taplin[42] and in an atlas by Frey *et al.*[43] which provides pleasing visual and textual information.

TREATMENT

The imidazoles – clotrimazole, miconazole, and econazole – are effective as topical agents in the treatment of infections due to dermatophytes. Used as a cream the various preparations should be applied 2 to 3 times daily as a thin film to the affected area and rubbed in gently. Improvement occurs within 10 to 14 days and treatment may continue for 2 to 8 weeks and preferably for 2 weeks after disappearance of cutaneous signs. On occasions, reddening of the skin and pruritus may occur, but this is seldom severe enough for the patient to stop treatment. Eradication of the infection may not be achieved by topical agents, although clinical effects are controlled.

Griseofulvin may be used orally in more severe cases and when there is folliculitis, but accurate diagnosis by microscopy and cultures is most desirable. It is taken up by keratin-forming cells and hair shafts, thus coming into intimate contact with the infecting dermatophyte. In tinea of the groin, treatment may be required for a period of 2 to 6 weeks, to be followed by careful re-examination and, if apparently clear, a follow-up after a month is desirable. It is prescribed as tablets, the adult dose is 0.5 g which may be sufficient if taken once daily after a meal. Itraconazole given in a dosage of 100 mg once daily by mouth for 14 days, or terbinafine 250 mg as a single oral dose given daily for 2 to 4 weeks are suitable alternatives to treatment with griseofulvin.

6. Erythrasma

Erythrasma is a mild chronic superficial infection of the skin, characterized by well-demarcated flat lesions caused by a group of closely related aerobic coryneform bacteria usually known as *Corynebacterium minutissimum*[44].

ETIOLOGY

C. minutissimum is a name that covers a complex of fluorescent diphtheroids, which may also be found on normal skin but which appear to be causative in erythrasma. The incidence is higher in children at boarding schools and patients in hospitals for those with learning difficulties[45].

CLINICAL FEATURES

Smooth and well-demarcated from the surrounding skin, the lesion is initially red in color. Scaling develops and as the lesion ages it becomes brown. Commonly it involves the toe clefts, but the groin is frequently affected, and the axilla or elsewhere occasionally. Usually there are no symptoms but, particularly in the groins, there may be mild pruritus.

DIAGNOSIS

Under Wood's light erythrasma shows a characteristic coral-red fluorescence which is attributable to coproporphyrin III[44]. Skin scales from the margin of the lesion should be examined and mounted in potassium hydroxide solution (see previous section) to exclude tinea cruris. Exclusion of tinea from the diagnosis should, preferably, include culture of skin scales as well as examination by microscopy. Skin scrapings may be stained with Giemsa's stain to detect the rods and filaments of *C. minutissimum*, and cultured to confirm the diagnosis.

TREATMENT

Without treatment the condition persists indefinitely with exacerbations and remissions. *Corynebacterium minutissimum* is sensitive to sodium fusidate *in vitro* and, in one small series, topical treatment for 2 weeks with 2% sodium fusidate ointment was curative[46]. Relapse appears to be more common when the toe web is affected.

Clotrimazole cream is effective in the treatment of erythrasma and in tinea cruris[47], although tendency to relapse is a characteristic of both conditions.

7. Lichen sclerosus

Lichen sclerosus, a condition of unknown etiology, is more common in women than in men. Although it may present in any age group other than the very young, it is most commonly found in the fifth or sixth decades of life.

ETIOLOGY

Genetic factors may predispose to lichen sclerosus, but the mechanisms are obscure. There is an association between lichen sclerosus and autoimmune disorders, especially in women, alopecia and vitiligo being the most common associated disorders[48]. At sites of trauma, the Koebner phenomenon can trigger lichen sclerosus, and the condition may recur around circumcision scars[49].

PATHOLOGY

The diagnostic histological feature is edema and homogenization of the dermal collagen, which occurs immediately beneath the epidermis in small islands or in a band of varying thickness. In these areas there is marked loss of elastic fibers. Similar changes occur in the dermal blood vessels. Immediately superficial to the altered collagen, the epidermis shows hyperkeratosis and atrophy of the stratum malpighii, resulting in flattening or absence of the rete pegs. Deep to the abnormal collagen there is a variable band of chronic inflammatory cells, mostly lymphocytes[50].

CLINICAL FEATURES

In women there may be no symptoms, the condition being detected at routine examination, or there may be persistent pruritus and soreness of the vulva and perianal regions[49]. Traumatic fissures may be associated with superficial dyspareunia, dysuria, and painful defecation. The signs (Figure 20.18) include areas of pallor that may occur in patches or in large plaques, atrophic and wrinkled skin with telangiectasia, purpura or erosions, tender fissures of the labia and perianal area, and occasionally hemorrhagic blisters. The labia may fuse, or there may be resorption of the labia, resulting in difficulties in sexual intercourse.

Prepubertal children can also be affected, the most common symptoms being pruritus and soreness. The signs may be confused with those of sexual abuse. Symptoms and signs of the disease often regress at menarche.

Men, in whom lichen sclerosus is often termed balanitis xerotica obliterans (BXO),

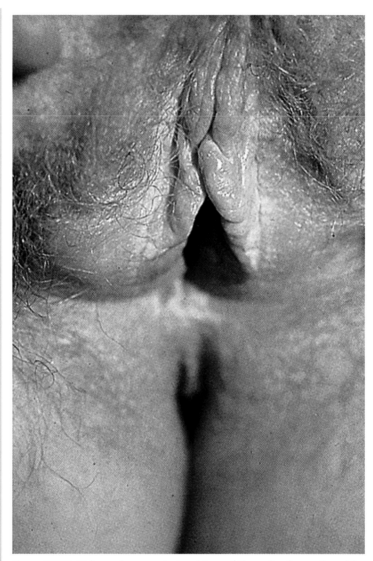

Figure 20.18 Lichen sclerosus et atrophicus of the vulva (reproduced from McMillan and Scott 2000[82])

may present with symptoms of a non-retractile prepuce, urinary obstruction, hematuria, pain and irritation of the penis, or a sub-preputial discharge[50]. The perianal region is not affected in the male. The lesions are characteristic ivory-white macules or confluent plaques on the surface of the glans and prepuce (Figure 20.19), usually occurring around the corona and extending a short way into the urethral meatus. The glans and prepuce, which may not be retractable, are thickened and fibrous. Involvement of the urethra is usually limited to the meatus and squamous epithelium of the fossa navicularis; in such cases there is a smooth white contracted meatal orifice and an atrophic meatal collar. Patients may be alarmed at

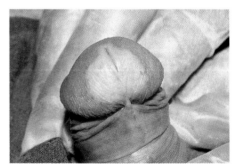

Figure 20.19 Lichen sclerosus of the penis (balanitis xerotica obliterans) (reproduced from McMillan and Scott 2000[82])

hemorrhagic bullae developing after intercourse and blood-stained urine if these lesions are at the meatus[51].

Although lesions are usually restricted to the penis in the male and anogenital area in women, unmistakable achromic papules of lichen sclerosus may, on occasions, be found elsewhere on the body as recorded by Laymon and Freeman[52] in 4 of 24 cases of BXO.

DIAGNOSIS

Diagnosis should be based on histological examination. As in any penile lesion, it is important to exclude syphilis and other sexually transmitted organisms which may cause balanitis and/or a urethritis.

TREATMENT

Anxiety about STIs may be relieved by satisfactory results in the tests taken to exclude such infections. The patient should be given written information about their condition, and, because of the small risk of malignancy, the importance of long-term follow-up should be stressed. Bland emollients should be used in place of soap for washing, and other irritants should be avoided. The use of lubricants may facilitate sexual intercourse.

Attempts may be made to control non-specific inflammation of the anogenital area. The topical application of a potent steroid such as clobetasol proprionate ointment (0.05% w/w) twice daily for 3 months can relieve symptoms and partially reverse the histological changes[53]. The application should then be gradually reduced and stopped. Further applications at weekly intervals may be used as required to control symptoms, but the excessive use of this agent (more than 30 g every 3 months) should be avoided to prevent the dermatological (atrophy) and systemic side effects (adrenal suppression from systemic absorption) from this potent drug[49].

Circumcision may be needed when the prepuce is involved and retraction difficult. If meatal stenosis causes urethral obstruction and the meatal lesion shows only non-specific changes on histological examination, then regular dilatation by urethral bouginage may be sufficient treatment. If the navicular fossa and urethral meatus show the changes characteristic of BXO then meatotomy or meatoplasty by a urologist may be necessary.

PROGNOSIS

Lichen sclerosus tends to progress, but sometimes this is at a very slow rate. Circumcision will only reduce the added effects of inflammation in the sub-preputial sac, and dilatation or meatotomy the effects of recurrent urinary obstruction. Carcinoma of the penis has been reported in some cases of BXO[54], and studies have shown that up to 5% of women with the condition develop squamous cell carcinoma of the vulva[55]. Whether or not lichen sclerosus is actually pre-malignant, however, is uncertain. Erosive lesions that fail to heal, or warty growths, however, should be biopsied to exclude the development of malignancy.

8. Erythroplasia of Queyrat

This is squamous cell carcinoma *in situ* of the penis of unknown etiology, presenting most commonly between the ages of 50 and 60 years; it is rare in those circumcised in infancy.

CLINICAL FEATURES

The condition appears as either single or multiple well-defined red plaques on the glans penis (Figure 20.20) or on the mucosal surface of the prepuce. The lesions have a velvety, shiny appearance, and may occasionally ulcerate. The lesions are commonly asymptomatic but may, on rare occasions, cause pruritus or discomfort. The disease is slowly progressive, invasive change being manifest as induration, ulceration, or warty growth.

DIAGNOSIS

Psoriasis, lichen planus, fixed drug eruption, fungal lesions, syphilis, and lichen sclerosus need to be carefully excluded in the differential diagnosis. Histological examination is essential for diagnosis.

The appearance on microscopy is characteristic: the epidermis is acanthotic with focal parakeratosis, atypical epithelial cells with hyperchromatic nuclei, and dyskaryotic cells. Mitosis is obvious in cells in the upper malpighian layer. The dermis is infiltrated with lymphocytes and plasma cells.

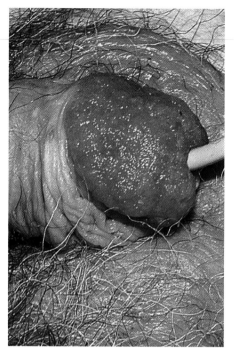

Figure 20.20 Erythroplasia of Queyrat (reproduced from McMillan and Scott 2000[82])

TREATMENT

Local excision may be effective[56], and the topical application of antimitotic agents such as 5-fluorouracil or the use of liquid nitrogen spray has produced excellent results in treatment[57, 58].

9. Peyronie's disease

In Peyronie's disease a chronic localized fibrous induration (commonly referred to as a plaque) involves the intercavernous septa of the penis, causing an angulation or curvature of the penis on erection. The disease, of unknown etiology, was first described by Francois de la Peyronie, court physician to Louis XIV. In the majority of cases it occurs in the fourth and fifth decades of life, although patients from 18 to 80 years of age have been affected[59].

ETIOLOGY

In the plaque of Peyronie's disease there is disordered collagen and abnormal deposition of elastic fibers. Although the precise etiology of Peyronie's disease is uncertain, trauma appears to be the initiating event[60]. In a case-control study of 134 Italian men with Peyronie's disease, patients who had had invasive procedures on the penis (transurethral prostatectomy, urethral catheterization, and cystoscopy) had a 16-fold increased risk over controls, and a threefold increase was noted in those men who had a history of genital or perineal trauma[61]. When there is flexion of the penis in the dorsoventral aspect, buckling may cause delamination of the layers of the tunica albuginea where the septal fibers are implanted. This may result in extravasation of blood into the intra-laminar space or shearing of septal fibers where they are interwoven with the inner circular fibers of the tunica albuginea. Fibrin deposition is found in plaque tissue from most patients with Peyronie's disease, consistent with the hypothesis that repetitive microvascular injury results in fibrin deposition in the tissues[62]. Buckling may result from diminution of the elasticity of the aging tissue in men susceptible to Peyronie's disease. The rapidity of loss of elasticity may be genetically determined, thereby explaining the observation that there is sometimes a family history of the condition (4% of men in the study by Carrieri et al.[61]). Fibrin deposition is said to stimulate fibroblasts with the resulting development of fibrosis.

As Peyronie's disease is often found in older men who have frequent sexual intercourse, it is postulated that repeated trauma leads to increasing fibrosis. An association with erectile dysfunction has been described, but, as this frequently pre-dates the onset of Peyronie's disease, a similar mechanism may be responsible. Interestingly, however, although an association between both Peyronie's disease and impotence and penile trauma was shown in the study by Jarrow and Lowe[63], men with Peyronie's disease had a lower frequency of attempting coitus with a partial erection than men without a history of impotence or Peyronie's disease. When sexual dysfunction has been evaluated, the main cause of impotence and loss of erection has been veno-occlusive dysfunction as shown by cavernosonography[64].

Although an association between Peyronie's disease and anti-hypertensive drugs, particularly β-blocking agents, the condition is known to be more prone to occur in the presence of atherosclerosis, so the link may be purely coincidental[65]. There is, however, an association with Dupuytren's contracture, 20% to 30% of patients with Peyronie's disease being affected[61, 60].

CLINICAL FEATURES

The symptoms of this disorder are pain and curvature on erection, the sensation of a cord within the penis, the palpation of a lump in the penis, decreased erection distal to the plaque, interference with coitus, and gradual impotence. Curvature of the penis is directed towards the lesion and a dorsal curvature is the most common.

The fibrotic plaque may range in size from a few millimeters to involvement of the entire dorsum of the penis. The plaque is usually located on the dorsum of the penis (about 70% of cases), the lateral aspect (about 20%), and occasionally on the ventrum (about 7%). Plaques may begin as multiple lesions and become confluent. There may be calcification on radiological examination in 20% of cases. The fibrosis tends to be self-limiting, but recent evidence from a postal questionnaire study suggests that spontaneous regression rarely occurs[66].

The differential diagnosis includes benign neoplasms, secondary thrombosis of the corpora, and leukemic infiltration of the corpora cavernosa[67].

TREATMENT

It is important to stress the benign nature of the condition, and it is often helpful to include the sexual partner in the discussions. The majority of patients with Peyronie's disease who have little pain and are able to have sexual intercourse do not require treatment.

Medical treatments in the form of X-ray radiation, diathermy, ultrasound, vitamin E, potassium para-aminobenzoate, and dimethylsulfoxide, have all been used without proof of value. Intralesional steroids have been popular, but there is often great difficulty in getting the fluid into the hard plaque, and the effectiveness of this treatment is uncertain[59]. A recent study of 38 men with Peyronie's disease showed that intralesional injections of the calcium-channel blocker, verapamil, given once every 2 weeks, is useful in achieving a reduction in pain and the degree of deformity in the majority of patients[68]. In a small study, a decreased plaque volume was reported by Rehman et al.[69], but there was no significant difference in the degree of penile curvature between men treated with verapamil and those given placebo. The results of larger studies of intralesional verapamil are awaited.

Surgical treatment may be required for more severely affected patients who have difficulties with sexual intercourse[60].

10. Lymphocele and localized edema of the penis (sclerosing lymphangitis of the penis)

This is a benign, transitory condition, first described in a patient with gonorrhea[70]. The etiology is unknown, although trauma, in the form of frequent or prolonged sexual intercourse, frequently antedates the appearance of the lesion by an interval varying between a few hours and several weeks.

Histological examination shows dilated lymphatic vessels with thickening of the wall due to hyperplasia of the smooth muscle cells and production of collagen and ground substance by fibroblasts[71]. Fibrin thrombi occlude the lumen of the vessel and recanalization may be seen in older lesions.

Characteristically there is a worm-like swelling in the coronal sulcus (Figure 20.21), parallel to the corona of the glans penis, sometimes completely encircling the penis, and on occasions involving the dorsal lymphatic vessels of the shaft. Edema of the prepuce may also be found. The swelling is neither painful nor tender, and on palpation it has a cartilaginous consistency. Within 3 weeks of its appearance, the lesion has usually resolved completely, and no treatment other than reassurance is required.

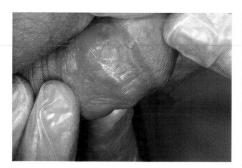

Figure 20.21 Lymphocele of the coronal sulcus

It is probable that there is wide variation in the presentation of this condition, varying between mild preputial edema, and the 'classical' lesion described[72]. A similar condition may affect the vulva[73].

11. Behçet's disease

Behçet's disease is a multisystem illness characterized by the triad of oral, genital, and eye lesions, and by its tendency to exacerbation and remission of unpredictable duration. Taking its name from the Turkish physician who, in 1937, described the triad of relapsing iridocyclitis with recurrent oral and genital ulceration, it affects males predominantly and although it shows its highest prevalence in the eastern Mediterranean basin and in Japan[74] cases are also to be found in mainland China, middle eastern countries, and north Africa[75]. A vasculitis appears to be the common histological lesion, and clinical features – present in most patients and considered to be diagnostic – are oral and genital ulcers, uveitis, and a variety of skin lesions. Clinical manifestations of the syndrome are protean but include particularly arthritis, thrombophlebitis, and various neurological states[76].

The prevalence of the human leukocyte antigen (HLA) B51 allele is high among patients with Behçet's disease who live along the old Silk Road (about 80% of cases), but not amongst Caucasians who live in western countries (13% of cases)[76]. It has been suggested that HLA-B51 is particularly related to ocular involvement, and it is well recognized that there is a very high incidence of ocular disease in Japanese and Turkish patients where the incidence of HLA-B51 is higher in the general population than in the UK[75]. The etiology is obscure, but heat shock proteins (Hsps) may play some role. Lymphocyte function is abnormal in patients with Behçet's disease, and proliferative responses to peptides derived from Hsp 60, which are homologous with bacterial Hsp 65, are found especially in those with ocular involvement[76]. The epitopes recognized by auto-reactive anti-Hsp T lymphocytes overlap with the B-cell epitopes of autoantibodies against Hsp in patients with Behçet's disease. There is clonal expansion of auto-reactive T cells specific for the peptide derived from Hsp 60. It is uncertain, however, whether this is a primary or secondary event.

CLINICAL FEATURES

Four common clinical patterns can be discerned

1. the *mucocutaneous* (MC) type, there are oral and genital lesions with or without skin manifestations which may be present also in all other types
2. the *arthritic* type
3. the *neurological* type with brain involvement
4. the *ocular* type[74].

Painful recurrent oral ulcers 2 to 10 mm in diameter (Figure 20.22) occur in half to three-quarters of all patients and are the most frequent initial manifestation. The ulcers are shallow or deep with a central yellowish necrotic base and they occur as single lesions or in crops affecting the mucosa anywhere from the lips to the larynx. The ulcers tend to persist for 1 to 2 weeks and recur after intervals of several days to several months.

Genital ulcers resemble those of the mouth both in appearance and in their tendency to persist, heal, and recur. They are located on the scrotum or the penis in men and on the vulva (Figures 20.23

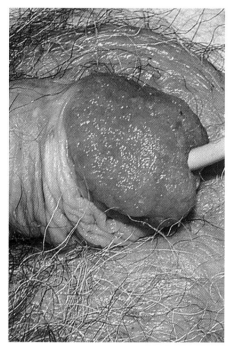

Figure 20.23 Vulval ulceration in Behçet's disease (reproduced from McMillan and Scott 2000[82])

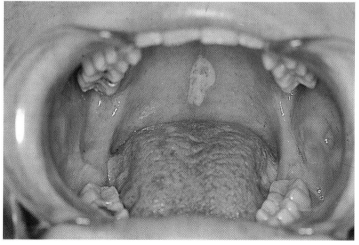

Figure 20.22 Oral ulceration in Behçet's disease (reproduced from McMillan and Scott 2000[82])

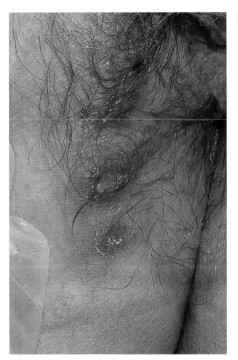

Figure 20.24 Vulval ulceration in Behçet's disease (reproduced from McMillan and Scott 2000[82])

and 20.24) or vagina in women. The ulcers are painful and disturbing to men but less troublesome to women. In the mouth or genitalia, fibrosis and scarring at sites of healed lesions produce a characteristic mottled appearance on naked-eye examination or with magnification, described as 'splash fibrosis'. Scarring and tissue loss develop particularly after scrotal ulceration[77].

Recurrent inflammation of the anterior segment of the eye usually shows itself as iridocyclitis and hypopyon. Posterior segment involvement may be found in about two-thirds of patients with lesions such as choroiditis, phlebitis, arteritis, and optic papillitis. Serious sequelae with blindness may result. It is important to exclude syphilis by means of the necessary tests (Chapter 15) otherwise it may be overlooked.

A variety of skin lesions also occur; these include particularly ulceration, erythema nodosum, and pustules, but erythema multiforme and thrombophlebitis migrans also occur[74]. Arthritis with synovial changes, which appear to be characteristic histologically[78], develops in about 40% of cases, the knees, ankles, and elbows being most commonly affected. Neurological complications occur after

some years and include transient or persistent brain-stem syndromes, intracranial nerve palsy, cerebellar and spinal cord lesions, and meningoencephalitis, all conditions that tend to regress over several months. Gastrointestinal involvement can cause abdominal pain, diarrhea, and melena. The ileocecal region is the most commonly affected part of the intestinal tract.

DIAGNOSIS

Diagnosis may be made in those with the 'complete' syndrome where three or four of the major features are present (oral and genital ulceration, ocular and skin lesions). Diagnosis in those with the 'incomplete' syndrome is often debatable[74]. An international study group proposed a set of diagnostic criteria, based on data from 914 patients, that required the presence of

---

Box 20.1 Criteria proposed by the International Study Group for the diagnosis of Behçet's Disease (International Study Group for Behçet's Disease 1990[80])

Recurrent oral ulceration – minor aphthous, major aphthous, or herpetiform ulceration observed by physician or patient, which recurred at least three times in one 12-month period.

plus two of

Recurrent genital ulceration – aphthous ulceration or scarring observed by physician or patient.

Eye lesions – anterior uveitis, posterior uveitis, or cells in the vitreous on slit-lamp examination; or retinal vasculitis observed by ophthalmologist.

Skin lesions – erythema nodosum observed by physician or patient, pseudofolliculitis, or papulopustular lesions; or acneiform nodules observed by physician in post-adolescent patients not on corticosteroid treatment.

Positive pathergy test – read by physician at 24 to 48 hours (see text for details).

---

oral ulcers plus any two of the features shown in Box 20.1.

In Behçet's disease the diagnostic usefulness of the 'pathergy' test has been reported in patients from Turkey and Japan but not in those from Britain. This test is based on a curious phenomenon, almost unique to Behçet's disease in some geographical localities, characterized by hyperreactivity of the skin to needle prick. In recording the result of the test an assessment is made 24 to 48 hours after one or ten needle pricks in different sites: for needle mark(s) only 0; for a papule 1+; for a small pustule 2+; and for a large pustule 3+[79]. In the individual case the value in diagnosis of a test for HLA-Bs is limited.

It is clearly important to exclude by appropriate tests an STI, including syphilis, not only because of the lesion in mucosal sites but also because the patient is often anxious about such possibilities.

TREATMENT

Evaluation of treatment is difficult because of the unpredictable natural course of the disease. Corticosteroids, immunosuppressants, or both are the basis of treatment for neurological, gastrointestinal and large-vessel lesions[76]. Ocular involvement should always be managed in conjunction with an ophthalmologist.

Local disease of the mouth or genitalia is not an indication for treatment with systemic corticosteroids, but the local application of corticosteroids – with added antimicrobial agents for the genital tract – has greatly improved the quality of life of those with Behçet's syndrome. As each ulcer is preceded by the development of a painful tender nodule under the mucous membrane or the skin, and under the mucosal surfaces, that lasts for 1 or 2 days before ulcerating, it may be aborted by local corticosteroids. In the mouth it may be felt with the tongue and identified by the patient, and it can be aborted or minimized by the local application of triamcinolone 0.1% in an adhesive oral paste after meals and last thing at night. On the genitalia hydrocortisone 0.5% (with nystatin 100 000 units/g, chlorhexidine hydrochloride 1%) in a water-miscible base may be applied. Colchicine, given orally in a dose of 0.5 to 1.5 mg/day may be helpful, and the authors have successfully used thalidomide in an oral dose of 100 to 300 mg/day.

12. Pyoderma gangrenosum[81]

This is a chronic destructive inflammatory condition of unknown origin. It may occur in isolation, or in association with other conditions that include ulcerative colitis, Crohn's disease of the colon, rheumatoid disease, Wegener's granulomatosis, plasma cell dyscrasias, and seronegative arthritis with paraproteinemia. The histology is not specific. There is venous and capillary thrombosis, hemorrhage, and necrosis and a chronic inflammatory infiltration of the tissues. The characteristic lesion is an ulcer that sometimes affects the vulva

(Figure 20.25); it is irregular in outline with a ragged, overhanging edge, a red edematous crater and a necrotic base. The lesions often persist for years. The differential diagnosis includes cutaneous amoebiasis, deep fungal infections, and tuberculosis. Any underlying condition should be treated appropriately, and high-dose steroids may be required to heal the ulceration.

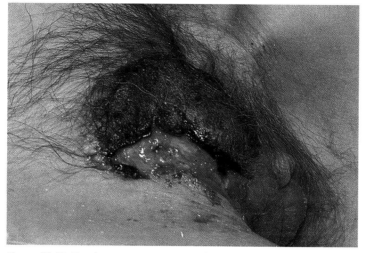

Figure 20.25 Pyoderma gangrenosum of the vulva (reproduced from McMillan and Scott 2000[82])

References

1 Wray D, Ferguson MM, Mason DK, Hutcheon AW, Dagg JH. Recurrent aphthae: treatment with vitamin B12, folic acid and iron. *Br Med J* 1975; **2**: 490–493.

2 Morson BC. Regional enteritis (Crohn's disease). In: Bockus HL (ed.) *Gastroenterology*, vol. 2. HL Saunders; Philadelphia: 1976, p. 550.

3 Cold CJ, Taylor JR. The prepuce. *Br J Urol* 1999; **83** (Suppl. 1): 34–44.

4 Deibert GA. The separation of the prepuce in the human penis. *Anat Rec* 1933; **57**: 387–399.

5 Gairdner D. The fate of the foreskin; a study of circumcision. *Br Med J* 1949; **2**: 1433–1437.

6 Oster J. Further fate of the foreskin. *Arch Dis Child* 1968; **43**: 200–203.

7 Burrows H. The union and separation of living tissues influenced by cellular differentiation. *Yale J Biol Med* 1944; **17**: 397–402.

8 Cooper GG, Thomson GJL, Raine PA. Therapeutic retraction of the foreskin in childhood. *Br Med J* 1983; **286**: 186–187.

9 Griffiths DM, Freeman NV. Non-surgical separation of the preputial adhesions. *Lancet* 1984; **ii**: 344.

10 Esscher T. Why not let preputial adhesions alone? *Lancet* 1984; **ii**: 581–582.

11 Pfaff G, Bolkenius M. Hands off the prepuce. *Lancet* 1984; **ii**: 874–875.

12 Kochen M 1980 Circumcision and the risk of cancer of the penis. A lifetime-table analysis. *Am J Dis Child* **184**: 484–486.

13 Frisch M, Friis S, Kjaer SK, Melbye M. Falling incidence of penis cancer in an uncircumcised population (Denmark 1943–90). *Br Med J* 1995; **311**: 1471.

14 Halperin DT, Bailey RC. Male circumcision and HIV infection: 10 years and counting. *Lancet* 1999; **354**: 1813–1815.

15 Van Howe RS. Circumcision and HIV infection: review of the literature and meta-analysis. *Int J STD AIDS* 1999; **10**: 8–16.

16 O'Farrell N, Egger M. Circumcision in men and the prevention of HIV infection: a 'meta-analysis' revisited. *Int J STD AIDS* 2000; **11**: 137–142.

17 Lavreys L, Rakwar JPN, Thompson ML, *et al.* Effect of circumcision on incidence of human immunodeficiency virus type 1 and other sexually transmitted diseases: a prospective cohort study of trucking company employees in Kenya. *J Infect Dis* 1999; **180**: 330–336.

18 Kelly R, Kiwanuka N, Wawer MJ, *et al.* Age of male circumcision and risk of prevalent HIV infection in rural Uganda. *AIDS* 1999; **13**: 399–405.

19 Berlin J, Laird NM, Sacks HS, Chalmers TC. A comparison of statistical methods for combining event rates from clinical trials. *Stat Med* 1989; **8**: 141–151.

20 Van Ulsen J, Stolz E, Van Joost Th, Guersen-Reitsma AM. Allergy to spermicidal lubricant in a contraceptive. *Contact Dermatitis* 1987; **17**: 115–116.

21 Birley HDL, Walker MM, Luzzi GA, *et al.* Clinical features and management of recurrent balanitis; association with atopy and genital washing. *Genitourin Med* 1993; **69**: 400–403.

22 Masfari AN, Kinghorn GR, Duerden BI. Anaerobes in genitourinary infections in men. *Br J Vener Dis* 1983; **59**: 255–259.

23 Kinghorn GR, Jones BM, Chowdhury FH, Geary I. Balanoposthitis associated with *Gardnerella vaginalis* infection in men. *Br J Vener Dis* 1982; **58**: 127–129.

24 Lucks DA, Venezio FR, Lakin CM. Balanitis caused by group B streptococcus. *J Urol* 1986; **135**: 1015.

25 Drusin LM, Wilkes BM, Ginigrich RD. Streptococcal pyoderma of the penis following fellatio. *Br J Vener Dis* 1975; **51**: 61–62.

26 Peutherer JF, Smith IW, Robertson DHH. Necrotising balanitis due to a generalised primary infection with Herpes simplex virus type 2. *Br J Vener Dis* 1979; **55**: 48–51.

27 Wikstrom A, von Grogh G, Hedblad M-A, Syrjanen S. Papillomavirus-associated balanoposthitis. *Genitourin Med* 1994; **70**: 175–181.

28 Watt L, Jennison RF. Incidence of *Trichomonas vaginalis* in marital partners. *Br J Vener Dis* 1960; **36**: 163–166.

29 Purpon I, Jiminez D, Engelking RL. Amebiasis of the penis. *J Urol* 1967; **60**: 372–374.

30 Kumar B, Sharma R, Rajagopalan M, Radotra BD. Plasma cell balanitis: clinical and histopathological features – response to circumcision. *Genitourin Med* 1995; **71**: 32–34.

31 Dockerty WG, Sonnex C. Candidal balano-posthitis: a study of diagnostic methods. *Genitourin Med* 1995; **71**: 407–409.

32 Hillman RJ, Walker MM, Harris JRW, Taylor-Robinson D. Penile dermatoses: a clinical and histopathological study. *Genitourin Med* 1992; **68**: 166–169.

33 Champion RH, Burton JL, Burns DA, Breathnach SM (eds). Rook/Wilkinson/Ebling. *Textbook of Dermatology* 6th edition. Oxford; Blackwell: 1998.

34 Schiff TA, Bodian AB, Buchness MR. Foscarnet-induced penile ulceration. *Int J Dermatol* 1993; **32**: 526–527.

35 Tanenbaum MH, Becker W. Papillae of the corona of the glans penis. *J Urol* 1965; **93**: 391–395.

36 Noble WC, Somerville DA. *Microbiology of Human Skin*. Saunders; London: 1774.

37 Rosman N. Infections with *Trichophyton rubrum*. *Br J Dermatol* 1966; **78**: 208–212.

38 Hay RJ, Moore M. Mycology. In: Champion RH, Burton JL, Burns DA, Breathnach SM (eds) Rook/Wilkinson/Ebling. *Textbook of Dermatology* 6th edition. Oxford; Blackwell: 1998.

39 La Touche CJ. Scrotal dermatophytosis. An insufficiently documented aspect of tinea cruris. *Br J Dermatol* 1967; **79**: 339–344

40 Davis CM, Garcia RL, Riordon JP, Taplin D. Dermatophytes in military recruits. *Arch Dermatol* 1972; **105**: 558–560.

41 Milne LJR, Barnetson RStC. Diagnosis of dermatophytoses using vinyl adhesive tape. *Sabouraudia* 1971; **12**: 162–165.

42 Rebell G, Taplin D. *Dermatophytes: their Recognition and Identification* 2nd edition. University of Miami Press; Coral Gables, FL: 1970.

43 Frey D, Oldfield RJ, Bridges RC. *A Colour Atlas of Pathogenic Fungi*. Wolfe Medical Publications; London: 1979.

44 Hay RJ, Adrianns BM. Bacterial infections. In: Champion RH, Burton JL, Burns DA, Breathnach SM (eds) Rook/Wilkinson/Ebling. *Textbook of Dermatology* 6th edition. Oxford; Blackwell: 1998.

45 Somerville DA, Seville RH, Cunningham RC, Noble WC, Savin J. Erythrasma in a hospital for the mentally subnormal. *Br J Dermatol* 1970; **82**: 355–360.

46 Macmillan AL, Sarkany I. Specific topical therapy for erythrasma. *Br J Dermatol* 1970; **82**: 507–509.

47 Clayton YM, Connor BL. Comparison of clotrimazole cream, Whitfield's ointment and nystatin ointment for the topical treatment of ringworm infections, pityriasis versicolor, erythrasma and candidiasis. *Br J Dermatol* 1973; **89**: 297–303.

48 Meyrick Thomas RH, Ridley CM, McGibbon DH, *et al*. Lichen sclerosus and autoimmunity – a study of 350 women. *Br J Dermatol* 1988; **114**: 377–379.

49 Powell JJ, Wojnarowska F. Lichen sclerosus. *Lancet* 1999; **353**: 1777–1783.

50 Bainbridge DR, Whitaker RH, Shepheard BGF. Balanitis xerotica obliterans and urinary obstruction. *Br J Urol* 1971; **43**: 487–491.

51 Ive FA. The umbilical, perianal and genital regions. In: Champion RH, Burton JL, Burns DA, Breathnach SM (eds). Rook/Wilkinson/Ebling. *Textbook of Dermatology* 6th edition. Oxford; Blackwell: 1998.

52 Laymon CW, Freeman C. Relationship of balanitis xerotica obliterans to lichen sclerosus et atrophicus. *Arch Dermatol Syphilol* 1944; **49**: 57–59.

53 Dalziel K, Wojnarowski F, Millard P. The treatment of lichen sclerosus with a very potent topical steroid (clobetasol proprionate 0.05%). *Br J Dermatol* 1991; **124**: 461–464.

54 Pride HB, Miller OF, Tyler WB. Penile squamous carcinoma arising from balanitis xerotica obliterans. *J Am Acad Dermatol* 1993; **29**: 469–473.

55 Meffert JJ, Davis BM, Grimwood RE. Lichen sclerosus. *J Am Acad Dermatol* 195; **32**: 393–416.

56 Mikhail GR. Cancers, precancers and pseudocancers on the male genitalia: a review of clinical appearances, histopathology, and management. *J Dermatol Surg Oncol* 1980; **6**: 1027.

57 Goette DK. Review of erythroplasia of Queyrat and its treatment. *Urology* 1976; **8**: 311–315.

58 Sonnex TS, Ralfs IG, Delanza MP, *et al*. Treatment of erythroplasia of Queyrat with liquid nitrogen cryosurgery. *Br J Dermatol* 1982; **106**: 581–584.

59 Billig R, Baker R, Immergut M, Maxted W. Peyronie's disease. *Urology* 1975; **6**: 409–411.

60 Jordan GH, Schlossberg SM, Devine CJ. Peyronie's disease. In: Walsh PC, Retik AB, Darracott Vaughan E, Wein AJ (eds) *Campbell's Urology* 7th edition. Philadelphia; WB Saunders: 1998.

61 Carrieri MP, Serraino D, Palmiotto F, Nucci G, Sasso F. A case-control study on risk factors for Peyronie's disease. *J Clin Epidemiol* 1998; **51**: 511–515.

62 Somers KD, Dawson DM. Fibrin deposition in Peyronie's disease plaque. *J Urol* 1997; **157**: 311–315.

63 Jarow JP, Lowe FC. Penile trauma: an etiologic factor in Peyronie's disease and erectile dysfunction. *J Urol* 1997; **158**: 1388–1390.

64 Weidner W, Schroeder-Printzen I, Weiske WH, Vosshenrich R. Sexual dysfunction in Peyronie's disease: an analysis of 222 patients without previous plaque therapy. *J Urol* 1997; **157**: 325–328.

65 Laake K. In: Dukes MNG (ed.). *Side Effects of Drugs*, Annual 7. Excerpta Medica; Amsterdam: 1983.

66 Gelbard MK, Dorey F, James K. The natural history of Peyronie's disease. *J Urol* 1990; **144**: 1376–1379.

67 Chesney J. Peyronie's disease. *Br J Urol* 1975; **47**: 209–218.

68 Levine LA. Treatment of Peyronie's disease with intralesional verapamil. *J Urol* 1997; **158**: 1395–1399.

69 Rehman J, Benet A, Melman A. Use of intralesional verapamil to dissolve Peyronie's disease plaque: a long-term single-blind study. *Urology* 1998; **51**: 620–626.

70 Hoffman E. Vortanschung primarer Syphilis durch gonorrhoische Lymphangitis (gonorrhoischer Pseudoprimaraffekt). *Munch Med Wochenschr* 1923; **70**: 1167–1168.

71 Marsch WCh, Stuttgen G. Sclerosing lymphangitis of the penis: a lymphangiofibrosis thrombotica occlusiva. *Br J Dermatol* 1981; **104**: 687–695.

72 Fiumara NJ. Nonvenereal sclerosing lymph-angitis of the penis. *Arch Dermatol* 1975; **111**: 902–903.

73 Stolz E, van Kampen WJ, Vuzevski V. Sklerosiesende Lymphangitis des Penis, der Oberlippe und des Labium minus. *Hautarzt* 1974; **25**: 231–237.

74 Lehner T, Barnes CG. Criteria for diagnosis and classification of Behçet's syndrome. In: Lehner T, Barnes CG (eds) *Behçet's Syndrome, Clinical and Immunological Features*. London; Academic Press: 1979.

75 Barnes CG. Behçet's syndrome. *J R Soc Med* 1984; **77**: 816–819.

76 Sakane T, Takeno M, Suzuki N, Inaba G. Behçet's disease. *N Engl J Med* 1999; **341**: 1284–1291.

77 Dunlop EMC. Genital and other manifestations of Behçet's disease seen in venereological practice. In: Lehner T, Barnes CG (eds) *Behçet's Syndrome, Clinical and Immunological Features*. Academic Press; London: 1979.

78 Vernon-Roberts B, Barnes CG, Revell P. Synovial pathology in Behçet's syndrome. *Ann Rheum Dis* 1978; **37**: 139–145.

79 Yazici H, Chamberlain MA, Juzun Y, Yurdakul S, Muftuoglu T. A comparative

study of the pathergy reaction amongst Turkish and British patients with Behçet's disease. *Ann Rheum Dis* 1984; **43**: 74–75.

80 International Study Group for Behçet's disease. Criteria for diagnosis of Behçet's disease. *Lancet* 1990; **335**: 1078–1080.

81 Ryan TJ. Cutaneous vasculitis. In: Champion RH, Burton JL, Burns DA, Breathnach SM (eds). Rook/Wilkinson/ Ebling Textbook of Dermatology. Oxford. Blackwell Science. 1998.

82 McMillan A, Scott GR. *Sexually Transmitted Infections, Colour Guide*. Churchill Livingstone; Edinburgh: 2000.

Index

Numbers in italics refer to figures and tables